OXFORD MEDICAL PUBLICATIONS

OXFORD TEXTBOOK OF PUBLIC HEALTH

EDITORS

ROGER DETELS
Professor of Epidemiology
UCLA School of Public Health
University of California, Los Angeles, CA 90024–1772, USA.

WALTER W. HOLLAND
Professor Emeritus of Public Health Medicine
Department of Public Health Medicine
United Medical and Dental Schools
St Thomas's Hospital
London SE1 7EH, England.

JAMES McEWEN
Professor, Department of Public Health
University of Glasgow
Glasgow G12 8QQ, Scotland.

GILBERT S. OMENN
Professor, Dean, School of
Public Health and Community Medicine
University of Washington,
Seattle, Washington 98195, USA.

OXFORD TEXTBOOK OF PUBLIC HEALTH

THIRD EDITION

VOLUME 2

The Methods of Public Health

Edited by

ROGER DETELS, WALTER W. HOLLAND,
JAMES McEWEN, and GILBERT S. OMENN

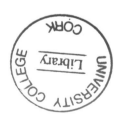

New York   Oxford   Tokyo
OXFORD UNIVERSITY PRESS
1997

Oxford University Press, Walton Street, Oxford OX2 6DP

Oxford   New York

Athens   Auckland   Bangkok   Bombay
Calcutta   Cape Town   Dar es Salaám   Delhi
Florence   Hong Kong   Istanbul   Karachi
Kuala Lumpur   Madras   Madrid   Melbourne
Mexico City   Nairobi   Paris   Singapore
Taipei   Tokyo   Toronto

and associated companies in
Berlin   Ibadan

Oxford is a trade mark of Oxford University Press

Published in the United States
by Oxford University Press Inc., New York

A catalogue record for this book is available from the British Library
(Data available)

Library of Congress Cataloging in Publication Data

ISBN 0 19 262553 5 (Three volume set).
ISBN 0 19 262550 0 (Vol. 1)
ISBN 0 19 262551 9 (Vol. 2)
ISBN 0 19 262552 7 (Vol. 3)

Typeset by Interactive Sciences Ltd, Gloucester
Printed in Great Britain by Butler & Tanner, Frome, Somerset

Contents
Volume 1 The scope of public health

Contents
Volume 2 The methods of public health

Contents
Volume 3 The practice of public health

List of Contributors

J.H. ABRAMSON
Emeritus Professor of Social Medicine, Hebrew University-Hadassah School of Public Health and Community Medicine, Jerusalem, Israel

Cross-sectional studies

MICHAEL ADLER
Professor of Genitourinary Medicine, Department of Sexually Transmitted Diseases, University College London Medical School, UK

Sexually transmitted diseases

EVA ALBERMAN
Emeritus Professor of Clinical Epidemiology, University of London, UK

Children

JOHN A.D. ANDERSON
Professor and Chairman, Department of Public Health and Occupational Medicine, University of the United Arab Emirates, Al Ain

Persons with physical disabilities

ROY ANDERSON
Linacre Professor of Zoology and Director of the Centre for the Epidemiology of Infectious Disease, University of Oxford, UK

Mathematical models of transmission and control

L.M. ARTZ
Birmingham, Alabama, USA

Objectives-based strategies for disease prevention

J.S.A. ASHLEY
Previously Deputy Chief Medical Statistician, Office of Population Censuses and Surveys, London, UK

Health information resources in the United Kingdom

JOAN AUSTOKER
Director, CRC Primary Care, Education Research Group, Department of Public Health and Primary Care, University of Oxford, UK

Screening

DEAN B. BAKER
Professor and Director, Center for Occupational and Environmental Health, University of California, Irvine, USA

Workers

A.E. BENJAMIN
Professor of Social Welfare, School of Public Policy and Social Research, University of California, Los Angeles, USA

Policies and strategies for health in the United States

RUTH L. BERKELMAN
Deputy Director, National Center for Infectious Diseases, Centers for Disease Control and Prevention (CDC), Atlanta, Georgia, USA

Public health surveillance

BONNIE BLANDER
Staff Research Associate, Southern California Injury Prevention Research Center, UCLA School of Public Health, Los Angeles, USA

Injury control: the public health approach

ANN BOSTROM
Assistant Professor, School of Public Policy, Georgia Institute of Technology, Atlanta, USA

Risk perception and communication

MARIE-HELENE BOUVIER-COLLE
Epidemiologist and Director of Research, Institut National de la Santé et de la Récherche Médicale, Paris, France

Cohort studies

LESTER BRESLOW
Professor of Public Health, School of Public Health, UCLA, Los Angeles, California, USA

Women's health

NORMAN E. BRESLOW
Professor of Biostatistics, University of Washington, Seattle, USA

Current scope and concerns in public health

JAMES W. BUEHLER
Associate Director for Science, Division of HIV/AIDS Prevention, Centers for Disease Control and Prevention, Atlanta, Georgia, USA

Public health surveillance

JULIE E. BURING
Associate Professor of Ambulatory Care and Prevention, Harvard Medical School and Deputy Director, Division of Preventive Medicine, Brigham and Women's Hospital, Boston, Massachusetts, USA

Methodology of intervention trials in individuals

SIR KENNETH CALMAN
Chief Medical Officer, Department of Health, Whitehall, London, UK

Ethical principles and ethical issues in health care

SUSAN K. COLE
Consultant in Public Health Medicine and Medical Adviser to the Registrar General (Scotland), UK

Health information resources in the United Kingdom

R.A. COUTINHO
Head of Department of Public Health, Municipal Health Service, Amsterdam, and Professor in the Epidemiology and Control of Infectious Diseases, University of Amsterdam, The Netherlands

Acquired immunodeficiency syndrome

FRANCES M. COWAN
Senior Lecturer in Genitourinary Medicine, University College London Medical School, UK

Sexually transmitted diseases

SHAN CRETIN
President, Shan Cretin and Associates, Santa Monica, California, USA

Operational and system studies

PETER R. CROFT
Professor of Epidemiology, Keele University, Staffordshire, UK

Musculoskeletal diseases

LISA CURTICE
Lecturer in Community Care Studies, Nuffield Centre for Community Care Studies, University of Glasgow, UK

The disadvantaged—their health needs and public health initiatives

G. DAVEY SMITH
Professor of Clinical Epidemiology, University of Bristol, UK

Meta-analysis and data synthesis in medical research

DON C. DES JARLAIS
Director of Research, Chemical Dependency Institute, Beth Israel Medical Center and Professor of Epidemiology, Albert Einstein College of Medicine, New York, USA

Alcohol and drug abuse

ROGER DETELS
Professor of Epidemiology, School of Public Health, University of California, Los Angeles, USA

Cohort studies

Current scope and concerns in public health

Epidemiology: the foundation of public health

CAM DONALDSON
Deputy Director, Health Economics Research Unit, University of Aberdeen, UK

Economic evaluation

R.S. DOWNIE
Professor of Moral Philosophy, University of Glasgow, UK

Ethical principles and ethical issues in health care

MATTHIAS EGGER
Senior Lecturer in Epidemiology, Department of Social and Preventive Medicine, University of Berne, Switzerland

Meta-analysis and data synthesis in medical research

MICHAEL J.G. FARTHING
Professor of Gastroenterology, St Bartholomew's and The Royal London School of Medicine and Dentistry, Queen Mary and Westfield College, University of London, UK

Gastrointestinal disease: public health aspects

ELAINE M. FAUSTMAN
Professor and Associate Chair, Department of Environmental Health, School of Public Health and Community Medicine, University of Washington, Seattle, USA

Risk assessment, risk communication, and risk management

ELIZABETH FEE
Chief, History of Medicine Division, National Library of Medicine, National Institutes of Health, Bethesda, Maryland, USA

The origins and development of public health in the United States

MANNING FEINLEIB
Research Professor, Department of Medicine, Georgetown University Medical Center, Washington DC, USA

Cohort studies

A.A. FILES
Acting Director, Health Benefits Division, Office of Budget, US Department of Health and Human Services, Washington DC, USA

Objectives-based strategies for disease prevention

BARUCH FISCHHOFF
Professor of Social and Decision Sciences and Professor of Engineering and Public Policy, Carnegie Mellon University, Pittsburgh, Pennsylvania, USA

Risk perception and communication

SEV S. FLUSS
Formerly Chief and currently Human Rights Coordinator, Health Legislation, WHO, Geneva

International public health law: an overview

WILLIAM H. FOEGE
Health Fellow, Carter Center, Emory University, Atlanta, Georgia, USA

Challenges to public health leadership

GODFREY FOWLER
Reader in General Practice, University of Oxford; Honorary Director, ICRF General Practice Research Group, Oxford, UK

Screening

RALPH R. FRERICHS
Professor of Epidemiology, University of California at Los Angeles, USA

Microcomputers and epidemiology

TOM FRYERS
International Consultant in Public Health, Kendal, Cumbria, UK and Distinguished Lecturer, New York Medical College, USA

Persons with mental handicaps

BERNARD D. GOLDSTEIN
Director, Environmental and Occupational Health Sciences Institute, a Joint Program of UMDNJ—Robert Wood Johnson Medical School and Rutgers University, Piscataway, New Jersey, USA

Toxicology and environmental health

LAWRENCE W. GREEN
Professor and Director, Institute of Health Promotion Research and Division of Preventive Medicine and Health Promotion, Department of Health Care and Epidemiology, University of British Columbia, Canada

Education and life-style determinants of health and disease

MICHAEL R. GREENBERG
Professor of Urban Studies and Community Health, Bloustein School of Planning and Public Policy, Rutgers University, New Brunswick, New Jersey, USA

Toxicology and environmental health

JOHN E. GREENE
Professor and Dean Emeritus, School of Dentistry, University of California, San Francisco USA

Dental public health

SANDER GREENLAND
   Professor of Epidemiology, UCLA School of Public Health, Los Angeles, California, USA

Concepts of validity in epidemiological research

Causation and causal inference

MICHAEL B. GREGG
   Private Consultant in Epidemiology, Disease Surveillance, and Epidemiological Training, Brattleboro, Vermont, USA

The principles of an epidemic field investigation

R. GRIFFITHS
   Professor of Public Health, University of Birmingham, UK

Reducing environmental risk

EMILY M.D. GRUNDY
   Reader in Gerontology, King's College London, UK

Populations and population dynamics

C.J. HAM
   Professor of Health Policy and Management, Health Services Management Centre, University of Birmingham, UK

Public health policies and strategies in the United Kingdom

JAMES A. HARRELL
   Deputy Director, Office of Disease Prevention and Health Promotion, US Department of Health and Human Services, Washington DC, USA

Objectives-based strategies for disease prevention

NICOLETTE HART
   Associate Professor, Department of Sociology, University of California, Los Angeles, USA

The social and economic environment and human health

A.J. HEDLEY
   Professor and Head of Department of Community Medicine, The University of Hong Kong

Respiratory disease

H.K. HEGGENHOUGEN
   Associate Professor of Medical Anthropology, Department of Social Medicine, Harvard Medical School; Associate Professor of Population Sciences, Department of Population and International Health, Harvard School of Public Health, Boston, Massachusetts, USA

Beyond quantitative measures: the relevance of anthropology for public health

CHARLES H. HENNEKENS
   John Snow Professor of Medicine and Professor of Ambulatory Care and Prevention, Harvard Medical School, and Chief, Division of Preventive Medicine, Brigham and Women's Hospital, Boston, Massachusetts, USA

Methodology of intervention trials in individuals

BASIL HETZEL
   Chairman, International Council for Control of Iodine Deficiency Disorders (ICCIDD), Women & Children's Hospital, North Adelaide, Australia

Endocrine and metabolic disorders

MICHAEL S.T. HOBBS
   Associate Professor, Department of Public Health, University of Western Australia, Nedlands

Medical care and public health

H. HOFFMEISTER
   Professor of Epidemiology and Director of the Robert Koch-Institute, Berlin, Germany

Community based intervention trials

WALTER W. HOLLAND
   Emeritus Professor of Public Health Medicine, London, UK

Public health—its critical requirements

Overview of policies and strategies

HANS HOUWELING
   Senior Scientist, Department of Infectious Diseases Epidemiology, National Institute of Public Health and the Environment (RIVM), Bilthoven, The Netherlands

Acquired immunodeficiency syndrome

ROBERT L. HUBBARD
   Senior Program Director for Substance Abuse Treatment Research, Research Triangle Institute, North Carolina, USA

Alcohol and drug abuse

DAVID J. HUNTER
   Professor of Health Policy and Management, University of Leeds; Director, Nuffield Institute for Health, Leeds, UK

Management science and planning studies: their application to public health

NAOKI IKEGAMI
   Professor, Department of Hospital and Medical Administration, School of Medicine, Keio University, Japan

International perspectives on public health policy

MARILYN JACOBS QUADREL
   Manager, Risk Management Program, Pacific Northwest National Laboratory, Richland, Washington, USA

Risk perception and communication

W.P.T. JAMES
   Director of the Rowett Research Institute, Bucksburn, Aberdeen, UK

Nutrition

KONRAD JAMROZIK
   Associate Professor in Public Health, Department of Public Health, University of Western Australia, Nedlands, Australia

Medical care and public health

JUEL JANIS
   Psychotherapist, Los Angeles Free Clinic, California, USA

Families

DEE JONES
   Director, Research Team for the Care of Older People, University of Wales College of Medicine, Cardiff, UK

Health maintenance for frail elderly people

M. PAULA J. KILBANE
Chief Executive, Eastern Health and Social Services Board, Belfast, Northern Ireland

Health information resources in the United Kingdom

ÅSA KILBOM
Professor of Work Physiology, Institute for Working Life, Solna, Sweden

What is ergonomics?

ROBERT J. KIM-FARLEY
World Health Representative to Indonesia, Jakarta, Indonesia

Control of infectious diseases

E.G. KNOX
Professor Emeritus, University of Birmingham, UK

Spatial and temporal studies in epidemiology

HELEN P. KOO
Senior Research Demographer, Research Triangle Institute, North Carolina, USA

Demography and public health

JESS F. KRAUS
Professor, School of Public Health, Department of Epidemiology, University of California at Los Angeles, USA

Injury control: the public health approach

TAI HING LAM
Reader, Department of Community Medicine, The University of Hong Kong

Respiratory disease

PHILIP J. LANDRIGAN
Professor and Chair of Community Medicine, Mount Sinai Medical Center, New York, USA

Workers

M.J.S. LANGMAN
Professor of Medicine, University of Birmingham, UK

Gastrointestinal disease: public health aspects

PHILIP R. LEE
Professor of Social Medicine Emeritus, School of Medicine, University of California, San Francisco; Assistant Secretary for Health, US Department of Health and Human Services, USA

Policies and strategies for health in the United States

KENNETH LEE
Professor and Director, Centre for Health Planning and Management, Keele University, Staffordshire, UK

International perspectives on public health policy

STEPHEN R. LEEDER
Professor of Public Health and Community Medicine, University of Sydney at Westmead Hospital, New South Wales, Australia

Measuring health needs

PAUL J. LIOY
Professor of Environmental and Community Medicine, Environmental and Occupational Health Sciences Institute, UMDNJ Roberts Wood Johnson Medical School, Piscataway, New Jersey, USA

The analysis of human exposures to contaminants in the environment

RICHARD F.A. LOGAN
Reader in Clinical Epidemiology, Department of Public Health and Epidemiology, University of Nottingham; Honorary Consultant Physician, University Hospital, Nottingham, UK

Gastrointestinal disease: public health aspects

ADETOKUNBO O. LUCAS
Adjunct Professor of International Health, Harvard School of Public Health, Boston, Massachusetts, USA

Policies and strategies for the developing world

DEBORAH R. MAIESE
Senior Prevention Policy Advisor, US Department of Health and Human Services, Office of Disease Prevention and Health Promotion, Washington, DC, USA

Objectives-based strategies for disease prevention

CARL F. MARRS
Associate Professor of Epidemiology, School of Public Health, University of Michigan, Ann Arbor, USA

Infectious agents

ICHIYO MATSUZAKI
Assistant Professor, Department of Environmental Health, Institute of Community Medicine, University of Tsukuba, Japan

The physical and chemical environment

NICHOLAS MAYS
Director of Health Services Research, King's Fund Policy Institute and Honorary Senior Lecturer, Department of Public Health and Policy, London School of Hygiene and Tropical Medicine, London, UK

Social policy and the welfare system

J. MICHAEL McGINNIS
Scholar-in-residence, National Academy of Sciences, Washington DC, USA

Objectives-based strategies for disease prevention

G.B.M. MENSINK
Head of Section for Risk Assessment Methods, General Epidemiology, Robert Koch Institute, Berlin, Germany

Community based intervention trials

ARNOLD S. MONTO
Professor of Epidemiology and International Health, School of Public Health, University of Michigan, Ann Arbor, USA

Infectious agents

GAVIN MOONEY
Professor of Health Economics, Department of Public Health and Community Medicine, University of Sydney at Westmead Hospital, New South Wales, Australia

Measuring health needs

MYFANWY MORGAN
Reader in Sociology of Health, United Medical and Dental Schools, St Thomas' Hospital, London, UK

Sociological investigations

ARNO G. MOTULSKY
Professor Emeritus (Active) of Medicine and Genetics, University of Washington, Seattle, USA

Human and medical genetics

J.A. MUIR GRAY
Director of Research and Development, Anglia and Oxford Regional Directorate, NHS, UK

Lessons and challenges

KENNETH MULLEN
Lecturer in Behavioural Science, Medical School, University of Glasgow, UK

The disadvantaged—their health needs and public health initiatives

MASATAKA MURAKAMI
Professor, Department of Environmental Health, Institute of Community Medicine, University of Tsukuba, Japan

The physical and chemical environment

MASAKI NAGAI
Professor, Department of Public Health, Saitama Medical School, Japan

Health information resources in Japan

TOSHITAKA NAKAHARA
Director, Department of Public Health, National Institute of Public Health, Japan

Public health policies and strategies in Japan

NORMAN D. NOAH
Professor of Public Health and Epidemiology, King's College School of Medicine and Dentistry, London, UK

Microbiology

D. JAMES NOKES
Royal Society University Research Fellow, Department of Biological Sciences, University of Warwick, Coventry, UK

Mathematical models of transmission and control

GILBERT S. OMENN
Dean, School of Public Health and Community Medicine, University of Washington, Seattle, USA

Risk assessment, risk communication, and risk management

WILLIAM Ll. PARRY-JONES
Professor of Child and Adolescent Psychiatry, University of Glasgow, UK

Adolescents

CALUM PATON
Professor of Health Policy, Centre for Health Planning and Management, Keele University, UK

International perspectives on public health policy

NANCY D. PEARCE
Statistician, Office of Applied Studies, Substance Abuse and Mental Health Services Administration, US Department of Health and Human Services, Rockville, Maryland, USA

Information resources in the United States

DUNCAN PEDERSEN
Lecturer, Department of Social Medicine, Harvard Medical School, Boston, Massachusetts, USA

Beyond quantitative measures: the relevance of anthropology for public health

CORINNE PEEK-ASA
Epidemiologist, Southern California Injury Prevention Research Center; Adjunct Professor, UCLA School of Public Health, Los Angeles, USA

Injury control: the public health approach

EDWARD B. PERRIN
Professor, Department of Health Services, University of Washington, Seattle, USA

Information systems for health outcome analysis

PETER O.D. PHAROAH
Professor of Public Health, Department of Public Health, University of Liverpool, UK

Children

ANDREW N. PHILLIPS
Reader in Epidemiology and Biostatistics, Royal Free Hospital School of Medicine, University of London, UK

Meta-analysis and data synthesis in medical research

MARY PIPER
Senior Registrar Public Health Medicine, North Thames Regional Health Authority, London, UK

Public mental health

DOROTHY PORTER
Senior Wellcome Lecturer in the History of Medicine, Department of History, Birkbeck College, University of London, UK

Public health and centralization: the Victorian British state

LOUISE POTVIN
Associate Professor of Social and Preventive Medicine, University of Montreal, Canada

Education and life-style determinants of health and disease

JEAN-PIERRE POULLIER
Head, OECD Policy Unit, Paris, France

Public health strategies in Europe – doing better and feeling worse

DEBORAH PROTHROW-STITH
Assistant Dean, Government and Community Programs and Professor of Health Practice, Harvard School of Public Health, Boston, Massachusetts, USA

Interpersonal violence prevention: a recent public health mandate

DENIS J. PROTTI
Professor, Health Information Science, University of Victoria, British Columbia, Canada

The application of information science, information technology, and information management to public health

VIRGINIE RINGA
Epidemiologist, INSERM, Villejuif, France

Women's health

LEON S. ROBERTSON
Lecturer in epidemiology and Public Health, Yale University, New Haven, Connecticut, USA

Injury control: some effects, principles, and prospects

RUTH ROEMER
Adjunct Professor Emerita, School of Public Health, University of California, Los Angeles, USA

Comparative national public health legislation

MILTON I. ROEMER
Professor of Health Services Emeritus, School of Public Health, University of California, Los Angeles, USA

Analysis of a national health system

GUSTAVO C. ROMÁN
Clinical Professor of Neurology, University of Texas at San Antonio: formerly Chief, Neuroepidemiology Branch, National Institute of Neurological Disorders and Stroke, National Institutes of Health, Bethesda, Maryland, USA

Neurology and public health

KENNETH J. ROTHMAN
Professor of Public Health, Boston University, Massachusetts, USA

Causation and causal inference

C. RUMEAU-ROUQUETTE
Director of Research, INSERM, Paris, France

Women's health

RODOLFO SARACCI
Director of Research in Epidemiology, National Research Council, Pisa, Italy and Scientific Adviser, International Agency for Research on Cancer, Lyon, France

Neoplasms

PATRICK SAUNDERS
Environmental Health Officer, Medical School, University of Birmingham, UK

Reducing environmental risk

MARIE-JOSEPHE SAUREL-CUBIZOLLES
Researcher in Social Epidemiology, INSERM Unit 149, Paris, France

Women's health

EGO SEEMAN
Associate Professor of Medicine, Austin and Repatriation Medical Centre, University of Melbourne, Australia

Endocrine and metabolic disorders

ROBERT D. SEGE
Assistant Professor of Pediatrics, Tufts University School of Medicine; Attending Physician, Floating Hospital for Children at New Boston, Massachusetts, USA

Interpersonal violence prevention: a recent public health mandate

BEATRICE J. SELWYN
Associate Professor of Epidemiology, Epidemiology Discipline and International and Family Health Module, University of Texas School of Public Health, Galveston, USA

Microcomputers and epidemiology

PHIL SHACKLEY
Research Fellow, Health Economics Research Unit, University of Aberdeen

Economic evaluation

P.S. SHETTY
Professor of Human Nutrition, London School of Hygiene and Tropical Medicine, University of London, UK

Nutrition

ALAN J. SILMAN
ARC Professor of Rheumatic Disease Epidemiology, ARC Epidemiology Unit, University of Manchester, UK

Musculoskeletal diseases

DENISE G. SIMONS-MORTON
Leader, Prevention Scientific Research Group, Division of Epidemiology and Clinical Applications, National Heart, Lung, and Blood Institute, Bethesda, Maryland, USA

Education and life-style determinants of health and disease

ROBERT A. SPASOFF
Professor of Epidemiology and Community Medicine, University of Ottawa, Canada

Public health policies and strategies in Canada

HOWARD SPIVAK
Associate Professor of Pediatrics and Community Health, Tufts University School of Medicine and Vice President for Community Health, New England Medical Center, Boston, Massachusetts, USA

Interpersonal violence prevention: a recent public health mandate

DONNA F. STROUP
Epidemiology Program Office, Centers for Disease Control and Prevention, Atlanta, Georgia, USA

Public health surveillance

C.M. SUCHINDRAN
Professor of Biostatistics and Fellow, Carolina Population Center, University of North Carolina at Chapel Hill, USA

Demography and public health

A.V. SWAN
Head of the PHLS Statistics Unit, Public Health Laboratory Service, London, UK

Statistical methods

HEIZO TANAKA
Professor, Department of Epidemiology, Medical Research Institute, Tokyo Medical and Dental University, Japan

Cerebrovascular diseases

KOZO TATARA
Professor of Public Health, Osaka University Medical School, Japan

The origins and development of public health in Japan

KEITH TONES
Professor of Health Education, Leeds Metropolitan University, UK

Health education, behaviour change, and the public health

HUGH TUNSTALL-PEDOE
  Professor and Director of Cardiovascular Epidemiology Unit, University
  of Dundee and Honorary Consultant Cardiologist and Specialist in
  Public Health Medicine, Dundee Teaching Hospitals NHS Trust, UK

Cardiovascular diseases

PETER TYRER
  Professor of Community Psychiatry, North West London Mental Health
  NHS Trust, UK

Public mental health

ARTHUR C. UPTON
  Clinical Professor of Environmental and Community Medicine,
  University of Medicine and Dentistry of New Jersey, Robert Wood
  Johnson Medical School, Piscataway, USA

Radiological sciences

ELIZABETH J. VAN HORN
  Clinical Research Fellow, Academic Department of Psychiatry, St Charles
  Hospital, London, UK

Public mental health

FRIEDRICH VOGEL
  Emeritus Professor of Human Genetics and Former Head of the
  Department of Human Genetics, University of Heidelberg, Germany

Human and medical genetics

MARK A. WEBER
  Associate Administrator for Communications, Substance Abuse and
  Mental Health Services Administration, US Department of Health and
  Human Services, Rockville, Maryland, USA

Policies and strategies for health in the United States

NOEL S. WEISS
  Professor, University of Washington and Member, Fred Hutchinson
  Cancer Research Center, Seattle, Washington, USA

Case-control studies

HIROSHI YANAGAWA
  Professor of Public Health, Jichi Medical School, Japan

Health information resources in Japan

TETSUJI YOKOYAMA
  Faculty Member, Department of Epidemiology, Medical Research
  Institute, Tokyo Medical and Dental University, Japan

Cerebrovascular diseases

PAUL ZIMMET
  Professor of Diabetes, Monash University, Melbourne, Australia

Endocrine and metabolic disorders

I Information systems and sources of intelligence

1 The application of information science, information technology, and information management to public health

Denis J. Protti

Introduction

The field of public health has greatly benefited in the past and will benefit even more in the future from the effective application of the principles of information science and information management and the effective implementation of information technology. Public health practitioners have at times been required to avail themselves of technology and systems designed to meet the requirements of the private sector or the acute care medical sector. As Friede *et al.* (1994) point out public health information requirements are different and their needs unique. In the traditional clinical setting, the focus is on the single patient; in the public health setting, the focus is on the population.

Numerical information systems developed for patient care or the clinical laboratory are typically oriented towards facilitating the entry and review of a single record or of several hundred records of subjects in a study. By contrast, public health practitioners often need to examine thousands of records, although they may not need detailed information for each individual but only summary information about the population. In addition, holders of data are often eager to share selections of their data with others, and to engage in collaborative studies.

Textual information systems that describe the experimental medical literature are easily accessed through MEDLARS and software packages such as Grateful Med. By contrast, searching the corresponding public health literature is difficult because government publications at all levels are not listed in Index Medicus, are not centrally stored, and have extremely variable formats and lengths. A further complicating factor is the paucity of public health oriented keywords in the Medical Subject Headings (MeSH) system; hence making the public health literature available in full text searchable form is an important way to provide access to it (Friede *et al.* 1994).

The data analysis needs of the clinically based epidemiologist often differ from those of public health professionals in health departments. While the clinically based epidemiologist collects and analyses data from chart reviews and clinical trials and needs software that supports non-parametric statistics and time–series analysis, the public health worker collects data from surveillance systems, population-based surveys, and outbreak reports and needs software that can be used to perform standardization, fit mathemat-ical models to disease patterns, analyse data from complex surveys, and draw maps.

However, the most significant difference is perhaps in the area of communications. The clinician needs to communicate with patients, with the clinical laboratory, and with colleagues who are typically close by. The amount of information to share is often small (a status, a recommendation) and urgency is often high; telephones and bleepers fit these needs. The public health practitioner on the other hand needs to communicate with colleagues in the state or district laboratory, with federal agencies, and with research collaborators at many geographically separated sites; large groups may be called upon to make decisions. The amount of information to share is often large but urgency is rarely high. Electronic mail and video-teleconferencing are often more appropriate technologies that fit these needs.

Information science

Before exploring the application of information management principles and the impact of information technology in the field of public health, it is important to first understand the foundations on which information science is built.

Information

The most universal definition of information comes from philosophy: information is knowledge for the purposes of taking effective action (Meadow 1979). In his original treatise on cybernetics, Wiener (1948) compared the acquisition and processing of information in human beings and animals with the similar activity in the control of machines and other activities. Many have attempted to define information, a few examples being:

1. an increment of knowledge;

2. an interpretation of external stimuli;

3. increasing the state of knowledge of a recipient;

4. a reduction in uncertainty, following communication;

5. any physical form of representation, or surrogate of knowledge, or of a particular thought, used for communication;

6. a measure of one's freedom of choice when one selects a message;

7. recorded experience that is, or can be, used in decision making.

The last definition is that of Churchman (1971) who postulated that recorded experience becomes information only when it is or can be applied to a decision process. Hence it is possible to have access to large amounts of descriptive raw data but yet have little or no information. In an engineering or information theory sense, information is the capacity of a communications channel, a measurable quantity which is independent of the physical medium by which it is conveyed. Applying this theory to Churchman's definition enables the measurement of the amount of information than can be obtained from a particular piece of raw data or descriptive material. In an 'information system' sense, information is generally considered to be data (raw material) that has been processed into a form that is meaningful to the recipient and is of real or perceived value in current or prospective decisions. Wiener regarded communication between the component parts of a community as vital to its activities. He saw an information system as the means by which the necessary communication can be established and maintained.

There appears to be no consensual definition of information. Information is a complex concept and simplistic views of it lead to simplistic decisions. In a world of uncertainty, information reduces uncertainty. It changes the probabilities attached to expected outcomes in a decision situation and therefore has value in the decision process. It is so closely related to the concepts of thought, values, knowledge, and environment, that it is often difficult to isolate and adequately define 'information'. Cybernetics, which is concerned with the use of information to effect certain control actions, is but one of many fields which claims to study information.

Information theory

Information theory was first suggested by Wiener (1948). His contention that any organism is held together by the possession of means for acquisition, use, retention and transmission of information denotes a biological sense of information. In their paper, 'A mathematical theory of communication', Shannon and Weaver (1960) provided the foundation for measuring information (in a non-semantic sense). Their concern was not with meaning, or the semantic aspects of information, but with the engineering problems of transmitting it. Information theory, as ascribed to by Shannon and Weaver, is only concerned with the factors that determine whether or not a message has been exactly or approximately transferred between a source and the destination. The principal elements of Shannon and Weaver's communications system can be delineated as follows:

1. Information source: the originator of the messages which are to be transferred to the destination. There is an almost unlimited variety of permissible message types. Typewriter-like systems use sequences of letters. Bank cheques are messages which are composed of letters and numbers.

2. Transmitter: operates on the message to transform it into a signal form which can be transmitted over the communication channel (path).

3. Channel: the communication path over which the signal is transmitted to the receiver.

4. Receiver: usually performs the inverse function of the transmitter to yield a reconstruction of the message.

5. Destination: the intended termination of the message transfer.

A noise source is included in the model as all systems are perturbed by unwanted signals in one form or another. There is a distinction between noise and distortion. Distortion is caused by a known (even intentional) operation and can be corrected by an inverse operation. Noise is random or unpredictable interference. Shannon and Weaver identified three levels of problems in a communication system, namely:

1. Technical Accuracy. Just how accurately are the message symbols transferred from the message source to the destination?

2. Semantic Accuracy. How accurately is the semantic meaning of the messages transferred from the message source to the destination? These semantic problems are concerned with how closely the destination interprets the knowledge conveyed by the message to the knowledge intended by the sender.

3. Effectiveness. How effectively does the received message control the system in the intended fashion?

The primary motivation for communication within a system is to instruct selected subsystems to take some course of action. Effectiveness is closely related to semantic accuracy, and the two problems cannot always be completely dissociated. In fact, it is not uncommon to discover situations in which it is either entirely impossible or meaningless to separate the three problem levels. No real communication can take place unless the transmitter and the receiver are making use of compatible codes or schemes for symbolic representation of information, for example a bridge player failing to 'catch' and respond to in an appropriate manner his partner's bidding signal.

Information science

Although information science is not a direct descendant of information theory many of its practitioners do, however, attempt to retain the spirit of information theory by making information the central concept and by providing precise definitions of what it is. In information theory, the concept of information was never meant to express the meaning of a message; Shannon and Weaver, in fact, clearly stated that semantic concepts were quite irrelevant to the problem. Yet to many, information science is interested in the meaningfulness of information and in the usefulness of information to the user. It is a field of study which investigates how systems, humans and/or machines, retrieve information rather than just receive information. Humans are active rather than passive, they search for information for a specific purpose and do not just wait to process it, should it happen to pass by (Radford 1978).

Webster's dictionary defines 'information science' as the collection, classification, storage, retrieval, and dissemination of recorded knowledge, treated both as a pure and an applied science. Although Webster's considers 'informatics' to be synonymous with information science, the literal translation of the French term 'informatique' and the German term 'informatik' is 'the rational scientific treatment, notably by computer, needed to support knowledge and communications in technical, economic, and social domains'. The significant difference between the English and European definitions is the latter's inclusion of the computer. It should also be noted that the European definitions of informatics make no explicit claim to being a science.

The field of information science is perhaps best exemplified by Meadow (1979) who views it as a study concerned with the:

1. nature of information and information processes;

2. measurement of information (including its value) and information processes;

3. communication of information between humans and information machines;

4. organization of information and its effect on the design of machines, algorithms and human perception of information;

5. human behaviour in respect to the generation, communication and use of information;

6. principles of design and measurement of the performance of algorithms for information processing; and

7. artificial intelligence applied to information processing.

Before discussing the broader concept of information science in public health, a historical review of the term medical informatics is in order.

Medical informatics

Over the past 25 years, many have published their impressions and opinions as to what constitutes the field of medical informatics. One of the first to use the term was Reichertz (1973), a physician, who defined medical informatics as the science of analysis, documentation, steering, control, and synthesis of information processes within the health care delivery system, especially in the classical environment of hospitals and medical practice.

Twenty years ago, Shires and Ball (1975) confidently wrote that 'The year 1975 will be noted as the year in which medical informatics became accepted as a legitimate term used to describe activities involved in assembling, correlating and making effective use of information and decision making in health care delivery'. Moehr et al. (1979) also observed that informatics as a science does not fit into the conventional classification of sciences: it neither belongs to the natural sciences – its objects are not phenomena of nature, nor is it a part of mathematics. It is not a human science nor is it one of the classical engineering sciences. In his opinion, informatics deals with investigating the fundamental procedures of information processing and the general methods of the application of such procedures in various application areas.

Another physician, Levy (1977) defined medical informatics as the acquisition, analysis, and dissemination of information in health care delivery processes. He concluded that on the grounds of relevance and direct appropriateness to modern medicine, informatics is a proper basic medical science. A similar view was expressed by van Bemmel (1984) who wrote that medical infor-

matics comprises the theoretical and practical aspects of information processing and communication, based on knowledge and experience derived from processes in medicine and health care. This definition is tempered somewhat by Hannah (1985) who reported that nurses continue to consider the term 'medical' to be synonymous with the word physician. A relatively new but highly related term is that of nursing informatics. In using the term, Hannah refers to the use of information technologies in relation to any of the functions which are within the purview of nursing and which are carried out by nurses. As evidenced by the above definitions, the term medical informatics on the one hand appears to be confined to the clinical practice of medicine while on the other it encompasses the broader notion of health and health care delivery. Perhaps the field of public health informatics will arise before too long!

Health information science

After an extensive review of the literature and a critical analysis of the aims and objectives of the University of Victoria's new baccalaureate degree programme in health information science, Protti (1982) defined health information science as the study of the nature of information and its processing, application and impact within a health care system. This definition was not intended to be unique and mutually exclusive of the work of others. It was rather an attempt to broaden the Reichertz domain of hospitals and medical practice to encompass all of health care. Health information science is to information science as health economics is to economics. An economist is one who specializes in the social science concerned chiefly with the description and analysis of the production, distribution and consumption of goods and services. A health economist, upon familiarizing himself with the institutions, participants, and concepts of health, illness, and disease, analyses economic phenomena in health care delivery and resource management settings. Similarly, a computer scientist is concerned with the science of properties, representation, construction and realization of algorithms. A medical computer scientist is concerned with the application of these concepts to medical science and medical practice. To be effective, he/she must have more than a passing acquaintance with concepts of diagnosis and treatment of disease. An engineer is concerned with the application of science and mathematics by which the properties of matter and the sources of energy in nature are made useful to man in structures, machines, products, systems, and processes. A biomedical engineer is concerned with the capacity of human beings to survive and function in abnormally stressing environments and with the protective modification of such environments.

In keeping with Meadow's views, a health information scientist or health informatician should therefore be concerned with:

1. the nature of information and information processes in all aspects of health promotion, detection and delivery of care;

2. the measurement of information and information processes;

3. the organization of information and its effect on the performance of health practitioners, researchers, planners and managers;

4. the communication of information between patients, health care providers, administrators, evaluators, planners, and legislators;

5. the behaviour of patients, health care providers, administrators, planners, and legislators, in respect to the generation, and use of information.

Many of health information science's conceptual foundations are borrowed from other fields such as mathematics, economics, psychology, engineering, sociology, and biology. It is a discipline which is not distinctively different from those in subject content, but different in outlook. Information science in health is concerned with the individual and group behaviour of health care personnel in their interaction with information and with the technology which processes information.

Information technology

What are the major issues surrounding this complex subject? Will information technology affect the public health profession over the next 20 years and if so in what ways? Rather than presume to have definitive answers, this section will raise questions, which readers will eventually have to answer for themselves.

The section is structured so as to develop the following premises:

1. Information technology is part of the larger domain of 'technology'.

2. The impact that informatics will have on public health can be seen by observing the impact technology is having on society.

Although technologies such as hydroponics, genetic engineering, and nuclear fission are important in the overall scheme of things, they will not be discussed in this section.

One must resist the temptation to predict unrealistically. Predictions of what the world will be like 30 to 40 years from now are easy, the predictor need not worry about being around to defend his/her views. The nearer to the present the more difficult the task for the political, social, economic, and emotional issues which influence change are much more apparent. This section will attempt to identify the issues which will probably affect public health over the next 5 to 10 years. The extent to which one agrees with someone else's view of the future is very much influenced by one's own view of the past and present. How each reader answers the questions will be governed by how well the individual understands the issues and is challenged or threatened by their implications. One consolation is that all health professionals are having to wrestle with the same questions.

The evolution of information technology

Information technology, is not a new phenomenon. It has been around since the beginning of time. It entails people communicating with each other, and recording their thoughts, ideas, and actions for others to read or hear. The broad definition of information technology includes:

- Computers (mainframes to workstations, desktop personal computers and multimedia)
- Telecommunications (switching systems to faxes)
- Networks (local area and wide area)
- Document reproduction
- Artificial intelligence and speed recognition expert systems.

In coming to understand information technology in a modern context, it is important to realize that the electronic computer is only one component in an elaborate and highly differentiated infrastructure. This infrastructure has grown through a succession of generations of computers, each of which represent a major change in technology. During the eight-year span of each computing generation (the first generation started in the late 1940s and the fifth in the early 1980s), revolutionary changes have taken place that correspond to those taking place over some seventy years or more in the aircraft industry. If we were to draw parallels to the rapid and massive advancements, aircraft would be able to go 100 times faster, a $200 000 home would cost $20 000, and colour televisions would cost $20.

The definition of generations in terms of electronic device technology captures important aspects of computing technology such as cost decreases, size decrease, power increases, and so on. However, it fails to account for the qualitative changes that have given computing its distinct character in each generation. The change from mechanical to electronic devices made it possible to store programs as data and enabled the use of computers as a general-purpose tool and then the development of programming language compilers. The transistor made reliable operation possible and enable routine electronic data processing and then interactive time-sharing. Integrated circuits reduced costs to the level where computers became commonplace and made possible the personal computer dedicated to the single user.

Each generation represents a revolution in technology with a qualitatively different impact. Each generation subsumes the capabilities of that preceding it, providing very much better facilities at very much lower cost, and adding new capabilities not possessed by the previous generations. One of the innovative new capabilities has been in the area of knowledge-based systems. The products stemming from breakthroughs in this area are expert systems which simulate some of the processes of the human mind, knowledge representation and inference, allowing expertise to be encoded for a computer and made widely available. This has generated a new industry based on creating expert systems to make the practical working knowledge of a human expert in a specific subject area such as medicine widely available to those without direct access to the original expert.

Technology and society

Society is experiencing its second major revolution in less than two hundred years. The first was the Industrial Revolution of the 19th century which saw the substitution of mechanical processes for human muscles. It changed the nature of work, though not the size of the workforce, and with it society's view of human values. The spinning jenny may have done the work of 1000 women, but hundreds of thousands were eventually needed in the mills. The automobile may have put the horse out of business, but Henry Ford saw to it that many more mechanics were needed than blacksmiths, many more oil industry personnel than haymakers. Although it had a significant impact on the nature of work, the Industrial Revolution did provide untold opportunities for the individual to hold a job at some level. Even if the job was classified as unskilled labour, the person still had an identity as a breadwinner, and could feel a sense of worth from that. If that industrial job was classified as skilled labour, the person had not only the benefits of the unskilled labourer, but in addition a higher job status. As a rule, every major technological advance destroys the civilization that existed at the time of its introduction into everyday life. The steam engine pushed us out of the fields and into the cities, the automobile out of the cities and into the suburbs. The movies gathered us in huge crowds in darkened halls, television returned us to our own darkened living rooms. The compass and chronometer made intercontinental travel possible, the airoplane makes it trivial, and advances in communications technology may make it unnecessary.

The second major revolution is the so-called electronic or information revolution in which electronic circuits are being substituted for human mental skills. The electronic revolution is replacing not only the mental processes of the unskilled labourer; it is creating a genuine human value dilemma for technologists, managers, and professionals. Technology is changing everyone's job. What is both exciting and frightening is that the rate of change does not appear to be diminishing.

The fundamental economic activities of our society – agriculture and the multitude of extractive, manufacturing, and service industries – continue, but they are increasingly influenced by a new decision-making process. Vastly more information (on markets, costs, techniques, other options) is being made available to decision-makers because of the information technology now available. This information is being eagerly sought because more informed decisions, be they in politics, operating factories, hospitals, public health agencies, or any organization, are likely to produce better results. The electronic revolution has made robotics a reality. The development and use of intelligent robots which perform delicate tasks that once could have been done by thinking human beings is increasingly commonplace in manufacturing sectors of society. Robotics are beginning to be introduced into health care. How long before they become commonplace?

While the industrial age found its symbol in the factory, the symbol of the information age is the computer, which can hold all the information in the Library of Congress in a machine the size of a small refrigerator. Alternatively, its proper symbol may be a robot, a machine capable of supplementing age-old manual labour and liberating human beings from the most arduous and repetitive tasks. Perhaps its symbol is the direct broadcast satellite, which can send television programmes directly into homes around the globe. Telephone companies the world over are joining forces under the banner of the Integrated Services Digital Network (ISDN), which is described as the key to linking all the elements of the information age. ISDN is several things at the same time, but it will allow every home and organization to receive simultaneously voice, computing, and video signals on a telephone line.

A popular way of looking at information technology is in terms of its utility. The most frequently used reasoning to justify purchases of information technology goes as follows: labour expenses are high and getting higher; computer expenses are low and getting lower; it then logically follows that one should always trade an expensive commodity, such as labour, for an inexpensive commodity, such as computers. One of the resulting dilemmas is

that 'value' has become less personal and more social or group-oriented. In a technological society, the individual has the potential of becoming insulated against ethical and moral decisions as these responsibilities are projected onto society itself. For people whose identities have been imbedded in their jobs, traditional culture provides no guidelines to help them value themselves after they have been more or less excluded from the productive parts of society.

The evolution of the health care industry

The future of the health care industry is not the same in all parts of the world. In many parts of the world, the health care industry is struggling to satisfy the most basic and fundamental of needs. In other parts of the world, the rapid advances in medical science are putting strains on governments to provide the best possible care, given the limited resources available. In the United States and the United Kingdom, the future of the health care industry is quite clear, the future is competition. Competition is not new, nor is it unique to the Americans and the British; competition has always existed in terms of institutional pride, quality of care, staff prestige, and reputation. In the United States and the United Kingdom, competition is being redefined to include price and marketing as important factors and the key to being competitive is how well information is provided and used.

The increasing emphasis on competition has spurred the movement toward 'alternate-site' medicine, that is the delivery of health care outside the traditional, and costly, hospital setting. Of particular interest is the role technology plays in this new movement. Diagnoses that were once run in the hospital or in the large clinical laboratories are now being performed in doctors' offices in minutes and at a fraction of the cost charged by the big automated laboratories. Increasingly, more and more surgical procedures are now performed routinely in outpatient day surgery units and in private surgicentres. Technological advances such as the lithotriptor, replace complex and costly major surgery, along with its 10 to 12 days hospital stay, with a 1 day procedure which 'shatters' rather than removes kidney stones. Medical costs are also being reduced by treatments that can be performed by many patients at home.

The market – which includes not only the drugs used in the treatment but also auxiliary equipment, such as small programmable pumps – now consists primarily of special nutritional products and services (aimed at patients with abnormal digestive systems), kidney dialysis, and continuous intravenous drug administration. Home therapies will almost certainly embrace such intractable disorders such as Alzheimer's disease and many forms of physical rehabilitation. One company markets a home chemotherapy system for cancer patients, many of whom would normally have to receive anticancer drugs in a hospital or physician's office. Patients who are healthy enough to live at home, can often use a continuously administered, pre-packaged drug or combination of drugs. The drugs are contained in a small plastic pouch that is attached to a catheter. A portable programmable pump delivers the drugs at a slow constant rate. One of the advantages to this approach is that the steady infusion of such drugs often eliminates the side-effects, such as nausea, that usually accompany large doses.

The benefits of such procedures, moreover, extend well beyond lower costs. Recovery or remission rates for many patients are dramatically reduced in the familiar and comfortable home environment. A lens implant in the eyes of a 75-year-old person allows her to continue to live independently in the home and community which is meaningful to her. The quality of life is infinitely 'better' than moving to a home for the blind in a nearby town or city. Neonatal intensive care units are allowing life to be continued in hundreds of cases in which death would have been a certainty 25 years ago. Microcomputing technology is providing artificial voices for those who cannot speak, workstations for the sightless, and communication for those paralysed by stroke. The elderly, handicapped people and others with high-risk medical conditions can find a new level of security when their hospitals use a computer and the telephone system to guarantee them almost instant response in an emergency. The list grows with each passing year. What are the implications of these trends on the public health practitioner?

Communications technology

Perhaps, the form of modern information technology which will most affect the public health practitioner in the future is communications technology. The advances in telecommunications are matching the speed of those of computing technology. More importantly the cost of this form of technology is now dropping – after years of overpricing. This drop in cost is no more evident than in the explosion of the Internet.

Internet – what is it?

What railroads were to America in the 19th century and superhighway systems were in the 20th, high bandwidth networks are to the 21st century.

Mitchell Kertzman, CEO
Powersoft Corporation

Ask for a definition of the Internet and, depending on whom you ask, you will get either a simplistic answer or one that is long, detailed, and mainly incomprehensible. The simplest way to describe the Internet is with one word – communication. The Internet is often called a network of networks (Plucauskas 1994). The Internet provides a vehicle for networks of all kinds and individual stand-alone computers to intertwine to form a global network which connects, as of late 1994, over 30 million users in over 40 countries. The number of users with access to the Internet is growing at 10 per cent per month; forecasts are that by the turn of the century there may be 1 million networks, 100 million computers, and 1 billion users on the Internet (Smith and Gibbs 1994).

The users are connected to small Local Area Networks (LANs) in their offices where they share files and electronic mail (e-mail). Increasingly, these LANs are being connected to form groups of thousands of computers that are linked across large areas sometimes referred to as Wide Area Networks (WANs). The speed at which one can do things on the Internet is remarkable; not because the Internet is particularly speedy, but because it enables one to travel around the world in seconds. The lure of the Internet is communication and access. People who want to exchange ideas and develop knowledge are increasingly doing it on the Internet (for example librarians – whose job it is to find documents, books, and

other materials – now share their catalogues through the Internet).

The system that has grown into the Internet was originally designed by the United States military in 1969 under the name ARPANET (Advanced Research Projects Agency). The first ARPANET configuration involved four computers and was designed to demonstrate the feasibility of building networks using computers dispersed over a wide area. Each computer communication point or node on the Internet is able to pass information on to the next node. Information on the Internet is controlled using a set of data communications standards know as the TCP/IP protocol. Protocols are agreed upon methods of communication used by computers – similar to the way people have protocols for communicating. The specifics of TCP are complex (and highly technical) and beyond the scope of this textbook. Let it be left to say that the TCP/IP protocol is designed to ensure that every piece of information finds the most direct route to its destination. The hundreds of thousands of nodes around the Internet form a web in which information can travel, thus eliminating the need for central communication switches and means that as long as at least two nodes are in contact, the network will remain operational.

There is no single owner, or even a formal coalition that actually 'owns' the Internet. The various sub-networks have owners who recognize that having connections to other networks either enhances their mission or makes their services more desirable. The only group that 'runs' the Internet is the Internet Society (ISOC). These volunteers freely give their time to support and promote the aims of the Internet. ISOC has many committees and working groups and is lead by the IAB, the Internet Architecture Board. The IAB is responsible for ratifying the standards (such as protocols and technologies) that the Internet will use. Another group – the Internet Engineering Task Force, or IETF – is a public forum that develops standards and resolves operational issues for the Internet. The IETF forms working groups to explore and evaluate issues and develops technical standards, which may be accepted by the IETF and sent to the IAB for ratification. Like ISOC, IETF is purely voluntary.

Internet tools

There are many different ways to send and receive information across the Internet. There are also many excellent publications that provide in-depth descriptions. Many are available for free around the Internet or can be purchased in the ever growing number of computer sections in bookstores. The ability to access different tools depends on the type of Internet account and the sophistication of the interfaces users employ to log on (connect) to the Internet.

E-mail and Usenet Electronic mail (e-mail) is and probably always will be the most common use of the Internet. It allows Internet users to send and receive messages from around the world. Requests for database searches and the result posted to an account can also be done by e-mail. E-mail is also used to join electronic mailing lists (called listservs) on specific topics of interest. E-mail is used to transfer text, program files, spreadsheets, and even photographic images. Messages can be sent and received in hours at most and often within minutes; it is no wonder that most e-mail users refer to the regular postal service as 'snail mail'.

E-mail is based on the fundamental concept of store-and--

forward technology. The store part refers to a message being added to a storage system by the message's originator. When the recipient is ready, the message is forwarded for retrieval. The beauty of this technique is that the recipient does not have to be available when the originator sends the message. This enables the e-mail system to select how the message will move from the place where it is first stored to the place where it is retrieved (forwarded to the user).

It is becoming increasingly easy to find anyone on the Internet – even if one does not know their e-mail address. Internet addresses are in two parts, a 'domain' name and a user name separated by an 'at (@)' sign. The domain name (more correctly called a hierarchical name) consists of the name of the machine on which the user has an account, along with the network groups and subgroups leading to that computer, thereby giving that machine a unique identification which enables the Internet software to determine where to deliver the message. Delivering the message to the addressee is then up to the named computer. The computer's name is chosen locally and is often colourful or thematic. User names can be cryptic. They are often composed of first initial and last name but can be shortened, a nickname, or identifying numbers. All Internet alphanumeric addresses are actually aliases for numeric addresses, such as 134.6.4.187. The alphanumeric addresses are used because, even though they can be hard to interpret, they are easier than the numeric names. The translation of alphanumeric names into numeric addresses is handled by machines on the Internet, called name servers. To get around the cumbersome Internet address of a person or persons, many mail programs enable users to create aliases. Aliases are particularly helpful when e-mail is sent to a group of people.

Electronic mail is such an inexpensive form of communication, and it is so easy to send copies of messages to long distribution lists, recipients may get much mail which is of little or no value to them. As a result, new filtering software is being developed to help sort the wanted from the unwanted mail. Users can develop their own filtering rules (such as if from 'boss', display immediately) and can modify them at any time. Techniques such as assigning points to messages to indicate their importance is another variation of the same theme to make e-mail communications among groups more effective – to get relevant information to the recipients with less waste of time on the part of both senders and recipients.

Usenet newsgroups are Internet bulletin boards that are similar to listservs but require the use of software known as a news reader. There are thousands of Usenet groups and listservs for discussion of medical and health related topics. A number of groups have already put up information relating to community and public health issues. The Institute of Maternal and Child Health Policy at the University of Florida has provided information through the Maternal and Child Health Network. The topics include items such as vaccination requirements, injury prevention summaries, school health information and child health policy documents. Internet resources for the hearing impaired including newsletters, software, and demographic data are available through a number if sites. As well as providing services for the hearing impaired, the Internet can be used as an enabling technology, especially for individuals who are homebound or live in an institution. Other types of community health information available includes breast cancer support and poison control information.

Telnet provides a tool by which users can log in to other computers around the Internet. Through Telnet a person can access other computer sites using their own computer as a terminal. This is particularly useful for accessing medical libraries and other health care database systems that are linked to the Internet.

FTP File Transfer Protocol (FTP) is the method by which specific computer data or files are transferred around the Internet. Files can be simple text – usually known as ASCII files, or more complex data such as graphics or computer programs – known as binary files. The ability to pull down a file to get data or run a program (if the file is executable) is vital for people doing research and development work. The Internet transfers files at a rate of millions of bytes per second, and with the coming of the National Research and Education Network (NERN), that will soon be upgraded to gigabytes (thousands of millions of bytes) per second. FTP can do more than just retrieve files. It can be used to transfer files to remote machines from a given computer. To make it a practical tool, FTP includes commands for listing directories, listing files in directories, changing directories, and getting information about what is being done and setting parameters for how the operations will be done. Many pieces of free software can be obtained from around the Internet via anonymous FTPs which allows users to log in to FTP sites where they do not have accounts. These anonymous FTP sites together contain millions of files that add up to terabytes of information.

Gopher Gopher is a menu driven service that allows people to seamlessly access information from around the Internet. Gopher was developed at the University of Minnnesota and gets its name from the university's mascot and from the fact that it allows individuals to tunnel through the Internet searching for information. Gopher and its counterpart WWW (see below) allows users to access information without ever needing to know its precise location. Links to other Internet tools such as telnet and FTP, can be made through Gopher. At the National Institutes of Health Gopher, for example, information can be found on NIH grants and contracts or a search can be performed on the NIH directory.

WWW World Wide Web (WWW) is the newest Internet service. It provides links to information via hypertext and for those who have the proper type of Internet access, it can bring multimedia Internet to the desktop. Hypertext provides links to other information sources through selected, or highlighted words within a text. A person simply chooses the highlighted word to get further facts on the topic of interest. The links could be to data located on the same machine or anywhere else on the Internet. Some WWW clients, or browsers as they are known, allow users the ability to incorporate graphics, sounds and even full motion video into a document. The most common of these browsers, Mosaic, is available from many sites around the Internet and is available in Windows 3.x, Macintosh or UNIX formats. Many groups have started to use multimedia Internet to produce medical education materials.

Internet search tools With so many potential sources of information, finding data on the Internet can be a daunting task. Fortunately, innovative ways of indexing and retrieving information is one of the fastest growing areas of the Internet. Finger and netfind are tools that can be used to search for e-mail addresses. A search tool known as Archie is available for searching titles of anonymous FTP software. The Archie interfaces, though a bit difficult for the novice, can become a useful method for tracking down where software is available. WAIS is a tool that can be used to index databases. Keyword and text searches of entire documents within WAIS databases can be performed. Veronica, the counterpart of Archie, is a WAIS-like tool that is used for searching Gopher-space. It performs text and Boolean searches on Gopher file and directory titles around the Internet and provides links to the information it finds.

Several sources on the Internet are particularly helpful for research:

1. CARL UnCover is a database through which citations to more than 10 000 journals can be accessed.

2. DIALOG enables one to get details about what businesses are doing, who runs them, etc.

3. OCLC is a library-oriented database.

4. ERIC is a database of interest to teachers, parents, and students.

Hooking up to the Internet

Not all Internet connections are the same; some allow users only to access certain types of Internet tools and are available in host-based dial up interfaces. Other, usually commercial, Internet connections can enable users to employ Windows or Macintosh based software to access the Internet. Although these commercial connections can be more expensive than other options, the ease of use that these interfaces offer make them an attractive option, especially for first time users. The three most common methods of accessing the Internet are: through a university affiliation; via a community access bulletin board know as Freenet; or through a commercial service provider.

Universities   Universities were the first large scale users of the Internet; thus virtually all schools within a typical university have some form of Internet connectivity. Students, faculty and groups with university affiliations may be eligible for some level of INTERNET connectivity through their institution. Most universities will give those who are eligible an account on a computer which has a connection to the Internet. University Internet accounts are generally accessed by dialing in to another machine at the university over a modem on a personal computer either at home or on campus. University accounts can be a good place to start to navigate the Internet, especially if they are available for free as part of a university affiliation – most universities do not expect their users to pay for the Internet access. However, difficulties mastering unfriendly interfaces and lack of user support have been known to cause problems for university based users.

Freenets   Freenets are community based electronic bulletin boards that allow users Internet access. Freenets are relatively new tools, but more are coming on-line every month. The Freenet system is menu driven and is set up with the novice user in mind. They are, as the name applies, free to use, however donations are strongly encouraged to help offset operating costs. As well as being able to attain local information, including health care resources, registered users can access e-mail and other Internet tools. Freenets are not intended for business or commercial ventures and users are limited in the scope of tools they can use. For example, the use of FTP and telnet are limited on most Freenets.

Commercial Internet accounts   Commercial service prices can vary greatly depending on the provider and the type of services used.

The four most common types of Internet access that commercial providers supply are:

1. Dial up Host Access – similar to a university account with access provided through a text based computing environment, however interfaces and user support may be better.

2. Dial up SLIP and PPP Access – Serial Line Internet Protocol (SLIP) and Point to Point Protocol (PPP) allow full Internet access over a modem and telephone line, thus users can employ interfaces that reside directly on their own computer. This is especially useful for neophytes because it means they can make use of Windows and Macintosh graphical interfaces, many of which are free, to access Internet tools. SLIP and PPP also can be used with multimedia Internet through the WWW and browsers such as Mosaic.

3. Dedicated SLIP and PPP Access – in this case a dedicated SLIP and PPP account is open for use 24 hours per day.

4. Dedicated Link – used to connect an entire LAN to the Internet and/or be connected to computer(s) which will act as Internet information servers. These links can be quite expensive and are usually only feasible at an organizational level.

Conclusion

The Internet was originally developed so that science and research could share resources. To a great extent, communications in the form of e-mail and discussion groups have overshadowed the Internet's use for resource sharing. Although the traditional methods of scholarly communication – presentations at conferences, publishing of papers in journals, and so on – have not been eliminated, they are being recognized as inadequate for current research needs. The Internet distributes information in a way that is infinitely more flexible and more timely. Findings, papers, and information can be instantly shared and discussed.

The Internet can provide an innovative solution for meeting a variety of communication needs within the public health community. As services and tools expand and improve, more ways of applying the technology will continue to be found; the Internet will probably become a service from the telephone company before too long. It is, however, important to remember that the Internet is not about technology, it is about people. The tools and applications are only as valuable as the people they enable and empower to communicate.

Group decision support technology

There are a varied and growing number of computer-based group support systems, including: computer conferencing, video and audio teleconferencing, document interchange services, meeting support tools and group decision support. Perhaps the most common group support system aimed at increasing the effectiveness of communication amongst individuals is computer conferencing.

Computer conferencing

Computer conferencing is a teleconference that uses computers, software and communications networks to allow groups of people to exchange ideas, opinions and information (McNurlin and

Sprague 1989). The people in a teleconference may all be located in the same building, or they can be scattered worldwide. Each user signs on to the teleconference (via a terminal or personal computer) at his or her own convenience; there is no need for members of the group to be using it simultaneously, although they may do so if they choose.

Although similar in some ways, computer conferencing systems are different from other types of computerized communication, such as electronic mail, bulletin boards, and information retrieval services. E-mail is essentially a one-to-one (or one-to-many) form of communication. Moreover, after a message has been read, it is generally deleted; there tends to be little or no storage of messages. Bulletin boards provide storage but are designed mainly for posting notices for other people to read, a one-to-many type of communication. Information retrieval services provide a stored database that users can retrieve from but cannot change.

Computer conferencing systems typically include not only electronic mail and bulletin boards but also many-to-many communications, by allowing all participants to join topics and enter comments on the subject being discussed. They provide storage; comments are not deleted after being read. In joining one or more conferences, each time the person logs on, the system tells them how many messages have been entered in those particular conferences since the last time they were logged in, and will deliver those messages, one at a time. If one gets tired of a conference, one can leave it and not get any more messages from it. Computer conferencing allows the setting up of subconferences for discussing some aspect of the general subject in more detail. Some systems also allow voting, to indicate consensus of opinion.

The benefits of computer conferencing include:

- fast exchange of information

- less formality

- encourages more stimulating ideas

- provides a written record of discussions

- convenient; use it at anytime

- non-interruptive

- avoids telephone tag and slowness of mail

- handles a dispersed group as easily as a local one

- branching allows for special interest discussions and limits junk mail

- late joiners can catch up easily

- users can settle matters without face-to-face meetings

- users like its collaborative nature

- supports group interaction; valuable for project management

- encourages chance meetings of people with shared interests

- fosters cross-fertilization of ideas

- managers can participate and be more proactive

- allows large numbers of people to interact as equals.

Video conferencing

Video conferencing technology is becoming an affordable reality that can substantially increase communications productivity. The products being developed to support 'personal conferencing' exploit the power and availability of the workstation and the capabilities of interfaces such as Microsoft Windows, Presentation Manager, and X Windows and Motif. They allow users on either end to share moving video images, voice communications, documents, and even applications across the 'new' digital ISDN phone service or over common high-speed LANs and WANs such as Ethernet or token ring. They now even work over public data networks such as Internet (Linthicum 1994). The multimedia revolution is making the presence of speakers and microphones on workstations commonplace. The new video cameras, the size of a stack of 10 silver dollars, are less intimidating than camcorders. The picture that these cameras produce and the sound quality from the audio equipment is surprisingly good. The price of these systems ranges from $500 to $20 000, depending on the features and the platform supported.

Video conferencing still has network problems and, until 1993 when desktop units came along, conference rooms systems went for upwards of $60 000; roll-abouts started at $25 000 (Strauss 1994). A research report estimated that there were just 14 000 desktop units installed worldwide at the end of 1993, but it expects that the number will soar to 1.96 million by the end of 1998. Even in view of AT&T's recently announced arrangement with Intel to create a personal conferencing gateway, universal video calling does not seem likely for a few years. However, innovative use of the technology is giving early users a competitive edge. As an example, most banks have television cameras at their automated teller machines for security purposes. Some are turning that camera into a two-way video conference application and staffing the bank remotely. They let customers interact with bank personnel and do all of their banking around the clock at considerably less expense than keeping branch offices open. MEDITrust Pharmacy, a Canadian mail-order pharmaceutical firm has created a virtual pharmacy. It put a video/phone/data kiosk in a convenience store, connects it to a pharmacist at a remote site over ISDN lines, and sends medicines by mail. The kiosk scans the prescription so that the pharmacist can give advice, stamps the prescription filled, and processes the credit card order. Medicine is sent to a customer's home by two day special mail service. The convenience store may be in a rural village too small to support a full pharmacy. Employers are considering offering their staff a similar service from the company offices.

Group decision support systems

Up until recently, most of the work in decision support systems has been to help individuals make decisions. However increasingly in all sectors, and particularly so in public health, decisions are not made by individuals; instead groups of people are involved. Rather than support only communication between members of groups, group decision support systems (GDSS) have features and functions that help these groups form a consensus or come to a decision (McNurlin and Sprague 1989).

The desired design of a GDSS typically includes several features or characteristics. Each participant is able to work independently of the others, and then publicly release or demonstrate his or her personal work. When personal work is released, all group members are able to retrieve and view it. Similarly, each member is able to retrieve and view any work performed by the group as a whole.

Elements of a GDSS include a database, a GDSS model base, specialized application packages, a good user interface, plus the 'people' component. The people include not only the participants but also a group facilitator who is responsible for the smooth operation of the group and who may also serve as the operator of the computerized system. Additional features typically include numerical and graphical summarization of ideas and votes, programs for specialized group procedures (such as calculating weights of different alternatives), anonymous recording of ideas, formal selection of a leader, handling progressive rounds of voting, and eliminating redundant input.

Undoubtedly the supporting of communications and decision-making will merge as researchers and developers from both areas begin supporting both. For example, rooms for video conferencing focus on communication support and seldom have workstations to support consensus building. Likewise, group decision rooms with workstations for each participant seldom have video conferencing capability to support dispersed groups. As the tools and technology improve, it is expected that group support will move beyond problems or decisions that are familiar to the participants to sensitive decisions, crisis decisions, confrontation decisions and even 'regular' day-to-day decisions.

Data capturing technology

When the first portable computers (now called notebooks or laptops) arrived on the scene 10 years ago, these 15 kg units were considered saviours for users that needed to take their computers with them. As size began to decrease and the portable computer's power began to increase, more and more people began to enjoy the benefits of computing on the go. The notebook is now full-featured enough to function as the main computer for many users – all in a package that can weigh approximately 2 kg. Future notebook users can expect to see more features added in with no gain in size or weight.

First lighter materials will be developed that will keep the weight down, and more functionality will be integrated into the motherboards, so that additional add-ons are not required. The monochrome screen will disappear as production yields increase and prices decrease on active-matrix colour LCD displays. Second, while nickel–metal hydride batteries are replacing traditional nickel–cadmium cells, lithium batteries are just emerging and are offering longer life and less weight.

One of the most important developments in notebooks is the advent of the PCMCIA (Personal Computer Memory Card International Association) card. PCMCIA presents a new paradigm of computing that extends the portability of notebook computers. These credit card sized devices offer plug-and-play convenience. They can also be inserted and removed without turning off the computer. PCMCIA cards are available for a variety of functions, including network cards, memory expansion, storage, fax/modems, sound cards, etc. PCMCIA cards will probably be a regular feature

on desktop machines as well. One future scenario has users simply moving their data and applications back and forth between machines on a PCMCIA. Another popular option is the notebook/docking station combination. The docking station will become more of a common accessory as users take the components out of their notebooks and plug them into the station at the office or home to obtain the benefits of a larger monitor, external keyboard, alternate pointing devices, better sound, or link onto a network.

One aspect of notebook computing is the palmtop computer which is an even smaller device capable of data collection in the field. This form of technology is already being used by nurses, physiotherapists, chiropodists and health visitors in the North West Anglia Healthcare Trust in Peterborough, England. Users, once they adjust their work patterns and behaviours, report that the palmtop leads to a more professional and business-like approach to the job, enabling one to rationalize the workload and manage one's time more efficiently, thereby offering a higher standard of patient care than was previously possible (Bradford 1994)

Finally, voice recognition is not far away. This technology has been used for sometime in the field of radiology and is now beginning to appear in other aspects of medicine. Computer systems are now being delivered with speech boards. Currently the voice recognition systems require more memory and disk space than is on most personal computers and require that the system processors be at least 486/66 MHz or the new Pentium chip. For dictation systems to run effectively requires a multi-tasking system that lets several programs run at the same time. One of the programs just sits and listens to what one is saying, looking for either command phrases or phrases to dictate. Physicians testing these new systems find the system accurate and capable of supporting dictation at 60 to 70 words per minute (Mullin 1994). They are finding that it saves time and provides more control over clinical notes, bypassing the normal transcription process.

Data storage and retrieval technology

The power of information technology rests in its ability to process instructions very quickly. One aspect of this quickness relates to a computer's ability to quickly store and retrieve data. Primary storage is part of the computer's central processing unit (CPU) and is generally referred to as memory. Secondary storage, on the other hand, is physically separated from the CPU. A type of secondary storage that is becoming increasingly common and affordable is optical disks (Hicks 1993)

One type of optical disk shares the same technology as the digital compact disk (CD) players used with stereo systems and is referred to as CD-ROM; the ROM referring to read-only-memory. Originally, data could be written on them only one time; however, there are now erasable versions. The primary advantage of optical disks is large storage capacity at low costs; some of them cost less than 10 dollars and hold 200 to 2000 megabytes (one gigabyte) of data. Five hundred megabytes is the equivalent of 300 000 double-spaced typewritten pages, or the entire Encyclopaedia Britannica several times over.

Optical disks are used for storing large volumes of data, including photographs, that are not changed often. The Medline CD-ROM available in most medical libraries is a well-known medical example. A number of medical specialties receive their journal references on CD-ROMs and access the material at home on their personal computers. SAM-CD is the CD-ROM version of Scientific American's reference book on Internal Medicine. Scientific American sends out a new CD-ROM every 3 months with the new data (including photos) in place and ready to use. The Compendium of Pharmaceuticals and Specialties (CPS) is available on CD-ROM, which offers users the power of the computer in conducting complex searches in a matter of seconds. New and more flexible software is being developed as CD-ROM technology will soon become a standard component of all personal computers, much as hard disks became standard in the late 1980s.

CD-ROM drives are, in the world of high-speed technology, considered slow; the average access time is one second and the average transfer rate is only 300 000 bits of data per second. The newer WORM (write-only-read-many) technology is being packaged in multifunction drives or 'jukeboxes' and has access times as fast as 45 milliseconds. Still, this is also 'too slow' and not far away is holography, a technique for recording and then reproducing a complete image of a three-dimensional object and the next great technology in data storage. In August 1994, researchers at Stanford University reported the first digital holographic storage system. The team believes 120 billion bytes can be stored per cubic centimetre using digital holographic storage and access rates will be significantly faster than today's technology.

Information management

Given the 'information revolution' our society is experiencing, it is not uncommon to assume that 'information' infers only the involvement of computers and communication technology. In organizational settings, one often further assumes that the major issue involved is the introduction of information technology within the organization. What is often overlooked is that the introduction of information technology in an organization is much more of a social process than it is a technical one. If the people involved in information management are to coordinate the acquisition and provision of information effectively, they must understand how people process information, both as individuals and as members of organized groups or units. The real challenges in implementing successful information systems are those of managing people and their perceptions.

Information systems

An information system collects, classifies, processes and stores data and retrieves, distributes and communicates data to decision makers. This processed data may or may not then be transformed into information by the human decision maker. In an organizational setting such systems are often called management information systems. This view was promulgated by Davis (1983) when he defined a management information system as an integrated, man/machine system for providing information to support the operations, management, and decision-making functions in any organization. The system uses computer hardware, software, manual procedures, management and decision models, and a database. In many ways, information systems are an extension of the study of organizations, organizational systems, organizational behaviour, organizational functions, and management. An organization is an administrative and functional structure of human resources, material, natural and information resources co-ordinated in some manner to achieve a purpose.

In the 1990s, the once traditional organization is quickly being replaced by the 'virtual' corporation (Davidow and Malone 1992). Whether real or virtual, any organization is held together by the methodologies of acquiring, processing, retaining, transmitting, and utilizing information. The purpose of an information system is to support managerial activities of all types at all levels of an organization. An organizationally based information system acquires, processes, stores and transmits raw material which is usually a mixture of (a) 'factual' data; (b) material that has been subjected to interpretation in its passage through the system; and (c) other content that is openly acknowledged to be the opinions, judgments, and observations of individuals both within the organization and outside it. The value of this material, that is information, depends upon the use to which it can be put. Measuring information, decision making, and productivity in information processing is an unresolved problem. Information is an essential commodity and a unique resource. It is often not depreciable and a 'purchaser' may not be able to determine the value of an information item without examining it. Information is not a 'free good'. It is a resource no less essential to the survival of an organization than are personnel, material and natural resources. Information is a resource that must be conserved, recycled and protected. As with any other resource it must be managed.

Increasingly, organizations are coming to accept this premise and hence look for people who view information management from an 'information science' versus a 'computer science' perspective. The two perspectives are related but by no means the same. People with computer science backgrounds tend to be more concerned with computer hardware and software. Their formal education had a strong theoretical and mathematical basis, with particular emphasis in algorithm development. They probably have a thorough grounding in the study of the implementation of algorithms in programming languages which operate on data structures in the environment of hardware. They usually have had little exposure to information requirements analysis and organizational considerations. They have greater expertise in programming, system software and hardware. People with such a technical background tend to be more machine and technology focused.

People with an information science background or orientation tend to be more concerned with people and the nature of information and information processes in the organization. They are more likely to assess the value of information and its effect on the performance of the decision makers within the organization. In a health care setting, they are more likely to be aware of how and why information is communicated between patients, clients, health care providers, epidemiologists, administrators, evaluators, and planners. The use to which these people put information is, in the end, the most critical criteria of success of information systems, be they computer based or not.

Managing information

If information is to be managed, someone has to be the information manager. The future will place new demands for information systems in public health environs. Information exchange between health care facilities, governments and other constituencies is becoming more prevalent, and the need for individuals within an organization to share and use the same information is becoming much more common. In this new climate, new professions are emerging, those of health information managers. These individuals will become active in planning, designing, implementing, managing and developing, and deploying information systems to meet the needs of rapidly changing health care systems. These information systems will vary in complexity from simple central registers, to hospital and/or community data abstracting and on to complex inter-institutional networked decisions support systems.

In health care settings information is needed to support decisions that relate to:

1. promoting wellness, preventing illness and curing or amelio-rating disease;

2. monitoring, evaluating, controlling and planning health care resources;

3. formulating health and social services policy; and

4. advancing knowledge through research and disseminating knowledge through education.

An information manager is any individual within an organiza-tion who has been given the responsibility to manage the organiza-tion's information. Given the information revolution that today's society is experiencing, it is not uncommon to assume that information infers the involvement of computers and communica-tion technology. In organizational settings, one often further assumes that the major issue involved is the introduction of information technology within the organization. What is sometimes overlooked is that the introduction of information technology is much more a social process than it is a technical one.

If information managers are to co-ordinate the acquisition and provision of information effectively, they must understand how people process information both as individuals and as members of organized groups or units. They will need to have excellent interpersonal skills in order to teach, motivate, convince and influence a variety of people. The real challenges in implementing successful information systems are those of managing people and their perceptions. Information managers will be change agents, a bridge between older systems and models, and newer technologies and techniques. No matter where they are positioned in the organization, they are usually expected to develop effective plan-ning processes for aligning all information systems to the strategic direction, objectives and structure of the organization. This entails co-ordinating all information systems within the organization including computing services, minicomputers and microcomput-ers, records rooms, office automation, management engineering, voice communication and other related areas. Determining the investment to be made in information systems and providing a rigorous and disciplined framework for evaluating information benefits versus information costs is also a part of the job. Specific standards and guidelines need to be established for the definition, measurement, use and disposition of information so that all segments within the organization are operating within the same framework. It is often left to the information manager to explain information technology and the need for new systems to staff at all levels of the organization. This critical educational role is often

carried out in conjunction with the development of policies and procedures that ensure the co-ordination and justification of requests for personal computers, terminals, office automation devices and various software packages.

These responsibilities can often be onerous, and those who succeed possess excellent interpersonal, written and verbal commu-nication skills (that is, an ability to function effectively at the board, senior and middle management and operational levels of the health care facility. Effective information managers understand the organ-ization's mission and the business that it is in. They also under-stand the complexity and dynamics of health care delivery, are able to function in multidisciplinary teams and environments, appre-ciate small 'p' and big 'P' politics and are able to assess political situations. To be effective information managers people have to be doers. They have to be able to demonstrate short-term success while making progress on the long-range information systems requirements. To do so they must understand the present and future capabilities of information technology, be technologically credible to their peers and staff and able to plan the effective use of information technology in the organization.

Information systems are people and information systems create change. Information managers must be able to manage change which includes a sincere appreciation of the effects of change on people. They must be willing and able to teach and educate a wide variety of individuals at all levels of the organization, none of which can be done without having a positive attitude towards users. Effective information managers demonstrate leadership through effective listening, team building and consensus building. They are creative, innovative and have a vision of the future. Most of all, they have an honest concern for the organization's most critical resource – its people.

The health of a nation depends to a certain extent on how well organizations use the resources available to them to promote wellness, prevent illness, and cure disease. The health of an organization depends to a large extent on the effectiveness of the decisions made by its staff; effective decisions require effective managers and information systems which produce reliable and useful information. The health of an information system is a function of how well it has been defined, designed, implemented, operated, and maintained. Keeping the organization's information systems healthy is the role of the information manager regardless of his or her title.

Organizational transformation

In 1991, Scott Morton and his colleagues at the Maasachusetts Institute of Technology's MIT's Sloan School of Management Research published a text entitled 'The Corporation of the '90s' (Scott Morton 1992). The work was as a 5 year, multimillion dollar research programme on 'How can organizations make better use of Information Technology (IT)?'

A consortium of MIT faculty and 12 corporate and public sector sponsors contributed financial resources, advice and their workplaces as experimental sites. The group's focus was about how new technologies are changing the way people work and the way organizations will collaborate and compete. The major findings have had a significant impact on a multitude of organizations in both the private and public sectors around the world, including the

United Kingdom's National Health Service. The MIT findings are summarized under the following six headings:

Information technology is enabling fundamental changes in the way work is done

The degree to which a person is affected is determined by how much their work is based on information; that is, information on what product to make or service to deliver and how to do it (production task), as well as when to do it and in conjunction with whom (co-ordination task). The impact on production work is apparent in:

1. Physical production – affected by robotics, process control, intelligent sensors;

2. Information production – affected by data processing computers for clerical tasks such as billings;

3. Knowledge production – affected by CAD (computer assisted design)/CAM (computer assisted manufacturing), workstations for building qualitative products such as loans.

What is less well known is that the new information technology is permitting a change in the economics and functionality of the co-ordinating process as distance can be shrunk toward zero as far as information flow is concerned. Time can shrink to zero or shift to a more convenient point. Organizational memory, as exemplified by the common database, can be updated by anyone and made available to all authorized users. New 'group work' and team concepts combine all three aspects of co-ordination: distance, time and memory.

The increasing availability of information technology can fundamentally change management work as relevant and timely information on changes in the external environment and the organization's view of the environment affects the direction dimension. Relevant and timely information on measuring the organization's performance against critical success factors affects the control dimension. The second aspect of control is interpreting such measures against the corporate plan and determining what actions to take.

Information technology is enabling the integration of business functions within and between organizations

Public and private telecommunication networks are making the principle of 'any information, at anytime, anywhere, and at anyway you want to look at it' economically feasible. The boundaries of organizations are becoming more permeable; where works gets done, when and with whom is changing. The electronic integration is showing up in the following forms:

1. Within the value chain – Land Area Networks permit 'teams' to work together on a common product;

2. End-to-end links of value chains between organizations – EDI (electronic data interchange) and JIT (just in time) systems are shifting the boundaries of an organization to include elements of other organizations thereby creating a 'virtual' organization;

3. Value chain substitution via subcontract or alliance – permit

an organization to take advantage (mutual) of economies of scale and unique skills of its partner organization.

Electronic integration is removing unproductive buffers and leveraging expertise.

Information technology is causing shifts in the competitive climate of many industries

Information technology is introducing unprecedented degrees of simultaneous competition and collaboration between firms. It is becoming increasingly important to know when to support standards and when to try to pre-empt competitors by establishing a proprietary *de facto* standard. The benefits do not flow from the mere use of information technology but arise from the human, organizational and system innovations that are added on to the original business benefit. Information technology is merely an enabler that offers an organization the opportunity to invest vigorously in added innovations if it wishes to stay ahead of its competitors.

Information technology presents new strategic opportunities for organizations that reassess their mission and objectives

Organizations are going to go through three distinctive stages as they attempt to respond to their changing environments:

1. Automate – reduce the cost of production, usually by reducing the number of workers. As an example, scanners, bar code and universal product codes are being introduced for more than identifying goods.

2. Informate – what happens when automated processes yield information as a byproduct. This necessitates that knowledge workers develop new skills to work with new information tools; it often entails new ways of thinking.

3. Transform – a stage characterized by leadership, vision and a sustained process of organization empowerment. It includes the broad view of quality but goes beyond this to address the unique opportunities presented by the environment and enabled by information technology.

Production workers will become analysers, a role offering a different level of conceptual skill from what was needed before as a doer or machine minder; it will require an ability to see patterns and understand the overall process rather than just looking at controlling information on a screen.

Successful application of information technology will require changes in management and organizational structure

Information technology is enabling a break-up or disintegration of traditional organizational forms; multiple skills can be brought together at an arbitrary point in time and location. The ability of information technology to affect co-ordination by shrinking time and distance permits an organization to respond more quickly and accurately to the marketplace. This not only reduces assets the organization has tied up but improves quality as seen by the customer. The 'metabolic' rate of the organization, that is, the rate at which information flows and decisions are made is speeding up and will get faster in the late 1990s. The measurements, the rewards, the incentives, and the required skills all require rethinking in the new information technology-impacted world.

A major challenge for management in the 1990s will be to lead their organizations through the transformation necessary to prosper in the globally competitive environment

Management must ensure that the forces influencing change move through time to accomplish the organization's objectives. Evidence to date is that at the aggregate level, information technology has not improved profitability or productivity. Some of the reasons are that:

- benefits are there but simply not visible

- improvement is in lower prices or better quality

- investment in information technology is necessary to stay in business

- the external world is demanding more

- use of information technology in low pay off areas

- information technology is laid on top of existing services

- no cost reduction, just cost replacement

To go successfully through the transformation process, organizations must have a clear business purpose and a vision of what the organization is to become; a large amount of time and effort must be invested to enable the organization to understand where it is going and why. The organization must have a robust information technology infrastructure in place, including electronic networks and understood standards; the organization must invest heavily and early enough in human resources – all employees must have a sense of empowerment. Last, but by no means least, understanding one's organizational culture and knowing what it means to have an innovative culture is the first key step in a move toward an adaptive organization.

Case study: the National Health Service – Information Management and Technology (NHS IM&T) Strategy

One public service organization which has adopted the MIT findings as a cornerstone to its corporate strategy is the United Kingdom's National Health Service (NHS). The business goal of the NHS Management Executive is to create a better health service for the nation in three ways:

1. Ensuring services are of the highest quality and responsive to the needs and wishes of patients.

2. Ensuring that health services are effectively targeted so as to improve the health of local populations.

3. Improving the efficiency of the services so that as great a volume of well targeted effective services as possible is provided from the available resources.

The July 1992 White Paper, the Health of the Nation identifies five priority areas and establishes key targets such as:

1. reducing deaths from coronary heart disease in the under-65 age group by at least 40 per cent by the year 2000;

2. reducing cervical cancer by at least 20 per cent by the year 2000;

3. reducing suicides by at least 15 per cent by the year 2000;

4. reducing gonorrhoea by at least 20 per cent by 1995;

5. reducing deaths from accidents among children under 15 by at least 33 per cent by 2005.

A strengthened information and research capability at central and regional levels is an essential component of the business plan. Expanded or new health surveys and epidemiological overviews to improve baseline statistics on the health of the population will be undertaken. A Central Health Outcomes Unit will lead on developing and co-ordinating work on assessment of health outcomes. Information systems which enable adequate monitoring and review will be developed including a Public Health Information Strategy (Ranade 1994).

The Information Management and Technology (IM&T) Strategy

Any Public Health Information Strategy will be a part of the NHS IM&T Strategy, was announced in December 1992, which responds to the business needs of the NHS to see best benefit and value for money from IM&T investment. It sets the direction for computerization and information sharing across the NHS into the next century. The Strategy is intended to ensure that the implementation of information systems in the NHS is co-ordinated and managed to achieve maximum potential benefits for patients, clinical staff, management and administrative staff.

The Strategy is intended to support better care and communication through the appropriate use of IM&T. It provides a framework for the collection and exchange of data (Keen 1994). The IM&T vision is of a health service where staff use information to improve continuously the service they provide, where an IM&T environment supports the controlled sharing of information across the NHS, and where information is handled and communicated securely, smoothly and efficiently. The Strategy supports the business goal of the National Health Service Management Executive (NHSME) through four strategic initiatives:

1. National facilitating projects, identifying the potential benefits of IM&T to NHS organizations, and pointing to common solutions and approaches to implementation;

2. The development of an infrastructure for NHS organizations;

3. Maximizing value for money – a framework to ensure that the NHS gets value for money from expenditure on information systems; and

4. Enabling people – the strategy recognizes the need for people to be trained and developed so that they apply IM&T imaginatively and effectively and thus obtain maximum benefit.

IM&T principles

The five key principles of the Strategy are:

1. Information will be person based. Priority will be given to person-based systems where data is collected as part of the process of care. Such systems will hold a health care record for each individual which can be uniquely referenced to that person's new English NHS number and thereby shared with other systems that use the same identifying key.

2. Systems are to be integrated. Wherever possible information should be entered into a computer only once; seamless care needs seamless information. After that it should be available to authorized NHS employees, with steps taken to protect confidential information from unauthorized access.

3. Information will be derived from operational systems. Whenever possible, information is to be captured at the point of delivery of care, from systems used by health care professionals in their day-to-day work. There should be little need for different systems to record management information. Information for management purposes (administrative, financial, research etc.) should be derived from operational point-of-care systems. Data not collected in a way that helps clinical professionals do their jobs better will not be clinically acceptable and will not be usable for other purposes.

4. Information must be secure and confidential. While recognizing the need for sharing and accessibility of information across organizations, all systems must recognize and respect the principles of privacy, security and confidentiality. Great care is being taken to ensure that all the data held in a computer will be available only to those who need to know it and are authorized to know it.

5. Information will be shared across the NHS. Common standards and NHS-wide networking will allow computers to communicate so that information can be shared between health care professionals and organizations, again subject to security and the safeguard of confidentiality.

The IM&T Strategy is acting as the transitional catalyst which is moving the NHS from its past state to its new emerging model. The well resourced IM&T Strategy has 23 projects to support the development of a national infrastructure and national standards.

One has to be impressed with the components of the IM&T infrastructure which will facilitate sharing, namely:

1. A unique identifier for all patients, clients, and customers. The new NHS number became the key to controlled sharing of data in person-based systems throughout the NHS in July 1995.

2. A repository of the key demographic data elements of each individual including the pointers to where other data on that individual resides; the new NHS Administrative Registers, using the Common Administrative Data Set Model provides the capability for purchasers and providers to share administrative data and facilitates the move to person-based systems.

3. A consistent and standard way of collecting and storing data;

the thesaurus of coded clinical terms and groupings underpins the essence of the clinical record throughout the NHS. Version 3 of the Read codes were fully mapped to ICD9 and OPCS4 in April 1994 and should have been mapped to ICD10 by April 1995.

4. A means by which data can be moved rapidly from one place to another in a consistent and meaningful way; the NHS-wide networking project and the standards for computer-to-computer communication using UN/EDIFACT messaging protocols assures that data can be exchanged accurately.

Public health practitioners have been encouraged to help implement the strategy by ensuring that local IM&T strategies take forward the national lead and exploit the opportunities presented by increased information sharing, subject to security and confidentiality safeguards, and that systems procured comply with national standards.

Conclusion — questions to be answered

Every individual has their own view, their own perception of the world around them. This view is a result of their individual backgrounds, cultures, education, and values. Everyone does not perceive that technology will affect them in the same way. A recent survey of nursing students found that over 95 per cent of them felt that they would never speak to a computer or use an expert system, yet voice recognition technology has moved out of the research laboratory and expert systems are routinely being used in financial investment circles.

We are witnessing not only the automation of clerical activities, but also the automation of thoughtful technical and clinical work. What are the consequences? Will the responsibility for the production of reliable information rest more with rules incorporated in equipment and on established procedures than on a health professional's judgment?

The acute care sector of health care is undergoing dramatic and radical changes in delivery and management, many of which are the result of new technologies and the realities of modern day fiscal conditions. The acute care sector is under increasing pressure to account for its actions, justify its decision making and its use of resources. Health care organizations are in the process of re-engineering and changing the way people do their work.

Is the same degree of change and accountability occurring in the public health sector? Will the public health information systems which currently support financial accounting and programme delivery be expected to allow costs to be matched to services provided and monitor productivity? Will the public health practitioner of the future be a multiskilled individual whose method of working is dramatically different than today? If not, why not?

References

Bradford, A. (1994). Palmtop Practitioners. *British Journal of Healthcare Computing*, **10**, 12–13.

Churchman, C. (1971). *The design of inquiring systems.* Basic Books, New York.

Davidow, W.H. and Malone M.S. (1992). *The virtual corporation: lessons from the world's most advanced companies.* Harper Business, New York.

Davis, G. (1983). *Evolution of information systems as an academic discipline. Administrative Sciences Association of Canada* Conference Proceedings, pp. 185–9.

Friede, A., *et al.* (1994). CDC WONDER: A co-operative processing architecture for public health. *Journal of Amercian Medical Informatics Association* **1** (4), 303–12.

Hannah, K. (1985). *Current trends in health informatics: implications for curriculum planning.* Computers in Nursing, North Holland, Amsterdam.

Hicks, J. (1993). *Management information systems: a user perspective.* West Publishing Co., New York.

Keen, J. (ed.) (1994). *Information management in health services.* Open University Press, Buckingham.

Levy, A.H. (1977). *Is informatics a basic medical science?* Medinfo 1977 proceedings, (ed. D. Shires and H. Wolfe), pp. 979–81. North Holland, Amsterdam.

Linthicum, D. (1994). Tommy, can you see me? *Open Computing*, September, pp. 67–8.

McNurlin, B.C. and Sprague, R.H. (1989). *Information systems in management practice.* Prentice Hall, New Jersey.

Meadow, C.T. (1979). Information science and scientists in 2001. *Journal of Information Science* **1**, 217–21.

Moehr, J.R. *et al.* (1979). *A specialized curriculum for medical informatics – review after 6 years of experience.* Proceedings of the International Conference in Medical Computing, Berlin.

Mullin, S. (1994). Start talking to your computer–three physicians rate IBM's speech recognition system. *Canadian Medical Informatics* **1** (3), pp. 16–17.

Plucauskas, M. (1994). Internet and medicine part II: hooking up and using Internet. *Canadian Medical Informatics* **1** (3), 28–30.

Protti, D.J. (ed.) (1982). *A new undergraduate program in health informatics.* AMIA Congress 1982 Proceedings, pp. 241–5. Masson Publishing, San Francisco.

Radford, K.J. (1978). *Information for strategic decisions.* Reston Publishers, New York.

Ranade, W. (1994). *A future for the NHS: health care in the 1990s.* Longman Group, London.

Reichertz, P. (1973). Protokoll der Klausurtangung Ausbildungsziele, inhalte und. *Methoden in der Medizinischen Informatik*, **2**, 18–21

Scott Morton, W. (ed.) (1992). *Corporation of the '90s.* Harvard University Press, Boston.

Shannon, C.E. and Weaver, W. (1960). *The mathematical theory of communication.* University of Illinois Press, Urbana, Illinois.

Shires, D. and Ball, M. (1975). *Update on educational activities in medical informatics.* Proceedings of the 5th Annual Conference of the Society for Computer Medicine. pp. 52–4.

Smith, R. and Gibbs, M. (1994). *Navigating the Internet.* SAMS Publishing. Indiana.

Strauss, P. (1994). Beyond talking heads: videoconferencing makes money. *Datamation.* 1 October, pp. 38–41.

van Bemmel, J.H. (1984). The structure of medical informatics. *Medical Informatics* **9**, 175–80.

Wiener, N. (1948). *Cybernetics.* Prentice Hall, Newark, New Jersey.

Information resources in the United States

Nancy D. Pearce

Introduction

Health information systems that provide data for routine monitoring of the health of the population of the United States are reviewed in this chapter. Since it is possible to discuss only a few of the existing systems, the material here represents a sampling of the total universe of data systems. Several criteria were applied in the selection of the systems to be included. Each system must be (i) national in coverage and representative of the situation in the country as a whole, (ii) currently operational, although it may be periodic in its collection of data (e.g. conducted biennially rather than continuously), (iii) operated by either the federal government or the private sector, and (iv) produce primary data rather than a secondary compilation of data from other sources. Systems excluded are those that provide data for specific programmes, with the exception of the Medicare programme statistical system which has been included because it covers virtually the entire population aged 65 years and older. Also excluded are programmes that operate at the state level, programmes that provide data only for a particular state and some or all of its subdivisions, and important and highly useful compendia that obtain highlights from a number of primary data sources. Examples of secondary data sources in the health area are the *Statistical abstract of the United States*, published annually by the US Bureau of the Census, and *Health, United States*, the annual report to Congress from the Secretary of the Department of Health and Human Services, which is prepared by the National Center for Health Statistics.

To provide a framework for the organization of these diverse data sources, they are presented in three broad groupings: **health status**, including morbidity and mortality, **health care resources** and their utilization, and **health economics**. Placement of individual data sources in the categories is somewhat arbitrary, but every effort was made to ensure that the placement is as logical as possible. For example, while the National Health Interview Survey produces information on both the utilization and financing of health care services, its primary purpose is provision of information on morbidity and so it is located in the section on health status.

The relative paucity of information on health care professionals is noteworthy. Numerous *ad hoc* studies have been conducted for several health occupations, but typically they have been limited to the membership of a particular national professional organization and conducted on an irregular basis. Anyone interested in the most recent data for any particular health occupation should contact the national professional association.

There are limited sources that meet the criteria for inclusion for health economic data because most health economics studies use secondary data, involve secondary analysis of data from various sources, or are based on single-time studies.

Typically, material for each data system is divided into two sections. The first section describes the purpose and scope of the system, and the second section provides an overview of the data collection procedures and data items. At the end of each description a reference is given to one or two sources for additional information about each system. Frequently the references also identify other data collection programmes of the respective organizations. In addition to published reports, most data systems have computerized public use data files, which can be obtained for direct manipulation in research activities, or special tabulations may be available upon user specification and appropriate reimbursement. Public use files and special tabulations are subjected to careful scrutiny prior to release in order to prevent inadvertent disclosure of respondent identity. Most of these publications are available at large libraries, particularly those at health care institutions.

The recent activity with regard to health care reform has subjected the design and content of many existing data systems to thoughtful scrutiny. There are major implications for change to existing health information systems even in the absence of structured health care reform at the national level. However, this is likely to be evolutionary, and resulting changes are undoubtedly a few years in the future.

Health status
National morbidity and mortality reporting systems
Purpose and scope
The United States Centers for Disease Control and Prevention (US CDC) maintain national surveillance programmes for selected diseases with the co-operation of state and local health departments. Over the years the surveillance systems maintained by these centres have expanded, and emphasis has shifted as certain diseases have lower incidence rates and other diseases have taken on new aspects. The data are used to identify outbreaks of communicable diseases and to monitor trends in those diseases.

In 1878 an act of Congress authorized the collection of morbidity reports by the Public Health Service for use in connection with quarantine measures against pestilential diseases such as cholera, smallpox, plague, and yellow fever. In the following year a specific appropriation was made for the collection and publication of reports of notifiable diseases, principally from foreign ports; in 1893, an act provided for the weekly collection of data from state and municipal authorities throughout the United States. To secure uniformity for the registration of these morbidity statistics, Congress enacted a law in 1902 directing the Surgeon General of the Public Health Service to provide forms for the collection, compilation, and publication of such data.

Data collection procedures and data items

Reports on notifiable diseases were received from very few states and cities prior to 1900, but gradually more states submitted monthly and annual summaries. In 1913 the state and territorial health authorities recommended weekly telegraphic reporting by states for a few diseases, but it was not until after 1925 that all states reported regularly. In 1950 the Association of State and Territorial Health Officers authorized a Conference of State and Territorial Epidemiologists for the purpose of determining the diseases that should be reported by the states to the Public Health Service. Following approval of the list of diseases by the Association of State and Territorial Health Officers, the first manual on reporting procedures was issued; since then recommendations and revisions made by this conference have been incorporated into the *Manual of procedures for national morbidity reporting and surveillance of communicable diseases.*

The following notifiable diseases are those agreed upon by the state and territorial epidemiologists and approved by state and territorial health departments: acquired immunodeficiency syndrome (AIDS), amebiasis, anthrax, aseptic meningitis, botulism, brucellosis, chancroid, cholera, diphtheria, encephalitis, gonorrhea, granuloma inguinale, *Haemophilus influenzae*, Hansen's disease (leprosy), hepatitis (A, B, non-A, non-B, unspecified), legionellosis, leptospirosis, Lyme disease, lymphogranuloma venereum, malaria, measles (rubeola), meningococcal infections, mumps, murine typhus fever, pertussis, plague, poliomyelitis, psittacosis, rabies (animal, human), rubella (German measles), congenital rubella syndrome, salmonellosis, shigellosis, syphilis, tetanus, toxic shock syndrome, trichinosis, tuberculosis, tularaemia, typhoid fever, and varicella (chickenpox). Physicians report cases of these diseases to their local city, county, or state health departments. Although notification of a case of one of the quarantinable diseases may have been made by telephone to the CDC, each case of cholera, plague, smallpox, and yellow fever is reported by the state epidemiologist to the CDC in the weekly morbidity report.

Completeness of reporting varies greatly, since not all cases receive medical care and not all treated conditions are reported by physicians. Thus the data should be interpreted with caution. Some diseases, such as plague and rabies, that cause severe clinical illness and are associated with serious consequences are probably reported quite accurately. However, diseases such as salmonellosis and mumps, which are clinically mild and infrequently associated with serious consequences, are less likely to be reported. Prior to the institution of the Measles Elimination Program in 1978, estimates of under-reporting were made by the CDC for two diseases—measles and viral hepatitis. At that time, it was generally accepted that about 10–15 per cent of cases of measles and about 15–20 per cent of all cases of viral hepatitis occurring in the United States were reported to the CDC. The degree of completeness of reporting is also influenced by the diagnostic facilities available, the control measures in effect, and the interests and priorities of state and local officials responsible for disease control and surveillance. Finally, factors such as the introduction of new diagnostic tests (e.g.

for hepatitis B) and the discovery of new disease entities (e.g. infant botulism and legionellosis) may cause changes in disease reporting independent of the true incidence of disease.

In addition to the weekly report of notifiable diseases, a weekly mortality report is made to the CDC by City Health Officers or Vital Statistics Registrars from 121 major cities. This report is in the form of a table in which total deaths by age are cross-classified by number of deaths assigned to pneumonia and influenza. An annual summary of the reported incidence of each listed, nationally notifiable disease is also submitted by each state and territorial health department to CDC for the previous calendar year.

Reference: US Centers for Disease Control and Prevention (weekly)

Drug Abuse Warning Network
Purpose and scope

The Drug Abuse Warning Network (DAWN) is operated by the Office of Applied Studies in the Substance Abuse and Mental Health Services Administration (SAMHSA) to monitor drug abuse trends and patterns, to identify licit and illicit drugs and new substances associated with drug abuse morbidity and mortality, and to provide data for national, state, and local drug abuse policy and programme planning. DAWN was initiated in 1972 by the Drug Enforcement Administration (DEA) under authorization of the Comprehensive Drug Abuse Prevention and Controlled Substance Act of 1970. Responsibility for the system was transferred to a SAMHSA predecessor agency in the Public Health Service in 1981.

Data collection procedures and data items

DAWN collects drug abuse information from a national probability sample of hospital emergency departments and from medical examiners located primarily in 27 primary metropolitan statistical areas throughout the continental United States.

Separate forms are completed by emergency departments and medical examiners. The data items collected concern specific drugs being abused, the magnitude of the abuse, abuse problems unique to certain specific geographic areas, the source of the abused substance, the form (e.g. tablet, capsule, powder) of the abused substance, and the age, race, sex, and employment status of abusers. No patient identifiers or names are ever transcribed on DAWN data collection forms. Data collection forms are completed for all drug-related events.

Eligible emergency departments are defined as those that are open 24 hours a day and seven days a week, and are located in non-federal short-stay general hospitals; eligibility is determined primarily from information in the American Hospital Association's *Guide to the health care field* and is updated with each new annual edition. In the 1986 redesign of the national sample of hospital emergency departments, hospitals in the frame were stratified by size, with hospitals reporting 80 000 or more annual emergency department visits assigned to a certainty stratum; additional strata were defined according to whether the hospital had an organized outpatient department or a chemical/alcohol inpatient unit. Twenty-one metropolitan statistical areas were designated for oversampling. The new sample of emergency departments included approximately 700 facilities located primarily in the 21 metropolitan statistical areas and a subset of the 27 primary metropolitan statistical areas in the former sample. Each year a sample maintenance procedure is used to make a random selection of 'newly eligible' hospitals from the annually updated sampling frame to keep the sample up to date and representative of the over 5000 DAWN-eligible hospitals. All medical examiners in the 27 metropolitan statistical areas in the old sample are considered eligible for continued participation; information on medical examiners is compiled from the organizational memberships lists of medical professional societies and other available sources.

Reference: Substance Abuse and Mental Health Services Administration (annual)

National Health Interview Survey

Purpose and scope

The National Health Interview Survey (NHIS) conducted by the National Center for Health Statistics (NCHS) is a principal source of information on the health of the population of the United States. The survey was initiated in July 1957 in response to the National Health Survey Act of 1956, which provided for a continuing survey and special studies to secure accurate and current statistical information, on a voluntary basis, on the amount, distribution, and effects of illness and disability in the United States and the services rendered for or because of such conditions.

The purpose of the survey is to provide national data on the incidence of acute illness and accidental injuries, the prevalence of chronic conditions and impairments, the extent of disability, the utilization of health care services, and other health-related topics. Data collected over the period of a year form the basis for the development of annual estimates of the health characteristics of the population and for the analysis of trends in those characteristics.

The survey covers the non-institutionalized civilian population of the United States alive at the time of the interview. Persons excluded are patients in long-term care facilities (data are obtained on patients in some of these facilities through the National Nursing Home Survey conducted by the NCHS), persons on active duty with the Armed Forces (although their dependents are included), United States nationals living in foreign countries, and persons who have died during the calendar year preceding interview.

Data procedures and data items

NHIS is a cross-sectional household interview survey which consists of continuous sampling and interviewing of the population. The sampling plan follows a multistage probability design that yields national estimates, although some estimates are obtained for the four geographic regions. The sample is redesigned following each decennial census; information from the 1990 census is the basis for the 1995 redesign implementation. In the 1995 sample redesign, the first stage consists of a sample of 358 primary sampling units drawn from approximately 2000 geographically defined primary sampling units that cover the 50 states and the District of Columbia. A primary sampling unit consists of a county, a small group of contiguous counties, or a metropolitan statistical area; within primary sampling units, smaller units called segments are defined in such a manner that each segment contains an expected eight households.

Households selected for interview each week are a probability sample representative of the target population. Beginning in 1995, all households are screened to identify those containing African Americans and Latin Americans in order to provide more precise estimates for these groups. Such households are oversampled, and a portion of households without a member of either group are retained in the sample. Each calendar year data are collected from approximately 41 000 households including about 107 000 persons. The annual response rate is usually at least 95 per cent of the eligible households in the sample; the 5 per cent who do not respond are divided equally between refusals and households where no eligible respondent could be found at home after repeated calls.

Data are collected through a personal household interview conducted by interviewers employed and trained by the Bureau of the Census according to procedures specified by NCHS. All adult members of the household (those aged 17 years and over) who are at home at the time of the interview are invited to participate and to respond for themselves; the mother is usually the respondent for children. For individuals not at home during the interview, information is provided by a responsible adult family member (age 19 years or older) residing in the household. On some occasions, a random subsample of adult household members is selected to respond to questions on selected topics. Follow-up supplements are sometimes completed for either the entire household or for individuals identified as having particular health problems. As required, these supplements are either left for the appropriate person to complete and return by mail, or the interviewer calls again in person or by telephone to secure the information directly.

On average, the interviews require about 80 minutes in the household. The questionnaire consists of two basic parts: (i) a 'core' set of health, socio-economic, and demographic items; (ii) one or more sets of 'supplemental' health items. The core items are repeated each year. The arrangement of core items complemented by rotating, as well as single-time supplements, allows the survey to respond to changing needs for data and to cover a wider variety of topics, while at the same time providing continuous information on fundamental topics.

The questionnaire includes the following type of core questions: the basic demographic characteristics of household members (including age, sex, race, education, and family income); disability days (including restricted activity and bed days) and work- and school-loss days occurring during the two-week period prior to the week of interview; physician visits occurring during the same two-week period; the acute and chronic conditions responsible for these days and visits; long-term limitation of activity resulting from chronic disease or impairment and the chronic conditions associated with the disability; short-stay hospitalization data (including the number of persons with hospital episodes during the past year and the number of discharges from short-stay hospitals); the interval since the last visit to a doctor. The questionnaire also includes six lists of chronic conditions; each concentrates on a group of chronic conditions involving a specific system of the body (e.g. digestive, circulatory, respiratory).

Supplements to the questionnaire change in response to current interest in special health topics. For example, throughout 1987 a cancer risk factor supplement was included, and in 1988 there were supplements on occupational health, medical device implants, child health, and AIDS knowledge and attitudes.

Suggestions and requests for special supplements are solicited and received from many sources, including university-based researchers as well as administrators of national organizations and programmes in the private and public health sectors and other parts of the Department of Health and Human Services. A lead time of at least 1 year is required to develop and pretest questions for new topics to include as special supplements.

A new questionnaire approach is planned for implementation in 1996. The content of the core questionnaire will be revised; some supplements will be identified for periodic use and other supplements responding to emerging public health needs will also be included. The new approach is likely to identify a sample adult and a sample child (if present) in each household about whom additional health status and health care behaviour and utilization information will be obtained.

References: National Center for Health Statistics (annual, 1989)

National Health and Nutrition Examination Survey

Purpose and scope

The first National Health and Nutrition Examination Survey (NHANES I) was initiated by the NCHS in 1970, with data collection beginning in April 1971. NHANES I was a modification and expansion of the earlier Health Examination Survey, which had been initiated a decade earlier and had carried out three separate programmes. The restructuring and modification of the Health Examination Survey reflected the assignment to the NCHS of an additional specific responsibility—the measurement of the nutritional status of the population and the subsequent monitoring of changes in that status over time. A second National Health and Nutrition Examination Survey (NHANES II) began in February 1976 and ended in February 1980. NHANES III began data collection in 1988 and ended in late 1994.

NHANES is designed to collect data that can be obtained best, or only, by direct physical examination, clinical and laboratory tests, and related measurement procedures. This information is of two kinds: (i) prevalence data for specifically defined diseases or conditions of ill health; (ii) normative health-related measurement data that show distributions of the total population with respect to particular parameters, such as blood pressure, visual acuity, or serum cholesterol level.

Successive surveys in the Health Examination Survey and NHANES programmes have been directed to different segments of the population and have had different sets of target conditions. The first Health Examination Survey 'cycle' involved examining a sample of adults with the focus primarily on selected chronic diseases. The second and third cycles were directed respectively to children between the ages of 6 and 11 years and youths between the ages of 12 and 17 years; both these surveys emphasized growth and development data and sensory defects. The nutrition component of the first NHANES programme was directed to a probability sample of the broad age range 1–74 years, while the detailed health examination component focused on the population between the ages of 25 and 74 years.

NHANES II was again directed to a broad population aged 6 months to 74 years, and the nutritional data collected can be used in conjunction with the earlier NHANES I data to monitor changes in nutritional status over time. A special health and nutrition examination survey directed to persons in families with one or more members of Latin American origin or descent who lived in areas with a high concentration of Latin Americans was conducted in 1983 and 1984. The study population for NHANES III was persons aged 2 months and older; African Americans and Latin Americans were oversampled, as were children and older persons.

Data collection procedures and data items

The samples for all the Health Examination Survey and NHANES programmes have been multistage highly clustered probability samples, stratified by broad geographic region and by population density grouping. Within strata the sampling stages employed have been the primary sampling unit, the census enumeration district, the segment, the household, and lastly the individual person. Until the household stage is reached, all sampling is carried out centrally.

The final stage of the sampling is conducted in the field in the particular chosen area. It involves interviewer visits and questionnaire completion at each one of the selected households, with the final selection of individuals included in the sample being dependent upon information elicited by the household interview questionnaire. The size of the sample in the survey programme has varied. The sample size was approximately 7500 persons in each of the three Health Examination Survey programmes.

In NHANES I the sample selected for the major nutrition components of the examination contained approximately 28 000 persons, of whom 21 000 were examined. A comparably sized sample for NHANES II again yielded approximately 21 000 examined persons. The sample for NHANES III is projected to be approximately 40 000 persons, of whom about 30 000 will be examined.

Data collection teams consist of specially trained interviewers and examiners, including physicians, nurses, dentists, dietitians, and medical and laboratory technicians. The examinations take place in the survey's specially constructed mobile examination centres, each consisting of three truck-drawn trailers, which are interconnected and which provide a standardized environment and equipment for the performance of specific parts of the examination. This standardized environment is necessary, for example for such components of the examination as audiometry which requires hearing chambers within which the ambient noise level conforms to the American Speech Association standards for acoustical measurements. In NHANES III, the inclusion of young infants down to 2 months of age and of significant numbers of elderly persons over age 75 (both subgroups with relatively lower response rates) resulted in the use of a home examination comprising a core set of questions and examinations.

The general pattern of data collection has meant that each survey has been conducted over a period of three or four years. This is due to the constraints that limit the number of persons examined in a given time span (e.g. the number of field teams and the number of sample areas). This imposes a limitation on the kinds of data to be collected by this mechanism, since conditions that might show marked year-to-year variation or seasonal patterns cannot be included. However, many important chronic diseases and health-related measurements are not subject to such changes in prevalence within short-run periods.

In the Health Examination Survey (HES) and National Health and Nutrition Examination Survey (NHANES) programmes much attention has been and continues to be devoted to the question of the response rate, which is the proportion of sample persons who are actually examined. Both previous NHANES programmes succeeded in obtaining household interview data on about 99 per cent of the sample population. More detailed health data appear in the medical history questionnaires; these were completed for 90 per cent of the selected sample persons in NHANES I, NHANES II, and NHANES. Overall, NHANES I, NHANES II, and NHANES averaged about a 74 per cent examination response rate. There is considerable ancillary information on most of the non-examined persons in the sample population, and it is possible to make use of that data in the process of imputation and analysis of non-response bias. Moreover, there is some evidence that data obtained through examinations, tests, and measurements such as used in these surveys are less susceptible to potential bias from a given rate of non-response than data provided by the individuals themselves.

The kinds of information collected in NHANES and other examination surveys are so varied and extensive that they are only illustrated here. With respect to nutrition, four types of data are included: (i) information concerning dietary intake (the mechanisms used have included 24-hour recall interviews and food frequency questionnaires, both administered by an interviewer who is a trained dietitian); (ii) haematological and biochemical tests (a sizeable battery of such tests has been performed; processing has been done at the mobile examination centres where necessary but, for the most part, at a central nutrition laboratory established at CDC); (iii) body measurements (the battery used is particularly important in connection with infants, children, and youths where growth may be affected by nutritional deficiencies); and (iv) various signs of high risk of nutritional deficiency, based on clinical examinations.

The health component of the NHANES programme includes detailed examinations, tests, and questionnaires which have been developed to obtain a measure of prevalence levels of specific diseases and conditions. These vary with the particular programme and have included such conditions as chronic rheumatoid arthritis and hypertensive heart disease. Important normative health-related measurements, such as height, weight, and blood pressure, are also obtained.

References: National Center for Health Statistics (annual, 1989)

National Electronic Injury Surveillance System
Purpose and scope

The Consumer Product Safety Commission, an independent regulatory agency established under the Consumer Product Safety Act of 1972 and activated in May 1973, is responsible for protecting the public against unreasonable risk of injury or illness associated with consumer products, to assist consumers in evaluating the comparative safety of consumer products, to develop uniform safety standards for consumer products, to minimize conflicting state and local regulations, and to promote research and investigation into causes and prevention of product-related deaths, illnesses,

and injuries. While the Commission relies on a number of sources to meet its data needs, its primary source of data is the National Electronic Injury Surveillance System (NEISS), which became operational in 1972 under the auspices of the Bureau of Product Safety of the Food and Drug Administration (which became the nucleus of the Consumer Product Safety Commission).

Data collection procedures and data items

NEISS operates at two levels and is designed and maintained as an intelligence-gathering system to provide decision-making data. As of 1 January 1991, the first level of the system, **surveillance**, comprised 91 hospital emergency departments (a statistical sample representative of all 50 states and United States territories). This represents an increase from a prior sample size of 65, and it provides for collection of approximately 40 per cent more injury cases annually, resulting in less time being needed to complete special studies and modest reductions in the associated sampling errors. The sample design is composed of four strata based on hospital size, measured by the annual number of emergency department visits; the hospital sample is redesigned and updated periodically to reflect the opening, closing, and changes in size of hospitals.

Each hospital participating in the system is expected to report all injuries treated within its emergency room that involved a consumer product in any way. It is the usual procedure in most emergency rooms to provide a brief description of the accident within the medical record, i.e. 'amputated finger on lawn mower'. However, the emergency department staff of each participating hospital is urged to provide an adequate description of any product involved. All emergency department records are reviewed daily, and a coded record is generated for those cases involving a consumer product. This record includes the following data: age of victim; sex of victim; up to two products involved in the accident; whether a third product was involved in the accident; type of injury (a simple 31-element coding scheme in which the injury is described in broad lay terms); body part injured; disposition of the patient after emergency department treatment; accident locale; fire/motor vehicle involvement; comments (space to provide a brief narrative description of the accident or other pertinent information such as product brand name); other supplementary data (a section of the record set aside to allow for coding specific information for defined accident types).

At the end of each day's coding, the coded data are entered into a computer terminal installed for this purpose. Simultaneously, the computer system edits the entered data and identifies errors for correction. A computer at Commission headquarters polls each hospital's NEISS computer in the early morning hours of each day, and data are uploaded to a mainframe computer and incorporated into the permanent database.

In 1994 operational coding rules were rewritten to define in-scope cases as those where the product normally falls under the Commission's jurisdiction. This means that farm equipment, medical devices, drugs (except childhood poisonings), pesticides, cosmetics, firearms, motor vehicles, aeroplanes, and trains are excluded.

This leads up to the second level of the system, **investigation**. When possible, effort is made to select cases representative of the NEISS surveillance data. Most cases assigned for investigation are selected to provide data for directing regulatory action, for monitoring existing standards, or for providing a basis for response to petitions submitted to the Consumer Product Safety Commission. Accident investigations are based on personal contact (on-site or telephone interviews) and provide information on the accident sequence, ways in which the product was being used, environmental circumstances related to the accident, and behaviour of the person or persons involved. Whenever possible, investigators document the product brand name, indicate the involvement of the product or its component parts in the accident, and include photographs and diagrams. Police, fire, and coroner's reports may be included as supplementary data. Abbreviated cases, generally conducted by telephone, contain most but not all of these items. None of the investigations includes identifying information on the victims or other respondents.

Reference: Consumer Product Safety Commission (1994)

Annual Survey of Occupational Injuries and Illnesses

Purpose and scope

The Annual Survey of Occupational Injuries and Illnesses is conducted by the Bureau of Labor Statistics in response to the requirements of the 1970 Occupational Safety and Health Act for the collection, compilation, and analysis of occupational safety and health statistics. The survey builds upon a record-keeping system, also mandated under the Act, that requires virtually all employers to keep records on all work-related deaths, illnesses, and those injuries that result in one or more of the following: loss of consciousness, restriction of work or motion, transfer to another job, or medical treatment beyond first aid.

The present annual survey produces data to reflect the job-related injury and illness experience of the work force as a whole. Survey data are solicited from a sample of employers with 11 employees or more in agriculture, forestry, and fishing, and from all employers in oil and gas extraction, construction, manufacturing, transportation and public utilities, and wholesale trade. Effective December 1982, low-risk industries in retail trade, finance, insurance, and real estate, and service industries are exempt from routine record-keeping of the log and supplementary record. The sample is selected to represent private industries in the states and territories. Data for employees covered by other federal safety and health legislation are provided by the Mine and Health Safety Administration of the Department of Labor and the Federal Railroad Administration of the Department of Transportation. The Occupational Safety and Health Administration is responsible for the collection and compilation of comparable data for federal agencies; state and local government agencies are not surveyed for national estimates. Self-employed persons are excluded because they are not considered to be 'employees' under the Act.

Data collection procedures and data items

The universe frame of employers is first stratified into industries and then into employment-size groups. Because the survey is a federal–state co-operative programme and the data must also meet the needs of participating state agencies, the universe is further stratified by state prior to sample selection. The Bureau of Labor Statistics designs and identifies the survey sample for each state and, through its regional offices, validates the survey results and

provides technical assistance to the state agencies on a continuing basis. In each state participating in the survey on an operational basis, an agency collects and processes the data, prepares state estimates, and provides the data from which the Bureau produces national results.

The national sample for the survey consists of approximately 250 000 sample units in private industry. Report forms are mailed to selected employers in February of each year to cover the previous calendar year's experience. Each employer completes a single report form, which is then used for national and state estimates. Information for the illness and injury portion of the report form is copied directly from the Log and Summary of Occupational Injuries and Illnesses, which is required record-keeping by each employer under the Act. For each recordable case, employers enter information into this log on the number of lost work days following the day of injury or onset of illness. The days are recorded as either days away from work or days of restricted work activity (days when the employee is assigned to another job on a temporary basis, works at a permanent job less than full-time, or works at a permanently assigned job but cannot perform all duties normally connected with it). The form also contains questions about the number of employee hours worked (needed in calculation of incidence rates), the reporting unit's principal products or activity, and average employment to ensure that the establishment is classified in the correct industry and employment size class.

Using a weighting procedure, sample units are made to represent all units in their size class for a particular industry. Data are further adjusted to reflect the actual employment in an industry during the survey year. Since the universe file that provides the sample frame is not current to the reference year of the survey, it is necessary to 'benchmark' the data to reflect current employment levels.

Although the reported data are carefully edited and reviewed, it is recognized that there are undoubtedly errors of interpretation, which are not uncovered, with regard to record-keeping definitions by employers. Therefore a quality assurance programme is conducted to evaluate the extent of this type of error in the records.

Beginning with the 1992 survey, details are obtained for more seriously injured and ill workers (those with days away from work) including the circumstances of the injury or illness. Work-related fatalities, which are relatively rare events, are no longer included in the survey; a new Census of Fatal Occupational Injuries has been established to capture this information.

Despite progress in identification, recording, and reporting of illnesses, there are some known limitations inherent in the system. These include the fact that cases are recorded only in the year in which they are diagnosed and recognized as work related. Many occupational illnesses may develop years after an employee has left the firm where he or she contracted the illness, and many illnesses that may be of occupational origin are not as yet commonly recognized as such.

Reference: Bureau of Labor Statistics (1988)

Basic vital statistics

Purpose and scope

Basic vital statistics provided through the registration system come from records of live births, deaths, fetal deaths, and induced terminations of pregnancy. Registration of these events is a local and state function, but uniform registration practices and use of the records for national statistics have been established over the years through co-operative agreements between the states and the NCHS and its predecessor agencies.

The purpose of the basic vital statistics programme is to formulate and maintain a co-operative and co-ordinated vital records and vital statistics system, in addition to promoting high standards of performance. The programme is nationwide in scope, covering the entire population of the United States.

Both provisional and final vital statistics are derived from the registration system. The provisional data are obtained from counts of vital records registered without reference to the date that the event occurred, and the final data are obtained from the record and its contents and are processed by date of occurrence of the event.

The civil laws of every state provide for a continuous and permanent birth, death, and fetal death registration system. In general, the local registrar of a town, city, county, or other geographic area collects the records of births and deaths occurring in the area, inspects, queries, and corrects these records if necessary, maintains a local copy, register, or index, and transmits records to the state health department. There, the vital statistics office inspects the records for promptness of filing and for completeness and consistency of information, queries if necessary, numbers, indexes, and processes the statistical information for state and local use, and binds the records for permanent reference and safe-keeping. Microfilm copies or machine-readable data of the individual records are transmitted to the NCHS for use in compiling the final annual national vital statistics volumes.

Provisional vital statistics are collected and published monthly and summarized annually. They are derived from monthly reports from the states to the NCHS giving the number of certificates accepted by the state for filing between two dates a month apart, without regard to the actual date of occurrence. These reports to NCHS are to be mailed on or before the 25th of the month following the data month. They are the source of the provisional vital statistics published in the *Monthly vital statistics report* and the annual summary of the monthly reports. Provisional data also include a 10 per cent sample of death certificates, known as the *Current mortality sample*, which provides provisional cause-of-death data on a monthly basis. The sample is selected by the NCHS from the regular data file of deaths for those states submitting their entire month's file by the end of the following month. Otherwise, the state is asked to provide a sample of records on a current basis. The sample is compiled by selecting each record that includes a given last digit in the certificate number.

To promote uniformity in the statistical information collected from states and local areas for national statistical purposes, the NCHS recommends standard certificates or reports for birth, death, fetal death, and induced termination of pregnancy. The standard certificates and reports are developed co-operatively with the states and local areas, taking into account the needs and problems expressed by the major providers and users of the data. They are reviewed about every ten years to ensure that they meet, to the fullest extent feasible, current needs as legal records and as sources of vital and health statistics.

The use of standard certificates and reports by states is voluntary. Although the form and content may vary according to the laws and practices of each state, the certificates and reports in most states closely follow the standard. For instance, the standard birth certificate includes information on the child's birth date and place of birth, the parents' state of birth, age, race, and educational attainment, previous pregnancy history of the mother, and data regarding the mother's prenatal care, any complications of pregnancy and labour, and any congenital malformations or anomalies noticed at birth. Items on the standard death certificate include the deceased's date and place of birth and death, place of residence, usual occupation, and immediate and underlying cause of death.

References: National Center for Health Statistics (annual, 1989)

Vital statistics follow-back surveys
Purpose and scope
National natality and mortality surveys are periodic data collections based on samples of registered deaths and births occurring during a calendar year. Mortality surveys were conducted by NCHS annually from 1961 to 1968, and natality surveys from 1963 to 1969 and in 1972 and 1985. A National Infant Mortality Survey was also conducted from 1964 to 1966. A National Natality Survey was conducted for 1980, which was expanded to include fetal mortality; a National Maternal and Infant Health Survey for 1988 was conducted, which had a 1991 Longitudinal Follow-up Survey component.

The national follow-back surveys extend, for statistical purposes, the range of items that are normally included on the vital records. They provide national estimates of births and deaths by characteristics not available from the vital registration system. They also serve as a basis for evaluating the quality of information reported on the vital records.

Data collection procedures and data items
The birth or death record serves as the sampling unit, and samples of these units are selected from a frame of records representing births or deaths registered during a given period (usually a calendar year). The sampling frame for the National Mortality Survey is the current mortality sample, i.e. the 10 per cent systematic sample of death certificates received each month by NCHS from the registration areas in the United States. The sample for the National Mortality Survey is subselected monthly from the current mortality sample. The sampling frame for the National Natality Survey is the file of birth certificates from each of the registration areas of the United States. Each registration area assigns a file number to each birth certificate; these file numbers run consecutively from the first to the last birth occurring in that area during that year. The survey samples are based on a probability design that makes use of these certificate numbers.

Data for all the followback surveys are collected primarily by mail. In the natality surveys, questionnaires are sent to the mother, to the physician who delivered the baby, and to the medical facility where the baby was born, using addresses given on the birth certificates. In addition, the 1980 and 1988 surveys obtained data from the medical sources that the woman had named as having given her radiation treatment or examination in the year prior to the delivery.

In the mortality surveys, a questionnaire is sent to the person who provided the funeral director with the decedent's personal information for recording on the certificate. This questionnaire requests socio–economic information about the decedent as well as the names and addresses of hospitals and institutions that might have provided care to the decedent at any time during the last year of life. If the death occurred in a hospital or institution, a hospital questionnaire is typically sent directly to the hospital or institution asking for information about the care provided and for the names and addresses of other medical facilities providing care.

The questionnaires for national mortality surveys have contained questions concerning the patient's last year of life. The surveys have included questions on hospital utilization, diagnoses, operations performed, institutions in which hospitalized, income, whether working or retired during most of the last year of life, household composition, education, health insurance, and the smoking habits of the deceased. The 1993 survey focused on socio-economic differentials in mortality, the potential for preventing premature death by inquiry about associations between risk factors and cause of death, access to and utilization of health care services during the last year of life, disability, and the reliability of certain items reported on the death certificate.

The questionnaire for the 1964–1966 National Infant Mortality Survey included questions on the hospital admission of the infant who died, information about other children of the mother, household composition, income, employment of mother, education of mother and father, and health insurance.

The national natality surveys collect information from mothers who had live births during a given year. They have gathered information on the medical and dental care and radiological treatment of the mother, employment and education of mother and father, family income, pregnancy history of the mother, expectations of having more children, household composition, income, whether this was a first or later marriage, whether the mother was employed and when during her pregnancy she stopped working, and health insurance coverage.

The 1980 and 1988 national natality surveys were broadened to include fetal mortality and the 1988 survey included infant mortality; these surveys included many of the same or similar questions as previous surveys to allow trend studies in the areas of smoking habits, marriage and pregnancy history, education, income, health status of mother and infant, sterilization, radiological treatment, employment, child-bearing expectations, and breast-feeding. Many new areas of study were added, such as alcohol consumption, electronic fetal monitoring, amniocentesis, additional maternal and infant health indicators, occupation of mother and father, and ethnicity. Furthermore, there was an oversampling of low-birth-weight infants in the natality survey, which will enable a more in-depth study of this high-risk group.

The 1991 Longitudinal Follow-up Survey had two components. There was a follow-up data collection to obtain information on the health and development of the live-birth cohort, including information on child care, health insurance coverage, household composition, and income. With the mother's permission, hospital and paediatric practitioner follow-up was conducted to obtain medical information not available from the mother. A subsample of women in the fetal and infant death cohorts was recontacted to obtain information on how they had coped with their loss, their subsequent fertility, and use of adoption and foster care.

References: National Center for Health Statistics (annual, 1989)

Health care resources and their utilization

National Health Provider Inventory

Purpose and scope

The National Health Provider Inventory (NHPI), compiled and updated periodically by the NCHS, is a comprehensive file of information on virtually all nursing and related care homes and hospices and home health agencies in the United States. It was initially established in 1991, and a 1996 update is planned. NHPI maintains files on facilities that provide medical, nursing, personal, or custodial care to groups of unrelated persons on an inpatient (at least overnight) basis. These include all types of nursing, personal, and domiciliary care facilities, not just those certified by Medicare or Medicaid; other facilities of a remedial or custodial nature are also included, such as homes or resident schools for the deaf, blind, mentally retarded, and emotionally disturbed, resident treatment centres for alcohol and drug abusers, and homes for unmarried mothers. Hospices and home health agencies are providers of nursing and personal care in non-institutional settings.

The NHPI is the only comprehensive source of information on the nation's long-term care services providers. Its major purpose is to provide data for the analysis of the supply, distribution, and utilization of health resources, and to serve as a sampling frame for probability sample surveys conducted among samples of providers.

Data collection procedures and data items

Generally, the data are collected by mail. The administrator of the facility or agency is sent a questionnaire and asked to complete and return it by mail.

Two mechanisms are used to keep the data in the NHPI as current as possible. The NCHS conducts a series of mail surveys (i) to ensure that the data on file on the basic characteristics of the facilities are accurate, and (ii) to identify and then delete those facilities that have gone out of business or are no longer eligible for inclusion. In addition, state licensing agencies, national voluntary associations, and other appropriate sources, send their most recent directories or lists of new facilities to the NCHS at regular intervals. These lists are then clerically matched with the most current NHPI file and entities not already included are added.

The NHPI contains the following types of data for the two categories of facilities:

- **Nursing and related care homes:** ownership; major type of service; licensed and staffed beds; beds certified for Medicare and Medicaid; admission policy with regard to age; patient census by age, race/ethnicity, and sex; inpatient days of care; staffing.

- **Hospices and home health care agencies:** ownership; major type of service; licensing; Medicare/Medicaid certification; number of active clients currently on the rolls; number of clients served and discharged during the prior calendar year; services offered to clients; staffing.

References: National Center for Health Statistics (annual, 1989)

Annual Survey of Hospitals
Purpose and scope
The Annual Survey of Hospitals is conducted by the American Hospital Association (AHA). The primary purpose of the survey, which has been conducted since 1946, is to provide a cross-sectional view of the hospital industry and to make it possible to monitor hospital performance over time; it also provides a sampling frame for other AHA surveys and special studies. Information is gathered from a universe of approximately 6700 hospitals in the country, and includes information on the availability of services, utilization, personnel, finances, and governance.

Data collection procedures and data items
The questionnaire for the annual survey is mailed to both AHA-registered and non-registered hospitals in the United States and associated areas (i.e. American Samoa, Guam, the Marshall Islands, Puerto Rico, and the Virgin Islands); United States government hospitals located outside the United States are not included.

Survey questionnaires are mailed in late October of each year. After follow-up, a response rate of about 90 per cent is achieved. Response rates vary among groups of hospitals categorized by size, ownership, service, geographic location, and membership status. For example, the response rate for community hospitals (defined as all non-federal short-stay general and other special hospitals) is generally higher than that of non-community hospitals. The response rate for AHA-registered hospitals averages about 90 per cent, while the rate for non-registered hospitals averages about 70 per cent (registered hospitals comprise approximately 98 per cent of the mailing universe).

When a questionnaire is incomplete or when the information provided does not pass specified edits, the individual hospital is contacted for clarification and confirmation. If it is not possible to obtain information from a hospital, estimates for most missing data items are generated on the basis of their values in the previous year, whether those values were actual or estimated, and on the basis of information reported by hospitals similar to the non-respondents in size, type of control, principal medical service provided, and length of stay (long or short term).

Since its inception, the survey questionnaire has been kept in the same format in order to provide continuity and to permit important time series and trend analysis. This means that similar definitions have been used, a similar arrangement of questions has been followed, and a relatively consistent data set has been collected.

The questionnaire is divided into several sections: reporting period; classification by governance and organizational structure; facilities and services available (provided by the hospital or under arrangement with another hospital or provider); beds set up and staffed within distinct inpatient service areas of the hospital and utilization of those units in terms of total inpatient days; total number of beds set up and staffed, admissions, discharges, inpatient days, discharge days, Medicare/Medicaid inpatient days and discharges, outpatient utilization, and inpatient and outpatient surgical operations for the entire reporting period; financial data on total patient and non-patient revenue, payroll and non-payroll expenses, restricted and unrestricted assets, and liabilities; full- and part-time hospital personnel, by occupational category, on payroll on the last day of the reporting period.

While the information gathered from the survey includes many specific services, it does not necessarily include all of each hospital's services and thus the data do not reflect an exhaustive list of all services offered by all hospitals. Similarly, although respondents are asked to provide data for a 12-month period beginning 1 October and ending 30 September of the following year, much of the survey data are not for that period; for example, in 1992 about one-third of responding AHA-registered hospitals used that reporting period, while about a quarter used a reporting period of July through June and the remainder used some other reporting period.

Reference: American Hospital Association (annual).

National Hospital Discharge Survey
Purpose and scope
The National Hospital Discharge Survey (NHDS) of the NCHS is the principal source of information on in-patient utilization of short-stay hospitals. Data collection began in 1965 and has been continuous since then.

The purpose of the NHDS is to produce statistics that are representative of the experience of the United States civilian non-institutionalized population discharged from short-term hospitals. Specifically, the survey provides information on the characteristics of patients, the lengths of stay, diagnoses, and surgical and non-surgical procedures, patterns of use of care in hospitals of different sizes and type of ownership in the four geographic regions of the country. The scope of the NHDS encompasses discharges from non-federal hospitals in the 50 states and the District of Columbia; only hospitals with six or more beds staffed for patient care and an average length of stay for all patients of less than 30 days are included in the sample. NHDS is the benchmark against which special programmatic data sources are most often compared.

Data collection procedures and data items
The unit of enumeration in the survey is a hospital discharge. Beginning in 1988, the NHDS sample includes a certainty stratum comprised of all hospitals with 1000 or more beds or 40000 or more discharges per year. The remaining sample is a stratified three-stage design. The first stage consists of primary sampling units (PSUs) used in the National Health Interview Survey; the second stage comprises systematic random samples of non-certainty hospitals selected in the sample PSUs with probability proportional to their annual numbers of discharges. The third stage is a systematic random sample of discharges from each hospital. Sampling rates at the third stage are determined by the hospital's sampling stratum and the system (manual or automated) used to collect data in the hospital. In 1992, the last year for which final data are available, the sample consisted of 528 hospitals from a universe of approximately 7000 short-stay hospitals. Of the 514 in-scope hospitals, information was collected from 494 participating hospitals (approximately a 96 per cent response rate) on approximately 274000 discharges.

Two data collection procedures for the survey were begun in 1985. The first is the traditional manual system of sample selection by hospital staff or representatives of NCHS; the daily listing sheet of discharges is used as the sampling frame. Sample discharges are selected by a random technique, generally using the terminal digit or digits of the medical record number for the patient. Data are then abstracted from the face sheet and discharge summary in the medical record. The second method involves purchase of data tapes from commercial abstracting services; this method is used in approximately a third of sample hospitals. For these hospitals, tapes containing machine-readable medical record data are purchased from abstracting service organizations, state data systems, or hospitals themselves, and are subjected to NCHS sampling, editing, and weighting procedures.

The medical abstract form contains items relating to the personal characteristics of the patient (including birth date, sex, race, and marital status, but not name and address), administrative information (including admission and discharge dates, discharge status, and medical record number), and medical information (including final diagnoses and surgical and diagnostic procedures). It takes an average of 5 minutes for medical records personnel to sample and complete each form. The contents of the medical abstract form did not change from the inception of the survey until 1977, when modifications were made so that it more nearly paralleled the Uniform Hospital Discharge Data Set. The items added to the abstract at that time were residence of patient (Zip code), expected source of payment, disposition of patient, and date of procedures.

References: National Center for Health Statistics (annual, 1989).

National Nursing Home Survey
Purpose and scope
Between 1963 and 1969, NCHS conducted surveys of nursing homes and their residents on an *ad hoc* basis. With the implementation of the Medicaid and Medicare programmes, the increased utilization of nursing homes, and the projected increases in the aged population, those who set standards for, plan, provide, and assess long-term care services needed comprehensive national data on a continuing basis. To meet their requirements, the National Nursing Home Survey (NNHS) was developed in 1972, with the initial survey conducted in 1973–1974, the second in 1977, and the third in 1985. Current plans are to establish the NNHS as an ongoing annual survey beginning in 1995.

This periodic data collection system is a series of nationwide sample surveys of nursing homes, their residents, and staff. The purposes of the surveys are to collect national baseline data on the characteristics, services, residents, and staff for all nursing homes in the nation, regardless of whether or not they are participating in federal programs such as Medicare or Medicaid, to collect data on the costs incurred by the facility for providing care by major components such as labour, fixed, operating, and miscellaneous costs, to collect data on Medicare and Medicaid certification (such as utilization of certified beds and the health of residents receiving programme benefits) so that all data can be analysed by certification status, and to provide comparable data for valid trend analyses on a variety of topics.

For the initial survey conducted in 1973–1974, the universe included only those nursing homes that provided some level of nursing care, regardless of whether or not they were participating in the Medicare or Medicaid programmes. Thus homes providing only personal or domiciliary care were excluded. Beginning with the 1977 survey, the universe was expanded to include all nursing, personal care, and domiciliary care homes, regardless of their participation in Medicare or Medicaid. Homes that provide room and board only are excluded. In all three surveys, homes in the universe included those that were operated under proprietary, non-profit-making, and government auspices and homes that were units of a larger institution (usually a hospital or retirement centre).

Data collection procedures and data items
The sample homes are selected from the NHPI which is maintained by the NCHS and contains basic information about the home (such as name, address, size, ownership, number of residents, and number of staff) that is needed to design efficient sampling plans.

Resident data are collected by reviewing medical records and questioning the nurse who usually provides care for the resident. Residents are not interviewed directly. Response rates for the surveys differ according to the type of questionnaire but range from 98 per cent for the resident questionnaires to 81 per cent for staff questionnaires. The initial survey, conducted from August 1973 to April 1974, had a nationally representative sample of 2100 nursing homes, with a subsample of 25 100 staff and 19 400 residents. The second survey, conducted from May to December 1977, had a total sample of 1700 nursing homes, with a subsample of 16 800 staff, 7100 residents, and 5300 discharged residents. The 1985 NNHS was conducted from August 1985 to January 1986 and had a total sample of about 1150 nursing and related care homes, 3400 registered nurses, 4600 current residents, and 6000 discharged residents.

The NNHS uses several questionnaires. The facility questionnaire includes questions on number of beds and residents, services provided, certification status, and various utilization measures. The expense questionnaire includes questions on the facility's expenses by major components such as labour, fixed, operating, and miscellaneous expenses. The staff questionnaire includes questions about the employee's demographic characteristics, work experience, education, and salary. The residents' questionnaire includes questions about demographic characteristics, health status, functional status, participation in social activities, monthly charge, and source of payment. The 1977 survey included a discharged resident questionnaire, with some of the same questions as the current resident questionnaire selected on the basis of their availability in the medical record.

A number of respondents in a home are surveyed with a combination of personal interviews and self-administered questionnaires. Facility information is secured through a 20-minute personal interview with the administrator. Expense data are collected on a self-administered questionnaire, requiring about 30 minutes to answer; this information is completed by the facility's administrator or by the staff accountant under authorization from the administrator. Sampled staff members (registered nurses in the 1985 survey) fill in a brief form that requires about 5 minutes to complete. Information on sampled current residents is secured through personal interviews, which require about 15 minutes per resident, with the nurses who provide care to the residents. The nurses may refer to medical records for information. For instance, beginning in the 1977 survey, information on the sampled discharged residents was secured by the interviewer in a personal interview with the nurse who was most familiar with the medical records and who referred to them for replying to all questions. In the 1985 survey, a telephone interview with next-of-kin of current and living discharged residents was conducted to obtain further information not available from the nursing home; this next-of-kin interview was repeated twice at approximately six-month intervals to obtain information on vital status, current living arrangements, and nursing home and hospital utilization.

References: National Center for Health Statistics (annual, 1989).

National Ambulatory Medical Care Survey / National Hospital Ambulatory Medical Care Survey

Purpose and scope

In May 1973, the National Center for Health Statistics inaugurated the National Ambulatory Medical Care Survey (NAMCS) on a continuing basis to gather and disseminate statistical data about ambulatory medical care provided to the United States population by office-based physicians. The National Hospital Ambulatory Medical Care Survey (NHAMCS) was initiated in December 1991 as a complement to NAMCS; it serves as a principal source of data on visits to hospital emergency and outpatient departments. Together, the two ongoing surveys provide nationally representative data on approximately 90 per cent of the ambulatory care rendered in the United States.

The NAMCS target population consists of all office visits within the conterminous United States made by ambulatory patients to non-federal physicians who are in office-based practice and engaged in direct patient care. Visits to hospital-based physicians, to specialists in anaesthesiology, pathology, and radiology, and to physicians who are principally engaged in teaching, research, or administration are excluded. Telephone contacts and other non-office visits are also excluded. Since about 70 per cent of all direct ambulatory medical care visits occur in physicians' offices, this office-based NAMCS design provides data on the majority of ambulatory care services. NAMCS was conducted annually from 1981 to 1985, and again annually beginning in 1989.

NHAMCS is conducted in a national probability sample of hospitals within a sample of clinics that provide ambulatory medical care under the supervision of a physician and under the auspices of the hospital in up to five emergency service areas. Clinics providing only ancillary services (such as diagnostic X-rays or radiation therapy) are out of scope, as are services provided in dental or dental surgery clinics, pharmacies, or other settings in which physician services typically are not provided. Free-standing clinics and ambulatory surgery centres are also out of scope, but ambulatory surgery centres were recently included in a new national survey by the NCHS.

Data collection procedures and data items

The NAMCS sampling frame is a list of licensed physicians in office-based patient care practice compiled from files that are classified and maintained by the American Medical Association (AMA) and the American Osteopathic Association. These files are continuously updated by both associations, making them as current and correct as possible at the time of sample selection.

For the years 1995 and 1996, the sample consists of approximately 3500 office-based physicians per year, with sample physicians randomly distributed across the 52 weeks of the year so that the resulting data reflect seasonal variations. Since the assignment of the reporting week is an integral part of the sample design, each physician is required to report during a predetermined period and no substitute reporting periods are permitted. Approximately 75 per cent of the eligible physicians in the sample participate in the survey.

The final stage involves sampling patient visits within a physician's practice. The sampling rate, determined at the time of the interviewer's appointment, is dependent on the number of days during the reporting week that the physician is in practice and the number of patients that he or she expects to see. In actual practice, the sampling procedure is handled through the use of a patient log.

Actual data collection for NAMCS is carried out by the participating physician, aided by office assistants when possible. The physician completes a patient record for a sample of patients seen during the assigned reporting week. Sampling procedures are designed so that patient records are completed on each day of practice for ten patient visits at most. Physicians expecting ten or fewer visits per day record data for all of them, while those expecting more than ten visits per day record data after every second, third, or fifth visit, observing the same predetermined sampling interval continuously. Each form requires only a few minutes to complete.

Two data collection forms are employed by the participating physician—the patient log and the patient record. The patient log is a sequential listing of patients, which serves as a sampling frame to indicate for which visits data should be recorded. The patient record contains the following items of information about the visit: date and duration; patient's date of birth; sex, race, and problem; expected sources of payment; whether the patient has been seen for the particular problem before and whether he or she was referred by another physician; length of time since the onset of the problem; diagnoses; diagnostic and therapeutic services; seriousness of the condition; disposition. Periodically, supplemental items are added to the basic patient record to investigate specific heath conditions or other aspects of ambulatory care. For example the 1995 survey includes pilot items to test addition of an item on total charges for the visit.

The NHAMCS universe and sampling frame are the same as for the NHDS. After initial sample selection from the 1991 data file, the sample is being updated every third year. Within the 490 sampled hospitals per calendar year, patient visits are systematically sampled over a four-week reporting period assigned to the hospital. A patient visit is defined as a direct personal exchange between an ambulatory patient and a physician, or a staff member acting under a physician's direction, for the purpose of seeking care and rendering health services; visits for purely administrative purposes, such as paying a bill, are out of scope. As with NAMCS, sampling rates are determined from the number of patients expected to be seen during the reporting period. On average, hospitals complete approximately 50 visit forms for the emergency department and 150 for the outpatient department. Names of patients are confidential and forms containing names remain in the hospital. Items on the patient visit form closely parallel those on the NAMCS form.

References: National Center for Health Statistics (annual, 1989)

Statistical system of the Medicare Programme
Purpose and scope

The Medicare programme, enacted on 30 July 1965 as Title XVIII of the Social Security Act, became effective on 1 July 1966. The programme, which is administered by the Health Care Financing Administration, makes available two separate but complementary health insurance programmes: (i) hospital insurance, covering nearly all persons age 65 years and over and disabled beneficiaries under age 65 years entitled to benefits for at least 24 consecutive months, and covered workers and their dependants with endstage renal disease who require renal dialysis or a kidney transplant; (ii) supplementary medical insurance, covering those persons who voluntarily pay the premiums. The hospital insurance programme, referred to as Part A, covers expenses for medical services furnished in institutional settings (e.g. hospital or hospice) or provided by a home health agency. The supplementary medical insurance, referred to as Part B, covers physician services, outpatient services, and certain other medical equipment and services.

The primary objective of the Medicare statistical system is to provide data to measure and evaluate programme operation and effectiveness. Benefit payment operations furnish information about the amount and kind of hospital and medical care service used by disabled persons and those aged 65 years and over, as well as the expenditures for such services. Applications to participate in the programme from hospitals, skilled nursing facilities, home health agencies, independent laboratories, and suppliers of portable X-ray and outpatient physical therapy services, as well as periodic survey updates, provide data on the characteristics of such providers of services. The health insurance claim number assigned to each individual serves as the link between the services used under Medicare and the demographic characteristics of individual beneficiaries.

System components and operation

All enrolment and entitlement data for persons who are or have been enrolled in Medicare are in the enrolment database files, which identify each aged and disabled person eligible for health insurance benefits and indicate whether he or she is entitled to hospital insurance benefits, supplementary medical insurance benefits, or both. The entitlement record provides the population data for each part of the programme and serves as the base for the computation of a variety of utilization rates. The enrolment database, which is updated daily, includes demographic data including age, sex, race, and state, county, and Zip code of residence. The database also contains information on date of death so that an important health outcome measure can be linked to records on use of services.

Each beneficiary is assigned to one of nine processing sectors for beneficiary and claims information handling. Each sector has a designated contractor host site and a number of satellite processing contractors. It is the host site that maintains the entitlement and utilization data, authorizes satellites to pay claims, and forwards claims data to the Health Care Financing Administration (HCFA) central office.

Every hospital, skilled nursing facility, home health agency, independent clinical laboratory, and supplier of portable X-ray or out-patient physical therapy services must apply for participation in the Medicare program; data on the application forms are stored in the central provider record and are updated as facilities are recertified periodically, as new facilities apply for participation, and as some leave the programme. When the information in the provider file is combined with utilization data, it relates the characteristics of facilities and agencies that provide care to the kinds and amounts of services used by the persons insured under Medicare. Information in the provider file includes the institution's size, location, and type of control. Just as each enrollee has a unique identification number, each institution also has a unique identification number.

Under the hospital insurance programme, fiscal intermediaries act as the link between the HCFA and institutional providers. The fiscal intermediaries review claims, pay providers for care rendered to beneficiaries, and assist the HCFA in the application of safeguards against unnecessary use of covered services. Utilization and benefit payment information is forwarded to the HCFA.

Supplementary medical insurance claims for home health services and outpatient hospital services are also processed by fiscal intermediaries. Claims for physician services are paid by contractors, referred to as carriers, who process and pay the claim. All claims are submitted to the host site, which pays, rejects, or recycles the claim for missing information. Upon authorization from the host site, the fiscal intermediary or carrier pays the claim. The host site also updates the beneficiary's utilization history and transmits the information to the HCFA. As part of this process, detailed information on diagnoses, surgical procedures, and services becomes part of the utilization database.

Reference: Bureau of Data Management and Strategy (1993)

Physician Masterfile
Purpose and scope

The AMA has maintained a masterfile of physicians since 1906. In the early days of its existence, the Physician Masterfile was primarily a listing of physicians maintained as a record-keeping device for membership and mailing purposes.

The AMA Physician Masterfile is considered the most comprehensive and complete source of physician data in the United States. It includes information on every physician in the country and on graduates of American medical schools who are temporarily practising overseas. The file includes both members and nonmembers of the AMA, and graduates of foreign medical schools who are in the United States and meet American education standards for primary recognition as physicians. Thus, all physicians in the total physician labour power pool are included on the AMA Physician Masterfile.

Data collection procedures and data items

A file is started on each individual who enters medical school or, in the case of foreign and Canadian graduates, upon entry into the United States. As a physician's training and career develop, additional information is added to the file (e.g. internship and residency training, licensing, board certification, professional affiliations, and other characteristics). These characteristics, while they may change over time, are not subject to constant change and are included in the historical portion of the masterfile.

There is also a current professional activities portion of each physician's record, which identifies current address, professional activity, specialties, and employment status. By definition, this current portion of the file is subject to constant change and is updated regularly. Between 1969 and 1985 mail surveys of all those in the masterfile were conducted approximately every four years by the AMA using a questionnaire entitled Record of Physicians' Professional Activities (PPA). From 1988, approximately a third of the physicians listed in the masterfile have received a PPA questionnaire each year.

Between periodic updates, a computerized updating system keeps the masterfile current. Each physician's record is updated to reflect the most recent change, which may be signalled by AMA mailings or publications, by physician correspondence, or by hospitals, government agencies, medical schools, medical agencies, medical societies, specialty boards, and licensing agencies. Any indication of a change in professional status or address triggers a questionnaire similar to the one used in the most recent census.

While the data collected from the PPA questionnaire represent a major input to the masterfile, data from other sources are also incorporated. These other data sources include medical schools, which provide information on year of graduation, name, address, place of birth, and date of birth of medical students, hospitals, which provide information on interns and residents, place of birth, and foreign medical graduates in training, the office of the Surgeon General of the United States, which provides annual information on physicians in government, American specialty boards, which provide data on board certification of physicians, professional societies, which provide information on membership in specialty, state, and county societies, and the Educational Commission for Foreign Medical Graduates, which provides data on foreign medical graduates.

Reference: American Medical Association (annual)

Health occupation data from the decennial census of population

Purpose and scope
The United States Constitution provides for an enumeration of the population every 10 years. It was quickly recognized that enumeration offered an opportunity to obtain important information on characteristics of the population. Therefore the first census, taken in 1790, included questions on the age and sex of each enumerated individual; over the years many additional items have been added to the census. Information on occupation was added in 1850 and has been included since. Beginning in 1940 many questions, including occupation, have been asked of only a sample of the households in the total population in order to reduce the burden on the public. The censuses of 1960 and 1970 obtained information on occupation for persons aged 14 years and over in the experienced labour force or in the labour reserve; the census of 1980 obtained information on occupation for each person aged 15 years and over in households that fell into the sample. For the 1990 census, essentially the same questions and procedures from 1980 were used.

Data collection procedures and data items
Like all information on the questionnaire, occupation is self-reported by household members in sample households where a long form of the questionnaire is received. Upon completion of the questionnaires in the households and their return to census field offices, the questionnaires are edited by hand for completeness and consistency. In 1990 occupation entries were processed first through data entry and computer software, which assigned codes to 38 per cent of the entries; remaining entries were referred for coding by clerical staff.

Persons queried about their occupation in the 1990 census were asked whether they had worked at all during the week prior to 1 April and, if so, how many hours they had worked that week at all jobs (if they worked at more than one job); they were also asked at what location they worked during that week in addition to a number of questions about the trip to work. Those who did not work at all in the prior week were asked other questions about their availability for employment in that week.

Specific occupation questions were asked of those who had worked during the prior week and of those who did not work in that week but had worked for at least a few days in the period from 1985 to 1990. If the person had more than one job activity or business during the prior week, the one at which the most hours were worked was to be described; if the person had no job or business that week, she or he was asked to provide information pertaining to the last job or business since 1985. These questions included the name of the company or employer for whom the person worked, the kind of business or industry, the kind of work performed, and the most important job duties. The respondents were asked whether they were employees of a private company for wages, salary, or commission, government employees (federal, state, or local), self-employed in their own business (either incorporated or unincorporated); or working without pay in a family business or farm.

The occupation classification system used in the 1990 census was similar to that used in each decennial census since 1940. However, the changes made for each of the censuses affect comparability of data from one census to another and require care in making such comparisons. There was a major change in the classification system used for coding occupations between the 1970 (441 specific categories) and 1980 (503 specific categories) censuses; in 1990 there were 501 specific occupational categories.

Prior to 1980, the Census Bureau used its own occupational classification system. The 1980 census was the first in which the Standard Occupational Classification system was used; this system was developed in 1977 for use by all federal agencies to provide greater comparability of occupation data among government agencies. Greatest occupational detail tabulations from the 1990 census are shown in a special subject report and on public use computer tape files.

Analysis of occupational data from the decennial census requires some caution, since the data are self-reported by individuals in response to open-ended questions. Since census data on occupations are based on a sample of the population, there is also sampling error associated with the estimates.

References: National Center for Health Statistics (1985) and Bureau of the Census (1992)

Health economics

National Medical Expenditure Survey

Purpose and scope

The 1987 National Medical Expenditure Survey (NMES), conducted by the National Center for Health Services Research (now named the Agency for Health Care Policy and Research), is a unique source of detailed national estimates on the utilization and expenditures for various types of medical care. The NMES builds on the experience of the former Current Medicare Survey, the National Health Interview Survey, the 1977 National Medical Care Expenditure Survey, and the 1980 National Medical Care Utilization and Expenditure Survey. Pretests are being conducted in 1995 for a similar survey planned for calendar year 1996.

The NMES was designed to be directly responsive to the continuing need for statistical information on the health care expenditures associated with health services utilization for the entire United States population. The 1987 survey was designed and conducted in collaboration with the HCFA to provide additional utilization and expenditure data for persons in the Medicare and Medicaid populations. The NMES provides estimates for the evaluation of the impact of legislation and programmes on health status, costs, utilization, and illness-related behaviour in the medical care delivery system. A separate household survey of American Indians and Alaska Natives (i.e. Aleuts and Eskimos) (SAIAN) was conducted under sponsorship of the Indian Health Service; SAIAN was designed to provide previously unavailable data on health services utilization and health care financing for these population subgroups. SAIAN used a probability sample of approximately 2000 households in a sample of the 482 counties served by the Indian Health Service. To be eligible for inclusion in the survey, a household had to include one or more American Indians or Alaska Natives eligible for services from the Indian Health Service.

Data collection procedures and data items

The NMES was composed of several related surveys. The household portion of the survey consisted of a national survey of approximately 14 000 households in the civilian non-institutionalized population and oversampled several population subgroups of particular policy interest—African Americans, Latin Americans, the poor and near poor, the elderly, and persons with functional limitations. The sample for this survey was a multistage area probability sample.

The household survey comprised a screening interview plus a series of five interviews over an approximately 18-month period in order to obtain all relevant data for calendar year 1987. The screening interview and interviews for rounds one, two, and four were conducted face to face; interviews for rounds three and five were conducted by telephone when possible.

Collection of data from the households was facilitated by the use of a calendar/diary and a summary. At the time of the first interview, the household respondent was given a calendar on which to record information about health problems and health services utilizations between interviews. Following each household interview, information about health provider contacts and the payment of charges associated with them was used to generate a computer summary of information provided. This summary was used by the interviewer to obtain information not available during a previous interview. In addition to a core questionnaire, each interview included supplements on topics such as functional limitations, health status, habits, and opinions, care-giving (for those living with or caring for functionally impaired persons within or outside the household), income during 1987, details of home ownership, and income tax filing status; and use of long-term care services.

A medical provider survey, a patient-identified physician survey, and a health insurance plans survey were also conducted as follow-back surveys to augment and enrich the person- and family-related data collected in the household surveys. Signed permission forms were obtained from individuals in the household surveys before conducting these other surveys to acquire additional information about their use of health care services or their health insurance coverage.

The **medical provider survey** had the purpose of adding data on charges and sources and amounts of payment where such information could not be provided by a household respondent or where experience had shown that household responses are not reliable; an additional purpose was to provide separate estimates of use and expenditures for validation of estimates derived from enriched household data. Information on the demographic and practice characteristics of physicians seen by participants in the household surveys was the focus of the **patient-identified physician survey**; for example, analysis focuses on mix of treatment by specialty and practice characteristics for different population subgroups. Through the **health insurance plans survey**, the private health insurance coverage of household survey participants is verified; information has also been obtained on the total premium costs of private health insurance, the division of these costs between employers and employees, the kinds of coverage and benefits held by privately insured persons, the availability of health insurance and other fringe benefits at the workplace, the extent of retiree health insurance benefits, and the degree to which employer-provided health insurance is self-insured. A Medicare records component was included to check the eligibility status and claims data for Medicare recipients in the household survey, in SAIAN, and in the institutional population component.

A separate institutional population component was developed to obtain, for the first time, information on the population in nursing and personal care homes and in facilities for the mentally retarded that would parallel and complement the information on the non-institutionalized population from the household survey. This institutional component surveyed about 13 000 sampled persons in a sample of eligible facilities. The universe for this survey was all persons in nursing homes and facilities for the mentally retarded for any part of 1987.

At the first visit to a sampled facility, the interviewer developed a sample of current residents as of 1 January 1987. Information for each of these individuals was obtained on their residential history in the facility, health status, and demographic characteristics. There were three subsequent quarterly visits to the facilities to update information on the January sample of residents and to select samples of new admissions during the preceding quarter. Information on facility charges and expenditures for other medical care services was obtained for each sampled resident. In addition, the interviewer identified a person outside the facility who was best able to answer questions about each sampled patient's life outside the institution—their residential history outside the facility, last household residence, health status before admission to the sampled facility, health insurance coverage, further demographic information, and 1986 income.

Reference: National Center for Health Services Research (1987)

Consumer Price Index
Purpose and scope
The Consumer Price Index (CPI) is a measure of the average change in prices over time for a fixed market basket of goods and services. The market basket is revised periodically to reflect changes in what Americans buy and in the way that they live. The CPI is not a cost-of-living index, since it does not reflect consumer changes in buying or consumption patterns in response to price changes.

The latest CPI revision, effective with the release of January 1987 data, continues a CPI for All Urban Consumers (CPI-U), which was introduced in 1978 and is representative of about 80 per cent of the total non-institutional population, and a CPI for Urban Wage Earners and Clerical Workers (CPI-W), which covers about 32 per cent of the non-institutional population. In addition to wage earners and clerical workers, the CPI-U includes groups such as professional, managerial, and technical workers, the self-employed, short-term workers, the unemployed, and retirees and others not in the labour force. The CPI includes an identifiable medical care component.

Effective with the 1978 revision, medical care represents a major expenditure group and is no longer a sublisting under health and recreation as it had been. However, the general definition of medical care continues to include both medical care services and other commodities. The medical care expenditure group is one of seven major groups, which are further divided into 69 expenditure classes; these, in turn, are divided into 184 item strata. Overall, the medical care component is relatively small, comprising only about 7 per cent of total expenditures as of December 1993.

Data collection procedures and data items
The CPI is based on prices of food, clothing, housing, transportation, medical care, entertainment, and the other goods and services that people buy for day-to-day living. Prices are collected by Census Bureau representatives for about 90 000 items in 85 urban areas across the country from persons in about 57 000 housing units and from about 19 000 retail and service establishments—grocery and department stores, hospitals, gasoline service stations, and other types of stores and service establishments.

In calculating the index, price changes for the various items in each location are averaged together with weights that represent their importance in the spending of the appropriate population group. Local data are then combined to obtain a United States city average. Price indexes are published by size of city and by region of the country, for cross-calculations of regions and population-size classes, and for 27 local areas.

The base period for the general-purpose federal index series is revised approximately every ten years. Base periods are changed in order to facilitate the visual comprehension of rates of change from a base period that is not too distant in time. Beginning with release of data for January 1988, the standard reference base period for both CPI-U and CPI-W is 1982–1984. An increase of 22 per cent, for example, is shown as 122.0. This change can also be expressed in dollars: the price of a base-period market basket of goods and services in the CPI rose from $10 in 1982–1984 to $12.20 in 1994.

The weights for items in the market basket were developed from the Consumer Expenditure Survey conducted for the Bureau of Labor Statistics by the Bureau of the Census during the period from 1982 to 1984. The 1982–1984 Consumer Expenditure Survey, conducted among a national sample of approximately 29 000 families, showed that, as a proportion of total consumption, the medical care services component was smaller than that of the most recent previous survey conducted in 1972–1973. The decrease reflects changes in the ways that consumers pay for medical care, with major medical expenses frequently paid for partially (and sometimes completely) by health insurance and with many insurance premiums fully or partially paid by employers or by government. Although medical care prices rose at a rapid rate over the decade, average consumer unit expenditures for medical care rose less rapidly because of these employer- and government-provided benefits.

The restructuring of the medical care component in 1987 created three new indexes by separating previously combined items: eye care was separated from other professional services, and in-patient and out-patient treatment were separated from other hospital and medical care services. Eye care has been combined with physicians' services, dental services, and other professional services to form the professional medical services index. The previous distinction between the purchase price of spectacles and contact lenses (commodities) and the charge for fitting spectacles and contact lenses (services) is increasingly difficult to make and so both eye care commodities and services are included in a single index in the medical care service component. Also, fees for laboratory tests and X-rays have now been moved from professional services and, along with emergency room charges, make up a new out-patient services category.

As of the 1987 revision, the expenditure weight for health insurance in the CPI reflects only payments that employees or consumer units make towards health insurance premiums. For computing CPI, contributions of employers are treated as income to consumers and not as a consumer expenditure. Changes in the price that consumers pay for health insurance are calculated through an indirect method, instead of through direct pricing.

References: Bureau of Labor Statistics (monthly), Ford and Sturm (1988), Mason and Butler (1987).

References

American Hospital Association (annual). *Hospital statistics.* AHA, Chicago, IL.

American Medical Association (annual). *Physician characteristics and distribution in the US.* AMA, Chicago, IL.

Bureau of the Census (1992). *Summary social, economic and housing characteristics: United States.* US Department of Commerce, Washington, DC.

Bureau of Data Management and Strategy (1993). *Data users' reference guide.* Health Care Financing Administration, Baltimore, MD.

Bureau of Labor Statistics (monthly). *CPI detailed report*. US Department of Labor and US Government Printing Office, Washington, DC.

Bureau of Labor Statistics (1988). *Occupational safety and health statistics: annual survey of occupational injuries and illnesses*, Bulletin 2285. US Department of Labor, Washington, DC.

Consumer Product Safety Commission (1994). *The NEISS sample (design and implementation)*. US Consumer Product Safety Commission, Washington, DC.

Ford, I.K. and Sturm, K. (1988). CPS revision improves pricing of medical care services. *Monthly Labor Review*, 111, 4.

Mason, C. and Butler, C. (1987). New market basket for the Consumer Price Index. *Monthly Labor Review*, **100**, 1.

National Center for Health Services Research (1987). *The 1987 National Medical Expenditure Survey: its design and analytic goals*. US Public Health Service, Rockville, MD.

National Center for Health Statistics (annual). *Catalog of publications of the National Center for Health Statistics*. US Public Health Service, Washington, DC.

National Center for Health Statistics (1985). *Decennial census data for selected health occupations, United States, 1980*, Department of Health, Education and Welfare Publication HRA 86–1826, US Public Health Service, Washington, DC.

National Center for Health Statistics (1989). *Data systems of the National Center for Health Statistics: Vital and Health Statistics*, Series 1, No. 23, Department of Health and Human Services Publication PHS 89–1325, US Public Health Service, Washington, DC.

Substance Abuse and Mental Health Services Administration (annual). *Data from the Drug Abuse Warning Network*, Series I. US Public Health Service, Rockville, MD.

US Centers for Disease Control and Prevention (weekly). *Morbidity and mortality weekly report*. Department of Health and Human Services, US Public Health Service, Atlanta, GA.

3 Health information resources in the United Kingdom

J. S. A. Ashley, Susan K. Cole, and M. Paula J. Kilbane

Introduction

The various sources of statistical information on health and social factors in the United Kingdom, excluding those that primarily contribute information about the health care, rather than the health, of the population, are described in this chapter. Thus we do not cover sources of data on health service activity or facilities, health personnel, or expenditure. Instead, we concentrate on the legislative history establishing the various health information resources, and we review matters relevant to the validity of the described data systems. In many cases the sources concerned have different characteristics within the different countries of the United Kingdom, and particular attention is drawn to such variation.

For many of the topics considered there may be access to additional analyses beyond those normally presented in the standard, and usually annual, publications. It may also be possible to consult unpublished supplementary tabular material or to request *ad hoc* analysis of the data. Many of the reports indicate whether these facilities are available, usually with the provision of a contract address. In some cases hard-copy publications are enhanced or supplemented by microfiche tables, which may provide greater detail.

The chapter is divided into four sections, the first of which provides a brief description of population statistics. These not only give a general overview of the demographic and social status of the population, but also provide the basic denominator material required for the calculation of appropriate rates from the event data covered in subsequent sections. The following section covers mortality statistics, including specific contributions relating to occupational and area mortality, and the availability of information from linked files.

In England and Wales, the Office of Population Censuses and Surveys (OPCS) is the central governmental department responsible for the collection and compilation of the census, most other population statistics, and mortality and other vital statistics. This was formerly the General Register Office with the Registrar-General as its director. Similarly there are General Register Offices in Scotland (GRO(S)) and Northern Ireland (GRO(NI)), directed by the respective Registrars-General.

The third section covers a range of morbidity statistics set out in approximate order of inauguration. It includes the notification of infectious disease, cancer registration, hospital discharge statistics, morbidity statistics from general practice, and the notification of congenital malformations and abortions. This order is used as it is not easy to classify the various sources by alternative means; they do not follow any particular pattern in terms of their contribution to morbidity information, nor do they relate to any logical sequence with respect to, for example, the age group to which they primarily refer.

OPCS and, to a lesser extent, GRO(S) AND GRO(NI) also collect and compile some of the available morbidity statistics. However, in other cases responsibilities lie with the appropriate health departments.

1. England: the Department of Health (formerly the Department of Health and Social Security (DHSS), previously the Ministry of Health).

2. Wales—the Welsh office.

3. Scotland—the Scottish Office Home and Health Department. A major role is also played by the Information and Statistics Division of the Common Services Agency of the Scottish Health Service.

4. Northern Ireland: the Department of Health and Social Services (DHSS(NI)).

The final section describes the General Household Survey and its Northern Ireland equivalent, which are designed as sources of a wide range of annual social information and which usually include data specifically related to health. In conclusion, brief mention is also made of other relevant sources.

Population statistics

The main United Kingdom sources of medical data, although important in their own right, are enhanced when combined with appropriate population statistics to give rates. Of special value are rates that take into account variation in the distribution of certain demographic characteristics in the base population from which the event data are derived.

Population data for the United Kingdom predate both mortality and mobility data; thus it is opportune to commence with a description of the national population censuses and the annual estimates of the population that emanate from them.

National population censuses

Background

In the middle of the eighteenth century, acknowledgement of the need for a count of the population led to the introduction of a Bill in Parliament, but this was allowed to lapse. However, the Population Act 1800 led to the first of four censuses (1801–1831) conducted under the guidance of the Clerk to the House of Commons. From 1841, when responsibility passed to the newly appointed Registrar-General, the method of enumeration was changed from a count of houses and persons by local Overseers of the Poor, to self-enumeration by household directed by the registration service.

By 1901 a standard legislative and administrative pattern had evolved. Authorization was by an Act of Parliament about a year before each census. The Registrars-General of England and Wales, Scotland, and Ireland were responsible for its conduct, with registrars organizing local arrangements. The head of each household was responsible for making the full return for the house, with the information being designated confidential and with prescribed penalties for disclosure. Subsequently, population figures were published for local government areas down to civil parishes.

The Census Act 1920 now governs the taking of censuses in Great Britain (England, Wales, and Scotland). Additionally, an Order in Council has to be laid before both Houses of Parliament and approved prior to submission to the Sovereign for each census. Apart from questions named in the 1920 Act, any others must have the purpose of ascertaining the 'social or civil conditions of the population'. In determining the frequency of censuses, the need for timely information about changes in the size, distribution, and structure of the population has to be balanced against the resources available, taking into account public attitudes to compliance. This has resulted in a decennial pattern, although an additional 'mid-term' census was carried out on a 10 per cent sample of dwellings in 1966. General descriptions of the development of censuses in England and Wales can be found in Redfern (1981) and Mills (1987). Plans for the 1991 census were published as a White Paper in 1988 (CM430) (Great Britain 1988*a*), and the census itself was carried out on 21 April 1991. A comprehensive overview and a full account of its administration and content are described by Dale (1993).

The situation in Northern Ireland is rather different. Until 1911 censuses in Ireland were organized from Dublin, but the Census Act (Northern Ireland) 1925 transferred responsibility to the Registrar-General for Northern Ireland. In consequence, the first census under the Act was carried out in 1926 and subsequently in 1937. From 1951 censuses were contemporaneous with those for Great Britain but, until more permanent legislation in the form of the Census (Northern Ireland) Act 1969, separate Acts preceded each census. The 1969 Act is still in force; however, it must be accompanied by an Order in Council for each subsequent census. The history of the census in Northern Ireland since 1926 has been fully described by Compton (1993).

Method and content

A similar procedure is used in both Great Britain and Northern Ireland. The census is usually carried out on a Sunday in April, and the vast majority of the population is counted in their (or someone else's) home. Each householder is required to complete a census schedule delivered by an enumerator before census day and subsequently collected.

Thus the household is the unit to which the census form normally relates, being defined since 1981 as one or more persons living at the same address with common housekeeping (with the implication that a dwelling may contain one or more households). Individuals may choose to make personal returns rather than have their data included on the household schedule. There are also arrangements for enumerating people present in communal establishments such as hospitals or prisons.

In Great Britain the range of topics on which information is collected was extended from the beginning of the century (Table 3.1). The number of topics reached a peak in 1971, decreased in 1981, and increased again in 1991. From the point of providing a denominator calculating rates, the main demographic items collected about individuals are as follows: sex, age, and marital status, including household composition; the educational level of all those who have left school; the occupation of those who are presently employed, temporarily out of work, or retired; migration within the United Kingdom; birth outside the United Kingdom, and other minor aspects such as travel to work. The household schedule also seeks information about accommodation and amenities.

Two new topics were included in the 1991 census: questions about ethnic group (Teague 1993) and limiting long-term illness. The results with respect to the latter are of particular interest to those planning health services, and are published in a separate census volume (OPCS and GRO(S) 1993) and summarized by Charlton *et al.* (1994).

The enumerator can help the householder to complete the schedule, if required, but in any case should identify the majority of missing answers and obtain the information. Some editing at punching occurs by checking that the values lie in an acceptable range. Further correcting of completion errors occurs with an auto-edit system, which replaces missing or unacceptable values of the simpler items by acceptable values using the last processed complete record with similar demographic or other characteristics. 'Hard-to-code' items, for example occupation and higher education, are clerically corrected where necessary.

Sampling was first used in the United Kingdom in 1951 when advanced tables of results were based on 1 per cent of households. In 1961, to reduce coding and processing costs, only 10 per cent of households were asked to complete a full-length questionnaire, involving 11 additional questions covering topics such as occupation. The mid-decade census of 1966 involved a different approach, with lists of all 1961 dwellings and valuation records of new buildings erected in the interim used to draw a 10 per cent sample. Since 1971 coding and processing of hard-to-code items has been predominantly on a 10 per cent sample of census schedules, all of which were fully completed.

The Welsh Office conducted a sample Intercensal Survey of Wales in 1986. Whilst some of its characteristics are those of the General Household Survey (see section on household surveys), in that it was conducted by interview, its content and aims were very similar to those of the national census. A 5 per cent sample of address was included, and a response rate of nearly 85 per cent was achieved. Tabulations covering population, housing amenities, and

Table 3.1 Various items collected in the population censuses in Great Britain, 1801–1991

Item	1801	1811	1821	1831	1841	1851	1861	1871	1881	1891	1901	1911	1921	1931	1951	1961	1971	1981	1991
Name	—	—	—	—	GB	GB	GB	GB	GB	GB	GB	GB	GB	GB	GB	GB	GB	GB	GB
Age	GB	GB	GB	GB	GB	GB	GB	GB	GB	GB	GB	GB	GB	GB	GB	GB	GB	GB	GB
Date of birth	—	—	—	—	—	—	—	—	—	—	—	—	—	—	—	—	GB	GB	GB
Marital status	—	—	—	—	—	GB	GB	GB	GB	GB	GB	GB	GB	GB	GB	GB	GB	GB	GB
Relationship to head of household	—	—	—	—	—	GB	GB	GB	GB	GB	GB	GB	GB	GB	GB	GB	GB	GB	GB
Usual address	—	—	—	—	—	—	—	—	—	—	—	—	—	GB	GB	GB	GB	GB	GB
Migration 1 year ago	—	—	—	—	—	—	—	—	—	—	—	—	—	—	—	GB	GB	GB	GB
Country of birth/birthplace	—	—	—	—	GB	GB	GB	GB	GB	GB	GB	GB	GB	GB	GB	GB	GB	GB	GB
Nationality	—	—	—	—	GB_a	GB_b	GB_b	GB_b	GB_b	GB_b	GB	GB	GB	GB	GB	GB	—	—	—
Ethnic group	—	—	—	—	—	—	—	—	—	—	—	—	—	—	—	—	—	—	GB
Education/scholar/student	—	—	—	—	—	GB	GB	GB	GB	S	S	GB_c	GB_c	—	GB_c	—	—	—	—
Employed/unemployed/retired	—	—	—	—	—	GB	GB	GB	GB	GB	GB	GB	GB	GB	GB	GB	GB	GB	GB
Employment status	—	—	—	—	—	GB_d	GB_d	GB_d	GB_d	GB	GB	GB	GB	GB	GB	GB	GB	GB	GB
Occupation	GB_e	—	—	GB	GB	GB	GB	GB	GB	GB	GB	GB	GB	GB	GB	GB	GB	GB	GB
Marriage and fertility	—	—	—	—	—	—	—	—	—	—	—	GB	—	—	GB	GB	GB	—	—
Infirmity deaf/dumb/blind etc	—	—	—	—	—	GB	GB	GB	GB	GB	GB	GB	—	—	—	—	—	—	—
Limiting long-term illness	—	—	—	—	—	—	—	—	—	—	—	—	—	—	—	—	—	—	GB
Number of rooms	—	—	—	—	—	—	S	S	S	GB_f	GB_f	GB	GB	GB	GB	GB	GB	GB	GB
Household amenities	—	—	—	—	—	—	—	—	—	—	—	—	—	GB	GB	GB	GB	GB	GB
Families per house	GB	GB	GB	GB	—	—	—	—	—	—	—	GB	GB	GB	GB	GB	—	—	—

GB, Great Britain; S, Scotland.
a Only for persons born in Scotland or Ireland.
b Whether British subject or not.
c Also whether full-time or part-time.
d Asked of farmers and tradesmen only.
e Limited question.
f Only required if under five rooms.

economic activity were presented in the report (Welsh Office 1987).

Validity of population censuses

In any census some individuals may be missed or others counted twice. Occasionally more serious difficulties arise. For example, the 1981 census of the Northern Ireland population had a degree of non-enumeration (estimated at 26 000–61 000) owing to problems of civil unrest (Morris and Compton 1985); however, much better coverage was achieved in the 1991 census (McMurray and Evans 1993).

On individual returns characteristics such as age or occupation can be wrongly recorded or incorrectly coded. Since 1961 it has become standard to carry out a post-census enumeration survey in England and Wales (Wiggins 1993). The two main areas checked by such surveys are the coverage and the quality of the replies entered on the schedule. The usual method is to attempt to repeat the enumeration for a sample of households shortly after census day using a skilled team of field staff. In Great Britain a most extensive programme was carried out and reported in both 1981 and 1991 (Britton and Birch 1985; Heady et al. 1994). The first Northern Ireland Census Validation Survey was carried out for the 1991 census.

Further aims of validation exercises are to allow users to appreciate the broad limits to which the data can be put (Marsh 1993a) and to give the Census Office some guidance on the topics and questions that may need attention in a future census (OPCS, Census Division 1985).

Annual population estimates
Background

The Census population provides the main source of detailed statistics suitable for use as denominators in calculating rates. Annual population estimates are then produced which take account of (i) the increment in age of the population, (ii) the occurrence of births and deaths, and (iii) estimates of migration into and out of the country or locality. These have been prepared for the country and large towns since the nineteenth century, and for local authority areas since 1911.

The method used in England and Wales for making subnational estimates is set out briefly in an occasional paper (OPCS 1991). It involves tuning the adjustment for ageing and the incorporation of births and deaths together with available data on migration. International migration is estimated from (i) the International Passenger Survey for countries outside the British Isles, (ii) the National Health Service (NHS) Central Register for movement to and from Scotland and Northern Ireland, and (iii) comparison of censuses for the Republic of Ireland and Great Britain. Similar sources of information are used to produce mid-year population estimates in Scotland and Northern Ireland. The International Passenger Survey has the difficulty of a sample; the NHS Central Register relies on initiation of action from individuals re-registering with doctors, and the census comparisons form a very approximate guide to Irish migration. None of these sources of information is adequate to provide local estimates of population movement. These have to be derived from changes in the size of the electoral roll, estimates of movements recorded at the NHS Central Register, and cohort comparison of certain education statistics.

Although of less direct relevance to the calculation of current rates, mention should also be made of the fact that the same parameters affect the projection of the future population, with the added complication of the need to make assumptions as to future trends in mortality, fertility, and migration. For a description of methods used for the projection of the United Kingdom population as a whole, see Daykin (1986) and Shaw (1994), and for local authority areas see Armitage (1986). Some of the difficulties of projecting mortality are described by Alderson and Ashwood (1985), and those relating to fertility are discussed by Werner (1983).

Validity of population estimates

The validity of the annual estimates will depend on the quality of the census enumeration (OPCS, Population Statistics 1993*a*), which is the base for the estimates; the process for rebasing the estimates as a result of the availability of 1991 census data has been fully described (OPCS, Population Statistics 1993*b*; Armitage 1994). Validity also depends on the precision with which changes in the population can be gauged. In this respect there is no cause for concern over births or deaths, but migration can be very difficult to quantify. This applies not only to movement across national boundaries but also to movement of persons from one locality to another. It is possible that statistics of internal migration have been affected recently by the computerization of the NHS Central Register (Hornsey 1993).

Publications relating to population

An abundance of census reports are published by OPCS, GRO(S), and GRO(NI). Many are relevant for use as denominators for calculating mortality rates or for preparing national or local population estimates. An innovation for the 1991 census has been the availability of a sample of anonymized records specially constructed so as not to conflict with confidentiality assurances given when collecting census information (Marsh 1993*b*). National population estimates for England and Wales, and those for local and health authorities, are published annually by OPCS (Series PP1), as are projections (Series PP2). Similar statistics are available for Scotland and Northern Ireland.

Mortality statistics

The most long-standing of health-related information is that pertaining to mortality. This has been available in England and Wales for over 150 years, and for well over a century in the rest of the United Kingdom. As it is based on a statutory process, without which there cannot be legal disposal of a body, there are few anxieties regarding its completeness, although there are some qualms as to certain aspects of its validity.

Legislative background and procedures

In England and Wales the registration of death dates from the Births and Deaths Registration Act 1836. This included provision for the recording of cause of death and came into operation on 1 July 1837. In consequence, the Registrar-General has collected and published mortality statistics since this date. Failure to register a death was initially neither subject to penalty nor was it a require-

ment that the cause should be supplied by a doctor, although a medical opinion as to this was sought wherever possible. With the enactment of the Births and Deaths Registration Act 1874, death registration was made compulsory, and a specific duty was placed on the medical practitioner who attended the deceased during the last illness to provide the cause of death unless there was an inquest.

Various subsequent modifying enactments were eventually consolidated into the Births and Deaths Registration Act 1953 and its companion legislation relating to the organization of the registration service—the Registration Service Act 1953. Current regulations are embodied in a Statutory Instrument (1987), although proposals for further changes to the registration services were made in a discussion document (CM531) issued in 1988 (Great Britain 1988*b*) and a subsequent White Paper in 1990 (CM939) (Great Britain 1990). One further important enactment affecting the provision and promulgation of mortality data is the Population Statistics Act 1938 and its revision in 1960, the history and provisions of which have been described by Whitehead (1987). These Acts follow the confidential collection at registration of certain additional items of information regarding the marital status of the deceased, which are not entered in the public record (the register) and may be used only by the Registrar-General for statistical purposes.

Registration of deaths in Scotland has occurred since the Registration of Births, Deaths and Marriages (Scotland) Act 1854. A new Act in 1965 relaxed some of the previous regulations, giving, for example, the Registrar-General for Scotland power to correct errors, which previously had been allowed only to a Sheriff. The current effective legislation in Northern Ireland is the Births and Deaths Registration (Northern Ireland) Order 1976, although births and deaths have had to be registered since 1864 following the passing of the Registration of Births and Deaths (Ireland) Act 1863. Throughout the United Kingdom, mortality data are derived from a certificate of cause of death, usually issued by a medical practitioner in combination with information given to the registrar by an informant. In England and Wales the regulation medical certificate currently required with respect to deaths after the neonatal period is similar to that presently recommended by the World Health Organization (WHO 1977). Furthermore, the format for the cause of death information—distinguishing diseases or conditions directly leading to death from other significant conditions contributing to death—differs in only minor detail from that initiated by the then General Register Office in 1927 (Swerdlow 1987). Also in line with WHO recommendations, provision is made for the supply of information as to the duration of each condition mentioned; however, unlike the basic cause information, this is not transcribed onto the public record.

After an initial pilot study (Gedalla and Alderson 1984), a new neonatal death certificate was introduced in 1986 for deaths occurring within the first 28 days of life. This also conforms with WHO recommendations and requires the certifier to distinguish between fetal and maternal contributions to the cause of death. In many cases this precludes the assignment of a single underlying cause of death normally associated with the traditional certificate of cause.

Both types of certificate include other items, again not for the public record, such as whether information from a postmortem has been taken into account or whether the death has been reported to the coroner. Neither Scotland nor Northern Ireland has introduced the alternative form of a neonatal death certificate, so that in both these countries the medical certificate of cause issued by a practitioner is similar to that issued in England and Wales at older ages. In Scotland the medical practitioner can indicate whether a postmortem has been carried out, or if one is proposed.

For deaths certified in England and Wales up to 1992, the certifier could indicate that further information regarding the cause of death was likely to be available at a later date. If such an offer was made, a standard enquiry form was then sent by the registrar at the time of registration of the death. On receipt of a reply (there was an 85 per cent response rate), the cause of death details were amended in the statistical system, where appropriate, but not in the public record. About 3 per cent of total deaths annually were affected in this way. In addition, there was a system whereby queries were sent by the OPCS to certifiers, seeking clarification when there were difficulties in coding the cause of death (accounting for a further 2.5 per cent of all deaths). Taken together, however, some causes were differentially affected in this way, particularly in the case of cancers (Swerdlow 1989). These arrangements are temporarily in abeyance in England and Wales, but not in Scotland where similar further enquiries are made by the GRO(S) if the doctor completing a death certificate indicates that further information may be available after a post-mortem has been performed (resulting in about a 65 per cent response rate). Another 6 per cent of deaths are subject to other enquiries seeking clarification of the medical diagnoses, to which there is a 90 per cent response rate.

In England and Wales the death certificate has to be delivered to the registrar of the subdistrict in which the death occurred. Registration districts and subdistricts are geographical subdivisions of local authority areas—a suitable arrangement since registrars are appointed and paid by local authorities. In Scotland registration of death is allowed in a district of choice or in the district of usual residence as a matter of convenience, although statistical analyses of death are attributed to the district of residence. The Registrar-General for Scotland also has power to instruct local registrars, but this is a more informal process than the comprehensive regulations governing local registrars in England and Wales.

In Northern Ireland deaths are registered by the registrar for the district in which the person died or in which he or she was ordinarily resident immediately before death. Since the 1973 reorganization of local government in Northern Ireland, each of the 26 districts has been administered by one registrar. This is in sharp contrast with the situation in 1864 when, as in England and Wales, registrars were assigned to areas based on the districts of the dispensary doctors of the Poor Law Unions, with approximately 120 registrars covering the area now known as Northern Ireland.

Those qualified as an informant of the death to the registrar are similarly defined throughout the United Kingdom. For example, in England and Wales he or she may be a relative of the deceased, a person present at death, the occupier of the institution in which death occurred or an inmate of the institution, or a person disposing of the body. Where death occurs in a public place, the informant may be the relative, any person present at death, any person who found the body, any person in charge of the body, or the person disposing of the body (i.e. the chain of responsibility stretches out until a responsible person is identified).

Table 3.2 Content of public record of death

Item	England and Wales	Scotland	Northern Ireland
Name of deceased	P	P	P
Maiden name if female	P	A	P
Usual address	P	P	P
Sex	P	P	P
Date of birth (and/or age)	P	P	P
Place of birth	P	A	P
Marital status	A	P	P
Details of spouse	A	P	A
Details of father	A	P	A
Details of mother	A	P	A
Occupation	P	P	P
Place of death	P	P	P
Date of death	P	P	P
Cause(s) of death	P	P	P
Details of informant	P	P	P
Details of certifier	P	P	A
Details of registrar	P	P	P
Date of registration	P	P	P

P, present; A, absent.

The informant is expected to provide information about the deceased for the public record and, if required, also confidentially for statistical purposes. The public record has a slightly different content in each of the different countries of the United Kingdom (Table 3.2).

Some categories of death must be notified to the appropriate legal authority who has the power to enquire into them. Thus, in England and Wales a registrar will report a death in one of the following categories to the coroner: (i) the deceased person was not attended by a medical practitioner during his or her last illness; (ii) the registrar has been unable to obtain a certificate of cause of death; (iii) the particulars of the certificate of cause of death indicate that the deceased was seen neither after death nor within 14 days before death by the certifying practitioner; (iv) the cause of death is unknown; (v) the registrar has reason to believe that death was due to an unnatural cause or violence, neglect, abortion, or from suspicious circumstances; (vi) death appears to have occurred from an operation or before recovery from an anaesthetic; (vii) from the contents of the certificate, it appears that death was due to industrial disease or poisoning. Doctors do not have a specific statutory duty to report deaths to coroners, although it is common practice for them to do so. However, a recent study (Start et al. 1993) highlighted several features of the coronial system that are poorly understood by clinicians.

The history of the development of the office of coroner is set out in the Brodrick Report (Brodrick 1971), and the coroner's particular role with regard to suicides has been described by Jennings and Barraclough (1980). The coroner may provide a notification of the cause of death without an inquest, having had a postmortem carried out in some circumstances. This will depend on the results of preliminary enquiries and decision as to whether death is free from natural causes.

In circumstances similar to those in England and Wales, the local registrar in Scotland must report certain deaths to the Procurator-Fiscal whose duty it is to enquire into cases that might be criminal and, also in the public interest, to eradicate dangers to health and life, to allay public anxiety, and to ensure that full and accurate statistics are compiled. The Procurator-Fiscal does not always decide to order an autopsy. If he or she is satisfied that death is due to natural causes and that there is no element of criminal negligence, the general practitioner or hospital doctor can be invited to complete a death certificate or, if they are unwilling to do so, the police surgeon can be asked to view the body and issue the certificate or advise whether an autopsy should be carried out.

In Northern Ireland the provisions of the Coroners' Act (Northern Ireland) 1959 are somewhat different. The coroner must be notified if a person has died either directly or indirectly (i) as a result of violence or misadventure, or by unfair means, (ii) as a result of an industrial disease of the lungs.

The proportion of deaths certified by coroners in England and Wales (24 per cent in 1987) is somewhat higher than for their counterparts elsewhere in the United Kingdom. In Scotland (in 1985) notifications to the Procurator-Fiscal comprised 19 per cent of deaths, whilst in Northern Ireland (in 1986) coroners considered 16 per cent of all deaths.

Despite a suggestion to a House of Commons Select Committee in 1893 (House of Commons 1893), stillbirths were first registrable in England and Wales in 1927 as a result of provisions in the Births and Deaths Registration Act 1926. Different documentation is used whereby a certifier, who may be the medical attendant or the midwife, completes a certificate where a child has been 'completely expelled or extracted from its mother after the twenty-fourth week of pregnancy and which did not at any time after such expulsion or extraction breathe or show any other evidence of life'. Throughout the United Kingdom the legal definition of a stillbirth was changed on 1 October 1992 from a baby born dead after 28 completed weeks gestation or more, to one born dead after 24 weeks gestation or more (Stillbirth (Definition) Act 1992). At present, statistics based on either definition are available.

Apart from the change in the legal definition, the current regulations date from 1968 and are as for deaths. However, the format of the certificate was revised in 1986 to be in line with the requirements for cause of death information for neonatal deaths. In addition to the cause particulars, the certifier is also asked to provide (not for the public record) the weight of the fetus and the estimated duration of pregnancy. It should also be indicated whether information has or will be obtained from postmortem.

In Scotland stillbirths have been registered since the beginning of 1939 under the provision of the Registration of Stillbirths (Scotland) Act 1938, which was superseded in 1965 by the Registration of Births, Deaths, and Marriages (Scotland) Act 1965. Registration of stillbirths in Northern Ireland began in 1961, following the passage of the Registration of Stillbirths Act (Northern Ireland) 1960, and is currently administered under the Births and Deaths Registration (Northern Ireland) Order 1976.

In both these countries the qualifications of certifiers and the requirements for certification are similar to those for England and Wales, but the cause of death information is not collected in the new format. However, in Scotland an annual national perinatal death enquiry (1983–1984) and stillbirth neonatal death enquiry (1985 to date) have been carried out by the Information and Statistics Division. These enquiries also led to the decision that there was no need to adopt the WHO recommended perinatal death certificate in Scotland, either for stillbirths or for neonatal deaths.

Validity of mortality statistics

Any routine data collection system is liable to incur inaccuracies. Alderson et al. (1983) identified many of the practical issues involved in death certification in response to a report on the medical aspects of certification by a joint working party of the Royal College of Physicians and the Royal College of Pathologists (1982).

Inaccuracies may occur at any of the several separate steps in the chain of events leading to the production of mortality statistics. These range from the allocation of a clinical diagnosis and the completion of a death certificate by a clinician, through the transcription of this information on to the death notification together with its classification and coding, to the processing, analysis, and interpretation of the statistics produced. Each of these processes may contribute factors that make mortality statistics difficult to interpret (Ashley and Devis 1992). For example, they contributed to the finding of Martyn and Pippard (1988) that death certificate data are not useful in exploring geographical variations in the frequency of dementia in England and Wales.

It is usual to examine the accuracy of the diagnostic information at the time of death by comparison of data derived from autopsy, as in a major study sponsored by the then General Register Office (Heasman and Lipworth 1966). However, one cannot assume the infallibility of the autopsy diagnosis or that differences found for hospital deaths can be extrapolated to the certification of persons dying at home. There is also evidence from Scotland that there may be some social class bias in the accuracy of diagnosis of the cause of death (Samphier et al. 1988). In a review of the literature on this topic, Alderson (1981) pointed out that some studies indicate a worrying degree of variation between autopsy and clinical diagnoses. Studies by Busuttil et al. (1981) and by Cameron and McGoogan (1981) in Scotland have used this approach.

The usual method of investigating variation in certification practice is to circulate 'dummy' case histories to clinicians and require them to complete 'mock' death certificates. Reid and Rose (1964) used this technique with the collaboration of physicians from Norway, the United Kingdom, and the United States. Similarly, in two related studies (Diehl and Gau 1982; Gau and Diehl 1982) a total of 25 fictitious case histories were circulated to samples of general practitioners and junior hospital doctors in England and Wales for 'certification'. The number of different causes of death assigned varied widely, as did the proportion designated 'refer to coroner', but there was no marked regional variation in certification habits. McGoogan and Cameron (1978) obtained information from clinicians via questionnaires on their attitudes to the value of an autopsy in different diagnoses. A variant of this method was used by Maudsley and Williams (1993) in a comparative study of house officers and general practitioners, which highlighted the variable knowledge of doctors regarding completion of the death certificate.

Others have compared death certificates with a review of

detailed case histories (Moriyama et al. 1958; Alderson 1965; Alderson and Meade 1967; Puffer and Griffith 1967; Pole et al. 1977; Clarke and Whitfield 1978). Edouard (1982) compared the clinical case notes with the certified cause of death for 200 stillbirths from 1973 to 1977. Using 14 categories of cause of death, there was concordance for 69 per cent of the stillbirths; the discrepancies were most frequently omission of particulars known at the time of death.

Linkage between two independent sources may be of help in the identification of validity issues in either or both systems. Goldacre (1993) linked death certificates and hospital records for people who died within four weeks and, for some diseases, one year of admission. He demonstrated a wide range of differences between the causes reported on the two separate systems. Cole (1989) compared the causes recorded on certificates of neonatal deaths with those assigned in the Scottish neonatal survey and found general agreement in the functional, if not the precise, cause of death. A more extensive validation study of deaths due to ischaemic heart disease was carried out in Belfast by McIlwaine et al. (1985). Relevant death certificates over a one-year period were verified not only from hospital sources and post-mortems, but also from the coroner's office, general practitioners, and ambulance service records. It was found that the number of deaths recorded as being due to this cause was numerically accurate but that most of the inaccurate certification occurred in hospital. Thus it was suggested that accuracy might improve if consultants issued deaths certificates in hospital or countersigned those completed by junior doctors. McCormick (1988) used a confidential reporting system to the Communicable Disease Surveillance Centre to assess the validity of mortality statistics for acquired immune deficiency syndrome (AIDS). He found that AIDS and human immunodeficiency virus (HIV) infection were considerably understated as a cause of death, which may be due to a variety of reasons, particularly sensitivity to having this disease or coming in contact with it.

The influence of coding was studied by Wingrave et al. (1981) using death data from the Royal College of General Practitioners study of oral contraception. The authors compared the coding by the Royal College with that of the OPCS and GRO(S) of 205 death certificates using the B list of 50 aggregated categories (WHO 1967). There was considerable agreement for non-violent deaths; however, some discrepancies occurred from using different sources of information. They also found that ten codes not in accordance with International Classification of Disease (ICD) rules were used; however, there have been observations that there are some shortcomings in these rules, and suggestions have been made for their improvement (Lindahl et al. 1990).

Because of the importance of coding and classification, the WHO Regional Office for Europe (1966) investigated coding consistency by circulating standard certificates amongst coders in different European vital statistics offices. It was suggested that there was considerable disagreement in the selection and coding of the underlying cause of death, both between coders in different countries and between these countries' coder and the appropriate WHO Centre for Classification. There was relatively less variation between coders working within the same office in each of the participating countries. It is to be expected that consistency will be greatly enhanced by the gradual international extension of auto-matic systems for coding causes of death statements and for selecting the underlying cause. Such a system is now in operation in England and Wales (Birch 1993).

Nearly all published national statistics are based on tabulations of single causes for individual deaths—the underlying cause of death—although from time to time in England and Wales multiple-cause coding of all diseases mentioned has been carried out (e.g. in 1985 and 1986). It has been pointed out a number of times that converting the information on the death certificate to a single cause of death may fail to identify the combination of different diseases that are or are not related but are thought by the certifier to contribute to death (Farr 1854; Moriyama 1952; Guralnick 1966; Markush 1968; Cohen and Steinitz 1969; Abramson et al. 1971).

It is generally accepted that, because of these problems, mortality statistics must be interpreted with caution. Obviously there are some conditions where the medical knowledge and facilities for diagnosis have altered markedly over time or vary from place to place. This will have a major impact on the interpretation of the data, as will major alterations in the ICD with the splitting or amalgamation of various cause groups.

Publications relating to mortality

From 1840 until 1974 the Registrar General published annual statistics for England and Wales. In recent times this consisted of three parts: Part I—medical tables. Part II—population tables, and Part III—a commentary volume. A range of detailed tables was provided which gave particulars of deaths and death-rates by cause, sex, age, locality, and a number of other variables. This series was replaced in 1974 by separate volumes incorporating subsets of the information. This mortality (DH) series now comes out in five parts: DH1—general, DH2—cause, DH3—childhood and maternity, DH4—accidents and violence, and DH5—area.

The main tables in the cause (DH2) volume present, at ICD three- and four-digit level, the numbers of deaths by age and sex; more limited analysis providing rates appear in the general (DH1) volume. The majority of published statistics by cause of death are based on underlying cause coding, although for years in which multiple coding of causes is carried out, it is usual to include a table of the number of mentions of each cause on the certificates in the DH2 volume.

Summary mortality statistics for England and Wales are made available by the OPCS in its quarterly journal *Population Trends*, which also includes articles on specific topics. In Scotland and Northern Ireland traditional series of annual reports on mortality are produced and published by the appropriate Registrar-General.

Geographical mortality

Place of usual residence is one of the items recorded at death registration, and regular analyses of mortality by area appear in publications of mortality statistics. Also included are basic rates using the appropriate estimates of the local populations as denominators. In addition, local mortality statistics are routinely made available to health and local authorities.

Around the period of each decennial census it is possible to examine the geographical pattern more closely than the annual data usually allow (Britton 1990). The census provides more detailed and more accurate figures of the size and distribution of the population at risk, and aggregation of deaths for several surrounding years can more often yield sufficient numbers of deaths to permit analysis of individual causes of death in relation to small local areas. Internal migration of ill (or healthy) people may affect the interpretation of such statistics, but Fox and Goldblatt (1982) suggested that differential migration of those with varying health is not a major source of bias in these area analyses.

Place of usual residence is not the only geographical variable associated with records of death. Both the location of death and the place of birth are potentially available for study, although they are not routinely coded. The former can be used to cast some light on the geographical distribution of treatment by residents of a particular locality, whilst the latter can contribute to studies of 'migrants'. However, it should be remembered that when a patient or resident dies in a long-stay institution (six months or longer), his or her usual area of residence is deemed to be that in which the institution is located even if he or she was originally admitted from elsewhere.

Decennial area mortality analyses have been produced for England and Wales since 1851. In recent times the publication of tabulations has been separated from the subsequent publication of a commentary. Area is also one of the variables used in tables for the decennial supplement on occupational mortality (see next section). No decennial area mortality analyses have been published for Scotland or Northern Ireland.

Occupational mortality

The first publication in the Registrar-General's decennial supplement on occupational mortality for England and Wales (1855) incorporated information from the 1851 census and the mortality returns for that year. In introducing the analyses, the Registrar-General suggested that 'the professions and occupations of men open a new held of enquiry, on which we are now prepared to enter, not unconscious, however, of peculiar difficulties that beset all enquiries in the mortality of limited, fluctuating and sometimes ill-defined sections of the population.' At approximately ten-year intervals since that time, tables have been produced showing the various mortality rates by occupation (the only gap in the series is due to the Second World War, as no census was carried out in 1941). Comparable reports in the Scottish series have appeared intermittently since 1895.

For many years it has been recognized that there are a number of difficulties in the circulation and presentation of occupational mortality rates, and each of the supplements on occupational mortality provides a careful discussion about the problems of collecting and interpreting this material.

The data for numerator and denominator in the rates are derived from two sources. The denominator is obtained from the record of current occupation inserted on the census schedule; the information from this is used to derive counts of males and females by age and occupation. The numerator is a count by occupation and cause of death for persons dying around the time of census. In 1951, for instance, the period on which the rates were based was extended to deaths occurring in a five-year period around the time of the census. Using these two sources, which are not necessarily statistically comparable, creates problems; the occupation recorded at census and the occupation recorded at death registration are provided under very different circumstances and are collected in rather different ways. For example, in describing a survey of the accuracy of occupational descriptions on records used for the calculation of indices of mortality and morbidity in the mining industry, Heasman et al. (1958) commented on errors in the descriptions of occupations used in the numerator and denominator of the rates, including errors introduced by the coding system.

A more generally based study, discussed in the General Report of the 1961 Census, concerned the matching of the information recorded at the death registration with the census schedule for a sample of deaths occurring shortly after the census. Of 2196 males, 63 per cent were assigned to the same occupation unit at death registration and at census, 10 per cent were assigned to different units within the same occupational order, and 27 per cent were assigned to different orders.

To overcome some of these problems, emphasis has also been given to the routine use of proportional mortality. Such analyses of the proportion of different causes of death within an occupational data set do not involve the potential biases introduced by using two different sources. Furthermore, the 1 per cent Longitudinal Study is proving to be a reliable source of secular occupational mortality material (see section on linked mortality records).

Another difficulty in the interpretation of the data concerns the situation where an individual has developed a fatal chronic disease (whether or not occupationally induced) and has had to change his or her occupation because of impaired ability. In such an instance, mortality will be shown against the final occupation. Should the change of job have been due to onset of occupationally induced disease, this will not be reflected in the mortality rate of the principal occupation; there will also be an erroneously high mortality rate for the final occupation.

A further particular problem relates to the classification of women at census. Single, widowed, or divorced women are classified by their own occupation; married women, who are recorded with their husbands, are classified by their husbands' occupations. Similarly, occupation is not systematically recorded for all married women at death registration. Thus indicators of 'way of life' rather than the environment of those married women who go out to work are included in analyses of occupational mortality.

Mention should also be made of analyses by social class, a traditional component of decennial occupational analyses since 1911. The history of this composite variable derived from occupational data has been critically reviewed by Jones and Cameron (1984), who advocated its abandonment. However, Alderson (1984) pointed to its ability to identify variation in exposure to hazard, use of health services, and risk of disease.

After the 1981 census, Scotland participated in the Great Britain occupational mortality study, and tables are also available showing Scottish results on their own. The Registrar-General for Northern Ireland arranged for an analysis of occupational mortality for the years 1960–1962, using the 1961 census as the denominator, but no official report was published. Age-standardized mortality ratios were calculated for males aged 15–64 years for 27 occupation orders and social classes for all causes as well as for four broad causes of death. Crude mortality rates were also shown for men and married women for 27 occupation orders. Park (1966) published these limited results, but emphasized that detailed tabulations were available upon request.

Linked mortality records

It has been recognized for many years that some of the limitations of analysis of event data can be overcome by linking records of events occurring to individuals. This was foreshadowed by some of the writings of Farr, particularly in relation to estimation of the outcome of care in different hospitals (Farr 1864) and in recommendations for health statistics to be compiled for the army (Farr 1861). Heady and Heasman (1959) examined the social and biological factors affecting stillbirth and infant mortality by linking data from the birth registrations for 1949 and 1950 to appropriate infant death details. A similar approach was used by Spicer and Lipworth (1966), who investigated regional and social factors influencing infant mortality for infant deaths during the period of 1 April 1964 to 31 March 1965 matched to appropriate birth registrations.

In England and Wales the national routine linkage of infant deaths to births commenced in 1975. This linkage, which uses the NHS number, sex, and date of birth as matching factor, extends the range of items by making available those recorded at birth and those recorded at death. Now, only a very small proportion of infant deaths cannot be matched with birth details. The cause of death can be tabulated against social class, place of residence, country of birth, mother's age and parity (for legitimate children), legitimacy, whether singleton or multiple birth, birth-weight, and certification. Annual statistical reports are now being made available from this infant linked file. In Scotland, birth and infant death registrations are linked within the GRO(S) but are not used for statistical analysis. However, since 1980 routine record linkage also occurs between infant deaths and hospital maternity records, covering 97 per cent of births in Scotland. These are used for statistical and epidemiological purposes only.

A major new venture began in England and Wales with the selection of a 1 per cent sample of respondents from the 1971 national census. Arrangements were made to assemble event data for the sample, including cancer registration, stay in a psychiatric hospital of more than two years duration, emigration, or death, into a cohort file. The sample was enhanced by 1 per cent of identified immigrants as well as 1 per cent of all births. The data set was later enhanced by the addition of data from the 1981 census. The outlines of the system, now known as the Longitudinal Study, were first described in 1973 (OPCS 1973a). A major category of analysis that the system permits is tabulation of mortality in relation to the variables recorded at the census. A comprehensive report (Fox and Goldblatt 1982) presented a wide range of results from mortality of the cohort over the period 1971–1975. Comparisons of mortality for subgroups of the population were presented, with each being derived from broad questions; this permitted examination of mortality in relation to economic activity (economic position the week before the census, alternative methods of classifying women, and transport to work), household structure (with emphasis on the elderly and those in non-private households), housing characteristics (tenure, density, amenities, etc.), marriage and fertility, education, area of residence, internal migration, and immigrants. Particular investigations were made of the influence of various forms of health-related selection of, for example, occupation, housing, and migration, of the influence of those who are 'permanently sick' upon subsequent mortality patterns, and of alternative ways of classifying individuals by non-occupationally derived socio-economic status.

Morbidity statistics

From the bedrock of mortality statistics, the then General Register Office extended its role in 1895 to become the national repository of a range of related morbidity information, which has, in general, been paralleled by similar arrangements in Scotland and Northern Ireland. Certain criteria have to be met for data collection systems to be included in this section. Each record has to relate to a single individual or client (with the obvious exception of maternity records) and should explicitly or implicitly include diagnosis (or other medical cause) as a parameter (Ashley and McLachlan 1985). There is no requirement that all national events of a particular character have to be covered, and various sample or selective schemes are included. Finally, the schemes are not easily classified and are considered roughly in chronological order of implementation.

Notification of infectious diseases

Compulsory notification of infectious disease was first introduced in England and Wales in Huddersfield in 1876; many other towns soon obtained local powers. The Infectious Diseases Notification Act 1889 provided a list of diseases that were to be notified and laid down how, when, and by whom they were to be notified. The original object of the Act was to provide powers to combat 'dangerous infectious disorders'. It was to apply immediately to London and to be extended to other areas thereafter. In 1895 the Registrar-General first included in his *Weekly Return* the numbers of cases of five infectious diseases that had been admitted to certain London hospitals.

Before 1922 the Ministry of Health compiled an unpublished document based on a weekly summary of returns from sanitary authorities. The Registrar-General's *Weekly Return* continued to include information about infectious diseases notified by the Metropolitan Asylum Board and the London Fever Hospital. In about 1920 proposals were made for publication, by the then General Register Office, of the material handled by the Ministry of Health, the first issue of which appeared in January 1922. Based on provisional weekly returns supplied by each Medical Officer of Health, these statistics were subject to amendment and did not show numbers of patients with infectious diseases by sex or age. However, beginning in 1944, Medical Officers of Health were asked to submit quarterly returns containing corrected figures grouped by sex and age (Registrar-General 1949), although this was not a statutory requirement.

Scotland's legislation is somewhat different, being based on the Infectious Disease (Notification) Act 1889 and the Public Health (Infectious Diseases) (Scotland) Act 1897; the latter Act made notification compulsory two years before similar legislation was introduced in England and Wales. Notification of infectious disease in Northern Ireland also dates from the Infectious Disease Notification Act 1889; the current legislation is the Public Health Act (Northern Ireland) 1967.

The list of notifiable diseases has enlarged with time, with some differences among the countries of the United Kingdom (Table 3.3). New or amended regulations were introduced through-

Table 3.3 Infectious diseases currently statutorily notifiable, with the date when first notifiable nationally

Disease	England and Wales	Scotland	Northern Ireland
Acute encephalitis	1915	Never notifiable	1949 a
Acute poliomyelitis	1912	1932	1913
Anthrax	1960	1960	1949
Chickenpox	Never notifiable	1988	1990
Cholera	1889	1889	1889
Continued fever	PN	1889	PN
Diphtheria	1889	1889	1889
Dysentry	1919	1919 b	1919
Erysipelas	PN	1889	PN
Food poisoning	1938	1956	1949
Gastroenteritis	Never notifiable	Never notifiable	1949 c
Legionellosis	Never notifiable	1988	1990 d
Leprosy	1951	PN	PN
Leptospirosis	1961	1975	1990 e
Malaria	1919	1919	1990 e
Measles	1915	1919	1949
Membranous croup	PN	1889	PN
Meningitis*	1912 f	1932 g	1949 a
Mumps	1988	1988	1988
Ophthalmia neonatorum	1914	PN	PN
Paratyphoid fever	1938 h	1889 i	1949 h
Plague	1900	1932	1949
Puerperal fever	PN	1889	PN
Rabies	1956	1976	1976
Relapsing fever	1889	1889	1889
Rubella	1988	1988	1988
Scarlet fever	1889	1889	1889
Smallpox	1889	1889	1889
Tetanus	1968	1988	1990
Tuberculosis	1911	1919	1909 j
Typhoid fever	1938	1889	1889
Typhus	1901	1889	1889
Viral haemorrhagic fever†	1976 k	1977 k	1976 l
Viral hepatitis	1968 m	1965 m	1949 n
Whooping cough	1939	1949	1949
Yellow fever	1968	1975 p	1949

PN, Previously, but not currently, notifiable.

* Variously named as cerebrospinal fever, meningococcal infection, acute meningitis, or meningococcal septicaemia.

† Viral haemorrhagic fevers include Argentine haemorrhagic fever (Junin), Bolivian haemorrhagic fever (Machupo), Chikungunya haemorrhagic fever, Congo/Crimean haemorrhagic fever, Dengue fever, Ebola virus disease, haemorrhagic fever with renal syndrome (Hantaan), Kyasanur Forest disease, Lassa fever, Marburg disease, Omsk haemorrhagic fever, and Rift Valley disease.

a Until 1990. Now separately as acute encephalitis/meningitis: bacterial or viral and meningococcal septicaemia.

b From 1988 as bacillary dysentery

c Until 1990; aged under 2 years only.

d As Legionnaires' disease.

e Previously notifiable and reintroduced in 1990.

f Currently as meningitis and meningococcal septicaemia without meningitis.

g Currently as meningococcal infection.

h From 1889 as enteric fever.

i As enteric fever; now includes paratyphoid fever.

j Differentiated into pulmonary and non-pulmonary.

k Until 1988 only Lassa fever and Marburg disease.

l Since 1990 includes Lassa fever and Marburg disease.

m Until 1988 as infective jaundice.

n Until 1990. Now as hepatitis A, hepatitis B, and hepatitis viral: unspecified.

p From 1988 yellow fever is included within viral haemorrhagic fevers.

out the United Kingdom in 1988 (Statutory Instruments 1988*a*, *b*; Statutory Rules 1988). Changes included the inclusion of mumps and rubella coincident with the national introduction of an immunization programme using measles, mumps, and rubella vaccine. In 1990 some further changes and additions were made in Northern Ireland (Statutory Rules of Northern Ireland 1990).

Notification by medical practitioners in England and Wales are to the proper officers (usually consultants in communicable disease control) of the local authority in which the disease is identified or suspected. In Scotland and Northern Ireland, notification is to the Director of Public Health for the area in which the case was diagnosed and for the area of residence respectively.

In England and Wales prior to 1982, the proper officers submitted a weekly statistical return to the OPCS, giving counts of the notifications that had been received during the week. This was followed at quarterly intervals by a statistical return giving extra details of the sex and age group of the cases and incorporating any corrections to the original weekly figures. Since 1982 a new reporting system has operated, whereby the proper officers continue to send in a weekly statistical summary and now also provide information about individual notifications. Sex and exact age, rather than age group, are included, as is extra detail for tuberculosis and food poisoning. The system retains the provisions of quarterly corrections and hence the data should be comparable with those for earlier years. Although individual records are now collected centrally, neither names nor addresses are included in the details submitted by proper officers.

In Scotland primary responsibility for the national collection and processing of the notifications lies with the Information and Statistics Division. In Northern Ireland the DHSS(NI) collates and publishes the information.

Other infectious diseases, although not notifiable under statute, have generated a need for specific reporting arrangements in relation to their surveillance—in particular, the systems set up for reporting AIDS and HIV infection. The Communicable Disease Surveillance Centre collates data for England and Wales, Northern Ireland, the Channel Isles, and the Isle of Man. In Scotland the Scottish Centre for Infection and Environmental Health operates a similar scheme. Three sources are used: the voluntary registration of AIDS cases by clinicians, laboratory reports of HIV-positive results, and death certificate data. Details of registered cases include age, sex, places of residence, diagnosis, mode of infection (if known), and certain clinical details (McCormick *et al.* 1987). Regular statistics from these systems are available through the Department of Health in England and are published both by the Scottish Office Home and Health Department and by Scottish Centre for Infection and Environmental Health in a supplement of the Communicable Disease Report.

In England and Wales the Royal College of General Practitioners collects data on patients with various infectious diseases (RCGP 1968). The College's Research Unit runs a surveillance system, which consolidates data on these and other conditions on a weekly basis of returns from a number of selected 'spotter' practices with a population of about 200 000 patients. It is acknowledged that these practices are not evenly spread throughout the country (they are predominantly concentrated in or near large conurbations), and the data are based on clinical diagnosis for most of the patients.

In Scotland a similar but somewhat larger surveillance system was established in 1971, principally to collect data on influenza incidence; information from general practices in 11 health boards is supplemented by information from laboratories, schools, and workplaces, with the returns collated by the Scottish Centre for Infection and Environmental Health. In a further development, Scotland has established an evolving list of infections 'reportable' by diagnostic laboratories, these data are published in the *Communicable Disease Report*.

Validity of notifications of infectious disease

The validity of statistics from notification has periodically been questioned; it is acknowledged that reporting is frequently far from complete, especially for the more common conditions. Therefore, although notifications may not give precise estimates of the incidence of individual infectious diseases, they do provide crude indicators of change in prevalence in the community.

Stocks (1949) compared notification statistics with data from the *Survey of Sickness* and various research reports on incidence or cumulative attack rates. He suggested that completeness varied with the illness, from fairly complete notification of acute poliomyelitis to only fractional notification of dysentery. A discussion by Taylor (1965) indicated that a number of Western countries have variable completion of notification of infectious disease and that notification is poor for some milder infections; this issue has also been discussed by Benjamin (1968*b*). A study from general practice (Haward 1973) suggested that there was substantial underreporting of certain infectious diseases.

Lambert (1973) used Hospital In-Patient Enquiry data to cross-check the statistics from notification of meningococcal infection. Assuming that the hospital data provide a fairly reliable estimate of the total number of cases, he suggested that notifications identify about half the total. Clarkson and Fine (1985) also used this source to assess the efficacy of measles and pertussis reporting in England and Wales and concluded that, whereas it was 40 to 60 per cent for measles, only between 5 and 25 per cent of cases of pertussis appeared to be notified. Goldacre and Miller (1976) used a variety of sources of information to study notification of acute bacterial meningitis in children in one hospital region between 1969 and 1973, concluding that only half the cases of meningococcal and less than a quarter of other types of bacterial meningitis had been notified.

Stewart (1980) suggested that there was strong circumstantial evidence to question the validity of whooping cough notification, partly because of confusion with infection from various respiratory viruses. He also pointed out that 18 per cent of the practitioners in Glasgow notified all the whooping cough cases reported between 1977 and 1979, with over one-third of the cases being reported by 2 per cent of the practitioners (Stewart 1981). In addition, many of the patients admitted to hospital were not notified. Davies *et al.* (1981) identified a number of problems with notification of tuberculosis, including duplicate notification, changes in diagnosis and definition of respiratory disease, and posthumous registration. They concluded that the OPCS statistics had an impressive level of accuracy, which they estimated as being within 10 per cent. Possible solutions for some of the problems were discussed.

Although influenza is not a notifiable disease, there is considerable interest in identifying epidemics of the infection. Tillett and

Spencer (1982) discussed the surveillance of routine statistics of the disease in England and Wales. They indicated that the use of the term influenza in death certification changed during the course of an epidemic. There was initial undercertification until it became common knowledge that an epidemic was in progress. As the epidemic waned, there was possible overcertification by way of 'compensation'. Paradoxically, therefore, the absolute numbers of death ascribed to influenza might be correct.

It is plausible that the same type of incorrectly timed rise and fall in reported numbers may occur with other acute infectious diseases. However, it is not clear that the overall reporting approximates the correct figures in every instance. When using notification to monitor progress of an epidemic, it must also be remembered that bank holidays result in a fall in the count of weekly notifications (by as much as 15–30 per cent), which may not be completely made up in succeeding weeks. It is impossible to validate information using laboratory reports because of the very biased referral for investigation of appropriate specimens. Where the infection is only rarely fatal, there is also no chance of cross-checking the statistics with those of mortality.

Publications relating to infectious diseases

For almost exactly 100 years, a principal source of infectious disease data was the *Registrar-General's Weekly Return for England and Wales*. Latterly, this return (identified by the serial WR) gave weekly statistics of notifications and deaths from the major infectious diseases in England and Wales as well as newly diagnosed episodes of communicable and respiratory disease supplied by 'spotter' general practices. Corrected data were provided in a quarterly report, which also included data from the Communicable Disease Surveillance Centre on the laboratory identification of various diseases within England and Wales.

Publication of the weekly return ceased at the end of 1994 when a change in arrangements was announced (OPCS 1995). The Communicable Disease Surveillance Centre now bears the responsibility for releasing weekly data on infectious disease in its *Communicable Disease Report*, which also includes data obtained from hospital laboratories and the Public Health Laboratory Service. These latter data refer to specific episodes of infection with bacterial confirmation, often providing background discussion of some detail of particular cases of interest.

The OPCS annual publication, *Communicable Disease Statistics* (series MB2), provides an appreciable number of tables on notifications and deaths from infectious disease, with some data on trends for the preceding years and a commentary from the Communicable Disease Surveillance Centre. In the foreseeable future, OPCS will also continue to produce quarterly reports of corrected data in the MB2 series of monitors.

The weekly report on communicable diseases in Scotland produced by the Scottish Centre for Infection and Environmental Health contains counts of notifications of infectious diseases and food poisoning by health board area, and includes 'current notes' on particular topics of interest. Data also appear in the weekly return of the Registrar-General, Scotland. Annual figures appear in the Scottish Office Health Statistics. In Northern Ireland statistics for 1935–1976 were published in the Annual Report of the Registrar-General; subsequently, they have been published by the DHSS(NI), which also publishes laboratory data, admissions to the infectious disease unit, and notifications in the *Communicable Disease Monthly Report*.

Cancer registration

Background

During the nineteenth century, a number of authorities pointed out the drawbacks of mortality data in studying malignant disease. In response, attempts were made at the beginning of the present century to collect morbidity data (Dollinger 1907). In 1923 the then Ministry of Health in England set up a system, through the national Radium Commission, for the follow-up of patients treated with radium. Their strategy was based on the premise that statistical information about such patients was essential for planning and operating cancer care services. The introduction of the NHS in 1948 was accompanied by further reaffirmation of this view, and the move toward a national cancer registration scheme was stimulated when the General Register Office took over responsibility for cancer records in 1947. Subsequently, it was suggested that studies of epidemiology and the cause of cancer should be considered as additional objectives of cancer registration (OPCS 1970).

Despite the desire for national registration at the introduction of the NHS, it was not until 1962 that all regions in England and Wales became incorporated in the national voluntary scheme, which relies initially upon co-operation at the clinic and hospital level. The data are then organized through regional cancer registries in England and the Welsh Office in Wales, which forward the material to the OPCS. Since 1971 patients registered with cancer have also been traced and flagged on the NHS Central Register. This permits automatic identification of the fact of death and permits calculation of survival statistics. Prior to this, the regional registries had to carry out *ad hoc* follow-up at hospital level or write to general practitioners. (For a full description of the organization of the cancer registration system in England and Wales, see Swerdlow (1986) and OPCS 1990).)

Scotland's cancer registration scheme, initiated by the Radium Commission in 1938, evolved similarly. Complete registration began in 1947 when reports were obtained from cancer treatment centres, but the scheme was reorganized and computerized in 1958. All hospitals, using local data obtained from medical records and pathology and radiology departments, now register cases with the five regional cancer registries. At the registries, additional material from case listings of cancer patients from the Scottish Hospital In-patient System and cancer deaths supplied by the GRO(S) are incorporated, and all the data are checked for accuracy. The registries then forward their data to the Information and Statistics Division for the production and publication of Scottish national statistics.

Since 1959 Northern Ireland has had limited information on cancers notified. A new system, which extracts information from pathology laboratories, hospital information systems, and other sources, was established at Queen's University, Belfast in 1994 and is expected to become operational by late 1995.

Validity of cancer registration data

Consideration has to be given to three different aspects of the validity of cancer registration from which statistics of survival are computed: the completeness of registration, the accuracy of the particulars registered, and the effectiveness of follow-up. Since 1948 the number of registrations in England and Wales has gradually risen, and it is difficult to determine what proportion of this rise is due to extension of the scheme, alteration in the efficiency of registration, or variation in the incidence of malignant disease. Benjamin (1968a) suggested that it was doubtful whether more than two-thirds of all malignant cases over the country as a whole were registered. Some studies have utilized morality data to check the validity of registration for persons dying from malignant disease; Faulkner *et al.* (1967) suggested that 3.1 per cent of individuals dying from a malignant disease were not known to the registry in Bristol.

Using various sources, Alderson (1973) concluded that about 10 per cent of patients might not be registered, a result comparable with that obtained by Gillis (1971) in an examination of the data for the western region of Scotland. Leck *et al.* (1976) reported a 7 per cent deficiency in the registration of childhood cancers in Manchester. Whilst many factors can be associated with 'failure to register', West (1973) and Alderson *et al.* (1976) found that the methods for organizing the system for cancer registration can also have an impact on the overall registration rate.

Turning to the validity of the items recorded, diagnosis is relatively accurate but errors and omissions of importance occur with items such as date of registration, place of birth, histology, and occupation. It appears that the major problem is variation in the completeness of registration rather than abstraction of particulars for patients who have been identified; thus interpretation of the data is still feasible (Alderson 1974; West 1976).

As far as survival statistics are concerned, Silman and Evans (1981) commented on the considerable variation of registration in different regions and suggested that this might be associated with systemic differences in the prognosis of the registered patients. They questioned whether differences in handling notification of cancer deaths could be a factor but did not specifically indicate all the possible variations in practice. They suggested that, when analysing survival, the rates based on post-death registrations should be distinguished from those of other patients. They also advocated that the national system should record stage of treatment as a classifying variate; this had been deleted from the national scheme in 1971 as a result of the Advisory Committee's Report in the previous year (OPCS 1970). This potential error in survival statistics has been discussed further in a publication from the Cancer Research Compaign (1982).

Publications on cancer registration data

In England and Wales there are annual OPCS national published statistics from cancer registration (series MB1) for registration and survival; since 1985 these have included detailed data on microfiche. The 1989 annual volume also contained a paper on trends with some international comparisons (Coleman and Esteve 1994). Recently, the Longitudinal Study (see the section on linked mortality records) has also been used for this latter purpose (Kogevinas 1990). Cancer registration for the countries as a whole and for individual registries also appear in the main international source book of cancer registration, *Cancer incidence in five continents* (Parkin *et al.* 1992). Scotland first achieved entry in the 1963–6

edition, lost it because of incomplete registration from 1967 to 1970, but thereafter has appeared in successive editions. The Northern Ireland cancer registry will provide regular reports on cancer incidence, trends, and mortality, thereby contributing to *Cancer incidence in five continents.* Cancer statistics particularly lend themselves to cartographic presentation; a recent atlas using registration data for England and Wales (Swerdlow and dos Santos Silva 1993) makes interesting comparison with an earlier atlas derived from mortality information (Gardner *et al.* 1983).

Hospital discharge statistics
Background

A leading article in the *Lancet* (1841) pointed out that data collection on hospital in-patients had been suggested in 1732. In the nineteenth century some developments were initiated by the Statistical Society (1842, 1844, 1862, 1866); another notable advocate of collecting and utilizing such data was Florence Nightingale (1863). Limited progress was made in the United Kingdom until the period between the two World Wars, which saw a reawakening of interest for large-scale analysis of hospital statistics (Spear and Gould 1937).

With the advent of the NHS in 1948, the opportunity arose to collect more extensive statistics relating to the morbidity aspects of patient care in hospital. After initial trials, the Ministry of Health and the General Register Office jointly set up two parallel schemes, one for mental hospitals and the other for the rest of the NHS hospitals, since it had been concluded that differences in length of stay dictated a separated mechanism for collecting data relating to mentally ill or mentally handicapped patients. The need for an enhanced data set for deliveries eventually led to a partially separate scheme for maternity patients. From 1955 to 1985 the Hospital In-Patient Enquiry collected and processed an anonymous 10 per cent sample of non-psychiatric discharges for England, with Wales also included until 1981. Initially, hospitals completed forms for individual patients and sent them directly to the General Register Office, but latterly the appropriate samples were drawn from Hospital Activity Analysis tapes held by Regional Health Authorities (for original descriptions of the Hospital Activity Analysis scheme, see Benjamin (1965) and Rowe and Brewer (1972)). Private patients in NHS hospitals were excluded until 1979, and day cases were accepted from 1974 but analysed and published separately from 1975.

The data collected centrally included demographic, administrative, and clinical items. Examples of demographic data were sex, age, marital status, and area of residence. The administrative particulars included the dates when entered on the waiting list, admitted, and discharged or died (hence, waiting time and length of stay), source of admission, category of patient (NHS or private), specialty, and disposal. The brief clinical particulars were the main condition treated together with other relevant conditions and the provision to record up to four surgical operations, with the principal one designated. Since 1982 similar data have continued to be collected from Wales.

From 1949 to 1960, an individual patient return was also sent to the General Register Office for each admission to, departure from, and death in the main designated hospitals for patients with mental disorder. Following the Mental Health Act 1959, the Ministry of

Health undertook the collection of psychiatric statistics for general planning and administrative purposes on an individual patient basis, with the General Register Office enquiry continuing in a modified form. From 1964 the two schemes were combined into the Mental Health Enquiry under the responsibility of the Ministry of Health, and all psychiatric hospitals and units were then included. This enquiry was in the form of a two-part submission. The first part was returned on admission and contained the demographic information, reference to previous psychiatric admissions, whether the admission was under the terms of the Mental Health Act, and some medical details. A second submission was completed on discharge and recorded further administrative details and the final diagnosis. The provision for some of the data set to be submitted on admission permitted analyses relating to hospital 'residents' to be carried out, an essential requirement for information on long-term care.

Although initially combined with the 'general' Hospital In-Patient Enquiry, an essentially separate enquiry (again on a 10 per cent basis) covered NHS hospitals and units exclusively treating maternity patients (but not admissions for abortion or other conditions in early pregnancy that were normally included in the non-maternity enquiry). As maternity patients were not routinely included in most regional Hospital Activity Analysis schemes, the data were assimilated from three different sources: a limited national maternity Hospital Activity Analysis scheme in selected hospitals provided about 20 per cent, a further 20 per cent came from other local detailed schemes, and the remainder were submitted directly to the OPCS on forms.

The particulars available included the standard demographic, administrative, and clinical items in the non-maternity system, augmented by maternal, delivery, and infant parameters. The maternal and delivery items included the date of the last menstrual period (and hence of gestation), previous pregnancies, diagnosis of general, antenatal, delivery, or puerperal complications, onset of labour, presentation, and mode and date of delivery. Items related to the infant included sex, birth-weight, outcome, and diseases or abnormalities present. Provision was also made to record such items separately for each of multiple births. (For a more detailed description of the scheme, see Ashley (1980).)

In England the first report of the Steering Group on Health Services Information (SGHSI 1982a) recommended unification of the three separate elements and a change in the 'unit of account' from stays in hospital to consultant episodes. Many data items were reclassified and all were precisely defined. With the emphasis being placed on the needs of local management, arrangements were suggested whereby there would be timely assimilation and availability of items after the 'transaction' to which they related. It was also recommended that a data set somewhat similar to Hospital In-Patient Enquiry should be submitted centrally for all consultant episodes. In a supplement to the first and fourth reports (SGHSI 1985), an appropriate data set for maternity episodes was also defined and, again, it generally resembled maternity Hospital In-Patient Enquiry. General implementation of the provisions of the first report was in April 1987, and the maternity provisions came into force in April 1988. This Hospital Episodes Statistics data set, as it is now called, is available for ad hoc analysis and yields a publication derived from a 25 per cent sample of completed episodes which do not identify individuals or the hospitals in which

they are treated. There is also an annual census of psychiatric patients.

In Scotland, general hospital and mental illness and mental handicap episode data were first collected in 1959. Anonymous summary data on all hospital admissions were collected by the Research and Intelligence Unit of the Scottish Home and Health Department, the precursor of the Information and Statistics Division. Maternity hospital episodes were first collected in 1969, and a neonatal discharge summary was started in 1975 by a paediatrician who ran it until it came under governmental management in 1980.

A record form (SMR1) is generated for each discharge or transfer to a different specialty or consultant within a hospital. Identifying data were added in 1968, and, beginning in 1975, the post-code was used to identify area of residence. In 1978 day cases were specifically collected for the first time. Prior to that year, information on day cases had been submitted unsystematically. Although there have been periodic revisions of the data items collected, currently, in addition to personal information, the demographic, administrative, and clinical details are similar to those for England and Wales. The mental illness and mental handicap return (SMR4) is a two-part form with similar context and method of transmission to that used with Mental Health Enquiry in England. Again, the file can be used to produce statistics on episodes and on current residents in hospital. The residents file is also periodically checked by a census.

The maternity discharge record (SMR2) is an episode record, which contains personal administrative and demographic data and a maternity-oriented section that is more comprehensive than either maternity Hospital In-Patient Enquiry or the implemented recommendations of the Steering Group on Health Services Information. The section on the past obstetric history also includes the number of previous perinatal deaths and the number of previous Caesarean sections. Data on the current pregnancy include the date of booking and type of antenatal care, the number of previous admissions during pregnancy, and maternal height and blood group. There is also a section for recording details of an abortive outcome to the pregnancy. Although the record of labour is similar to that for England, the details for the baby are enhanced to include Apgar scores as well as the baby's case reference number to facilitate linkage to the neonatal discharge record. If the baby dies, the underlying cause of death is also recorded. As well as being capable of analysis on an episode basis, records that include delivery details can be segregated to give pregnancy-based statistics. (For a fuller description, see Cole (1980).)

The Scottish neonatal discharge record (SMR11) is an individual record, started at birth and continued until the infant is discharged from the neonatal service of a maternity hospital. It includes personal and administrative data (for instance birthweight) as well as the maternal case reference number to facilitate linkage to the SMR2. There are data on the condition at birth and whether resuscitation was required. Head circumference is recorded, and transfer to special care and length of stay are noted, as is the need for transfer to another neonatal unit. Other clinical observations additional to diagnostic data include the presence of jaundice and its severity, in addition to the presence or absence of significant hypotonia, convulsions, recurrent apnoea, assisted ventilation lasting longer than 30 minutes, or feeding difficulties.

Northern Ireland has a Hospital In-Patient System covering acute and maternity services. A new mental health system for both mental illness and mental handicap inpatient admissions was implemented in 1995, and a system to collect outpatient information is being developed.

Validity of hospital discharge data

Comprehensive studies of hospital discharge data (Lockwood 1971; Martini et al. 1976) have demonstrated a high level of accuracy for demographic and administrative items, although Gruer (1970) and Ashley (1972) questioned the quality of geographical data before the use of post-codes for this purpose. Thus most exercises that have checked the accuracy of hospital discharge data have concentrated on the diagnostic information. Alderson and Meade (1967) compared hospital discharge data with mortality statistics for patients who had died in hospital, and suggested that there were appreciable errors in the principal conditions treated for about 13 per cent of completed forms. Dunnigan et al. (1970) examined 1093 Scottish hospital records where the discharge diagnosis had been coded to 'heart disease specified as involving coronary arteries' and judged 92 per cent to be appropriately assigned. Other studies on the accuracy of such data have produced a range of opinions. McNeilly and Moore (1975) observed appreciable errors in codes for a small sample of Welsh patients. Patel et al. (1976) suggested that there was a considerable proportion of errors in Scottish morbidity data in Glasgow, but Parkin et al. (1976) seriously questioned some of their conclusions. Martini et al. (1976) quantified the errors for patients treated in the Nottingham area and pointed out that the statistics were almost as good as the clinical notes from which they were derived. Cameron et al. (1977) contrasted autopsy findings with data from the medical records and indicated that fresh findings might arise at autopsy that were not incorporated in the Scottish statistical system.

Turning to other parameters, a series of small studies (Crawshaw and Moss 1982; Hole 1982; Rees 1982; Whates et al. 1982) quoted appreciable error rates for specific operative data in Hospital Activity Analysis, but Butts and Williams (1982) questioned some of the rather general conclusions reached. Forster and Mahadevan (1981) compared the data on the Mental Health Enquiry forms of 824 mental health patients in the north of England with those in their records; there were serious discrepancies for source of referral (20.5 per cent), outcome (10.8 per cent), and previous psychiatric care (6.3 per cent). In checking the validity of Scottish maternity data, Cole (1980) identified some clerical misconceptions from internal inconsistency in the computer-held data. In a comparison between the statistical return and research data abstracted from 1000 records, there was close agreement (97–98 per cent) on factual items such as past obstetric history, but about 70 per cent of discrepancies on items such as 'certainty of gestation'.

Perhaps as a result of the equivocal nature of the evidence about the accuracy of hospital morbidity data, much more emphasis is now placed on the audit of data quality as envisaged by the Steering Group on Health Services Information (SGHSI 1982b). In consequence, the volumes of published statistics often draw attention to the quality of the information that is included. In England the recent publications of Hospital Episodes Statistics (e.g. Department of Health 1994) identify deficiencies of completeness and

make estimates to correct for these. Nevertheless, however competent such estimates are, they can never totally compensate for lack of completeness in the data.

Linkage of repeat events

Reference has already been made to the value of record linkage event data and the general concept applies equally to linkage of morbidity records. Acheson (1967) has described the history of medical record linkage and the pioneering efforts in assembling a cumulative record of hospital admissions in the Oxford Region, with the ability to link to mortality information derived from death certificates (Goldacre 1993). He described the system used as well as the medical care and other epidemiological studies that could be facilitated by such work. The only element of linkage involving morbidity records that occurs nationally in England and Wales is the tracing of individuals with cancer registered in the NHS Central Register so as to identify deaths that occur and permit calculation of survival rates (see background notes in the section on cancer registration).

The medical record linkage facility developed in Scotland has been described by Heasman and Clarke (1979) and Kendrick and Clarke (1993). The objectives are (i) to provide economical collection of events occurring to an individual to permit statistical analysis, (ii) to enable individuals to be followed up, and (iii) to produce person-based statistics. The Scottish system includes (i) general hospital discharge records from 1968, (ii) obstetric discharge records from 1970, (iii) mental and mental deficiency hospital admissions and discharges from 1963, (iv) cancer registrations from 1968, (v) school entrant and leaver medical examinations from 1967, (vi) handicapped children's register from 1973, and (vii) death and stillbirth registrations from 1968. An important point is that the system contains linkable records but only assembles a linked file for a particular (restricted) purpose, such as for epidemiological and health services research, and for follow-up of specific groups of individuals. Although the intention is to facilitate production of person-based statistics, these have yet to be published as a routine; however, it is thought that the system would enable examination, for example, of length of stay for either consecutive spells in different hospitals or multiple admissions into the same hospital. The authors stressed the importance of considering the issues of privacy and steps taken to ensure confidentiality of the data.

Publication of hospital discharge data

The division between 'acute', maternity, and psychiatric events was reflected in the publication policy for England and Wales. Latterly, the data relating to the first two of these types of events were published as Hospital In-Patient Enquiry jointly by the DHSS and OPCS (and by the Welsh Office until 1981) in annual OPCS volumes in the MB4 series. Psychiatric events were published by the DHSS as the Mental Health Enquiry within its Statistics and Research Report Series. Hospital Episode Statistics, which replaced Hospital In-Patient Enquiry and the Mental Health Enquiry from 1987, are published by the Department of Health annually on a financial year (April to March) basis. The general content of the tabular material presented is very similar to that issued previously as Hospital In-Patient Enquiry, with tables by diagnoses, operations, and demographic, geographic, and administrative parameters. A separate volume is dedicated to waiting times by diagnoses, operations, and specialties.

Corresponding publications for Scotland are produced by the Information and Statistics Division, and data for Wales since 1982 can be obtained from the Welsh Office. Information on the use of acute and maternity services in Northern Ireland is available on request from DHSS(NI), as are standard reports from the mental health inpatient system. Annual mental health publications will be produced when the new system is implemented.

Morbidity statistics from general practice

Background

A pilot study was launched in 1951 to test methods for collecting and analysing medical records kept by a small number of general practitioners. From this work, Logan (1953) concluded that it was possible, without exceptional difficulty, to keep records over a 12-month period that were suitable for analysis. Various alternative methods of recording were advocated; however, when this study was extended to 1954, a specially modified NHS continuation card was used.

The Royal College of General Practitioners, in conjunction with the General Register Office, initiated what was to become the first National Morbidity Study (1955–1956), involving 171 doctors and 106 practices in England and Wales. A standard method of recording limited particulars was used for each patient contact, including identification particulars of the individual, date of birth, diagnosis, date of consultation, and date of admission to hospital if this occurred.

A second National Morbidity Study was carried out in 1970–1971, with the aim of collecting data compatible with the 1955–1956 study (RCGP et al. 1974). In addition to morbidity information, particulars about the use of community and hospital facilities were recorded, and the patients' consultation patterns were identified. For each episode of care, the name and date of birth were recorded together with the date of first consultation and the episode type. Up to six face-to-face consultations could be coded on the same line of the record sheet, with continuation if required. Referral to other agencies was also identified. Fifty-four practices were initially involved, although one withdrew during the survey. Unlike the previous study, diagnostic and other information was coded at practice level rather than centrally, using the Royal College of General Practitioners classification for coding morbidity. This classification was modified to conform to the eighth revision of the ICD, having been derived initially from the seventh revision.

A linkage exercise with the census was also carried out to relate census variables to morbidity rates. Using census schedules for the enumeration districts that represented the catchment area of the practices, computer matching was carried out without access to full names of the subjects in the study (RCGP et al. 1982). The non-matches from the age–sex registers were then examined clerically and possible matches were added to the computer file. This resulted in a 65 to 75 per cent initial match for most practices, with up to a further 20 per cent added by the clerical exercise. The number of enumeration districts was extended for the few practices

with a low match rate. The final proportion of the practice register population that could be matched was 78 per cent. Tabulations were presented on morbidity in relation to population characteristics, marital status, country of birth, urban/rural residence, social class, occupation order, housing tenure, and household amenities.

The third National Morbidity Study (RCGP et al. 1986) took place in 1981–1982 and involved 48 practices providing care for over 300 000 patients. Information similar to the previous studies was collected, but the diagnostic classification was modified to conform with the ICD. Linkage of patient records to census data was again carried out for a proportion of the practices.

A fourth national study to provide morbidity statistics from general practice (MSGP4) was conducted in England and Wales in 1991–1992 (McCormick et al. 1995). Sixty computerized general practices collaborated, covering a population that represented almost half a million person-years at risk. As nurses now perform some duties which ten years previously would have been carried out by doctors, MSGP4 also included face-to-face contacts with practice-employed nurses. This allowed the provision of more comparable 'consultation' information. The scope of the information collected was very similar to that in the previous studies. However, there were some other differences: collection of socio-economic data from patients was by interview, and an enhanced categorization of disease 'severity' was used. A validation study was carried out, which demonstrated a generally high level of completeness and accuracy.

A number of other studies from general practice have collected data on contact with patients; these vary from pioneer efforts where individual doctors or groups of doctors have invested effort to codify material on the patients they see, to major collaborative studies such as that carried out by 68 doctors in South Wales in 1965–1966 (Williams 1970). The various surveys have included mainly practices from England and Wales. Although there has been no input from Scotland throughout, three practices from Northern Ireland (representing a population of 15 000) took part in the second national study.

Validity of data

A vital element in such studies is the count of the number of individuals on the doctor's NHS practice list and their age distribution; this is required as the denominator in calculating rates. Lees and Cooper (1963) identified problems of definition and net change in the practice list. The first National Morbidity Study initially showed practice list inflation of 1.1 per cent, although this was reduced to 0.7 per cent on investigation. Other studies have identified variations of 20 per cent (Backett et al. 1954) and 14 per cent (Morrell et al. 1970). Less extreme variation was found by Fraser (1978) and by Fraser and Clayton (1981). Another issue is the extent to which contact with a general practitioner indicates the prevalence of morbidity in the population. A number of studies have indicated that there is a varying degree of self-care and undetected disease (Horder and Horder 1954; Last 1963; Kessel and Shepherd 1965; Cartwright 1967; Wadsworth et al. 1971).

Equally important is the validity of data recording, as the accuracy of the analyses may be constrained by errors in the capture, coding, or processing of the material. This has been discussed by Morrell and his colleagues in a series of papers

(Morrell *et al.* 1970, 1971; Morrell 1972; Morrell and Kasap 1972; Morrell and Nicholson 1974), and other aspects have been investigated by Kay (1968), Clarke and Bennett (1971), Dawes (1972), Hannay (1972), Farmer *et al.* (1974), and Munroe and Ratoff (1973). The effect of different systems of classification has been examined by Martini *et al.* (1976), who highlighted the contrast between presenting problems and underlying morbidity.

In the second National Morbidity Study, the validity of the practice registers was checked, indicating a true inflation of about 1.1 per cent (RCGP *et al.* 1974). An attempt was made to check the morbidity data, which indicated some diagnostic problems and variation between the practices; coding errors resulted in only marginal variation in the recorded morbidity. It appeared that about 3.5 per cent of consultations and 2.4 per cent of episodes recorded on practice records were not on the computer records, whilst 0.35 per cent of the events on the computer file could not be identified in the practice notes. There was no independent check of the diagnostic labels used as specific contacts in any of the practices. A similar post-study evaluation exercise was carried out on the third National Morbidity Study (RCGP *et al.* 1986), with broadly similar results. Consultations were under-reported by 2.2 per cent and episodes were under-reported by 0.8 per cent; there were greater discrepancies for home visits and referrals.

It is not known how typical are studies which involve volunteer general practitioners. For example, among the general practitioners who volunteered for the second National Morbidity Study, there was a slight excess from practices with more than four principals and from those with large list sizes, as well as from younger doctors and those practising from health centres or with ancillary help. Crombie (1973) has suggested that the diagnostic patterns and differences in the case mix that a family doctor draws toward him or her can have some influence. Provided that the number of doctors is sufficiently large, the overall population that is served approximates closely to the general population. One report examined some of the characteristics of the practices participating in the second survey and concluded that morbidity rates were likely to vary in relation to the location of the practice, the size of the partnership, the doctor's age, and the availability of ancillary staff (RCGP *et al.* 1979).

The exercise whereby data from the second National Morbidity Study were linked to the census also facilitated a check of the representativeness of the study sample. The matched sample showed some deviation from the characteristics of the total study sample: the older age groups were slightly under-represented, as were the widowed and divorced. In contrast, social classes I, II, and III non-manual, and those in owner-occupied housing, were over-represented. It was concluded that these differences were insufficient to introduce bias such that the consultation rates of the census-matched sample were appreciably distorted.

Crombie and Fleming (1986) compared consultation rates for the second National Morbidity Study with those derived from the General Household Survey of 1971. They found a broad level of agreement, despite the different approaches of the two surveys.

Publications of general practice morbidity

The results from the first National Morbidity Study appeared in three reports (Logan and Cushion 1958; Logan 1960; Research Committee of the Council of the College of General Practitioners 1962). Later publications were issued jointly by the Royal College of General Practitioners, the OPCS and the DHSS.

Congenital malformations
Background

Two pioneering local schemes for collecting information about congenital malformations began in Birmingham in 1949 (Charles 1951) and in Liverpool in 1960 (Smithells 1962). Together, these covered only about 20 000 births in each year, but were sufficient to study the more common serious abnormalities.

Stimulated in part by the thalidomide epidemic in 1960, a national scheme was launched in England and Wales in 1964 in which the doctor or midwife notifying a birth to the local Medical Officer of Health was asked to include particulars about any identifiable congenital abnormality. A standard form was completed by the Medical Officer of Health with respect to every child with an observable malformation identified at birth or within 7 days thereof. Each Medical Officer of Health forwarded to the General Register Office forms relating to mothers resident in their area, with appropriate arrangements being made where the mother was resident elsewhere.

The process was described in detail by Weatherall (1978) and, subject to changes in the channels of communication resulting from various reorganizations of the NHS, the method of data acquisition is essentially unchanged. As well as descriptions of all abnormalities present, details required include maternal date of birth, whether a multiple birth, live birth, or stillbirth, length of gestation, birth-weight, and place of birth.

A similar scheme was initiated in Northern Ireland in 1964. Since 1989 the four Health and Social Services Boards receive information from the Northern Ireland Child Health system via a notification of birth form, a maternal/neonatal hospital discharge form, and the results of routine developmental examinations. Information is sent monthly to the Department of Medical Genetics at Queen's University, Belfast. In Scotland there is no separate reporting scheme, but a congenital malformation register, started in 1988 by the Information and Statistics Division, uses data from SMR11 supplemented by information derived from records of hospital episodes for infants aged less than one year.

As the main aim of the schemes is to monitor trends, there are two separate aspects of the analysis of malformation data: (i) the routine tabulation of the data for the publication of statistics, and (ii) the statistical examination of the material to identify significant variations in reporting. In England and Wales tabulations relating to reported malformations are sent monthly to each District Health Authority, which is also warned if the actual numbers of a particular malformation are greater than the expected number derived from the rate for that malformation in that month in the country as a whole. A comparison is also made with the numbers of the same malformation reported from the locality in the previous time period. Once a given malformation has been identified as having increased, the level in the locality is reviewed monthly for the following 11 months; if the reporting remains significantly higher, a further warning is automatically generated within a further three months.

Validity of congenital malformation data

As one objective is to detect 'epidemics' by finding changes in reporting, some degree of incompleteness does not materially affect the value of this work. However, it is of obvious importance to know the degree to which malformations are identified and also whether diagnoses are appropriately classified. By comparing the notification of anencephaly with the number of deaths recorded for this condition, Weatherall (1969) suggested that notification was fairly complete for this (serious and obvious) condition.

A more thorough investigation of the child population in Exeter and Devon has indicated that the proportion of malformations found and reported in the national scheme varies with the type of malformation. The levels detected for all but a few internal malformations were thought to be sufficient to expose any increase in incidence (Vowles *et al.* 1975). In a case–control study Greenberg *et al.* (1975) found that further enquiry by the local health authority indicated that 77 out of a sample of 2867 notifications were normal babies who should not have been included. Ericson *et al.* (1977) compared the information provided by (i) specific notifications of congenital malformations, identified at birth, and (ii) computer records of routine birth diagnosis for all infants. Both systems appeared to 'lose' about 20 per cent of the malformed infants, but the quality of diagnostic information was better for the specific notification system and the speed of data transmission was greater.

Publications on congenital malformations

Initially, annual volumes were not published by the OPCS for this topic for England and Wales, as quarterly and annual material was issued in the monitor series (MB3). However, there were occasional analyses covering a longer period; the latest volume covered the quinquennium 1981–1985 (OPCS 1988) with tabular material and maps provided for each malformation, which give notification rates by a variety of parameters. Commencing with the information for 1987, this has now become an annual volume.

Until 1975 some material for Northern Ireland appeared in the annual reports of the Registrar General and, until 1984, material was published by the DHSS(NI) in its annual Health and Personal Social Service Statistics. Recently, information on selected abnormalities has been published annually by Area Boards and in the annual report of the Chief Medical Officer, Northern Ireland. All United Kingdom countries contribute to the European Registration of Congenital Anomalies (EUROCAT), from which regular reports are produced (e.g. EUROCAT 1993). An informal international monitoring system (International Clearing House for Birth Defects 1981) also exists, to which data from England and Wales are contributed and from which an annual report is produced (International Clearing House for Birth Defects 1985).

Abortion

Background

The Abortion Act 1967 came into force in Great Britain in April 1968, but there is no corresponding Act in Northern Ireland. This Act requires notifications of termination of pregnancy to be made within seven days on a standard form (as presented in subsequent regulations, for example Statutory Instruments (1968)), which is sent to the Chief Medical Officer of England, Wales, or Scotland.

Amendment regulations were made in 1969 (Statutory Instruments 1969) and 1976 (Statutory Instruments 1976). Further amendments in 1980 (Statutory Instruments 1980*a*, *b*) made certain adjustments to the content of the notification forms both for England and Wales and for Scotland.

Section 37 of the Human Fertilization and Embryology Act (1990) made some changes to the Abortion Act, in particular to the statutory grounds for termination and to the time limits associated with these grounds. These changes came into effect on 1 April 1991 and affected the content and presentation of the statistics from that date.

The aim of the information notified to the Chief Medical Officers is primarily to ensure that the requirements of the Act are being properly observed but provision is also made for subsequent processing by the OPCS (for England and Wales) and the Information and Statistics Division (for Scotland), acting as agents. This enables basic epidemiological and demographic data about women undergoing terminations to be collected and published regularly. It is interesting to note that in this system the particulars are recorded in the unit where the termination takes place and the forms are transmitted directly to central government, with no provision for collating or checking the material at the local or regional level.

The notification forms for England and Wales and for Scotland are similar. They include such items as the age of the woman, her place of residence, marital status, and the number of her previous children. Also included are the length of gestation, the statutory grounds for termination, and the method used. These items are utilized in a range of cross-tabulations.

Publications on abortion

Preliminary information for England and Wales is published quarterly by the OPCS as an Abortion Monitor (AB series), which provides relatively quick issue with limited tables. More detailed statistics are presented in an annual publication in the AB series. Material for Scotland, which includes terminations carried out in England and Wales on Scottish residents, is published in the Scottish Health Statistics and in the Annual Report of the Registrar General for Scotland.

Household surveys

Routine information about morbidity derived from the kind of events described in the previous section has the built-in disadvantage that it is mostly associated with a contact between a patient and a health professional, usually a doctor. Thus it fails to cover minor or other illnesses not associated with consultation, information about which can be obtained only by direct enquiry of population sample. Thus, household interview surveys traditionally conducted within the United Kingdom have included such enquiries in recent years. Furthermore, the opportunity can be taken to use this mechanism to provide corroborative evidence regarding the accuracy of alternative sources of information about the use of health services, such as outpatient consultations.

Background

From 1944 to 1953 a monthly survey of sickness was carried out in England and Wales, questioning a sample of people about their health in the preceding two to three months (Stocks 1949). The sample size was initially 2500 persons aged from 16 to 64 years, but it increased to 4000 with the addition of those aged over 64 years.

The final report of the survey (Logan and Brooke 1957) had a considerable section devoted to some of the problems of the survey, with a detailed examination of the bias introduced by the memory factor. This was followed by a general critical appraisal, which considered the validity and general usefulness of the data that were obtained. One interesting issue is the comment that the tables provided became heavily weighted with data on minor and trivial illness and, in particular, that it was unrewarding to examine for time trends. Apart from the number of comments about interpretation of the data, it was emphasized that the survey's positive contribution was to identify the large amount of ill-health that people suffer for which no medical advice is sought. It was concluded that the main contribution of such a survey should not be to provide a permanent operation identifying the total load of ill-health; it is more appropriate, as the need arises, to quantify items of information on illness and its effects that cannot be readily obtained in a routine way.

A major alteration occurred in the collection of data in Great Britain with the initiation of a General Household Survey in 1971 (OPCS 1973b). The aim of this survey was to provide a substantially improved flow of social statistics to complement the wide range of routine material then processed by central government and to develop an instrument to examine the interaction among different policy areas. The intention was to create a survey that was developed in close collaboration with a number of government departments in order to link their needs for information on population, housing, employment, education, health, and social services. Consideration of the predominant objective of the survey indicated that a very long interview would be required with all respondents; at the same time, there were constraints on resources available. These two factors markedly influenced the study design. It was essential that respondents co-operated willingly in order to obtain the detailed answers called for in the interview.

A nationally representative sample was required. The sample design was two-stage rotating and stratified, with electoral wards forming the primary sampling units. The sampling was similar for the whole of Great Britain, but the number of households contacted was doubled for Scotland to provide the minimum of precision thought necessary for separate analysis. The sampling procedure identified addresses from the electoral register; the interviewer converted the list of addresses to the identification of households. For addresses containing more than one household, set procedures were used to try to ensure that there was the correct probability of selection of multi-households (OPCS 1982). The initial report provided considerable detail on the sampling errors of the survey; further detailed consideration of this appeared in the report for 1976 (OPCS 1978).

This social survey used a detailed structured interview, which was tested in pilot trials during the development phase; throughout, the interviewers were carefully trained and supervised. There appeared to be marked stability in the response rate, but modest variation occurred across the country. The reports regularly provide comment on the quality of the information provided. The simplest checks that can be carried out on the data are by comparison with other material or by examination of internal

consistency of response. For example, comparison with the 1971 census data suggested that the General Household Survey provided a good representation of the population in private households. However, an appreciable proportion of the morbidity in the total population is amongst residents in institutions.

An analogous Continuous Household Survey, based on a sample of the general population resident in private households in Northern Ireland, has been running since 1983. The nature and aims of the Continuous Household Survey are similar to those of the General Household Survey, covering the subject areas of population, housing, employment, education, health, and use of health services. In addition to these 'core' areas, which are covered each year, there are 'periodic' sections, which are repeated on a regular basis, and 'ad hoc' sections, which have been included irregularly or only once to date. Examples of subjects covered by periodic sections include smoking habits, drinking habits, sport, physical activity, and entertainment. Examples of ad hoc sections include the elderly, carers, diet, and European languages.

The Continuous Household Survey is designed primarily to provide information for the government, but there are plans to make the data sets accessible to academics and other researchers through the Economic and Social Research Council (ESRC) Data Archive within the next year.

The sample for the Continuous Household Survey is drawn from the domestic properties identified on the Rating Valuation List; a set sample of 4500 addresses is drawn from the list annually as a simple random sample from three strata. The first of these is the Belfast District Council area. The other two are formed by dividing the remainder of the province into east and west along district council boundaries. The 4500 addresses selected in the sample are visited by interviewers throughout the year, and information is collected from households living at the addresses. Interviews are conducted with each person aged 16 and over in the household.

The intention was always to change the items included in the General Household Survey in response to users' requirements. Over time, the health section has collected data on activity limitation caused by acute or chronic sickness and contacts with health and personal social services. These have regularly included questions on consultations with doctors, and patient attendance at hospitals and details of in-patient care. In some years, questions on the use of other health and personal social services by the elderly have also been included, as have enquiries regarding sight and hearing. Also of direct relevance to health has been the establishment of patterns of smoking and alcohol consumption. The main changes in content are detailed cumulatively in the published volumes and those for the past decade are summarized in Table 3.4, which also shows the general compatibility of regular and occasional topics between the General Household Survey and the Continuous Household Survey. Each annual volume of the General Household Survey includes the questionnaire used, from which the exact nature of definitions can be determined.

An important point to emphasize is that the nature of the General Household Survey provides a powerful analytical tool by virtue of its ability to cross-tabulate the health data against the wide range of terms collected on 'social' topics. Some of these topics overlap with material collected at census so as to provide continuous information, and include demographic particulars about

Table 3.4 Major items covered in the health section of the General Household Survey, Great Britain, 1977–1992, and the Continuous Household Survey, Northern Ireland, 1983–1994/5

Item	1977	1978	1979	1980	1981	1982	1983	1984	1985	1986	1987	1988	1989	1990	1991	1992
Great Britain																
Chronic sickness	−	−	+	+	+	+	+	+	+	+	+	+	+	+	+	+
Acute sickness in the last 2 weeks	−	−	+	+	+	+	+	+	+	+	+	+	+	+	+	+
Health in general in the last 12 months	+	+	+	+	+	+	+	+	+	+	+	+	+	+	+	+
GP consultation in the past 2 weeks	+	+	+	+	+	+	+	+	+	+	+	+	+	+	+	+
Outpatient attendance in the past 3 months	+	+	+	+	+	+	+	+	+	+	+	+	+	+	+	+
Inpatient stays in the past year	−	−	−	−	−	+	+	+	+	+	+	+	+	+	+	+
Day patient in the past year	−	−	−	−	−	−	−	−	−	−	−	−	−	−	−	+
Use of various health/welfare services in the past month	−	−	(+)	(+)	(+)	(+)	(+)	(+)	(+)	−	−	−	−	−	(+)	−
Difficulty with sight	+	+	+	(+)	+	+	−	−	(+)	−	−	−	−	−	(+)	−
Difficulty with hearing	+	+	+	(+)	+*	−	−	−	(+)	−	−	−	−	−	(+)	−
Dental health	−	−	−	−	−	+	−	+	−	+	−	+	−	+	−	−
Smoking	−	+	−	+	−	+	−	+	−	+	−	+	−	+	−	+
Alcohol consumption	−	+	−	+	−	+	−	+	−	+	−	+	−	+	−	+
Accidents	−	−	−	−	+	−	−	+	−	−	+	+	+	−	−	−

Northern Ireland	1983	1984	1985	1986	1987	1988	89/90	90/91	91/92	92/93	93/94	94/95
Chronic sickness	+	+	+	+	+	+	+	+	+	+	+	+
Acute sickness in the last 2 weeks	+	+	+	+	+	+	+	+	+	+	+	+
Health in general in the last 12 months	+	+	+	+	+	+	+	+	+	+	+	+
GP consultation in the past 2 weeks	+	+	+	+	+	+	+	+	+	+	+	+
Outpatient attendance in the past 3 months	+	+	+	+	+	+	+	+	+	+	+	+
Inpatient stays in the past year	+	+	+	+	+	+	+	+	+	+	+	+
Day patient in the past year	−	−	−	−	−	−	−	−	−	+	+	+
Use of various health/welfare services in the past month	−	(+)	(+)	−	−	−	−	−	−	−	−	(+)
Difficulty with sight	−	−	(+)	−	−	−	+	+	+	+	+	+
Difficulty with hearing	−	−	(+)	−	−	−	−	−	+	−	−	(+)
Dental health	−	−	+	−	+	−	+	−	+	+	+	(+)
Smoking	−	+	−	+	−	+	−	+	−	+	−	+
Alcohol consumption	−	+	−	+	−	+	−	+	−	+	−	+
Accidents	−	+	−	−	+	+	+	−	−	−	−	+

+ Included
− Not included
() Included only for the elderly
* Additional information collected on tinnitus

the population as well as information on housing, employment, education, income, and family structure.

Validity of General Household Survey data

All material is collected by direct questioning and no independent validation of the data occurs (such as detailed study of a subsample of the respondents, including medical investigations). The influence of memory bias in probing for events in the past has been indicated above. Obviously some of the general points about validity of surveys that record morbidity statistics apply. (For a review of this topic, see Alderson and Dowie (1979).)

A Scandinavian study of the validity of health contact data showed false-positive reporting of 12.8 per cent and false-negative reporting of 13.4 per cent (Brorsson and Smedby 1982). The misclassification of reported visits varied with age and self-reported state of health, but it is not known whether this applies equally to the United Kingdom.

Publications from the General Household Survey

The General Household Survey, with sections relating to each of the topics covered, is published annually by the OPCS. On occasion there has been a special supplement on a health-related topic, for example that on drinking in 1986 (Green 1989). This report also describes the methods used to classify drinking behaviour between 1978 and 1984, in comparison with a new method introduced from 1986. Publication from the Continuous Household Survey is by way of monitors issued by the Policy and Planning Research Unit of the Department of Finance and Personnel in Northern Ireland.

Other surveys

An innovation in 1991 was the introduction of the Health Survey for England, commissioned by the Department of Health and carried out by OPCS. The general aim of the survey is to monitor trends in the nation's health, initially focusing primarily on cardiovascular disease with an additional component of nutrition. It was designed to measure all the main risk factors for cardiovascular disease in a nationally representative sample of adults living in England.

The survey includes an interview questionnaire covering present health, illness history, cardiovascular symptoms, use of health services, smoking, alcohol consumption, eating habits, and family history of heart disease. Measurements are taken of height and weight, and a nurse visits to obtain information on prescribed medicine, to take blood pressure readings, and to draw blood for cholesterol, haemoglobin, and other analytes.

A sample of 3242 adults was obtained in 1991 (White et al. 1993) and a sample of 4018 was obtained in 1992. The main aim of the 1992 survey was to contribute to a larger sample size for the provision of baseline data. In future it is hoped that it will be possible to monitor changes over time (Breeze et al. 1994).

The OPCS has also developed a multipurpose 'omnibus' survey for use by government departments and other public bodies on topics too brief to warrant a survey of their own. A health-related example of this approach was a prevalence survey of back pain in 1993 (Mason 1994).

Other information sources

Some aspects of information sources have not been covered in this chapter. For example, the definition of the United Kingdom has been taken to include only England, Wales, Scotland, and Northern Ireland. Some of the sources mentioned have counterparts in the Channel Isles and the Isle of Man. In fact, regular censuses are carried out on each island, the most recent being in 1981 on the Isle of Man and in 1986 on both Jersey and Guernsey. Similarly, regular mortality information can be found in the annual reports of the Medical Officers of Health of the Channel Isles and the Chief Registrar of the Isle of Man.

Over time some other national, but limited, sources of morbidity information have been available, such as occupational disease and injury data (issued by the Health and Safety Executive) and sickness absence statistics (hitherto published by DHSS).

Similarly, a wide range of sources of social information with some relevance to health exists; for example, the OPCS National Food Survey and the Family Expenditure Survey give food and nutrition data. Also, information is available on occupation from the OPCS Labour Force Survey, which may contribute information either in its own right or provide appropriate denominators. Many of the more topical aspects of these kinds of information are presented annually in the Central Statistical Office's publication *Social trends*.

References

Abramson, J.H., Sacks, M.I., and Cahana, E. (1971). Death certification data as an indication of the presence of certain common diseases at birth. *Journal of Chronic Diseases*, **24**, 417–31.

Acheson, E.D. (1967). *Medical record linkage*. Oxford University Press, London.

Alderson, M.R. (1965). The accuracy of the certification of death, and the classification of underlying cause of death from death certificate. Unpublished MD thesis, University of London.

Alderson, M.R. (1973). Cancer registration. In *Cancer priorities* (ed G. Bennette), p. 101. British Cancer Council, London.

Alderson, M.R. (1974). Central government routine health statistics. In *Reviews of United Kingdom statistical sources* (ed. W.F. Maunder), Vol. II, p. 1. Heineman, London.

Alderson, M.R. (1981). *International mortality statistics*. Macmillan, London.

Alderson, M.R. (1984). A comment on social class analysis. *Community Medicine*, **6**, 1–3.

Alderson, M. and Ashwood, F. (1985). Projection of mortality rates for the elderly. *Population Trends*, **42**, 22–9.

Alderson, M.R. and Dowie, R. (1979). *Health surveys and related studies*. Pergamon Press, Oxford.

Alderson, M.R. and Meade, T.W. (1967). Accuracy of diagnosis on death certificates compared with that in hospital records. *British Journal of Preventive and Social Medicine*, **21**, 22–9.

Alderson, M.R., Bradley, K., Rushton, L., and Thacker, P. (1976). Cancer registration as a by-product of hospital activity analysis. *Hospital and Health Service Review*, **72**, 118–21.

Alderson, M.R., Bayliss, R.I.S., Clarke, C.A., and Whitfield, A.G.W. (1983). Death certification. *British Medical Journal*, **287**, 444–5.

Armitage, B. (1994). Retrospective revisions to population estimates for 1981–1990. *Population Trends*, **77**, 33–6.

Armitage, R.I. (1986). Population projections for English local authority areas. *Population Trends*, **43**, 31–40.

Ashley, J.S.A. (1972). Present state of statistics from hospital in-patient data and their uses. *British Journal of Preventive and Social Medicine*, **26**, 135–47.

Ashley, J.S.A. (1980). The maternity hospital in-patient enquiry. In *Perinatal audit and surveillance* (ed. I. Chalmers and G. McIlwaine), p. 61. Royal College of Obstetricians and Gynaecologists, London.

Ashley, J. and Devis, T. (1992). Death certification from the point of view of the epidemiologist. *Population Trends*, **67**, 22–8.

Ashley, J. and McLachlan, G. (ed.) (1985). *Mortal or morbid? A diagnosis of the morbidity factor*. Nuffield Provincial Hospitals Trust, London.

Backett, E.M., Heady, J.A., and Evans, J.C.G. (1954). Studies of a general practice. The doctor's job in an urban area. *British Medical Journal*, i, 109–15.

Benjamin, B. (1965). Hospital activity analysis. *Hospital*, **61**, 221–8.

Benjamin, B. (1968a). *Demographic analysis*. Allen and Unwin, London.

Benjamin, B. (1968b). *Health and vital statistics*. Allen and Unwin, London.

Birch, D. (1993). Automatic coding of causes of death. *Population Trends*, **73**, 36–8.

Breeze, E., Maidment, A., Bennett, N., et al. (1994). *Health survey for England, 1992*. HMSO, London.

Britton, M. (ed.) (1990). *Mortality and geography. A review in the mid-1980s, England and Wales*. HMSO, London.

Britton, M. and Birch, F. (1985). *1981 Census: Post enumeration survey—an inquiry into the coverage and quality of the 1981 Census in England and Wales*. HMSO, London.

Brodrick, N. (1971). *Report of the Committee on Death Certification and Coroners* (Cmd 4810). HMSO, London.

Brorsson, B. and Smedby, B. (1982). Validity of health survey interview data concerning visits to doctors at Swedish health centres. *Stat Tidsksrift*, **1**, 31.

Busuttil, A., Kemp, I.W., and Heasman, M.A. (1981). The accuracy of medical certificates of cause of death. *Health Bulletin*, **39**, 146–52.

Butts, M.S. and Williams, D.R.R. (1982). Accuracy of hospital activity analysis data. *British Medical Journal*, **285**, 506–7.

Cameron, H.M. and McGoogan, E. (1981). A prospective study of 1152 hospital autopsies. *Journal of Pathology*, **133**, 273–83.

Cameron, H.M., Wilson, B., McGoogan, E., Clarke, J., and Melville, A. (1977). Autopsies and medical records. *Health Bulletin*, **35**, 113–14.

Cancer Research Campaign, Cancer Statistics Group (1982). *Trends in cancer survival in Great Britain*. Cancer Research Campaign, London.

Cartwright, A. (1967). *Patients and their doctors—a study of general practice*. Routledge & Kegan Paul, London.

Charles, E. (1951). Statistical utilisation of maternity and child welfare records. *British Journal of Social Medicine*, **5**, 41–61.

Charlton, J., Wallace, M., and White, I. (1994). Long term illness: results from the 1991 census. *Population Trends*, **75**, 18–25.

Clarke, C. and Bennett, A.E. (1971). Problems in the measurement of hospital utilisation. *Proceedings of the Royal Society of Medicine*, **64**, 795–8.

Clarke, C. and Whitfield, A.G.W. (1978). Death certification and epidemiological research. *British Medical Journal*, ii, 1063–5.

Clarkson, J.A. and Fine, P.F.M. (1985). The efficiency of measles and pertussis morbidity reporting in England and Wales. *International Journal of Epidemiology*, **14**, 153–68.

Cohen, J. and Steinitz, R. (1969). Underlying and contributory causes of death of adult males in two districts. *Journal of Chronic Diseases*, **22**, 17–24.

Cole, S. (1980). Scottish maternity and neonatal records. In *Perinatal audit and surveillance* (ed. I. Chalmers and G. McIlwaine), p. 39. Royal College of Obstetricians and Gynaecologists, London.

Cole, S.K. (1989). Evaluation of a neonatal discharge record as a monitor of congenital malformations. *Community Medicine*, **11**, 1–8.

Coleman, M.P. and Esteve, J. (1994). Trends in cancer incidence and mortality in the United Kingdom. In *Cancer statistics: registrations, 1989*, p. 8. HMSO, London.

Compton, P.A. (1993). Population censuses in Northern Ireland 1926–1991. In *The 1991 census user's guide* (ed. A. Dale and C. Marsh), p. 330. HMSO, London.

Crawshaw, C. and Moss, J.G. (1982). Accuracy of Hospital Activity Analysis operation codes. *British Medical Journal*, **285**, 210.

Crombie, D.L. (1973). Research and confidentiality in general practice. *Journal of the Royal College of General Practitioners*, **23**, 863–79.

Crombie, D.L. and Fleming, D.M. (1986). Comparison of Second National Morbidity Study and General Household Survey 1970–71. *Health Trends*, **18**, 15–18.

Dale, A. (1993). An overview, and the content of the 1991 census: change and continuity. In *The 1991 census user's guide* (ed. A. Dale and C. Marsh), p. 1. HMSO, London.

Davies, P.D.O., Darbyshire, J., Nunn, A.J., *et al.* (1981). Ambiguities and inaccuracies in the notification system for tuberculosis in England and Wales. *Community Medicine*, **3**, 108–18.

Dawes, K.S. (1972). Survey of general practice records. *British Medical Journal*, iii, 219–23.

Daykin, C. (1986). Projecting the population of the United Kingdom. *Population Trends*, **44**, 28–33.

Department of Health (1994). *Hospital Episode Statistics England: financial year 1991–1992*. Government Statistical Service, London.

Diehl, A.K. and Gau, D.W. (1982). Death certification by British doctors: a demographic analysis. *Journal of Epidemiology and Community Health*, **36**, 146–9.

Dollinger, J. (1907). Statistique des personnes attientes de cancer. *Publication Statistique Hongerie, Nouvelle Serie 19*. Budapest.

Dunnigan, D.G., Harland, W.A., and Fyfe, T. (1970). Seasonal incidence and mortality of ischaemic heart disease. *Lancet*, ii, 793–7.

Edouard, L. (1982). Validation of the registered underlying cause of stillbirth. *Journal of Epidemiology and Community Health*, **36**, 231–4.

Ericson, A., Kallen, B., and Winberg, J. (1977). Surveillance of malformations at birth: a comparison of two record systems run in parallel. *International Journal of Epidemiology*, **6**, 35–41.

EUROCAT (European Registration of Congenital Anomalies and Twins) (1993). *Surveillance of congenital anomalies, 1980–1990* (ed. EUROCAT Working Group), EUROCAT Report No. 5. Institute of Hygiene and Epidemiology, Brussels.

Farmer, R.D.T., Knox, E.G., Cross, K.W., and Crombie, D.L. (1974). Executive council lists and general practitioner files. *British Journal of Social and Preventive Medicine*, **28**, 49–53.

Farr, W. (1854). Letter to the Registrar General. In *13th Annual Report of the Registrar-General of Births, Deaths and Marriages in England*, p. 129. HMSO, London.

Farr, W. (1861). *Report of the Committee on the Preparation of Army Medical Statistics, and on the Duties to be Performed by the Statistical Branch of the Army Medical Department*. British Parliamentary Papers XXXVII.

Farr, W. (1864). Hospital mortality. *Medical Times Gazette*, i, 242–3.

Faulkner, K., Leyland, L., and Wofinden, R.C. (1967). Cancer registration. *Medical Officer*, **118**, 147–8.

Forster, D.F. and Mahadevan, S. (1981). Information sources for planning and evaluating adult psychiatric services. *Community Medicine*, **3**, 160–8.

Fox, A.J. and Goldblatt, P.O. (1982). *Longitudinal study: socio-economic mortality differentials, 1971–75, England and Wales*. OPCS, London.

Fraser, R.C. (1978). The reliability and validity of the age–sex register as a population denominator in general practice. *Journal of the Royal College of General Practitioners*, **28**, 283–6.

Fraser, R.C. and Clayton, D.G. (1981). The accuracy of the age–sex registers, practice medical records and family practitioner committee registers. *Journal of the Royal College of General Practitioners*, **31**, 410–19.

Gardner, M.J., Winter, P.D., Taylor, C.P., and Acheson, E.D. (1983). *Atlas of cancer mortality in England and Wales, 1968–1978*. Wiley, Chichester.

Gau, D.W. and Diehl, A.K. (1982). Disagreement among general practitioners regarding cause of death. *British Medical Journal*, **284**, 239–41.

Gedalla, B. and Alderson, M.R. (1984). Pilot study of revised stillbirth and neonatal death certificates. *Archives of Diseases in Childhood*, **59**, 976–82.

Gillis, R.C. (1971). *9th Annual Report of the Regional Cancer Committee for 1968*. Western Regional Hospital Cancer Registration Bureau, Glasgow.

Goldacre, M.J. (1993). Cause specific mortality: understanding uncertain tips of the disease iceberg. *Journal of Epidemiology and Community Health*, **47**, 491–6.

Goldacre, M.J. and Miller, D.L. (1976). Completeness of statutory notification for acute bacterial meningitis. *British Medical Journal*, ii, 501–3.

Great Britain (1988a). *1991 Census of Population* (CM430). HMSO, London.

Great Britain (1988b). *Registration: a modern service* (CM531). HMSO, London.

Great Britain (1990). *Registration: proposals for change* (CM939). HMSO, London.

Green, H. (1989). *Drinking—General Household Survey 1986*, GHS No. 16, Supplement A. HMSO, London.

Greenberg, G., Inman, W.H.W., Weatherall, J.A.C., and Adelstein, A.W. (1975). Hormonal pregnancy tests and congenital malformations. *British Medical Journal*, ii, 191–2.

Gruer, R. (1970). Hospital discharges in relation to area of residence. *British Journal of Preventive and Social Medicine*, **24**, 124–8.

Guralnick, L. (1966). Some problems in the use of multiple causes of death. *Journal of Chronic Diseases*, **19**, 979–90.

Hannay, D.R. (1972). Accuracy of health-centre records. *Lancet*, ii, 371–3.

Haward, R.A. (1973). Scale of under notification of infectious diseases by general practitioners. *Lancet*, i, 873–5.

Heady, J.A. and Heasman, M.A. (1959). Social and biological factors in infant mortality. In *General Register Office studies on medical and population subjects*, No. 15. HMSO, London.

Heady, P., Smith, S., and Avery, V. (1994). *1991 Census validation survey: coverage report*. HMSO, London.

Heasman, M.A. and Clarke, J.A. (1979). Medical record linkage in Scotland. *Health Bulletin*, **37**, 97–103.

Heasman, M.A. and Lipworth, L. (1966). Accuracy of certification of cause of death. In *General Register Office studies of medical and population subjects*, No. 20. HMSO, London.

Heasman, M.A., Liddell, F.O.K., and Reid, D.D. (1958). The accuracy of occupational vital statistics. *British Journal of Industrial Medicine*, **15**, 141–6.

Hole, R. (1982). Accuracy of Hospital Activity Analysis operation codes. *British Medical Journal*, **285**, 210.

Horder, J. and Horder, E. (1954). Illness in general practice. *Practitioner*, **173**, 177–88.

Hornsey, D. (1993). The effects of computerisation of the NHS central register on internal migration statistics. *Population Trends*, **74**, 34–6.

House of Commons (1893). *First and Second Reports from the Select Committee on Death Certification*. HMSO, London.

International Clearing House for Birth Defects (1981). A communication from the International Clearing House for Birth Defects monitoring systems. *International Journal of Epidemiology*, **10**, 245–6.

International Clearing House for Birth Defects (1985). *Annual report 1985*. International Clearing House for Birth Defects, San Francisco, CA.

Jennings, C. and Barraclough, B. (1980). Legal and administrative influences on the English suicide rate since 1900. *Psychological Medicine*, **10**, 407–8.

Jones, I.G. and Cameron, D. (1984). Social class analysis—an embarrassment to epidemiology. *Community Medicine*, **6**, 37–46.

Kay, C.R. (1968). A comparison of two methods of determining social status. *Journal of the Royal College of General Practitioners*, **16**, 162–6.

Kendrick, S. and Clarke, J. (1993). The Scottish record linkage system. *Health Bulletin*, **51**, 72–9.

Kessel, W.I.N. and Shepherd, M. (1965). The health and attitudes of people who seldom consult a doctor. *Medical Care*, **3**, 6–10.

Kogevinas, E. (1990). *Longitudinal Study 1971–83. Socio-demographic differences in career survival*, Series LS, No. 5. HMSO, London.

Lambert, P.M. (1973). Recent trends in meningococcal infection. *Community Medicine*, **129**, 279–81.

Lancet (1841). Hospital physicians and surgeons. *Lancet*, i, 649–53.

Last, J.M. (1963). The iceberg: 'completing the clinical picture' in general practice. *Lancet*, ii, 28–31.

Leck, I., Birch, J.M., Marsden, H.B., and Steward, J.K. (1976). Methods of classifying and ascertaining children's tumours. *British Journal of Cancer*, **34**, 69–82.

Lees, D.S. and Cooper, M.H. (1963). The work of the general practitioner. *Journal of the College of General Practitioners*, **6**, 408–35.

Lindahl, B.I.B., Glattre, E., Lahti, R., *et al.* (1990). The WHO principles for registering causes of death, suggestions for improvement. *Journal of Clinical Epidemiology*, **43**, 467–74.

Lockwood, E. (1971). Accuracy of Scottish Hospital morbidity data. *British Journal of Preventive and Social Medicine*, **25**, 76–83.

Logan, W.P.D. (1953). General practitioners' records. In *General Register Office studies on medical and population subjects*, No. 7. HMSO, London.

Logan, W.P.D. (1960). Morbidity statistics from general practice, Vol. II (occupation). In *General Register Office studies on medical and population subjects*, No. 14. HMSO, London.

Logan, W.P.D. and Brooke, E.M. (1957). The survey of sickness—1943–1952. In *General Register Office studies on medical and population subjects*, No. 12. HMSO, London.

Logan, W.P.D. and Cushion, A.A. (1958). Morbidity statistics from general practices, Vol. I (general). In *General Register Office studies on medical and population subjects*, No. 14. HMSO, London.

McCormick, A. (1988). Trends in mortality statistics in England and Wales with particular reference to AIDS from 1984 to April 1987. *British Medical Journal*, **296**, 1289–92.

McCormick, A., Tillett, H., Bannister, B., and Emslie, J. (1987). Surveillance of AIDS in the United Kingdom. *British Medical Journal*, **295**, 1466–9.

McCormick, A., Fleming, D., and Charlton, J. (1995). *Morbidity statistics from general practice: fourth national study 1991–1992*, Series MB5, No. 1, HMSO, London.

McGoogan, E. and Cameron, H.M. (1978). Clinical attitudes to the autopsy. *Scottish Medical Journal*, **23**, 19–22.

McIlwaine, W.J., Donnelly, M.D.I., Chivers, A.T., *et al.* (1985). Certification of death from ischaemic heart disease in Belfast. *International Journal of Epidemiology*, **14**, 560–5.

McMurray, R. and Evans, T. (1993). 1991 census of population for Northern Ireland. *Population Trends*, **74**, 24–6.

McNeilly, R.H. and Moore, F. (1975). The accuracy of some hospital activity analyses data. *Hospital and Health Services Review*, **71**, 93–5.

Markush, R.E. (1968). National chronic respiratory disease mortality study. *Journal of Chronic Diseases*, **21**, 129–41.

Marsh, C. (1993a). The validation of census data—general issues. In *The 1991 census user's guide* (ed. A. Dale and C. Marsh), p. 155. HMSO, London.

Marsh, C. (1993b). The sample of anonymised records. In *The 1991 census user's guide* (ed. A. Dale and C. Marsh), p. 295. HMSO, London.

Martini, C.J.M., Hughes, A.O., and Patton, V.J. (1976). A study of the validity of the Hospital Activity Analysis. *British Journal of Preventive and Social Medicine*, **30**, 180–6.

Martyn, C.N. and Pippard, E.C. (1988). Usefulness of mortality data in determining the geography and time trends of dementia. *Journal of Epidemiology and Community Health*, **42**, 134–7.

Mason, V. (1994). *The prevalence of back pain in Great Britain*. HMSO, London.

Maudsley, G. and Williams, E.M.I. (1993). Death certification by house officers and general practitioners—practice and performance. *Journal of Public Health Medicine*, **15**, 192–201.

Mills, I. (1987). Developments in census-taking since 1841. *Population Trends*, **48**, 37–44.

Moriyama, I.M. (1952). Needed improvements in mortality data. *Public Health Reports*, **67**, 851–6.

Moriyama, I.M., Baum, W.S., Haenszel, W.M., and Mattison, B.F. (1958). Inquiry into diagnostic evidence supporting medical certifications of death. *American Journal of Public Health*, **48**, 1376–87.

Morrell, D.C. (1972). Symptom interpretation in general practice. *Journal of the Royal College of General Practitioners*, **22**, 297–309.

Morrell, D.C. and Kasap, H.G. (1972). The effect of an appointment system on demand for medical care. *International Journal of Epidemiology*, **1**, 143–51.

Morrell, D.C. and Nicholson, S. (1974). Measuring the results of changes in the method of delivering primary medical care—a cautionary tale. *Journal of the Royal College of General Practitioners*, **24**, 111–18.

Morrell, D.C., Gage, H.G., and Robinson, N.A. (1970). Patterns of demand in general practice. *Journal of the Royal College of General Practitioners*, **19**, 331–42.

Morrell, D.C., Gage, H.G., and Robinson, N.A. (1971). Referral to hospital by general practitioners. *Journal of the Royal College of General Practitioners*, **21**, 77–85.

Morris, C. and Compton, P. (1985). 1981 census of population in Northern Ireland. *Population Trends*, **40**, 16–20.

Munroe, J.E. and Ratoff, L. (1973). The accuracy of general practice records. *Journal of the Royal College of General Practitioners*, **23**, 821–6.

Nightingale, F. (1863). *Notes on hospitals* (3rd edn). Longman, Longman, Roberts and Green, London.

OPCS (Office of Population Censuses and Surveys) (1970). *Report of the Advisory Committee on Cancer Registration*. OPCS, London.

OPCS (Office of Population Censuses and Surveys) (1973a). Cohort studies: new developments. In *Studies on medical and population subjects*, No. 25. HMSO, London.

OPCS (Office of Population Censuses and Surveys) (1973b). *General Household Survey: introductory report*. HMSO, London.

OPCS (Office of Population Censuses and Surveys) (1978). *General Household Survey: 1976*. HMSO, London.

OPCS (Office of Population Censuses and Surveys) (1982). *General Household Survey: 1980*. HMSO, London.

OPCS (Office of Population Censuses and Surveys) (1988). *Congenital malformation statistics—notification, England and Wales 1981–1985*, Series MB, No. 2. HMSO, London.

OPCS (Office of Population Censuses and Surveys) (1990). *Review of the national cancer registration system. Report of the Working Group of the Registrar General's Medical Advisory Committee*, Series MB1, No. 17. HMSO, London.

OPCS (Office of Population Censuses and Surveys) (1991). *Making a population estimate in England and Wales*, Occasional paper No. 37. OPCS, London.

OPCS (Office of Population Censuses and Surveys) (1995). *Registrar General's Weekly Return for England and Wales week ended 30 December 1994* (WR 94/52). OPCS, London.

OPCS (Office of Population Censuses and Surveys), Census Division (1985). Census evaluation programme. *Population Trends*, **40**, 21–7.

OPCS (Office of Population Censuses and Surveys), Population Statistics (1993*a*). How complete was the 1991 census? *Population Trends*, **71**, 22–5.

OPCS (Office of Population Censuses and Surveys), Population Statistics (1993*b*). Rebasing the annual population estimates. *Population Trends*, **73**, 27–35.

OPCS and GRO(S) (Office of Population Censuses and Surveys and General Register Office (Scotland)) (1993). *1991 census: limiting long term illness—Great Britain*. HMSO, London.

Park, A.T. (1966). Occupational mortality in Northern Ireland (1960–1962). *Journal of the Statistical Society and Inquiry Society of Ireland*, **21**(4), 24–42.

Parkin, D.M., Clarke, J.A., and Heasman, M.A. (1976). Routine statistical data for the clinician. Review and prospect. *Health Bulletin*, **34**, 279–84.

Parkin, D.M., Muir, C.S., Whelan, S.L., *et al*. (ed.) (1992). *Cancer incidence in five continents*, Vol. VI. International Agency for Research on Cancer, Lyon.

Patel, A.R., Gray, G., Lang, G.D., *et al*. (1976). Scottish hospital morbidity data. 1: Errors in diagnostic returns. *Health Bulletin*, **34**, 215–20.

Pole, D.J., McCall, M.G., Reader, R., and Woodings, T. (1977). Incidence and mortality of acute myocardial infarctions in Perth, Western Australia. *Journal of Chronic Disease*, **30**, 19–27.

Puffer, R.R. and Griffith, W.G. (1967). *Patterns of urban mortality*. Pan American Health Organization, Washington, D.C.

RCGP (Royal College of General Practitioners) (1968). Returns from general practice. *British Medical Journal*, iv, 63.

RCGP (Royal College of General Practitioners), Office of Population Censuses and Surveys, and Department of Health and Social Security (1974). Morbidity statistics from general practice, Second National Study, 1970–71. In *Studies on medical and population subjects*, No. 26. HMSO, London.

RCGP (Royal College of General Practitioners), Office of Population Censuses and Surveys, and Department of Health and Social Security (1979). Morbidity statistics from general practice 1971–72, Second National Study. In *Studies on medical and population subjects*, No. 36. HMSO, London.

RCGP (Royal College of General Practitioners), Office of Population Censuses and Surveys, and Department of Health and Social Security (1982). Morbidity statistics from general practice 1970–71: socio-economic analyses. In *Studies of medical and population subjects*, No. 46. HMSO, London.

RCGP (Royal College of General Practitioners), Office of Population Censuses and Surveys, and Department of Health and Social Security (1986). *Morbidity statistics from general practice 1981–1982: Third National Study*, Series MB5, No. 1. HMSO, London.

Redfern, P. (1981). Census 1981—an historical and international perspective. *Population Trends*, **23**, 3–15.

Rees, J.L. (1982). Accuracy of hospital activity analysis data in estimating the incidence of proximal femoral fracture. *British Medical Journal*, **284**, 1856–7.

Registrar-General (1949). *The Registrar-General's statistical review of England and Wales for the six years 1940–45, Text: Medical, statistics of infectious diseases*, Vol. I, p. 85. HMSO, London.

Reid, D.D. and Rose, G.A. (1964). Assessing the comparability of mortality statistics. *British Medical Journal*, ii, 1437–9.

Research Committee of the Council of the College of the General Practitioners (1962). *Morbidity statistics from general practice: diseases in general practice*, Vol. III. HMSO, London.

Rowe, R.G. and Brewer, W. (1972). *Hospital Activity Analysis*. Butterworth, London.

Royal College of Physicians and Royal College of Pathologists (1982). Medical aspects of death certification. *Journal of the Royal College of Physicians, London*, **16**, 205–18.

Samphier, M.L., Robertson, C., and Bloor, M.J. (1988). A possible artifactual component in specific cause mortality gradients. *Journal of Epidemiology and Community Health*, **42**, 138–43.

SGHSI (Steering Group on Health Services Information) (1982*a*). *First Report to the Secretary of State* (Chairman E. Korner). HMSO, London.

SGHSI (Steering Group on Health Services Information) (1982*b*). *Converting data into information*. King's Fund, London.

SGHSI (Steering Group on Health Services Information) (1985). *Supplement to the First and Fourth Reports to the Secretary of State* (Chairman M.J. Fairey). HMSO, London.

Shaw, C. (1994). Accuracy and uncertainty of the national population projections for the United Kingdom. *Population Trends*, **77**, 24–32.

Silman, A.J. and Evans, S.J.W. (1981). Regional differences in survival from cancer. *Community Medicine*, **3**, 291–306.

Smithells, R.W. (1962). The Liverpool Congenital Abnormalities Register. *Developmental Medicine and Child Neurology*, **4**, 320–4.

Spear, B.E. and Gould, C.A. (1937). Mechanical tabulation of hospital records. *Proceedings of the Royal Society of Medicine*, **30**(1), 633–44.

Spicer, C.C. and Lipworth, L. (1966). Regional and social factors in infant mortality. In *General Register Office studies on medical and population subjects*, No. 19. HMSO, London.

Start, R.D., Delargy-Aziz, Y., Dorries, C.R., *et al*. (1993). Clinicians and the coronial system: ability of clinicians to recognise reportable deaths. *British Medical Journal*, **306**, 1038–41.

Statistical Society (1842). Report of the Committee on Hospital Statistics. *Journal of the Statistical Society*, **5**, 168–76.

Statistical Society (1844). Second Report of the Committee on Hospital Statistics. *Journal of the Statistical Society*, **7**, 214–31.

Statistical Society (1862). Statistics of general hospitals of London 1861. *Journal of the Statistical Society*, **25**, 348–88.

Statistical Society (1866). Statistics of metropolitan and provincial general hospitals for 1865. *Journal of the Statistical Society*, **29**, 596–605.

Statutory Instruments (1968). *Medical Profession. The Abortion Regulations 1968*, SI No. 390. HMSO, London.

Statutory Instruments (1969). *Medical Profession. The Abortion (Amendment) Regulations 1969*, SI No. 636. HMSO, London.

Statutory Instruments (1976). *Medical Profession. The Abortion (Amendment) Regulations 1976*, SI No. 15. HMSO, London.

Statutory Instruments (1980*a*). *Medical Profession. The Abortion (Amendment) Regulations 1980*, SI No. 1724. HMSO, London.

Statutory Instruments (1980*b*). *Medical Profession. The Abortion (Scotland) (Amendment) Regulations 1980*, SI No. 1964 (S169). HMSO, London.

Statutory Instruments (1987). *Registration of births, deaths, marriages, etc. England and Wales. The Registration of Births and Deaths Regulations 1987*, SI No. 2088. HMSO, London.

Statutory Instruments (1988*a*). *Public Health, England and Wales. The Public Health (Infectious Diseases) Regulations 1988*, SI No. 1546. HMSO, London.

Statutory Instruments (1988*b*). *Public Health, Scotland, The Public Health (Notification of Infectious Diseases) (Scotland) Regulations 1988*, SI No. 1550 (SI55). HMSO, London.

Statutory Rules (1988). *Public Health. The Public Health Notifiable Diseases Order (Northern Ireland) 1988*, SR No. 319. HMSO, Belfast.

Statutory Rules of Northern Ireland (1990). *Public Health Notifiable Diseases Order (Northern Ireland) 1990*, SR No. 66. HMSO, Belfast.

Stewart, G.T. (1980). Whooping cough in the United Kingdom, 1977–78. *British Medical Journal*, **281**, 451–2.

Stewart, G.T. (1981). Whooping cough in relation to other childhood infections in 1977–79 in the United Kingdom. *Journal of Epidemiology and Community Health*, **35**, 139–45.

Stocks, P. (1949). *Sickness in the population of England and Wales 1944–47*. HMSO, London.

Swerdlow, A.J. (1986). Cancer registration in England and Wales: some aspects relevant to interpretation of the data. *Journal of the Royal Statistical Society*, **149**(2), 146–60.

Swerdlow, A.J. (1987). 150 years of Registrar-Generals' medical statistics. *Population Trends*, **48**, 20–6.

Swerdlow, A.J. (1989). Interpretation of England and Wales cancer mortality data: the effect of enquiries to certifiers for further information. *British Journal of Cancer*, **59**, 787–91.

Swerdlow, A. and dos Santos Silva, I. (1993). *Atlas of cancer incidence in England and Wales*. Oxford University Press.

Taylor, I. (1965). The notification of infectious disease in various countries. In *Trends in the study of normality and morbidity*, WHO Public Health Papers 27, p. 17. World Health Organization, Geneva.

Teague, A. (1993). Ethnic group: first results from the 1991 census. *Population Trends*, **72**, 12–17.

Tillett, E. and Spencer, I.L. (1982). Influenza surveillance in England and Wales using routine statistics. *Journal of Hygiene*, **88**, 83–94.

Vowles, M., Pethybridge, R.J., and Brimblecombe, F.S.W. (1975). Congenital malformations in Devon, their incidence, age and primary source of detection. In *Bridging in health—reports on studies for health services in children*, p. 201. Nuffield Provincial Hospitals Trust, Oxford.

Wadsworth, M.E.J., Butterfield, W.J.H., and Blaney, R. (1971). *Health and sickness: the choice of treatment*. Tavistock, London.

Weatherall, J.A.C. (1969). An assessment of the efficiency of notification of congenital malformations. *Medical Officer*, **121**, 65–8.

Weatherall, J.A.C. (1978). Congenital malformations: surveillance and reporting. *Population Trends*, **11**, 27–9.

Welsh Office (1987). *Welsh intercensal survey, 1986*. Welsh Office, Cardiff.

Werner, B. (1983). Family size and age at childbirth: trends and projections. *Population Trends*, **33**, 4–13.

West, R.R. (1973). Cancer registration by means of Hospital Activity Analysis. *Hospital and Health Services Review*, **69**, 372–4.

West, R.R. (1976). Accuracy of cancer registration. *British Journal of Preventative and Social Medicine*, **30**, 187–92.

Whates, P.D., Birzgalis, A.R., and Irving, M. (1982). Accuracy of hospital activity analysis operation codes. *British Medical Journal*, **284**, 1857–8.

White, A., Nicolaas, G., Foster, K., *et al.* (1993). *Health survey for England 1991*. London, HMSO.

Whitehead, F. (1987). The use of registration data for population statistics. *Population Trends*, **49**, 12–17.

WHO (World Health Organization) (1967). *Manual of the International Statistical Classification of Diseases, Injuries and Causes of Death (8th revision)*. World Health Organization, Geneva.

WHO (World Health Organization) (1977). *Manual of the International Statistical Classification of Diseases, Injuries and Causes of Death (9th revision)*. World Health Organization, Geneva.

WHO (World Health Organization) Regional Office for Europe (1966). *Studies of the accuracy and comparability of statistics on causes of death*. Unpublished WHO Document EURO–215, 1/16. World Health Organization, Copenhagen.

Wiggins, R. (1993). The validation of census data: post enumeration survey approaches. In *The 1991 census user's guide* (ed. A. Dale and C. Marsh), p. 129. HMSO, London.

Williams, W.O. (1970). A study of general practitioners' workload in South Wales, 1965–66. In *Reports from General Practice*, No. 12. Royal College of General Practitioners, London.

Wingrave, S.J., Beral, V., Adelstein, A.M., and Kay, C.R. (1981). Comparison of cause of death coding on death certificates with coding in the Royal College of General Practitioners Oral Contraceptive Study. *Journal of Epidemiology and Community Health*, **35**, 51–8.

4 Health information resources in Japan

Hiroshi Yanagawa and Masaki Nagai

Introduction

Health information systems that periodically provide population data on health and social factors in Japan are reviewed in this chapter. The criteria for selection of information systems in this review are (1) national coverage, (2) currently operational, (3) periodic data collection, (4) operated by governmental organizations, and (5) primary data rather than data compiled from other sources. For each system, we describe the background, the method of data collection, and the resulting official publications.

Population census

Population censuses have been conducted every five years in Japan since 1920, except for the suspension of 1945 census owing to the confusion at the end of the Second World War. In its place, an extraordinary census was carried out in 1947.

The censuses conducted every ten years, starting in 1920, are comprehensive, whereas those conducted between each decennial census are simplified. The items investigated in the simplified censuses were originally limited to basic characteristics of population. However, the items included after the Second World War, such as in 1955, 1965, and 1975, were expanded in response to the demand from users in various fields. The census covers the whole territory of Japan excluding the islands ruled by foreign countries.

Method of data collection

The whole area of Japan is divided into about 820 000 enumeration districts comprising 50 households on average. The census is carried out by about 750 000 census enumerators and census supervisors who are temporarily appointed by the Director-General of the Management and Co-ordination Agency of the Japanese Government. The enumerators distribute the census questionnaires, which the head of household is required to fill in as of 1 October of the census year. The Statistics Bureau of the Management and Co-ordination Agency of the Government takes charge of the tabulation of the results. The items investigated in the 1990 census are shown in Table 4.1.

The census supervisors take responsibility for the training and supervision of enumerators as well as for the inspection of the census document. Therefore the validity of the Japanese census is higher than that of any other set of national statistics.

Table 4.1 Items investigated in the 1990 Japanese census

Household members
Name
Sex
Year and month of birth
Relationship to the head of the household
Marital status
Nationality
Place of residence five years previously
Education
Type of activity
Name of establishment and classification of business
Type of occupation
Employment status
Place of work or location of school
Commuting time to the place of work or school

Households
Type of household
Number of household members
Source of household income
Type and tenure of dwelling
Number of dwelling rooms
Area of floor space of dwelling rooms
Type of building and number of storeys

Official publications

The official publications of the census are as follows.

1. The preliminary counts of the population by sex, by prefecture (47 prefectures), and by municipality (about 3300 cities, towns, and villages) are published two months after the survey. These counts are based on the entries on the summary sheets of the census, which are prepared by prefectures and municipalities. The title of this report is *Preliminary counts of the population on the basis of summary sheets.*

2. A prompt tabulation is made of the principal statistics based on a 1 per cent sample of the households. This is published as the *Population census of Japan, prompt report of the basic findings (results of one per cent sample tabulation).*

3. The final counts of population and households for the entire country and the prefectures and municipalities are published as *Population and households (final counts)*.

4. The first complete tabulation is of the basic characteristics of population and households. This is published in *Population census of Japan, Volume 1—Total population, and Volume 2—Results of the first basic complete tabulations: Part 1—Japan; Part 2—Prefectures and municipalities*. The second complete tabulation includes basic statistics on economic structure within the municipalities. The publications are *Population census of Japan, Volume 3—Results of the second basic complete tabulation: Part 1—Japan; Part 2—Prefectures and municipalities*. The third tabulation includes basic statistics on the occupational structure of population at the level of municipalities as well as statistics on specific households such as single elderly person households and mother–child households. The publications are *Population census of Japan, Volume 4—Results of the third basic complete tabulation: Part 1—Japan; Part 2—Prefectures and municipalities*.

5. A detailed tabulation of statistics covering the whole country is carried out for a 20 per cent sample of households. Statistics on detailed classification of industry and occupation, and on socio-economic groups, are included. These are published in *Population census of Japan, Volume 5—Results of detailed sample tabulation: Part 1—Whole of Japan; Part 2—Prefectures*.

6. Statistics on place of work or location of school are published by sex, age, occupation, and place of work. This tabulation identifies the daily movement of workers and students between their homes and places of work or study, and the daytime population of each locality. Data are published in *Population census of Japan, Volume 6—Commutation: Part 1—Place of work or schooling of population by sex, age and industry; Part 2—Place of work or schooling of population by occupation; Part 3—Place of work or schooling of population by industry and occupation*.

Vital statistics report

Vital statistics in Japan date from 1872. The statistics are compiled from the notification of birth, death, stillbirth, marriage, and divorce. They are nationwide, cover the entire population of Japan, and are collected for promoting health services.

Method of data collection

The local health centres (municipal facilities for personal and environmental health services established under the jurisdiction of Community Health Act) collect vital statistics records from legal documents: birth, death, stillbirth, marriage, and divorce certificates. These records are sent to the Prefectural Health Department every month and then to Ministry of Health and Welfare of the Japanese Government. Statistical analyses are made by the Statistics and Information Department of the Ministry. The five record forms compiled in Japan and their principal items are listed in Tables 4.2 to 4.6. Statistics for people in Japan (Japanese and other nationalities) and for Japanese people abroad are analysed.

Table 4.2 Items included in birth records

Name
Names of parents
Sex
Legitimacy of birth
Date of birth
Address
Age of parents at birth
Date of marriage
Nationality
Occupation of head of household
Weight at birth
Plurality
Place of delivery
Length of gestation
Number of previous births
Attendant at birth

Table 4.3 Items included on death records

Name
Sex
Address
Date of birth
Date of death
Nationality
Marital status
Occupation of household
Place of death
Causes of death

Table 4.4 Items included on fetal death records

Name of parents
Age of parents
Marital status
Date of delivery
Address of mother
Occupation of head of household
Number of previous live births and fetal deaths
Length of gestation
Weight of fetus
Place of delivery
Plurality
Type of delivery
Attendant at birth
Cause of fetal death

Table 4.5 Items included on marriage records

Names of bride and groom
Dates of birth
Address of groom
Nationality
Date of marriage
Marriage order
Occupation of household heads before marriage

Table 4.7 Contents of annual *Vital statistics reports*

Volume 1 (summary)

Volume 2 (detailed statistics)
Live births
Deaths
Infant deaths
Fetal deaths
Perinatal deaths
Marriages
Divorces
Appendix (vital statistics for foreigners in Japan and Japanese in foreign countries)

Volume 3 (detailed statistics)
Cause of death
Cause of infant death
Cause of fetal death
Cause of perinatal death
Appendix (cause of death of foreigners in Japan and Japanese in foreign countries)

All Japanese citizens are registered by the family registration act and are required to notify to the local government changes of registration status brought about by birth, death, stillbirth, marriage, and divorce. Therefore the validity of the vital statistics in Japan is very high except for the cause of death in certain diseases. Improvement in this area is expected as a result of the tenth revision of International Classification of Disease (ICD).

Official publications

Annual *Vital statistics reports* (three volumes) are published not more than eighteen months after the end of the year of data collection. The contents of the reports are summarized in Table 4.7.

Monthly vital statistics reports, which include basic monthly statistics and cumulative data of the year, are published no later than six months after data collection. A special series of vital statistics reports tabulated for socio-economic factors is published every year, and those for occupation and industry are published every five years. These series are based on sampling surveys.

Statistics on age-adjusted mortality rate, by sex and prefecture, for leading causes of death have been published every five years since 1960.

Communicable disease statistics

Weekly statistics of communicable disease were first compiled in 1880. The diseases included in this series are those listed by the Infectious Disease Prevention Act, recently the Venereal Disease Prevention Act, the Tuberculosis Prevention Act, the Leprosy Prevention Act, and the AIDS Prevention Act.

The infectious diseases currently included are shown in Table 4.8. The purpose of notification is to examine trends in communi-

cable diseases and to facilitate the planning and evaluation of control programmes.

Method of data collection

Based on the Acts relating to infectious disease prevention, physicians who diagnose the diseases mentioned above are required to notify their local health centre. The director of each local health centre reports to the Prefectural Health Department. The records are sent to the Statistics and Information Department, Ministry of Health and Welfare, by the end of the following month.

Doctors complete one of the three different notification forms that are used according to which diseases are diagnosed. One is for the majority of infectious diseases but excludes tuberculosis,

Table 4.6 Items included on divorce records

Names of husband and wife
Dates of birth of husband and wife
Nationality
Legal type
Number of children
Date of marriage
Date of divorce
Address before divorce
Main sources of income in the family before divorce

Table 4.8 Diseases included in statistics of communicable diseases

Cholera	Dysentery (amoebic or bacillary)
Typhoid fever	Paratyphoid fever
Smallpox	Typhus
Scarlet fever	Diphtheria
Epidemic encephalomyelitis	Plague
Japanese encephalitis	Poliomyelitis
Lassa fever	Influenza
Rabies	Anthrax
Infectious diarrhoea	Whooping cough
Measles	Tetanus
Malaria	Tsutsugamushi disease
Filariasis	Yellow fever
Relapsing fever	
Syphilis	Gonorrhoea
Chancroid	Lymphogranuloma inguinale
Tuberculosis	Leprosy
AIDS	

Table 4.9 Items included on the communicable disease notification form

Name of disease
Date of onset
Date of doctor's visit
Date of diagnosis
Method of diagnosis
Date of death
Name
Sex
Date of birth
Address
Present location of patient
Occupation
Name and occupation of household head
Doctor's name and address

Table 4.10 Items included on the tuberculosis and leprosy notification form

Name of disease
Date of onset
Date of doctor's visit
Date of diagnosis
Name
Sex
Date of birth
Address
Present location of patient
Occupation of household head
Doctor's name and address

Table 4.11 Items included on the venereal disease notification form

Name of disease
Type and stage (syphilis and gonorrhoea only)
Sex
Age
Occupation
Occupation of the infection source person
Name of facility
Doctor's name and address

leprosy, and venereal diseases. The items on this form are shown in Table 4.9. The items on the form for tuberculosis and leprosy are shown in Table 4.10. Items on the venereal disease notification form are shown in Table 4.11.

The notification rates range widely between diseases, with lower rates found in reporting common mild diseases (influenza, scarlet fever, whooping cough, measles, infectious diarrhoea, etc.).

Official publications

A report is published every year by the Statistics and Information Department, Ministry of Health and Welfare. Numbers and case rates of each disease are tabulated by year, month, sex, age, and prefecture. Detailed tabulations are made for certain diseases. For example, a table by group of bacillus is made in shigellosis. Tabulation by stage is made for cases of syphilis.

Infectious disease surveillance

The surveillance of infectious diseases based on notification from monitor clinics and hospitals throughout Japan started in 1981, and the on-line computer database system started in 1987.

Methods of data collection

Weekly data on specified infectious diseases are collected from monitor facilities. The monitor facilities, which consist of four types of clinics or departments in hospitals, are selected in each health centre district in proportion to population size. The monitor facilities for the diseases mainly prevalent in children are selected from paediatric facilities, those for ophthalmological diseases are from ophthalmological facilities, and those for sexually transmitted diseases are from urological or gynecological facilities. Data from these three types of monitor facilities are collected on a weekly basis. The last type is for the diseases mainly treated in hospitals. The monitor facilities for this type are selected from hospitals. Data from the last type are collected on a monthly basis. Lists of diseases according to each category of monitor station are shown in Table 4.12.

The monitor stations are usually selected intentionally and therefore do not necessarily represent the local situation correctly in some health centre districts. The frequency of patients in certain districts is measured on a number of patients per station basis. While this system provides good estimates of temporal trends, it does not provide good estimates of incidence rates and area differences.

Official publications

Weekly reports on the on-line computer system are available at the health centres by the following Thursday morning and monthly reports by the fourth day of the following month.

A summary report is published every year by the Bureau of Health and Medical Care, Ministry of Health and Welfare. Numbers of reported cases per monitor facility are tabulated by month and week.

Food poisoning statistics

Statistics on cases of food poisoning in Japan have been available since the reporting system for food poisoning and misapplication of drugs was established in Japan in 1952. The Food Sanitation Act, which was enacted in 1947, made it compulsory for doctors to report cases of food poisoning.

Method of data collection

Doctors who diagnose food poisoning notify local health centres. On notification, the health centre investigates the causative food

Table 4.12 Lists of diseases notified according to type of monitor station

Paediatric facilities
Measles
Rubella
Chickenpox
Mumps
Pertussis
Streptococcal infection
Atypical pneumonia
Infectious (viral and bacterial) gastroenteritis
Infantile vomiting and diarrhoea
Hand–foot–mouth disease
Erythema infectiosum
Exanthema subitum
Herpangina
Influenza
Kawasaki disease (mucocutaneous lymph node syndrome)

Ophthalmological facilities
Pharyngoconjunctival fever
Epidemic keratoconjunctivitis
Acute haemorrhagic conjunctivitis

Hospitals
Meningitis (septic and aseptic)
Encephalomyelitis
Viral hepatitis
Kawasaki disease (mucocutaneous lymph node syndrome)

Urological or gynaecological facilities
Gonorrhoea
Genital chlamydial infection
Genital herpes
Condyloma acuminatum
Trichomoniasis

Health centres
Tuberculosis

Table 4.13 Items included on the food poisoning notification form

Type of food poisoning
Date of onset
Date of doctor's visit
Date of diagnosis
Method of diagnosis (bacteriological, serological, clinical examination)
Date of death
Name
Sex
Date of birth
Address
Present location of patient
Occupation
Name and occupation of household head
Doctor's name and address

and pathogenic substance, and completes a food poisoning investigation form for each individual patient and a summary report of the food poisoning episode. The report is submitted to the Statistics and Information Department, Ministry of Health and Welfare. Items included on the notification form are shown in Table 4.13, and those additional items on the investigation form are listed in Table 4.14.

Many food poisoning cases are mild, and physicians hesitate to notify them to local health centres. The actual numbers of cases are estimated to be far more than the numbers notified.

Official publications

A report is published every year by the Statistics and Information Department, Ministry of Health and Welfare. The pathogenic agents in the report are classified as shown in Table 4.15.

Health Administration Survey

The Health Administration Survey was conducted annually from 1953 until 1985. Its purpose was to collect basic information on the structure of households and the socio-economic background of household members. The basic sampling frame was the same as

that used for the national health and disease surveys conducted by the Ministry of Health and Welfare.

Method of data collection

About 88 000 households (280 000 household members) in 1800 areas randomly sampled from census tracts with stratification were investigated. The questionnaire was completed by an interviewer who visited the households. The forms were collected by health centres and sent to the Statistics and Information Department, Ministry of Health and Welfare, through the prefectural governments. The principal items collected for each family member and household are shown in Table 4.16. The data collection is virtually complete.

Official publications

The report of the Health Administration Survey was published every year from 1953 to 1985. The results are available for all households and specified households such as those with elderly people, children, or a fatherless or motherless family. The survey was incorporated into the Basic Survey on Living Conditions, which was established in 1986.

National Health Survey

The National Health Survey is the principal source of information on levels and distribution of illness and impairment, and on treatment. The purpose of the survey is to provide national data on the prevalence of illness and impairment, and on the utilization of

Table 4.14 Items included on the food poisoning investigation form

Name of causative food
Place where the causative cooking was undertaken
Type of cooking of causative food
Microbiological examination
Prognosis
Principal symptoms
Description of place of occurrence
Type of food poisoning

Table 4.15 Pathogenic substances classified in the report

Bacteria
Salmonella species
Staphylococcus aureus
Clostridium botulinum
Vibrio parahaemolyticus
Escherichia coli (pathogenic)
Clostridium perfringens
Bacillus cereus
Yersinia enterocolitica
Campylobacter jejuni/coli
Non-0$_1$ *Vibrio cholerae*
Others

Chemical substances
Methanol
Others

Natural poisons
Poisonous plants
Poisonous animals

Unknown

medical facilities. The survey was initiated in 1948 and continued until 1985. It was incorporated into the Basic Survey on Living Conditions in 1986.

Method of data collection

Sampling followed two stages. The first stage was the sampling frame for the Health Administration Survey (1800 areas). The second stage used 700 of these areas, in which 16 000 households were located.

Before the interview survey, a calendar on which to record information about illness and impairment over a three-day period of investigation was distributed to the households. All household members in the survey areas were interviewed by interviewers who were trained and supervised by local health centre officials in the district. The survey forms consisted of a household summary sheet and an individual sheet for family members with disease during the

Table 4.16 Items included on the Health Administration Survey form

Family members
Relation to the family head
Date of birth
Sex
Marital status
Type of social insurance and pension
Occupation
Type of employment

Household
Type of household
Monthly household expenditure
Size of area under cultivation (farmers only)

Table 4.17 Items included on the National Health Survey form

Items for household summary sheet (all family members)
Sex
Date of birth
Type of health insurance
Occupation
Days of bed rest in a year
Days under treatment at medical institutions in a year

Items for individual personal sheet
Name of illness
Duration of illness
Type of treatment
Bed rest and sickness absence

specified three-day observation period. The items included on these two forms are listed in Table 4.17. The data collection is virtually complete.

Official publications

A report was published every year until 1985. Since 1986 the report has been included in the Basic Survey on Living Conditions.

Daily Life Survey

The Daily Life Survey, which started in 1962, was intended to collect information on family income, housing conditions, and various other aspects of family life. The questions on income were included every year, but other questions varied between years. The information obtained in this survey was useful for the planning of social security and social welfare.

Method of data collection

About 9000 households in 360 areas taken from the sample frame for the Health Administration Survey (approximately 1800 areas) were investigated by trained interviewers. The items studied in the 1985 survey, for example, included source of family income, taxation, participation in community affairs, and balance of the household economy. The data collection is virtually complete.

Official publications

The report was published every year from 1962 until 1985. Publications include a detailed report of income levels.

Basic Survey on Living Conditions

The Health Administration Survey, National Health Survey, and Daily Life Survey were incorporated into the Basic Survey on Living Conditions in 1986. The results of this survey provide fundamental data on levels of health, utilization of medical care, social welfare, pension, income, and life-styles. The surveys that are conducted every three years are comprehensive, whereas those conducted in the intervening years are simplified.

Method of data collection

In the 1992 survey, 250 000 households (780 000 household members) in 5240 areas sampled from 1990 census tracts were studied.

The questionnaires on incomes and savings were supplied to 40 000 households sampled from above the areas. Each household was visited by an interviewer who completed the form. The items studied are listed in Table 4.18. The questionnaire forms concerning private matters (such as income and bank account balances) are collected on a form with a sealed cover. The data collection is virtually complete.

Official publications

The results of the Basic Survey on Living Conditions are published annually.

Patient Survey

The Patient Survey is the principal source of information on utilization of hospitals and clinic services on one specified day and on hospital discharges over a one-month period. It provides information on the numbers and distribution of patients, their diagnosis, and the type of health insurance plan utilized.

Beginning in 1953, the Patient Survey was carried out annually on a sampling basis. About one in a hundred medical and dental clinics and one in ten hospitals were randomly selected and stratified by prefecture. The purpose of the study was to obtain fundamental information on patients treated in medical institutions. In 1984 the sampling frame of the survey was enlarged by a factor of three so that estimates could be made for 47 prefectures, and the frequency of the survey was reduced to once every three years.

Total numbers of medical facilities sampled for the 1993 survey were 6865 hospitals, 5884 medical clinics, and 983 dental clinics.

Method of data collection

Inpatients and outpatients on one specified day (One-Day Patient Survey) and in-patients who were discharged during one specified

Table 4.18 Items included in the Basic Survey on Living Conditions

Type of housing
Household expenses
Household structure
Sex
Date of birth
Marital status
Type of health insurance
Type of pension
Occupation
Bedridden or not
In hospital or not
Symptoms
Name of illness
Effects on daily activities
Participation in health examination
Knowledge on health
Total income by type
Total tax
Premium for social insurance
Total savings
Total loans

Table 4.19 Items included in Patient Surveys

One-day patient survey
Sex
Date of birth
Address
Type of treatment (inpatient or outpatient)
Name of illness or injury
Specialty of medical facility
Type of health insurance
Time of last visit
Route of consultation

One-month discharge survey
Sex
Date of birth
Address
Name of illness or injury
Specialty of medical facility
Type of health insurance
Date of hospital admission
Date of discharge
With or without surgical operation

month (One-Month Discharge Survey) in randomly sampled medical facilities stratified by prefecture throughout Japan are the subjects for this survey. The items included are listed in Table 4.19.

The response rate to the survey is almost 100 per cent. In some medical facilities, the questionnaire forms are filled out by clerical staff, which may cause some diversity in describing diagnoses. Sometimes the weather on the specified day influences the behaviour of the patients.

Official publications

The report of this survey was published every year until 1983. Since 1984, when the method of data collection changed, the report has been published once every three years. In 1993 the report consisted of three volumes: data for all Japan, data for prefectures, and data for medical service districts. Estimated numbers and rates of admissions and discharged patients according to ICD standards were tabulated for the items observed. The average length of hospital stay for discharged patients was also routinely assessed.

Tuberculosis statistics

Tuberculosis statistics were first collected in 1961 when the registration of this disease was introduced by the revision of Tuberculosis Control Act. Physicians who diagnose tuberculosis are required to notify the case to local health centres. Confirmed tuberculosis cases are registered and followed up by the health centre. Medical expenses for the treatment of tuberculosis are publicly subsidized by authority of the Tuberculosis Control Act.

The registration of tuberculosis cases ensures the availability of basic epidemiological data on this disease (such as incidence and prevalence rates according to the type of disease by sex, age, and prefecture, as well as type of treatment). The data are useful for evaluating countermeasures for tuberculosis provided by the Tuberculosis Control Act.

Table 4.20 Items included in the statistical tables for tuberculosis registration

Diagnostic category
Sex
Age
Address
Bacteriological finding
In hospital or not
Social health insurance

Method of data collection

Health centres are responsible for the registration of tuberculosis patients. Statistics on newly registered cases in a year and total registered cases at the end of the year are reported by health centres to the Statistics and Information Department, Ministry of Health and Welfare, through the prefectural government. The items included in the statistical tables are shown in Table 4.20. The registration rate is high because the medical expenses for notified tuberculosis cases are subsidized by the government.

Official publications

The Ministry of Health and Welfare publishes tuberculosis data every year. The tables included in the report are tabulated for prefectures and selected large cities.

Medical facility statistics

Statistics on medical facilities provide fundamental data for the analysis of the supply and geographical distribution of hospitals, medical clinics, and dental clinics. The survey first started in 1948.

Method of data collection

All hospitals, medical clinics, and dental clinics that are newly established, closed, or altered are required to submit a notification form (Table 4.21) to the governor of their prefecture.

Official publications

The Ministry of Health and Welfare publishes a yearly report on medical facilities. The number of hospitals, medical clinics, and

Table 4.21 Items included on the form for medical facility statistics

Name of the institution
Address
Ownership
Type of medical service offered
Medical specialty
Number of licensed beds
Number of staff (medical and paramedical)
Type of social health insurance accepted

dental clinics are tabulated by prefecture, ownership, medical specialty, and size of facility.

Hospital patient statistics

The data were first collected in 1945 and published as a weekly report of hospital patients; since 1948 reports have been monthly. At present, monthly statistics of hospital patients and the number of working staff at 1 October every year are collected.

Method of data collection

Information is gathered from all the hospitals in the country. Hospitals are required to submit a monthly report of hospital patients and an annual report of hospital employees. Table 4.22 shows the data collected on the monthly and yearly report forms. The collection of data is virtually complete.

Official publications

The Ministry of Health and Welfare publishes yearly reports. The average daily and monthly number of patients are calculated. These numbers are tabulated by type of hospital and prefecture. The occupancy rate and average length of patient stay in hospital is tabulated by type of bed and prefecture.

The numbers of hospital employees based on the annual reports are tabulated as number per 100 beds. The tabulation for each specialty is made on type of hospital, size of hospital, prefecture, and ownership.

Survey of physicians, dentists, and pharmacologists

The purpose of this survey is to obtain basic information on the number and distribution of physicians, dentists, and pharmacologists in Japan, and thus to aid medical administration. The reporting of physicians and dentists began in 1948 when the Medical Act and the Dentist Act became effective. The reporting

Table 4.22 Items included on the report forms for hospital patient statistics

Monthly report form
Cumulative number of monthly outpatients
Cumulative number of monthly inpatients
Number of newly admitted patients
Number of newly discharged patients
Number of hospital beds
Type of hospital
Ownership
Number of newborn babies

Yearly report form
Number of physicians
Number of dentists
Number of pharmacologists
Number of nurses
Number of assistant nurses
Number of midwives
Number of medical social workers
Number of other medical staff members
Number of clerical workers

of pharmacologists started six years later when the Drugs, Cosmetics, and Medical Instruments Act became effective. The reporting was primarily on an annual basis, but was revised to take place in alternate years beginning in 1982.

Method of data collection

Physicians, dentists, and pharmacologists are required to report their professional activities for the year to the local health centres. The items included in the forms are shown in Table 4.23. The reporting rates are usually over 90 per cent.

Official publications

Until 1982 a report of this survey was published every year by the Statistics and Information Department, Ministry of Health and Welfare. It is now produced biannually. Data on employment status, sex, age, specialty, and prefecture are also available.

National Nutrition Survey

The National Nutrition Survey has been conducted every year since 1952 under the Nutrition Improvement Act. The purpose of the survey is to investigate the intake of nutrients and health status in order to obtain fundamental data to improve nutrition.

At the beginning of the survey, the main object was the assessment of malnutrition. The dietary habits of the Japanese have changed greatly with the increase in national income levels. The intake of fat and animal protein has increased sharply. The current nutritional aims in Japan are to improve dietary habits, notably to prevent hypertension, stroke, and heart diseases.

Method of data collection

All households and household members in about 300 areas taken from the Japanese census are studied. The numbers of households and household members studied in 1993 were 5500 and 17 000, respectively. The survey consists of three parts: physical examination, a nutrient intake survey, and a dietary habit survey.

The physical examination surveys focus on chronic diseases of adults such as hypertension and heart diseases. The measurements taken in the 1993 survey were height, weight, skinfold thickness, blood examination (red cell count, haemoglobin, total cholesterol, triglyceride, HDL-cholesterol, total protein, and blood sugar), blood pressure, and physical fitness level.

Nutrient intake was estimated by recording the total food intake

---

Table 4.23 Items included on the physician, dentist, and pharmacologist report form

Name
Address
Address of legal residence
Registration number
Type of licence
Type of professional activities
Specialties
Name of institution
Address of institution

Table 4.24 Functions of health centres

Health education
Matters concerning vital statistics
Improvement in nutrition and food hygiene
Environmental health
Community activity of public health nurse
Medical social services
Maternal, child, and adult health
Dental health
Laboratory examination for personal and environmental health
Mental health
Control of communicable diseases
Other functions regarding community health

---

of each household for three consecutive days. Nutritionists specially trained for the survey visited each household at least once a day during the survey period and checked the records.

The dietary habit surveys vary between years. The 1993 survey included items on daily frequency and amounts of consumption of selected foods (such as confectionery, coffee, and tea), the time of taking the evening meals, the frequency of meal-taking after regular supper or dinner, and so on.

Since the measurement of the nutrient intake is on a household basis, it has a major disadvantage in the estimation of individual nutrient intake.

Official publications

The yearly reports are published by the Ministry of Health and Welfare. The average amount of energy, food, and nutrient intake per capita are calculated from the food intake records. These data are tabulated by geographical area, income level, whether the area is urban or rural, and the size and type of household. The weight, height, blood pressure levels, and skinfold thickness are tabulated by age and occupation.

Data on health centre activity

Health centres that are run by prefectural or city governments are core institutions in disease prevention and health promotion for the people in the community. The function of health centres is shown in Table 4.24.

When the Health Centre Act was first enforced in 1948, health centres were asked to submit a monthly report of their activities. In 1954 the format of the report was revised, and it has continued in this form, with minor revisions, to the present. Statistics are collected in order to obtain fundamental information on the activities of health centres and on the status of public health in the population of each administrative area.

Methods of data collection

Statistical tables covering the whole spectrum of health centre activities are prepared by the Ministry of Health and Welfare based on data supplied every year by the directors of health centres (some of the data are supplied quarterly). The tables are collected and tabulated at the Statistics and Information Department, Ministry of Health and Welfare. The forms of the statistical tables are shown

Table 4.25 Tables included in the report of health centre activity statistics

Number of health examinations
    Mental disorders, stomach and uterine cancers, hypertension, pregnant women, newborn babies, three-year-old children, and other examinations

Number of pregnancies notified

Amount of health guidance for mothers and children

Amount of guidance for disabled people

Number of consultation and home visits by public health nurses
    Mental disorders, medical social work, health education

Number of vaccinations

Activities on tuberculosis control

Number of bacteriological examinations

Number of parasitological examinations

Number of food hygiene inspections

Number of environmental sanitation inspections

Number of drinking water examinations

Table 4.26 Information required from local government for the Report on Health Services for the Elderly

Number of health record books issued

Number of health consultations

Number of health education sessions

Number of fundamental health examinations
    Basic and detailed examinations for hypertension, liver disorders, diabetes, and anaemia

Number of cancer examinations
    Early detection for stomach, uterine, lung, breast, and colon cancer

Amount of functional training

Number of visits for guidance (mainly by public health nurses)

in Table 4.25. This is an administrative report ordered by the government: therefore the reporting rate is 100 per cent.

Official publications

The report, which is published annually, describes all the activities of more than 800 health centres throughout Japan. The statistical tables are given by prefecture and for selected large cities.

Statistics on health services for the elderly

With the enforcement of Health and Medical Services Act for the Elderly in 1983, a variety of health services for the elderly were provided by local governments throughout Japan (about 3300 cities, towns, and villages). The Report on Health Services for the Elderly is intended to provide fundamental statistics regarding health activities directed at the ageing population.

Method of data collection

Local governments are required to submit details of health activities for the elderly for each fiscal year, using a form prepared by the Ministry of Health and Welfare. The information required is shown in Table 4.26. This is an administrative report ordered by the government, and therefore the reporting rate is 100 per cent.

Official publications

The Report on Health Services for the Elderly is published every year and information is given by prefecture. The number of staff by specialty engaged in each activity is also tabulated for each prefecture.

Statistics on health care facilities for the elderly

These statistics give information on the distribution and function of health care facilities that provide medical care and daily living assistance to the bedridden elderly. The facilities are implemented and financially subsidized by the public under the authority of the Health and Medical Services Act for the Elderly. The statistics were first collected in 1988.

Methods of data collection

Health care facilities for the elderly are required to submit reporting forms to the Ministry of Health and Welfare through the prefectural government. The information required is shown in Table 4.27. This is an administrative report ordered by the government, and therefore the reporting rate is 100 per cent.

Official publications

The report on health facilities for the elderly is published every year and information is given by prefecture. Statistics on the

Table 4.27 Items for the statistics on health care facilities for the elderly

Institution form
Location
Capacity
Service fee
Working status of the employees

User form
Sex
Age
Reason for using the facility
Type of illness
Physical and mental condition
Activities of daily life
Type of health insurance

Table 4.28 Items for the eugenic operation and induced abortion forms

Eugenic operation form
Name
Sex
Address
Reason for operation
Date of operation
Type of operation

Induced abortion form
Age
Address
Week of pregnancy
Date of abortion
Reason for abortion
Public assistance of medical expense

---

facilities for the elderly, patients under care, and personnel in the facilities tabulated by prefecture are available.

Eugenic protection statistics

These statistics provide information on eugenic operations (tubal sterilization, vasoligation, vasectomy) and induced abortions as well as a survey of maternal health. The statistics were first collected in 1948 by monthly reporting of eugenic operations and induced abortions. The present system of yearly collection of statistics began in 1969.

Method of data collection

Physicians who perform eugenic operations are required to submit a report form to the local health centre under the Eugenic Protection Act. Each prefecture collects all the reports from local health centres and prepares a yearly report. The Statistics and Information Department, Ministry of Health and Welfare, summarizes the reports from all prefectures. The items required for the eugenic operation form and the induced abortion form are shown in Table 4.28. No information on the reporting rate is available. It is believed that the actual number of eugenic operations is far greater than the number reported.

Official publications

The Ministry of Health and Welfare publishes a yearly report summarizing these data. The number and rate per unit population of eugenic operations and induced abortions by reason, sex, age, prefecture, and week of pregnancy (induced abortion only) are tabulated.

National medical care expenditure estimates

National medical care expenditure is the total amount of money paid to hospitals, medical and dental clinics, midwives, pharmacies, and other medical institutions. Medical care expenditure in Japan has continued to expand at a faster pace than the increase in national income. The factors affecting this increase include the increase in chronic diseases owing to the aging of the population,

popularization of highly developed medical techniques, and the high percentage of pharmaceutical expenses in the total medical expenditure.

Method of estimation of medical care expenditure

Annual national medical care expenditure is estimated from the annual amount of medical care carried out at public expense under the Daily Life Security Act, Tuberculosis Control Act, Mental Health Act, etc., social insurance (medical care insurance, national health insurance), medical services for the elderly, and personal expenses. Statistics from the Patient Survey are also used. Since the estimation is based on actual medical expenditures for each medical care system, reliability is high.

Official publications

The report on medical care expenditure is published every year and includes tables of the total amount, the percentage increase, expenditure per capita, proportion of gross national product and of national income, amount according to public liability of cost, amount by type of medical care, and amount by classification of disease.

Age-adjusted mortality rate—a special vital statistics report

Since 1960 the Statistics and Information Department, Ministry of Health and Welfare, has published age-adjusted mortality rates as a Special Report of Vital Statistics every five years. The aging of the population varies widely among prefectures in Japan. Therefore this report is useful for comparison of mortality rates among prefectures and between years.

Official publications

The report includes age-specific age-adjusted mortality rates by prefecture for selected causes. The standard population of this series was the 1960 Japanese population by sex for prefectural observation and the 1935 population for yearly observation. Because of the recent increase in the proportion of aged in the Japanese population, a new standard population based on the 1985 national census was introduced and the age-adjusted mortality rates were recalculated.

Life-tables

The first complete Japanese life-tables were calculated based on death for the period 1891–1898, and were published in 1902. Since then, the life-tables have been calculated seventeen times, approximately every five years. Since 1948 an abridged life-table has been calculated every year.

The latest complete life-table in Japan was constructed on the basis of mortality data from the vital statistics of 1990 and on the census population on 1 October 1990. The latest abridged life-table was calculated on the basis of mortality data and estimated population on 1 October 1994.

Official publications

The complete life-tables are published every five years, and the abridged life-tables are published every year.

Table 4.29 Items on inclusion and exclusion forms for public assistance recipients

Inclusion form
Type of household
Past recipient
Reason
Duration of unemployment
Source of income
Type of assistance
Housing conditions
Medical assistance
Family members

Exclusion form
Date of starting assistance
Reason for assistance and for stopping
Type of assistance
Medical assistance
Family members

National survey of public assistance recipients

This survey provides a unique source of data on the number and distribution of households that receive public assistance under the Daily Life Security Act. The report was begun in 1956.

Method of data collection

The report is based on two forms—the inclusion form and the exclusion form. The inclusion form is for households that start to receive public assistance, and the exclusion form is for those that have stopped receiving assistance. Local social welfare organizations complete the survey forms. The items in the inclusion and exclusion forms are shown in Table 4.29. This is an administrative report, and reliability is high.

Official publications

The report is published every year by the Statistics and Information Department, Ministry of Health and Welfare. Yearly changes, type of household, reasons for giving assistance and its withdrawal, period of assistance, type of assistance, and distribution by prefecture are described in the report summary.

Summary table

All the information sources described in this chapter are summarized in Table 4.30.

Concluding comments

All the information described in this chapter is prescribed by various statutes. Therefore data collection is almost perfect. However, some of the surveys based on notification by physicians are less reliable. Details regarding this point are provided in each section. The health information is used by health personnel in public health centres, health administrators in central and local health departments, and medical researchers. Access to this

Table 4.30 List of official publication of health and social information*†

Population census of Japan (published every five years, 1920–)*†
Preliminary counts of population on the basis of summary sheets
Prompt report of the basic findings (results of 1 per cent sample tabulation)
Population and households (final counts)
Basic complete tabulation
   Volume 1—Total population
   Volume 2—Results of the first basic complete tabulation
   Volume 3—Results of the second basic complete tabulation
   Volume 4—Results of the third basic complete tabulation
Detailed sample tabulations
Tabulation on place of work or location of school

Vital statistics report (yearly, 1872–)
   Volume 1—Summary of the results
   Volume 2—Birth, total death, fetal death, perinatal death, marriage, and divorce
   Volume 3—Death, infant death, fetal death, and perinatal death by cause
Special series of vital statistics
   Socioeconomic characteristics (every year)
   Age-adjusted mortality rate (every five years)
   Statistics according to occupation and industry (every five years)

Communicable disease statistics (yearly, 1880–)

Infectious disease surveillance (yearly, 1981–)

Food poisoning statistics (yearly, 1880–)

Health administration survey (yearly, 1953–1985)
   Included in *Basic survey on living conditions* since 1986

National health survey (yearly, 1948–1985)
   Included in *Basic survey on living conditions* since 1986

Daily life survey (yearly, 1962–1985)
   Included in *Basic survey on living conditions* since 1986

Basic survey on living conditions (yearly, 1986–)

Patient survey (yearly, 1953–1983; every three years, 1984–)

Tuberculosis statistics (yearly, 1961–)

Medical facility statistics (yearly, 1948–)

Hospital patient statistics (yearly, 1948–)

Survey of physicians, dentists, and pharmacologists (yearly, 1948–)

National nutrition survey (yearly, 1952–)

Data on health centre activity (yearly, 1948–)

Report of health services for the elderly (yearly, 1983–)

Report of health care facilities for the elderly (yearly, 1988–)

Eugenic protection statistics (yearly, 1948–)

National medical care expenditure estimates (yearly, 1954–)

Life-tables (complete life-table about every five years, 1981–; abridged life-table yearly, 1948–)

National survey of public assistance recipients (yearly, 1956–)

---

* All publications are available from the Statistics and Information Department, Ministry of Health and Welfare of the Japanese Government, unless otherwise stated.

† Available from Statistics Bureau, Management and Coordination Agency of the Japanese Government.

information is easily obtainable in governmental offices, university libraries, and other places in Japan. All these reports can be purchased at bookstores and through the Government Printing Office.

5 Information systems for health outcome analysis

Edward B. Perrin

Introduction

The past decade has seen a rapid growth in the use of outcomes analysis for the purpose of decision making in public health. Although there has been a resurgence of interest, many of the ideas employed in these analyses are not new. The growth of activity in this area has been marked, however, by a significant broadening of the concept of outcomes of health care to include a richer mix of what could be characterized as non-clinical, patient-based outcome variables. Further, this broadening in scope has been accompanied by the development of several useful instruments for the measurement of these newly defined health outcome variables.

In this chapter we will examine a definition of health outcomes and present a framework for relating health outcomes to the relevant components of health care. We will discuss the most commonly observed types of health outcomes and will examine the methods available for their measurement. Finally, we will present examples of the use of outcome analysis in studying the health of populations and in evaluating the effect of public health interventions in those populations.

Health outcomes: definition and framework

Health outcomes are defined as the effects of health care or health service activity on the health and well being of individuals and populations. The successful application of this general definition depends, of course, on the specification of such important ideas as health and the effects of health service activities. Much of the recent research in outcomes has indeed been on the further development and measurement of the concepts of health and health effects that are basic to the application of health outcomes analysis (Wennberg 1990).

Perhaps the most useful model for relating health outcomes to the component elements of health services and for understanding the key role of health outcomes in the evaluation of health services is that presented by Donabedian (1966, 1985) in his work on the assessment and assurance of quality of health care. Donabedian (1966, 1985) suggested that the elements of health services can be divided into three major components: structure, process, and outcome. He defined structure as the human, physical, and financial resources available to provide the health services. The structure of health services would include such elements as, for example, the number, distribution, and qualification of professional personnel, the number and size of hospitals and other facilities, etc. He defined process as the care or health service provided to the patient or population in question and outcome as the resulting effect on the health of the individual or population.

The key element in Donabedian's (1966, 1985) model is the assertion that a fundamental functional relationship exists between these components of health services, as follows:

Structure → Process → Outcome

That is, the structure in which the health service is provided influences the process of care and the structure and process taken together affect the outcome. Thus, the health outcome is viewed as the end product of the health services system and the structure and process of health services are seen as potentially controllable components causally related to outcome.

Recognizing that this model is a simplified version of reality, Donabedian (1985, p. 84) stated that 'the three part division is a somewhat arbitrary abstraction from what is, in reality, a succession of less clearly differentiated, but causally related, elements in a chain that probably has many branches'. None the less, this representation has proved useful in organizing our thinking about the elements of health services and providing a framework for an evaluation process.

The Donabedian (1966, 1985) model is helpful in that it provides a means of illustrating the logic of health outcomes analysis and of emphasizing an important point, that is that there are two critical steps in carrying out an outcomes analysis and that both steps must be accomplished for a successful analysis. The steps are as follows.

1. The definition and measurement of the health outcome variables of interest.

2. The explication of the assumed causal relationship between the structure and process (that is, intervention) variables and the related health outcome variables.

This point, although seemingly an obvious one, requires emphasis because there is a tendency to feel that an outcome analysis is complete once the measurement of the outcome has been accomplished. In fact, the second step is critical if we are to achieve our objective, that is to make the appropriate inferences about the effectiveness of the process and structure (intervention) variables, the variables over which one usually has some programmatic control.

In this chapter we will be primarily concerned with the presentation of methodologies for defining and measuring health outcome variables and examples of their use. The methods for inferring the relationship between the outcomes and the process and structure variables in the case where that relationship is not known or not assumed to be known are, of course, the accepted methods of scientific inference (for example, randomized clinical trials, case–control studies, cohort studies, etc.), examples of which have been explored extensively elsewhere (for example, Cochrane 1972) and will be covered in more detail in the next section of this volume (e.g., Chapters 11 and 12). It can be said in this context, however, that health (or health services) research is usually characterized by a broader specification of outcome variables and more broadly defined and less easily measured and controlled structure and process variables (that is, interventions) than are found in purely clinical research. This, therefore, often renders the inference concerning the relationship of structure, process, and outcome more difficult, although none the less important, in this type of research.

Types of health outcomes

A health outcome is defined as the effect of a health services activity on the health and well being of an individual or population. It is most useful operationally to regard a health outcome as a change (either positive or negative) or maintenance in the health state or health status of an individual or population. Thus, the availability of measures of health status becomes important in the conduct of outcomes analysis.

In their report on the results of the Medical Outcomes Study (**MOS**), Tarlov et al. (1989) defined four classes of health outcomes as follows.

1. Clinical endpoints: signs and symptoms, laboratory values, and death.

2. Functional status: physical functioning, mental functioning, social functioning, and role functioning.

3. General well being: health perceptions, energy/fatigue, pain, and life satisfaction.

4. Satisfaction with care: access, convenience, financial coverage, quality, and general.

Other similar outcomes classification schemes exist (Lohr 1988; Kaplan 1989; FHSR 1994). Although some argue that patient satisfaction with care should not be considered a health outcome (Doessel and Marshall 1985), there is general agreement concerning the use of clinical endpoints and measures of functional status and general well being as outcome measures and an increasing acceptance of patient satisfaction as a goal of the health services system.

The use of clinical endpoints as outcomes measures has long been a tradition in medical and health services research. The clinical endpoints, the signs and symptoms of disease, physiological measurements, and the alive/dead state, have historically been the most frequently studied outcomes, for example in clinical trials and case–control studies. Whether one considers death as a clinical endpoint or a profound change in functional status, as one might,

death remains one of the most important, most easily defined and measured, most frequently recorded, and, therefore, most useful endpoints to the public health practitioner, of all health outcomes.

Changes in the frequency of the signs and symptoms of disease (that is, morbidity) are also important health outcomes, whether the desired outcome is the elimination of existing cases of disease or the prevention of new ones. In the final section we will discuss examples of current efforts at formalizing the analysis of mortality and morbidity outcomes as part of the practice of public health.

Much of the recent advance in the definition and measurement of health outcomes has been in the refinement of the concepts of functional status, well being, and satisfaction (Hunt et al. 1986; Smith 1988; Stewart and Ware 1992; Patrick and Erickson 1993). There has been an increased recognition of the centrality of the patient's view in the evaluation of health services outcomes (Geigle and Jones 1990) and an acceptance that the goal of health services is the achievement of a more effective life and the preservation of functioning and well being for individuals and populations (Schroeder 1987).

The terms 'health status' and 'quality of life' or, more precisely, 'health-related quality of life', are often used interchangeably in the study of health outcomes (Lohr 1989). Health status and quality of life, although significantly overlapping concepts, are not strictly equivalent in the sense that quality of life more clearly invokes the notion of value (Bergner 1990). For example, Patrick and Erickson (1992, p. 22) defined health-related quality of life as 'the value assigned to duration of life as modified by impairment, functional status, perception and social opportunities that are influenced by disease, injury, treatment or policy.' Others have written extensively on the importance of quality of life as a measure of the effectiveness of health services (Katz 1987; Walker and Rosser 1988; Baldwin et al. 1990; EuroQol Group 1990; Fallowfield 1990).

Similarly, the quantity (that is, duration of survival) and quality of life of individuals are distinct but related concepts. There has been much progress in recent years in developing methods to capture these two concepts in a single measure (Rosser 1990; Spilker 1990; Patrick and Bergner 1990; Feeny et al. 1991; Patrick and Erickson 1992), since both the quality and duration of life play an important role in the evaluation or the outcomes of health services.

Years of healthy life (**YHL**) is an example of a measure combining the quality and duration of life considerations. Briefly, the YHL of an individual during any period is defined as the duration of life of that individual during that period weighted by a fraction between 0 and 1 that estimates the quality of life of that individual during that period. For example, if during any one year an individual is estimated to have a quality of life 80 per cent of what would be considered optimal (that is, the quality of life is assigned a weight of 0.80), the individual would be credited with 0.80 of a YHL for that period. YHL can, of course, either be observed during the lifetime of an individual or predicted for future years using life table or cohort analysis estimation procedures. The calculation always requires an estimate of the relative quality of life of the individual during the period in question. It is worth noting that the concepts of YHL and quality-adjusted life years (**QALY**) are essentially equivalent and interchangeable and examples of both abound in the literature. Figure 5.1 illustrates the use of the YHL

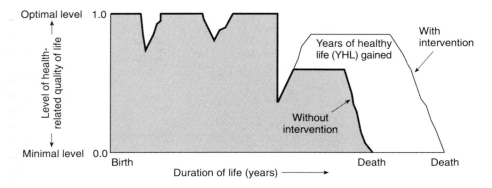

Fig. 5.1 Years of healthy life added by intervention for a prototype individual. (Reproduced from Torrance and Feeny (1989), with permission.)

measure in evaluating the outcome of an intervention on a prototype individual.

Measures of health status and quality of life

Employing a health outcomes measure appropriate to the process or intervention being studied is, of course, a key to a successful health outcomes analysis. As suggested, simple morbidity and mortality measures have been useful in the past and, indeed, retain their usefulness today. There has, however, been a need to extend the range of available measures to cover the recently refined concepts of health status and quality of life. For example, as we have seen above, such measures are necessary if we are to employ the concept of YHL or QALY in a refinement of a simple survival analysis. During the past three decades researchers have succeeded in developing many measures of health status and quality of life and they are well catalogued (McDowell and Newell 1987; Bowling 1994). We will review only a few of the more widely used measures here.

Health status and quality of life assessment instruments can, in general, be classified along many dimensions, but perhaps two of the most important are the range of populations or domain for which the instrument is intended and the type of score produced on the application of the instrument. In the case of the domain, there are two major subclasses: generic (applies across all disease and population groups) and disease specific (applied to a specific disease or condition grouping only). With respect to the type of score produced there are three major subclasses: single indicator numbers, profile of interrelated scores, and a battery of independent scores. Almost all available health status and quality of life assessment instruments can be classified in this taxonomy and there are advantages and disadvantages to each class of instruments. For example, a generic measure is more broadly applicable than a disease-specific measure but in some cases may be less responsive to change in that disease-specific population. Similarly, a single indicator may be more useful for population monitoring than a profile of interrelated scores but, in turn, may be less responsive to change. The selection of a particular measure will, of course, depend on the needs of the investigator. A more complete discussion of the strengths and weaknesses of these various categories of measures can be found in Patrick and Erickson (1993, pp. 113–42).

The Sickness Impact Profile (**SIP**) is one of the earliest developed (Gilson *et al.* 1975) and, until recently, most extensively used (for example, Deyo 1986) of the generic health profile class of assessment instruments. The SIP uses responses to 136 items to assess sickness-related dysfunction in 12 different areas of activity along the dimensions of independent, physical, and psychosocial functioning. It was developed to provide a measure of perceived health status that would be sensitive enough to detect changes or differences in health status that might occur over time or between groups. A major strength of the SIP is its broad coverage of the concept of quality of life and its sensitivity in a wide variety of situations. A British–English version of the SIP, known as the Functional Limitations Profile (**FLP**), is available (Charlton *et al.* 1983*b*).

A similar generic health profile instrument, the Nottingham Health Profile (**NHP**), has been used extensively and proved useful in evaluating health interventions in Britain and Western Europe (Jenkinson *et al.* 1988) and has been translated into a number of languages (for example, Alonso *et al.* 1990). The NHP instrument consists of two parts and can be used to produce scores for each of 13 domains of experience, including, for example pain, physical mobility, and social isolation.

A shorter health profile instrument, the short-form health survey or the **SF-36**, so named because it contains only 36 items, has become available in the past few years (Ware and Sherbourne 1992), has been translated to and validated in several languages and is increasingly becoming the patient-based outcomes measurement instrument of choice. The SF-36 was developed from measures used in the Health Insurance Experiment (Brook *et al.* 1979). It was the assessment instrument employed in the MOS (Tarlov *et al.* 1989), a study designed to determine whether variation in health outcomes could be explained by differences in organization of care delivery, clinician specialty, or the clinician's technical and interpersonal style. The SF-36 includes one multi-item scale measuring each of eight health concepts: physical functioning; role limitations because of physical health problems, bodily pain, social functioning, general mental health (psychological distress and psychological well being), role limitations because of emotional problems, vitality (energy/fatigue), and general health perceptions. Thus, the SF-36 permits scoring of a set of eight scales displayed as a profile of health status concepts. Figure 5.2, for example, shows the difference observed in the average profile of a group of 638 chronically ill but relatively well patients when compared with 168 severely

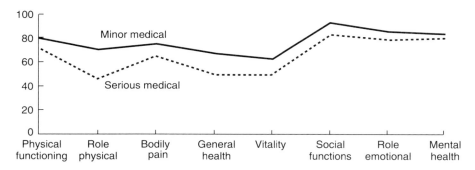

Fig. 5.2 SF-36 Profile for patient groups with minor versus serious medical conditions. (Source: Ware, J.E., *et al.* (1993) *SF-36 Health Survey Manual and Interpretation Guide.* The Health Institute, New England Medical Center, Boston, MA.)

chronically ill patients on the eight scales measured by the SF-36 (McHorney *et al.* 1993).

The SF-36 can be self-administered in approximately 3 min, the scores are readily computed, and considerable information on population norms has been accumulated in the use of the instrument thus far. For widespread application in large populations, even shorter forms, for example the SF-12, are now available (Ware *et al.* 1996).

In addition to generic health profile measures such as those cited above, there are a large number of disease or condition-specific measures of health status and quality of life which can be useful in measuring health outcomes in special populations. Examples of instruments of this type are the EORTC—Quality of Life Questionnaire for Cancer Patients (Aaronson *et al.* 1993), the Quality of Life Questionnaire for Asthma (Townsend *et al.* 1991), and the McMaster–Toronto Arthritis Patient Preference Disability Questionnaire (**MACTAR**) (Tugwell *et al.* 1983). A more complete listing of these condition-specific instruments can be found in Patrick and Erickson (1992) or Bowling (1994). As noted, these instruments are sometimes especially useful in measuring changes in health status, that is health outcomes, in condition-specific populations and often can be used in conjunction with generic measures.

Although the trend has most recently been towards using profiles of measures for examining health status such as those cited above, there has been a tradition of attempting to define single indicators or summary measures of health status that could be useful in the evaluation of health outcomes. An example of a disease-specific single indicator that has long been in use is the Karnofsky Performance Status Scale for Cancer (Karnofsky and Burchemal 1949). Similarly, an example of a generic single index is the Quality of Life (**QWB**) Index (Kaplan *et al.* 1984) which produces a score summarizing different health status and quality of life dimensions. Mortality and morbidity rates can also be thought of as either generic or disease-specific single indicators of health status and, while relatively crude measures, can, as we shall see in the next section, be of value to the public health practitioner in the evaluation of health outcomes.

Information systems for assessing population health outcomes

The more sophisticated health status and quality of life measurement instruments, such as the SF-36, are proving very useful in

clinical trials and other special studies on the outcomes of medical care (Spilker 1990; Feeny *et al.* 1991; Patrick and Erickson 1992). Unfortunately, these methods are of relatively recent development and may involve more costly and time-consuming data collection techniques than can reasonably be applied on a large scale, at least until the use of shorter instruments such as the SF-12 becomes more widespread. Thus, information on health status using these measures has not generally been available for populations of significant size, that is for county, state, or regional populations, for example, or even for the parts of those populations which have been diagnosed as having a particular disease or condition. The exception to this has been the inclusion of measures of general health perception, activity restriction, and physical impairment in national sample surveys such as the National Health Interview Survey (**NHIS**) and the National Health and Nutrition Examination Survey (**NHANES**) in the United States (NCHS 1992). However, the relatively small sample sizes and the cross-sectional nature of these surveys have thus far limited their usefulness in the study of health outcomes.

Recently, an organized effort to obtain outcomes information for a special set of conditions in a larger population was mounted by the US Department of Health and Human Services in its Medical Treatment Effectiveness Program (**MEDTEP**) (AHCPR 1990; Maklan *et al.* 1994). In this programme patient outcomes research teams (**PORTS**) were created at research institutions in the United States to investigate health services outcomes for a set of 14 conditions or diagnoses: back pain, ischemic heart disease, prostate disease, cataracts, diabetes, pneumonia, knee replacement, hip replacement, acute myocardial infarction, biliary tract disease, childbirth management, stroke, schizophrenia, and low birth weight. The emphasis in these PORTS has been not in the generation of new data sets but in the use of available data for 'developing and disseminating scientific information regarding the effect of presently used health care services and procedures on patient survival, health status, functional capacity and quality of life' (AHCPR 1990, p. 1). In addition to using the methodology of meta-analysis to summarize previous research findings in the area, much effort has been put into investigating the use of automated administrative and survey databases to study the outcomes of care for these conditions (AHCPR 1991; Grady and Schwartz 1992). Deyo *et al.* (1994) have, for example, examined methods for identifying episodes of low back pain and for quantifying the severity of unrelated, comorbid medical conditions from administrative data sets and studied the potential for using these methods in outcomes analysis.

In another population-based system, investigators in Manitoba, Canada, have embarked upon a programme to develop methods for using the administrative data sets of that province to study health outcomes (Roos *et al.* 1988). They report success in using administrative data sets in populations to develop control groups and adjust for case severity, important steps in health outcomes studies (Roos 1989).

Perhaps the most significant effort to date in adapting existing national data sets for use in assessing outcomes in populations had its beginnings in the work of Charlton *et al.* (1983*a*) and the European Community (**EC**) Concerted Action Project in Health Services and Avoidable Deaths and resulted in the publication of the *European Community atlas of avoidable death* (Holland 1993). The work of this group has been significantly expanded in both scope and concept under the direction of the Department of Health in Britain, leading to the publication of a feasibility study defining the theoretical basis for suggested population health indicators, including morbidity indicators, for the National Health Service (**NHS**) (McColl and Gulliford 1993) and a consultation document for use by regional and district health authorities (University of Surrey 1993) in applying these indicators to outcomes analysis.

The idea of defining certain deaths and diseases in the population as 'avoidable' and regarding the occurrence of these avoidable deaths and diseases as negative health outcomes is, of course, widely accepted in the practice of public health (Mackenbach *et al.* 1990). Infant deaths, for example, have often been regarded in this manner and the causes actively investigated. Similarly, many communicable diseases, for example tuberculosis and poliomyelitis, now fall into that category in various countries of the world. A theoretical framework for viewing 'unnecessary disease and disability and unnecessary untimely death' as measures of quality of health care, that is as negative health outcomes, was presented by Rutstein *et al.* (1976). In their presentation the authors argued that, although caution should be exercised in ascribing cause and effect, an excessive number, perhaps even a single one, of these unnecessary events (outcomes) could serve as a warning signal of possible shortcomings in the health services system. Rutstein *et al.* (1976) presented a list of what they considered unnecessary and untimely health events.

The *European Community atlas of avoidable deaths* (Holland 1993) provides an example of the use of national vital statistics systems as a data source for the study of health outcomes based on this model. Having as its roots a list of relevant disease categories developed in the study of geographical variations in England and Wales (Charlton *et al.* 1987), the EC atlas presents data on mortality in the following 17 disease groups (each defined by a discrete set of ICD–8 codes):

1. tuberculosis;

2. malignant neoplasm of cervix uteri;

3. malignant neoplasm of cervix and body of uterus;

4. Hodgkin's disease;

5. chronic rheumatic heart disease;

6. all respiratory diseases;

7. asthma;

8. appendicitis;

9. abdominal hernia;

10. cholelithiasis and cholecystitis;

11. hypertensive and cerebrovascular diseases;

12. maternal deaths (all causes);

13. perinatal mortality;

14. infectious diseases;

15. malignant neoplasm of trachea, bronchus, and lung;

16. cirrhosis of liver;

17. motor vehicle accidents.

Data for the most recent time period available are presented in the atlas in tabular form and as standard mortality ratios in a series of maps of the entire EC region and of the countries individually. This provides an opportunity to view both between- and within-country variation in what might be considered 'avoidable mortality' in each of these disease groupings.

The step of relating observed variation in health outcome (avoidable mortality) to variation in process (for example, personal or public health services), cited previously as being such an important part of this analysis, must be approached with considerable care in this non-experimental situation. In fact, the authors of the atlas quite correctly state in the introduction to the first edition that 'the interpretation of the relationship between health service inputs, indicators of social conditions and avoidable deaths is complex and requires further research' (Holland 1993, p. 2). They see two uses of the avoidable death indicators in the atlas. The first is to examine whether significant geographic variations in mortality outcome exist for specific areas of health service activity in a region. The second is to identify problems to be investigated by local studies in an effort to identify health services which might be improved. These are modest but useful objectives and the EC atlas provides a good illustration of a type of outcomes analysis which can be of value in regions of the world where routinely collected mortality data are available.

In its development of population health indicators for use by the NHS of England and Wales (McColl and Guilliford 1993; University of Surrey 1993), the Faculty of Public Health Medicine of the Royal College of Physicians, London, while including nine of the avoidable death indicators from the EC atlas, expanded the concept of population health indicators significantly by defining a new set of 30 indicators, not necessarily mortality based, in the following 12 clinical areas:

1. breast cancer;

2. diabetes mellitus;

3. peptic ulcer;

4. osteoporosis and hip fracture;

5. unplanned pregnancy and termination of pregnancy;

6. congenital abnormalities;

7. skull fracture and intracranial injury;

8. childhood immunizations;

9. early orchidopexy for cryptorchidism;

10. acceptance rate for renal replacement therapy;

11. suicide;

12. schizophrenia.

In selecting these 12 clinical areas the goal of the developers was to create a set of outcome indicators for the NHS which would reflect effective health service intervention, be based on routinely collected reliable data, and reflect local health service intervention.

The following information was developed and presented in the feasibility study for each of the 12 clinical areas and for the 9 avoidable death indicators from the EC atlas:

1. definition of the basic health problem;

2. expectation of change;

3. definition of outcome objective;

4. definition of service/intervention required;

5. definition of indicator(s);

6. definition of data;

7. constraints in using the indicator;

8. extent to which an indicator reflects local health service provision.

In the area of osteoporosis and hip fracture, for example, the outcome objective was defined in the NHS document as the reduction of the incidence of hospital admissions and deaths from hip fractures and the following three indicators were defined for measuring progress toward that objective.

1. Annual admission rates for hip fracture per 10 000 regional and district residents over the age of 65 years.

2. District and regional standardized mortality ratios for deaths between the ages of 65 and 84 years inclusive caused by fracture of proximal femur.

3. District and regional standardized mortality ratios for deaths over the age of 85 years caused by fracture of proximal femur.

Similarly, the outcome objective identified in schizophrenia was the reduction of premature deaths in people with that condition. The outcome indicator was defined as the regional standardized mortality ratios for deaths mentioned as associated with schizophrenic psychoses under the age of 75 years.

As indicated, the presentation of information in each of these clinical areas in the NHS report includes a discussion of such important issues as the definition of the intervention required, the change to be expected, etc. This approach can be seen to be similar in some ways to the approach of the US Public Health Service (1991) in its development of its health objectives for the year 2000, but is much more complete in its discussion of the assumed

relationship between intervention (process) and outcome of the issues of data availability and the special constraints in applying the methodology.

The Department of Health for England and Wales regards its effort at creating population health outcome indicators from currently available information as the starting point of a longer term programme to establish data sets that are specifically designed to evaluate the extent of the NHS's success in improving health. The developers of the indicators cite the difficulty in inferring cause and effect relationships from aggregate data but suggest (McColl and Gulliford 1993, p. 1) that 'nevertheless, for carefully selected conditions, outcome indicators based on aggregated data are of practical use because it is argued that effective health services should influence the value of the indicator.'

An important next step in the development of information systems for population health outcomes analysis is the integration of hospital and community information systems, an accomplishment that would be of considerable importance to the public health practitioner. We can, in fact, expect to see an emphasis in the next decade on the integration of inpatient, outpatient, and public health data systems for the purpose of evaluating health outcomes, led by efforts such as those of the NHS and incorporating the newly developed methods of measuring health status and quality of life.

References

Aaronson, N.K., Ahmedzai, S., Bergman B., *et al.* (1993). The European Organization for Research and Treatment of Cancer QLQ-C30: a quality of life instrument for use in international clinical trials in oncology. *Journal of the National Cancer Institute*, **85**, 365–76.

AHCPR (1990). *AHCPR program note: medical treatment effectiveness research.* Agency for Health Care Policy and Research, Rockville, MD.

AHCPR (1991). *The feasibility of linking research-related data bases to federal and non-federal medical administrative data bases.* Agency for Health Care Policy and Research, Rockville, MD.

Alonso, J., Anto, J.M., and Moreno, C. (1990). Spanish version of the Nottingham Health Profile: translation and preliminary validity. *American Journal of Public Health*, **80**, 704–8.

Baldwin, S., Godfrey, C., and Propper, C. (1990). *Quality of life: perspectives and policies.* Routledge, London.

Bergner, M. (1990). Advances in health status measurement: the potential to improve experimental and non-experimental data collection. In *Medical innovation at the crossroads*, vol I: *modern methods of clinical investigation* (ed. A. Gelijns), pp. 23–32, National Academy Press, Washington, DC.

Bowling, A. (1994). *Measuring disease: a review of disease-specific quality of life measurement scales.* Open University Press, Buckingham, UK.

Brook, R.H., Ware, J.E., Davies-Avery, A., Stewart, A.L., Donald, C.A., Rogers, W.H. *et al.* (1979). Overview of adult health status measures fielded in Rand's health insurance study. *Medical Care*, **17** (Suppl.), 1–131.

Charlton, J.R.H., Hartley, R.M., Silver, R., and Holland, W.W. (1983*a*). Geographical variation in mortality from conditions amenable to medical intervention in England and Wales. *Lancet*, i, 691–6.

Charlton, J.R.H., Patrick, D.L., and Peach, H. (1983*b*). Use of multivariate measures of disability in health surveys. *Journal of Epidemiology and Community Health*, **37**, 296–304.

Charlton, J.R.H., Holland, W.W., Lakhani, A., and Paul, E.A. (1987). Variations in avoidable mortality and variations in health care. *Lancet*, i, 858.

Cochrane, A.L. (1972). *Effectiveness and efficiency.* National Provincial Trust, London.

Deyo, R.A. (1986). Comparative validity of the Sickness Impact Profile and shorter scales for functional assessment in low-back pain. *Spine*, **11**, 951–4.

Deyo, R.A., Taylor, V.M., Diehr, P., Conrad, D., Cherkin, D.C., Ciol, M. *et al.*

(1994). Analysis of automated administrative and survey databases to study patterns and outcomes of care. *Spine*, **19**, 20835–915.

Doessel, D.P., and Marshal, J.V. (1985). A rehabilitation of health outcomes in quality assessment. *Social Science and Medicine*, **21**, 1319–28.

Donabedian, A. (1966). Evaluating the quality of medical care. *Milbank Memorial Fund Quarterly*, **44**, (Suppl.), 166–204.

Donabedian, A. (1985). *Explorations in quality assessment and monitoring (volume I: the definition of quality and approaches to its assessment)*. Health Administration Press, Ann Arbor, MI.

EuroQol Group (1990). EuroQol—a new facility for the measurement of health-related quality of life. *Health Policy*, **16**, 199–208.

Fallowfield, L. (1990). *The quality of life: the missing measurement in health care*. Souvenir Press, London.

Feeny, D., Guyatt, G., and Patrick, D. (ed.) (1991). Proceedings of the international conference on the measurement of quality of life as an outcome in clinical trials. *Controlled Clinical Trials: Design, Methods, and Analysis*, **12** (Suppl.), 1–280.

FHSR (1994). *Health outcomes research: a primer*. Foundation for Health Services Research, Washington, DC.

Geigle, R., and Jones, S.B. (1990). Outcomes measurement: a report from the front. *Inquiry*, **27**, 7–13.

Gilson, B.S., Gilson, J., Bergner, M., Bobitt, R.A., Kressel, S., Pollard, W.E. *et al.* (1975). The Sickness Impact Profile: development of an outcome measure of health care. *American Journal of Public Health*, **65**, 1304–10.

Grady, M.L., and Schwartz, H.A. (1992). *Medical effectiveness research data methods*. Agency for Health Care Policy and Research, Rockville, MD.

Holland, W.W. (ed.) (1993). *European Community atlas of avoidable death*. Oxford University Press, New York.

Hunt, S.M., McEwan, J., and McKenna, S.P. (1986). *Measuring health status*. Croom Helm, London.

Jenkinson, C., Fitzpatrick, R., and Argyle, M. (1988). The Nottingham Health Profile: an analysis of its sensitivity in differentiating illness groups. *Social Science and Medicine*, **27**, 1411–14.

Kaplan, R.M. (1989). Health outcome models for policy analysis. *Health Psychology*, **8**, 723–35.

Kaplan, R.M., Atkins, C.J., and Timms, R.M. (1984). Validity of a Quality of Well-Being Scale as an outcome measure in chronic obstructive pulmonary disease. *Journal of Chronic Diseases*, **37**, 85–95.

Karnofsky, D.A., and Burchemal, J.H. (1949). The clinical evaluation of chemotherapeutic agents. In *Evaluation of chemotherapeutic agents*, C.M. MacLeod, pp. 191–4. Columbia University Press, New York.

Katz, S. (ed.) (1987). The Portugal conference: measuring quality of life and functional status in clinical and epidemiologic research. Proceedings. *Journal of Chronic Diseases*, **40**, 459–650.

Lohr, K.N. (1988). Outcome measurement. *Inquiry*, **25**, 37–50.

Lohr, K.N. (1989). Conceptual background and issues in quality of life. In *Quality of life and technology assessment* (ed. F. Mosteller, and J. Falotico-Taylor), pp 1–6. National Academy Press, Washington, DC.

McColl, A.J., and Gulliford, M.C. (1993). *Population health outcome indicators for the NHS: a feasibility study*. HMSO, London.

McDowell, I., and Newell, C. (1987). *Measuring health: a guide to rating scales and questionnaires*. Oxford University Press, London.

McHorney, C.A., Ware, J.E., and Raczek, A.E. (1993). The MOS 36–item short form health survey (SF-36): II psychometric and clinical tests of validity in measuring physical and mental health constructs. *Medical Care*, **31**, 247–63.

Mackenbach, J.P., Bouvier-Colle, M.H., and Jouqla, E. (1990). Avoidable mortality and health services: a review of aggregate data studies. *Journal of Epidemiology and Community Health*, **44**, 106–111.

Maklan, C.W., Green R., and Cummings, M.A. (1994). Methodological challenges and innovations in patient outcomes research. *Medical Care*, **32**, JS13–21.

NCHS (1992). *Sample Design: Third National Health and Nutrition Examination Survey*. DHHS Pub. No. (PHS) 92–1387. US Government Printing Office, Washington, DC.

Patrick, D.L., and Bergner, M. (1990). Measurement of health status in the 1990s. *Annual Review of Public Health*, **11**, 165–83.

Patrick, D.L., and Erickson, P. (1992). Assessing health-related quality of life for clinical decision making. In *Quality of life assessment: key issues in the 1990's*, (ed. S.R. Walker, and R.N. Rosser), pp. 11–62. Kluwer Academic Publishing, London.

Patrick, D.L., and Erickson, P. (1993). *Health status and health policy: quality of life in health care evaluation and resource evaluation*. Oxford University Press, New York.

Roos, N.P. (1989). Using administrative data from Manitoba, Canada to study treatment outcomes: developing control groups and adjusting for case severity. *Social Science and Medicine*, **28**, 109–13.

Roos, N.P., Roos L.L., Mossey, J., and Havens, B. (1988). Using administrative data to predict important health outcomes: entry to hospital, nursing home, and death. *Medical Care*, **26**, 221–39.

Rosser, R.M. (1983). Issues of measurement in the design of health indicators: a review. In *Health indicators: an international study for the European Science Foundation*, (ed. A.J. Culyer), pp. 34–87. St Martin's Press, New York.

Rosser, R.M. (1990). From health indicators to quality-adjusted life years: technical and ethical issues. In *Measuring the outcomes of medical care* (ed. A. Hopkins and B. Costain), pp. 1–17, Royal College of Physicians, London.

Rutstein, D.D., Berenberg, W., Chalmers, T.C., Child, C.G., Fishman, A.P., and Perrin, E.B. (1976). Measuring the quality of medical care. *New England Journal of Medicine*, **294**, 582–8.

Schroeder, S.A. (1987). Outcome assessment 70 years later: are we ready? *New England Journal of Medicine*, **316**, 160–2.

Smith, G.T. (ed.) (1988). *Measuring health: a practical approach*. John Wiley and Sons, New York.

Spilker, B. (ed.) (1990). *Quality of life assessments in clinical trials*. Raven Press, New York.

Stewart, A.L., and Ware, J.E. (ed.) (1992). *Measuring functioning and well-being*. Duke University Press, Durham, NC.

Tarlov, A.R., Ware, J.E., Greenfield, S., Nelson, E.C., Perrin, E.B., and Zubkoff, M. (1989). The Medical Outcomes Study: an application of methods for monitoring the results of medical care. *Journal of American Medical Association*, **262**, 925–30.

Townsend, J., Feeny, D., Guyatt, G., Furlong, W., Seip, A., and Dolovich, J. (1991). Evaluation of the burden of illness for pediatric asthmatic patients and their parents. *Annals of Allergy*, **10**, 403–8.

Tugwell, P.X., Bomardier C., Buchanan, W., Grace, E., Southwell, D., Bianchi, F., and Hannah, B. (1983). The ability of the MACTAR disability questionnaire to detect sensitivity to change in rheumatoid arthritis. *Clinical Research*, **31**, 239A.

US Public Health Service (1991). *Healthy people 2000: national health promotion and disease prevention activities*. DHSS, Washington.

University of Surrey (1993). *Population health outcome indicators for the NHS: a consultation document* HMSO, London.

Walker, S.R., and Rosser, R.M. (ed.) (1988). *Quality of life: assessment and application*. MTP Press, Lancaster, UK.

Ware, J.E., and Sherbourne, C.D. (1992). The MOS 36–Item Short-form Health Survey (SF–36). 1. Conceptual framework and item selection. *Medical Care*, **30**, 473–83.

Ware, J.E., Kosinski, M., and Keller, S. (1996). A 12-Item Short Form Health Survey: Construction of Scales and Preliminary Tests of Reliability and Validity. *Medical Care*, **34**, 220–3.

Wennberg, J.E. (1990). What is outcomes research? In *Medical innovation at the crossroads, vol. I: modern methods of clinical investigation* (ed. A. Gelijns), pp. 33–46, National Academy Press, Washington, DC.

II Epidemiological and biostatistical approaches

6 Epidemiology: the foundation of public health

Roger Detels

Detailed discussions of the principles and methods of epidemiology are presented in the subsequent chapters in this section. In this introductory chapter, an attempt is made to define epidemiology, to present ways in which epidemiology is used in the advancement of public health, and finally to discuss the range of applications of epidemiological methodologies.

What is epidemiology?

There are probably as many definitions of epidemiology as there are epidemiologists, although every epidemiologist will know exactly what it is that he or she does. Defining epidemiology is difficult primarily because it does not represent a body of knowledge, as does anatomy, for example, nor does it target a specific organ system, as does cardiology. Epidemiology represents a philosophical method of studying a health problem and can be applied to a wide range of problems, from transmission of an infectious disease agent to the design of a new strategy for health care delivery. Furthermore, that methodology is continually changing as it is adapted to a greater range of health problems and more techniques are borrowed and adapted from other disciplines such as mathematics and statistics.

Maxcy, one of the pioneer epidemiologists of this century, offered the following definition: 'Epidemiology is that field of medical science which is concerned with the relationship of various factors and conditions which determine the frequencies and distributions of an infectious process, a disease, or a physiologic state in a human community' (Lilienfeld 1978). The word itself comes from the Greek *epi*, *demos*, and *logos*; literally translated it means the study (*logos*) of what is among (*epi*) the people (*demos*). All epidemiologists will agree that epidemiology concerns itself with populations rather than individuals, thereby separating itself from the rest of medicine and constituting the basic science of public health. Following from this, therefore, is the need to describe health and disease in terms of frequencies and distributions in the population. The epidemiologist relates these frequencies and distributions of specific health parameters to the frequencies of other factors to which populations are exposed in order to identify those that may be causes of a disease or promoters of good health. Inherent in the philosophy of epidemiology is the idea that ill health is not randomly distributed in populations, and that elucidating the reasons for this non-random distribution will provide clues regarding the risk factors for disease and the biological mechanisms that result in loss of health. Because epidemiology

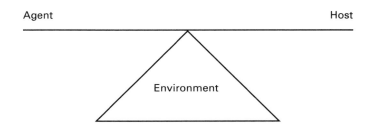

Fig. 6.1. The triadic relationship between agent, host, and environment in epidemiology.

usually focuses on health in human populations, it is rarely able to provide experimental proof in the sense of Koch's postulates, as can often be done in the laboratory sciences. Epidemiology more often provides an accumulation of increasingly convincing indirect evidence of a relationship between health or disease and other factors. This process can be referred to as causal inference (Rothman 1988). Veterinary epidemiologists, of course, focus on disease in animal populations, often with important implications for disease in human populations.

Although epidemiologists will differ on the exact definitions of epidemiology, most will agree that they try to characterize the relationship between the agent, the environment, and the host (usually human). The epidemiologist considers health to represent a balance among these three forces, as shown in Fig. 6.1.

Changes in any one of these three factors may result in loss of health. For example, the host may be compromised as a result of treatment with steroids, making him or her more susceptible to agents that do not ordinarily cause disease. Alternatively, a breakdown in the water supply system may result in an increased exposure of people to hepatitis A, as happened some years ago when the main water supply of New Delhi, the River Jumna, was drastically reduced by drought. Finally, some agents may become more or less virulent over time —often because of the promiscuous use of antibiotics—thereby disturbing the dynamic balance between agent, host, and environment. Two examples are the recent cases of acute necrotizing fasciitis caused by *Streptococcus* A (Communicable Disease Surveillance Centre 1994) and the development of multidrug-resistant tuberculosis (Chapman and Henderson 1994).

The epidemiologist uses another triad to study the relationship of agent, host, and environment: time–place–person. Using various epidemiological techniques described in subsequent chapters, the epidemiologist describes the loss of health in terms of characteristics of time (for example, trends, outbreaks, etc.), agent (transmissibility, the usual reservoir, host range, etc.), and host (demographic, sociological and biological characteristics, susceptibility, immune response, etc.). By describing the agent, host, and environment in terms of time, place, and person, the epidemiologist is often able to elucidate the causative agent, the natural history of the disease, and risk factors that increase the likelihood that the host will acquire the disease. With this information the epidemiologist is able to suggest ways to intervene in the disease process to prevent disease or death.

Epidemiology has been described as the 'art of the possible'. Because epidemiologists work with human populations, they are rarely able to manipulate events or the environment as can the laboratory scientist. Therefore they must exploit situations as they exist naturally to advance knowledge. They must be both pragmatic and modest (realistic). They must realize both what is possible and the limitations of the discipline. Morris has said that the 'epidemiologic method is the only way to ask some questions . . . , one way of asking others and no way at all to ask many' (Morris 1975). The art of epidemiology is to know both when epidemiology is the method of choice and how to use it to answer the question.

Applying the epidemiological method to resolve a health question successfully can be compared to constructing a memorable Chinese banquet. It is not enough to have the best ingredients and to know the various Chinese cooking methods. The truly great Chinese chef must be able to select the appropriate ingredients and cooking methods for each individual dish and, further, must know how to construct the correct sequence of dishes to excite the palate without overwhelming it. He creates the memorable banquet by adding his creative genius to the raw ingredients and the established cooking methods. Similarly, it is not enough for the epidemiologist to know the various strategies and methods of epidemiology; he or she must be able to apply them creatively to obtain the information needed to understand the natural history of the disease. It is not enough to know what a cohort study is; the epidemiologist must know when the cohort design is the appropriate design for the question at hand, and then must apply that design appropriately and creatively. It is that essential skill that makes epidemiology more than a methodology. It is this opportunity for creativity and innovation that provides excitement for the practitioner and makes the successful practice of epidemiology an art.

For example Imagawa et al, (1989) identified probable transient HIV-1 infection in men by focusing their viral isolation studies on relatively few HIV-1-antibody-negative homosexual men who had many different sexual partners. A simple cohort study of antibody-negative individuals would have required a cohort of thousands of men rather than the 133 studied. The effects of passive smoking were demonstrated by performing cohort studies of non-smoking family members of smokers. The effects of passive smoking/second-hand smoking were demonstrated in nursing students by comparing the reported symptoms in room-mates of smokers and non-smokers who kept diaries of their symptoms. The room-mates of the smokers had a 1.8 times greater risk of episodes of phlegm than room-mates of non-smokers (Schwartz and Zeger 1990). Colley et al. (1974), Tager et al. (1979), and Tashkin et al. (1984)

demonstrated that children of smokers had lower levels of lung function than children of non-smokers. All these investigators used the traditional study designs, but demonstrated their creativity by applying that design to specific populations which were most likely to reveal a relationship if it existed.

Epidemiological studies rarely provide 'proof' of a causal relationship. Thus there is continuing debate among epidemiologists about what constitutes adequate criteria for inferring a causal relationship from epidemiological studies (Rothman 1988). Hill (1965) suggested the following criteria for establishing a causal relationship: strength of association (statistical probability and risk ratio), consistency of findings across multiple studies, specificity of the relationship, temporality (outcome follows causation), biological gradient (a dose–response relationship), plausibility, coherence (consistency with prior knowledge), experimental evidence, and analogy (relationship hypothesized similar to that in known relationships). Susser has added to these criteria the ability of the observed relationship to predict other relationships correctly (Rothman 1988). The debate goes on, but the principle is the same: epidemiological studies seldom provide 'proof' of a causal relationship in the sense of Koch's postulates, but can be used to reveal a possible relationship and build a case that this relationship is causal.

Uses of epidemiology in support of public health

Epidemiology is the basic science of public health because it is the health science that describes health and disease in populations rather than in individuals, information that is essential for the formulation of effective public health initiatives to prevent disease and promote health in the community. Epidemiology can be used in the following applications.

Describe the spectrum of the disease

Disease represents the end-point of a process of alteration of the host's biological systems. Although many disease agents are limited in the range of alterations that they can initiate, others such as measles can cause a variety of disease end-points. For example the majority of infections with rubeola (the measles virus) result in the classical febrile blotchy rash disease, but the rubeola virus can also cause generalized haemorrhagic rash and acute encephalitis. Years after initial infection, measles can also cause subacute sclerosing panencephalitis, a fatal disease of the central nervous system. Measles virus is also suspected of being a causative factor in multiple sclerosis (Alter 1976; Sullivan et al. 1984).

Various types of epidemiological studies have been used to elucidate the spectrum of disease resulting from many agents and conditions. Cohort studies have been used to document the role of high blood pressure as a major cause of stroke, myocardial infarct, and chronic kidney disease. For rare diseases such as subacute sclerosing panencephalitis and multiple sclerosis, case–control studies have been useful in identifying the role of the rubeola virus (Detels et al. 1973; Alter 1976). Knowing the spectrum of disease that can result from specific infections and conditions allows the public health professional to design more effective intervention strategies; for example, education, screening, and treatment programmes to reduce the prevalence of high blood pressure will also reduce the incidence of myocardial infarct, stroke, and chronic kidney disease (Hypertension Detection and Follow-up Program Cooperative Group 1979).

Describe the natural history of disease

Epidemiological studies can be used to describe the natural history of disease and to elucidate the specific alterations in the biological system in the host. For example cohort studies of individuals who were infected with HIV, the AIDS virus, revealed that a drop in the level of T lymphocytes having the CD4 marker was associated with infection with HIV, and that a further decline in CD4 cells was associated with the development of clinical symptoms and AIDS (Detels *et al.* 1987; Polk *et al.* 1987). This observation stimulated immunologists to focus their research on the interaction of the immune system and HIV. From a clinical perspective, clinicians can target HIV-antibody-positive individuals who have declining CD4 cells for prophylactic treatment when it is most likely to be effective. Thus describing the natural history of AIDS has assisted researchers to focus their studies and clinicians to use the limited treatment modalities available more effectively (Phair *et al.* 1992).

Identify factors that increase or decrease the risk of acquiring disease

Some factors increase the probability that individuals will develop disease. These 'risk factors' may be social (smoking, drinking), genetic (ethnicity), dietary (saturated fats, vitamin deficiencies), and so on. Knowing these risk factors can often provide public health professionals with the necessary tools to design effective programmes to intervene before disease occurs. For example, descriptive, cross-sectional, case–control, cohort, and intervention studies have all shown that smoking is the largest single risk factor for ill health because it is a major risk factor for cardiovascular disease, chronic respiratory disease, and many cancers (for example cancers of the lung, nasopharynx, and bladder). Thus, smoking is the leading cause of disability and death in developed countries, if not the world. Health education campaigns to stop or reduce smoking are now a major public health initiative in most countries.

Predict disease trends

The ability to predict future epidemics provides the public health professional with the opportunity to muster the most effective forces to combat the disease. Descriptive studies of many infectious diseases, such as measles, poliomyelitis, and influenza, have revealed a periodicity of pandemics and epidemics caused by them. Knowledge of these disease patterns has been useful to public health officials in preparing for these epidemics.

More recently, studies of the trends of HIV infection in high-risk groups and of changing frequency of high-risk activities have permitted epidemiologists and statisticians to develop models that predict the number of cases of AIDS likely to occur in five to ten years (Brookmeyer and Damiano 1989; Taylor 1989; Chin *et al.* 1990). This information is particularly useful for public health professionals who must anticipate future health care needs.

Elucidate mechanisms of disease transmission

Understanding the mechanisms of disease transmission can suggest ways in which public health professionals can protect the public by stopping transmission of the disease agent. Epidemiological studies of the various types of arboviral encephalitides have incriminated certain species of mosquitoes as the vectors of disease and specific animals as the reservoirs for the virus. For example, public health efforts in California to prevent western equine encephalitis have concentrated on eradication of the mosquito vector and vaccination of horses, which are the reservoir of the virus. Although an effective vaccine for smallpox had been available for almost 200 years, eradication of the disease was not achieved until the recognition that the low infectivity of the varicella virus and the relatively long incubation for development of smallpox could be used to develop a strategy of surveillance for cases, with identification and immediate vaccination of all susceptible contacts (containment). A worldwide effort using this containment strategy based on epidemiological principles resulted in the eradication of smallpox in less than ten years (Fenner *el al.* 1988).

Test the efficacy of intervention strategies

A primary objective of public health is to prevent disease through intervention in the disease process. However, a vaccine or other intervention programme must be proved to be effective before it is used in the community. Epidemiological studies (double-blind placebo-controlled trials) are a necessary step in developing an intervention programme, whether that programme is administration of a new vaccine or a behavioural intervention strategy to stop smoking. Although it may be argued that injection of saline is no longer considered ethical, a proven vaccine, such as the poliomyelitis vaccine, can often be used as a placebo for a trial of a new vaccine for a different disease, as was done for trials of rubella vaccines in Taiwan (Detels *et al.* 1969). Widespread use of an intervention strategy not subjected to epidemiological studies of efficacy may result in implementation of an ineffective intervention programme at great public expense, and may actually result in greater morbidity and mortality because of an increased reliance on the favoured but untested intervention and a reduced use of other strategies which are thought to be less effective but which are actually more effective.

To evaluate intervention programmes

Although an intervention such as a vaccine may have been demonstrated to have efficacy in double-blind trials, it may fail to provide protection when used in the community. Double-blind trials may demonstrate the 'biological efficacy' of the vaccine, but if it is not acceptable to the majority of the public, they will refuse to be vaccinated and its 'public health efficacy' will be very low. For example, the typhoid vaccine provides some protection against the agent, but the frequency of unpleasant side-effects and the need for multiple injections influence many people against being vaccinated (Hornick 1982).

Another problem of inferring public health efficacy from small vaccine trials is that volunteers may not be representative of the general public which needs to be protected against a specific disease. Thus broad-based intervention trials also need to be carried out to demonstrate the acceptability and public health efficacy of a vaccine or other intervention to the population in need of protection.

Since adverse side-effects are associated with any vaccine, ongoing evaluations of the cost–benefit relationship of specific vaccines are important. By comparing the incidence of smallpox with the incidence of adverse side-effects from the vaccine, Lane *et al.* (1969) demonstrated that in the United States more disease resulted from use of the vaccine than from the import of cases.

Several epidemiological strategies are available for ongoing evaluation of intervention programmes. Serial cross-sectional studies can be used to determine if there has been a change in the prevalence of disease or of indicators of health status over time. The cohort design can be used to compare incidence of disease in comparable populations receiving and not receiving the prevention programme. The case–control design can be used to determine if there are differences in the proportion of cases and non-cases who received the intervention programme.

Identify the health needs of a community

To be effective in promoting the health of a community or country, health agencies must know what the major health problems of that community are and which subgroups in it are most affected. Cross-sectional studies will reveal the prevalence of disease in the community as well as in specific subgroups of the population, while surveillance programmes can identify trends in disease, infection, and/or health status over time. For example, the prevalence of untreated high blood pressure is high in most developed countries, but is disproportionately high in some subgroups such as African Americans and the poor. With this information, many health departments are now focusing their education and screening programmes for high blood pressure on African Americans and the poor.

Evaluate public health programmes

Departments of health are engaged in a variety of activities to promote the health of the community, ranging from vaccination programmes to clinics for the treatment of specific diseases in the needy. Ongoing evaluation of such programmes is necessary to ensure that they continue to be cost effective. Periodic review of routinely collected health statistics can provide information about the effectiveness of many programmes. For those programmes for which relevant statistics are not routinely available, cohort studies and serial cross-sectional studies of the incidence and prevalence of the targeted disease in the populations who are the intended recipients of these programmes can measure whether they have had an impact and are cost effective.

Applications of epidemiology

Specific epidemiological study designs are used to achieve specific public health goals. These goals range from identifying a suspected exposure–disease relationship to establishing that relationship, designing an intervention to prevent it, and, finally, assessing the effectiveness of that intervention. The usual sequence of study designs in the identification and resolution of a disease problem are as follows:

- descriptive studies
- cross-sectional (prevalence) surveys
- case–control studies
- experimental studies

However, there are many exceptions to the application of this sequence of study designs, depending on such things as the prevalence and virulence of the agent and the nature of the human response to the agent.

The earliest suspicion that a relationship exists between a disease and a possible causative factor is frequently obtained from observing correlations between exposure and disease in existing data such as mortality statistics and surveys of personal or national characteristics. These can be correlations observed across geographical areas (ecological studies), or over time, or a combination of both. Many of the initial epidemiological investigations into chronic bronchitis used vital statistics data, particularly data on mortality. Case–control studies identified smoking as a possible causal factor for chronic bronchitis. Subsequent prevalence studies confirmed the relationship, as have cohort studies. Finally, a decline in the respiratory symptoms of chronic bronchitis and a slower decline in lung function have been observed in individuals who cease smoking (Colley 1991).

Although the sequence given above is the usual sequence in which the various epidemiological study designs are applied, there are exceptions. Furthermore, all study designs are not appropriate to answer all health questions. Therefore the usual applications of each of the different epidemiological study designs and the limitations of each are presented briefly below.

Ecological studies

The use of existing statistics to correlate the prevalence or incidence of disease with the frequency or trends of suspected causal factors in specific localities or over time has often provided the first clues that a particular factor may cause a specific disease. However, these epidemiological strategies document only the co-occurrence of disease and other factors in a population; the risk factors and the disease may not be occurring in the same people. These types of descriptive studies are cheap and relatively easy to perform, but the co-occurrence observed may be due merely to chance. For example, the incidence of both heart disease and lung cancer has increased concurrently with the prevalence of automatic dishwashers in the United States. However, few people, would attribute the increase in these two diseases to the use of automatic dishwashers. Thus, descriptive studies usually only provide a rationale for undertaking more expensive analytical studies.

Cross-sectional/prevalence surveys

Cross-sectional/prevalence surveys establish the magnitude of disease and other factors in a community. However, since they require the collection of data, they can be expensive. They are useful for estimating the number of people in a population who have the disease and can also identify the difference in frequency of disease in different subpopulations. This descriptive information is particularly useful for health administrators who are responsible for developing appropriate and effective public health programmes. Cross-sectional studies can also be used to document the co-occurrence of disease and suspected risk factors not only in the population but also in specific individuals within the population. The cross-sectional study design is useful for studying chronic diseases such as multiple sclerosis and chronic bronchitis, which have a high prevalence but an incidence that is too low to make a cohort study feasible (Detels *et al.* 1978). However, they are not useful for studying diseases that have a low prevalence, such as subacute sclerosing panencephalitis. Cross-sectional studies are subject to problems of respondent bias, recall bias, and undocumented confounders. Further, unless historical information is obtained from all the individuals surveyed, the time relationship between the factor and the disease is not known. Further, prevalence surveys identify people who have survived to that time point with disease and thus under-represent people with a short course of disease.

Case–control studies

The case–control study compares the prevalence of suspected causal factors in cases and controls. If the prevalence of the factor in cases is significantly different from that in controls, this suggests that this factor is associated with the disease. Although case–control studies can identify associations, they do not measure risk. However, an estimate of risk can be derived by calculating the odds ratio (Volume 2, Chapter 10). Case–control studies are often chosen as the initial analytical study design used in the investigation of a suspected association. Compared with cohort and experimental studies, they are usually relatively cheap and easy to perform. Cases can often be selected from hospital patients and controls either from hospitalized patients with other diseases or by using algorithms or formulae for selecting community (neighbourhood) or other types of controls, although selection bias is often a problem, especially when using either hospitalized cases or controls. The participants are seen only once, and no follow-up is necessary. Although time sequences can often be established for factors elicited by interview, this is not usually possible for laboratory test results. Thus, an elevation in factor B may be causally related, or it may be a result of the disease process and not a cause. Furthermore, factors elicited from interview are subject to recall bias; for example, patients are often better motivated than controls for recall of events because they are concerned about their disease. The case–control study is particularly useful for exploring relationships noted in observational studies. However, a hypothesis is necessary for case–control studies. Relationships will be observed only for those factors studied. Case–control studies are not useful for determining the spectrum of health outcomes resulting from specific exposures, since a definition of a case is required in order to perform a case–control study. However, case–control studies are the method of choice for studying rare diseases. They are often indicated when a specific health question needs to be answered quickly.

Cohort studies

Cohort studies have the advantage of establishing the temporal relationship between an exposure and a health outcome, and thus they measure risk directly. Because the population studied is defined on the basis of its exposure to the suspected factor, cohort studies are particularly suitable for investigating health hazards associated with environmental or occupational exposures. Further, cohort studies will measure more than one outcome of a given exposure and therefore are useful for defining the spectrum of disease resulting from exposure to a given factor. Occasionally, a cohort study is performed to elucidate the natural history of a disease when a group can be identified that has a high incidence of disease but in which specific risk factors are not known. Although this cohort is not defined on the basis of a known exposure, questions are asked and biological specimens are collected from which exposure variables can be identified concurrently or in the future. Unfortunately, cohort studies are both expensive and time consuming. Unless the investigator can define a cohort from some time in the past and can be assured that the cohort has been completely followed up for disease outcome in the interim, the cohort design can take years or decades to yield information about the risks of disease resulting from exposure to specific factors. Ensuring that participants remain in a cohort study for such long periods of time is both difficult and expensive. Further, the impact of those who drop out of follow-up must be taken into account in the analysis and interpretation of cohort studies. Finally, exposures may vary over time, complicating the analysis of their impact. Because of the cost and complexity of cohort studies, they are usually performed only after descriptive, cross-sectional, and/or case–control studies have suggested a causal relationship. The size of the cohort to be studied is dependent in part on the anticipated incidence of the disease resulting from the exposure. For diseases with a very low incidence, cohort studies are often not feasible in terms of the logistics or the expense of following very large numbers of people, or both. Cohort studies establish the risk of disease associated with exposure to a factor but do not 'prove' that the factor is causal. The observed factor may merely be very closely correlated with the real causative factor, or may even be related to the participants' choice to be exposed.

Experimental studies

Experimental studies differ from cohort studies because the investigator makes the decision about who will be exposed to the factor based on the specific design factors to be employed (for example randomization, matching, etc.). Therefore confounding factors that may have led to the subjects' being exposed in the cohort studies are not a problem in experimental studies. Because epidemiologists usually study human populations, there are few opportunities for an investigator to expose participants deliberately to a suspected factor. However, intervention studies of individuals randomly assigned to receive or not receive an intervention programme that demonstrates a reduction in a specific health outcome do provide strong evidence, if not proof, of a causal relationship. Because of the serious implications of applying an intervention that may alter the biological status of an individual, intervention studies are not undertaken until the probability of a causal relationship has been well established using the other types of study designs.

The uses and limitations of the various epidemiological study designs have been presented to illustrate and emphasize the fact that the successful application of epidemiology requires more than a knowledge of study designs and epidemiological methods. These designs and methods must be applied both appropriately and innovatively if they are to yield the desired information. The field of epidemiology has been expanding dramatically over the last two decades as more epidemiologists have demonstrated new uses and variations of traditional study designs and methods. We can anticipate that the uses of epidemiology will expand even more in the future as increasing numbers of creative epidemiologists develop new strategies and techniques of epidemiology.

Summary

Epidemiology is the basic science of public health because it is the science that describes the relationship of health or disease to other factors in human populations. Furthermore, epidemiology can be used to generate much of the information required by public health professionals to develop and implement effective intervention programmes for the prevention of disease and the promotion of health. Finally, it is the best strategy for evaluating the effectiveness of public health programmes.

Unlike pathology, which constitutes a basic area of knowledge, and cardiology, which is the study of a specific organ, epidemiology is a medical philosophy or methodology that can be applied to learning about and resolving a very broad range of health problems. The art of epidemiology is knowing when and how to apply epidemiological methods creatively to answer specific health questions; it is not enough to know what the various study designs and statistical methodologies are. Used innovatively, epidemiology can be one of the most effective tools available to science to combat disease and promote health.

References

Alter, M. (1976) Is multiple sclerosis an age-dependent host response to measles? *Lancet*, i, 456–7.

Brookmeyer, R. and Damiano, A. (1989). Statistical methods for short-term projections of AIDS incidence. *Statistics in Medicine*, 8, 23–24.

Chapman, S.W. and Henderson, H.M. (1994). New and emerging pathogens multiply resistant *Mycobacterium tuberculosis*. *Current Opinion in Infectious Diseases*, 7, 231–7.

Chin, J., Sato P., and Mann, J. (1990). Projections of HIV infections and AIDS cases to the year 2000. *Bulletin of the World Health Organization*, 68, 1–11.

Colley, J.R.T. (1991). Major public health problems; respiratory system. In *Oxford textbook of public health* (2nd edn), (ed. W. W. Holland, R. Detels, and G. Knox), Vol. 3, pp. 227–48. Oxford University Press.

Colley, J.R.T., Holland, W.W., and Corkhill R.T. (1974) Influence of passive smoking and parental phlegm on pneumonia and bronchitis in early childhood. *Lancet*, ii (7888), 1031–4.

Communicable Disease Surveillance Centre (1994). Invasive group A streptococcal infections in Gloucestershire. *Communicable Disease Report (England/Wales)*, 4, 97–100.

Detels, R., Grayston, J.T., Kim, K.S.W., *et al.* (1969). Prevention of clincial and subclinical rubella infection: efficacy of three HPV-77 derivative vaccines. *American Journal of Diseases of Children*, 118, 295–300.

Detels, R., McNew, J., Brody, J.A., and Edgar, A.H. (1973). Further epidemiological studies of subacute sclerosing panencephalitis. *Lancet*, 819, 11–14.

Detels, R., Visscher, B.R., Haile, R.W., *et al*, (1978). Multiple sclerosis and age at migration. *American Journal of Epidemiology*, 108, 386–93.

Detels, R., Visscher, B.R. Fahey, J.L., *et al.* (1987). Predictors of clinical AIDS in young homosexual men in a high-risk area. *International Journal of Epidemiology*, 16, 271–6.

Fenner, F., Henderson, D.A., Arita, I., *et al*, (1988). *Smallpox and its eradication*. World Health Organization, Geneva.

Hill, A.B. (1965). The environment and disease: association or causation? *Proceedings of the Royal Society of Medicine*, 58, 295–300.

Hornick, R.B. (1982) Typhoid fever. In *Bacterial infections of humans: epidemiology and control* (ed. A. S. Evans and H. A. Feldman), pp. 659–76. Plenum, New York.

Hypertension Detection and Follow-up Program Co-operative Group (1979). Five-year findings of the hypertension detection and follow-up program. I. Reduction in mortality of persons with high blood pressure, including mild hypertension. *Journal of the American Medical Association*, 242, 2562–71.

Imagawa, D.T., Lee, M.H., Wolinsky, S.M., *et al.* (1989). Human immunodeficiency virus type 1 infection in homosexual men who remain seronegative for prolonged periods. *New England Journal of Medicine*, 320, 1458–62.

Lane, J.M., Ruben, F.L., Neff, J.M., and Millar, J.D. (1969). Complications of smallpox vaccination, 1968: national surveillance in the United States. *New England Journal of Medicine*, 281, 1201–8.

Lilienfeld, D.E. (1978). Definitions of epidemiology. *American Journal of Epidemiology*, 107, 87–90.

Morris, J.N. (1975). *Uses of epidemiology* (3rd edn). Churchill Livingstone, London.

Phair, J., Jacobson, L., Detels, R., *et al.* (1992). Acquired immune deficiency syndrome occurring within 5 years of infection with human immunodeficiency virus type-1: the Multicenter AIDS Cohort Study. *Journal of Acquired Immune Deficiency Syndromes*, 5, 490–6.

Polk, B.F., Fox, R., Brookmeyer, R., *et al.* (1987). Predictors of the acquired immunodeficiency syndrome developing in a cohort of seropositive homosexual men. *New England Journal of Medicine*, 316, 61–6.

Rothman, K.J. (ed.) (1988). *Causal inference*. Epidemiology Resources, Chestnut Hill, MA.

Schwartz, J., and Zeger, S. (1990). Passive smoking, air pollution, and acute respiratory symptoms in a diary of student nurses. *American Review of Respiratory Disease*, 141, 62–7.

Sullivan, C.B., Visscher, B.R., and Detels, R. (1984). Multiple sclerosis and age at exposure to childhood diseases and animals: cases and their friends. *Neurology*, 34, 1144–8.

Tager, I.B., Weiss, S.T., Rosner, B., and Speizer, F.E. (1979). Effect of parental cigarette smoking on the pulmonary function of children. *American Journal of Epidemiology*, 110, 15–26.

Tashkin, D.P., Clark, V.A., Simmons, M., *et al.* (1984). The UCLA Population Studies of Chronic Obstructive Respiratory Disease: VII. Relationship between parental smoking and children's lung function. *American Review of Respiratory Disease*, 129, 891–7.

Taylor, J.M.G. (1989). Models for the HIV infection and AIDS epidemic in the United States. *Statistics in Medicine*, 8, 45–58.

7 Spatial and temporal studies in epidemiology

E. G. Knox

Fundamentals

Classical epidemiology was concerned almost entirely with communicable disease; the now dominant interest in chronic diseases developed only within the last three or four decades. The scope of epidemiology is now recognized as universal and encompasses both themes, but the subject remains divided in terms of its professional activities and scientific methodologies. Epidemiologists tend to specialize in one field or the other, to rely upon different supporting disciplines, and to employ different analytical repertoires.

The division of the subject is, indeed, better expressed in methodological terms than in terms of the original subject matters. The technical division is between the epidemiology of **events** and the epidemiology of **states**. The first is associated with temporal graphs and plots on maps, and the second with contingency tables. States and events are dimensionally different, and the clue to understanding the different technical requirements of different investigations lies in understanding this distinction. It is this that dictates the observational and analytical techniques that must be employed. Events are necessarily dimensioned in time, while states, whether categorical or quantitative, are not. Records of either, at the investigator's option and according to the objectives of the enquiry, may also be located in space.

We elaborate on these points as follows.

Dimensionalities

States (whether measured values or categorical) exist over a period of time. They are unchanging. The appropriate adjective is 'static'! Observers can intercept and observe a state at any single point in time between its onset and its termination. They need to visit only once; there is no point in visiting twice. Consequently, the frequency of a state is expressed as a **point prevalence** (or **point prevalence rate**), which in technical terms is a simple proportion, undimensioned in time. This is as befits a record based upon a single observation, without the benefit of a clock and without the measurement of passing time.

Events (deaths, traffic accidents, onsets of measles) occur at a point in time. Unlike states, they cannot be intercepted by observers who themselves attend only at a single point in time. To intercept and record an event, the investigators must observe over a period of time. They must observe continuously or else return repeatedly. Frequencies of events are expressed as an event-rate (or 'attack-rate', 'incidence', or 'incidence-rate') which is expressed per unit time as well as per thousand population. This befits a period of observation between two declared points in time, whose duration must be measured.

The inversion of the relationship between points and periods is important. A time-extended phenomenon demands a point observation; a point phenomenon demands time-extended observation. We should note that it is the dimensionality of the observing mode that imposes the dimensionality of the frequency measure, not the duration of the phenomenon itself.

Events and states are related to each other through processes analogous to mathematical integration and differentiation. If a constant incidence rate is multiplied by the time during which it operates, the result is a **prevalence** or, more properly, a **prevalence increment**. Thus the multiplication by time (t) of a unit initially measured per unit time (t^{-1}), results in a cancelling out of the time element; the resulting prevalence is dimensionless. Where the incidence varies over time, the accumulation process corresponds to integration rather than simple multiplication, but the dimensionality consequences are the same. Conversely, where the state of an individual is ascertained at two different times, and where the state has changed, we can claim to have detected an event without actually having seen it happen. The analogy here is with algebraic differentiation.

We can see that an event is formally definable as a **change of state**. When an event is observed indirectly, as above, it is usual to locate it arbitrarily at a point in time midway between the two observations. It is possible through the use of record-linkage operations to create a file of point-in-time observations from which the occurrence of many events can be inferred without any having been directly witnessed. For a series of such paired observations, and through a differencing process (to ascertain the change of state and to measure the period of time), we generate a time-dimensioned **incidence-rate**. However, this is so only if the original observations are accurately dated.

Our concern in this chapter is more with the pragmatic solution of practical problems than with the syntax of medical and scientific observations. However, we begin with this formal differentiation of different kinds of observation because it provides an orderly framework within which to locate a varied constellation of epidemiological questions. Epidemiologists are constantly bombarded with questions relating to incidence and prevalence, to disease events and disease states, and to questions relating to temporal and geographic patterns. The supposed patterns may take the form of trends or cycles or steps or irregular clusters. They may be presented as 'pure' phenomena, without reference to anything else on the map or on the calendar, or they may be presented in conjunction with putative hazards, thus raising questions of covariations and cause. These questions may also relate to space and time jointly—a conceptual distribution of events and hazards within a space–time block.

In all these circumstances it is necessary to distinguish legitimate analytical operations from illegitimate, and to distinguish what it is about a particular question that demands one technical approach as opposed to another, or what it is about a particular data set that entirely denies the possibility of answering a particular question. This is a major preoccupation of this chapter.

Real and random

A second necessary preoccupation is to distinguish between 'real' and 'random' phenomena in space, in time, or in space and time jointly. As in other branches of epidemiology, this is subsumed within the subject matter of 'sampling theory'. We ask whether the phenomena displayed in our sample are the products of the sampling process alone or whether they reflect real world phenomena in the universe from which the sample was drawn.

Styles of analysis

Investigators analysing chronic disease states and exploring aetiologies through the medium of contingency tables seldom pay much attention to the timing or the geographic spacing of their observations. These analyses concentrate upon measuring the frequencies of coexistence of different pairs of states (smokes, has cancer) within the same subject. 'Events', as recorded in this kind of study, are generally represented as static attributes: has *had X* (e.g. has had previous tonsillectomy, has had recent poliomyelitis). Contingency analyses such as these have formed a very large proportion of the corporate epidemiological effort reported in the scientific literature over the last 40 years. This style of working, both the collection of data and the subsequent analysis, is quite different from the methods addressed in this chapter. Why should this be? What is the technical basis of the distinction?

The clue to its understanding is in the formal file and record operations used in each style of working. Briefly, one style of analysis is concerned with **intra**-record relationships and the other with **inter**-record relationships.

Contingency analysis depends upon the simultaneous coexistence of different attributes within the same record; where these attributes are noted in separate records, a major element of such investigations lies in bringing them together within a new record through record-linkage procedures. The technical basis of contingency studies, the **consolidated medical record**, first became available on a large scale through the use of such devices as the Hollerith card and (later) by efficient record-handling computer systems. These processes have been well supported by the development of statistical tabulation processes and multivariate analysis methods (e.g. in SPSS and GLIM) imported from other disciplines. In contrast, spatial/temporal investigations study the relationships between records, distances apart and times apart, and the dispersion of different recorded observations to different locations and different dates on the calendar. In studying infective

transmission processes, in particular, the different records note the same class of event in different people, as opposed to the same record noting different classes of events in the same person.

Inter-record operations invoke complexities beyond those encountered in intra-record analyses. In record-linkage operations, for example, n records offer n^2 relationships between different pairs of records, far greater than for the types of record-linkage (strictly file–merging) operations referred to earlier. If we are dealing with larger groupings, for example triplets and quadruplets of events, the analytical task is very onerous indeed (see Knox and Lancashire (1991) for an example involving sibship assembly).

There is also a serious problem when we try to relate records through matching personal identifiers. Problems of these kinds arise in kindred studies, including the assembly of sibships, and in the investigation of contacts in the study of communicable diseases. For simple file-merging operations, we can usually cope with a proportion of near-miss matches and with varied spelling and clerical errors, but for intrafile inter-record linkage operations, a very large number of false-positive near-miss matches can readily outnumber and bury the true links.

Finally, investigators are faced with model-fitting problems relating to natural histories, disease transmission, latent intervals, and contact/diffusion mechanisms of daunting complexity. These are far more difficult to formalize within generalized software systems than those commonly encountered within the framework of multivariate analysis.

Geographic display and analysis

The majority of geographic patterns are interpreted intuitively, at least in the first instance. This is commonly referred to as 'eyeball' epidemiology. The most pervasive restriction upon the display and interpretation of geographically located morbidity is the uneven distribution of the populations at risk. This nearly always forces us to use rates (prevalences, incidences, etc.) so that we take simultaneous account of the distribution of denominators as well as numerators.

The most characteristic forms of presentation are the choropleth map, the isopleth (or isoline) map, and the spot map. We also frequently need to use a technical procedure described as 'map on map' in which (for example) a disease-distribution map is overlaid upon a hazard distribution map. (See McGlashan (1972) for a discussion of geographic techniques.)

Choropleth mapping

This most familiar of all geographic formats uses geopolitical or other boundaries related to known populations at risk. Attack rates of events, or prevalences of states, are calculated for each subarea. The different rates are represented by differential shading, hatching, or colouring. (See Gardner *et al.* (1983) for a good example.)

There is a hazard of interpretation. A large sparsely populated rural area will tend to catch the eye of the investigator, while a small densely populated city may almost escape notice. A useful modification to correct for this is the **demographic** map in which the different zones are shrunk or expanded so that their areas are proportional to the populations at risk.

For sparse observations, individual events can be marked as

spots on the map. On a demographic map the exact locations can be difficult to identify, but once achieved, there are some special advantages. Appearances of spot clusters on a non-demographic map chiefly represent the uneven distribution of the population at risk; but on a demographic map they represent genuine concentrations of risk.

Distances on demographic maps do not represent physical distances (e.g. kilometres), and so biological interpretation is not straightforward. As always, the form of presentation must depend upon the biological model under investigation. Distance deformation will be a disadvantage in examining the data for the presence of a 'toxic cloud' diffusion model in relation to a suspected point source; however, these maps provide an advantage in the study of a case-to-case infection hypothesis. People (and animals such as foxes) tend to travel further for their social contacts when they live in sparsely populated areas than they do when they live at high densities. The rate of geographic spread of rabies by foxes is almost independent of the density of foxes.

Isopleth mapping

An isopleth (or isoline) map uses contours of equal disease density. Its form is not then dependent upon geopolitical outlines. It looks like an ordinary elevation contour or an isobar or isotherm map. The mapping technique draws its own lines and does not rely upon arbitrary boundaries. Isopleth mapping avoids dependence upon a direct knowledge of local populations by using a series of 'control observations' as well as the disease observations. For example, it compares the distribution of malformed births against a sample of normal births. It can use one or several normal controls for each abnormal observation.

This technique can be used where adequate civil data do not exist at all, as in socially underdeveloped regions, but it is also useful where the epidemiological hypothesis under investigation is not easily expressed in terms of the available geopolitical divisions. For example, if we wished to see whether anophthalmos occurred to excess in localized inner-city industrial zones, or whether leukaemia registrations were relatively frequent near motorways, or whether hydrocephalus tended to occur in small clusters irrespective of any recognizable map feature, we might find that available census or electoral divisions were entirely unsuited to our purposes.

Choropleth presentations cannot show fine detail, whereas an isopleth map can, in principle, display small clusters as concentric nests of closely spaced isolines. In practice, however, isopleth maps have a serious disadvantage. They are often based upon small numbers of control observations compared with the large denominators frequently available for choropleth rates. This leads to a loss of resolution. Suspected disease concentrations visible coarsely on a choropleth map can disappear altogether within the noise of sampling variations on an isopleth map.

A register of population denominators, set out in small areas in order to permit flexible reassembly and backed by their geographic coordinates and other characteristics, offers the best of both worlds. There is mounting pressure from many fields for the establishment of such geographic information systems (GIS). At present, however, the various small areas—electoral wards and constituencies, electoral lists, health districts and hospital budgeting areas, general practice populations, census enumeration districts, post-codes,

social survey samples, etc.—are almost entirely uncoordinated, each reflecting its own idiosyncratic functions (Raper et al. 1992). In the United Kingdom, automatic map referencing of post-codes from the existing Central Post-code Directory provides a basis for locating address-specified events on the map and ultimately for space–time studies and for isopleth mapping at resolutions of a few hundred metres. However, their accuracies are sometimes poor and the post-codes are very variable in their population-size. Post-code identification of health data also compromises confidentiality, to a degree that has already resulted in epidemiologists being denied access to important public health data (Knox and Gilman 1992a, b; Knox 1994). Commercial pressures for marketing information, which seems to be less susceptible to such objections, have already led to the mapping of individual United Kingdom addresses at high levels of resolution in computer-processable form (Draper 1991), but national coverage is incomplete. Furthermore, neither the commercial nor the post-code systems have yet been linked with electoral, census, or other demographic boundaries.

Map-on-map techniques

We have not yet considered what else may be found on the map apart from disease observations and the populations at risk. Yet we frequently need to bring disease observations into visual apposition with atmospheric pollution levels, income distributions, other indices of affluence and poverty, power stations, high-tension transmission lines, roads, railways, canals, or recreation areas. To do this at the visual level, we have to combine two maps. The method depends upon the formats of the original maps.

If death rates from chronic bronchitis and a range of socio-economic indices, such as car ownership statistics, are both available on a congruent choropleth basis, then we can find a means of expressing them side by side, or we might even redraw the mortality map as a ratio of observed to expected mortality. However, in relating bronchitis deaths to particulate smoke deposition, we might find that the pollution data had been set out in isopleth form, having been derived from a large number of measuring stations that were geographically unrelated to electoral population boundaries. We might then simply superimpose the pollution contours upon the choropleth map and interpret them visually as best we can.

The problems of relating different map formats in any strictly formal manner are extremely difficult. It is usually necessary to fall back upon parallel correlation analyses with no intrinsic geographic dimension. The problems are heightened because disease phenomena are not always represented best as single points; the biological model under investigation will then itself dictate the necessary mode of presentation. In childhood leukaemia we may be interested in several alternative points, namely the address at birth, the address at onset, and the address at death. For tuberculosis we will be interested in a complete trace of addresses at different ages. For suspected legionnaires' disease we would trace in great detail all the journeys undertaken and all the places visited within a restricted period of time.

The choice of format for representing map-features also presents many options, but the choice is not entirely arbitrary. In general, map features representing hazards come in three main forms, namely (a) points (for example nuclear processing plants),

(b) linear features (canals, roads, power lines), and (c) areal features (zones of affluence, high/low pollution zones). For points and for linear features we will be chiefly interested in 'distance from'; for areal features we will be chiefly interested in 'within or without.'

Because of these difficulties, many investigators have had to coerce reconciliations between different types of map-on-map plots. For example, background radiation levels collected at scattered points and subsequently converted into an isopleth map have been related to choropleth data for childhood cancer death rates whose distribution is set out in quite another manner (for example civil registration areas). Both distributions were forced into yet another mode, namely the 10 km squares of the National Cartographic Grid (Knox *et al.* 1988). In other examples, civil-area data on leukaemias and populations at risk have been forced into a correspondence with circles of different radii centred upon nuclear processing plants (Cooke-Mozaffari *et al.* 1987).

Computer-generated displays

Geographers, who see their brief as essentially descriptive, use a wide variety of map-on-map techniques at a purely visual level. Epidemiologists, seeking to identify causal connections, suspicious of intuitive interpretations, and still wistful about the possibilities of formal inference, have in the past been less prolific in devising or using them. However, the availability of computers, and particularly microcomputers with coloured screens and relatively inexpensive colour-pen plotters, has generated forms of presentation that at least follow formal rules. We are likely to see a growth in the use of these methods in the immediate future. For example, there are now formal algorithms for converting an ordinary choropleth map into a demographic map. There is no longer any need to construct them on a trial-and-error basis using large quantities of graph paper (Selvin *et al.* 1987).

There is an also an engaging format of display for congruent choropleth maps of two different variables, one set over the other. One variable is represented as a shaded colour system graded from yellow (low incidence) through intermediate shades (orange) to red. The other variable is shaded from yellow (low social index) through shades of green to blue. Finally, the two systems are overlaid to create a combined map in which each combination of levels on the two scales is shown as a unique colour mix. The 'key' to the map is set out as a chequer-board matrix of rows and columns showing all the colour mixes, with one gradation set in horizontal bars and the other overlaid as vertical bars. One diagonal shows shades ranging from yellow to purple and the other from red to blue. If the two variables are positively correlated, the predominant colours will stretch along the yellow-to-purple diagonal; if they are negatively correlated, then they will stretch along the red-to-blue diagonal.

With a little practice, this permits immediate recognition of the type of correlation (positive or negative), without any necessary reference to numerical data, and at the same time locates the particular zones of greatest positive or negative association. It also instantly shows the atypical outliers. A large number of combinations of different social, physical, and morbidity variables can be inspected seriatim.

Isopleth presentations can be performed on simple monochrome devices such as dot matrix printers, but the ideal device is the colour-pen graph-plotter. The value to be plotted, and represented by the isolines, is the **relative density** of cases and controls. There are several alternative algorithms for estimating relative density. One uses the sums of the inverse squared distances from the map point in question to the locations of all the events and to the locations of all the controls. The granularity of the resulting map derived from all these points can then be smoothed and the contours traced in order to separate the different density zones. For isopleth-on-isopleth plots, the two sets of lines can simply be traced in different colours for inspection. Commercial packages for calculating isopleths exist, but none has yet won a routine place in epidemiological analysis.

A computer-generated cluster-display method described by Openshaw *et al.* (1988) that is used to study childhood leukaemias is based upon a hybrid presentation. The denominators (populations) are derived from choropleth data while the numerators consist of exactly located events. Every point on the map is scanned. Circles of different radii around each point are used to estimate alternative 'populations at risk', and significant departures of the associated event-counts from a random expectation are marked. The authors use the drawn perimeter of the circle itself as the map 'marker', and clusters are displayed as sets of concentric/overlapping circles. The algorithm displays points of statistical significance rather than points of high incidence *per se*.

Spot maps, clustering, and proximity analyses

Where large numbers of events are available for mapping, such that predefined subareas can have prevalences attached to them, the map can be set out in choropleth format. We can then apply correlation techniques to the rates in adjacent and non-adjacent pairs of subareas to see whether the former exhibit relative similarities (Kemp *et al.* 1985). Such an approach will detect geographic heterogeneities that have a granularity of substantially larger diameter than the individual areas themselves. For example, the prevalences of emphysema in electoral wards might show adjacency correlations which reflect the systematically raised prevalences in large urban areas compared with rural areas.

However, geographic plots of disease events or disease states may be so sparse that we can scarcely think of them in terms of continuous variables such as prevalences or incidences. They arrive in distinct quanta. We must then base our analyses upon the measured distances between pairs of events, pairs of controls, and case–control pairs. For example, we might plot a distribution of the distances between all possible pairs of cases and another between all possible pairs of controls. If the proportional distributions differ, such that there is a relative excess of short inter-pair distances among the cases, we can conclude that there is a relative degree of geographic clustering.

If we wish to study distance relationships among cases, controls, and putative hazards, we compare the distributions of control-to-hazard distances with case-to-hazard distances. We refer to this as a **proximity analysis**. In effect, we follow the perimeter of an expanding circle centred on the position of the hazard and plot the progressive accumulation of cases as the radius enlarges. We do the same for controls and plot the two incremental curves on a single graph. If there is more than one hazard point, then we expand the radii simultaneously around each of these points, accumulating cases and controls as we do so. If the hazard is a linear feature, such

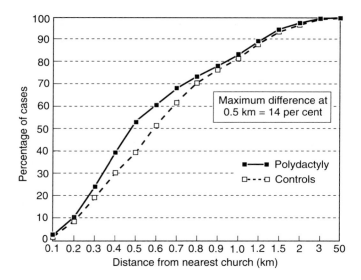

Fig. 7.1 Polydactyly and churches in Birmingham.

as a high-voltage power line, we drop perpendiculars from the positions of the events and the controls to the nearest point of the nearest element of the linear feature in question. Again, we compare the cumulative acquisition curves for the cases and the controls as we move away from the suspected hazard. We should use several different sets of controls. If the tested hypothesis is correct, then the case curve will differ from the control curves (Fig. 7.1).

Two main tests of significance for such differences are available. One seeks and tests the significance of the **maximum ratio** between the cumulative observed and the cumulative expected values (Stone 1988); the other is a version of the Kolmogorov–Smirnov statistic, which seeks and tests the significance of the **maximum difference** between two separate curves (see Siegel (1956) for details of this and related tests). The Stone method is probably best suited to the testing of precisely postulated diffusion hazards, for example occurrences of childhood leukaemias at different distances from nuclear processing plants. The second method is probably best suited to demonstrating less specific proximity hypotheses; for example the increased birth prevalence of polydactyly close to churches in Birmingham, as shown in Fig. 7.1, probably reflects the high prevalence among Afro-Caribbean immigrants and their geographic concentration in dense mid-nineteenth-century housing areas with plenty of churches.

For areal map features we may be interested either in the distance from the boundary (for example lakes, uninhabited wooded areas) or, alternatively, in whether the events and controls occur inside or outside the boundary (for example polluted zones). The distinction between 'inside' and 'outside' turns out to be an intractable philosophical question. The simplest route to its pragmatic solution in programming terms seems to be through the use of Jordan's theorem. An arbitrary point is declared as outside—for example the grid origin of the map—and a line is drawn from it to each event and to each control. We count the number of points where this line crosses a boundary segment of any of the areas in question. If the number is even, then the test point is also outside all of them; if it is odd, then it is inside one of them.

Temporal patterns

The temporal scale is one-dimensional, and it is used to seek one-dimensional phenomena. It is usual first to seek (a) linear trends (upwards or downwards) and (b) cycles (hour of day, month of year, etc.). Trends, sometimes referred to as secular trends, may extend across the full range of the time period, or they may be quite localized (usually referred to as steps). Curvilinear as well as linear trends may be sought. Finally, investigators look for non-linear, non-cyclical, and non-random residual phenomena. This is often referred to as **clustering**, which tends to be regarded as something to be sought after the more systematic forms of variation have been detected and excluded (i.e. de-trended or de-cycled).

Basic formats

There are two basic formats for representing a time series of events. First, we can set a series of rates or integer values on different dates, or in different weeks, or in other short periods. The durations of the periods are arbitrary. The representation is analogous with a choropleth map. Second, we can simply record a series of exact dates and times, to whatever resolution we wish, and we can measure the time intervals between successive pairs or between all possible pairs. The point format can be converted to the period format, at the cost of some loss of information, but the reverse operation is not possible.

Trends

Trends are usually sought using the first of the two formats; each time-period records a number of events (for example cases of meningitis in each week). A simple linear regression coefficient can be calculated using the numbers or rates as the y-variable and the sequence number of the time periods (for example weeks) as the x-variable. The line of best fit is calculated and drawn, and a standard significance test is applied. Residual variations of frequency ('de-trended' values) can be calculated as the differences between the observed values and those predicted from the regression line.

With calendar data it is often sufficient to operate on absolute counts. However, if the population at risk varies over the period of investigation, or is suspected of varying, then we must convert the absolute frequencies to attack rates through reference to the appropriate denominators.

Cycles

Periodicities are also generally sought using the first basic format. Often we can use absolute numbers or, perhaps, de-trended numbers, although it is safer to use rates based upon appropriate denominators. For example, mortality from cerebrovascular accident in the United Kingdom has in recent years exhibited both a steady year-by-year decline and a well-marked seasonal variation. The curve can be de-trended using the first technique, and periodicities displayed on the basis of the residual variations. The raw numbers should be sufficient here, since equal numbers of persons are at risk each month. However, if we were examining the birth prevalence of a malformation, and if we knew or suspected that the numbers of all births varied seasonally, then we would need to calculate the rates for each month. Edwards (1961) devised a method for testing departure from an even non-cycling distribution of uncorrected numerators. A modification devised by Walters and Elwood (1975) incorporated a consideration of varying denominators.

Steps

Steps, which in truth are very short trends, are frequently of interest in relation to environmental hazards. One particular detection procedure, with a long tradition of industrial usage, has been adapted to monitor the frequency of congenital malformations; this is the so-called Cusum procedure (Weatherall and Haskey 1976). An incremental curve of acquisitions of events is simultaneously decremented at each 'tick of the clock' by the expected increase. The cumulative curve of net acquisition, the balance between increment and decrement, is then represented as a horizontal line. Any stepwise change in the level of risk occurring during the period of surveillance causes the horizontal curve to take off at an upward or downward angle from its previous course. Formal tests have been developed for optimizing the sensitivity and specificity of decision criteria and to adjust the ratio of true alarms and false alarms to particular needs; the main virtue of this approach is probably the sensitive and immediate visual trigger that it supplies when plotted on a wall chart. However, it is not particularly useful for the detection of short-term alternations of risk of the switch-up–switch-back variety.

General analyses

As we saw earlier, investigators seeking cyclical phenomena can nominate a particular periodicity in advance (day of week, hour of day, month of year) and test for its presence. However, there are more general approaches, which do not require such prior nomination, for which efficient analytical programs are now available for microcomputers. The first general method is known as Fourier analysis and the second is polynomial analysis.

Fourier analysis programs decompose a curve of any complexity into a series of sine waves of successive integer frequencies, and they calculate a coefficient (i.e. a weighting) and a significance test appropriate to each of these cycles. By an **integer frequency** $(1,2,...,n)$, we mean a wave form with $1,2,...,n$ complete cycles within the total period of observation. Frequency is the reciprocal of the length of the cycle, expressed as a fraction of the total period of observation. We can extend the integer-frequency analysis to include all frequencies up to the point where n is half the total number of data-containing cells within the total observation period. It is possible to reconstruct the original curve exactly from these coefficients or, alternatively, to construct an approximation to it from a limited number of statistically significant coefficients.

The second method, polynomial analysis, is generally simpler to use. The curve is expressed in the form

$$y = a + bx + cx^2 + dx^3 + ex^4 + \ldots + tx^n.$$

This is an extension of linear and quadratic regression; however, it provides a more flexible curve which can be fitted to more complex serial data sets. The maximum number of coefficients is one less than the number of data points. The fitting is done by minimizing the least-squares deviation of the observations from the regression line. This method is capable, using a few coefficients, of providing a concise summary of the basic waveforms underlying a curve with a large amount of random variation. It is purely descriptive, has no specific biological interpretation apart from its capacity to exclude a purely random explanation, and cannot be extrapolated beyond the limits of the data.

These techniques are for special cases, and such generality of analysis is not often justified. We usually have sufficient prior indications of cyclical patterns or other forms of variation to know in advance the form that we have to test.

Clusters in time

A series of integers representing events in successive time intervals (period format above) can be treated, under the terms of the null hypothesis, as elements of a Poisson distribution. The observed frequency distribution of time periods with $0,1,2,\ldots,n$ events can be compared with a calculated Poisson distribution to see whether the observed pattern differs from it. For a reasonably large average value per interval (for example $n > 8$), we can use the theorem that the variance of a Poisson distribution is equal to its mean and the standard deviation of the sampling distribution is the square root of the variance. Therefore we do not expect individual values to depart very often from n by more than $2\sqrt{n}$ in either direction.

Alternatively, we can calculate a chi-square value for departures from the mean monthly expectation, attaching $n - 1$ degrees of freedom for n time periods. For example a weekly count of infants diagnosed with congenital dislocation of the hip over a ten-year period gave a chi-square of 603.7, with 521 degrees of freedom (df). We use a normalizing transformation to estimate significance. First, we calculate $\sqrt{(2X^2)}=34.75$; then we calculate the random expectation for this value from $\sqrt{(2df-1)}=32.2$. The latter value has unit variance (and unit standard error), from which we see that the observed transformation (34.75) is 2.54 standard errors outside the null expectation.

These methods are commonly used, but this is an intrinsically weak form of examination. It takes no account of any 'order', and loses all information relating to sequence. It will frequently fail to demonstrate genuine non-randomness, and negative findings cannot be trusted.

However, in this kind of work positive findings are almost as difficult to interpret as negative ones. Suppose that in a series of 80 serial values we encountered two cells with 'significant' excesses of cases ($p < 0.05$). This is what we would expect by chance. Suppose now that one of them was quite exceptional, with $p = 0.001$. If this particular cell had been nominated for testing in advance, we would regard the excess as significant. However, the question we really have to ask is the probability that such an event will occur by chance among any of the 80 values.

First, we note that the probability that so many events will not occur in a single nominated cell is $(1 - p)$. Therefore, the probability that it will not occur in any of 80 cells is $(1 - p)^{80}$. Finally, the probability that it will occur in any cell is $1 - (1 - p)^{80}$. Then, $p = 1 - 0.999^{80} = 0.077$. We now see that, while this is still a rather unusual observation on a purely random basis, it is not so unusual that we would feel compelled to accept it as a 'cluster.'

It is not too difficult to 'manufacture' significant findings in such situations. We might double up the weeks to fortnights, or measure the weeks from Thursday to Wednesday instead of

Monday to Sunday, or some such procedure. Of course, this is illegitimate. It would be better to recognize from the beginning the difficulties that will be encountered, both with respect to false negatives and false positives, and to use instead a form of investigation that makes use of 'sequence' information right from the start.

Sequence-based tests

The **sliding window** technique was devised in order to evade the problem of locating the boundaries of successive time intervals in a particular way. Suppose that we have records of a sparse set of events, located to individual days, and that we wish to search for the 'maximum seven-day period' without committing ourselves to the day of the week on which this might begin. Probability calculations based upon an arbitrary (for example Monday-to-Sunday) week would not then be legitimate. The sliding-window method is an extension of the probability conversion technique described above. An exact mathematical solution for this manoeuvre has, indeed, been found, but the time required for its computation is impractical on existing computers (Naus 1965).

Approximations have been worked out to relieve this problem (Knox and Lancashire 1982), but yet another problem appears. Although the window may be located at any position, it is still a window of predefined size. Unless we have good prior information as to what that size might be, the real problem is to look for clusters of an undefined length at any position. This is not the relatively simple question that the sliding-window test answers, and its extended generality increases the mathematical difficulty and reduces further the efficiency of the search method. For obvious reasons, these methods are not widely used.

This example has been discussed at disproportionate length because it illustrates a very general point, namely that in the absence of a good prior epidemiological model, the questions arising in such situations are almost always of such generality and so lacking in specificity as to defeat the significance test approach altogether. The best to be expected from an initial approach is a clarification of the question, so that it can be asked again more precisely on another occasion, using fresh data.

There are other kinds of sequencing tests from which to choose, but they all run into similar problems. For example, the **runs test** classifies successive intervals as containing more than or less than the median value (for example coded + or −). There is a very simple test for measuring the probability that n consecutive runs of pluses or minuses might be encountered. This test will detect periods of increased or decreased incidence spanning, for example eight or more intervals; a greater length of run reduces the total number of runs, and it is this reduction that we test. However, the runs test would be of little use if an epidemic oscillation of higher frequency produced something approaching an alternation of short and long intervals. A number of other tests (for example the Kolmogorov–Smirnov test) also interact with cyclical or clustering frequencies; this particular test will detect slow long-term changes but is unsuitable for detecting other forms of heterogeneity, including tight clusters. The technique of serial correlation, in which the number of events (or the rate) in one time period is correlated with the number in the next, is another test which is sometimes useful, but it is also susceptible to interactions between the periodicities of the measuring scale and of the underlying process.

An analogous method is to calculate 'parallel' correlations between two separate series of events. For example, if we wished to examine the hypothesis that outbreaks of meningococcal meningitis are triggered by inhibitory cross-immunity reactions involving a particular form of *Escherichia coli*, then we would set week-by-week isolations of the two organisms alongside each other and look for cross-correlations between the two. We might also wish to experiment with a series of time offsets between the two data sets.

Exact timings and the detection of clusters

In the previous section, time was generally presented as the x co-ordinate and the number of events as the enumerated value. In this section we consider the alternative class of presentation, where the lengths of the intervals between the events are treated as a quantitative independent variable x and the number of intervals of different lengths as the enumerated value y. This is the natural mode of presentation for calendar plots with sparse distributions of events, such that most of the days contain no events at all and the remainder contain only one each.

For a first approach, the observed distribution of interval lengths between successive pairs can be set against a calculated negative-exponential distribution. This is the natural form of the frequency distribution of spells between randomly occurring events. Clustering, and indeed any heterogeneity of frequency, would be represented here as an excess of observed over expected at both the left-hand (short) and the right-hand (long) ends of the scale. This approach may sometimes be fruitful but is *a priori* inefficient. It fails to use any of the information contained in the adjacency or non-adjacency of different short/long intervals, i.e. it wastes information about sequence.

The runs test can again be used in this context to repair some of this deficiency (Siegel 1956). The intervals are classified according to whether they are greater than (+) or less than (−) the median interval, and the numbers of alternating 'runs' of pluses and minuses are counted. However, as mentioned earlier, it is not a good test for the detection of isolated or sparsely repeated tight clusters of (say) two to five events.

An alternative and more fruitful method of taking account of sequential relationships between shorter and longer intervals is to construct a distribution of intervals between all possible pairs of events rather than (as earlier) between successive events. The form of the distribution turns out to be quite simple. It is triangular in shape, high to the left and tapering downward toward the right. For a series of indefinite duration, it approaches the form of a rectangular flat-topped distribution. A plot of the observed distribution of interval lengths between all possible pairs, set against an expected set of values, clearly contains much more information relevant to infective and toxic models than does a distribution of intervals between successive pairs alone. This kind of display is capable, in principle, of displaying not only an excess of the very shortest intervals (such as we might expect from a point-source infective epidemic or a 'toxic cloud' escape) but also of intervals of other 'preferred' lengths (such as might occur in the onward transmission of an infective process through secondary and tertiary waves, each separated by one latent interval).

For a period of D days with n events, and $n(n-1)/2$ possible pairs of events, the number of pairs separated by less than t days is

$$\frac{n(n-1)}{2}(1-v^2) \text{ where } v = \frac{D-t}{D-0.5}$$

Time on time

Exactly as for our initial discussions on geographic distributions, we have so far considered temporal distributions mainly *in vacuo*, without reference to anything else that might have been marked on the calendar. Exactly as for geographic distributions, there may be considerable advantages in setting one temporal plot upon another. As with geographically distributed hazards, the representation of temporal hazards may take different forms ranging from point events (such as earthquakes), through point events with extended subsequent exposures to a continuing risk (such as Chernobyl), to prolonged periods of exposure with well-defined or ill-defined onsets and terminations (such as the marketing of thalidomide or the practice of taking radiographs of pregnant women). For short exposures we must introduce a concept with no clear geographic analogue, namely the concept of the latent period. If we have prior evidence as to what that latent interval might be, the power of the examination is greatly increased. Otherwise, we must investigate parallel correlations between putative hazards and effects by using a series of different offsets. Unfortunately, this introduces additional degrees of freedom to any prior hypotheses that we wish to test. Thus the tests themselves are degraded. In practice, we find ourselves returning to a now familiar problem; we must use a first data set only to formulate hypotheses and a second independent set of data to test them.

Interactions

In addition to detecting and interpreting heterogeneities of disease frequency according to place, time, or person, epidemiologists may wish to seek interactions between these different forms of heterogeneity. Such interactions are among the most fruitful of analytical tools. We can, in principle, ask three general questions.

1. Is a geographic heterogeneity constant in time or does it change? Conversely (but equivalently) formulated, is the temporal heterogeneity constant everywhere, or does it differ in extent or in its configuration in different places? Put briefly, is there evidence of a space–time interaction?
2. Is the temporal distribution constant for different kinds of affected persons or does it differ? Conversely, but equivalently, do different kinds of affected persons display the same form and the same degree of temporal heterogeneity? Put briefly, is there evidence of a person–time interaction?
3. Is the geographic heterogeneity constant for different kinds of affected persons or does it differ? Conversely, do different kinds of persons display the same or a different geographic pattern? Put briefly, is there evidence of a person–place interaction?

The last two interactions are mentioned here only for the purpose of completeness and for illustrating the generality of the interaction concept. We pursue the examination of space–time interactions (question 1 above) in greater detail below.

Space–time interaction

The main application of space–time analysis is to detect sparse mobile clusters. Each individual cluster is conceived as being located within the three dimensions of an extended space–time block and is, itself, defined in terms of its joint geographic and temporal limits. Several clusters, located in different parts of the extended block, are conceived as having similar spatial and temporal sizes, reflecting a common interaction between some biological process and the socio-demographic structure of the local population. The initial problem is not so much to identify a particular cluster as to demonstrate the phenomenon of clustering within a data set bounded by defined time and geographic limits.

If a narrow time slice is taken from such a time–space block, then any space–time clusters will appear as a simple geographic–cluster pattern. Alternatively, if a sufficiently small geographic subarea is examined, then these space–time clusters will appear as a temporal–cluster pattern. A space–time cluster pattern can be regarded as either a time-dispersed set of different geographic patterns—a series of maps—or a spatially dispersed set of time cluster patterns—a group of non-synchronous time plots. It is possible to simplify a space–time distribution by collapsing the time dimension, thereby producing a simple map. Alternatively, the geographic dimensions can be collapsed, and the result then projected onto the time-scale alone. Thus, so far as events are concerned, each of the simple cluster formats already presented——temporal and geographic—can be seen as condensations of this more general format.

The 'subslice' and 'collapsing' techniques do raise a problem, however. If a sufficiently small time period is taken, then there may be insufficient cases for the observer to be reasonably sure that the geographic clustering is real. If a wider time slice, incorporating more months and years, is taken, then the inconstant position of the clusters may effectively 'even out' the geographic heterogeneities. The phenomenon, even though it is real, will disappear. Conversely stated, a sufficiently small geographic area may contain insufficient cases for the observer to be sure that the temporal clustering is real. If the geographic area is enlarged, then the out-of-phase nature of the different temporal cluster components may 'even out' the total, so that the phenomenon again dissipates.

One solution consists of an expansion of the 'all possible pairs' treatment of time sequences, which was described earlier. The 'all possible pairs' are categorized simultaneously in terms of time apart and distance apart. These differencing operations create new variables with new spatial and temporal dimensionalities. Distance, which is non-directional, effectively removes both the geographic coordinate scales. A two-dimensional table of observations relating to pairs of events is constructed in order to display the relative numbers of pairs with different combinations of long and short time separations, and long and short distance separations.

The overall distribution of temporal intervals can be expected to be triangular (for a constant overall incidence), but the distribution of spatial intervals is idiosyncratic and depends upon the geography of the particular population. The expected values for the cells of the table can be obtained from the marginal totals (time intervals and distance intervals) and compared with the observed values.

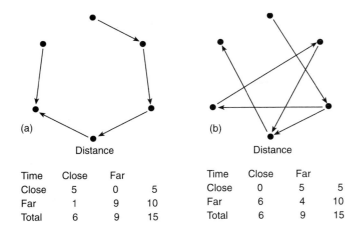

Time	Distance Close	Far	
Close	5	0	5
Far	1	9	10
Total	6	9	15

Time	Distance Close	Far	
Close	0	5	5
Far	6	4	10
Total	6	9	15

Fig. 7.2 Stylized space–time interactions for six events. (Source: Shore, R.E., Hemplemann, L.H., Kowaluk, E., *et al.* (1977). Breast neoplasms in women treated with X-rays for acute postpartum mastitis. *Journal of the National Cancer Institute*, **59**, 813.)

Short-distance short-time clustering is displayed as an excess of observed pairs over expected pairs in the short-distance short-time cells. A positive finding means that, following the occurrence of an index case, any subsequent cases appearing within a short period of time are more likely than otherwise to occur within a short distance as well.

The interaction format is illustrated in Fig. 7.2. We imagine six events located at the vertices of a regular hexagon. These six events generate 15 possible pairs, six of which are adjacent on the perimeter and can be classified as 'close', while the remaining nine pairs are 'distant.' These considerations determine the grand total and the column totals of the tabular representations. In Fig. 7.2(a) we imagine a contagious process in which events at times 1,2, . . . ,6 form a 'contagious' pattern, with each event following on at the position closest to the previous event. In Fig. 7.2(b) we envisage an 'anti-contagious' process in which successive events consistently skip the nearest position and strike at the next. Inspection of the figures and the derived tables clearly illustrates the manner in which these two hypothetical sequences produce different numerical interactions within a table whose marginal totals are fixed by the circumstances.

This form of analysis offers an unexpected benefit to the analyst. Because it is designed to display only interactions, it can operate upon the absolute numerators rather than rates, and the observed-to-expected ratios can be obtained from marginal totals without reference to the population at risk. The technique is effectively 'denominator free'. This freedom also allows the analyst to pursue higher levels of interaction. For example, in the investigation of childhood cancers we may first of all seek evidence of interaction among all possible pairs irrespective of the type of cancer. We then repeat the analysis for leukaemia–leukaemia pairs, and again for solid tumour–solid tumour pairs; finally, by subtracting the last two tabulations from the first, we display an interaction pattern for leukaemia–solid tumour pairs.

The author has also experimented with the reproduction of epidemics in compressed real time on a map drawn on the screen of a microcomputer. The objective was to see whether 'eyeball real time' techniques were capable of picking up space–time cluster

patterns intuitively when the actual epidemic was displayed in this manner. In general, this has not proved to be a successful approach to detection. For example, occurrences of congenital hydrocephalus raised no intuitive suspicions when displayed in this way, yet showed a clear space–time interaction when analysed formally (Knox and Lancashire 1991).

Different applications of the space–time principle have used different modes of display and analysis. The simplest (the Knox method, as described above) uses simple contingency tables (Knox 1963, 1964). The Mantel method (Mantel 1967; Klauber 1971) is based upon parametric statistics and is essentially a correlative representation of the associations between the time and space intervals. However, because of the non-normal distribution of the time and distance intervals, the Mantel method first converts times and distances to their reciprocals (which values can be referred to as 'closeness'), converting the original asymmetric distributions to forms more appropriate to testing through standard correlative/ regression methods.

However, there is a special problem in testing significance for any method based on all possible pairs. The pairs are not independent of each other; each of the n individual events has been incorporated into $(n-1)$ of the $n(n-1)/2$ pairs. This can invalidate the use of methods based on the Poisson distribution (such as the chi-square statistic), which are based upon the premise of independence. These tests are valid only when the dichotomies between short and long times and between short and long distances are sufficiently asymmetric to render the short-time short-distance pairs effectively independent of each other. The parametric method partly overcomes this difficulty by circumventing the problems of what dichotomies to choose, but can be less efficient at distinguishing highly localized (very short time, very short distance) clustering from within a large number of more widely spaced pairs. As with other choices between alternative modes of presentation and testing, some techniques are more effective in one situation and others are more effective elsewhere.

Space–time interactions do not have to be based upon pairs alone. They can be based upon an examination of all possible triplets, all possible quadruplets, . . . ,n-tuplets . . . , using some composite value of spatial and temporal distance for purposes of tabulation. For example the mean distance and the mean time interval between all possible pairs within the n-tuplet can be used for an overall space–time tabulation. These methods are expensive in computer time, and the tabulation must usually be restricted to a search for interactions within one part of the total tabulation, setting upper limits to the n-tuplet times that will be incorporated within the analysis. The interaction is then sought, in effect, within a moving time window. Moving narrow time limits are also useful in pair analyses pursued over extended time periods during which the spatial population distribution may itself have shifted, and where an unrestricted search may superimpose a demographic artefact upon the disease-pair findings (a method used by Knox and Gilman (1992a)).

Spatial and temporal models

There is a constant pressure upon investigators of spatial/temporal data to move beyond the scope of traditional statistical analysis and into the domain of model construction, model validation, and the estimation of model parameters. This arises partly from the limited relevance and validity of sampling theory in this field, and the limited value that can be placed upon significance tests and the calculation of confidence limits. It is reflected in the wide usage of 'eyeball interpretation', for example in the inspection of maps. Such interpretations usually depend upon investigators bringing external knowledge and externally derived theoretical constructs to bear upon their data. Indeed, this is the main point of drawing maps and plotting graphs. If analysis could be handled entirely through formal techniques, then plotting for visual inspection would not be necessary at all.

Another area where model fitting, whether intuitive or formal, seems obligatory is in the study of natural histories. For example, cervical cancer screening policies still suffer from the inadequacy of the available natural history formulations. It was recognized many years ago that much of this problem arose from the manner in which screening services had become focused upon the individual test result, and from the technical and operational difficulties of assembling these observations into sequences. Clearly, a 'natural history' was dimensioned in time, and it was not possible to infer the natural history of this disease until time-dimensioned records of the process had been assembled through large-scale linking of the results and the dates of successive examinations in the same women. However, even when this was achieved, how was a natural history to be calculated from temporally linked data? Where was the computational algorithm for doing this?

Except for the simplest components of a natural history, the only practical way of handling this problem is to 'propose' a natural history model, to set it out in the form of a matrix of transfer rates between different stages of the disease, and to adjust the values until the calculated consequences successfully match the observed age-specific prevalences and incidences of the different pathological states. Several quite different models may be capable of achieving this! That is to say, the data might be incapable of distinguishing between these alternative models. This can be something of a shock to planners of preventive services; however, to scientists it may indicate what kinds of data must next be collected and analysed in order to solve a problem now recognized as unsolved.

A modelling approach also permits a more satisfactory definition of a cluster than that afforded by effectively defining the phenomenon as a residual statistical heterogeneity after the exclusion of trends and cycles. Negative definitions are seldom of much use, yet this is a position into which many investigators have been forced. In 'model' terms, we can define a cluster in an alternative and positive manner as a temporally and/or spatially bounded set of events that are related to each other through some biological or social mechanism, or that have a common relationship with some other event or circumstance. Declared in this way, the definition itself owes nothing to probability theory or random distributions or to departures from them. It does not mention statistical criteria at all. This has the advantage that we are now entitled to use statistical methods to decide when such clustering might be present, without becoming embroiled in the circularities that occur when we use statistical concepts for both our definition and our decision process. It also serves as a reminder that, once our suspicions are aroused, we must still seek to uncover the biological or social mechanisms,

and that the 'reality' or otherwise of our clusters depends ultimately upon our success in doing this.

References

Cooke-Mozaffari, P.J., Ashwood, F.L., Vincent, T., *et al.* (1987). *Cancer incidence and mortality in the vicinity of nuclear installations: England and Wales, 1950–1980.* Studies on Medical and Population Subjects No. 51. HMSO, London.

Draper, G. (1991). *The geographical epidemiology of childhood leukaemia and non-Hodgkin lymphoma in Great Britain, 1966–1983.* Office of Population Censuses and Surveys, London.

Edwards, J.H. (1961). The recognition and estimation of cyclic trends. *Annals of Human Genetics*, 25, 83–7.

Gardner, M.J., Winter, P.D., Taylor, C.P., and Acheson, E.D. (1983). *Atlas of cancer mortality in England and Wales, 1968–78.* Wiley, Chichester.

Kemp, I., Boyle, P., Smans, M., and Muir, C. (ed.) (1985). *Atlas of cancer in Scotland 1975–1980: incidence and epidemiological perspective.* IARC Scientific Publications, Vol. 72. IARC, Lyon.

Klauber, M.R. (1971). Two-sample randomization tests for space–time clustering. *Biometrics*, 27, 129–42.

Knox, E.G. (1963). Detection of low intensity epidemicity: application to cleft lip and palate. *British Journal of Preventive and Social Medicine*, 17, 121–7.

Knox, E.G. (1964). Epidemiology of childhood leukaemia in Northumberland and Durham. *British Journal of Preventive and Social Medicine*, 18, 17–24.

Knox, E.G. (1994). Leukaemia clusters in childhood: geographical analysis in Britain. *Journal of Epidemiology and Community Health*, 48, 369–76.

Knox, E.G. and Gilman, E.A. (1992a). Leukaemia clusters in Great Britain: 1. Space–time interactions. *Journal of Epidemiology and Community Health*, 46, 566–72.

Knox, E.G. and Gilman, E.A. (1992b). Leukaemia clusters in Great Britain: 2. Geographical concentrations. *Journal of Epidemiology and Community Health*, 46, 573–6.

Knox, E.G. and Lancashire, R.J. (1982). Detection of minimal epidemics. *Statistics in Medicine*, 1, 183–9.

Knox, E.G. and Lancashire, R.J. (1991). *Epidemiology of congenital malformations.* HMSO, London.

Knox, E.G., Stewart, A.M., Gilman, E.A., and Kneale, G.W. (1988). Background radiation and childhood cancers. *Journal of Radiological Protection*, 8(1), 9–18.

McGlashan, N.D. (ed.) (1972). *Medical geography.* Methuen, London.

Mantel, N. (1967). The detection of disease clustering and a generalised regression approach. *Cancer Research*, 27, 209–20.

Naus, J.L. (1965). The distribution of the size of the maximum cluster of points on a line. *Journal of the American Statistical Association*, 60, 532–8.

Openshaw, S., Craft, A.W., Charlton, M., and Birch, J.M. (1988). Investigation of leukaemia clusters by use of a geographical analysis machine. *Lancet*, i, 272–3.

Raper, J.F., Rhind, D.W., and Shepherd, J.W. (1992). *Postcodes: the new geography.* Longman, Harlow.

Selvin, S., Shaw, G., Schulman, J., and Merrill, D.W. (1987). Spatial distribution of disease: three case studies. *Journal of the National Cancer Institute*, 79(3), 417–23.

Siegel, S. (1956). *Nonparametric statistics for the behavioural sciences.* McGraw-Hill, New York.

Stone, R.A. (1988). Investigations of excess environmental risks around putative sources: statistical problems and a proposed test. *Statistics in Medicine*, 7, 649–60.

Walters, S.D. and Elwood, J.M. (1975). A test for seasonality of events with a variable population at risk. *British Journal of Preventive and Social Medicine*, 29, 18–21.

Weatherall, J.A.C. and Haskey, J.C. (1976). Surveillance of malformations. *British Medical Bulletin*, 32, 39–44.

8 Cross-sectional studies

J.H. Abramson

Introduction

This chapter deals with prevalence and other cross-sectional studies, i.e. with surveys of the situation existing at a given time (or during a given period) in a group or population or a set of groups or populations. These surveys may be concerned with:

- the presence of disorders, such as diseases, disabilities, and symptoms of ill-health;
- dimensions of positive health, such as physical fitness;
- other attributes relevant to health, such as blood pressure and body measurements;
- factors associated with health and disease, such as exposure to specific environmental factors, defined social and behavioural attributes (including health practices and attitudes to health and health services), and demographic characteristics; the correlates may be determinants, predictors, or effects of health and disease states.

Such a study may be descriptive, analytical, or both. At a descriptive level it yields information about a single variable (acquired immunodeficiency syndrome, haemoglobin concentration, capacity to work, cigarette smoking, etc.) or about each of a number of separate variables, in a total study population or in specific population groups. At an analytical level, it provides information about the presence and strength of associations between variables, permitting the testing of hypotheses about such associations.

Most cross-sectional studies are individual-based, i.e. they seek information about the individuals in the group or sample studied. There are also group-based surveys, which seek information about groups or populations. As an example, Poikolanen and Eskola (Poikolanen and Eskola 1988) found that mortality rates from various causes in 25 developed countries had strong negative associations with the per capita gross domestic product (a measure of economic development), but not with the numbers of doctors, nurses, or hospital beds per 10 000 population or with health expenditure per head. Analytical group-based surveys are sometimes referred to as ecological or correlational studies.

Cross-sectional studies may be contrasted with incidence and other 'time-span' studies that require information relating to two or more points of time. The latter studies, which are discussed in later chapters, measure changes in status (e.g. disease onset, growth, changes in blood pressure) or examine associations between variables with a defined temporal relationship, e.g. between childhood experiences and health in adulthood, or between treatment and subsequent survival. The difference between cross-sectional surveys and these studies is often likened to the difference between snapshots and motion pictures.

This distinction is not, however, a rigid one. Although the essential feature of cross-sectional surveys is that they collect information relating to a single specified time, they are often extended to include historical information that can be easily collected at the same time. This may lead to the demonstration of statistical associations with past experience, e.g. a relationship between varicose veins and the number of pregnancies (Maffei et al. 1986) and a negative association (in women) between weight and the frequency of drinking alcohol during the previous year (Williamson et al. 1987). Field investigations of epidemics (see Volume 2, Chapter 9) typically combine a cross-sectional approach (case-finding and the investigation of environmental and other hazards) with the collection of historical information (about possible exposures to infection). Case–control comparisons that are confined to current (and not historical) information can be regarded as cross-sectional studies, but are conveniently considered with other case–control studies see Volume 2, Chapter 10.

Unless historical information is collected, cross-sectional studies are generally non-directional, in the sense that specific variables cannot necessarily be considered as causes or effects when associations between variables are analysed and construed. The temporal relationships of the variables (which came first?) may be uncertain. Sometimes, however, data that refer to a single point in time can be treated as if they referred to different times, and it is reasonable to consider a causal relationship in a specific direction. In a study of behavioural problems in school, for example, the lead content of the schoolchildren's milk teeth was used as an indicator of lead poisoning in early childhood (Needleman et al. 1979).

If cross-sectional studies are repeated they may be used for the purpose of health surveillance, to observe changes in the population's health status and its determinants. If there are enough surveys extending over a long enough period they may be used to reconstruct the lifetime experience of birth cohorts. An analysis of successive surveys of smoking habits in Norway, for example, demonstrated the differences between the smoking habits of people born in different periods and the changes that occurred in specific birth cohorts (Ronneberg et al. 1994). Such appraisals are generally based on a comparison of graphs based on a rearrangement of the age-specific findings of successive studies. Ages at the time of the study are converted to birth-dates, and birth-cohort graphs are then constructed by bringing together the data for each birth cohort and plotting them against age; also, the data for each age group can be plotted against year of birth or year of death

(McMahon and Pugh 1970). Birth-cohort effects can also be investigated by the median polish procedure (Selvin 1991)—a very simple exploratory data analysis technique that shows whether age and time trends alone can explain the findings—as well as by more elaborate statistical procedures.

The uses of cross-sectional studies can be categorized as follows:

1. The findings may be used to promote the health of the specific group or population studied; i.e. the study can be used as a tool in community health care.

2. The study may contribute to clinical care.

3. The study may provide 'new knowledge'—generalizable inferences that can be applied beyond the specific group or population studied. This knowledge may relate, for example, to the aetiology of a disease or the value of a type of health care.

These uses are, of course, not mutually exclusive; a single study may fulfil more than one purpose.

This chapter briefly considers the terms prevalence and incidence, and then reviews the methods used in cross-sectional studies, paying special attention to rapid epidemiological appraisal (cluster surveys and rapid methods of data collection) and to statistical measures, including prevalence rates of various kinds. The next three sections give consideration to the uses listed above. The first of these sections, on uses in community health care, considers community diagnosis, surveillance, community education and community involvement, and the evaluation of a community's health care. The subsection on community diagnosis deals with studies of health status, determinants of health and disease, associations between variables (including the measurement of impact, risk markers, and community syndromes), and the identification of groups requiring special care. The section on uses in clinical practice briefly describes applications in individual and family care and in community-oriented primary care. The section on studies yielding new knowledge reviews studies of growth and development, studies of aetiology, and programme trials.

Prevalence and incidence

Prevalence refers to the number of individuals who have a given disease or other defined attribute at a specific time, as opposed to incidence, which refers to the number of events that occur within a given period. The event may be the onset of a new disease, death, and so on.

The prevalence of a disease in a population at any point in time depends on the prior incidence of new cases and on the average duration of the disease from onset to recovery or death. This relationship is outlined in Fig. 8.1, in which the contents of the container represent prevalence, and the time spent in the container is the duration of the disease.

If incidence and the average duration have remained constant over a long period (a condition seldom encountered in real life), the point prevalence rate (defined below) is the product of the incidence rate of new cases per time unit t and the average duration of the disease (mean t per case). For a disease that runs an episodic course, the point prevalence rate of active disease is (under certain assumptions) the product of the incidence rate, the average

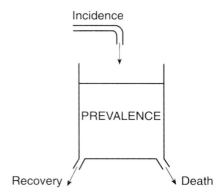

Fig. 8.1 Relationship between prevalence and incidence.

duration of an episode, and the average number of episodes per case (Von Korff and Parker 1980).

Methods

Like any other kind of study, a cross-sectional study can yield useful findings only if sound methods are used. At all stages—in the planning phase, during the collection of data, and when the data are processed and interpreted—there is a need for detailed attention to methods (Abramson 1990), so as to minimize bias and ensure that the results will be as accurate as practical constraints permit. Simple rapid methods may be called for if resources are limited or speedy results are needed (see below).

A cross-sectional study may be performed in a total target group or population, or in a representative sample. Simple random sampling or systematic, stratified, or cluster sampling may be used (Cochran 1977).

Methods of collecting information may be broadly classified as follows:

1. Clinical examinations, special tests, and other observations.

2. Interviews and questionnaires. The subjects themselves may be questioned, or proxy respondents, e.g. household informants, may be used.

3. Clinical records and other documentary sources. Sources of information on the prevalence of diseases include hospital and other medical records, disease registers, records of routine examinations (in schools, prenatal clinics, army induction centres, health insurance schemes, etc.), and published statistics based on these or other records.

Disease prevalence may be studied in two stages, by using a screening test to identify people who are likely to have a given disease, and then subjecting them to more elaborate and specific tests.

Each method of data collection has its own advantages and limitations and carries its own possible biases. If information on the prevalence of a disease is obtained from hospitals, for example, people with mild disease are likely to be under-represented. The degree of bias may vary for different categories of the study population as a result of variation in the accessibility or use of health services, or of differences between clinical services in their diagnostic and recording procedures. In a rural region in the United States, Anderson *et al.* (Anderson *et al.* 1988) found that 42 per cent of the cases of Parkinson's disease found in a survey based on screening questions and subsequent neurological examinations had not been diagnosed previously, and would have been missed by a survey based on medical records. Had people in institutions been omitted from the survey, a quarter of the cases would have been overlooked.

Since any method of case-finding may miss cases, it is often recommended that prevalence surveys should use more than one method, and combine the findings. The cases can be cumulated, or the total (including cases not found by any method) can be estimated by the 'capture–recapture' and related techniques (Hook and Regal 1993; McCarty *et al.* 1993). These are methods used in estimating animal populations, where they are based on marking and releasing a batch of captured animals, and then seeing how many are recaptured in the next batch of animals caught. Applied to two independent case-finding procedures that identify A and B cases respectively, with C cases common to both procedures, the formula for the estimated 'ascertainment-corrected' total number of cases is

$$[(A + 1)(B + 1)/(C + 1)] - 1.$$

The estimated variance is

$$[(A + 1)(B + 1)(A - C)(B - C)]/[(B + 1)^2(B + 2)].$$

In a study of childhood diabetes in Madrid, 451 cases were identified—432 by one procedure and 138 by another, with 119 common to both. The estimated total by the above formula was 501; the 95 per cent confidence interval (by the above variance formula) was 472 to 530 or (by a more conservative formula suggested by Hilden 1994) 451 to 552. But case-finding procedures are usually not independent, and cases ascertained by one method are often especially likely to be identified by another method also. The calculated total will then be an underestimate; the total will be an overestimate if cases ascertained by one method are likely to be missed by the other.

This bias can be largely controlled by log-linear modelling (the multiple recapture census). This is a more elaborate technique that takes account of the observed dependencies between procedures (Fienberg 1972; Bishop *et al.* 1975), and can be used if there are three or more case-finding methods; a computer is required. Frischer *et al.* (Frischer *et al.* 1991) used this technique to estimate the number of injecting drug users in Glasgow, where 2006 cases were ascertained from three sources. The computed 'ascertainment-corrected' total was 13 050, a number that the authors reduced to 9424 to compensate for possible false-positive reports (95 per cent confidence interval = 6964–11 884). These methods of estimation are useful, although they do not completely answer the problem of incomplete ascertainment (Fienberg 1972; Armstrong and Hayes 1992; Kiemeney *et al.* 1994). If, for example, a certain type of case is 'uncatchable'—i.e. systematically missed by *all* procedures—no manipulation can estimate their number; or if all cases have in fact been found, the computed total will be an overestimate.

Associations observed in the group studied may differ from those in the general population if admission rates to the study group are connected with the variables whose associations are studied. This is a common form of bias (berksonian bias) in studies of hospital or clinic patient and autopsy samples.

In addition to selection bias, where the individuals for whom data are available are not representative of the target population (generally because of failure to choose a representative sample, or incomplete coverage of the sample or study group), there may be information bias, caused by shortcomings in the gathering or handling of information. A catalogue of biases, most of them applicable to cross-sectional studies, has been published by Sackett (Sackett 1979).

In cross-sectional studies that set out to examine causal associations, bias is commonly caused by the respondents' or investigators' knowledge that there has been exposure to the putative cause (a source of bias in cohort studies also) or that the putative effect is present (a source of bias in case–control studies also). In a study of the association between coffee drinking and digestive symptoms, for example, a respondent who drinks much coffee and believes that this beverage causes digestive upsets may be more likely to recall and report symptoms, or an interviewer may tend to be more persistent when asking such a respondent about symptoms. Also, subjects who have symptoms and believe these are caused by coffee may tend to provide a fuller (or exaggerated) account of their consumption of the beverage, and interviewers may tend to be especially persistent when questioning subjects whom they know to have symptoms. The subjects' awareness of their symptoms may also have led them to avoid coffee. These and other kinds of bias can be minimized by suitable survey procedures.

Some biases can be avoided, measured, or corrected during the analysis. Others cannot, but must still be taken into account when inferences are drawn from the findings.

When analysing the findings of a cross-sectional study, the exploration of cause–effect relationships may be based on the retrospective ('backward-looking') approach that characterizes most case–control studies (e.g. comparing the coffee consumption of people who do and do not have symptoms) or on the prospective ('forward-looking') approach used in cohort studies (comparing the prevalence of symptoms in coffee drinkers and non-drinkers). Cross-sectional studies in which a direction of effect is assumed may be called quasiretrospective or quasiprospective (Abramson 1990). As in other epidemiological studies, causal effects can be inferred from the findings of cross-sectional studies only after careful consideration has been given to the possibility of fortuitous and artefactual associations and confounding effects (Susser 1973; Rothman 1988; Abramson 1994). For example, associations between moderate or vigorous sports activities and low levels of blood pressure and other cardiovascular risk factors, observed in three cross-sectional surveys in Germany, could be taken as evidence for the preventive role of physical activity only after the effects of age, social class, body mass index, overall health, treatment for hypertension, activity at work, and other variables had been taken into account in the analysis (Helmert *et al.* 1994).

The results of group-based (correlational) studies may be especially difficult to interpret, since they are usually based on official statistics, which may not provide satisfactory measures, and confounding may be difficult to control. Moreover, associations found at a group level may not exist at the individual level; there is more malaria in poor countries than in rich countries, but it does not follow that poor people will be at higher risk than better-off people in the same village (the so-called 'ecological fallacy').

Rapid epidemiological assessment

Simple, undemanding, and inexpensive methods can often supply information that will adequately meet the study's purpose. Such methods are particularly useful if financial, and human or other resources are limited, as in developing countries. They also have special relevance in situations (in both developed and developing countries) where it is important to obtain results rapidly as a basis for programme decisions, particularly in the health care of specific communities or regions.

The evolution and use of rapid assessment methods are reviewed by Smith (Smith 1989), who points out that the introduction of these methods was a major factor responsible for the worldwide eradication of smallpox. Rapid assessment is especially important in mass emergencies, where health needs should be appraised within 24 to 48 h (Guha-Sapir 1991).

Simple methods will generally provide information that is less detailed and less accurate than would be provided by more elaborate methods. This does not matter, provided that the information meets the study's purposes. At the same time, special care should be taken to avoid unnecessary inaccuracy, e.g. by due attention to the training of data collectors, and checks on completed questionnaires and the accuracy of data entered into computers.

Aspects of rapid survey methodology that are of relevance to cross-sectional studies—cluster surveys and simplified methods of data collection—are discussed below. In addition, the appropriate use of computers can greatly speed up the performance and analysis of surveys. In developed countries, where most people have telephones, random-digit dialling (Waksberg 1978) can facilitate sample selection, and computer-assisted telephone interviewing (Birkett 1988) can make data collection faster; samples selected by random digit dialling have been reported to be reasonably representative of the general population. As computers decrease in cost and their portability and capabilities increase, they will become increasingly useful as survey tools in developing countries (Bertrand 1985; Byass 1989a, b; Frerichs and Tar 1989) as well as developed ones. Uses of microcomputers are described elsewhere.

Cluster surveys

Two-stage cluster sampling has been advocated by the World Health Organization's (WHO's) Expanded Programme on Immunization since 1978 as a rapid, cheap, and accurate basis for surveys of immunization coverage (Lemeshow and Robinson 1985). The method has been adopted for studies of specific diseases, service coverage, health service needs, and other topics, and a great number of such studies have been done. Cluster surveys have a special role in emergency situations. In the public health disaster that followed civil disturbances in Rwanda in 1994, for example, when over half a million Rwandans fled to Zaïre, such surveys, combined with morbidity surveillance, provided a basis for a programme that was well co-ordinated and was associated with a steep decline in deaths of refugees by the second month of the crisis (Goma Epidemiology Group 1995).

In cluster sampling, a simple random sample is selected not of individual subjects, but of groups or clusters of individuals. This is easier than simple random sampling because there is no need for a list of all potential subjects for use as a sampling framework, and (if the clusters are defined geographically) the selected subjects do not have to be sought in widely scattered locations. Since clusters may contain people with similar characteristics, a representative sample requires a reasonably large number of clusters. If the probability of a cluster's inclusion is proportional to its size, and in the second stage the same number of subjects is selected from each cluster, the sample is a 'self-weighting' one, i.e. one in which each individual has an equal chance of entering; the findings as they stand can therefore be generalized to the target population.

Cluster surveys following the Expanded Programme on Immunization pattern are based on the random selection of 30 or more villages, towns, sectors of cities, etc., the probability of inclusion being proportional to the cluster's size (it is possible for a large cluster to be selected more than once). This requires reasonably accurate population estimates; a simple method of making the selection is described by Bennett et al. (Bennett et al. 1991). Strictly speaking, the subjects in each cluster should be chosen randomly, using a census. But for simplicity, Expanded Programme on Immunization surveys use a modified method. One household in each cluster is randomly selected, preferably using a list or map; alternatively, the investigator can start at a central point, count the number of households (H) in a randomly chosen direction (a spinning top or pencil can be used) from the central point to the border of the area, and then randomly choose a number from 1 to H to identify a household for selection. A preset number of subjects (e.g. children of a defined age) is then studied in each cluster, starting with the selected household and moving on to the next one (the residence whose front door is closest) or (say) the fifth nearest household until the quota is filled.

The number required in each cluster is decided by applying the usual method of estimating sample size for simple random sampling (Cochran 1977; Gahlinger and Abramson 1995) and then multiplying the result by the 'design effect' and dividing it by the number of clusters. The design effect, which expresses the difference in precision between a cluster sample and a simple random sample of the same size, may be estimated from previous surveys (Bennett et al. 1991) or arbitrarily taken as 2. Typical Expanded Programme on Immunization cluster surveys, which aim to provide an immunization coverage rate that is within 10 percentage points of the true rate, with 95 per cent confidence, use seven non-randomly chosen subjects in each of 30 clusters. Computer simulation has shown that although this method yields overall results that are more biased and variable than those based on simple random sampling, it meets the above requirement in over 95 per cent of replications (Henderson and Sundaresan 1982; Lemeshow and Robinson 1985, Lemeshow et al. 1985). The results in specific clusters or in subsets of clusters can of course not be relied on; analyses of a particular cluster are warranted only if the sample is large and not based on non-random selection. Comparisons of subsets of clusters may be feasible, as in an Indian survey that showed a higher level of immunization coverage in urban than in periurban areas and an especially low level in rural areas (Balraj et al. 1993). In a study of disease prevalence, the extent to which the disease is clustered within sampling clusters may be of interest; a survey in Tanzania, for example, revealed clustering of trachoma within neighbourhoods in villages, not explicable by known risk factors (West *et al.* 1991).

Computer simulations suggest that, in view of its ease and cheapness, cluster sampling with non-random selection in the second stage may be 'a reasonable alternative' to simple random sampling even in analytical studies that use the ratio of two prevalence rates (e.g. in people exposed and unexposed to a risk factor) to measure the strength of an association. But if the rates are large and their ratio is high, simple random sampling is much more successful in yielding a ratio within 0·1 of the true value and a confidence interval that includes the true value (Harris and Lemeshow 1991).

Approximate incidence rates can sometimes be derived from the prevalence findings. For example, lame children can be identified in a cluster survey, and the prevalence of lameness attributable to poliomyelitis can then be calculated, using criteria such as the presence of flaccid paralysis and intact sensation, with a history of an acute onset. Correction factors can then be applied to allow for the omission of upper limb paralysis, lethal cases, and complete recovery, and approximate poliomyelitis incidence rates can be computed (LaForce *et al.* 1980). Such a survey in Nigeria led to the estimate of at least 33 300 paralytic poliomyelitis cases annually between 1979 and 1983, before an immunization programme was introduced (Babaniyi and Parakoyi 1991). In Burkino Faso, a cluster survey of this sort led to the conclusion that incidence had decreased significantly between 1984 and 1988, possibly because of immunization (Schwoebel *et al.* 1992). Incidence rates may also be estimated by obtaining a history of diseases or fatal conditions (e.g. neonatal tetanus) that occurred in the households included in the clusters (Rothenberg 1985).

If a large sample size is required and clusters of equal size can be defined, a self-weighting sample can be achieved by selecting a random sample of clusters and then including all eligible individuals, or using the same sampling ratio, in each cluster. Stratification and multistage sampling may be used in cluster surveys. Simple methods of analysis, including the use of simple spreadsheets, are described by Bennett *et al.* (Bennett *et al.* 1991) and Frerichs (Frerichs 1989).

Simplified methods of data collection

Data collection may be simplified in various ways. The most obvious way is to restrict the variables to those that are essential to meet the study's purposes. In a questionnaire survey, questions can be reduced to the minimum, and made as simple as possible to ask and answer. It may be decided to use proxy measures instead of more expensive or elaborate ones, e.g. arm circumference as an easy and cheap index of malnutrition in children (Velzeboer *et al.* 1983*a*, *b*), or night blindness as a relatively easily measured surrogate for vitamin A deficiency (Sommer *et al.* 1980), or a characteristic depigmentation pattern ('leopard skin') as an index of the endemicity of onchocerciasis (Edungbola *et al.* 1987). If measures are simple, it is easy to train health workers or others in their use. Schoolteachers can measure weight and height with adequate precision, assistants can be taught simple cataract recognition (Venkataswamy *et al.* 1989), and traditional midwives have been taught to identify low birth weight babies by using a hand-held scale that shows a coloured signal if the weight is below 2·5 kg

(Ritenbaugh *et al.* 1989). In Tanzania, a simple questionnaire on diseases and symptoms was administered by teachers to children in 245 schools; a comparison with urine tests showed that reports of haematuria or schistosomiasis had a high validity (Lengeler *et al.* 1991).

It may also be possible to choose sources that are easily accessible. Available records may, despite their deficiencies, supply information accurate enough to obviate the need for a more elaborate survey, and patients attending a health facility may be deemed sufficiently representative of the total community to warrant their use (with reservations) as a study sample.

Where appropriate, qualitative (as opposed to quantitative) methods may be used. These are methods, widely used by anthropologists, whose findings are described in words rather than numbers. They are especially useful in the investigation of knowledge, attitudes, and practices—'beliefs and perceptions regarding health, the prevention and treatment of illness, and the utilisation of traditional and biomedical health resources' (Scrimshaw and Hurtado 1987). In this context, these techniques have been termed 'rapid ethnographic assessment' (Smith 1989), 'rapid assessment procedures' (Scrimshaw and Hurtado 1987) and 'social research methods' (Smith and Morrow 1991).

Qualitative methods, which (except in their simplest applications) require special training, may be based on (a) interviews and conversations with key informants and other members of the community, in which people can express their attitudes, perceptions, motivations, feelings, and behaviour; (b) observations in health-care facilities and the community at large; (c) focus group discussions, in which a small group of informants talk freely and spontaneously about themes considered important to the investigator (Khan *et al.* 1991); and (d) other methods. Guidelines for the collection of data on topics related to health and health care are provided by Scrimshaw and Hurtado (Scrimshaw and Hurtado 1987).

Qualitative methods provide 'culture specific maps [that] can help to improve the "fit" of programmes to people'. These maps show the presence of beliefs and behaviours, but not their numerical prevalence in the population (Scrimshaw and Hurtado 1987). Qualitative and quantitative approaches may be regarded as complementary (Kroeger 1983). In a study of the reasons for incomplete childhood immunization in Haiti, for example, ethnographic methods were used to identify barriers to the use of preventive services, and these were then measured in a quantitative survey (Coreil *et al.* 1989). Qualitative methods have also been used as a follow-up to a quantitative study, to explain and expand the findings.

The nominal group technique, which was developed by Van de Ven and Delbecq (Van de Ven and Delbecq 1972), may be used to obtain a semiquantitative picture of the opinions of a number of experts (Abramson 1990). The technique is so called because although the participants sit together, direct interaction is permitted only during specified phases of the process; hence during most phases this is a group 'in name only'. If professionals and/or laypeople who are especially well informed about a specific community are brought together, this simple technique can provide a ranking of the community's perceived problems, or of proposed solutions. The Delphi procedure (Linstone and Turoff 1975) is a much more elaborate method.

The WHO is currently giving emphasis to the development of rapid evaluation methods that can provide timely information on the population's health status and the performance of health-care services, as a basis for immediate adjustments to care programmes; critical tables required by health service managers are generally available within 7 to 10 days, and a draft report in a few weeks (WHO 1993). The approach is essentially the performance of a set of cross-sectional studies using rapid methods, carried out mainly in health-care facilities, with the aim of identifying and solving operational problems. Depending on the issues studied, information may be obtained from the community, e.g. leaders, mothers, or people attending for care (clinic exit interviews), or from health workers, using interviews or focus group discussions, as well as from direct observations of activities in clinics, checks on clinic facilities and supplies, and (rarely) household interviews (Anker *et al.* 1993).

Statistical measures

The statistical measures used to summarize the findings of descriptive cross-sectional studies include means and standard deviations, medians, percentiles, and other quantiles, measures of prevalence (see below), and other proportions. Ratios other than proportions are occasionally used, e.g. the sex ratio (usually the male to female ratio) of people with a specific disease. Separate statistical measures may be provided for specific sex and age categories, ethnic groups, social classes, regions, etc. Measures of association commonly used in analytical cross-sectional studies are described below.

If the study is based on a random sample, confidence intervals may be calculated in order to obtain an interval that has a high probability of containing the true value of the measure in the total target population. Confidence intervals are also often calculated, even in the absence of a 'chance' process such as random sampling, to permit generalization to a broad 'reference' population, e.g. 'the nation's children', but in this instance the procedure is open to criticism.

Measures of prevalence

A measure of prevalence, or prevalence rate, expresses the relative frequency of a disease or other qualitative attribute in a group or population; it is a proportion. It should be noted that this use of the convenient term 'prevalence rate', which conforms with common usage by many epidemiologists, is disparaged by many experts who prefer to confine the term 'rate' to measures of the rapidity of change, and therefore use 'prevalence' or 'prevalence proportion' rather than 'prevalence rate', claiming that the latter is an impossible concept (Elandt-Johnson 1975).

There are different kinds of prevalence rate. When the term is used without qualification it usually refers to a point prevalence rate, i.e. the prevalence at a specified point of time. The point prevalence rate of a disease per 1000 population, for example, is calculated by the formula:

$$\frac{\text{Number of individuals with the disease at a specified point of time}}{\text{Population at that time}} \times 1000.$$

The numerator of this rate is the total number of people who have the disease at the stated time, irrespective of when the disease

commenced. The denominator is the total population (actual or estimated) at that time, including affected and unaffected people. A multiplier of 1000 or any other convenient or conventional multiple of 10 is used (as in other rates) in order to eliminate awkward decimals—a rate of 6·5 per 100 000 is easier to comprehend than the equivalent 0·000065.

The point of time to which prevalence refers need not be a fixed calendar time. The reference may be to a fixed point in the experience of each individual, e.g. birth, entry to a job or army service, immigration, death, or (in a prevalence survey where interviews or examinations are staggered over a period) the date of examination. In such instances the formula is:

$$\frac{\text{Number of individuals with the disease at the time the individual is studied}}{\text{Number of individuals studied}} \times 1000.$$

A rate expressing the frequency of a finding in an autopsy study is a point prevalence rate that refers to the time of death. Such a rate is especially useful to indicate the prevalence of a disorder whose presence does not affect the risk of dying or the probability of an autopsy. Autopsy studies showed, for example, that 45 per cent of young American soldiers killed in battle had coronary atherosclerotic lesions (MacNamara *et al.* 1971).

Like other rates, the point prevalence rate may express the findings in a specific subgroup of the population; when so used, the numerator and denominator must both refer to the same population category. As an example of a sex- and age-specific rate, the point prevalence rate of a disease per 1000 men aged 45 to 64 years is calculated by the formula:

$$\frac{\text{Number of men aged 45 to 54 years with the disease at a specified point in time}}{\text{Total number of men aged 45 to 54 years in the population at that time}} \times 1000.$$

Paradoxically, there are some point prevalence rates that can be accurately measured only by a longitudinal study. An example is the rate of congenital anomalies per 100 live births. This may be regarded as a point prevalence rate referring to the moment of birth. Many anomalies become manifest only weeks, months, or years after birth, so that reasonably full case-finding requires long-term follow-up.

A period prevalence rate measures prevalence not at a single point in time but during a defined period (usually a specific year). The period prevalence rate (persons) represents the proportion of the population manifesting the disease at any time during the period. The formula is:

$$\frac{\text{Number of individuals manifesting the disease in the stated time period}}{\text{Population at risk}} \times 1000.$$

The numerator is the number of people with the illness during the specified period, including those whose illness started earlier. The denominator is the average size of the total population during the specified period. It is often estimated by using the population at the middle of the period, or by averaging the size of the population at the beginning and end of the period. Other methods may be needed if the change in population size during the period was large and did not occur at an approximately even pace. It is usually more helpful to know the point prevalence rate at the beginning of the period and the incidence rate of new cases during the period, than the period prevalence rate.

There is also a type of period prevalence rate that refers not to a defined calendar period but to a defined period of the individual's life, e.g. the period of pregnancy. A study of a sample of healthy pregnant women in an American city, for example, revealed that the prevalence of reported physical battering during the current pregnancy was 8 per cent (Helton *et al.* 1987).

The numerator of the little-used period prevalence rate (spells) is the number of episodes of an illness observed during the specified period (including episodes that commenced before the start of the period); the same person may be ill more than once. The denominator is the population at risk. For a short-term disease, this rate is usually similar to the incidence rate (spells).

A lifetime prevalence rate is a period prevalence rate referring to the whole of the subject's prior life. It differs from the point prevalence rate only if the disorder is one that does not always persist. It refers to the presence of the disorder or of a scar, antibodies, or other evidence that the disorder was present in the past. The formula is:

$$\frac{\text{Number of individuals with evidence of the disorder (past or present)}}{\text{Number of individuals studied}} \times 1000$$

This rate is usually useful only if it refers to a specific age, and if valid information on prior occurrence is available. As an example, a cross-sectional study in Jerusalem revealed that the point prevalence rate of inguinal hernia among men aged 65 to 74 years was 30 per cent, whereas the lifetime prevalence rate (including men with scars of hernia repair operations) was 40 per cent (Abramson *et al.* 1978). It could be inferred that in this cohort the risk of developing a hernia, among men surviving to the age of 65 to 74 years, was 40 per cent. Such information would be of little value if the disorder were one with an important association with survival, such as cancer.

The lifetime prevalence rate of a disorder among the blood relatives of an index case may be used as a measure of familial risk, especially in genetic studies.

Measures of association

In analytical cross-sectional studies, associations between variables (e.g. between the presence of a disease and exposure to a supposed causal factor) may be measured by correlation and regression coefficients, differences between means, and other statistics. The most commonly used measures in such studies, applicable if both variables are dichotomies, are odds ratios, rate ratios (i.e. ratios of proportions, for example of prevalence or exposure rates) and rate differences (i.e. differences between proportions, for example the prevalence difference and the exposure difference). These common measures are defined in Table 8.1, illustrated by fictional data on the association between exposure to fumes and headaches, based on a cross-sectional study in Denmark that found that reported exposure to fumes or chemicals at work was associated with the

Table 8.1 Measures of association and impact (study of a population). Fictional data on headaches and exposure to fumes

Exposure to fumes	Disease present (headaches)	Disease absent (no headaches)	Total
Factor present	$a = 10$	$b = 90$	$a + b = 100$
Factor absent	$c = 50$	$d = 850$	$c + d = 900$
Total	$a + c = 60$	$b + d = 940$	$n = 1000$

Odds ratio = ad/bc = 1.89; this is the formula for both the disease odds ratio and the exposure odds ratio, which have the same value. Can also be calculated as bc/ad = 0.53 (the reciprocal of 1.89).

 Disease odds ratio = the ratio of a/b (one disease odds) to c/d (another); or the ratio of c/d to a/b.

 Exposure odds ratio = the ratio of a/c (one exposure odds) to b/d (another); or the ratio of b/d to a/c.

Rate ratios

 Prevalence ratio = $[a/(a+b)]/[c/(c+d)]$ = 1.8 or $[c/(c+d)]/[a/(a+b)]$ = 0.56 (the reciprocal of 1.8).

 Exposure ratio = $[a/(a+c)]/[b/(b+d)]$ = 1.74 or $[b/(b+d)]/[a/(a+c)]$ = 0.57 (the reciprocal of 1.74).

Rate differences

 Prevalence difference = $a/(a+b) - c/(c+d)$ = 0.04

 Exposure difference = $a/(a+c) - b/(b+d)$ = 0.07

Measures of impact

If the factor is a risk factor:

 Excess risk among exposed = $a/(a+b) - c/(c+d)$ = 0.04

 Population excess risk = $(a+c)/n - c/(c+d)/0.004$

 Attributable fraction (exposed) = $[a/(a+b) - c/(c+d)]/[a/(a+b)] \times 100$ = 44.4%

 or (prevalence ratio − 1)/prevalence ratio × 100 = 44.4 per cent

 Attributable fraction (population) = $[(a+c)/n - c/(c+d)]/[(a+c)/n] \times 100$ = 7.4 per cent

 or [(prevalence ratio − 1) × E]/{1 + [(prevalence ratio − 1) × E]} × 100 = 7.4 per cent (where E = exposure rate in population)

If the factor is a protective factor:

 Excess risk among unexposed = $c/(c+d) - a/(a+b)$

 Population excess risk = $(a+c)/n - a/(a+b)$

 Prevented fraction (exposed) = $[c/(c+d) - a/(a+b)]/[c/(c+d)] \times 100$

 (This is also the preventable fraction per cent among the unexposed).

 Prevented fraction (population) = $[c/(c+d) - (a+c)/n]/[c/(c+d)] \times 100$

 Preventable fraction (population) = $[(a+c)/n - a/(a+b)]/[(a+c)/n] \times 100$

prevalence of reported headaches (migraine or tension-type headaches in women and tension-type headaches in men) during a 1-year period (Rasmussen 1992).

An odds is the ratio of the probability that something is so or will occur, to the probability that it is not so or will not occur; in table 1, a/b is an odds in favour of the presence of headaches. An odds ratio is the ratio of one odds to another; if the variables are exposure to some factor and the presence of a disease, an odds ratio (ad/bc) of 1·89 means that the odds in favour of headaches are 1·89 times as high among people exposed to fumes (odds = a/b) as they are among those not exposed (odds = c/d); this is the disease odds ratio. The odds ratio of 1·89 also means that the odds in favour of exposure are 1·89 times as high among people with headaches (a/c) as they are among people free of headaches (b/d); this is the exposure odds ratio. A prevalence ratio of 1·8 means that the prevalence of the disease in exposed people is 1·8 times as high as in unexposed people. An exposure ratio of 1·74 means that exposure is 1·74 times as prevalent among people with the disease as it is among those free of it.

Odds ratios are more difficult to understand than rate ratios, and opinions of their utility vary widely (Greenland 1987; Kahn and Sempos 1989; Selvin 1991; Lee 1994). But they have useful statistical properties and other desirable features. Among their advantages (using the example in Table 8.1 where possible) are the following:

1. Use of the odds ratio facilitates comparisons of results from different kinds of study. Odds ratios with the same value can be expected in a study of a total population (or representative sample), a comparison of representative samples of people exposed and not exposed to fumes (yielding the disease odds ratio), and a comparison of a representative sample of people who have headaches with a representative sample of control subjects free of headaches (yielding the exposure odds ratio, which has the same value as the disease odds ratio). The sampling fractions do not affect the value of the odds ratio; for example, the ratio remains 1·89 if the numbers in the 'factor absent' group are reduced to one-tenth ($c = 5$, $d = 85$). Disease rate ratios cannot be used in the same way, since (unless additional information is available) a case–control comparison can yield only a ratio of exposure proportions, which can be very different from the ratio of disease rates. Under certain conditions, odds ratios from cross-sectional studies can be compared with odds ratios from time-span studies.

2. The odds ratio for freedom from the disease is the reciprocal of the disease odds ratio. The disease odds ratio in Table 8.1 is 1·89, and the ratio of the odds in favour of freedom from headaches in exposed people (90/10) to the corresponding odds in unexposed people (850/50) is 0·53, which is 1/1·89. This does not hold true for the rate ratio: the disease prevalence ratio is 1·8, but the ratio of the 'healthy' (freedom from headaches) rates, i.e. the ratio of 90/100 to 850/900, is 0·95—which gives the impression of very little difference between exposed and unexposed people.

3. Observations in different population groups or strata are often combined by the Mantel–Haenszel procedure, multiple logistic regression analysis, or other techniques, on the assumption that the association has the same strength in each group. There is no problem with this concept if odds ratios are used to measure the association. But if rate ratios are used the concept of a common value may be untenable if rates are high (Kahn and Sempos 1989). The prevalence rate ratio in Table 8.1 is 1·8. In a different stratum where the rate in the unexposed was 70 per cent, a rate ratio of 1·8 would be impossible—the highest possible ratio would be 100 per cent/70 per cent, or 1·4.

4. The regression coefficients yielded by logistic regression analyses are the natural logs of odds ratios, and the odds ratios derived from them render the findings easy to understand. Multiple logistic regression analysis yields adjusted odds ratios that control for the effects of the other variables included in the model, and confounding can be appraised by comparisons with the odds ratios based on the crude data.

5. In aetiological studies of disease, the measure of interest is the ratio of the incidence in persons exposed and unexposed to a putative causal factor. The prevalence ratio can serve as an indicator of the risk ratio (cumulative incidence-rate ratio) in some cross-sectional studies of the association between a disease and a risk factor that is no longer active, e.g. a study of non-lethal birth defects in relation to some prenatal factor, or other studies of diseases with short and well-defined periods of risk, e.g. of an epidemic of diarrhoeal illness after a social gathering (Kleinbaum et al. 1982; Rothman 1986). The prevalence ratio may not be available if the study compares cases (or a sample of cases) with a sample of control subjects free of the disease. But an odds ratio is a good estimator of a rate ratio if the rates of the characteristic or event are low, and in such studies it can therefore be used as an estimator of the risk ratio, from which the person–time rate ratio can (if required) be calculated. Selvin (1991) suggests that 'low' here means a rate of under 10 per cent in each of the groups that are compared. The odds ratio and prevalence ratio in Table 8.1 are fairly close (1·89 and 1·8); they would be closer (the odds ratio would also be 1·8) if the prevalence of headaches was only 1·8 per cent in exposed and 1 per cent in unexposed people. Greenland (Greenland 1987) provides a correction factor: to obtain the rate ratio $[a/(a + b)]/[c/(c + d)]$ in a 2×2 table like Table 8.1, multiply the odds ratio by $(1 + c/d)/(1 + a/b)$. He offers a simple rule of thumb for use in more complicated instances, e.g. when there are a number of strata and an adjusted 'common rate ratio' is estimated: if the highest odds in any stratum is x, the error in the rate ratio will not exceed $100x$ per cent. The odds ratio may be a biased estimator of the risk ratio if the proportion of the population exposed to risk changed much during the risk period (Greenland and Thomas 1982).

6. The odds ratio can sometimes be interpreted as an incidence ratio even if the disease is not rare (Breslow 1982; Miettinen 1985; Rothman 1986; Pearce 1993). This applies to cross-sectional or case–control studies of exposure to some factor in which cases of a disease with a long risk period (like most chronic diseases) are compared with disease-free controls who are representative of the population from which the cases developed, and who at the time they are studied can be regarded as possible future cases. In a cross-sectional study in which prevalent cases are compared with non-cases from the same population who are still at risk of the disease at the time of the study, the odds ratio is equivalent to the ratio of person–time incidence rates, provided that exposure can be assumed to precede the onset of the disease, exposure does not affect the duration of the disease, and the disease does not affect exposure status; this equivalence does not apply within narrow age categories, or if aetiological factors have changed in the course of time. The odds ratio can also be interpreted as the ratio of person–time incidence rates in a study comparing cases that develop during a given time with control subjects selected at the same times as the cases, and as a risk ratio if controls are sampled from the whole population at the beginning of follow-up.

Critics of the use of odds ratios are concerned mainly with their role in aetiological studies of disease (Lee 1994). Greenland (Greenland 1987) states that the controversy arises from the inherent disadvantages of the odds ratio for biological inference and its inherent advantages for statistical inference; in his opinion, 'odds ratios are useful only when they serve as incidence-rate estimates, and logistic and log-linear models are useful only insofar as they provide improved (smoothed) estimates of incidence differences or rates'.

Odds ratios and prevalence ratios based on samples tend to overestimate the true odds and prevalence ratios in the population sampled. This bias may be marked if the sample is small, and the use of estimators that offset the bias has been suggested. Jewell's low-bias estimator of the odds ratio is $ad/[(b + 1)\ (c + 1)]$ or (inversely) $bc/[(a + 1) (d + 1)]$ (Jewell 1986). For the fairly large numbers in Table 8.1 the disease odds ratio becomes 1·83, instead of 1·89 by the usual formula. A disadvantage of this method is that the odds ratio for freedom from the disease is no longer the reciprocal of the disease odds ratio (Walter and Cook 1991); in this instance it is 0·48, which is 1/2·11. Jewell's low-bias point estimate of the prevalence ratio is $[a/(a + b)]/[(c + 1)/(c + d + 1)]$ or (inversely) $[c/c + d]/[(a + 1)/(a + b + 1)]$ (1·77 or 0·51 in this instance).

Odds and rate ratios are generally used in studies of causal relationships, and differences between proportions, especially the prevalence difference, may be preferred when interest lies in the magnitude of a public health problem, e.g. if we wish to estimate how many people in a population have headaches because of exposure to fumes, or to use this information in estimating treatment costs or impact on productivity.

Measures of the impact of the factor on the prevalence of the disease (assuming a causal association) are also shown in Table 8.1. They will be discussed below.

In analytical cross-sectional studies that aim to explain as well as to describe associations, a variety of measures and techniques may be used to control confounding factors and determine whether other variables modify the association. These procedures range in complexity from stratification and standardization to sophisticated multivariate techniques that permit the simultaneous consideration of a large number of variables and their relationships. The findings in separate strata (e.g. sex and age groups) are frequently combined by the Mantel–Haenszel or similar procedures, to obtain adjusted odds ratios, rate ratios and rate differences (controlling for the effects of the stratifying variable or variables); these methods should be used only after appraising the homogeneity of the findings in order to see whether they can be validly combined (Fleiss 1981; Selvin 1991; Gahlinger and Abramson 1995).

Uses in community health care

Cross-sectional studies can fulfil important functions in the health care of a community. They can contribute to the planning of services, to the effective implementation of care, and to decision-making on the continuation and modification of services. In this discussion, 'community' may be taken to refer to any aggregation of people for whose care a physician, health care team, agency, or authority is responsible; it may be a nation or region, a local neighbourhood, a list of registered patients, a defined group of schoolchildren or workers, inmates of an institution, and so on.

Attention will be given to the use of cross-sectional studies in community diagnosis, in ongoing surveillance, in community health education and the promotion of community involvement, and in the evaluation of the community's health care.

Community diagnosis

Cross-sectional studies can provide a major part of the epidemiological foundation for community diagnosis, i.e. for determining the health status of a community and the factors that influence it. They can supply information on the nature, extent, and impact of health problems, as a basis for the identification of priorities and the planning of intervention. Such studies may relate to a broad spectrum of health states and their correlates, or may be limited in their scope.

Health status

Cross-sectional studies may yield useful information on a variety of dimensions of health and disease, including self-appraised health, mental health status, growth and development, physical fitness, the distribution of blood pressures, and so on. The following remarks refer only to the prevalence of disorders; the cross-sectional method for the study of growth and development is discussed later in this chapter. It must be remembered that prevalence studies, especially point prevalence studies, may provide an incomplete picture because of the under-representation of conditions with a short duration. These include not only the acute non-fatal diseases that constitute a considerable load for the health services, and acute episodes of long-term or recurrent diseases, but also severe and rapidly fatal conditions, such as fatal strokes and sudden deaths from coronary heart disease. This bias was strikingly illustrated during a famine in Chad in 1973, when a rapid assessment displayed no severe malnutrition in children, and it was concluded that serious malnutrition did not exist; in fact many children were affected, but they died too fast to be included in the survey (Guha-Sapir 1991).

The most direct evidence of a need for improved secondary and tertiary prevention, at least for long-term diseases that are not rapidly fatal, is an unduly high prevalence of remediable disease that has not been diagnosed or that is untreated or inadequately treated. Prevalence surveys providing such information may be based on examinations, interviews, clinical files or other documentary sources, or a combination of these. In Italy, a survey based on the Registry of the Blind showed that the rate of blindness was much higher in the south of the country than in the north; possible causes for the difference in blindness due to treatable conditions such as cataract and glaucoma included a regional difference in the quality or accessibility of care (Nicolosi et al. 1994).

Needs for primary prevention can be inferred from the presence of preventable disorders, i.e. those whose incidence can be reduced by known preventive measures. For this purpose too, the prevalence data should be supplemented by data on incidence and mortality, both because diseases with a high fatality rate will otherwise be under-represented and because prevalent cases may be long-standing ones that do not reflect present preventive needs. A high prevalence of crippling due to poliomyelitis does not necessarily mean that current preventive procedures are ineffective. Information on the recent incidence of new cases is to be preferred for this purpose. If prevalence data are to be used, information should be sought on the duration of the disorder, so that the prevalence of disease of recent onset can be measured. In institutional settings where people who develop a disorder are especially likely to remain in the institution, prevalence data may overestimate the need for primary prevention. In a hospital, for example, patients who develop nosocomial infections are for this reason likely to have a longer hospital stay. A prevalence survey of such infections in a hospital may thus give an exaggerated idea of the need for primary prevention.

The use of highly valid measures of the presence of a disease often presents practical difficulties, and reliance may be placed on a proxy measure that is simple, cheap, and acceptable; a screening test may be used for this purpose. The confidence interval of the prevalence of the disease can be estimated from the prevalence of the proxy attribute (Rogan and Gladen 1978; Gahlinger and Abramson 1995).

Determinants of health and disease

Information on the prevalence of modifiable factors that are known to affect health is of obvious relevance to the planning of health care. These may be factors that affect the community's health in a general way, e.g. dietary, infant rearing and family planning practices and (presumably) the use of health services, and they may be factors that affect the risk of developing specific disorders. They may be risk factors, which increase the risk of ill health, or protective factors, e.g. physical activity or specific immunity (natural or acquired) to a pathogenic agent.

Associations between variables

When associations are investigated in a cross-sectional study in the context of community health care, the dependent variable is usually the presence of a disease or disability or other health characteristic. The aim of such analyses is usually to throw light on determinants or predictors. The dependent variable may also be a supposed risk factor or protective factor, as in studies of the determinants of cigarette smoking, the use of a health service, or compliance with medical advice. Attention may also be paid to associations among diseases or other dimensions of health, or among determinants of health.

In the context of community health care, analyses of associations with diseases are usually undertaken in order to determine what causal factors or correlates (of those known to be potentially important) are active in the specific community, and to measure their impact. The primary aim is to obtain information that will be useful in practice, not to generate new knowledge about aetiology, although this may be a secondary gain.

Measurement of impact In a situation where it is believed that an association of a risk factor with the prevalence (or incidence) of a disease expresses a causal relationship, the factor's impact may be measured by the attributable (or aetiological) fraction in the population. This is the proportion of the disease in the population that can be attributed to exposure to the factor (see Table 8.1). Among workers aged 20 to 64 years in a community in Jerusalem, for example, the fraction of the prevalence of varicose veins that could be attributed to work involving much standing was 16 per cent in each sex, after controlling for effects connected with age, region of birth, weight and height (Abramson *et al.* 1981*b*). Such values must be interpreted with caution, as part or all of the apparent causal effect may be due to other (uncontrolled) factors associated with the apparent causal factor. The attributable fraction among the exposed may also be of interest; 31 per cent of the prevalence of varicose veins in men whose work involved much standing could be attributed to their work posture; for women, this fraction was 32 per cent.

For a protective factor, the corresponding measures (see Table 8.1) are the prevented fraction, which is the proportion of the hypothetical total prevalence that has been prevented by exposure to the factor, and the preventable fraction, which is the proportion of the observed prevalence that would be prevented if everyone was exposed to the factor. These fractions are sometimes termed the 'efficacy' of the protective factor, particularly with respect to vaccines.

Attributable, prevented, and preventable fractions in the population are influenced by the factor's prevalence.

Risk markers Interest may not be confined to cause–effect relationships. Any attribute or exposure that is strongly associated with a disease or other disorder, even non-causally, has potential value as a predictor, provided there is reason to believe that it precedes the appearance of the disorder. Such predictors may be used as risk markers to identify vulnerable individuals or groups. The risk marker may be a factor that itself influences the risk, or a precursor or early manifestation of the disorder, or it may be secondarily associated with the disorder because it is associated with a cause or precursor of the disorder.

Risk markers are best identified by longitudinal studies, but can also be detected by cross-sectional ones. A cross-sectional study in Singapore, for example, showed that over 80 per cent of people with corneal arcus (a grey circle around the cornea) at the age of 30 to 49 years had high serum low-density lipoprotein cholesterol levels (Hughes *et al.* 1992). In the Netherlands, a cross-sectional study showed that divorced people were less healthy than single, married or widowed people, controlling for age, sex, living arrangements (alone, cohabiting, etc.), and other variables (Joung *et al.* 1994). The reasons for the associations with corneal arcus and divorced status are of interest, but irrelevant to the decision whether to use these characteristics as risk markers.

The value of a risk marker or combination of risk markers depends on the following considerations:

1. Is its use practical? Questions of cost, resources, acceptability, safety and convenience must be considered.

2. Is detection of high risk likely to be beneficial? Are resources and techniques available for reducing the risk? Does the benefit outweigh any harm that intervention may cause? What is the predictive value of the risk marker, i.e. what proportion of people with the marker are likely to have or develop the disease?

3. How prevalent is the risk marker? If more than half of the children in a community fall into a high-risk group, might it not be more efficient and possibly more effective to modify the routine care programme so as to give extra attention to all children?

4. What is the marker's sensitivity as a predictor? That is, what proportion of the individuals with the disorder will it identify? If it can identify only a small minority its value is limited.

The answers to these questions may vary in different contexts, as may the associations between specific factors and diseases. A given risk marker may be useful in one setting but not in another.

Community syndromes The term 'community health syndrome' may be used to refer to diseases or other health characteristics found to occur together in a community. Examples described by Kark (Kark 1974, 1981), who introduced the community syndrome concept and has emphasized its potential importance for the development of community health programmes, are (a) a syndrome of malnutrition, communicable diseases, and mental ill-health in a poor rural community undergoing rapid change; and (b) the syndrome of hypertension, coronary heart disease, and diabetes frequently found in affluent communities characterized by nutritional imbalance and excesses, limited physical activity, and a drive for achievement.

The components of a syndrome may occur together because they possess shared or related causes, or because they are themselves causally inter-related. The syndrome indicates a nexus of causal processes in the community. Even if this nexus is not completely understood, a health programme directed at the syndrome as a whole may be more effective and efficient than an endeavour to deal separately with the individual components.

Associations between diseases or other health states may be detected at a population level or (more convincingly) at an individual level, i.e. by finding a tendency to affect the same persons. As an example of the latter approach, a study of coprevalence in Jerusalem revealed clustering of migraine and other common disorders characterized by complaints (rather than objective signs) (Abramson et al. 1982). These disorders were frequently associated with emotional symptoms and with family disharmony or other stressful situations, and people with one or more components of the syndrome made heavy use of medical services. This syndrome represented a considerable burden of discomfort for many individuals and their families, and there was no organized programme to deal with it.

Identification of groups requiring special care

Community diagnosis may focus not only on the community as a whole but also on its component groups. Comparisons may identify groups for whom special care may be needed. This identification may be based on the presence of disorders, on screening tests that point to a high probability of having a disorder, on the presence of modifiable risk factors, and/or on the presence of known risk markers indicative of vulnerability and a need for preventive care.

A differential approach in community diagnosis is of basic importance for the identification of priorities and the allocation of resources. Sometimes simple descriptive findings suffice for these purposes, and in other circumstances the planning of effective care requires an understanding of the reasons for the differences found, requiring the use of analytical epidemiological techniques.

The detection of a high-risk or high-morbidity group does not, of course, necessarily mean that special care is indicated; this depends on the likely benefits, on what proportion of the community's cases or prospective cases is concentrated in the group, and on practical and other considerations.

Surveillance

Ongoing surveillance permits the identification of changes in health status and its determinants in the community, and updating of the community diagnosis. Cross-sectional as well as incidence studies have a role in surveillance. For some purposes, e.g. to detect changes in a community's health habits or blood pressure distributions, the only practicable method of surveillance is the performance of repeated cross-sectional studies. For this purpose, surveys of different representative samples may be advisable, rather than repeated investigations of the same sample, to avoid the possibility that participation in a survey may have effects on the subjects' behaviour, including their participation in health programmes and

their responses in a later survey (Kroeger 1985; Puska 1991). In North Karelia, during 3 years of operation of a cardiovascular risk factor programme, men who were followed up longitudinally decreased their smoking by 11 per cent, whereas a comparison of the baseline data with a new representative sample showed a drop of only 7 per cent (Puska 1991). Repeated cross-sectional studies, including those of the WHO's multinational monitoring of trends and determinants in cardiovascular disease (MONICA) project, have yielded much information about changes in cardiovascular risk factors in various countries (e.g. Vartiainen et al. 1994).

Surveillance of the prevalence of chronic disorders may be based on repeated prevalence surveys, or on the use of a case register that is updated as new cases are found or old ones recover, die, or leave. Changes in the prevalence of chronic disorders may be important as an indication of changing needs for curative and rehabilitative care facilities.

Changes in the prevalence of a chronic disease cannot, however, be glibly taken to indicate changes in the risk of developing the disorder; for this purpose, incidence data should be used. There are a number of possible reasons for changes in prevalence. As illustrated in Fig. 8.1, the changes reflect the interplay of incidence, recovery, and fatality rates. They may be caused by changes in the demographic characteristics of the population, as a result of ageing or inward or outward migration. Especially in studies of small local communities, prevalence may be influenced by a tendency of affected persons to leave or enter the neighbourhood. Often, apparent changes in prevalence are artefacts caused by changes in methods of case identification (e.g. the introduction of a case-finding programme), in the use of medical services, in diagnostic procedures or definitions, or in recording, notification or registration practices. They may also be caused by incomplete updating of a case register.

Community education and community involvement

Community surveys can be used as tools for community health education. This may be done not only by communicating the findings and their implications to the community and its leaders, but also by using the educational potential of the survey situation itself, e.g. by explaining to participants why the collection of specific information is important. If accurate results are required, such explanations should preferably be given after the information has been collected, to minimize bias in the responses.

An example is provided by the 'Know Your Body' programme, which aims at motivating schoolchildren to adopt a healthier lifestyle (Williams et al. 1977). An essential component of the programme is a set of measurements of chronic disease risk factors, yielding a picture of their prevalence. Each child receives a feedback of results in a 'health passport', together with explanations of desirable ranges for each test, in the hope that this may enhance the effect of the curriculum. Trials indicate that this programme effectively modifies knowledge and beliefs (Marcus et al. 1987), and can favourably affect blood pressure and smoking (Walter et al. 1987), and serum lipids and body mass index (Tamir et al. 1990).

Involvement of key community members in the planning and conduct of a health survey may be a useful way to motivate them to a more active participation in the promotion of their community's health. A community's interest and involvement in its own health care may find expression in the performance of community self-surveys, even without the participation of professional health workers. Such surveys are usually simple descriptive ones, and may not collect very accurate or sophisticated information.

Evaluation of a community's health care

In the context of community health care, the purpose of an evaluative study is to yield a factual basis for decisions concerning the provision of care to a specific community. This kind of evaluative study, the programme review, can be contrasted with the programme trial, which aims to provide generalizable inferences about the value of a given type of health programme. In programme reviews, considerable attention is given to evaluation of the process of care (the performance of activities by providers and recipients of care), as well as to measurements of desirable and undesirable effects, especially more immediate outcomes.

Certain findings that are used in the process of community diagnosis as indicators of needs for health care, such as a high prevalence of preventable or remediable disorders, may by the same token be seen as indicators of the value of past health care. In some instances a prevalence survey may reveal more direct evidence of the quality of previous care; for example, the quality of the dental work in subjects' mouths may be appraised, or the presence of inguinal hernia recurrences may be recorded (in one study, 1 in 5 operated hernias showed evidence of recurrence; Abramson et al. 1978).

Evaluative judgements that relate to the subjects' prior health care as a whole, however, may be less helpful than those relating to recent or current health care, and especially to care in the context of a specific health programme or service. Studies might deal, for example, with compliance with medical advice (what proportion of hypertensive patients are taking the medicines prescribed for them?), with satisfaction with medical care, or with immunization status.

In these as in other studies, separate attention is usually paid to various population subgroups. The impact of a health programme often varies with age, sex, social class, and other characteristics. In Beirut, nutritional surveys of children of displaced families showed more undernutrition in 1991 than in 1986, although a large food-aid programme for needy families was instituted after the first survey, and despite government subsidy of bread and partial wage correction to counter monetary inflation and rises in food prices. The children of semiskilled and unskilled fathers (whose families received more food aid) had a significantly better nutrient intake than other children in 1991 (Shaar and Shaar 1993).

Evidence of change in health status or practices may be provided by repeated cross-sectional studies as well as by incidence and other longitudinal studies. Surveys of the contraceptive practices of postnatal women in a Jerusalem neighbourhood, for example, revealed that during a 6-year period the proportion using contraceptive pills, an intrauterine device, or condoms increased from 33 to 62 per cent (Kark 1981). It is usually assumed that such changes (or their absence) are, at least to some extent, reflections of programme effectiveness, and not attributable only to outside influences. At the very least, the findings may indicate whether there is a need for more detailed evaluative study.

More rigorous proof that the change is attributable to the programme requires a comparison with control subjects. For example, in a community where a breast feeding promotion programme was instituted, the prevalence of breast feeding among infants aged 26 weeks rose from 10 to 29 per cent in a 7-year period. Confidence that this was attributable to the programme and not to a secular change was enhanced by the finding that in a neighbouring community with no such programme the corresponding proportion at the end of the period was 12 per cent (Palti et al. 1988).

Uses in clinical practice

Epidemiological studies serve important functions in clinical care. The role of cross-sectional studies in individual and family care, and in community-oriented primary care, is considered.

Individual and family care

Textbooks of clinical epidemiology emphasize that epidemiology is a basic science for clinicians (Sackett et al. 1985; Weiss 1986). 'A great many routine clinical decisions about individual patient care relating to matters such as the choice of diagnosis and treatment options, and advice on prognosis can only be based upon information from properly designed and executed studies in groups or populations' (Roberts 1977). The systematic use of properly appraised information as a basis for clinical decisions is the central feature of what is increasingly becoming known as 'evidence-based medicine' (Evidence-Based Medicine Working Group 1992).

For the clinician who bases decisions on epidemiological facts rather than on dogma or impressions, the required information may be derived from any epidemiological studies whose results can validly be generalized to the population in which the clinician works. If information about this specific population is available, it is of course of especial value. Such information (usually largely based on cross-sectional studies) may deal with the prevalence of diseases and their causes, the frequency distributions of biochemical and other measurements in the population in patients with specific disorders, patterns of child growth, health practices, and so on. This information is, of course, seldom the fruit of the clinician's own labours. Sometimes, however, even a physician concerned only with individual patients may conduct a small-scale (usually cross-sectional) epidemiological survey, e.g. of a patient's contacts for evidence of a communicable disease, if only to reduce the patient's risk of reinfection.

A family physician, responsible for the care of whole families, may need to perform such investigations more often. Whenever a patient is found to have a disease with a known tendency to 'run in families' (e.g. rheumatic heart disease, diabetes, amoebiasis or acquired immuno-deficiency syndrome) this may be seen as a signal that the whole family should be surveyed.

Family diagnosis

The process of appraising a family's health status and the factors that affect it (Kark and Kark 1962; Medalie 1978) is an exercise in small-group epidemiology. Its aim is to determine a family's health needs as a basis for the planning of a family health programme. This involves the elucidation of the health of the family's members and appraisal of relevant features of the family life situation, e.g. the family's structure and composition, the role performance and health-relevant behaviour of its members, relationships, material resources and their use, and the family's social and physical environment. At an analytical level, it involves assessment of the ways in which individuals' health may be affected by other family members and by the family life situation.

Community-oriented primary care

Community-oriented primary care refers to the integration of the health care of a defined community and of its individual members, in a single practice (Kark 1981; Kark et al. 1994). The practitioner or team providing primary clinical care for the individuals in the community also initiates or participates in specific programmes that deal in a systematic way with the community's main health problems. There is a growing awareness of the potential of this form of integrated practice for improving health in both developing and developed countries (Connor and Mullan 1983; Nutting 1987; Gillam et al. 1994; Tollman and Friedman 1994).

Epidemiology is an indispensable basis for the planning, development, and evaluation of the community health programmes that characterize community-oriented primary care. The uses listed above of cross-sectional studies in community health care and in individual and family care are relevant to this form of practice.

The integration of individual-oriented and community-oriented functions in the same primary care setting carries important implications for the conduct of epidemiological studies. An important feature is that much of the information needed for community diagnosis, surveillance, and evaluation can be obtained in the course of routine clinical care. The collection of data thus serves a double function. When a child is weighed, a question is asked about smoking, or a diagnosis is made, the results may be used both in the management of the patient and as data for subsequent analysis at a group level. Such information may be derived either from routine clinical procedures or from questions or tests specially added for epidemiological purposes. In a practice where periodic health examinations are conducted, these provide an especially useful opportunity for the collection of data for analysis.

This use of clinical data demands careful attention to methods of obtaining, recording, and retrieving data, to make the information as accurate and complete as possible. Standardized procedures are required, and definitions and diagnostic criteria should be standardized as rigorously as possible.

The performance of a cross-sectional study in this way (of the sort based on interviews or examinations staggered over a period) may, of course, extend over a considerable span of time. There may be a need for supplementary survey procedures to obtain information about members of the community who have not attended for clinical care. These people may be invited to attend, visited at home, or asked for information by mail or telephone. In population groups with very high attendance rates (say infants and their mothers, pregnant women, and the elderly), there may be little bias if non-attenders are excluded.

For chronic diseases, a common technique is the maintenance of a case register (this may be a list, a card index, or a computerized database). Such a register, like other practice records, has a dual purpose. At a group level, it permits the calculation of prevalence rates or other epidemiological indices, and may assist in monitoring the performance of tests and other activities; and at an individual level, it can be used as a tool for ensuring that patients receive the care they need.

If resources are available, information may also be obtained by special surveys. For some purposes (say to measure smoking habits) it may be satisfactory to investigate a representative sample. But surveys in the context of community-oriented primary care usually aim to identify individuals who need care, as well as providing information at a community level, and the use of a sample may not meet this purpose. The WHO has published a practical guide to the conduct of simple epidemiological surveys at a district level (Vaughan and Morrow 1989).

A survey that has obvious relevance to health may be a useful means of stimulating the community's interest and involvement in its own health care. The purpose of the survey should be explained to the community, and feedback of results supplied to community leaders and the community at large. In some community-oriented primary care practices, focus groups have proved to be a valuable means not only of collecting data, but as a means whereby the community recognizes its needs and subsequently mobilizes to meet them (Plaut et al. 1993).

Sackett and Holland (Sackett and Holland 1975) have contrasted the roles of epidemiological surveys, screening, and 'case-finding' in the detection of disease. They define epidemiological surveys as studies of carefully selected samples, aimed at generating new knowledge and implying no health benefits to the participants. Screening involves the testing of apparently healthy people invited for examination, and carries an implicit promise of benefit. 'Case-finding' is performed among patients who seek health care, and is concerned with tests to reveal disorders that may be unrelated to their complaints. Such distinctions become blurred or vanish in the community-oriented primary care context, where an epidemiological survey may aim to provide information that will benefit individual participants as well as providing a basis for decisions about care at a community level, and may be conducted in a clinical setting. In a community-oriented primary care practice, people are seldom invited to attend solely for screening purposes—screening tests may be performed routinely when patients attend for care, or incorporated in health examinations that provide an opportunity for appraising the individual's health status and life situation and for counselling, not only for screening.

The collection of data by care providers in a care setting carries advantages and disadvantages. On the one hand, it may be relatively easy to obtain answers to awkward questions, and to achieve a high response rate. On the other hand, there may be bias. The respondents may be aware of what replies are acceptable to care providers, and their desire to please may influence their responses. Also, care providers who are evaluating the care they themselves provide may tend to make biased observations and inferences—bias should be reduced by using objective measures when possible, and by obtaining the help of independent observers or investigators.

Denominator data, i.e. information about the number of people in the community and their demographic characteristics, may be available from censuses or other official sources, from the registration system used by the practice for administrative or fiscal purposes, or from other records (Nutting 1987). In countries that have computerized databases, techniques of small area analysis (United States Department of Health and Human Services 1990) may provide useful information about a community's hospital use, morbidity, and other characteristics, as well as about its size and composition. Various mathematical models have been proposed for estimating denominator characteristics from data on attenders, but these have limited value (Cherkin *et al.* 1982). If appropriate demographic data are not available, the health service may have to devise its own data-gathering mechanism. One approach is to incorporate the collection of demographic data in a broader household health survey, confined to a sample if necessary. Demographic surveillance often becomes one of the functions of voluntary or other community health workers. An incremental approach may be used, by starting data collection in an 'initial defined area' and gradually expanding the defined segment of the practice population (Kark 1966; Nutting 1987).

Studies yielding 'new knowledge'

Many cross-sectional studies are performed to expand the horizons of knowledge, rather than solely to promote the health of the specific group or population studied. They are 'research' studies that aim to yield generalizable inferences that are of broad applicability and not relevant only to a specific local context.

We will briefly consider studies of growth and development and of aetiology, and programme trials. Other research topics include the natural history of health and disease (usually better investigated by time-span studies) and methodological issues. Cross-sectional studies are commonly used to examine the effects of differences in operational definitions or study methods and to appraise the validity of screening tests and proxy measures.

Studies of growth and development

Growth and development, and age trends in the prevalence of disorders, can be studied cross-sectionally as well as longitudinally. The cross-sectional method compares different age groups observed at one point of time, whereas the longitudinal method makes repeated observations of a single cohort as its age changes. The cross-sectional method is simpler, but has limitations. It can provide information about average changes, but not about intra-individual changes or interindividual differences.

The main limitation of the cross-sectional method is that the age groups that are compared may differ in respects other than age, so that the effects of age and other influences may be confounded. There is always potential confounding of age changes with differences between birth cohorts, as the age groups that are compared must belong to different cohorts. Cohort differences in growth may be negligible, but they may be significant if cohorts were exposed to very different circumstances, e.g. different infant feeding or child-rearing practices, changes in economic prosperity, or war. As a result the cross-sectional method may yield a misleading picture. If there has been a secular increase in height, a cross-sectional study may show a decrease in average height throughout adult life; but young adults will be taller because they belong to a more recently born generation, not because they are younger. If a series of cross-sectional studies has been done, suitable rearrangement of the data may permit examination and comparison of the longitudinal changes in different cohorts.

In studies that include middle-aged and elderly people, selective survival may be important. The mean blood pressure may be lower in the very old, not because blood pressure tends to drop with age, but because hypertensive people are more likely to have died and thus left the study sample. Also, the validity of measures may vary with age. The results of a memory test in elderly people may reflect hearing ability, attentiveness, or depression, rather than memory capacity.

Studies of aetiology

Cross-sectional studies often provide useful guides to aetiological processes, especially with respect to influences on long-term disorders and relatively stable measurements and health habits. They have two features, however, that often restrict their value for the testing of causal hypotheses.

First, any associations they reveal are with the presence, not the appearance, of the disorder or other variable studied. Transient or rapidly fatal cases are inevitably under-represented. The causes that determine the appearance of the disorder are confounded with those that influence its duration, and it may be difficult to draw clear inferences about either set of causes. As an example, a high frequency of the A2 human lymphocyte antigen was found in children with acute lymphocytic leukaemia, suggesting that this was a risk factor; but later studies showed that the antigen lengthened the children's lifespan, which was why prevalent cases included a high proportion who had the antigen (Rogentine *et al.* 1972, 1973; cited by Newman *et al.* 1988). Such confounding is relatively unimportant if the disorder studied is seldom fatal and has high chronicity, or data on lifetime prevalence are used. In such instances the main difficulty in a cross-sectional study is that the causal factors may no longer be apparent because of the time-lag since the initiation of the disease.

Second, in a strictly cross-sectional study the absence of information on time relationships may render it difficult to separate effects on a dependent variable from effects of the dependent variable. The influence of blood pressure, serum cholesterol, and cigarette smoking on the occurrence of myocardial infarction, for example, may be confounded with changes ensuing from the disease episode. The demonstration in a cross-sectional study that fat abdomens (based on a comparison of waist with hip size) are associated with hypertension, hypertensive heart disease, and diabetes (controlling for sex, age, and ponderal index) is difficult to interpret without knowing which came first, the fat abdomen or the disease (Gillum 1987). The discovery of an inverse association in San Francisco's bus drivers between hypertension and reported job-related problems—a relationship that was not explained by confounding factors and was specific to hypertension (gastro-intestinal, respiratory and musculoskeletal problems were positively associated with the self-reported stressors)—was given two competing explanations. On the one hand, 'emotional states or coping mechanisms . . . may play a role in the pathogenesis of hypertension through the repression of anger and hostility . . . ' On the other, 'the hemodynamic consequences of elevated blood pressure may lead to a physiologic alteration of perception . . . elevation in blood pressure reduces reactivity to noxious stimuli' (Winkleby *et al.* 1988). There is of course no 'chicken-or-egg' (time-sequence) problem if the variable in question is blood type or some other genetically determined characteristic, or a long-past exposure or long-lived acquired attribute that can be assumed to precede the onset of the latent period of the disease being studied.

The value of a cross-sectional study in the search for causes and precursors is limited whenever there is a possibility that the disease may change the subject's lifestyle, bodily functions and characteristics, or circumstances. To throw light on time sequences, cross-sectional studies are often extended to include historical information on times of disease onset or of other occurrences. Repeated cross-sectional studies of the same population can sometimes establish the order of events.

Cross-sectional studies frequently demonstrate unexplained associations that can form a basis for causal hypotheses for testing in subsequent epidemiological or other studies. As an example, the most striking finding in a study of the prevalence of human T-lymphotropic virus type 1 infection in seven villages in Gabon (where this infection is endemic) was that Kota-Obamba residents had a very much higher infection rate than members of other ethnic groups (Le Hasran et al. 1994). They also had a somewhat higher seroprevalence rate for syphilis, but there was no significant relationship (controlling for age) between human T-lymphotropic virus type 1 and syphilis, and sociological and ethnographic studies provided no clues to behavioural differences that might explain the rate of human T-lymphotropic virus type 1 infection. Associations of this kind pose important aetiological riddles—findings awaiting an explanation.

A cross-sectional study may form the first stage of a time-span study, for which it provides baseline measurements of dependent and independent variables, and sometimes a sampling base. If the study is concerned with the incidence of a long-term disease, the baseline prevalence study identifies affected people, who may be followed up in order to study the natural history of the disease, but must be excluded from the population at risk of subsequently developing the disease. A cluster survey in a region of Tanzania, for example, provided information on the prevalence of human immunodeficiency virus infection in adults aged 15 to 34 years (the prevalence was 10 per cent, reaching 24 per cent in an urban zone), and seronegative individuals were re-examined 2 years later in order to determine the rate and correlates of seroconversion (this demonstrated an annual incidence rate of 1·4 per 100 person-years) (Killewo et al. 1993).

Programme trials

A simple way of testing the effectiveness of a health programme is to compare the status of people who have and have not been exposed to the programme. In eight clinics in Lesotho, for example, a children's growth monitoring and nutrition education programme was evaluated by means of a cross-sectional study in which maternal knowledge about infant feeding was measured, and mothers were classified according to whether or not they had previously attended the clinic. Women who had attended were found to be more knowledgeable about the introduction of animal protein foods, the use of oral rehydration salts, and the method of weaning (Ruel et al. 1992). But an evaluative study based on simple comparison of the findings or changes seen in people who voluntarily participate or do not participate in a programme is generally not convincing, as the comparison may be confounded by differences between the groups. It is difficult to be sure that the difference in the findings can be attributed to the difference in exposure to the programme. Maybe women who were more knowledgeable, or more educable, were also more likely to attend the clinics. The possible confounding effects are not easy to control. In this study, the difference in knowledge remained apparent when a few easily measured possible confounders—maternal education, working status, parity, and the child's age—were controlled in the analysis. The authors correctly limited their conclusion to the statement that previous clinic attendance 'appeared to be' beneficial.

A similar approach is used in case–control studies that aim to evaluate preventive and therapeutic procedures or programmes by comparing people who have experienced an unfavourable outcome with control subjects, to see whether they differ in their prior exposure to the procedure or programme. Such studies offer a relatively simple and rapid approach to evaluation (Smith 1989). But they present problems, particularly the possibility that the cases and control subjects may have differed in their initial characteristics (including prognostic factors), or eligibility for the procedure or programme, and care is required to control for confounding and other biases (Horwitz and Feinstein 1981).

To obtain convincing evidence of the effectiveness of a health programme that aims to modify the distribution of a characteristic in a population or to reduce the prevalence of a disease, it is necessary to measure the change in the population and to demonstrate that this can be attributed to the programme rather than to other causes. A trend shown by repeated cross-sectional studies adds to the force of the evidence—e.g. in a population where the prevalence of anaemia in pregnant women was originally 12·0 per cent, and the introduction of an intervention programme was followed by a progressive drop to 8·8, then 3·3, then 1·6 per cent (Kark 1981). But the cause and effect relationship between a programme and its apparent outcome is always difficult to substantiate without observations of a comparison or reference population not exposed to the programme.

In trials of programmes directed at populations, it is unfortunately seldom possible to randomize. There is often little or no choice as to which population will be exposed to the programme under trial, and a restricted choice concerning a control population. Most programme trials are therefore quasiexperimental, in which the control group or groups are selected so as to be as similar as possible to the intervention group, and it remains necessary to control for possible confounders in the analysis. In an evaluation of the CHAD (Community syndrome of Hypertension, Atherosclerosis and Diabetes) programme for the control of cardiovascular risk factors in a Jerusalem neighbourhood, for example, where cross-sectional studies revealed a significantly greater decrease in the prevalence of some risk factors in the exposed population than in a neighbouring control population, the confounders that were controlled included age, sex, education, and region of birth (Abramson et al. 1981a). The prevalence of some risk factors declined in the control population as well, apparently as a result of changes in awareness and health care—underlining the need for comparison groups in such studies. Difficulties in the evaluation of community programmes are discussed by Blackburn (Blackburn 1991), who stresses the need for studies involving more communities (possibly smaller), and preferably randomized.

The use of population samples in surveys designed to evaluate health programmes is discussed by Salonen et al. (Salonen et al. 1986), who compare the pros and cons of surveying separate samples on each occasion, compared with repeated surveys of the same samples.

Summary

This chapter has reviewed uses, methods, strengths, and weaknesses of cross-sectional studies. The essential feature of such surveys is that they collect information relating to a single specified time, but a time dimension is often introduced by the inclusion of easily collected historical information or by comparing successive studies so as to appraise changes in health status and its determinants, and their sequence.

Like other epidemiological studies, cross-sectional studies (descriptive and analytical) can both contribute to the health care of a specific group or community and serve as a research method for the attainment of generalizable new knowledge. These purposes, especially the first, can sometimes be met by the use of simple, undemanding and inexpensive methods, such as cluster sampling; 'rapid epidemiological assessment' is especially relevant in situations (in both developed and developing countries) where resources are limited or results are required as a basis for programme decisions.

Cross-sectional surveys may be used in community diagnosis, ongoing surveillance, community health education, and the promotion of community involvement, and evaluation of the community's health care, and they can contribute to the planning of services, the effective implementation of care, and decision-making on the continuation and modification of services.

In clinical practice, information derived from prevalence studies of the population in which the clinician works is of special pertinence. The performance of cross-sectional studies is often integrated with clinical care in the provision of community-oriented primary care, where (with other sources of information) they play an essential role in the planning, development, and evaluation of community health programmes.

Cross-sectional studies can contribute new knowledge on growth and development, birth-cohort effects, aetiology, the effectiveness of health programmes, the validity of screening tests, and other topics. In some circumstances a prevalence study can yield a ratio expressing the effect of a putative causal factor on the incidence of a disease. But uncertainties concerning time relationships limit the value of cross-sectional studies in aetiological research, unless the causal factors are genetically determined ones, long-past exposures, or long-lived acquired attributes that can be assumed to precede the onset of the latent period of the disease under study. Cross-sectional studies are a fruitful source of causal hypotheses for subsequent testing in other studies. A cross-sectional study may form the first stage of a longitudinal study, for which it provides baseline measurements of dependent and independent variables, and sometimes a sampling base.

References

Abramson, J.H. (1990). *Survey methods in community medicine: epidemiological studies, programme evaluation, clinical trials*, (4th edn). Churchill Livingstone, Edinburgh.

Abramson, J.H. (1994). *Making sense of data: a self-instruction manual on the interpretation of epidemiologic data*, (2nd edn). Oxford University Press, New York.

Abramson, J.H., Gofin, J., Hopp, C., Makler, A., and Epstein, L.M. (1978). The epidemiology of inguinal hernia. *Journal of Epidemiology and Community Health*, 32, 59.

Abramson, J.H., Gofin, R., Hopp, C., Gofin, J., Donchin, M., and Habib, J. (1981a). Evaluation of a community program for the control of cardiovascular risk factors: the CHAD program in Jerusalem. *Israel Journal of Medical Sciences*, 17, 201.

Abramson, J.H., Hopp, C., and Epstein, L.M. (1981b). The epidemiology of varicose veins: a survey in western Jerusalem. *Journal of Epidemiology and Community Health*, 35, 213.

Abramson, J.H., Gofin, J., Peritz, E., Hopp, C., and Epstein, L.M. (1982) Clustering of chronic disorders—a community study of co-prevalence in Jerusalem. *Journal of Chronic Diseases*, 35, 221.

Anderson, D.W., Schoenberg, B.S., and Haerer, A.F. (1988). Prevalence surveys of neurologic disorders: methodological implications of the Copiah County study. *Journal of Clinical Epidemiology*, 41, 339.

Anker, M., Guidotti, R.J., Orzeszyna, S., Sapirie, S.A., and Thuriaux, M.C. (1993). Rapid evaluation methods (REM) of health services performance: methodological observations. *Bulletin of the World Health Organization*, 711, 15.

Armstrong, J.R.M. and Hayes, R. (1992) Estimating prevalence of injecting drug use in an urban population: limitations of the three-sample estimation procedure. *International Journal of Epidemiology*, 21, 613.

Babaniyi, O. and Parakoyi, B. (1991). Cluster survey for poliomyelitis and neonatal tetanus in Ilorin, Nigeria. *International Journal of Epidemiology*, 20, 515.

Balraj, V., Mukundan, S., Samuel, R., and John, T.J. (1993). Factors affecting immunisation coverage levels in a district of India. *International Journal of Epidemiology*, 22, 1146.

Bennett, S., Woods, T., Liyanage, W.M., and Smith, D.L. (1991). A simplified general method for cluster-sample surveys of health in developing countries. *World Health Statistics Quarterly*, 44, 98.

Bertrand, W.E. (1985). Microcomputer applications in health population surveys: experience and potential in developing countries. *World Health Statistics Quarterly*, 3, 91.

Birkett, N.J. (1988). Computer-aided personal interviewing: a new technique for data collection in epidemiologic surveys. *American Journal of Epidemiology*, 127, 684.

Bishop, Y., Fienberg, S., and Holland, P. (1975) *Discrete multivariate analysis: theory and practice*. MIT Press, Cambridge, Massachusetts.

Blackburn, H. (1991). Community programmes in coronary heart disease prevention and health promotion: changing community behaviour. In *Coronary heart disease epidemiology: from aetiology to public health* (ed. M. Marmot and P. Elliott), p.495. Oxford University Press, Oxford.

Breslow, N. (1982). Design and analysis of case–control studies. *Annual Reviews of Public Health*, 3, 29.

Byass, P. (1989a). Choosing and using a microcomputer for tropical epidemiology. I. Preliminary considerations. *Journal of Tropical Medicine and Hygiene*, 92, 282.

Byass, P. (1989b). Choosing and using a microcomputer for tropical epidemiology. II. Study implementation. *Journal of Tropical Medicine and Hygiene*, 92, 330.

Cherkin, D.C., Berg, A.O., and Phillipa W.R. (1982). In search of a solution to the primary care denominator problem. *Journal of Family Practice*, 14, 301.

Cochran, W.G. (1977). *Sampling techniques*, (3rd edn). Wiley, New York.

Connor, E. and Mullan, F. (ed.) (1983). *Community oriented primary care: new directions for health service delivery*. National Academy Press, Washington, D.C.

Coreil, J., Augustin, A, Holt, E., and Halsey, N.A. (1989). Use of ethnographic research for instrument development in a case–control study of immunization use in Haiti. *International Journal of Epidemiology*, 18, S33.

Edungbola, L.D., Alabi, T.O., Oni, G.A., Asaolu, S.O., Ogunbanjo, B.O., and Parakoyi, B.D. (1987). 'Leopard skin' as a rapid diagnostic index for estimating the endemicity of African onchocerciasis. *International Journal of Epidemiology*, 16, 590.

Elandt-Johnson, R.C. (1975). Definitions of rates: some remarks on their use and misuse. *American Journal of Epidemiology*, 102, 261.

Evidence-Based Medicine Working Group (1992). Evidence-based medicine: a new approach to teaching the practice of medicine. *Journal of the American Medical Association*, 268, 2420.

Fienberg, S.E. (1972). The multiple recapture census for closed populations and incomplete 2*k* contingency tables. *Biometrics*, **59**, 591.

Fleiss, J.L. (1981). *Statistical methods for rates and proportions*, (2nd edn). Wiley, New York.

Frerichs, R.R. (1989). Simple analytic procedures for rapid microcomputer-assisted cluster surveys in developing countries. *Public Health Reports*, **104**, 24.

Frerichs, R.R. and Tar, K.T. (1989). Computer-assisted rapid surveys in developing countries. *Public Health Reports*, **104**, 14.

Frischer, M., Bloor, M., Finlay, A., Goldberg, D., Green, S., Haw, S., *et al.* (1991). A new method of estimating prevalence of injecting drug use in an urban population: results from a Scottish city. *International Journal of Epidemiology*, **20**, 997.

Gahlinger, P.M. and Abramson, J.H. (1995). *Computer programs for epidemiologic analysis: PEPI: Version 2*. USD, Inc., Stone Mountain, Georgia.

Gillam, S., Plamping, D., McClenaham, J., Harries, J., and Epstein, L. (1994). *Community-oriented primary care*. King's Fund, London.

Gillum, R.F. (1987). The association of body fat distribution with hypertension, hypertensive heart disease, diabetes and cardiovascular risk factors in men and women aged 18–79 years. *Journal of Chronic Diseases*, **40**, 421.

Goma Epidemiology Group (1995). Public health impact of Rwandan refugee crisis: what happened in Goma, Zaire, in July, 1994? *Lancet*, **345**, 339.

Greenland, S. (1987). Interpretation and choice of effect measures in epidemiologic analysis. *American Journal of Epidemiology*, **125**, 761.

Greenland, S. and Thomas, D.C. (1982). On the need for the rare disease assumption in case–control studies. *American Journal of Epidemiology*, **116**, 547.

Guha-Sapir, D. (1991) Rapid assessment of health needs in mass emergencies: review of current concepts and methods. *World Health Statistics Quarterly*, **44**, 171.

Harris, D.R. and Lemeshow, S. (1991). Evaluation of the EPI survey methodology for estimating relative risk. *World Health Statistics Quarterly*, **44**, 107.

Helmert, U., Herman, B. and Shea, S. (1994). Moderate and vigorous leisure-time physical activity and cardiovascular disease risk factors in West Germany, 1984–1991. *International Journal of Epidemiology*, **23**, 285.

Helton, A.S., McFarlane, J., and Anderson, E.T. (1987). Battered and pregnant: a prevalence study. *American Journal of Public Health*, **77**, 1337.

Henderson, R.H. and Sundaresan, T. (1982). Cluster sampling to assess immunisation coverage: review of experience with a simplified sampling method. *Bulletin of the World Health Organization*, **60**, 253.

Hilden, J. (1994). Ascertainment corrected rates: applications of *capture-recapture* methods. *International Journal of Epidemiology*, **23**, 865.

Hook, E.B. and Regal, R.R. (1993). Effect of variation in probability of ascertainment by sources ('variable catchability') upon 'capture–recapture' estimates of prevalence. *American Journal of Epidemiology*, **137**, 1148.

Horwitz, R.I. and Feinstein, A.R. (1981). The application of therapeutic-trial principles to improve the design of epidemiologic research: a case–control study suggesting that anticoagulants reduce mortality in patients with myocardial infarction. *Journal of Chronic Diseases*, **34**, 575.

Hughes, K., Lun, K.C., Sothy, S.P., Thai, A.C., Leong, W.P., and Yeo, P.B. (1992). Corneal arcus and cardiovascular risk factors in Asians in Singapore. *International Journal of Epidemiology*, **21**, 473.

Jewell, N.P. (1986). On the bias of commonly used measures of association for 2×2 tables. *Biometrics*, **42**, 351.

Joung, I.M.A., van de Mheen, H., Stronks, K., van Poppel, F.W.A., and Mackenbach, J.P. (1994). Differences in self-reported morbidity by marital status and by living arrangement. *International Journal of Epidemiology*, **23**, 91.

Kahn, H.A. and Sempos, C.T. (1989). *Statistical methods in epidemiology*, (2nd edn). Oxford University Press, New York.

Kark, S.L. (1966). An approach to public health. In *Medical care in developing countries* (ed. M. King), p.5:1. Oxford University Press, Nairobi.

Kark, S.L. (1974). *Epidemiology and community medicine*. Appleton-Century-Crofts, New York.

Kark, S.L. (1981). *The practice of community-oriented primary health care*. Appleton-Century-Crofts, New York.

Kark, S.L. and Kark, E. (1962). A practice of social medicine. In *A practice of social medicine: a South African team's experience in different African communities* (ed. S.L. Kark and G.W. Steuart), p.3. Churchill Livingstone, Edinburgh.

Kark, S.L., Kark, E., Abramson, J.H., and Gofin J (ed.) (1994). *Atencion Primaria Orientada a la Comunidad (APOC)*. Ediciones Doyma S.A., Barcelona.

Khan, M.E., Anker, M., Patel, B.C., Barge, S., Sadhwani, H., and Kohle, R. (1991). The use of focus groups in social and behavioural research: some methodological issues. *World Health Statistics Quarterly*, **44**, 145.

Kiemeney, L.A.L.M., Schouten, L.J., and Straatman, H. (1994). Ascertainment corrected rates. *International Journal of Epidemiology*, **23**, 203.

Killewo, J.Z.J., Sandstrom, A., Raden, U.B., Mhalu, F.S., Biberfeld, G., and Wall, S. (1993). Incidence of HIV–1 infection among adults in the Kagera Region of Tanzania. *International Journal of Epidemiology*, **22**, 528.

Kleinbaum, D.G., Kupper, L.L., and Morgenstern, H. (1982). *Epidemiologic research: principles and quantitative methods*. LifeTime Learning Publications, Belmont, California.

Kroeger, A. (1983). Health interview surveys in developing countries: a review of the methods and results. *International Journal of Epidemiology*, **12**, 465.

Kroeger, A. (1985). Response errors and other problems of health interview surveys in developing countries. *World Health Statistics Quarterly*, **38**, 15.

LaForce, F.M., Lichnevski, M.S., Keja, J., and Henderson, R.H. (1980). Clinical survey techniques to estimate prevalence and annual incidence of poliomyelitis in developing countries. *Bulletin of the World Health Organization*, **58**, 609.

Lee, J. (1994). Odds ratio or relative risk for cross-sectional data? *International Journal of Epidemiology*, **23**, 201.

Le Hasran, J.Y., Delaporte, E., Gaudebout, C., Trebuck, A., Schrijvers, D., Josse, R., *et al.* (1994). Demographic factors associated with HTLV-I infection in a Gabonese community. *International Journal of Epidemiology*, **23**, 812.

Lemeshow, S. and Robinson, D. (1985). Surveys to measure programme coverage and impact: a review of the methodology used by the Expanded Programme on Immunization. *World Health Statistics Quarterly*, **38**, 65.

Lemeshow, S., Tserkovnyi, A.G., Tulloch, J.L., Dowd, J.E., Lwanga, S.K., and Keja, J. (1985). A computer simulation of the EPI survey strategy. *International Journal of Epidemiology*, **14**, 473.

Lengeler, C., Mshinda, H., de Savigny, D., Kilima, P., Morona, D., and Tanner, M. (1991). The value of questionnaires aimed at key informants, and distributed through an existing administrative system, for rapid and cost-effective health assessment. *World Health Statistics Quarterly*, **44**, 150.

Linstone, H.A. and Turoff, M. (ed.) (1975). *The Delphi method: techniques and applications*. Addison-Wesley, Reading, Massachusetts.

McCarty, D.J., Tull, E.S., Moy, C.S., Twoh, C.K., and LaPorte, R.E. (1993). Ascertainment corrected rates: applications of capture–recapture methods. *International Journal of Epidemiology*, **22**, 559.

MacMahon, B. and Pugh, T.F. (1970). *Epidemiology: principles and methods*. Little, Brown, Boston.

MacNamara, J.J., Molot, M.A., Stremple, J.F., and Cutting, R.T. (1971). Coronary artery disease in combat casualties in Vietnam. *Journal of the American Medical Association*, **216**, 1185.

Maffei, F.H.A., Magaldi, C., Pinho, S.Z., Lastoria, S., Pinho, W., Yoshida, W.B., *et al.* (1986). Varicose veins and chronic venous insufficiency in Brazil: prevalence among 1755 inhabitants of a country town. *International Journal of Epidemiology*, **15**, 210.

Marcus, A.C., Wheeler, R.C., Cullen, J.W., and Crane, L.A. (1987). Quasi-experimental evaluation of the Los Angeles 'Know Your Body' program: knowledge, beliefs, and self-reported behaviours. *Preventive Medicine*, **16**, 803.

Medalie, J.H. (ed.) (1978). *Family medicine: principles and applications*. Williams & Wilkins, Baltimore.

Miettinen, O.S. (1985), *Theoretical epidemiology: principles of occurrence research in medicine*. Wiley, New York.

Needleman, H.L., Gunnoe, C., Levison, A., Reed, R., Pereshie, H., Maher, C., *et al.* (1979). Deficits in psychologic and classroom performance of children with elevated dentine lead levels. *New England Journal of Medicine*, **300**, 689.

Newman, T.B., Browner, W.S., Cummings, S.R., and Hulley, S.B. (1988). Designing a new study: II. Cross-sectional and case–control studies. In *Designing clinical research* (ed. S.B. Hulley and S.R. Cummings). Williams & Wilkins, Baltimore.

Nicolosi, A., Marighi, P.E., Rizzardi, P., Osella, A., and Miglior, S. (1994). Prevalence and causes of visual impairment in Italy. *International Journal of Epidemiology*, **23**, 359.

Nutting, P.A. (ed.) (1987). *Community oriented primary care: from principle to practice*. Health Resources and Services Administration, Public Health Services, Washington, D.C.

Palti, H., Adler, B., Flug, D., Shamir, Z., and Kark, S.L. (1977). Community diagnosis of psychomotor development in infancy. *Israel Annals of Psychiatry*, **15**, 223.

Palti, H., Valderama, C., Pogrund, R., and Kurtzman, H. (1988). Evaluation of the effectiveness of a structured breast feeding program integrated into the Maternal and Child Health services in Jerusalem. *Israel Journal of Medical Sciences*, **24**, 731.

Pearce, N. (1993). What does the odds ratio estimate in a case–control study? *International Journal of Epidemiology*, **22**, 1189.

Plaut, T., Landis, S., and Trevor, J. (1993). In *Successful focus groups* (ed. D.L. Morgan). Sage Publications, Beverly Hills.

Poikolanen, K. and Eskola, J. (1988). Health services resources and their relation to mortality from causes amenable to health care intervention: a cross-national study. *International Journal of Epidemiology*, **17**, 86.

Puska, P. (1991). Intervention and experimental studies. In *Oxford textbook of public health*, (2nd edn) (ed. W.W. Holland, R. Detels and G. Knox), p.177. Oxford University Press, Oxford.

Rasmussen, B.K. (1992). Migraine and tension-type headache in a general population: psychosocial factors. *International Journal of Epidemiology*, **21**, 1138.

Ritenbaugh, C.K., Said, A.K., Gaslal, O.M., and Harrison, G.G. (1989) Development and evaluation of a colour-coded scale for birthweight surveillance in rural Egypt. *International Journal of Epidemiology*, **18**, S54.

Roberts, C.J. (1977). *Epidemiology for clinicians*. Pitman Medical, Tunbridge Wells.

Rogan, W.J., and Gladen, B. (1978). Estimating prevalence from the results of a screening test. *American Journal of Epidemiology*, **107**, 71.

Rogentine, G.N., Yankee, R.A., Gart, J.J., Nam, J., and Trapani, R.J. (1972). HL-A antigens and disease: acute lymphatic leukemia. *Journal of Clinical Investigation*, **51**, 2410.

Rogentine, G.N., Trapani, R.J., and Henderson, E.S. (1973). HL-A antigens and acute lymphocytic leukemia: the nature of the HL–A2 association. *Tissue Antigens*, **3**, 470.

Ronneberg, A., Lund, K.E., and Hafstad, A. (1994). Lifetime smoking habits among Norwegian men and women born between 1890 and 1974. *International Journal of Epidemiology*, **23**, 267.

Rothenberg, R.B. (1985). Observations on the application of EPI cluster survey methods for estimating disease incidence. *Bulletin of the World Health Organization*, **63**, 93.

Rothman, K.J. (1986). *Modern epidemiology*. Little, Brown, Boston, Massachusetts.

Rothman, K.J. (ed.) (1988). *Causal inference*. Epidemiology Resources, Chestnut Hill, Massachusetts.

Ruel, M.T., Habicht, J.–P., and Olson, C. (1992). Impact of a clinic-based growth monitoring programme on maternal nutrition knowledge in Lesotho. *International Journal of Epidemiology*, **21**, 59.

Sackett, D.L. (1979). Bias in analytic research. *Journal of Chronic Diseases*, **33**, 51.

Sackett, D.L., and Holland, W.W. (1975). Controversy in the detection of disease. *Journal of Chronic Diseases*, **33**, 51.

Sackett, D.L., Haynes, K.B., and Tugwell, P. (1985). *Clinical epidemiology: a basic science for clinical medicine*. Little, Brown, Boston, Massachusetts.

Salonen, J.T., Kottke, T.E., Jacobs, D.R.Jr., and Hannan, P.J. (1986). Analysis of community-based cardiovascular disease prevention studies—evaluation issues in the North Karelia Project and the Minnesota Heart Health Program. *International Journal of Epidemiology*, **15**, 176.

Schwoebel, V., Dauvisis, A.–V., Helynck, B., Gomes, E., Drejer, G.F., Schlumberger, M., *et al.* (1992). Community-based evaluation survey of immunisations in Burkino Faso. *Bulletin of the World Health Organization*, **70**, 583.

Scrimshaw, S.C.M., and Hurtado, E. (1987). *Rapid assessment procedures for nutrition and primary health care: anthropological approaches to improving programme effectiveness*. UCLA Latin American Center Publications, Los Angeles, California.

Selvin, S. (1991). *Statistical analysis of epidemiologic data*. Oxford University Press, Oxford.

Shaar, K.H., and Shaar, M.A. (1993). The nutritional status of children of displaced families in Beirut. *International Journal of Epidemiology*, **22**, 348.

Smith, G.S. (1989) Development of rapid epidemiologic assessment methods to evaluate health status and delivery of health services. *International Journal of Epidemiology*, **18** (Supplement 2), S1.

Smith, P.G., and Morrow, R.H. (1991). *Methods for field trials of interventions against tropical diseases: a 'toolbox'*. Oxford University Press, Oxford.

Sommer, A., Hussaini, G., Muhilal, T.I., Susanto, D., and Saroso, J.S. (1980). History of nightblindness: a simple tool for xerophthalmia screening. *American Journal of Clinical Nutrition*, **33**, 887.

Susser, M. (1973). *Causal thinking in the health sciences: concepts and strategies in epidemiology*. Oxford University Press, New York.

Tamir, D., Feurstein, A., Brunner, S., Halfon, S.-T., Reshef, A., and Palti, H. (1990). Primary prevention of cardiovascular diseases in childhood: changes in serum total cholesterol, high density lipoprotein, and body mass index after 2 years of intervention in Jerusalem schoolchildren aged 7–9 years. *Preventive Medicine*, **19**, 22.

Tollman, S. and Friedman, I. (1994). Community-orientated primary health care—South African legacy. *South African Medical Journal*, **84**, 646.

United States Department of Health and Human Services (1990). *Outline of proceedings of consensus conference: small area analysis* DHHS Publication No. HRS-A–PE 91.1(A). United States Department of Health and Human Services, Washington D.C.

Van de Ven, A.H., and Delbecq, A.L. (1972). The nominal group as a research instrument for exploratory health studies. *American Journal of Public Health*, **62**, 337.

Vartiainen, E., Puska, P., Jousilahti, P., Korhonen, H.J., Tuomilehto, J., and Nissinen, A. (1994). Twenty-year trends in coronary risk factors in North Karelia and in other areas of Finland. *International Journal of Epidemiology*, **23**, 495.

Vaughan, J.P., and Morrow, R.H. (ed.) (1989). *Manual of epidemiology for district health management*. World Health Organization, Geneva.

Velzeboer, M.I., Selwyn, B.J., Sargent, F., Pollitt, E., and Delgado, H. (1983*a*). Evaluation of arm circumference as a public health index of protein energy malnutrition in early childhood. *Journal of Tropical Paediatrics*, **29**, 135.

Velzeboer, M.I., Selwyn, B.J., Sargent, F., Pollitt, E., and Delgado, H. (1983*b*). The use of arm circumference in simplified screening for acute malnutrition by minimally-trained health workers. *Journal of Tropical Paediatrics*, **29**, 159.

Venkataswamy, G., Lepkowski, J.M., Ravilla, T., Brilliant, G.E., Shanmugham, C.A.K., Vaidyanathan, K., Tilden, R.L. and the Aravind Rapid Epidemiologic Assessment staff (1989). Rapid epidemiologic assessment of cataract blindness. *International Journal of Epidemiology*, **18**, S60.

Von Korff, M., and Parker, R.D. (1980). The dynamics of the prevalence of chronic episodic disease. *Journal of Chronic Diseases*, **33**, 79.

Waksberg, J. (1978). Sampling methods for rapid digit dialing. *Journal of the American Statistical Association*, **73**, 40.

Walter, S.D. and Cook R.J. (1991). A comparison of several point estimators of the odds ratio in a single 2×2 contingency table. *Biometrics*, **47**, 795.

Walter, H.J., Hofman, A., Barrett, L.T., Connelly, P.A., Kost, K.L., Walk, E.H., *et al.* (1987). Primary prevention of cardiovascular disease among children: three years' results of a randomised intervention trial. In *Cardiovascular risk factors in childhood: epidemiology and prevention* (ed. B.S. Hetzel and G.S. Berenson), p.161. Elsevier, Amsterdam.

Weiss, N.S. (1986). *Clinical epidemiology: the study of the outcome of illness.* Oxford University Press, New York.

West, S.K., Munoz, B., Turner, V.M., Mmbaga, B.B.O., and Taylor, H.R. (1991) The epidemiology of trachoma in Central Tanzania. *International Journal of Epidemiology*, **20**, 1088.

WHO (World Health Organization) (Division of Epidemiological Surveillance and Health Situation and Trend Analysis) (1993). News from the World Health Organization: rapid evaluation methods in health services. *International Journal of Epidemiology*, **22**, 578.

Williams, C.L., Arnold, C.B., and Wynder, E.L. (1977). Primary prevention of chronic disease beginning in childhood, the 'Know Your Body' program: design of study. *Preventive Medicine*, **6**, 344.

Williamson, D.F., Forman, M.R., Binkin, N.J., Gentry, E.M., Remington, P.L., and Trowbridge, F.L. (1987). Alcohol and body weight in United States adults. *American Journal of Public Health*, **77**, 1324.

Winkleby, M.A., Ragland, D.R., and Syme, S.L. (1988). Self-reported stressors and hypertension: evidence of an inverse association. *American Journal of Epidemiology*, **127**, 124.

9 The principles of an epidemic field investigation

Michael B. Gregg

Introduction

This chapter contains a simple, practical, and essentially non-technical discussion of how to prepare for and perform an epidemic field investigation, that is the practice of field epidemiology. We focus attention on a presumed point-source (common-source) epidemic, recognized and reported by local health authorities to a regional or state health department. This frequent and typical scenario highlights some key operational and public health issues. The discussion describes the tasks to perform, but attention is also directed towards important operational and public health policy concerns. Although this chapter centres about an acute infectious disease epidemic in a community, the epidemiological and public health principles apply equally well to non-infectious diseases.

Background considerations

Definition of field epidemiology

Although no medical or epidemiological dictionary has yet to include the words field epidemiology in their texts, a definition has been proposed which applies directly to our discussion of investigating an epidemic in the field (Goodman *et al.* 1996).

The four ingredients that together comprise the essential elements of field epidemiology are:

1. The problem is unexpected.

2. An immediate response may be necessary.

3. Public health epidemiologists must travel to and work on location in the field.

4. The extent of the investigation is likely to be limited because of the imperative for timely intervention.

These elements, indeed, characterize the scenario of this entire chapter, and, hopefully, place the actions of the investigative team into an understandable perspective.

Overall purposes and methodology

As mentioned in earlier chapters, the purposes of epidemiology are to determine the cause(s) of a disease, its source, its mode of transmission, who is at risk of developing disease, and what exposures predispose to disease. With answers to these questions, the epidemiologist hopes to control and prevent disease. Clearly, these purposes also apply to field investigations of infectious diseases. Fortunately, in many outbreak investigations, the clinical

syndromes are easily identifiable, the agents can be readily isolated and characterized, and the source, mode of transmission, and risk factors of the disease are usually well known and understood. Therefore, the epidemiologists are often quite well prepared for their field investigations. However, when the clinical diagnosis and/or laboratory findings are unclear, the task becomes much more difficult. Careful consideration of the clinical presentation of disease is needed in order to obtain key information regarding the source, mode of spread, and population(s) at risk of disease. For example, bacterial contamination of food or water is usually manifested by signs and symptoms referable to the gastrointestinal tract. Pathogenic agents transmitted in air often affect the respiratory tract and sometimes the skin, eyes, or mucous membranes. Skin abrasions or lesions may suggest animal or insect transmission. So the clinical manifestations of disease may serve as critical leads for epidemiologists who may at times have no other information to guide them. Regardless of how secure the clinical diagnosis may be, the thought process must include clinical, laboratory, and epidemiological evidence. Together these provide leads and pathways to take or reject, so that ultimately the natural history of the epidemic will be understood.

Although epidemiologists perform several separate operations (which are listed below), in broad strokes they really do two things. First, they collect information that describes the setting of the outbreak, namely, over what time period people became sick, where they acquired disease, and what the characteristics of the ill people were. These are the descriptive aspects of the investigation. Often, simply by knowing these facts (and the diagnosis), the epidemiologist can determine the source and mode of spread of the agent and can identify those primarily at risk of developing disease. Common sense will often give these answers, and relatively little, if any, further analysis is required.

However, on occasion, it will not be readily apparent where the agent resided, how it was transmitted, who was at risk of disease, and what the risk factors were. Under these circumstances, a second operation, analytic epidemiology, must be used, hopefully to provide the answers. As has been described in other chapters, epidemiological analyses require comparisons of persons – ill and well, exposed and not exposed. In epidemic situations, the epidemiologist usually compares ill and well people – both believed at risk of disease – to determine what exposures ill people had that well people did not. These comparisons are made using appropriate statistical techniques. If the differences between ill and well are greater than one would expect by chance, the epidemiologist can draw certain inferences regarding the transmission of and exposure to the disease.

The pace and commitment of a field investigation

An underlying theme woven through this chapter emphasizes the need to act quickly, to establish clear operational priorities, and to perform the investigation responsibly. This should not imply the haphazard collection and inappropriate analysis of data, but rather the use of simple and workable case definitions, case-finding methods, and analyses. If at all possible, one should collect data, perform analyses, and make recommendations in the field as part of the investigation. There is often a strong tendency to collect what is believed to be the essential information in the field and then retreat to 'home base' for analysis – particularly with the availability of computers. However, such action may be viewed as lack of interest or concern or even possessiveness by the local constituency. Equally important, premature departure also makes any further collection of data or direct contact with study populations and local health officials difficult, if not impossible. Once home, the epidemiology team has lost the urgency and momentum to perform, the sense of relevancy of the epidemic, and, most of all, the totally committed time for the investigation. Every field investigation should be completed not only to the team's satisfaction, but particularly to the satisfaction of the local health officers as well. Contemplate what the local health department must face if the team leaves without providing reasonably final results and firmly based recommendations.

The unique aspects of field epidemiology

The epidemiological methods used in most field investigations suffer to a greater or lesser degree from several limitations that result from the need to respond rapidly (Goodman *et al.* 1990). First, field investigations usually rely on a variety of data sources that often are incomplete, less than accurate, or are collected for other purposes. Second, epidemiologists in the field are often faced with analysing small numbers, significantly decreasing the statistical power of their studies. Third, because one often arrives late in the epidemic or, indeed, 'after the fact', there may be no specimens to collect for analysis or acute blood samples to test. Fourth, there may be a modest amount of publicity surrounding the investigation. As a result, members of the community may have preconceived ideas of what happened and who was responsible, making collection of unbiased data difficult. Fifth, because vested interests are commonly involved, there will often be some reluctance to participate. In common-source outbreaks this is particularly true where restaurants, other public establishments, industry, or health care providers may have been the source or cause of the epidemic. Lastly, there commonly will be conflicting pressures to intervene. All too often the field investigators will be forced by the community or others to make recommendations for prevention and control before all the evidence is in or before the completion of a scientifically acceptable investigation.

Thus, in every field investigation the pressures of time and necessary action will always be balanced against the need for good science.

Recognition and response to a request for assistance

The report

The regional health officer may learn of an epidemic from a variety of sources such as the local health department, a private physician, a hospital administrator, a concerned citizen, or perhaps even the news media. Generally, the most direct and reliable source of information is a local health official. There will be a 'working' diagnosis, an estimate of the number of cases, the background expected number of cases, and the affected population. Reports of a possible or real epidemic from others such as private physicians, hospitals, etc. may reveal only a segment of the overall picture of the epidemic or may, indeed, not reflect the existence of an epidemic at all. Therefore, when reports such as these are received at the regional level, the regional official should contact the local health officials and inform them of the reports. Local officials will usually try to verify such reports and, if verified, they will often investigate the epidemic themselves. Even if no epidemic is ultimately recognized or no request for assistance results, the regional health official has clearly discharged an important responsibility by reporting back to the local health department.

The request

However, if local health officials request assistance, the regional epidemiologist, before making any decision, should try to acquire as much information as possible regarding the diagnosis, the normal occurrence of disease, and the population primarily affected. Quite frequently local health departments will have performed a preliminary and sometimes relatively extensive investigation before calling for assistance. They will be able to provide a considerable amount of valuable information which can be used in planning for the investigation.

It is important to find out exactly why the request for assistance is forthcoming. Does the local health department simply need an extra pair of hands to perform or complete the investigation? Has it been unable to uncover the nature or source of infection or the mode of spread, thereby limiting adequate control or prevention? Perhaps the health department wants to share the responsibility of the investigation with a more seasoned and knowledgeable health authority so as to be relieved of local political or scientific pressure. Occasionally, legal or ethical issues may have become prominent in the early investigation. Those responding to requests for help must be aware of these possibilities. Rarely, an epidemic may even be declared or announced by local authorities or citizens. Assistance is then requested in order to publicize perceived adverse health conditions, to awaken regional or national health leaders, or even to secure funds. Regardless of the motivation behind a call for assistance, there must be an established official basis for such a request and official local permission for an epidemiological investigation. Many a field study has been aborted simply because either those requesting assistance had no authority to do so or state, regional, or national teams were investigating without local permission.

The response and the responsibilities

The relationships between regional and local health departments vary not only from region to region within countries but also from country to country. In general, the larger health districts help serve the smaller in time of need. Yet the sensitivities between these two authorities are frequently delicate, particularly as they relate to perceived competence, local jurisdiction, and ultimate authority. The regional health officer must decide – on the basis of prevailing local-provincial amenities and agreements and his best judgement – the most appropriate response. There are several important reasons why requests for a field investigation should be answered, if not encouraged:

1. to control and prevent further disease;

2. to provide agreed upon or statutorily mandated services;

3. to derive more information about interactions among the human host, the agent, and the environment;

4. to assess the quality of epidemiological surveillance at the local level;

5. to maintain or improve such epidemiological surveillance by personal and direct contact;

6. to establish a new system of epidemiological surveillance;

7. to provide training opportunities in practical field epidemiology.

If the regional health officer decides to provide field assistance, both he or she and the local health official should discuss and hopefully agree upon (i) what resources (including personnel) will be available locally; (ii) what resources will be provided by the regional team; (iii) who will direct the day-to-day investigation; (iv) who will provide overall supervision and ultimately be responsible for the investigation; (v) how will the data be shared and who will be responsible for their analysis; (vi) will a report of the findings be written, who will write it, to whom will it go; and (vii) who will be the senior author of a scientific paper, should one be written. These are extremely critical issues, some of which cannot be totally resolved before the investigative team arrives on the scene. However, they must be addressed, discussed openly, and agreed upon as soon as possible.

Preparation for the field investigation

No attempt is made here to describe in detail what personnel or equipment should be deployed for the field investigation. These decisions will clearly depend upon the presumed cause, magnitude, geographical extent of the epidemic, and the local and regional resources available. Rather, the emphasis focuses upon the necessary collaborative relationships between health professionals at the regional office and key instructions to the investigating team before they depart.

Collaboration and consultation

Virtually all infectious disease outbreaks require the support of a competent laboratory. Even if local laboratories are capable of processing and identifying specimens, the regional epidemiological team should immediately, upon being informed of the proposed investigation, contact their counterparts within their regional laboratories. These microbiologists should be requested to provide any needed guidance and laboratory assistance. Now is the time to

obtain assurance of cooperation and commitment rather than during the field investigation or near the end when specimens have already been collected and await testing. Not only must the microbiologists schedule the processing of specimens, but they should be asked to recommend what kinds of specimens to collect and how they should be collected and processed. There also may be substantive basic or applied research questions that could be appropriately addressed and answered during the field investigation. These issues should be discussed in detail with the microbiologists and every effort made to enlist and support their interest.

Advice on statistical methods may also be sought at this time as well. The same philosophy applies also to contacting other health professionals, such as veterinarians, mammalogists, or entomologists, whose expertise can be crucial to a successful field investigation. Moreover, serious consideration should be given to including such professionals on the investigative team. It is important to determine whether such scientists should be part of the initial team so that appropriate information and, particularly, specimens can be collected concomitantly with other relevant epidemiological information.

Other persons who can be extremely important in the overall management of a field investigation are information specialists. When large outbreaks of disease are to be investigated that will probably attract even moderate local or regional attention in the news media, the presence of an experienced and knowledgeable information officer who can respond to public inquiries and meet with the news media on a regular basis can be invaluable. Some consideration should be given to including secretarial and/or administrative personnel on the investigating team – not only in order to utilize their services but to expose them to a real-life investigation. By such experience they will return home with a better understanding of fieldwork and an increased ability to support technical personnel in the regional offices.

Basic administrative instructions

Once the field team has been designated, certain key instructions should be emphasized:

1. Identify the team leader and the person to whom he or she should report regularly at the regional level.

2. Specify when and how communications should be established with the regional home base for information and guidance. Do not permit the investigating team to notify, at their convenience, the regional supervisors of the progress of the investigation. Instead establish within reason fixed times and places for regular communication regardless of whether new facts or findings have been uncovered. There may be just as important reasons for the home base to communicate with the field team as the reverse.

3. Emphasize the need for the team to meet with appropriate local health officials immediately upon arriving in the field. If the local official has not already been identified, instruct the team leader to determine as soon as possible who at the local level will be in charge. Encourage the team to identify and meet with all persons they may need cooperation from in the investigation. Such persons include: local health department directors and/or chiefs of epidemiology, laboratory services, vital statistics, nursing, and maternal and child health. Other important persons would often include the mayor, the local medical society, or hospital administrators and

staff. It is highly preferable to take the day or so needed to meet these persons initially – so that key doors will be opened – than to spend valuable time later in the investigation mending bridges.

4. Have the team leader identify the appropriate local person to speak for the entire investigative team when necessary. In general, the regional team should try to avoid direct contact with the news media and should always defer to local health officials. The investigative team is usually working at the request and under the aegis of the local health authorities. Therefore, it is the local officials who not only know and appreciate the local aspects of the epidemic but are the appropriate persons to comment on the findings of the investigation. In the most practical sense, the less the news media make contact with the investigative team, the more can be done at the pace and discretion of that team.

5. Before leaving to conduct an investigation, the team leader or preferably his immediate supervisor should write a memorandum. It should summarize how and when the region was contacted, what information was provided by the local health department, what the proposed response by the region is, what the agreed upon commitments of both local and regional health authorities are, who is on the field team, and when the latter is expected to arrive in the field. This memorandum should be distributed to key supervisors in both regional and local health offices and to others who may have need to know.

The field investigation

Before the actual field activities are discussed, it should be borne in mind that the order of the tasks should not be considered fixed or binding but rather logical in terms of field operations and epidemiological thinking. The epidemiologist may perform several of these functions simultaneously or in different order during the investigation and may even institute control and prevention measures soon after beginning the investigation on the basis of intuitive reasoning and/or common sense. No two epidemiologists will take the same pathway of investigation. Yet, in general, the data they collect, the analyses they apply, and the control and prevention measures they recommend will probably be similar.

Since, by definition, the epidemic in question has resulted from a point source and may be continuing or nearly over before the field team arrives, the investigation will be retrospective in nature. This should alert the epidemiologist to some fundamental aspects of any investigation that occurs after the fact. First of all, because many illnesses and critical events have already occurred, virtually all information acquired and related to the epidemic will be based upon memory. Health officers, physicians, and patients are likely to have different recollections, views or perceptions of what transpired, what caused the disease, and even who or what was responsible for the epidemic. Information may conflict, may not be accurate, and certainly cannot be expected to reflect the precise recounting of past events. Yet, just as the clinician may ask patients what they think is making them sick, the epidemiologist will do well to ask members of the affected community what they think caused the epidemic.

For the young, inexperienced medical epidemiologist steeped in the tradition of molecule and millimole determinations, the 'more-or-less' measurements of the field epidemiologist can initially be major hurdles to the successful field investigation. However lacking in accuracy these data may be, they are the only data available, and must be collected, analysed, and interpreted with care, imagination, and caution.

Determine the existence of an epidemic

In most instances, local health officials will know whether more cases of disease are occurring than would normally be expected. Since most local health departments have ongoing records of the occurrence of communicable disease, comparisons by week, month, and year can be made to determine whether the observed numbers exceed the normally expected level. Although strict laboratory confirmation may be lacking at this time, an increase in the number of cases of a disease reasonably accurately reported by local physicians should stimulate further inquiry. However, the terms 'epidemic' and 'outbreak' are quite subjective, not only depending upon how local health officials view the expected rises and falls in disease incidence, but upon whether such changes merit investigation. One must be acutely aware of artefactual causes of increases or decreases in numbers of reported cases, such as changes in local reporting practices, increased interest in certain diseases because of local or national awareness, or changes in methods of diagnosis. Even the presence of a new physician or clinic in the community may lead to a substantial increase in reported numbers of cases, yet not represent a true increase above normal.

In certain situations, however, it may be difficult to document the existence of an epidemic rapidly. One may need to acquire information from such sources as school or factory absentee records, out-patient clinic visits, hospitalizations, laboratory records, or death certificates. Sometimes a simple survey of practising physicians will strongly support the existence of an epidemic, as would a similar rapid survey of households in the community. Frequently, such quick assessments, entail asking about signs and symptoms rather than about specific diagnoses. For example, such inquiry might involve asking physicians or clinics if they are treating more people than usual with sore throats, gastroenteritis, fever with rash, etc., in order to obtain an index of disease incidence. Although not specific for any given disease, such surveys can often document the occurrence of an epidemic. Sometimes it is extremely difficult to establish satisfactorily the existence of an epidemic. Yet because of local pressures, epidemiologists may be obliged to continue the investigation even if they believe that no significant health problem exists.

Confirm the diagnosis

Every effort possible should be made to confirm the clinical diagnosis by standard laboratory techniques such as serology and/or isolation and characterization of the agent. One should not attempt to apply newly introduced, experimental, or otherwise not broadly recognized confirmatory tests – at least not at this stage in the investigation. If at all possible, visit the laboratory and verify the laboratory findings in person.

Not every reported case has to be confirmed. If most patients have the expected or similar clinical signs and symptoms and, perhaps, 15 to 20 per cent of the cases are laboratory confirmed, one does not need more confirmation at this time. This should be ample confirmatory evidence. One should try to examine several representative cases of the disease as well; clinical assumptions should not be made. The diagnosis should be verified by a physician member of the team. Nothing convinces epidemiologists and responsible health officers more than an eyewitness confirmation of clinical disease by the investigating team.

Create a case definition and determine the number of cases

Now the epidemiologist must create a workable case definition, decide how to find cases, and count cases. The simplest and most objective criteria for a case definition are usually the best (for example, fever, radiographic evidence of pneumonia, white blood cells in the spinal fluid, number of bowel movements per day, blood in the stool, skin rash, etc.). However, be guided by the accepted, usual presentation of the disease, with or without standard laboratory confirmation, in the case definition. Where time may be a critical factor in a rapidly unfolding field investigation, a simple, easily applicable definition should be used – recognizing that some cases will be missed and some non-cases included. Some factors that can help determine the levels of sensitivity and specificity of the case definition are the following:

1. What is the usual apparent-to-inapparent clinical case ratio?

2. What are the important and obvious pathognomonic or strongly clinically suggestive signs and symptoms of the disease?

3. What isolations, identification, and serological techniques are easy, practicable, and reliable?

4. How accessible are the patients or those at risk; can they be recontacted after the initial investigation for follow-up questions, examination, or serology?

5. In the event that the investigation requires long-term follow-up, can the case definitions be applied easily and consistently by individuals other than the current investigating team?

6. Is it absolutely necessary that all patients be identified during the initial investigation or would only those seen by physicians or hospitalized suffice? Would a sample of the affected population be acceptable?

These considerations and others will probably play an important role in how cases will be defined and how intensive case investigation will be. However, no matter what criteria are used, the case definition must be applied equally and without bias to all persons under investigation.

Methods for finding cases will vary considerably according to the disease in question and the community setting. In many field investigations the techniques for identifying cases will be relatively self-evident. Most outbreaks involve certain clearly identifiable groups at risk. It is simply a matter of intensifying reporting from physicians, hospitals, laboratories, or school and industrial contacts, or perhaps using some form of public announcement to identify most of the remaining, unreported cases. However, there may be times when more intensive efforts – such as physician, telephone, door-to-door, culture or serological surveys – may be necessary to find cases. Regardless of the method, some system(s) of case identification must be established for the duration of the investigation and perhaps for some time afterwards.

In the vast majority of instances, simply determining the number of cases does not provide adequate information. Control and prevention measures depend upon knowing the source and mode of spread of an agent as well as the characteristics of ill patients. Therefore, the process of case finding should include collecting pertinent information likely to provide clues or leads to the natural history of the epidemic and, particularly, relevant characteristics of the ill. First, one should collect basic information about each patient's age, gender, residence, occupation, date of onset, etc., to define the simple and basic descriptive aspects of the epidemic. However, if the disease under investigation is usually water- or food-borne, one should ask questions about exposure to various water and food sources. If the disease is most frequently transmitted by person-to-person contact, one should seek information that will help determine the frequency, duration, and nature of personal contacts. If the nature of the disease is not known or cannot be comfortably presumed, the epidemiologist will need to ask a variety of questions covering all possible aspects of disease transmission and risk.

Orient the data in terms of time, place, and person

Having now reasonably accurately counted cases and determined the order of magnitude of the epidemic, the field epidemiologist should now record the descriptive aspects of the investigation. Characterize the epidemic in terms of when patients became ill, where patients resided or became ill, and what characteristics the patients possess. There may be a tendency to wait until the epidemic is over or until all likely cases have been reported before performing such an analysis. This tendency should be strongly avoided because further inclusion of a proportionately small number of cases will usually not affect the analysis or recommendations. Moreover, the earlier one can develop ideas of why the epidemic started, the more pertinent and accurate data one can collect.

Time

In most instances, it will be very valuable to describe the cases by time of onset by constructing a graph that depicts the occurrence of cases over an appropriate time interval (Fig. 9.1). This 'epidemic curve' as it is frequently called, can give a considerably deeper appreciation for the magnitude of the outbreak, its possible mode of spread, and the possible duration of the epidemic than would a simple listing of cases. A remarkable amount of information can be inferred from a pictorial representation of times of onset of disease. If the incubation period of the disease is known, relatively firm inferences can be made regarding the likelihood of a point-source exposure, person-to-person spread, or a mixture of the two. Also, if the epidemic is in progress, one may be able to predict, using the epidemic curve, how many more cases are likely to occur. Finally, a pictorial representation of cases over time serves as an excellent way of ready communication to non-epidemiologists, administrators, and the like who need to grasp in some fashion the nature and magnitude of the epidemic. The epidemic curve in Fig. 9.1 portrays cases of Pontiac fever (subsequently confirmed as legionnaires' disease) that occurred in Pontiac, Michigan, July and August 1968, by day of onset (Glick *et al.* 1978). The epidemic was explosive in

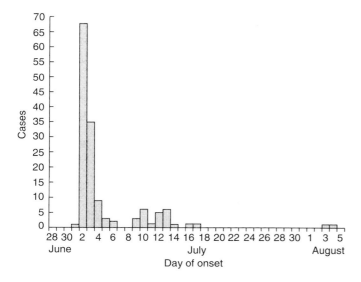

Fig. 9.1 Cases of Pontiac fever, by day of onset, Oakland County (Michigan) Health Department, 28 June to 5 August 1968.

onset suggesting (i) a virtually simultaneous common-source exposure of many persons, (ii) a disease with a short incubation period, and (iii) a continuing exposure spanning several weeks.

Place

Not infrequently, exposures to microbial agents occur in unique locations in the community, which, if properly depicted and analysed, may provide major clues or evidence regarding the source of the agent and/or the nature of exposure. Water supplies, milk distribution routes, sewage disposal outflows, prevailing wind currents, air-flow patterns in buildings, and ecological habitats of animals may play important roles in disseminating microbial pathogens and determining who is at risk of acquiring disease. If cases are plotted geographically, a pattern of distribution may emerge that approximates these known sources and routes of potential exposure that may help identify the vehicle or mode of transmission.

Figure 9.2 illustrates the usefulness of a 'spot map' in the investigation of an outbreak of shigellosis in Dubuque, Iowa, in 1974 (Rosenberg *et al.* 1976). Initially the investigation revealed that cases were not clustered by area of residence or age or gender. A history of drinking water gave no useful clue as to a possible source and mode of transmission. However, it was later learned that many infected persons had been exposed to water by recent swimming in a camping park located on the Mississippi River. As can be seen in Fig. 9.2, the river sites where 22 culture-positive persons swam within three days of onset of illness strongly suggested a common source of exposure. Ultimately, the epidemiologists incriminated the Mississippi River water by documenting gross contamination by the city's sewage treatment plant five miles upstream and by isolating *Shigella sonnei* from a sample of river water taken from the camping park beach area.

Person

Lastly, the epidemiologist should examine the character of the patients themselves in terms of a variety of attributes, such as age, gender, race, occupation, or virtually any other characteristic that

may be useful in portraying the uniqueness of the case population. Some diseases primarily affect certain age groups or races; frequently, occupation is a key characteristic of people with certain infectious diseases. The list of human characteristics is nearly endless. However, the more the investigators know about the infectious disease in question (the reservoir, mode(s) of spread, persons usually at greatest risk), the more specific and pertinent information they can seek from the cases to determine whether any of these characteristics predisposes to illness.

Determine who is at risk of becoming ill

It is at this time in the investigation that epidemiologists may begin to apply analytical techniques. They now know the number of people ill, when and where they were when they became ill, what their general characteristics are, and usually they will have a firm diagnosis or a good 'working' diagnosis. These data frequently provide enough information for the field team to feel relatively sure how and why the epidemic started. For example, often this information will strongly suggest that only people in a particular community supplied by a specific water system were at risk of getting sick, or that only certain students in a school or workers in a single factory became ill. Perhaps it was only a group of people who attended a local restaurant who reported illness. In other

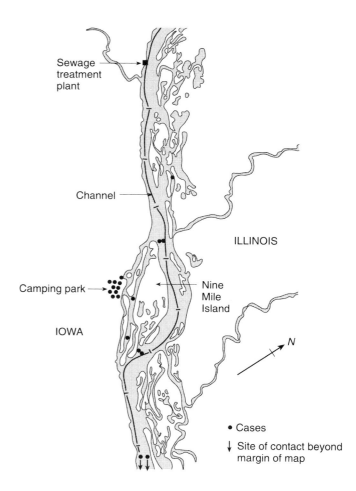

Fig. 9.2 Mississippi River sites where 22 culture-positive cases swam within 3 days of onset of illness.

words, the simple descriptive aspects of the epidemic frequently identify those most likely at risk of disease. However, no matter how obvious it might appear that only a single group of persons were at risk, the epidemiologist should apply analytical methods to support this conclusion.

For example, if fever, abdominal cramps, and diarrhoea occur among 35 residents of a housing subdivision 'A' (presumably caused by water contaminated with *Shigella*) and no similar illness was reported from subdivision 'B' over the same time period, one would logically conclude that only subdivision 'A' residents were at risk of developing disease. However, only after a proper survey is applied to the residents of subdivision 'B' or even elsewhere in the community, looking for the same illness and comparing illness rates in such groups, can one legitimately infer that the at-risk population were all residents of subdivision 'A'.

Develop an hypothesis that explains the specific exposure that caused disease and test this hypothesis by appropriate statistical methods

The next analytical step is often the most difficult one to perform. By now the epidemiologists should have an excellent grasp of the epidemic and an overall feel for the most likely source and mode of transmission. However, they must still determine the most likely exposure that caused disease. A classic example of what is meant here would be an investigation of an outbreak of nausea, vomiting, and diarrhoea among people who had attended a church supper presumedly caused by staphylococcal contamination of food(s) eaten at the supper. Since the disease was most likely acquired by eating something (because of the signs and symptoms) and because no other cluster of similar disease had occurred elsewhere in the community, the investigators focused attention only on those who attended the supper. The hypothesis posed was that the exposure necessary to develop nausea, vomiting, and diarrhoea was consumption of some food(s) contaminated with staphylococcal enterotoxin. Therefore, the ill people were asked what they had eaten at the church supper (that is, what they had been exposed to) and their food histories were compared with those people who had not become ill but had also attended the church supper. Comparisons of food histories (eating rates) between the ill and the well participants were made and statistically analysed. The food histories—'exposures'—were found to be similar between the two groups except for one single food item where many more ill persons had eaten this item than well persons. Since such a difference was very unlikely to occur simply by chance alone, the inference was drawn that that particular food item was the exposure that caused the illness.

Several other examples of epidemiological investigations of infectious diseases may serve to emphasize the importance of developing hypotheses and testing them.

In August 1980, a community hospital in the State of Michigan recognized seven cases of group A steptococcal postoperative wound infections which had occurred over the previous four months (Berkelman *et al.* 1982). This represented more cases than usual, and an investigation was started. Using a standard case definition the epidemiologists ultimately identified 10 cases that had occurred over this time period, all of whom were patients on several surgical wards. This geographical clustering plus the fact that the infections developed within one or two days following surgery suggested a common source of exposure, presumably in the operating rooms. Although streptococcal disease can rarely be transmitted by inanimate objects, within the hospital setting, the most frequent source of streptococci is man, and the most common mode of spread is person-to-person. Therefore, the epidemiologists hypothesized that the probable risk factor unique to these patients was contact with or exposure to an infected or colonized member of the hospital's professional staff sometime during surgery. After selecting appropriate non-streptococcal-infected post-surgical patients as controls, the investigators compared both ill and well in regard to what exposure they had had with a total of 38 surgeons, anaesthetists, and nursing staff during surgery for the epidemic period. Exposure rates were not statistically different between cases and controls except for one nurse. Samples from this nurse were cultured and she was found to be an anal and vaginal carrier of a strain of β-haemolytic streptococci identical to the epidemic strain. Following appropriate treatment this strain of streptococci could no longer be cultured from her. She returned to work and six months later two more cases of postoperative β-haemolytic streptococcal infection occurred, caused, however, by a different serotype. Samples from the nurse were cultured again and she was found to be a vaginal and anal carrier of this different strain.

The investigation of an epidemic of *Listeria monocytogenes* is a classic example of how the epidemiological method, simple inferences, and persistent re-examination of data can point to a hitherto unknown source and mode of spread of disease. Thirty-four cases of perinatal listeriosis and seven cases of adult disease occurred between 1 March and 1 September, 1981, in several maritime provinces of Canada (Schlech *et al.* 1983). These cases represented a several-fold increase over the number of cases diagnosed in previous years suggesting some common exposure. Although *L. monocytogenes* is a common cause of abortion and nervous system diseases in cattle, sheep, and goats, the source of human infection has been obscure. The epidemiologists therefore undertook an investigation to determine if infected persons had had contact with one another or whether there had been a common environmental source which would explain their disease. Cases could not be linked together by person-to-person contact; they shared no common water source; and food exposures, as determined from a general food history, were not different between cases and controls. However, a second, more detailed food history and subsequent intensive interrogation of infected and non-infected persons revealed that there was a statistically significant difference between cases and controls regarding exposure to coleslaw. Even though this food had never been previously incriminated as a source of listeria, it was the only food item statistically incriminated and essentially the only lead the investigators had at the time. Armed with this association, the epidemiologists subsequently found a specimen of coleslaw in the refrigerator of one of the patients which grew out the same serotype of listeria found in the epidemic cases. No other food items in the refrigerator were positive for listeria. The coleslaw had been prepared by a regional manufacturer who had obtained cabbages and carrots from several wholesale dealers and many local farmers. Although environmental cultures from the coleslaw plant failed to reveal listeria organisms, two unopened packages of coleslaw from the plant subsequently grew *L. monocytogenes* of the same epidemic serotype. A review of the sources of the vegetable ingredients was made, and a single farmer was identified who had grown cabbages and also maintained a flock of sheep. Two of his sheep had previously died of listeriosis in 1979 and 1981. Also, he was in the habit of using sheep manure to fertilize his cabbage.

It cannot definitely be proven that this particular farm was the source of the listeria organisms that caused the epidemic. However, the hypothesis that coleslaw was the source and the statistical test which supported this hypothesis provided the necessary impetus to continue the investigation. Ultimately a single highly suggestive source of the bacteria was discovered. These findings strongly implied listeriosis as a zoonotic infection transmitted from infected animals via contaminated vegetables to man.

Lastly, a similar logic in a much more difficult situation was applied to an outbreak of legionnaires' disease among persons attending an American Legion convention in Philadelphia, Pennsylvania, in July 1976 (Fraser *et al.* 1977). From the very beginning to the end of the field investigation, neither the clinical presentation nor laboratory results provided the epidemiologists with a diagnosis. However, initially it appeared and was epidemiologically established that disease was not transmitted from person to person. Yet being a delegate who stayed at or visited the Bellevue Stratford Hotel in Philadelphia conferred an increased risk of disease, although this conclusion did not provide enough information about the source or mode of spread of the agent to be particularly useful. In other words, simply the person's presence in the Bellevue Stratford did not help explain what the specific exposure was or how the disease was acquired. A legionnaire could easily have eaten a meal, consumed water from the hotel, or simply breathed in the hotel – all possible exposures to the agent that could place a person in a high-risk category of becoming ill. Therefore, a series of hypotheses were proposed to determine whether eating meals, drinking water, or simply being in the hotel conferred increased risk of developing illness among the legionnaires. When the final analysis was done, there was no significant difference between ill and well legionnaires in terms of eating or drinking at the hotel. However, spending at least one hour in the hotel lobby conferred a much greater risk of disease than would have been expected by chance alone. Therefore, the investigators inferred that being in the lobby of the hotel was the necessary exposure for acquiring disease. This, coupled with the clinical features of the disease (pneumonia), implied that the agent was airborne and was transmitted through the air-conditioning system. Although the bacterium responsible for legionnaires' disease was not isolated from the Bellevue Stratford Hotel's air-conditioning system at that time, it was later recovered from lung tissue of several diseased legionnaires. Moreover, subsequent investigations of similar epidemics of legionnaires' disease elsewhere have not only confirmed the epidemiological pattern of this disease, but *Legionella* bacteria have been isolated from similar air-conditioning systems.

Again, this phase of the investigation clearly will pose the greatest challenge to epidemiologists. They must review their findings carefully, weigh the clinical, laboratory, and epidemiological features of the disease, and hypothesize possible exposures that could plausibly cause disease. In other words, they must seek, from the patients' histories exposures that could conceivably predispose to illness. If exposure histories for ill and well are not significantly different, the epidemiologist must develop new hypotheses. This may require imagination, perseverance, and sometimes resurveying those at risk to obtain more pertinent information.

Compare the hypothesis with the established facts

Having determined by epidemiological and statistical inference the probable exposure responsible for disease, the epidemiologist still must 'square' the hypothesis with the clinical, laboratory, and other epidemiological facts of the investigation. In other words, do the proposed exposure, mode of spread, and population affected fit well with the known facts of the disease? For example, if in the gastroenteritis outbreak referred to above the analysis incriminated an uncooked food left at room temperature for 18 to 24 hours and previously known to promote growth of staphylococci, the hypothesis fits well with our understanding of staphylococcal food poisoning. However, if the analysis incriminated coffee or water – highly unlikely sources of staphylococcal enterotoxin – the epidemiologist must then reassess the findings, perhaps secure more information, reconsider the clinical diagnosis, and certainly pose and test new hypotheses.

In a field investigation, when the disease is undiagnosed, the epidemiologist will clearly find it very difficult to fit a hypothesis to the natural history of the disease in question. All that can be hoped for is that the clinical, laboratory, and epidemiological findings portray a coherent, plausible, and physiologically sound series of findings and events that make sense.

Plan a more systematic study

The actual field investigation and analyses may be completed by now, requiring only a written report (see below). However, because there may be a need to find more patients, to define better the extent of the epidemic, or because a new laboratory method or case-finding technique may need to be evaluated, the epidemiologists may want to perform more detailed and carefully executed studies. With the pressure of the investigation somewhat removed, the field team may now consider surveying the population at risk in a variety of ways to help improve the quality of data and answer particular questions. Perhaps the most important reasons to perform such studies are to improve the sensitivity and specificity of the case definition and establish more accurately the true number of persons at risk, that is to improve the quality of numerators and denominators. For example, serosurveys coupled with a more complete clinical history can often sharpen the accuracy of the case count and define more clearly those truly at risk of developing disease. Moreover, repeat interviews of patients with confirmed disease may allow for rough quantification of degrees of exposure or dose responses – useful information in understanding the pathogenesis of certain diseases.

Preparation of a written report

Frequently, the final responsibility of the investigative team is to prepare a written report to document the investigation, the findings, and the recommendations. It is beyond the scope of this chapter to provide a detailed set of guidelines on scientific report writing. However, in most instances there are several important reasons why a report should be written and as soon as possible.

Administrative/operational purposes

A document for action Frequently, control and prevention efforts will only be taken when a report of all relevant findings has been written. This can and should place a heavy but necessary burden on the epidemiologists to complete their work quickly. Even if all possible cases have not yet been found or some laboratory results are still pending, reasonable written assumptions and recommendations can usually be made without fear of retraction or subsequent major change.

A record of performance In this day of input and output measurements, programme planning, programme justifications, and performance evaluations, there is often no better record of accomplishment than a well-written report of a completed field investigation. The number of investigations performed and the time and resources expended not only document the magnitude of health problems, changes in disease trends, and the results of control and prevention efforts, but serve as concrete evidence of programme justification and needs.

A document for potential medical/legal issues Presumably, epidemiologists investigate epidemics with objective, unbiased, and scientific purposes and similarly prepare written reports of their findings and conclusions objectively, honestly, and fairly. Such information may prove absolutely invaluable to consumers, practising physicians, or local and provincial health department officials in any legal action regarding health responsibilities and jurisdictions. In the long run, the health of the public is best served by simple, careful, honest documentation of events and findings made generally available for interpretation and comment.

Scientific/epidemiological purposes

Enhancement of the quality of the investigation Although not fully explained and rarely referred to, the actual process of writing and viewing data in written form often generates new and different thought processes and associations in the mind of the epidemiologist. The discipline of committing to paper the clinical, laboratory, and epidemiological findings of an epidemic investigation almost always will bring to light not only a better understanding of the natural unfolding of events, but their importance in terms of the natural history and development of the epidemic. The actual process of creating scientific prose, summarizing data, and creating tables and figures representing the known established facts forces one to view the entire series of events in a balanced, rational, and explainable way. This is considerably more so than an oral report given to the local health department the day of departure from the field. Occasionally, previously unrecognized associations will emerge from a careful and step-by-step written analysis that may be critical in the final interpretation and recommendations. The exercise of writing what was done and what was found will sometimes uncover facts and events that were more or less assumed to be true but not specifically sought for during the investigation. This in turn may stimulate further inquiry and fact finding in order to verify these assumptions.

An instrument for teaching epidemiology There would hardly be disagreement among epidemiologists that the exercise of writing the results of an investigation constitutes an essential building block in learning epidemiology. Much the way a lawyer prepares a brief or the physician organizes a case presentation, the epidemiologist should know how to fashion and present in logical sequence the important and pertinent findings of an investigation, their quality and validity, and the scientific inferences that can be made by their written presentation. The simple, direct, and orderly array of facts and inferences will not only reflect on the quality of the investigation itself but on the writer's basic understanding and knowledge of the epidemiological method.

Execute control and prevention measures

It is not the purpose of this chapter to elaborate on this aspect of the investigation. Nevertheless, the underlying purposes of all epidemic investigations are to control and/or prevent further disease.

Conclusion

In summary, the process of performing a thorough and successful epidemic field investigation has two major components. The first is the operational aspect that includes knowing why the investigation should be performed, who are the principal health officers involved, and who will assume the primary responsibility for data collection, interpretation, and implementation of prevention and control measures. The epidemiologist must also identify other health professionals who will provide the necessary laboratory and field support early in the planning stage.

Second, the field investigation is a direct application of the epidemiological method yet with unique limitations that relate to a balance between timely intervention and good science. With a relatively circumscribed timetable, this forces the investigative team (i) to establish workable case finding techniques, (ii) to collect data rapidly but carefully, and (iii) to describe these cases in a general sense regarding the time and place of occurrence and those primarily affected. Usually, the infectious agent is known and its sources and modes of transmission are well established, allowing the epidemiologist to identify the source and mode of spread rapidly. However, when the clinical disease is obscure and/or the origin of the agent ill-defined, one may be hard pressed to create an hypothesis that will not only identify the critical exposure and show statistical significance, but will logically explain the occurrence of the epidemic.

Scientific proof of causation in the strictest sense will not be established by such retrospective investigations, and, indeed, there will often be some reservations regarding the methods used and the validity of the data. Yet in most instances the careful development of epidemiological inferences coupled with persuasive clinical and laboratory evidence will almost always provide convincing evidence of the source and mode of spread of disease.

References

Berkleman, R.L., Martin D., Graham, D.R., *et al.* (1982). Streptococcal wound infections caused by a vaginal carrier. *Journal of the American Medical Association*, **247**, 2680.

Fraser, D.W., Tsai, T.R., Orenstein, W., *et al.* (1977). Legionnaires' disease. Description of an epidemic of pneumonia. *New England Journal of Medicine*, **297**, 1189.

Glick, T.H., Gregg, M.B., Berman, B., *et al.* (1978). Pontiac fever. An epidemic of unknown etiology in a health department: I Clinical and epidemiological aspects. *American Journal of Epidemiology*, **107**, 149.

Goodman, R.A. and Buehler, R.A. (1996) Field epidemiology defined. In *Field Epidemiology*. (ed. M. B. Gregg). pp. 3–8. Oxford University Press.

Goodman, R.A., Buehler, J.W., and Koplan, J.P. (1990). The epidemiological field investigation. Science and judgment in public health practice. *American Journal of Epidemiology*, **132**, 91.

Rosenberg, M.L., Hazlet, K.K., Schaefer, J., *et al.* (1976). Shigellosis from swimming. *Journal of the American Medical Association*, **236**, 1849.

Schlech, W.F. III, Lavigne, P.M., Bortobussi, R.A., *et al.* (1983). Epidemic listeriosis – evidence for transmission by food. *New England Journal of Medicine*, **308**, 203.

10 Case–control studies*

Noel S. Weiss

In 1971 Herbst *et al.* reported that the mothers of seven of eight teenage girls diagnosed with clear cell adenocarcinoma of the vagina in Boston between 1966 and 1969 claimed to have taken a synthetic hormone, diethylstilboestrol, while their daughters were *in utero*. None of the mothers of thirty-two girls without vaginal adenocarcinoma, matched to the mothers of cases with regard to hospital and date of birth, had taken diethylstilboestrol during the corresponding pregnancy. Within a year, a New York study of five cases and eight girls without vaginal cancer obtained similar results (Greenwald *et al.* 1971). The introduction of the use of prenatal diethylstilboestrol into obstetrical practice in the United States during the 1940s and 1950s, followed by the appearance of this hitherto unseen form of cancer some 20 years later, supported a causal connection between *in utero* exposure to diethylstilboestrol and vaginal adenocarcinoma. The means by which *in utero* diethylstilboestrol exposure might predispose to the occurrence of clear cell vaginal adenocarcinoma was unknown in 1971; at present, it is believed that diethylstilboestrol acts by interfering with the normal development of the female genital tract, resulting in the persistence into puberty of vaginal adenosis in which adenocarcinoma can arise (Ulfelder and Robboy 1976). None the less, a causal inference was made at that time by the United States Food and Drug Administration, which specified pregnancy as a contraindication for diethylstilboestrol use.

The investigation by Herbst *et al.* was a case–control study: a comparison of exposures or characteristics of ill or injured persons (cases) that preceded the occurrence of the outcome with those of persons at risk for the illness in the population from which the cases arose. Generally, the prior experience of persons at risk is estimated from observations on a sample of that population (controls). A difference in the frequency or levels of exposure between cases and controls (i.e. an association) may be a reflection of a causal link.

At first glance the case–control approach appears to proceed backwards, from consequence to potential cause. None the less, if a case–control study enrols cases and controls from the same underlying population at risk of the outcome and can measure exposure status validly in them, the results obtained will be identical to those from a properly performed cohort study. A case–control, cohort, or any other form of non-randomized study has the potential to identify associations that are not causal, either because of chance or because of the influence of some other factor

associated with both exposure and outcome. Even so, the evidence that is provided by well-done case–control studies can carry great weight when evaluating the validity of a causal hypothesis. Indeed, a number of causal inferences have been based largely on the results of case–control studies. These include, in addition to the diethylstilboestrol–vaginal adenocarcinoma relationship, the connection between aspirin use in children and the development of Reye's syndrome, and the use of absorbent tampons and the incidence of toxic shock syndrome.

One of the criteria used to assess the validity of a causal hypothesis is the 'strength' of the association between exposure and disease, usually as measured by the ratio of the incidence rate in exposed and non-exposed persons. Generally, in case–control studies the incidence is measured in neither exposed nor non-exposed persons. None the less, it is usually possible to estimate closely the ratio of the incidence rates from the frequency of exposure observed in cases and controls.

To understand how this can be done, consider a cohort study in which exposed and non-exposed persons are followed for a certain period of time. The table below summarizes their experience with regard to a particular disease:

	Disease		
Exposed	Yes	No	
Yes	a	b	$a + b$
No	c	d	$c + d$

The cumulative incidence of the disease in exposed and non-exposed persons over a given period of follow-up is $a/(a + b)$ and $c/(c + d)$ respectively. The relative risk (RR) is the ratio of these:

$$RR = \frac{a/(a + b)}{c/(c + d)}$$

If the incidence of the disease is relatively low during the follow-up period in both exposed and non-exposed persons, then a will be small relative to b, and c will be small relative to d. Therefore

$$RR = \frac{a/(a + b)}{c/(c + d)} \approx \frac{a/b}{c/d} = \frac{a/c}{b/d}$$

In this expression the numerator a/c is the odds of exposure in persons who develop the disease and the denominator b/d is the odds of exposure in persons who remain well. The odds ratio (OR) is given by

* The author is indebted to Lisa Herrinton, Julie Marshall, and Thomas Koepsell for their comments on an earlier draft of this chapter.

$$OR = \frac{a/c}{b/d}$$

The numerator can be estimated from a sample of cases, while the denominator can be estimated from a sample of non-cases. Neither estimate is influenced by the proportion of cases among the subjects actually chosen for study.

In the following hypothetical example, assume that 100 of 10 000 persons exposed to a particular substance or organism developed a disease, in contrast with 300 of 90 000 non-exposed persons:

	Disease		
Exposed	**Yes**	**No**	
Yes	100	9 900	10 000
No	300	89 700	90 000

$$RR = \frac{100/100\,000}{300/90\,000} = 3.00$$

If a case–control study including 50 per cent of cases but only 1 per cent of non-cases had been performed, the following results would have been obtained:

	Disease	
Exposed	**Yes**	**No**
Yes	$100 \times 0.5 = 50$	$9900 \times 0.01 = 99$
No	$300 \times 0.5 = 150$	$89\,700 \times 0.01 = 897$

$$RR \approx OR = \frac{50/150}{99/897} = 3.02$$

When controls are chosen in this way—from persons who had not developed the disease by the end of the same time period during which other persons (the cases) had developed it—the less common the disease in both exposed and non-exposed persons during the period, the better the odds ratio will estimate the ratio of cumulative incidence. In the previous example, only 1 per cent and 0.33 per cent of exposed and non-exposed persons respectively developed the illness, and so the relative cumulative incidence and odds ratio were in close correspondence (3.00 versus 3.02). However, it is also possible to choose controls from persons free of disease only until the corresponding cases have been diagnosed; a person can appear in the study first as a control and later as a case. If this approach is used, the odds ratio will be a valid estimate of the ratio of incidence rates (i.e. number of cases divided by the person-time at risk) irrespective of the disease frequency (Greenland and Thomas 1982; Pearce 1993).

Retrospective ascertainment of exposure status in cases and controls

Epidemiological studies seek to obtain information on exposures present during an aetiologically relevant period of time. That period varies across aetiological relationships. For example, while excess consumption of alcohol predisposes to both motor vehicle injuries and cirrhosis of the liver, it does so during considerably different time intervals prior to the occurrence of the injury or the onset of the illness.

Some case–control studies are nested within cohort studies in which specimens (e.g. blood, urine) have been obtained prior to diagnosis on all cohort members but have not yet been analysed for the exposure(s) in question. When these analyses are performed on cohort members who developed a particular illness and on controls selected from the cohort, the results obtained cannot have been influenced by events occurring following the diagnosis of the illness. (In order to avoid the possibility of occult illness in cases influencing levels of a suspected aetiological factor, many studies of this type exclude from the analyses specimens obtained within the period prior to diagnosis that might correspond to the duration of the preclinical stage of disease.) Also, among the large majority of case–control studies in which exposure status is not measured until the illness or injury has been diagnosed, some are concerned only with an exposure or characteristic that would have been the same at all times in a person's life. This is true for a genetically determined characteristic such as ABO blood type or the absence of glutathione transferase M1 activity (an enzyme that metabolizes several potentially carcinogenic constituents of cigarette smoke). Clearly, these studies are no less valid for having had to measure exposure in retrospect.

However, most case–control studies are required to consider explicitly how best to assess in retrospect the exposure status of subjects during one or more possible aetiologically relevant time periods. Possible data collection methods may include interviews or questionnaires, available records, or physical or laboratory measurements.

Interviews and questionnaires

For many exposures, a subject's memory is an excellent window to the past. A number of important aetiological relationships have been identified through interview-based case–control studies. As a general rule, study participants will report longer-term and more recent experiences with the greatest accuracy. Attention to the ways in which questions are asked (Armstrong et al. 1992), together with the use of visual aids when appropriate (for example pictures of medicines or of containers of household products, and calendars for important life events to enhance recall of the timing of other exposures), will maximize the accuracy of the information received. These efforts, together with the use of the same questions for cases and controls asked in the same way, will also minimize the potential for bias that could result from the subject's or interviewer's awareness of case or control status.

One virtue of exposure ascertainment via interview or questionnaire is that information can be sought for multiple points in the past. It is possible that a given exposure plays an aetiological role only if present at a certain age, for a certain duration, or at a certain time in the past. Because there is often little guidance before a study starts to suggest the most relevant age, length, or recency, key exposures are often elicited throughout the subject's lifetime. However, care must be taken not to include exposures that took place after the illness began. An instructive example was provided by Victora et al. (1989) in a case–control study of infant death from diarrhoea in relation to type of feeding. They asked mothers whether their child was or was not being breast-fed immediately prior to the onset of the fatal illness (mothers of controls were queried about type of feeding prior to a comparable point in time). Mothers were also asked if there had been any subsequent changes in type of feeding, which often occur following the onset of diarrhoea. Infants who were supplemented with powdered or cow's milk prior to their illness had about four times the risk of diarrhoeal death relative to infants who were solely breast-fed. However, the authors showed that if one inappropriately considered the feeding method that was present during the illness, about a 13-fold increase in risk associated with supplementation would have been estimated.

Records

Case–control studies have exploited the presence of vital, registry, employment, medical, and pharmacy records, to name only some, as a means of obtaining information on exposures. However, because the information contained in the records will usually have been assembled for purposes other than epidemiological research, it may not provide precisely that information desired by the epidemiologist. For example, a death certificate or an occupational record may state an individual's job, but often will not give his or her actual exposure to the substance(s) of interest to the study. Similarly, a pharmacy record will indicate that a prescription has been filled, but not necessarily whether the patient took the medication on a given day or took it at all. This sort of imprecision will impair a study's ability to discern a true association between an exposure and a disease—the greater the imprecision, the greater the impairment. None the less, some very strong associations have been identified through record-based case–control studies. For example, Daling et al. (1982) conducted a tumour-registry-based case–control study to test the hypothesis that homosexual men have a relatively high incidence of anal cancer. While registry data do not specify a man's sexual preference, they do contain information regarding his marital status. The investigators found that three times more men with anal cancer than controls (men with a colon or rectal cancer) had never been married. Of course, being single is far from a perfect predictor of homosexuality. None the less, the presence of such a large case–control difference, given the very poor means of gauging the relevant exposure, was a stimulus to conducting interview-based studies that could elicit information regarding sexual history with greater precision. The latter studies showed an exceedingly strong association (odds ratio of 50) (Daling et al. 1987).

In case–control studies in which medical records are used to characterize exposure status, care must be taken to restrict the information obtained to that which preceded the case's diagnosis (and the presence of symptoms, if any, that led to the diagnosis). The records of controls must be truncated at similar points in time. Without this safeguard, it is possible that bias will arise because there are systematically more records available to review on cases than controls, particularly if the illness has stimulated an inquiry by medical personnel into the case's history.

Physical and laboratory measurements

The recognized limitations of interviews and records in characterizing a variety of potentially relevant exposures have stimulated the conduct of epidemiological studies that use laboratory and other methods of measurement for this purpose. A woman cannot tell an investigator the level of her reproductive hormones, the concentration of various micronutrients in her blood, or whether her cervix is infected with human papillomavirus, while laboratory tests can. Unfortunately, such tests provide these data for the time at which the specimens have been obtained. For some exposures, there will be a high correlation between the measured level following case and control identification and that present during the aetiologically relevant time period. For example, lead enters and does not leave the dentine of teeth. Therefore lead dentine levels in young school-age children are an indicator of cumulative lead exposure, a good portion of which could be relevant to the development of intellectual impairment and other adverse neurological outcomes. In contrast, one would not rely on serum levels of reproductive hormones of postmenopausal cases of breast cancer and controls to indicate their premenopausal levels, much less their hormonal status during their very early reproductive years (at which time it is plausible that hormones are exerting their greatest impact on future risk of breast cancer).

Case definition

Ideally, the cases in a case–control study would comprise all (or a representative sample of) members of a defined population who develop a given health outcome during a given period of time. For studies of disease aetiology, that outcome is disease incidence. For studies that seek to determine the efficacy of early disease detection or treatment, the outcome is generally the occurrence of complications of the disease or mortality; such studies have recently been described in detail elsewhere (Selby 1994; Weiss 1994) and will not be discussed further here.

The population from which cases are to be drawn may be defined geographically or on the basis of other characteristics, such as membership of a prepaid health care plan or an occupational group. The identification of all newly ill persons in a defined population can be facilitated by the presence of a reporting system, such as a cancer or malformation registry, that seeks to accomplish this identification for other purposes. On occasion, care for the condition being studied may be centralized, so that it will be necessary to review the records of only one or a few institutions to identify all cases in the population in which those institution are located. However, in many instances it is not feasible to identify all cases that occur in a given population, and therefore case–control studies are often based on cases identified from hospital records or from the records of selected providers from whom patients had sought health care. The study of vaginal adenocarcinoma by Herbst et al. (1971) was of this type. Whether or not the cases are derived from a defined population, it is necessary that they be drawn in an unselected manner with regard to exposure status (for example, by including in the study all otherwise eligible cases diagnosed or receiving care during a defined time period).

While the aim of a case–control study of aetiology is to enrol incident cases, under some circumstances it may be necessary to enrol prevalent cases at a particular point in time, irrespective of when the illness of each subject had begun. For some conditions, the date of occurrence may simply not be known. For example, in the absence of very close sero-monitoring, one generally cannot determine when a person acquired an HIV infection. Second, for uncommon diseases of long duration, an incidence series may yield too few cases for meaningful analysis. The disadvantages of using prevalent cases in a case–control study relate in part to the added problems of accurate exposure ascertainment. For prevalent conditions whose date of diagnosis is known, pre-illness exposure information on study subjects must be obtained for more distant points in the past, on average, than would be necessary for an incident series. For prevalent conditions whose date of occurrence is unknown (e.g. HIV infection), there will be uncertainty as to the best point in time before which one should elicit exposure information. Also, by studying persons remaining alive with a given condition, one is studying at the same time not only aetiological factors, but also those that influence survival from the condition.

Ideally, objective criteria of high sensitivity and specificity for the disease should be used to identify and select individual cases for study. Specificity is of particular concern, since the inadvertent inclusion of persons without the disease in the case group will generally obscure any true association with exposure. With this in mind, in the case–control study of Reye's syndrome in relation to antecedent analgesic use conducted by the United States Centers for Disease Control and Prevention (Hurwitz et al. 1985), only cases with a substantial degree of neurological impairment (stage 2 or higher) were included. The use of this criterion minimized the chances that children with diseases other than Reye's syndrome (diseases that would generally have a lesser degree of severity) would be included in the case group. It was also intended to serve as protection against selective misclassification of Reye's syndrome based on knowledge of exposure status, since the hypothesis that aspirin was associated with Reye's syndrome was well known by the time that the study took place. Conceivably, the knowledge that the child had consumed aspirin could have led some physicians to diagnose Reye's syndrome in cases with an atypical illness.

Control definition

The function of a control group in a case–control study is to estimate the frequency and degree of exposure that would have taken place among cases in the absence of an exposure–disease association. Thus an ideal control group would consist of individuals:

1. who are selected from a population whose distribution of exposure is that of the population from which the cases arose;

2. who are identical with the cases with respect to their distribution of all characteristics that (a) influence the likelihood and/or degree of exposure, and (b) independent of their relation to exposure, are also related to the occurrence of the illness under study or to its recognition;

3. in whom the presence of the exposure can be measured accurately and in a manner that is identical to that used for cases.

If all the criteria listed above are not met in a particular study then selection bias, confounding bias, or information bias respectively will be present.

Minimizing selection bias

If the cases identified in the study are all or a sample of those that occurred in a defined population, one can seek to achieve comparability by choosing as controls persons sampled from that same population. A number of different methods of sampling have been used for geographically defined populations, including random

digit dialling of telephone numbers, area sampling, neighbourhood sampling, voters' lists, population registers, motor vehicle licenses, and birth certificates. When cases are members of a prepaid health care plan who develop an illness or injury, a sample of persons who were members of the health plan when the illness or injury occurred can serve as controls. When cases are ill or injured members of an employed population, controls can be selected from that same group of employees.

If cases have not been selected from a definable population at risk for the disease, but rather from persons treated for a particular illness at one or a few hospitals or clinics, then selection bias may be introduced if (i) controls are not chosen from persons who, had they developed the illness under study, would have received care at these hospitals or clinics, and (ii) persons who do and do not receive care from these sources differ with regard to their frequency or level of exposure.

Therefore, when cases are chosen from a narrow range of providers of health care, controls are often chosen from other ill persons treated by these providers. Such ill controls may also be used if, irrespective of the source of cases, there is no feasible way of sampling from the population at large, or if sampling from the population at large would be likely to result in a substantial level of non-response or information bias (see below). For these reasons, in some studies of fatal illness exposures in persons with a given cause of death are compared with exposures in a sample of persons who died for other reasons.

However, the choice of ill or deceased controls can itself give rise to selection bias if the illnesses (or causes of death) represented in the control group are in some way associated with the exposure of interest. For example, ill or recently deceased persons tend to have been smokers of cigarettes more often than other persons (McLaughlin et al. 1985), since smoking is associated with a variety of causes of illness and death. Because smoking histories of ill persons overstate the cigarette consumption of the population from which the cases arose (even if that population cannot be defined), the odds ratio associated with smoking based on the use of ill persons as controls will be spuriously low.

To minimize selection bias related to having chosen ill or deceased controls, an attempt can be made to omit potential controls with conditions known to be related (positively or negatively) to the exposure. For example, in the analysis of a hospital-based case–control study of bladder cancer in relation to prior use of artificial sweeteners, the investigators excluded from their control group persons who were being treated for obesity-related diseases (Silverman et al. 1983). They showed that without this restriction, the control group would have a spuriously high proportion of users of artificial sweeteners relative to the actual population from which their cases had come. This approach will succeed to the extent that one judges correctly which conditions are truly related to exposure and how accurately the presence of those conditions can be determined. For many exposures this may pose few problems, and judicious exclusion will yield a control group capable of providing an unbiased result. For others, such as cigarette smoking or alcohol drinking, it has been shown that admitting diagnoses or statements of cause of death are incapable of identifying all persons with illnesses related to these exposures (McLaughlin et al. 1985).

Occasionally, controls are chosen from individuals who are

tested for the presence of the disease under study and are found not to have it. For example, persons demonstrated to have coronary artery occlusion on coronary angiography have been compared with angiography patients without occlusion with regard to potential risk factors (Thom *et al.* 1992). It may be inexpensive to select controls in this way, and it is also possible to achieve case–control comparability with regard to the choice of a health care provider (and the correlates of that choice). This approach can have an impact on the validity of the study if the frequency or degree of exposure differs between otherwise comparable members of a population who do and do not receive the test. It will increase the validity if the disease being investigated is generally asymptomatic, and so would not be detected in the absence of testing. Thus the relation of the use of oral contraceptives to the incidence of *in situ* cancer of the cervix is best studied in women who have received cervical screening, by comparing oral contraceptive use between cases of *in situ* cancer and women with a negative screen. This is because, in most societies, screening is more commonly administered to women who use oral contraceptives than women who do not, and *in situ* cancers are asymptomatic and will not be identified in the absence of cervical screening. Therefore, if controls are chosen from women in general who may or may not have received cervical screening, an apparent excess of oral contraceptive users would be present among cases of *in situ* cancer even if no true association were present.

However, the choice of test-negative controls will detract from the validity of a study if the large majority of persons who develop the disease would soon be diagnosed whether or not the test was administered. There was a controversy in the late 1970s regarding the suitability, in case–control studies of postmenopausal oestrogen use and endometrical cancer, of a control group restricted to women with no evidence of cancer on endometrial biopsy. Among women without endometrial cancer, oestrogen use differs greatly between those who had and had not undergone biopsy since oestrogen use predisposes to uterine bleeding of non-malignant causes that often leads to endometrial biopsy. Those investigators who believed that there was a great prevalence of occult endometrial cancer in the population suggested that the optimal control group ought to be women undergoing endometrial biopsy and found not to have cancer (Horwitz and Feinstein 1978). However, the majority of investigators believed that no such large pool of prevalent occult disease existed, and that choosing biopsy-negative controls would lead to a spuriously high estimate of oestrogen use in the population at risk and thus a spuriously low odds ratio (Shapiro *et al.* 1985).

No matter how controls are defined in a case–control study, selection bias may be introduced to the extent that exposure information is not obtained on all who have been selected to take part. This can also occur if information is not obtained on all eligible cases. The magnitude of the bias will increase in relation to the frequency of missing data and the degree to which exposure frequencies or levels differ between study subjects on whom exposure status is and is not known. The problem of incomplete ascertainment of exposure on study subjects is particularly common in interview- or questionnaire-based case–control studies. Strategies for minimizing the degree of non-response in case–control studies are discussed in detail elsewhere (Armstrong *et al.* 1992).

Minimizing confounding bias
Characteristics of confounding variables in case–control studies

Confounding is present when the estimate of the relation between an exposure and disease is distorted by the influence of another factor. In any study design, confounding will occur to the extent that the other factor is associated with both exposure (though not as a result of the exposure) and the occurrence of the disease or its recognition. In case–control studies specifically, a factor may confound even if it is not associated with an altered risk of disease if the proportions of cases and controls vary across levels or categories of the factor. For example, in a collaborative study of ovarian cancer in relation to use of oral contraceptives (Weiss *et al.* 1981), an attempt was made to identify and interview all incident cases during a period of several years in two American populations. In one of the populations (western Washington State) several controls per case were interviewed, whereas the control-to-case ratio in the other (Utah) was 1.0. Since the use of oral contraceptives was more common in Washington women than in Utah women, failure to take into account the state of residence in the analysis (e.g. by adjustment) would have led to a spuriously high estimate of the frequency of oral contraceptive use in controls relative to that in cases.

Means of controlling for confounding

One straightforward way of preventing confounding is to restrict cases and controls to a single category or level of the potentially confounding variable. For example, in their study of physical activity in relation to primary cardiac arrest, Siscovick *et al.* (1982) excluded persons with conditions that could both predispose to cardiac arrest and might be expected to alter level of activity (such as clinically recognized heart disease). A second way is to obtain information on exposures or characteristics that may differ between cases and controls, and then to make statistical adjustments for those that are also found to be related to the exposure or characteristic under investigation (Rothman 1986).

Finally, it is possible to match one or more controls to each case's category or level of a potentially confounding factor. It is appropriate to match under the following conditions.

1. The variable is expected to be strongly related to both exposure and disease. Thus, in a case–control study of breast cancer in relation to use of hair dye, it would make sense to match on gender (if the study had not already been restricted to women) since (a) in most cultures use of hair dye is more common in women than in men, and (b) in the absence of matching the case-to-control ratio would be very uneven between women and men. While confounding by gender could be prevented even without matching by adjustment in the analysis, the statistical precision of the unmatched study would be substantially reduced relative to that of a case–control study with a more similar proportion of female cases and controls.

2. Information on possible matching variables can be obtained inexpensively. There are some means of control selection in which information regarding some confounders can be obtained at no cost. For example, from voters' lists or prepaid health plan membership records it would generally be

possible to choose directly one or more controls who were identical with a given case's age. However, if a population-sampling scheme such as random digit dialling were being employed, the age of the respondent would not be known in advance of approaching him or her. Rather than omitting already contacted controls who did not match a particular case's age, the matching can be done much more broadly. Additional control for finer categories of age can be accomplished in the data analysis.

3. Information on exposure status cannot be obtained inexpensively. The higher the cost of exposure ascertainment, the greater is the incentive to limit the number of control subjects to the number of cases. In particular, case–control differences regarding confounding factors will reduce the statistical power of a study that does not have a surplus of controls. Enriching the group of controls selected with persons more similar to the cases with regard to confounding factors (i.e. matching) can prevent this loss of statistical power.

It should be remembered that matching alone is not sufficient to eliminate a variable's confounding influence: failure to consider a matching variable in the analysis of the study can lead to a biased result (Rothman 1986). Analyses of studies that have matched controls to cases on a given characteristic can adjust for that characteristic as if no matching had taken place. Alternatively, these analyses can explicitly consider cases and controls as matched sets. In the instance of matched case–control pairs and a dichotomous exposure variable, the following table can be constructed:

	Control	
Case	Exposed	Non-exposed
Exposed	a	b
Non-exposed	c	d

Only the b pairs, in which the case was exposed but not the matched control, and the c pairs, in which the reverse was true, would enter the analysis. The odds ratio would be calculated as b/c. When there is more than one control per case, the odds ratio can also be calculated (Breslow and Day 1980).

Minimizing information bias

In case–control studies in which information on exposure status is sought via an interview or questionnaire, the chief safeguards against information bias entail asking questions (i) about events that are salient to the respondent, (ii) that are framed in an unambiguous way, and (iii) that are presented identically to both cases and controls. However, employment of these safeguards will not prevent differential accuracy of reporting between cases and controls in all circumstances. Some past exposures or events will simply be more salient to persons with an illness, who might have dwelt on the possible reasons for its occurrence, than to persons without that illness. Other exposures may be viewed as socially undesirable, and there may be a difference between cases and healthy controls in their willingness to admit to them. If the anticipated difference in the quality of information between cases and otherwise appropriate controls is too great, a control group that is less than ideal in other respects may be selected instead so as to minimize the potential for

information bias. For example, some studies of prenatal risk factors for a particular congenital malformation that utilize maternal interviews as the source of exposure data have selected as controls infants with other malformations (Rosenberg et al. 1983). This control group will provide a more valid result than a control group that consists of infants in general if (i) mothers of malformed and mothers of normal infants report prenatal exposures to a different degree even in the absence of an association, and (ii) the exposure in question is not associated with the occurrence of the malformations present in control infants.

There will rarely be any firm knowledge of the truth of either of the conditions above, and so the choice of the most appropriate control group will be very much a subjective one. None the less, there are data to suggest that differences in the accuracy of reporting can indeed occur for some exposures. For example, in a study of karyotypically normal spontaneous abortions (Kline et al. 1991), mothers of cases interviewed after the abortion reported a higher degree of heavy caffeine consumption (≥ 225 mg per day) during the first weeks of pregnancy than did women registered for prenatal care from the same providers who had been interviewed at the corresponding point in the pregnancy (risk relative to that of very low caffeine consumers, 1.9; 95 per cent confidence interval, 1.3–2.6). However, when the comparison group consisted instead of women who had a karyotypical abnormal spontaneous abortion, there was virtually no difference in reported caffeine intake (relative risk, 1.2; 95 per cent confidence interval, 0.8–1.8). The distribution of caffeine consumption around the time of conception was similar among women with either type of spontaneous abortion and the women registered for prenatal care. These data suggest that there was more accurate reporting of heavy caffeine intake during pregnancy by mothers with a spontaneous abortion than by other pregnant women—probably it was spuriously low in the latter group—since caffeine consumption after conception could not have had a bearing on the occurrence of a chromosomal abnormality that led to a miscarriage. (It should be noted that, in another setting, interviews with women at the outset of pregnancy and after delivery produced largely comparable information regarding coffee consumption early in pregnancy both in those who did and those who did not sustain an adverse pregnancy outcome (Mackenzie and Lippman 1989).)

When the exposure under consideration is sufficiently imprecise or is open to subjective interpretation, there may not be any control group that will provide information comparable to that provided by cases. An instructive example comes from a case–control study of Down's syndrome (Stott 1958) conducted shortly before the chromosomal basis for its aetiology had been established. The study sought to determine whether emotional 'shocks' during pregnancy might be a risk factor. The author interviewed mothers of children with Down's syndrome with regard to the occurrence of a 'situation or event [that would be] stress- or shock-producing if this would have been its expected effect on an emotionally stable woman.' Identical interviews were administered to mothers of normal children, and also to mothers of retarded children who did not have Down's syndrome. Even though it is not possible that an emotional shock in pregnancy could play any aetiological role in a condition already determined at conception, a far higher proportion of mothers of cases of Down's syndrome reported an emotional shock than did mothers of normal controls (relative risk estimated from the data, 17.0). The use of other retarded children as controls only partially reduced the spuriously high relative risk to a value of 4.3.

When conducting an interview-based study of a rapidly fatal disease or a disease that impairs a person's ability to provide valid interview data, it is necessary to obtain information from at least some surrogate respondents. Typically, these respondents are close relatives of the cases. In general, for purposes of comparability, similar information ought to be obtained from surrogates of controls, even though the controls themselves would be expected to provide more accurate data.

Results of case–control studies based on exposure information provided by surrogate respondents need to be interpreted with particular caution. Though by no means present in every instance (Nelson *et al.* 1990), there can be a large difference in the validity of the responses given by case and control surrogates. For example, Greenberg *et al.* (1985) investigated the basis for an apparent strong association between cancer mortality and 'nuclear' work among employees of a naval shipyard that had been found in a comparison of work histories provided by surrogates of men who died from cancer and of men who died of other conditions. They observed that, regarding work in the nuclear part of the industry, surrogates of the cases generally provided information similar to that contained in employment records of the shipyard. In contrast, the surrogates of controls substantially misclassified the nature of their relative' jobs as not involving radiation. When the data provided by employment records, which included individual radiation dosimetry (Rinsky *et al.* 1981), were used, little or no association was present between radiation exposure and cancer mortality.

What was undoubtedly a spuriously negative association was found in a case–control study of lung cancer and passive cigarette smoking in which information obtained from surrogate respondents was used for one analysis (Janerich *et al.* 1990). In this analysis, the relative risk of lung cancer among non-smokers associated with a spouse's having smoked was 0.33 (i.e. a 67 per cent reduction in risk); this would almost certainly seem to be due to a spurious minimization or denial of smoking by spouses of cases, who may have feared that their habit caused their spouse to develop lung cancer.

Incomparable assessment of exposure status between cases and controls is not confined to interview- or questionnaire-based studies. Most laboratory-based studies seek to prevent this by testing samples blind to case/control status. If feasible, it is desirable to do this blinding as well in studies in which exposure is to be determined from medical or other records. However, there are instances in which the nature of the information available in records has already been influenced by whether the subject is a case or a control. For example, it was found that among 100 infertile women who underwent laparoscopy (Strathy *et al.* 1982), 21 had endometriosis. Only 2 per cent of 200 women undergoing laparoscopy for another indication, tubal ligation, were noted in the records of their procedure to have endometriosis. However, the interpretation of this association is unclear, since the identification and/or recording of endometriosis in cases and controls (women undergoing tubal ligation) may well have been incomparable—only in the infertile women was the laparoscopy expressly performed as a diagnostic tool to investigate the possible presence of conditions such as endometriosis.

Estimating the attributable risk from results of case–control studies

Occasionally, a case–control study identifies a large odds ratio relating an exposure and a disease, and for this and other reasons a causal influence of the exposure may be suspected. The decision to seek to limit or eliminate that exposure requires weighing its negative and positive consequences. This weighing must be done in absolute rather than relative terms, since the same relative increase (or decrease) in risk is of far greater consequence for common than for rare outcomes. The absolute increase in the risk of disease believed to be due to the exposure, sometimes referred to as the attributable risk (AR), can be estimated directly from data gathered in cohort studies or randomized trials as the difference between the incidences I_e and I_n in exposed and non-exposed persons respectively. The term $I_e–I_n$ can be rewritten as $RR(I_n)–I_n$, or as $I_n(RR-1)$. Since the RR can be estimated from the results of a case–control study by means of the odds ratio, the only additional piece of information needed to estimate the AR is an estimate of I_n. For the population in which the study has been conducted, I_n can be estimated if (i) the overall incidence I of the disease in that population is known or can be approximated, and (ii) the frequency of exposure p_e in the controls selected for study reasonably reflects that of the population that gave rise to the cases. Given (i) and (ii),

$$I = I_e(p_e) + I_n(1 - p_e)$$
$$= I_n\, RR(p_e) + I_n(1 - p_e)$$
$$= I_n[p_e\,(RR-1) + 1]$$

and so

$$I_n = \frac{I}{p_e\,(RR - 1) + 1}\,.$$

Therefore

$$AR = \frac{I\,(RR-1)}{p_e\,(RR-1) + 1} = \frac{I}{p_e + \dfrac{1}{(RR-1)}}$$

For example, consider a disease with an incidence rate of 10 per 100 000 per year in a population in which 5 per cent of persons have been exposed during a relevant period of time. The following table summarizes data from a case–control study conducted in that population:

Exposed	Cases	Controls	OR
Yes	15%	5%	3.35
No	85%	95%	1

The AR that corresponds to the estimated 3.35-fold increase in risk is

$$\frac{10/100\,000}{0.05 + \dfrac{1}{(3.35-1)}} = 20.2 \text{ per } 100\,000 \text{ per year.}$$

From the results of case–control studies that suggest a causal relation, it is also possible to estimate the percentage of exposed persons with the disease who developed it because of their exposure, rather than through one or more causal pathways not involving the exposure. This measure, often termed the attributable risk per cent (AR%) among exposed persons, is defined as $\frac{(I_c - I_n)}{I_c} \times 100\%$. It can be described in terms of the RR alone:

$$AR\% = \frac{I_c}{I_c} - \frac{I_n}{I_c} = 1 - \frac{1}{RR} = \frac{RR - 1}{RR} \times 100\%$$

Therefore the results of a case–control study that provide a valid estimate of the RR (via the OR) can provide the AR% as well, with no additional assumptions or sources of data. It is also possible to estimate the percentage occurrence of a disease in the population as a whole that resulted from the actions of a given exposure. This measure, the population attributable risk per cent (PAR%) or aetiological fraction, is simply the AR% reduced by the proportion p_c of cases in that population who were exposed:

$$PAR\% = AR\% (p_c) \times 100\%.$$

In the example above,

$$AR\% = \frac{(3.35 - 1)}{3.35} = 70.1\%, \text{ and } PAR\% = 70.1\% \times 0.15 = 10.5\%.$$

When should we look to results of case–control studies for answers to questions of disease aetiology?

Randomized trials will not be able to answer all our questions regarding the reasons that diseases occur. Many potential disease-causing or disease-preventing exposures cannot be manipulated at all (e.g. most genetic characteristics) or in any practical way for the purposes of a study. For many exposure–disease relationships, either the disease is too uncommon or the induction period is too long to conduct a randomized trial that is not infeasibly large in size or long in duration. Finally, in general it will not be possible to conduct separate randomized trials to measure the impact of all potential types, amounts, and durations of a class of exposure.

Also, it is not possible to rely solely on cohort studies for answers. Just as with randomized trials, the disease outcome being studied may be too rare to allow a cohort approach to be useful. This explains why the aetiologies of vaginal adenocarcinoma and Reye's syndrome, for example, have been evaluated exclusively by case–control studies; these diseases are simply too uncommon for most cohort studies to generate any cases, even in 'exposed' individuals. Prospective cohort studies are also of limited use when the induction period for the exposure–disease relationship is either very short or very long. If the induction period is very short and the exposure status of an individual varies over time, a cohort study would need to assess exposure status repeatedly among cohort members. For this reason, studies of alcohol consumption in relation to the occurrence of injuries are typically case–control in nature. Similarly, unless information on exposure status can be ascertained retrospectively at the time that the cohort is formed, it would not be feasible to initiate a cohort study of a suspected

aetiological relation that requires a very long time (e.g. several decades) to manifest itself.

While case–control studies may be of particular value in the evaluation of the aetiology of uncommon diseases, they may have difficulty in obtaining statistically precise results if the frequency of the exposure in the population under study is either extremely common or extremely uncommon (Crombie 1981). Thus only an association as strong as the one between cigarette smoking and lung cancer could have emerged reliably from case–control studies of several hundred British men conducted in the late 1940s (Doll and Hill 1950), given that well over 90 per cent of that population were cigarette smokers. For very uncommon exposures (for example occupational exposure to a specific substance suspected of posing a risk to health, or an infrequently prescribed drug), barring a strong observed association based on a large number of subjects, even the best designed case–control study will usually offer no more than a suggestion of the presence or absence of a relation with regard to the occurrence of a given illness.

References

Armstrong, B.K., White, E., and Sarucci, R. (1992). *Principles of exposure measurement in epidemiology*, Chapters 6 and 7. Oxford University Press, New York.

Breslow, N.E. and Day, N.E. (1980). *Statistical methods in cancer research*, Vol. 1, *The analysis of case–control studies*. IARC Scientific Publication 32, Lyon.

Crombie, I.K. (1981). The limitations of case–control studies in the detection of environmental carcinogens. *Journal of Epidemiology and Community Health*, 35, 281–7.

Daling, J.R., Weiss, N.S., Klopfenstein, L.L., *et al.* (1982). Correlates of homosexual behaviour and the incidence of anal cancer. *Journal of the American Medical Association*, 247, 1988–90.

Daling, J.R., Weiss, N.S., Hislop, T.G., *et al.* (1987). Sexual practices, sexually transmitted diseases, and the incidence of anal cancer. *New England Journal of Medicine*, 317, 973–7.

Doll, R. and Hill, A.B. (1950). Smoking and carcinoma of the lung. *British Medical Journal*, 2, 739–48.

Greenberg, E.R., Rosner, B., Hennekens, C., *et al.* (1985). An investigation of bias in a study of nuclear shipyard workers. *American Journal of Epidemiology*, 121, 301–8.

Greenland, S. and Thomas, D.C. (1982). On the need for the rare disease assumption in case–control studies. *American Journal of Epidemiology*, 116, 547–53.

Greenwald, P., Barlow, J.J., Nasca, P., *et al.* (1971). Vaginal cancer after maternal treatment with synthetic estrogens. *New England Journal of Medicine*, 285, 390–3.

Herbst, A.L., Ulfelder, H., and Poskanzer, D.C. (1971). Adenocarcinoma of the vagina: association of maternal stilbestrol therapy with tumor appearance in young women. *New England Journal of Medicine*, 284, 878–81.

Horwitz, R.I. and Feinstein, A.R. (1978). Alternative analytic methods for case–control studies of estrogens and endometrial cancer. *New England Journal of Medicine*, 299, 1089–94.

Hurwitz, E.S., Barrett, M.J., Bregman, D., *et al.* (1985). Public Health Service Study on Reye's syndrome and medications: report of the Pilot Phase. *New England Journal of Medicine*, 313, 849–57.

Janerich, D.T., Thompson, W.D., Varela, L.R., *et al.* (1990). Lung cancer and exposure to tobacco smoke in the household. *New England Journal of Medicine*, 323, 632–6.

Kline, J., Levin, B., Silverman, J., *et al.* (1991). Caffeine and spontaneous abortion of known karyotype. *Epidemiology*, 2, 409–17.

Mackenzie, S.G. and Lippman, A. (1989). An investigation of report bias in a case–control study of pregnancy outcome. *American Journal of Epidemiology*, 129, 65–75.

McLaughlin, J.K., Blot, W.J., Mehl, E.S., *et al.* (1985). Problems in the use of dead controls in case–control studies. II. Effect of excluding certain causes of death. *American Journal of Epidemiology*, **122**, 485–94.

Nelson, L.M., Longstreth, W.T., Koespell, T.D., *et al.* (1990). Proxy respondents in epidemiologic research. *Epidemiologic Reviews*, **12**, 71–86.

Pearce, N. (1993). What does the odds ratio estimate in a case–control study? *International Journal of Epidemiology*, **22**, 1189–92.

Rinsky, R.A., Zumwolde, R.D., Waxweiller, R.J., *et al.* (1981). Cancer mortality at a naval nuclear shipyard. *Lancet*, **i**, 231–5.

Rosenberg, L., Mitchell, A.A., Parsells, J.L., *et al.* (1983). Lack of relation of oral clefts to diazepam use during pregnancy. *New England Journal of Medicine*, **309**, 1282–5.

Rothman, K.J. (1986). *Modern epidemiology*. Little, Brown, Boston, MA.

Selby, J.V. (1994). Case control evaluations of treatment and program efficacy. *Epidemiologic Reviews*, **46**, 90–101.

Shapiro, S., Kelly, J.P., Rosenberg, L., *et al.* (1985). Risk of localized and widespread endometrial cancer in relation to recent and discontinued use of conjugated estrogens. *New England Journal of Medicine*, **313**, 969–72.

Silverman, D.T., Hoover, R.N., and Swanson, G.M. (1983). Artificial sweeteners and lower urinary tract cancer: hospital vs. population controls. *American Journal of Epidemiology*, **117**, 326–34.

Siscovick, D.S., Weiss, N.S., Hallstrom, A.P., *et al.* (1982). Physical activity and primary cardiac arrest. *Journal of the American Medical Association*, **248**, 3113–17.

Stott, D.H. (1958). Some psychosomatic aspects of casualty in reproduction. *Journal of Psychosomatic Research*, **3**, 42–55.

Strathy, J.H., Molgaard, C.A., Coulam, C.B., *et al.* (1982). Endometriosis and infertility: a laparoscopic study of endometriosis among fertile and infertile women. *Fertility and Sterility*, **38**, 667–72.

Thom, D.H., Grayston, J.T., Siscovick, D.S., *et al.* (1992). Association of prior infection with *Chlamydia pneumoniae* and angiographically demonstrated coronary artery disease. *Journal of the American Medical Association*, **268**, 68–72.

Ulfelder, H. and Robboy, S.J. (1976). The embryologic development of the human vagina. *American Journal of Obstetrics and Gynecology*, **126**, 769–76.

Victora, C.G., Smith, P.G., Vaughn, J.P., *et al.* (1989). Infant feeding and deaths due to diarrhea. *American Journal of Epidemiology*, **129**, 1032–41.

Weiss, N.S. (1994). Application of the case–control method in the evaluation of screening. *Epidemiologic Reviews*, **16**, 102–8.

Weiss, N.S., Lyon, J.L., Liff, J.M., *et al.* (1981). Incidence of ovarian cancer in relation to the use of oral contraceptives. *International Journal of Cancer*, **28**, 669–71.

11 Cohort studies

Manning Feinleib, Norman E. Breslow, and Roger Detels

Introduction

The cohort study is an observational epidemiological study which, after the manner of an experiment, attempts to study the relationship between a purported cause (exposure) and the subsequent risk of developing disease. As in other observational epidemiological studies, and unlike experimental studies, the suspected causal factor or exposure is not randomly assigned to the study population. However, the cohort study follows the same time direction as an experiment in that the suspected exposure is identified as having or not having occurred in the study population before the occurrence of disease is investigated. Thus, certain biases that may occur in other forms of epidemiological studies can be avoided, specifically those concerned with ascertaining the exposure status of the population. Furthermore, because disease occurrence is identified subsequent to enumeration of exposure groups, this type of study allows direct estimation of the risk of developing disease and how risk varies with time since exposure.

Cohort studies have been given a variety of names including incidence studies, prospective studies, follow-up studies, longitudinal studies, and panel studies, although the latter two terms have more generally been applied to studies involving repeated measurements of the same variables over time. They are similar to the usual scientific experiment in that they proceed from the suspected cause or aetiological agent to the disease outcome with controls or comparison groups selected on the basis of absence of exposure to the putative cause. As a type of observational study, there is no randomization to exposure classes nor is there any attempt to manipulate the exposure. In contrast, case–control studies (also known as case–referent studies and, formerly, as retrospective studies) have no counterpart in experimental science since they work from the outcome event back towards the supposed aetiological factor. Indeed, case–control studies are often viewed conceptually in terms of sampling data from an ongoing (and possibly fictitious) cohort study.

Cohort studies offer the possibility of studying the full range of effects of the suspected aetiological factor. Frequently the suspected aetiological factor is not only related to the occurrence of the disease of primary interest, but may influence the natural history of the disease and may be related to a variety of other health conditions that may not have been suspected at first. A particularly important aspect of cohort studies is that they provide direct estimates of the risk of disease for each exposure group separately. These separate estimates of risk can then be used to estimate a variety of measures of interest to epidemiologists such as the attributable risk, the relative risk, and the aetiological fraction.

(These measures of risk are discussed in the section on analysis below and in Table 11.3). Although these risks can often be estimated from other types of studies when certain assumptions are made or ancillary information is available, cohort studies permit direct estimates of these measures from the data obtained in the study itself.

The disadvantages of cohort studies are primarily logistic and administrative. Often, relatively large populations have to be followed for long periods of time, thus entailing considerable expense in terms of funding and professional resources. If the disease outcome of interest is rare, the sample sizes required for concurrent studies may be prohibitively large. If the follow-up period is long, which is often the case for chronic diseases, the problem of attrition of the study group due to loss from follow-up, migration, competing causes of death, or gradual deterioration of interest in participation may present serious analytical problems that might negate the value of the overall study. Longitudinal follow-up requires careful attention to maintaining standardized diagnostic methods and criteria. Finally, of course, the longer the study is continued, the more difficult it is to maintain a committed investigative team and stable funding for the project.

In the first part of this chapter we discuss the major methodological aspects of cohort studies: forms of cohort studies, selection of study cohorts, gathering of baseline information, follow-up, and analysis. To illustrate these points we use examples from three studies: a historical cohort study of artificial menopause and breast cancer using available hospital and death certificate information (Feinleib 1968), a prospective cohort study, using mail questionnaires, of cigarette smoking and mortality among British doctors (Doll and Peto 1976), and a prospective cohort study of heart disease in Framingham, Massachusetts, using periodic medical examinations (Kannel *et al.* 1961; Dawber *et al.* 1963). In the second part of the chapter we present the various types of bias that can confound interpretation of cohort studies and suggests ways of identifying, reducing, and/or resolving these biases. In this section examples are drawn from a wider range of studies.

Design of cohort studies
Forms of cohort studies

Cohort studies may take a variety of forms. The key distinction that has been established in the past is based primarily on the availability of data. In **prospective (or observational) cohort studies**, data on exposure status and disease outcome are not available at the outset of the study; they must be ascertained through the direct efforts of the investigator in the future. In **ambispective cohort** studies, data on exposure status have been collected in the past and are available from existing records while disease outcome is unknown or incompletely known; the investigator is obliged to follow the cohort for subsequent occurrence of the disease. In **historical (or non-concurrent) cohort studies**, data on exposure status and disease outcome have been collected in the past and are available from existing records; the investigator's efforts are devoted primarily to linking the relevant data files.

A form of cohort study that has been used increasingly in studies of HIV and AIDS is the 'nested case–control study'. Nested case–control studies are useful when specimens and/or data sources have been collected prospectively and preserved during a cohort study. Cases are selected from among members of a cohort who have developed disease and controls from members of the cohort who have not developed disease. Evaluating the entire population prior to knowing who would become cases, as would be necessary in an observational cohort study, would be very expensive. Therefore the advantage of the nested case–control study is that the measurement of the exposure variables can be made after the identity of the cases and non-cases is known but reflects the level before diagnosis of the disease, thereby reducing the number of samples that must be evaluated. Another advantage is that information elicited from interviews that were conducted without knowledge of the disease outcome eliminates the recall bias inherent in classical case–control studies.

Each type of study involves certain basic steps, which will be described below (with the exception of the nested case–control study, which basically uses a case–control study approach discussed in the chapter on case–control studies). These steps include selecting the study and comparison groups, obtaining baseline information with regard to exposure and initial health status, follow-up of the members of the cohort and surveillance for disease outcome, and analysis of the results.

Selection of the study cohorts
Objective
There are two approaches to the selection of representative samples of exposed and non-exposed groups to be followed in a cohort study.

1. The identification of a **special exposure group** defined because of (i) unusual exposure to a suspected causative (aetiological factor) or (ii) unusual life-style or work experience.

2. Using a **general population sample** in which there is heterogeneity of exposure to the suspected aetiological factor.

Where the study group is a special exposure group, it is necessary to find appropriate comparison groups or the means to make comparisons with the general population. When the general population sample is used as a starting point, the various levels of exposure within the study group provide the basis for internal comparisons. Each approach also takes into consideration various logistic constraints; for example accessibility and co-operativeness of the study groups, availability of medical and other records, and anticipated completeness and cost of end-point surveillance.

Example 1—A historical cohort study of the relation between artificial menopause and breast cancer
Seven case-control studies performed between 1926 and 1962 all reported that artificial menopause (surgical removal of the uterus and/or ovaries) occurred significantly less frequently among breast cancer patients than among a variety of controls. Because the case–control studies did not present information about the extent of surgery (the effect of removal of only the uterus versus removal of the ovaries) or the effects of the age at which the artificial menopause occurred, it was decided to investigate these issues by means of a cohort study. The disadvantage of using a prospective cohort method in elucidating the relation between artificial menopause and breast cancer is that there is a long interval between the gynaecological procedure and the appearance of the disease in appreciable frequency. To reduce this delay it was decided to use the historical cohort approach. The cohorts were selected from the records of two technical hospitals in the Boston area. The study cohorts included all eligible patients seen at these hospitals from 1920 to 1940. Women aged 55 years or younger were eligible for inclusion in the study if they had undergone any of the following procedures as determined from surgical and pathological records: (i) hysterectomy; (ii) unilateral oophorectomy; (iii) bilateral oophorectomy; (iv) radium or X-ray treatment of the ovaries or uterus; (v) cholecystectomy. The last group served as a control cohort.

Certain patients were excluded from the study: (i) women who had a prior mastectomy or a prior breast malignancy or who had undergone castration as part of the treatment for an existing breast tumour; (ii) women treated for pelvic malignancies; (iii) women who had previous removal of their ovaries or a history of natural menopause before the age of 40 years; (iv) women who did not survive their index admission; (v) all who were not residents of Massachusetts at the time of their index procedure. At the final editing of the study abstract forms and the elimination of duplicate records, there were 8387 patients in the study populations. They were subdivided into four 'exposure' categories.

1. Natural menopause—1479 women (including 953 women who underwent cholecystectomy and 526 women who were post-menopausal at the time of the gynaecological procedures for benign conditions).

2. Hysterectomy and bilateral oophorectomy—3241 women (this constitutes the surgically castrated group who were believed to have no residual ovarian activity).

3. Those undergoing hysterectomy and/or unilateral oophorectomy who, as far as could be ascertained from the surgical and pathological records, retained at least one intact ovary—2149 women (referred to as the 'partial surgery' group).

4. Radiation-induced artificial menopause—1518 women.

The partial surgery group constituted a second control cohort and 'sham operations' with which to contrast the women subjected to hysterectomy and bilateral oophorectomy.

It should be noted that it is not possible to relate the actual cohort studies to a clearly definable population. Although in this case adequate records were available for virtually every woman admitted to these hospitals who was eligible for the study, it is not known from what source population these women came. However, it is assumed that the reasons for coming to these particular hospitals were not correlated with both the type of procedure and the subsequent risk of developing breast cancer, i.e. they were not confounding factors (see section on biases).

Example 2—A prospective cohort study of the relation between cigarette smoking and mortality: the British Doctors Study (Breslow and Day 1987, Appendix IA)

By 1950 several case–control studies had been published and were in agreement in showing that a larger proportion of lung cancer patients had been heavy cigarette smokers and a smaller proportion had been non-smokers than patients with other diseases. Because of the possibility of a variety of biases in these case–control studies, a prospective study was launched in 1951 among the members of the medical profession in the United Kingdom. This group was chosen because it was felt that physicians would respond to mailed questionnaires, would report their smoking histories accurately, and could be followed economically through the death records of the Registrars-General and through the registries of the General Medical Council and the British Medical Association. It was felt that the relation of smoking to health among physicians would be similar to that in the general population. A simple questionnaire was mailed out on 31 October 1951 to 59 600 men and women on the Medical Register.

The replies received from 40 637 doctors were sufficiently complete to be used—34 445 from men and 6192 from women. From a one-in-ten random sample of the register, it was estimated that this represented answers from 69 per cent of the men and 60 per cent of the women alive at the time of the inquiry. The degree of self-selection in those who replied was assessed in terms of the overall mortality using this one-in-ten sample. The standardized death rate of those who replied was only 63 per cent of the death rate for all doctors in the second year of the inquiry and 85 per cent in the third year. In the fourth to tenth years the proportion varied about an average of 93 per cent and there was no evidence of any regular change with the further passage of years. Evidently the effect of selection did not entirely wear off, but after the third year it had become slight.

Example 3—A prospective cohort study of risk factors for heart disease: the Framingham Heart Study

The Framingham Heart Study is a long-term follow-up study of a sample of adults who lived in the town of Framingham, Massachusetts, in 1950. The first participants were actually examined in 1948 as part of an effort to conduct a demonstration programme in the detection and natural history of cardiovascular diseases. In 1950, however, the study was reconstituted as a long-term epidemiological investigation of coronary heart diseases, and the original voluntary participants were incorporated into a random sample drawn from all adults aged 30–60 years living in the town. Of the eligible random sample of 6507 persons, 4469 (68.7 per cent) participated in the examinations. When this number was supplemented with the volunteers, a total cohort of 5209 was obtained. The possible effects of supplementing the cohort to replace the originally selected participants who refused to participate in the reconstituted study are discussed in Example 9.

Although it was recognized from the outset that the town of Framingham could be considered neither a random nor a completely representative sample of the United States, the town did have certain characteristics that made it extremely suitable for a long-term epidemiological study. The town was of adequate size (28 000) to provide enough individuals in the desired age range. It was sufficiently compact that the study population could be observed conveniently by means of an examination at a single examining facility, and most of the residents received their hospital care at a single central hospital in the town. Owing in part to a relatively stable economy supported by a diversity of employment opportunities, the population was relatively stable so as to enable adequate follow-up for a long period of time. Both the general community and the medical profession of the town were felt to be co-operative. The town was not believed to be 'grossly atypical in any respect that appeared relevant'.

Since only 68.7 per cent of the eligible random sample participated in the 1950 examinations, it is possible that they might not be representative of the total population. This is a serious concern in all epidemiological studies where participation is voluntary and may be subject to self-selection. In this study it was felt that reasons for not participating were not appreciably related simultaneously to both the characteristics to be studied in the investigation and the risk of developing heart disease (see the section on biases).

Gathering of baseline information
Objectives
There are multiple objectives to be achieved in gathering baseline information.

1. Valid assessment of the exposure status of the members of the cohort groups.

2. Define the individuals 'at risk'; exclude those individuals with known disease at baseline.

3. Establish a basis for follow-up: obtain identifying data, informed consent, commitment to co-operate in the follow-up (for example, permission to contact family members and physicians, and to obtain hospital and employment records).

4. Obtain data on important covariables (i.e. other exposures that may be associated with the risk of acquiring the disease) so that adjustments can be made for their contribution to the incidence of disease in analysis (see section on confounding variables).

Sources of baseline information

Existing records Baseline information about the cohorts can be obtained from a variety of sources such as available records from hospitals or employment records, interviews of the cohort members or other informants, direct medical and other special examinations, and indirect measures of exposure estimated from investigations of the environment. The availability of written records such as medical or employment records may provide useful information to select and define the cohort. If high-quality records are available, they may permit the study to begin from the point of the recording of the information, thereby adding a considerable period of follow-up time before the actual initiation of the investigation. Studies based on such records with follow-up of patients from such a prior point in time to the present have been given special names such as retrospective cohort studies, non-concurrent cohort studies, and historical prospective studies. There are several other advantages for using previously recorded information. The data are apt to be free from certain biases since they are recorded before any knowledge of the particular study for which they are used. Written records may provide information that is not fully known to the subject, such as details on medical conditions or actual levels of exposure. However, such records may also have certain drawbacks. Records may not be uniformly available for all cohort members. Even when available, the detail and quality of the data in the records are not controllable by the investigator and it is difficult to verify the accuracy of questionable items.

Interviews   One of the more common methods of obtaining information is to interview the cohort members or other informants. A variety of techniques can be used: direct personal interviews, mailed questionnaires, telephone interviews, having the subject complete a questionnaire administered by computer, and using a tape recorder and headphones for asking intimate questions in a crowded setting. When approaches are made to individual cohort members, there are varying rates of response to requests to participate in the study. A wide variety of cohort studies has reported response rates of approximately 65–75 per cent for direct interviews. Mail questionnaires, depending on the length of the questionnaire and motivations of the group, often have appreciably lower rates of response. The advantages of interviewing the cohort members include the ability to obtain information on a wide variety of topics. Interviews can provide data on attitudes and permit quite complex questions to be asked with the possibility of probing to ensure accurate recording of responses (such as eliciting histories about diet, exercise, or measures of stress). However, interview data may not always be reliable because the subject may fail to recall information or may not be aware of his or her own habits or history. There is also the possibility that the information may be biased by the subject's knowledge of the aims of the investigation.

Examinations   Medical and other special examinations are necessary to obtain information of which the subject cannot be expected to be aware. Direct examination is often necessitated by the nature of the aetiological factor to be investigated and may be the only way to obtain biologically meaningful information. Subjects often appreciate the availability of an examination, and this may enhance the response rate to certain types of investigations. However, special examinations are usually expensive and require attention to standardization of procedures, training of appropriate observers or laboratory personnel, and quality control across observers and over time. It has also been reported that response rates to medical examinations tend to be biased towards subjects who are relatively free from disease. Direct examination can also be used to validate information obtained from interviews. For example, testing for urinary thiocyanate has been a useful adjunct to smoking studies.

Measure of environment   The fourth type of baseline information is that obtained for each of the groups as a whole, particularly when one is dealing with special exposure groups. Thus it might be appropriate to measure air pollution, exposure to radiation or other toxicological substances, or exposures on the job for an entire group of workers and to apply this measure to each of the individuals in the group. Although this type of information is usually quite useful, particularly when individual measures of exposure cannot be obtained directly, one should be aware that it essentially constitutes 'ecological data', i.e. the measurement of a mean or modal value for a group, which may conceal individual variability within the group.

Example 4—Artificial menopause and breast cancer

All the baseline information for this investigation was obtained from the available surgical and pathological records already filed in the record rooms of two hospitals between 1920 and 1940. The data were felt to be adequate for providing a valid assessment of the exposure status of the members of the cohorts in terms of whether or not they had received the indicated operation. Furthermore, as indicated above, those individuals with known disease could be identified from the available records. In part, the high quality of the records was due to the fact that the hospitals chosen were teaching hospitals for a major medical school, and the records were generally filled out by medical students and interns who provided careful and detailed histories. However, if there was no mention of existing or pre-existing breast cancer, there was no means of confirming this independently of the available records. Likewise, the existence of breast cancer was based solely on the report of the patient to the interviewing physician. Covariables that were available from the hospital records were the age at the time of the index procedure and the parity of the women. Other covariables of possible interest, since they could have been related to both the risk of cancer and the risk of gynaecological procedures, were not available from the records. These included body weight, history of breast-feeding, and exposure to diagnostic X-rays.

Example 5—The British Doctors Study

The initial mail questionnaire was intentionally kept short and simple to encourage a high proportion of replies. The doctors were asked to classify themselves into one of three groups: (i) whether they were, at that time, smoking; (ii) whether they had smoked but had given it up; (iii) whether they had never smoked regularly (i.e. had never smoked as much as one cigarette a day, or its equivalent in pipe tobacco, for as long as one year). Present smokers and ex-smokers were asked additional questions. The former were asked the age at which they had started smoking, the amount of tobacco that they were currently smoking, and the method by which it was consumed. The ex-smokers were asked similar questions, but relating to the time just before they had given up smoking.

> In a covering letter, the doctors were invited to give any information on their smoking habits or history that might be of interest, but, apart from that, no information was sought on previous changes in habit (other than the amount smoked prior to last giving up, if smoking had been abandoned). The decision to restrict question on amount smoked to current smoking habits was based mainly on the results of [an] earlier case– control study . . . [which showed] that the classification of smokers according to the amount that they had most recently smoked gave almost as sharp a differentiation between the groups of patients with and without lung cancer as the use of smoking histories over many years—theoretically more relevant statistics, but clearly based on less accurate data (Breslow and Day 1987, Appendix IA).

Example 6—The Framingham Heart Study

On the basis of an initial examination and detailed interview, the sample was characterized according to a variety of 'risk factors': blood cholesterol, blood pressure, cigarette smoking status, body mass index, and the presence of a variety of other diseases and conditions. Careful attention was given to standardization of the examination procedures and the structure of the interview.

On the basis of a medical history and examination, an electro-cardiogram, and other medical tests, it was found that 82 individuals in the base cohort of 5209 had a cardiovascular event before the baseline examination. Thus the cohort of individuals 'at risk' for the key cardiovascular end-point of coronary heart disease numbered 5127.

To establish the basis for follow-up, each of the subjects was advised at the initial interview that it was intended to re-examine him [or her] at two intervals, and that he [or she] would be approached directly at the appropriate time. The names of a relative, a friend, and the family physician were all recorded so that the subject would be traced in case he [or she] moved during the interval. An abstract of the initial examination was sent to the family physician and the subject was advised by letter as to whether the physician should be consulted or not. The objective of this procedure was to provide some tangible benefit to the subject other than the knowledge of his [or her] contribution to medical science. At the same time, care was taken not to become involved in the medical management of the subjects and to avoid interfering in any way with the relationship between the subject and his [or her] physician. This helped to maintain rapport, not only with the subjects themselves, but with the medical community as well (Dawber *et al.* 1963).

Follow-up
Objectives

There are multiple objectives to be achieved in follow-up.

1. Uniform and complete follow-up of all cohort groups.

2. Complete ascertainment of outcome events.

3. Standardized diagnosis of outcome events.

One of the key criteria by which the quality of a longitudinal incidence study can be judged is the extent to which the investigator achieves complete ascertainment of outcome events in all exposure classes. Although a variety of methods are available for follow-up, it is desirable that the follow-up methods be independent of the method used to classify the exposure category in order to ensure uniform ascertainment across all subgroups. Methods of follow-up include correspondence with the subject and other informants, periodic re-examination of the subjects, and indirect surveillance of hospital records and death certificates. (Some countries such as the United Kingdom, the United States, and some Scandinavian countries maintain central death registers which facilitate efficient and complete mortality follow-up.) The duration of follow-up will be governed primarily by the natural history of the disease and the length of the incubation period between exposure and the onset of illness. It is important that the criteria for diagnosis of end-points be standardized early in the follow-up period. Although criteria for the end-points may change in the clinical community during the study, it is important that some criteria remain stable over time so that the incidence of cases occurring early in the period of follow-up can be compared with similar cases occurring later on in the observational period. Attention should be paid to criteria to verify the absence as well as the presence of the study end-points (i.e. to minimize both false-positive and false-negative diagnoses).

Unequal loss of follow-up across different exposure categories presents serious problems in the analysis, and every method possible should be used to ensure uniform surveillance of each group. Because of the possibility of ascertainment bias resulting from knowledge of the exposure class, it is often desirable to have objective end-point criteria which can be measured by 'blinded' observers. Information used in these criteria should be sought with equal diligence in all exposure classes. This is particularly important when the exposure class is defined by a variable that may lead to different degrees of medical observation, particularly medical examinations that are not under the direct control of the study investigators. For example, if in a study of cardiovascular diseases there is a tendency for participants with high cholesterol levels to receive more frequent electrocardiograms or other examinations by cardiologists, there may be a tendency to diagnose more cardiovascular events, particularly milder events, in this group than in the group with low cholesterol levels. Repeat examination of the subjects, besides providing standardized information on the illnesses under investigation, can often yield additional information about covariables that may be of importance and also allows studies of longitudinal changes in the exposure status.

Example 7—Artificial menopause and breast cancer

All patients in the study were followed from their index admission to 1 December 1961 so that the potential period of observation ranged from 21 to 42 years. The follow-up information was obtained from three sources, of which the first was the hospital records. All information relating to a given patient from any and all admissions to either hospital in the study was located and the data for each patient were then combined into a single record. The second source was the death certificates registered at the Massachusetts Division of Vital Statistics from 1 January 1920 to 31 December 1961. Alphabetical listings of the names of the study patients were compared with those in the index of vital records. Whenever a possible match was obtained, the death certificate was located and the information on the certificate and the identifying data obtained from the hospital chart were compared according to a prescribed set of criteria designed to minimize false matches. Therefore there may have been increased risk of discarding acceptable matches owing to some discrepancies in the available identifying information. All conditions mentioned on the death certificates were coded according to a uniform system. In addition, the underlying cause of death was coded according to the revision of the International Classification of Diseases in use at the State Division of Vital Statistics at the time of the patient's death. Thus direct comparison could be made with published mortality statistics. The third source of follow-up information was the Massachusetts Tumor Registry, a unit of the Bureau of Chronic Disease Control of the Massachusetts Department of Public

Health. Since 1927 this registry had recorded all patients diagnosed with, or treated for, malignancies at State or State-aided cancer clinics. Possible matches were obtained according to rules similar to the criteria for death certificate matching. With regard to mortality follow-up, the assumption was made that all patients dying during the study period should be registered at the Division of Vital Statistics. If no death certificate was located, one of three situations may have occurred: (i) the patient was still alive; (ii) before death she had emigrated from the State and was not a resident of Massachusetts at the time of death; (iii) she had died, but no record could be located because of reporting or matching errors (misspellings, changes of name, failure to file a death certificate, etc.). From the three sources of information the status of 19 per cent of the women was known as of January 1962. It was noted that those receiving pelvic radiation had slightly more complete follow-up to death than those surgically treated—20 per cent versus 18.9 per cent. This difference was statistically significant but there was no significant difference in completeness of follow-up among the surgically treated groups. The relative success of the follow-up procedure was estimated by comparing the percentages of those in the cohorts known to have died before 1962 with those expected on the basis of published mortality rates and estimated migration rates. It was estimated that the observed deaths would comprise 72.8 per cent of the expected number after allowance for migration.

With the advent of automated data files in hospitals and the creation of national automated databases, including central death registries, follow-up of cohorts such as these should become easier and more complete. Although, as in this study, only a small proportion of the original cohort may be known to have died, if one is confident that those known are nearly all of those who had died and there is no bias for better ascertainment of deaths in one group compared with the other, the results should be valid for mortality end-points. The British Doctors Study (Example 8) is an illustration of the use of multiple questionnaires, linkage to other files (physician registries), and other forms of contact to ensure that complete follow-up has been attained. It should be noted that the artificial menopause study, using historical records, took less than three years to complete, while the next two examples of prospective studies took several decades to achieve similar follow-up.

Example 8—The British Doctors Study
The following quotations are from Breslow and Day (1987, Appendix IA).

> During the study, further questionnaires were sent out on three separate occasions to men and on two occasions to women. The purpose was partly to obtain detailed information on smoking habits, in particular giving up smoking, and also to ask additional questions, the relevance of which had emerged during the period of follow-up. Degree of inhalation was asked in these questionnaires, and the use of filter-tipped or plain cigarettes asked in the last questionnaire.

> Information about the death of doctors was obtained at first directly from the Registrars-General of the United Kingdom, who provided particulars of every death as referring to a medical practitioner. Later, lists of deaths were obtained from the General Medical Council, and these were complemented by reference to the records of the British Medical

Association and other sources at home and abroad. Some deaths came to light in response to the questionnaires. Others were discovered in the course of following up doctors who had not replied to or who had not been sent subsequent questionnaires. Of the 34 440 men studies, 10 072 were known to have died before 1 November 1971, 24 265 were known to have been alive at that date, and 103 (0.3 per cent) were not yet traced.

Many of the 103 untraced doctors were not British, and 67 (65 per cent) were known to have gone abroad. It was felt unlikely that more than about a dozen deaths relevant to the study could have been missed.

Information on the underlying cause of death in the 10 072 doctors known to have died before 1 November 1971 was obtained for the vast majority from the official death certificates. Except for deaths for which lung cancer was mentioned, the certified cause was accepted and (unless otherwise stated) the deaths classified according to the underlying cause. (In only four cases was no evidence of the cause obtainable.) The underlying causes were classified according to the seventh revision of the International Classification of Disease . . . except that a separate category of 'pulmonary heart disease' was created.

Cancer of the lung, including trachea or pleura, was given as the underlying cause of 467 deaths and as a contributory cause in a further 20. For each of the 487 deaths, confirmation of the diagnosis was sought from the doctor who had certified the death and, when necessary, from the consultant to whom the patient had been referred. Information about the nature of the evidence was thus obtained in all but two cases. Doubtful reports were interpreted by an outside consultant, with no knowledge of the patient's smoking history. As a result, carcinoma of the lung was accepted as the underlying cause of 441 deaths and as a contributory cause of 17.

Example 9—The Framingham Heart Study
The key method of follow-up in the Framingham Heart Study was through repeated medical examinations on a two-year cycle. The greatest loss due to drop-out occurred between the first and second examinations, and those who came in most reluctantly for the initial examination (i.e. towards the end of the recruitment period) seemed to have the highest drop-out rate during the next 30 years. During the first 14 years of follow-up, more than 85 per cent of the participants who were still alive at any examination cycle came in for their examinations. During the subsequent 12 years the examination rates fell to about 80 per cent of the surviving cohort. The chief reasons for non-examination were believed to be the increasing numbers of people who were physically incapacitated or had migrated from the Framingham area.

Indirect follow-up through secondary sources of information was also pursued. The Framingham Union Hospital, the major source of hospital care for the Framingham community, identified each of the Framingham Heart Study participants and notified the study staff of admissions of participants to the hospital. This is particularly important for allowing standardized examination of stroke cases while symptoms of the disease are still present.

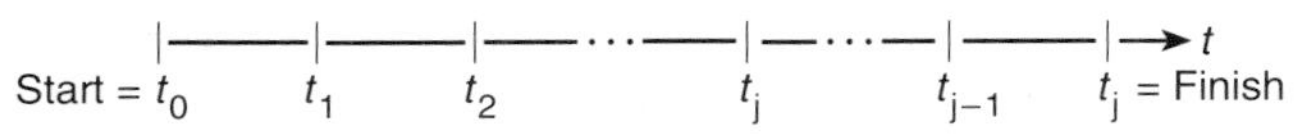

Fig. 11.1 Division of the study period time *j* time intervals.

Mortality follow-up was maintained through regular perusal of vital records at the Town Registrar and following up of obituary notices in newspapers. Mortality follow-up after 30 years was virtually complete with the vital status of less than 2 per cent of the cohort being unknown.

The criteria for diagnosis of cardiovascular and other end-points investigated in the Framingham Heart Study have been precisely defined, and the utility of the various sources of information in providing diagnostic information according to the study criteria has been investigated. Throughout the follow-up period the core criteria for the major cardiovascular end-points have remained fixed and all potential cases are reviewed by a panel of trained medical reviewers.

It should be noted that the rate of disease occurrence in this cohort might have been altered by the subjects' continued participation in the biennial series of examinations. Although no direct advice or treatment was offered to the participants, they were informed through their physicians of abnormal findings such as high blood pressure. If effective preventive measures were instituted in such subjects, then rates of overt cardiovascular diseases would be lowered and would interfere with estimating the 'true' effects of the risk factors. It was felt that during the early period of the study such treatment was not widely offered in this population.

Analysis

If a cohort study has been appropriately designed according to the principles given above, the analysis of the results is relatively straightforward. The first step is to estimate the incidence of the disease of interest for the cohort as a whole and, if the study was designed to make internal comparisons, in the 'exposed' and 'non-exposed' subgroups. If the follow-up period is relatively short and there is little or no loss to follow-up due to death from other conditions, a simple estimate of risk is easily calculated as the number of new (incident) cases diagnosed during the study period divided by the total population at risk at the beginning of the period. Persons who already have the disease at the outset of the study (prevalent cases) are eliminated from the population at risk. For studies of longer duration, however, the risk of disease may change over the course of the study and there may be appreciable losses from the population at risk due to death from other causes, loss from follow-up, or the occurrence of the illness of interest itself. Then it is advantageous to divide the study period into a number of intervals (Fig. 11.1) and to estimate the incidence rate of disease as outlined in Tables 11.1 and 11.2.

Disease risk refers to the probability of developing the disease during the study period (or some subinterval). As a probability it is a dimensionless quantity that must range in value between zero and unity. The incidence rate, however, is a measure of the frequency of the occurrence of disease per unit time relative to the size of the population at risk. Crude incidence is the ratio of the disease risk

Table 11.1 Notation for cohort analysis

$l_j = t_j - t_{j-1}$	Length of *j*th interval, $j = 1, \ldots, J$
N_j	Number of subjects being followed at time t_j
D_j	Number of new disease cases diagnosed in the *j*th interval
T_j	Total observation time for all subjects during the *j*th interval
$D_+ = \Sigma D_j$	Total number of cases
$T_+ = \Sigma T_j$	

during a time interval to the length of the interval. Instantaneous incidence, also known as the hazard rate of force or morbidity, measures the rate of diagnosis of new cases per unit time relative to the size of the disease-free population at risk at time *t*. The units for incidence rates are $(time)^{-1}$ and they have no upper limit quantitatively. Owing to limitations of the available data, it is not possible to estimate precisely the incidence rate at each time *t*. Instead, estimates are made of the average rates over the study period or over each subinterval by dividing the number of new cases diagnosed in the interval by the total person-years of observation time accumulated during the interval (Table 11.2, eqns. (11.1) and (11.2)). Accurate estimation of the person-years denominators requires, for each individual in the study, knowledge of the exact duration of follow-up from the start of the study until diagnosis of the disease of interest, death from a competing cause, or loss from further observation. The contributions from each individual at risk during the *j*th interval are summed to yield the totals T_j shown in Table 11.1. If such data are not available, various methods can be used to approximate the person-years of observation. For example, the estimated size of the population at the mid-point of the interval can be multiplied by the interval length.

Table 11.2 Measures of incidence and risk

Equation 11.1	$I = D_+ / T_+$	Average incidence rate over the entire study period
Equation 11.2	$I = D_j / T_j$	Average incidence rate over the *j*th interval
Equation 11.3	$CI_j = \sum_{j=1}^{i} I_j l_j$	Cumulative incidence rate to time t_j
Equation 11.4	$CI = CI_j$	Cumulative incidence rate over the entire study period to time $= t_j$
Equation 11.5	$CR = 1 - \exp(-cl)$	Cumulative disease risk over the entire study period (adjusted for intercurrent mortality and loss to follow-up)
Equation 11.6	$CI(t) = \sum_{tj \le t} D_j / N_j$	Cumulative incidence to time *t* (non-parametric estimate)*
Equation 11.7	$CR(t) = 1 - \prod (1 - D_j / N_j)$	Cumulative risk to time *t* (non-parametric estimate)*

* Assumes the intervals are so fine that diagnosis are made *only* at times t_j.

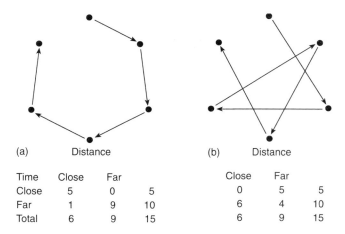

Time	Distance		
(a)	Close	Far	
Close	5	0	5
Far	1	9	10
Total	6	9	15

(b)	Close	Far	
	0	5	5
	6	4	10
	6	9	15

Fig. 11.2 Cumulative breast cancer morbidity curves for women treated with X-rays for post-partum mastitis (7) and a control group (t), adjusted to the age distribution of the control group. (Source: Shore, R.E., Hemplemann, L.H., Kowaluk, E., *et al.* (1977). Breast neoplasms in women treated with X-rays for acute postpartum mastitis. *Journal of the National Cancer Institute* **59**, 813).

Another useful measure of disease occurrence, known as the **cumulative incidence rate**, is obtained by summing the products of incidence rate and interval length over a series of intervals (eqns. (11.3) and (11.4)). The cumulative incidence rate over a specified interval, which is a dimensionless quantity with no upper limit, is related via the exponential function to the disease risk over the interval (eqn. (11.5)). If the disease is rare or the study period is short (so that the cumulative risk is no more than 5 per cent), cumulative incidence and risk are nearly equal. Both can be estimated non-parametrically as a function of time t by choosing the intervals to be so fine that the interval end-points occur exactly at the times of disease diagnosis (eqns. (11.6) and (11.7)). Plots of cumulative incidence over time provide a powerful graphic tool for examining the evolution of disease risk in the exposed and non-exposed subgroups. As an example, Fig. 11.2 shows that breast cancer incidence in a cohort of women treated with radiation for post-partum mastitis paralleled the incidence in the control population until some 16–20 years after treatment, but then increased to substantially higher levels.

Although the preceding definitions used time on study as the basic time-scale for estimation of instantaneous incidence, other choices may be more appropriate in some circumstances. The possibilities include age, calendar time, and, for studies where exposure starts before entry into the study, time since initial exposure. With these other time-scales the population at risk changes due not only to the loss from observation of subjects who die or develop the disease of interest, but also to the entry into the cohort of other subjects depending, for example, on their age or the calendar year at the time that they join the study. All the definitions and formulae continue to apply with these alternative time-scales. More advanced statistical analyses often consider several time-scales simultaneously, using a multidimensional classification of incident cases and person-years denominators according to age, calendar year, time on study, and other fixed and time-varying factors.

Cohort studies also facilitate the estimation of various measures of association between the exposure of interest and the occurrence

of disease. The **standardized morbidity ratio** (SMR) is frequently used in occupational cohort studies to estimate the ratio of cohort rates to standard rates obtained from national health statistics registers or other standard sources. As shown in eqn. (11.8) (Table 11.3), the SMR is simply the ratio of the number of cases of disease observed to the number of cases expected from the standard rates as applied to the age/time-specific person-years of observation. Dose–response trends may be evident from SMRs that are estimated separately for subcohorts defined by levels of cumulative exposure (Table 11.4). However, doubts about the comparability of the cohort and the standard population, coupled with the fact that the ratio of SMRs for two or more subcohorts may not adequately summarize the ratios of age/time-specific rates, have led many investigators to discard the SMR in favour of measures of association that do not depend on external rates. The Mantel–Haenszel rate ratio (eqn. (11.11)) summarizes the ratios of the age/time-specific rates for the exposed versus the non-exposed members of the cohort. It is closely related to the Mantel–Haenszel relative risk measure that is widely used to summarize tables of exposure/disease odds ratios in case–control studies (see Volume 2, Chapter 10). This is the preferred measure of association when, as is often the case, the rate ratios are relatively constant over time but the rate differences are not. The cumulative risk difference (eqn. (11.12)), which is also known as the attributable risk or excess risk, provides an absolute measure of the effect of exposure, which is useful for public health workers.

Data from cohort studies can also be used to measure the potential impact of the removal of a suspected aetiological factor. This is measured either in terms of the estimated effect of removal on disease incidence or on the cumulative risk over the study period. The most direct measure of potential impact is known as the aetiological fraction, defined here using risk (eqn. (11.13)) rather than incidence. It represents the proportion of all new cases

Table 11.3 Measures of association †

Equation 11.8   SMR $= D_+/ST_j\,I_j^*$ Standardized morbidity ratio

Equation 11.9 $RR_j = I_j^E/I_j^O$ Rate ratio in the jth interval

Equation 11.10 $RD^j = I_j^E - I_j^O$ Rate difference in the jth interval

Equation 11.11 $RR_{MH} = \dfrac{SD_j^E T_j^O (T_j^E + T_j^O)}{SD_j^O T_j^E I(T_j^E = T_j^O)}$ Mantel–Haesnzel summary rate ratio

Equation 11.12 $RD = CR^E - CR^O$ Cumulative risk difference (attributable risk)

Equation 11.13 $RR^E = CR^E/CR^O$ Relative risk (crude)

Equation 11.14 $AF = (CR - CR^O)/CR$ Aetiological fraction

$$= \frac{P^E\,(RP^E - 1)}{P^E\,(RR^E - 1) + 1}$$

† the superscripts refer to the exposed subcohort (E), the non-exposed subcohort (O), and the external standard population (*), respectively. Non-superscripted quantities refer to the entire cohort. P^t denotes the proportion of the population that is exposed.

Table 11.4 Lung cancer mortality by cumulative radiation exposure among Canadian fluorspar miners*

Cumulative WLM†	No. of person-years at risk	No. of lung cancer deaths		SMR (O/E ratio)‡
		Observed	Expected	
0	13 567.8	7	7.00	1.00
1–9	3 045.5	3	2.02	1.49
10–239	9 510.5	13	7.22	1.80
240–599	5 105.5	10	3.87	2.58
600–1979	7 107.0	6	1.71	3.51
1980–2039	2 415.5	25	1.54	16.23
≥ 2040	2 889.0	40	1.07	37.38

* Committee on the Biological Effects of Ionizing Radiations (1988). In *Health risks of radon and other internally deposited alpha-emitters*, National Academy Press, p. 471.
† WLM, working level months of radon daughter exposure.
‡ SMR, standardized mortality ratio; O, observed; E, expected.

of disease that can be considered to be due to the exposure and therefore that are potentially preventable if the exposure were to be completely removed. Equation (11.14) shows how it may be represented using two parameters: the proportion P^E of the total population with the exposure, and the risk ratio RR^E. Although useful for studies of short duration involving a single risk factor, serious conceptual difficulties arise when attempts are made to extend the definition of aetiological fraction for use with multiple interacting risk factors or in situations where a long study period is needed in order to ascertain the temporal aspects of the exposure–disease association.

Example 10—Artificial menopause and breast cancer

Some of the results of this study are shown in Table 11.5. For the four 'exposure' categories of women who were less than 40 years old at the time of admission into the cohort, 37 cases of breast cancer were discovered to have occurred during the follow-up period. Several difficulties in applying the usual estimates of incidence and risk are readily apparent.

1. Because of migration and incompleteness of follow-up, the observed cases are known to be an undercount.

2. The time of onset for each malignancy was not usually known (those ascertained from death certificates did not usually state age at onset).

3. The duration of follow-up for most of the women was not precisely known.

However, by making several assumptions it is possible to obtain some reasonable estimates of the association of breast cancer occurrence with the extent of pelvic surgery. The basic assumption is that whatever inadequacies there were in the follow-up procedures, they occurred uniformly in each of the exposure groups (for example the women with natural menopause were no more likely to have migrated than those with surgical menopause), and therefore any cases of breast cancer were equally likely to be ascertained in each group. Another problem is that the frequency with which the various procedures were performed varied considerably during the 21 years of potential admission to the study (for example pelvic irradiation was more frequent in the 1920s than later). Thus the women in the radiation group tended to have longer potential periods of follow-up than those in the surgical groups. This was handled by examining the specific dates of entry into the study for each woman.

The fourth column of Table 11.5 gives an estimate of the crude risk of developing breast cancer. For the reasons given above, this is a very poor estimate. The next column gives an estimate of the cumulative incidence rate of breast cancer over the average 30-year follow-up period, which was obtained by estimating the person-years contribution of each woman. Because of the inadequacies in follow-up mentioned above, the estimates shown are undoubtedly

Table 11.5 Breast cancer in patients with and without artificial menopause

Exposure group	Number in group (No)	Number of cases (D+)	Crude rate (D+/No)	Estimated cumulative risk	RR (relative risk)
Cholecystectomy	400	6	0.0150	0.0198	1.00
Unilateral oophorectomy	1635	20	0.0122	0.0210	1.06
Hysterectomy and bilateral oophorectomy	1278	6	0.0047	0.0054	0.27
Radiation	468	5	0.0107	0.0106	0.54

Table 11.6 Deaths from coronary heart disease (CHD) among British male doctors*

Age group (years) j	No. of person-years (1000s)		No. of CHD deaths		CHD rates†		Rate ratio RR_j	Rate difference† RD_j
	Non-smokers T_j^O	Smokers T_j^E	Non-smokers D_j^O	Smokers D_j^E	Non-smokers I_j^O	Smokers I_j^E		
35–44	18.790	52.407	2	32	0.11	0.61	5.73	0.50
45–54	10.673	43.248	12	104	1.12	2.40	2.14	1.28
55–64	5.710	28.612	28	206	4.90	7.20	1.47	2.30
65–74	2.585	12.663	28	186	10.83	14.69	1.36	3.86
75–84	1.462	5.317	31	102	21.20	19.18	0.90	− 2.02
Total	39.220	142.247	101	630	2.58‡	4.43‡	1.72	1.85

* From Doll and Hill (1966) as quoted by Breslow and Day (1987).
† Per 1000 person-years
‡ Average rates I^O and I^E over entire age range.

lower than the true rates. However, provided that the under-ascertainment was approximately equal in the different exposure groups, there should be less bias in the estimates of relative risk shown in the last column. The cholecystectomy group was considered to be the 'unexposed' or control group. Using eqn. (11.13), the relative risk for the women with unilateral oophorectomy is 1.06, which is not statistically different from the standard group. The relative risk for the women with hysterectomy and bilateral oophorectomy is 0.27, which is significantly less than the standard group. The women receiving irradiation also had a low relative risk for developing breast cancer (0.54), but because this group is small the risk is not statistically significant.

Because of the problems in estimation of the cumulative incidence rates in this study, no attempt was made to obtain estimates of the aetiological fraction.

Example 11—Coronary heart disease and smoking among British doctors

Table 11.6 shows the numbers of deaths from coronary heart disease and corresponding person-years denominators for smokers and non-smokers observed during the first ten years of follow-up of the British Doctors Study. The coronary heart disease rates increase markedly with age, but less so for smokers than for non-smokers. Since the rate ratios for smokers versus non-smokers decline sharply with age, whereas the rate differences generally increase, this is an example where neither the Mantel–Haenszel rate ratio nor the cumulative rate difference is very useful in summarizing the age-specific quantities. Either the age-specific rates themselves, or variations in the rate ratios or differences with age, are needed to describe the results of the study adequately. Nevertheless, using the age-specific rates, it can readily be calculated that the cumulative mortality rate in the 35–74 years age group is 17.0 per cent for non-smokers and 24.9 per cent for smokers. The corresponding cumulative risks are $CR^E = 1 - \exp(-0.170) = 15.6$ per cent and $CR^O = 1 - \exp(-0.249) = 22.0$ per cent for a risk ratio of $RR^E = 1.41$ and an attributable risk of $RD = 6.4$ per cent. Assuming that $P^E = 83$ per cent of British doctors were smokers at the beginning of the study period, the aetiological fraction is $AF = (0.83 \times 0.41)/(0.83 \times 0.41 + 1) = 25$ per cent. However, this number should be interpreted cautiously for the

reasons mentioned earlier. The aetiological fraction is much smaller when the coronary heart disease deaths occurring at ages 75–84 years are also taken into account. The Mantel-Haenszel rate ratio for the entire 50-year age span is $RR_{MH} = 1.42$, the attributable risk is $RD = 3.9$ per cent, and the aetiological fraction is $AF = 9$ per cent.

Example 12—The Framingham Heart Study

During the first three decades of its existence, the Framingham Heart Study generated more than 300 publications. Many involved quite sophisticated methodological applications, which are beyond the scope of this presentation.

An example of the relation between the occurrence of coronary heart disease and serum cholesterol based on six years of follow-up is shown in Table 11.7. Data are shown for men who were aged between 40 and 59 years and were free from coronary heart disease at entry. There were 1333 men with measured cholesterol levels and follow-up was complete for six years for nearly all of them. These men were classified into tertiles on the basis of their initial serum cholesterol levels as shown in the first column of the table. Person-years of observation were estimated for each tertile based on the assumption that each of the men who developed coronary heart disease was followed on average for half the study period, whereas the other men were followed for the entire six years. (It would be better to count those who developed coronary heart disease plus those who died from other causes as contributing three years each.) Thus, for example, the average annual incidence for the entire cohort was estimated from eqn. (11.1) as $I = 96/[(1333 - 48) \times 6] = 0.0125$. The cumulative risks determined from eqn. (11.5) are virtually identical in this instance to the crude risks (number of cases divided by number of persons at risk at the start of the period). The relative risks associated with high cholesterol levels are shown in the next column, where the men with cholesterol levels lower than 210 mg per 100 ml are taken as the standard or unexposed group. Men with cholesterol levels between 210 and 244 mg per 100 ml have 1.81 times the risk of developing coronary heart disease compared with men with lower cholesterol levels, and men with cholesterol levels above 244 mg per 100 ml have risks 3.43 times greater. The attributable risks RD associated with higher cholesterol levels are shown in the last column.

Table 11.7 Six-year incidence of coronary heart disease according to initial serum cholesterol in men aged 40–59 years

Serum cholesterol (mg/100 ml)	Number in group	Number of cases	I (average annual incidence)	CR (cumulative risk)	RR^E (relative risk)	RD (attributable risk)
< 210	455	16	0.0060	0.0352	1.00	0.000
210–244	455	29	0.0107	0.0637	1.81	0.0285
≥ 245	423	51	0.0214	0.1207	3.43	0.0855
Total						

If men could be prevented from having cholesterol levels above 244 mg per 100 ml, the potential impact upon the incidence of coronary heart disease can be estimated from the aetiological fraction (eqn. (11.14)). The combined group of men with cholesterol levels below 245 mg per 100 ml is considered to be the unexposed groups with a (crude) risk of $CR^0 = (16 + 29)/(454 + 455) = 0.0495$. Then $AF = (0.0720 - 0.0495)/0.0720 = 0.31$, i.e. the risk of coronary heart disease among men could potentially be lowered by 31 per cent if none of them had cholesterol levels over 245 mg per 100 ml. A similar calculation showed that if all the men had cholesterol levels below 210 mg per 100 ml, the aetiological fraction would be 51 per cent, i.e. half of the cases of coronary heart disease could potentially be prevented. This illustrates the strong dependence of the aetiological fraction on the rather arbitrary specification of the baseline level for a continuous-valued risk factor. Furthermore, since whatever intervention was undertaken to reduce the serum cholesterol levels might have unpredictable effects on the coronary heart disease rates, it is clear that 'potential impact' as used here must be interpreted in terms of statistical association rather than causation.

Types of bias and their resolution

In this section the different types of bias that may occur in cohort studies are presented and discussed. Because all the different types of bias are not necessarily present in the same study, we draw examples from additional studies as well as from two of the three studies presented earlier.

Factors related to the selection of the study population, response rate, collection of information, methodologies used, and analytical strategies employed often introduce biases which, if not anticipated, can lead to incorrect conclusions concerning a possible relationship between an exposure (independent variable) and a disease (outcome variable). Such biases are inherent in all types of epidemiological studies. In this section we shall confine our discussion to the types of biases that affect cohort studies.

There are five broad categories of bias that are operative in cohort studies. These are selection bias, follow-up bias, information bias, confounding bias, and *post hoc* bias. Each of these is discussed separately below. These biases can cause systematic errors, which affect the internal validity of a study. This is in contrast with random errors, which may not affect the internal validity of the study but will reduce the probability of observing a true relationship. A true bias (i.e. a systematic error that is introduced into one group or subgroup to a greater extent than in other subgroups) often leads to the observation of a relationship that is not a true

relationship or, vice versa, leads to the conclusion that there is no relationship when, in fact, there is a true relationship between the independent and outcome variables. Errors that occur with equal frequency in all subgroups usually do not affect the validity of a relationship. However, because a certain proportion of the measurements in all the subgroups will be erroneous, the probability of observing a true relationship is diminished and the true magnitude of the relationship may be underestimated.

While internal validity is paramount, it is often important to have external validity in cohort studies as well. External validity refers to the degree to which an association observed in the study populations also holds true in the general population. In order to ensure external validity, the population studies must be representative of the population to which the results of the study will be generalized. In many cohort studies, it is necessary for various reasons to study some subpopulation of the general population. This subpopulation may represent a non-random sample of the general population, such as an occupational group, a group selected from a particular health plan, etc. If such subpopulations are used, external validity may be reduced.

Selection bias

Selection bias may occur when the group actually studied does not reflect the same distribution of factors (such as age, smoking, race, etc.) as occurs in the general population. This may be because some of the members of the cohort selected originally refuse to participate or, in a non-current cohort study, because records on some individuals are missing or incomplete. Therefore the response rates among the various subgroups invited to participate in the study differ. In some studies particular subgroups may be used for convenience and may not be representative of the general population for other reasons.

Example 13—Effects of volunteering

An example of selective non-response to recruitment was observed and documented in the Framingham studies cited earlier in this chapter (Example 1). It was found that individuals who agreed to participate in these cohort studies were healthier than individuals who did not agree to participate. While this would not affect the internal validity of the study, since the groups to be followed were characterized on the basis of factors present at baseline, it would be likely to reduce the incidence of the disease of interest, particularly in the first few years of the study. Thus the external validity would be diminished, but the internal validity should not be affected for those independent variables defined at baseline. However, because the incidence of disease might be lower in this healthier group that is being followed up, the probability of finding significant relationships would be somewhat diminished. In occupational cohort studies, this type of selection bias has been termed 'the healthy worker effect'.

Example 14—Spectrum of independent variables in study groups

A second problem with selection non-response is associated with the extent to which the population that agrees to participate in the study actually represents the true spectrum of the independent variable.

Early studies of the relationship of dietary cholesterol and saturated fat intake to coronary heart disease in the United States gave inconclusive results. This may have been due, in part, to the fact that very few Americans have dietary cholesterol and saturated fat intakes in the lower ranges, whereas residents of less affluent countries have a higher proportion of individuals with these low levels of intake. If there exists a threshold level of the independent variable necessary to produce disease and the respondents include only individuals with levels of the independent variable that are above the threshold level, then no relationship will be seen between the variable and the disease under study. Thus some of the comparisons of the incidence of coronary heart disease among Americans with higher levels of cholesterol and fat in the diet may not have shown a relationship because the threshold level of dietary fats was below the levels consumed in the study population. Even in situations where there is no threshold level, inclusion of individuals at only one end of the spectrum of the independent variable will reduce the likelihood that a dose–response relationship will be observed. Thus non-response or non-inclusion of participants in the cohort who represent one or the other extreme of the independent variable may affect the internal validity of the study and lead to a false observation that there is no relationship.

Example 15—Presence of incipient disease

Another problem of selection bias occurs when individuals who have incipient disease are included in the cohort. Individuals with the disease of interest should be excluded from the study population at the time of recruitment. However, with many chronic diseases that have a long induction period such as cancer and heart disease, it is difficult to identify individuals with incipient disease. Their inclusion in the study population may lead to an observation of associations that are, in fact, a result of the disease process rather than a risk factor for the disease.

An association between low cholesterol and risk of cancer has been observed in several cohort studies. The induction period for cancer is probably one or more decades. Individuals who develop cancer in a follow-up period of less than the induction period probably had incipient disease at the time of the formation of the cohort. Thus a low cholesterol level in these individuals may have been a result of the cancer process rather than a risk factor for it.

Example 16—Distribution of covariables

A final example of selection bias occurs when the distribution of covariables that may be related to disease incidence is not equally represented in the study cohorts.

Smoking is related to a number of diseases. In some, it is the probable major cause whereas in others, such as coronary heart

disease, it represents only one of several risk factors that increase the probability of developing disease. Thus, if the non-respondents include a higher proportion of smokers than non-smokers, the total incidence of coronary heart disease in the study cohort would be lower than if smokers were appropriately represented in the cohort. However, the effect would be not only to make the observed incidence of coronary heart disease lower in the study population than in the general population, but also to lead to a false estimate of the proportion of coronary heart disease that is associated with smoking (the aetiological fraction). Specifically, the incidence of coronary heart disease among the smokers would be correct, but the proportion of the total numbers of cases that were associated with smoking would be smaller than actually exists because the proportion of smokers in the study population would be lower than in the general population. Thus any estimates of the aetiological fraction of coronary heart disease due to smoking would be too low.

Follow-up bias

One of the major problems in cohort studies is to accomplish the successful follow-up of all members of the cohort. If the loss to follow-up occurs equally in the exposed and unexposed groups, the internal validity should not be affected. Of course, this assumes that the rate of disease occurrence is the same among those lost to follow-up as among those not lost to follow-up within each group. However, if the rate of disease is different among those lost to follow-up, then the internal validity of the study may be affected (i.e. the relationship between exposure and outcome may be changed).

Example 17—Bias resulting from differential incidence in those lost to follow-up

If the rate of lung cancer is higher in those smokers who are lost to follow-up than in those who remain in the study, the observed incidence of lung cancer in those smokers who remain in the study will be lower than the actual incidence of lung cancer in the entire cohort of smokers. The effect will be to observe a lower association between lung cancer and smoking than actually exists (provided that the incidence of lung cancer is the same in non-smokers who were and were not followed). If the lung cancer incidence rate is lower in smokers who are not followed up than in those who are, the reverse effect would occur (i.e. the observed association would be greater than the true association).

Usually the incidence of disease is not known among those lost to follow-up, making it difficult to look for this type of bias. If possible, the occurrence and cause of death should be sought in those who are lost to follow-up. This is easier in the United States now that there is a National Death Registry. If the death rate is similar between those lost and not lost to follow-up within each group, the occurrence of a different incidence of disease in the two groups is less likely.

Another strategy is to compare the known characteristics at baseline of those lost and not lost to follow-up. The more similar the two groups are, the less likely it is that a different incidence of disease occurred in them.

Neither of these strategies guarantees that the incidence was the same in both those followed and those not followed. Therefore the best strategy is to reduce the number lost to follow-up to the lowest level possible.

Example 18—Bias resulting from loss to follow-up of individuals under observation for the independent variable

Another possible source of bias may be observed in studies in which the independent variable is being documented concurrently with the development of the outcome variable, presenting the opportunity for misclassification resulting from loss to follow-up.

In evaluating the relationship between a decline in lung function test results and concurrent levels of exposure to photochemical oxidants at place of residence, a problem arises in considering how to evaluate individuals who have moved from the study area to other areas (Detels *et al.* 1991). In some instances they will have moved to areas with lower levels of exposure to photochemical oxidants and in other instances to areas with higher levels. It is not feasible to maintain constant monitoring for levels of photochemical oxidants in all the areas to which these individuals have moved. If there is indeed a relationship between levels of exposure to photochemical oxidants and decreasing lung test performance, the inclusion in analyses of individuals who have moved to a cleaner area, as if they had remained in the area of high exposure, will lead to misclassification bias and thus to an underestimate of the relationship. However, if individuals who moved to a dirtier area are included, this will lead to misclassification bias with the reverse effect.

Another potential bias is introduced if the individuals who have moved are excluded from the analysis to avoid misclassification bias. Individuals who have moved out of the study area may have done so because of the high level of exposure to photochemical oxidants and their awareness of their declining respiratory ability. This would result in an observed relationship in those not moving that is lower than the true relationship.

While this type of bias is almost impossible to prevent, there are several pieces of information that can assist the investigator in evaluating the magnitude of the bias that may be introduced. First, the investigator may compare lung function test results at baseline among those who remained and those who moved away. Any difference between those re-tested and those not re-tested would provide information about the direction, and possibly about the magnitude, of the bias that occurred.

Second, it is often possible to send a mail questionnaire to individuals who have moved away from the study area, which should include questions regarding reasons for moving. If it is found, for example, that many of the respondents moved because of the development of respiratory symptoms, the probability of potential bias can be recognized. In addition, the ascertainment of diagnosed respiratory impairment among those not re-tested would also indicate the presence of bias.

Although there is no completely satisfactory solution to this problem resulting from loss to follow-up, awareness of the potential for bias will enable the investigator to explore various methods to evaluate its effect.

Example 19—Unequal observation

Smoking is associated with a wide range of adverse health outcomes. Any one of these adverse health outcomes is more likely to result in smokers being seen by a physician, thus increasing the likelihood that the disease of interest may also be diagnosed at that time. That is to say, there would be an earlier diagnosis of disease in the smoking individual than in a comparable non-smoking individual who would be less likely to come under medical scrutiny. As a result, there would be an overestimate of the association of the disease of interest with the smoking variable. This overestimate would occur when a crude relative risk analysis (eqn. (11.13)) is used since cohort studies usually have a defined follow-up period. It would also occur when a summary rate ratio based on person-years (eqn. (11.11)) is used since the individual would appear as a case after fewer years of follow-up than would normally occur if he or she were not brought to medical attention as a result of smoking.

Information (misclassification) bias

Information bias occurs when there is an error in the classification of individuals with respect to the outcome variable. This may result from measurement errors, imprecise measurement, and misdiagnosis for whatever reason. Information bias is also termed misclassification bias. If the misclassification occurs equally in all the subgroups of the study population, the internal validity of the study will not be affected, but the precision or probability of being able to demonstrate a true relationship is reduced and the true magnitude of the relationship is likely to be underestimated.

Example 20

If the proportion of cases under- or over-reported in a cohort study of the risk of coronary heart disease is equal among smokers and non-smokers, no change in the observed risk ratio for smoking would occur and the internal validity of the study would be unaffected. However, if the misclassification occurs to a greater extent among either smokers or non-smokers, the observed risk will be altered, thereby affecting the relative risk and incidence difference and, as a result, the internal validity of the study.

Confounding bias

Confounding occurs when other factors that are associated with both the outcome and exposure variables do not have the same distribution in the exposed and unexposed groups. Two common confounders in cohort studies are smoking and age. The risk of disease varies with age for almost all diseases. Likewise, smoking increases the risk of acquiring a wide range of diseases.

Example 21

In a cohort study to determine the risk of coronary heart disease among individuals who drink and do not drink, the prevalence of individuals who smoke is likely to be higher among those who drink than those who do not drink. If one does not take into account the prevalence of smoking in the two groups, there will be a higher incidence of coronary heart disease in the drinking group than in the non-drinking group, which is, in fact, ascribable to smoking rather than to drinking. A false association or non-association also might be observed if the age distributions were not the same in the drinking and non-drinking groups since the incidence of coronary heart disease increases with age.

Confounding bias can result in either an overestimate or an underestimate of the relative risk of an independent variable with disease. Estimates of the effect of confounding variables in a cohort study usually require primarily the use of the investigator's

judgement, although the application of specific statistical procedures can help in reducing the effects of recognized confounders
(see Volume 2, Chapter 14).

Post hoc bias

Another source of potential bias is the use of data from a cohort
study to make observations that were not part of the original study
intent. Thus interesting relationships that were not originally
anticipated are often observed in cohort studies. These findings
should be treated as hypotheses that are an appropriate subject for
additional studies. Such fortuitous findings should not be considered to have established the validity of a relationship and in no
circumstance should the same data be analysed to test hypotheses
arising from that data.

Resolution of bias

There are various strategies for reducing the presence of bias in
cohort studies. Selection bias can be reduced by careful selection of
individuals for inclusion in the study and by making every attempt
to characterize differences that may exist between respondents and
non-respondents. Although consideration of characteristics that
may be more frequent in non-respondents will not eliminate bias,
it may permit the investigator to assess the directionality and
degree of bias that may have resulted from specific selection
procedures. Information bias can be reduced by using well-defined
precise measurements and classification criteria for which the
sensitivity and specificity have been determined. Follow-up bias
can be reduced by intensive follow-up of all study participants and
by establishing criteria for follow-up that will assure that all
members of the cohort have an equal opportunity for being
diagnosed as having the outcome variable. Comparison of the
characteristics present at baseline among those lost to follow-up
and those successfully followed up may provide information upon
which estimates of the nature and degree of bias that may have been
introduced through loss to follow-up may be based.

Confounding bias can be reduced in the analysis stage by careful
stratification and/or adjustment procedures. However, fine stratification for multiple potential confounders may result in a loss of
information, which reduces the likelihood of observing a significant
difference. Thus careful consideration should be given to whether
proposed adjustment factors are clearly related to the disease
outcome. If not, it is usually better not to attempt to restrict the
selection of participants or to adjust during analysis. The identification and resolution of bias is primarily a matter of epidemiological
judgement. Statistical and analytic techniques designed to reduce

bias should be applied only to factors that, in the judgement of the
investigators, are potential sources of bias.

We have discussed the major sources of bias in a cohort study.
However, this list is far from exhaustive, and additional types of
bias will surely be described in the future for which investigators
should be alert. More detailed discussions of the problems of
cohort studies are given by Kleinbaum et al. (1982), Rothman
(1986), Breslow and Day (1987), and Hennekens and Buring
(1987).

Summary

Cohort studies are usually the best type of studies for demonstrating the association between an exposure and a disease because it is
possible to derive relative and attributable risks and often incidence
measures from them. However, they are usually expensive to carry
out and large cohorts are required for rare diseases. In addition,
there are very significant problems associated with the selection of
appropriate groups to be studied and with complete ascertainment
of disease occurrence in them. Usually it is necessary to compromise the ideal, thus providing the opportunity for various types
of bias to occur that can result in incorrect conclusions. The
success of a cohort study often depends on the care of the
investigator in recognizing and correcting for these biases.

References

Breslow, N.E and Day, N.E. (1987). *Statistical methods in cancer research*. Vol. 2,
    The design and analysis of cohort studies. International Agency for Research
    on Cancer, Lyon.
Dawber, T.R., Kannel, W.B., and Lyell, L.P. (1963). An approach to longitudi-
    nal studies in a community: the Framingham Study. *Annals of the New York
    Academy of Sciences*, **107**, 539–56.
Detels, R., Tashkin, D.P., Sayre, J.W., *et al.* (1991). The UCLA Population
    Studies of CORD: X. a cohort study of changes in respiratory function
    associated with chronic exposure to SO_x, NO_x, and hydrocarbons. *American
    Journal of Public Health*, **81**, 350–9.
Doll, R. and Peto, R. (1976). Mortality and relation to smoking: 20 years'
    observations on male British doctors. *British Medical Journal*, **2**(6051),
    1525–36.
Feinleib, M. (1968). Breast cancer and artificial menopause: a cohort study.
    Journal of the National Cancer Institute, **41**, 315–29.
Hennekens, C.H., and Buring, J.E. (1987). *Epidemiology in medicine*. Little,
    Brown, Boston, MA.
Kannel, W.B., Dawber, T.R., Kagan, A., *et al.* (1961). Factors of risk in the
    development of coronary heart disease—six year follow-up experience. The
    Framingham Study. *Annals of Internal Medicine*, **55**, 33–50.
Kleinbaum, D.G., Kupper, L.L., and Morgenstern, H. (1982). *Epidemiologic
    research*. Lifetime Learning, Belmont, CA.
Rothman, K. (1986). *Modern epidemiology*. Little, Brown, Boston, MA.

12 Community based intervention trials

H. Hoffmeister and G.B.M. Mensink

Health promotion of large populations

The major health concerns of industrial societies today are a few chronic diseases, in particular cardiovascular diseases, cancer, adult-onset diabetes, arthropathies, and chronic diseases of the respiratory tract and the liver. The main characteristic of these diseases is their development over a long period of time without severely influencing a person's quality of life. In the early stages no symptoms appear and the subjective health status is not necessarily altered because the body can compensate for the effects of the disease by physiological and metabolic changes.

The risk of developing one of these diseases early in life depends considerably on an individual's health behaviour. Habits such as smoking, alcohol consumption, unbalanced nutrition, physical inactivity, and incorrect posture are likely to result in elevated risk factor levels, for example increased blood lipid levels, high blood pressure, overweight, atherosclerotic lesions of blood vessels, chronic inflammations, and musculoskeletal disorders. These, together with other risk factors such as age and genetic predisposition, play an important role in the initiation and progression of chronic diseases.

Strategies to enhance the population's health

Preventive medicine basically uses two approaches to reduce the population's risk of getting one of these diseases.

The medical or high-risk approach

This approach mainly consists of screening for risk factors and individual treatment of people at high risk by members of the medical profession. The identification of high-risk individuals, their consequent medical treatment, and the repeated advice to change their lifestyle is one way to enhance the individual health and thereby the health of the population. Several controlled intervention studies and experimental studies have shown successful reduction of risk factors as will be described in the next section. Successes were particularly achieved in the reduction of high blood pressure and in the treatment of hypercholesterinaemia, disorders of carbohydrate metabolism, and subsequent cardiovascular diseases. This approach has limitations and disadvantages. A large proportion of these chronic diseases occur in the segment of the population that does not show extreme risk factor levels. Screening, drug treatment, and individual health counselling are expensive and, in addition, serious undesired side-effects of drugs have been observed.

The public health approach

The public health approach is directed towards general populations in communities, regions, or whole countries rather than to individuals. It is concerned with creating a healthy life-style, convincing the population to avoid health risks, and teaching skills to lower or avoid drug consumption and to cope with difficult life situations. This approach tries to enhance knowledge about risky and profitable health behaviour as well as to change unhealthy attitudes. It is the public health answer in the fight against civilization-associated diseases and the promotion of the population's health. Various uncontrolled activities and programmes are carried out in communities, on a regional and state level, using different ways to enlarge health knowledge and influence attitudes and health behaviour of community inhabitants. While it can be assumed that all these activities have no adverse effects, it is not clear whether they really work. Sufficient knowledge about the most effective intervention strategies is missing and often the cost-effectiveness has not been taken into account appropriately.

Ascertainment of the impact of community intervention

Considering this, scientific evidence is needed which shows that the community approach to promote public health is effective. The different aspects and elements of underlying theories (such as social cognition theory and persuasive communication theory) must be tested in studies and evaluated with respect to their health impact. The evaluation should also be used as a feedback for the development of life-style intervention methods. This is a difficult and expensive scientific task. The aspects of community health are so complex that there is neither a general definition nor an agreement about a set of indicators to measure it. The changes in knowledge, attitudes, and health behaviour (that is, knowledge about the danger of smoking and alcohol consumption, health trends such as jogging, or increased vegetable consumption) can be observed early by 'process evaluation'. Such changes, however, do not provide certainty that health improvement will occur. The process of determining the physically measurable outcomes of intervention is complicated by the fact that a certain time delay in changes in risk factor levels occurs. Changes in morbidity and mortality rates are usually not detectable until several years have passed.

During the last 20 years only a few large, community-oriented, intervention studies have been conducted in the United States and in Europe (see Table 12.1). The objective of these studies was to reduce the occurrence of cardiovascular diseases and some other

Table 12.1 Community trials on cardiovascular disease prevention

Study		Net risk factor changes		

North Karelia Project (Vartiainen *et al.* 1994)

		After 20 years		
Start/duration:	1972; 10 years intervention		Men	Women
Population:	180 000 inhabitants, ages 25–59 years	Cholesterol	4.0%	−1.4%
Intervention:	comprehensive community intervention, reduction of cardiovascular risk factors	Smoking	−14.0%	−2.7%
		SBP	−0.7%	−3.3%
Design:	one intervention, one (later two) reference group(s)	DBP	2.1%	−1.0%
Evaluation:	three (later five) independent samples			
Results:	after 20 years still a decline in risk factors observed; initially stronger decline in total mortality, after 15 years similar as rest of Finland			

Coronary Risk Factor Study (CORIS) (Rossouw *et al.* 1993)

		After 4 years		
Start/duration:	1979; 4 years intervention			Men	Women
Population:	11 700 white persons, ages 15–64 years	Cholesterol	L	−0.4%	−0.6%
Intervention:	comprehensive community intervention, small mass media and		H	1.5%	1.5%
	interpersonal (high intense) intervention; reduce cholesterol BP, smoking,	Smoking	L	1.8%	−17.4%
	stress, increase physical activity		H	1.7%	−22.9%
		SBP	L	−2.0%	−2.4%
			H	1.9%	−1.1%
Design:	two intervention groups (one low intensity, one high intensity intervention),	DBP	L	−4.3%	−3.7%
	one reference group		H	−5.2%	−3.2%
Evaluation:	independent and cohort samples before and after	BMI	L	−0.4%	−2.0%
	intervention, surveys at 4-year intervals planned		H	−0.4%	−1.2%
Results:	low intensity intervention achieves as much reduction of risk factors as high intensity, mortality evaluation pending				

Stanford Five City Project (Farquhar *et al.* 1990)

		After 6 years		
Start/duration:	1980; 5 years intervention		Cohort	Independent
Population:	122 800 persons, ages 12–74 years			
Intervention:	comprehensive community intervention; reduce cholesterol,	Cholesterol	−2%	−2%
	BP, smoking, weight, increase physical activity	Smoking	−13%	0%
		SBP	−4%	−4%
Design:	two intervention groups, two reference groups, one for mortality and morbidity	DBP	−5%	−5%
	trend monitoring, based on Three Communities Study	BMI	−0%	−2%
		Pulse	−3%	−3%
Evaluation:	2 year distances independent and cohort samples			
Results:	reduction in some risk factors and total mortality risk score—15%, not significant in independent samples			

Minnesota Heart Health Program (Luepker *et al.* 1994)

		After 7 years		
Start/duration:	1980; 5–6 years intervention		Cohort	Independent
Population:	231 000 adults			
Intervention:	improve health behaviour,	Cholesterol	1.4%	0.5%
	reduce cholesterol, 7 mg/dl, BP 2 mmHg,	Smoking		
	smoking 3%, increase physical activity	Men	9.5%	−1.2%
	50 kcal/day, reduce cardiovascular disease morbidity and	Women	3.2%	−12.1%
	mortality 15%	SBP	1.1%	0.7%
Design:	three intervention groups, three reference groups, matched on size,	DBP	0.8%	−0.3%
	type, and distance from Minneapolis	BMI	0.1%	−1.2%
Evaluation:	independent and cohort samples	PA	9.4%	6.3%
Results:	not successful in reducing risk factors more than favourable secular	Risk score	3.4%	2.8%
	trends, mortality evaluation pending			

Pawtucket Heart Health Study (Carleton *et al.* 1995)

		After 8.5 years		
Start/duration:	1981; 7 years intervention		Cohort	Independent
Population:	72 000 working class people			
Intervention:	community activation	Cholesterol	−0.7%	0.1%
Design:	one intervention group, one reference group	Smoking	−4.1%	0.9%
Evaluation:	formative and process evaluation,	SBP	0.5%	−2.1%
	six biennial household surveys	DBP	−0.9%	−1.6%

Study	Net risk factor changes		

Results:	small insignificant reductions in chol and BP; not successful in maintaining CVD risk reduction	BMI	0.0%	−0.8%
		Risk score	−25.6%	−21.7%

German Cardiovascular Prevention Study (Hoffmeister *et al.* 1995)

After 7 years

			Men	Women
Start/duration:	1984; 7 years intervention			
Population:	500 000 persons target population,	Cholesterol	−1.9%	−1.8%
	ages 25–69 years	Smoking	−9.7%	−1.8%
Intervention:	comprehensive community intervention;	SBP	−1.6%	−2.4%
	reduce cholesterol 3.5%, BP 1.5%	DBP	−1.6%	−2.3%
	smoking 7.5%, BMI 1%, mortality 8%,	BMI	0.4%	−0.3%
Design:	six intervention groups (pooled representative for Germany), one reference group (total of Germany)			
Evaluation:	three independent samples			
Results:	significant reductions of risk factors except BMI, risk score lowered, mortality evaluation pending			

Kilkenny Health Project (Shelley *et al.* 1995)

After 8 years

			Men	Women
Start/duration:	1985; 8 years intervention			
Population:	70 000 persons	Cholesterol	5.8%	−0.7%
Intervention:	comprehensive community intervention	Smoking	6.2%	−8.8%
Design:	one intervention, one reference	SBP	0.0%	−0.7%
Evaluation:	independent samples	DBP	7.2%	2.4%
Results:	(preliminary) not successful through stronger changes in reference and too weak intervention, although some reduction of risk factors in women	BMI	−2.2%	−3.5%

Washington Heights–Inwood Healthy Heart Program (Shea *et al.* 1992)

Duration:	7 years intervention
Population:	240 000 Hispanics in New York
Evaluation:	process evaluation

Eberbach–Wiesloch Study (Nüssel 1985)

Design:	two intervention groups, one reference group

Pennsylvania County (Community) Health Improvement Project (CHIP) (Schechter, *et al.* 1982)

Design:	one intervention group, one reference group

North Coast Project (Australia) (Egger *et al.* 1983)

Duration:	4 years intervention
Design:	two intervention groups, one reference group; reduce smoking

Swiss National Research Program (Gutzwiller *et al.* 1985)

Duration:	3 years intervention
Design:	two intervention groups, two reference groups

Martignacco Project (Italy) (Feruglio *et al.* 1983)

Duration:	15 years intervention
Design:	one intervention group, one reference group, cohort evaluation only
Results:	SBP −5 (mmHg), DBP −3 (mmHg), cholesterol −14 (mg/dl), BMI −0.36 (kg/m²), total CHD risk −30%, successful but strong cohort effects and small population

Di.S.Co. Project (Italy) (Giampaoli *et al.* 1991)

Population:	25 706 males and females, ages 20–69 years
Design:	one intervention group, one reference group

WHO European Multifactorial Prevention Trial (World Health Organization European Collaborative Group 1983)

Duration:	6 years intervention
Population:	63 000 male employees, ages 40–59 years, from England and Wales, Belgium, Italy, Poland, and Spain
Intervention:	community plus high-risk approach (medications)

Net change = (level intervention last year/level intervention first year − level reference last year/level reference first year) × 100.
Significance levels are not provided because the studies used different statistical test, making a direct comparison difficult.
SBP, systolic blood pressure; DBP, diastolic blood pressure; BMI, body mass index; PA, physical activity; BP, blood pressure; L, low risk; H, high risk.

chronic diseases in large populations by means of primary prevention. These studies represent a logical consequence of the modern understanding of 'civilization disease' patterns and their development in industrial societies. Nevertheless, many intervention studies report only limited changes in indicators of risk, morbidity, and mortality. This is not necessarily due to a general failure of community-based intervention. More research is needed considering the most effective and efficient ways to change the population's health behaviour. In addition, in some studies the apparent lack of success may result from methodological problems.

The final evaluation of an intervention trial should not only be focused on outcome variables but should include issues such as social and structural characteristics of the intervention communities which determine strongly the outcome of intervention. The intensity and density of the intervention and the statistical power of the samples should be optimized. Variances in health indicators within the communities should be estimated before initiation of the trial. The main concerns in the design and the evaluation of community intervention trials will be elucidated below.

Rationale of community intervention trials

Health promotion within the structure of communities or regions seems to be a good strategy to reduce civilization diseases. It is hypothesized that this approach has advantages compared to both individual treatment and to large national programmes (which often lack components that fit to the individual). In this context several statements have to be considered.

1. Most people in a community need a greater knowledge about health issues before they are likely to change unhealthy behaviour.

2. A change to a healthier lifestyle is beneficial, not only for high-risk persons but for all inhabitants of a community.

3. In Western societies most people have one or more elevated risk factors for cardiovascular (and other chronic) diseases. A reduction of these risk factors is likely to have a large impact on the health status of populations.

4. Programmes and activities to promote health will not only prevent the diseases focused for intervention but will also affect many other disease outcomes. For example, healthy lifestyle campaigns directed towards smoking cessation, reduction of alcohol consumption, increased vegetable consumption, and physical activity are useful in preventing many civilization diseases (cardiovascular diseases, major forms of cancer, adult onset diabetes, and the chronic diseases of the respiratory and digestive tract).

5. An action centre implemented in the community initiating, conducting, and co-ordinating health-oriented programmes is an important tool to improve the health status of a community.

6. Structures already existing within communities such as schools, sports grounds, clubs, health facilities, and community leaders will facilitate health promotion and preventive

measures and make them more cost-effective compared to health promotion only focused on individuals.

7. An individual is usually influenced by the community in which he or she lives. Health improving activities within the community will encourage personal involvement in health-related issues.

8. A broad public acceptance of health programmes and projects supported by the local opinion leaders will enhance confidence in the benefit of such activities and will make it easier for individuals to accept and use them.

Objectives of community intervention trials

The typical conditions of social life and the environment in a community often determine the objectives and the likelihood for success of community intervention. The overall health in such a community is influenced by many aspects such as knowledge, awareness, and behaviour of the individuals, health facilities, and provisions within the communities (health-oriented activity groups, hospitals, sports grounds, etc.) and the specific risk profile of this community (mean risk factor levels and specific morbidity and mortality). Since these aspects interact with each other, the community intervention measures should try to influence all necessary aspects to improve health.

A positive preventive climate has to be created within a community. This process of changes in particular health aspects should be followed in intervention trials (in subsequent time periods). In community intervention trials this 'process evaluation' has not often been used, although it could give a deeper insight into the influence of intervention on the process and determinants of health changes than solely measuring the outcome does. The achievement of the objectives can be observed by specific outcome measurements, which reflect the changes of various health aspects (see Fig. 12.1).

Improvement of health knowledge, health attitudes, and health behaviour

Instead of concentrating on an individual's behaviour, community intervention is concerned with the manipulation of health knowledge, health attitudes, and health behaviour in whole communities. Thus, an important goal of community intervention is to achieve a favourable change in these health aspects in the whole population or larger groups within the population.

A primary target of community intervention studies is a verifiable improvement of health knowledge in the community which should be maintained for a long period of time. This does not guarantee improved health, but it supports all the other efforts to achieve a better health behaviour. A change in health knowledge within the community is one of the earliest detectable effects of community intervention.

Changes in attitudes and beliefs are further aims of community intervention. Attitudes and beliefs are not always in accordance with the prevailing knowledge. Although many attitudes may be based on a certain knowledge, such a knowledge is not a necessary condition for health attitudes and beliefs. A community can have developed certain health attitudes (such as 'too much coffee is bad for your heart') without knowing why the behaviour is unhealthy (it increases serum cholesterol level). On the contrary, a gain of

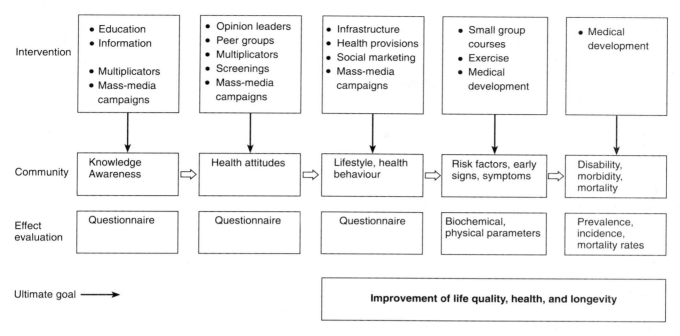

Fig. 12.1. Elements, pathways, and outcomes of community intervention.

knowledge does not always change a person's attitude. Although a certain behaviour (such as smoking) may be generally accepted as harmful, it is not necessarily regarded as a risk for oneself ('my grandfather smoked his whole life and lived until 90'). Changes in attitudes and beliefs can also be observed as early effects in intervention populations.

The most difficult to achieve objective of intervention actions and programmes is to gain significant influence on the health behaviour of a larger part of the population in a community. Although a change in knowledge and attitude could be reached, the past experience of community intervention trials shows that changes in behaviour with a high impact on health (such as smoking, alcohol drinking, nutritional habits, and physical activity) are difficult to achieve and are even more difficult to maintain over a long period of time.

Societal conditions

An improvement of health knowledge, health attitudes, and health beliefs does not inevitably lead to changes in behaviour. These changes can only occur if the community's health infrastructure is appropriate (that is, enough health-related information sources, courses to stop smoking or other drug consumption, availability of fresh vegetables, low fat products, sports grounds, and so on). If the infrastructure is not sufficient, an improvement in it should be an additional target of intervention. Societal characteristics of a community should therefore be analysed and taken into account before starting with a community intervention project.

Behaviour changes are difficult to achieve even in communities with a well-established infrastructure to enhance and maintain health. This becomes obvious by looking at smoking behaviour. The majority of people are aware that active smoking is the most dangerous single health risk of advanced societies. Still, a large number of people in our population smoke. This discrepancy between health knowledge and attitudes was also observed in a German study examining pupils. All of the pupils who smoked on a regular basis knew about the main diseases caused by smoking. However, despite this knowledge 20 per cent of the subjects wanted to continue smoking. Those 80 per cent answering they would like to stop smoking or reduce it are more susceptible to programmes, courses, and other community activities about smoking cessation.

Risk factors, early signs, and symptoms

Altered behaviour should lead to a measurable change in physical risk factors. Changes in classical risk factors such as obesity, high blood pressure, hypercholesterolaemia, unfavourable levels of specific liver enzymes (as indicators of alcohol consumption), and a high resting heart rate (as an indicator of poor physical fitness) can give important indications of the success of intervention. To achieve favourable changes in risk factors is the most common and verifiable goal of community intervention. It is assumed that a favourable change of risk factor levels or of early signs and symptoms of diseases will improve the health of a population. A community intervention trial is needed to prove this assumption.

The interdependency of risk factor changes and sometimes contrasting impacts on different disease outcomes, complicates the determination of overall success. An improvement of certain risk factors may induce an undesirable trend in others. Several studies observed an increase in body mass index among people who stopped smoking. Measures to reduce a risk factor may not be beneficial for the prevention of all diseases. Individuals with high levels of cardiovascular risk factors have an increased risk of developing coronary heart disease and premature death. Replacing a high amount of saturated fatty acids by polyunsaturated fatty acids in the diet leads to lowered serum cholesterol levels. This is a favourable change concerning the development of atherosclerosis and cardiovascular diseases, but the results of several long-term studies suggest that there is an increased cancer rate among individuals who eat a higher amount of polyunsaturated fatty acids.

Another controversial issue is the moderate intake of alcohol, in particular red wine, which seems to reduce the chance of getting ischaemic heart disease. On the other hand, alcohol consumption is assumed to increase the risk of certain cancers.

Several hypotheses about causal links between certain risk factors and the development of disease have been suggested but many could not be confirmed. The objective to achieve a reduction of risk factor levels solely should therefore be handled with caution. For example, at present, there is controversy among health scientists whether a regular intake of higher amounts of antioxidants (such as tocopherol, vitamin C, provitamin A, and selenium) has a preventive effect on cancer and cardiovascular diseases. As long as convincing evidence for a causal link is missing, it is not regarded as necessary to recommend a higher daily antioxidant intake.

Morbidity and mortality rates

The improvement of a healthy lifestyle and of risk factors is just a necessary step on the way to the crucial objective. The final success of a community intervention programme has to be analysed on the basis of changes in disability, morbidity, and mortality rates. At the community level, these outcomes are usually measured by prevalence rates, incidence rates, lost years of life, mean age at onset of disease, or mean age at death from a specific disease. Improvement of the quality of life may be measured as well as the mean years of disease-free life of a population. Changes in specific mortality rates as well as in morbidity rates and premature disabilities are important outcomes of community intervention. These outcomes are often overlooked in the evaluation of community trials, although they can largely contribute to healthy life expectancy.

In addition, the intervention should have a positive impact on total mortality. A successful reduction of coronary heart disease mortality through intervention should, for example, not be accompanied by higher cancer mortality rates. A real improvement of health can only be ascertained if total mortality rates are decreased and life expectancy is improved.

Most civilization diseases occur at older ages. To reach this group of people through community intervention and to have an essential influence on the morbidity and mortality of very old people, seems hardly possible. For example, high mortality rates of cardiovascular diseases occurring at old age in a society are not alarming but, on the contrary, provide an indication of superior health status and medical care in this society. Health promotion cannot prevent all diseases and will not lead to immortality. The purpose of the intervention measures is to reduce the occurrence of diseases and deaths early in life. In the Western world this means a reduction of mortality and morbidity before reaching the age of 70 to 80 years. Thus, this should be a criterium to measure the success of intervention, which is possible in a well-designed trial.

Early estimate of mortality outcome: the multiple logistic function

As mentioned before, the final evaluation of success of community trials should be based on the changes in premature morbidity and mortality of the disease(s) of interest and total mortality. In practise, this can only be evaluated after a long time period in which the detectable changes in disease rates will occur. Changes in risk factor levels will occur much earlier. For example, the elevated risk of smoking on lung cancer will remain for approximately 10 to 20 years after smoking cessation (for cardiovascular disease, the risk will drop faster). Consequently, most researchers want to summarize risk factor changes to predict changes in morbidity or mortality in the long run. The project financiers and health politicians are also eager to get an early estimate of the success of the intervention programme.

A classical tool to summarize the changes in risk factor levels is the 'multiple logistic function'. Such a function weighs the changes in major risk factors according to their importance as contributors to mortality risk. The weighting factors are derived from multiple logistic regressions of longitudinal mortality data. Multiple logistic functions are applied by many epidemiologists to estimate mortality risk from measured risk factors.

Although these functions are widely used for a summary evaluation of risk factor changes, one has to be careful when applying them. The estimated weights (from a different population) may not reflect the impact of risk factors on mortality in the observed population. The logistic model does not consider follow-up time and censoring (due to unfinished observation times for drop-outs and individuals still alive). Basically, a multiplicative effect of risk factors is assumed, which is, for instance, not appropriate for coronary heart disease (CHD) risk factors. Inclusion of new risk factors will therefore change the estimates of the others. The estimated function is likely to be more a reflection of the model than of the data. Recent multiple logistic functions are based on more sophisticated proportional hazard models (Cox and Oakes 1984).

Intervention in communities

The development of chronic, civilization-associated diseases early in life may result from unhealthy behaviour patterns and unfavourable life conditions. A major fraction of the population shows such behaviours. Therefore, health promotion and disease prevention programmes try to manipulate these behaviours and try to establish structures which support a healthy lifestyle.

Communities as the field of intervention activities

Communities play a key role in the realization of intervention measures. They are the field in which most events of social life take place. They provide the structures and institutions for daily life. The local media are, for example, effective instruments to spread health-related information. Churches, schools, sports clubs, and other organizations meeting regularly are important institutions in creating a positive intervention climate and establishing norms and reinforcing them frequently. The health system and the food supply system can also be used for purposes of health promotion.

Available health structures, information resources, and persons and groups with influence and credibility within the community are important tools in reaching the study goals in community intervention trials. They will provide the conditions by which a larger population can be exposed to messages about healthy lifestyles, get involved in health topics, and experience the advantages of improved health behaviour. Different methods of communication, education, and advertising concerning health issues can be

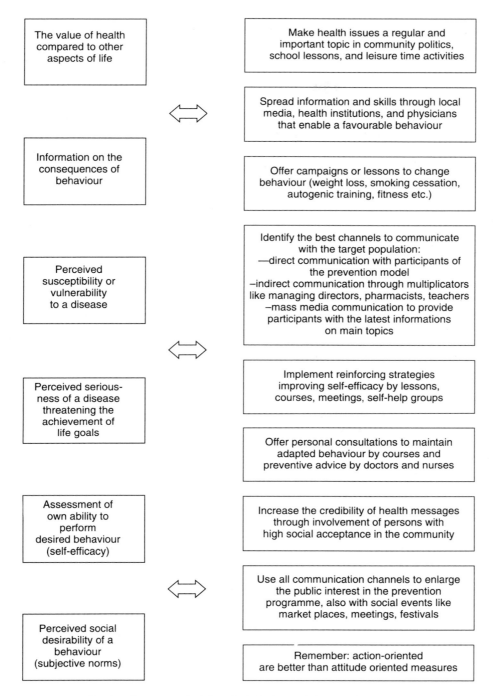

Fig. 12.2. Focus points for influencing behaviour and elements of intervention.

used to achieve an improvement in health knowledge, health attitudes, and health behaviour.

Theories and frameworks focused on community intervention trials

Intervention methods and activities in community studies should have a theoretical foundation. Social science research has provided profound experience about the psychological and sociological mechanisms by which new norms in daily life can be achieved and propagated, new fashions can be created, and more involvement in

health issues can be generated in populations. Different social theories and frameworks attempt to explain individual behaviour as well as trends and fashions of populations. All of these general behaviour theories can be applied to health-relevant issues. They should be used to define a set of measurements in a community intervention study. Important points and elements applicable to community intervention are listed in Fig. 12.2.

One of the earliest and most often applied theories is the 'social cognition theory' (formerly social learning theory) (Bandura 1986). The focal point of this theory is that a change of behaviour can be achieved through intensive exposure to important models (ideals and archetypes, such as pop stars and sport stars). Self-efficacy (for which elements are self-esteem, self-regard, self-respect, self-confidence, competence, and effective functioning) and group efficacy play an important role in changing behaviour. It is influenced by own, observed, or otherwise transferred experiences. Further, according to this theory, for maintenance of a newly adapted behaviour, a supportive social setting and the development of skills are needed.

To adopt this framework for health purposes, opinion leaders in a community (for example, the mayor, the medical professionals, and a local sport star) should be involved in intervention management. They should convincingly and repeatedly appeal to the public about smoking cessation, less fat consumption, more physical activity, and so on. In addition, skill training should be organized within communities.

The 'theory on reasoned action' later 'theory of planned behaviour', which analyses and predicts behaviour, was mainly developed by Ajzen and Fishbein and extended by Ajzen and Madden (1986). This framework concentrates on establishing the credibility of persons distributing information about (health) issues, favourable life-style, and disease prevention measures. The theory suggests that individuals pass through a series of steps from awareness, attitudes, and knowledge, acquisition through motivation and skill development, and, finally, take action and change behaviour. The prevailing subjective norms in the community have a high impact on health behaviour of its members. Perceived behaviour control is the ability to cope with difficulties by adapting positive behaviour. To sustain adapted behaviour, skills for self-management have to be learned. The theory can be used in community intervention trials by regularly distributing information about healthy lifestyles in media with high credibility (such as local press and television).

'Persuasive communication' campaigns (McGuire 1984) try to convince individuals to take more responsibility for their own health maintenance. Based on psychological theories concerning communication, attitudes, and behaviour, it proposes a seven-step procedure. These seven steps are

1. reviewing the realities;

2. axiological analysis;

3. surveying the sociocultural situation;

4. mapping the mental matrix;

5. teasing out the target themes;

6. construction of the communication;

7. evaluating the effectiveness.

The sixth step is the crucial one, because it is the practical application. It uses a communication set containing aspects such as credibility, attractiveness, and power. Elements mediating the communication such as exposure, skill acquisition, and motivation are also implemented in this framework.

The 'precede–proceed model' (**P**redisposing, **R**einforcing, and **E**nabling **C**onstructs in **E**ducational–**e**nvironmental **D**iagnosis and **E**valuation and **P**olicy, **R**egulatory and **O**rganizational **C**onstruct in **E**ducational and **E**nvironmental **D**evelopment; Green and Kreuter 1991) for educational intervention is a framework to plan and administer health education programmes. It begins with five phases in the precede process: social, epidemiological, behavioural/environmental, educational/organization, and administration/policy diagnosis. The proceed process follows with implementation, process, impact, and outcome evaluation. This plan of action covers the multidimensionality of health and its large number of collaborators.

'Social marketing theories' analyse the needs of a target population (Kotler and Clarke 1987). They then offer the adequate products and define the costs and benefits for provider and consumer. Preventive health services are products, for which the audience has to be defined, messages should be developed, and most effective channels for acceptance have to be selected. These theories combine and apply elements of the theories and frameworks mentioned before.

Study design

The community intervention study has a quasi-experimental design. It is experimental in the sense that the observer manipulates the intervention community with public health programmes and observes the changes in the population against a reference (without such manipulation). It is quasi-experimental in so far as the observer cannot control for every exposure or health-related change in the intervention or in the reference community.

A well-chosen study design can partly prevent such unwanted confounding exposures and will control more efficiently for unknown or unexpected influences on the population's health. Observing several intervention versus reference communities which are spread over the region of interest is one possibility of ruling out initial inequalities and lowering the chance of unexpected confounding trends between the intervention and reference areas. This can also be achieved by taking 'embedded' intervention communities out of a larger region which may serve as a reference.

The choice of intervention and reference populations

Theoretically, a design for a community intervention trial should consist of a group of communities randomly chosen out of a country or region of interest. The chosen units should by chance be assigned as intervention or reference units.

If the findings of an intervention programme are intended to be applied to a larger population in future, they should reflect this population. The units must represent the main health relevant differences within the country or region. Depending on the infrastructure of the country it should include rural regions, middle-sized towns, and (parts of) large towns. Inhabitants within those units should reflect socio-economic groups and the variety in life-style. The samples of such intervention and reference regions then would allow generalization of the outcomes of intervention measures to the total population. From a health policy perspective this would be an important aspect of a community intervention study. This type of study would have the additional advantage of avoiding a wrong interpretation of results due to unknown secular trends and variance of outcome variables.

Such a design, although desirable from a scientific perspective, is often not feasible for many practical reasons. It requires a complex organization and logistical support and would be very expensive. After a long period of intervention and evaluation no major health impact might be visible and the cost-effectiveness might be unfavourable.

Therefore, in most conducted trials, one or only a few regions were taken as intervention and reference areas. Table 12.1 shows the main characteristics of the major cardiovascular disease community intervention studies. The number of selected communities, size of intervention populations, intervention and observation period, and other typical issues are described. In most of the conducted community intervention trials between one and three cities or parts of cities were chosen as intervention units and one or two as reference cities.

In such a situation, it is even more important to ensure that the reference community resembles the intervention community as closely as possible. Both regions should be identical in respect to socio-demographic structure, initial risk factor levels, and mortality risks. In practice, however, the researcher is not free to choose appropriate communities. Reasons for this can be the need for intervention due to high cardiovascular mortality risk, the near distance to the intervention centre or research group, or the pressure to conduct intervention from the public or community leaders of a certain region.

The appropriate reference should also be chosen carefully. The need for similarity with the intervention community often makes it necessary to find a region in proximity, although this may raise specific problems. Unexpected changes in health status or health perspectives can occur due to other interventive measures in the reference community. Spill-over of information and cognition from the intervention population, changes in socio-economic conditions such as increasing unemployment, changes in the health care system or improvement of medical diagnoses, and spontaneous lifestyle change due to health-relevant events can occur in the reference community. For example, when a local individual or team becomes a sport champion in a certain sport and gains popularity, many inhabitants may start to participate in this sport. Such changes can also occur in the intervention population, independently of the intervention efforts.

Secular trends in the reference population could differ from the intervention population. Such differences cannot be detected from initial levels of risk factors. Several of these unwanted coinciding changes are unlikely to occur when a nested design is chosen. This can be realized, if the pre- and post-surveys are representative independent samples of the whole nation and the intervention population is an independent representative (clustered) sample of the total population of this nation. This was the case in the German Cardiovascular Prevention Study (**GCP**) (see Table 12.1; Hoffmeister *et al.* 1996). In this study, six intervention communities and rural regions scattered over the country were selected. The pooled intervention units closely represent the German population by age, gender, and socio-economic status. The risk factor means of the pooled intervention regions were nearly identical to those of the national reference at the start of the study. Although there were differences in the initial levels between the six single regions, the close resemblance of the risk factor means between the pooled intervention regions and the reference shows convincingly that the chosen regions together represent the German health conditions. Figure 12.3 gives an impression of the magnitude of differences

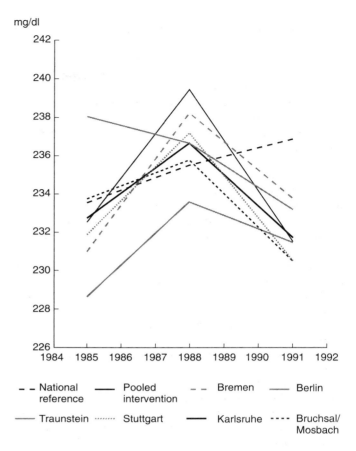

Fig. 12.3. Changes in mean total serum cholesterol values (GCP study 1984–92).

occurring between communities or regions due mainly to socio-economic and cultural settings. The mean levels of total serum cholesterol in the six intervention regions of the GCP are presented as an example (corrected for differences in age and gender distribution). The figure also shows that for this risk factor the intervention had a delayed impact. Often the financial aspects of such a widespread reference will force projects to use a different reference design. National representative surveys, however, can also be used as national health surveys.

Survey sampling

Population surveys should be conducted before, during (often at midtime), and after the intervention programme. An additional survey, some years after the end of intervention measures, could give insight into the endurance and implementation of improved health behaviour. The surveys should preferably be independent samples with the same age and socio-economic distributions. Ideally, the samples for both intervention and reference communities should be random, representative, or stratified samples of the community. In a situation where intervention programmes focus on certain risk groups (age, ethnic, or socio-economic), it might be more effective to restrict the sample to this target population. Usually community intervention is directed towards the whole population but the disease of interest is only restricted to a certain group (for example 40- to 60-year age groups for coronary heart disease). Then again it would be appropriate to sample just this group.

The researcher should make a great effort to achieve maximal response rates in the survey samples. To avoid a substantial bias, the response rate should be at least 70 per cent. Non-respondents can differ considerably from (primary) respondents in health behaviour and sensitivity to health intervention programmes. For a valid evaluation of the intervention-related changes it is therefore most important to achieve a high response rate. Non-respondents should be contacted repeatedly to persuade them to participate in the surveys. At the least, minimal information about non-respondents should be gathered, for instance through a short questionnaire. This should provide some information about the difference between non-respondents and the participants.

The attempts to enlarge the response rate should be equal in both the intervention and the reference communities. If response rates between the intervention and reference communities differ considerably, this response bias could have major consequences for the evaluation of the intervention trial. In the German national health surveys, for example, the smoking prevalence among spontaneous respondents (first 50 per cent of the sample) was 1 to 2 per cent lower compared to the next 20 per cent of respondents. Fortunately, the non-respondents did report a no higher smoking prevalence in a short questionnaire.

The use of a cohort sample may have a serious impact on observed risk changes, which possibly restricts the intervention evaluation. Repeated screenings are powerful intervention measures themselves. They induce a strong version of the so-called 'Hawthorne' effect. People aware that they are under study are likely to change their behaviour in a positive way. The screening effect of the cohort survey thus can affect the health behaviour of the participants independent of the intervention programme or could make them react differently to the intervention programme. Therefore, an unbiased estimate of the impact of intervention on the total community is not possible.

On the other hand, in contrast to cross-sectional independent samples, cohort samples may provide information about the persons who are susceptible to intervention. In this way, a better evaluation of the intervention programme is possible because the subpopulations which have responded to intervention can be identified. It may also give information about the parts of the intervention programme which were most effective. Ideally, a cohort sample is drawn in combination with independent cross-sectional samples, so the advantages of both designs can be used.

An attempt to minimize the effect of repeated screenings among cohorts was made in the Minnesota Heart Health Study (Luepker et al. 1994) by repeating the surveys for one half of the cohort after 2 years and for the other half after 4 years (midtime samples). Finally, the complete cohort sample was remeasured after 7 years of intervention. Whether this really eliminates a cohort screening effect, however, is not clear. This study additionally included independent cross-sectional samples.

Problems with secular trends

For several risk factors as well as for specific morbidity and mortality rates, a gradual up- or downward trend over long periods of time (decades) occurs in various countries and regions. This phenomenon is referred to as the secular trend.

Health behaviours, for example smoking prevalences, will also follow trends, although they have rarely been documented. The outcome variables in community intervention trials therefore have to be controlled for such trends. An intervention programme has to be successful in modifying these secular trends in a favourable direction. An intervention effect will be validated by comparing it with the secular trend estimated from the reference communities. In the GCP study, risk factor changes of the six pooled intervention regions were corrected for the national secular trends by using the total nation as the reference population. The magnitude of a secular trend in a large population can be seen from the reference trend in Fig. 12.3.

In the case of small communities a good estimate of secular trends may be a problem. An observer should have carefully gathered information about the secular trends in life-style and risk factors they want to modify before the initiation of the intervention programme. If there is already a very sharp decline in their levels, it will be difficult to modify this change additionally by intervention.

In the North Karelia Project (see Table 12.1), the Finnish North Karelia region was chosen as an intervention area because it had the highest cardiovascular mortality rates worldwide at the beginning of the study. The public awareness of and concern about this fact might have had an influence on the life-style and health behaviour changes of the North Karelian inhabitants. This already initiated favourable secular trend cannot be separated from the intervention effects. In North Karelia the favourable trend in risk factors as well as in cardiovascular morbidity and mortality rates continued several years after the intervention measures had stopped. The occurrence of cardiovascular diseases was lower in the reference region and it is not assumed that there was such a strong decreasing secular trend in the reference region (Kuopio). Differences in secular trends in the outcome variables (risk factors, cardiovascular morbidity, and mortality rates) observed between North Karelia and Kuopio should therefore be considered as possible explanations in addition to an intervention effect.

Nevertheless, a population being aware of its high cardiovascular disease risk might be more susceptible to health issues and intervention. Thus, it is possible that the intervention is responsible for the downward trends. The design of this project does not allow for relying on a single explanation, although from a public health view the study was very successful.

In contrast to a multicommunity intervention trial or a nested intervention trial, a study based on only one or two matched intervention–reference pairs should be matched for more criteria than described above. The pairs should have the same starting levels of risk factors, morbidity, and mortality rates. If these parameters differ initially, it is an indication of inequalities concerning lifestyles and living conditions between those communities. These differences could also be caused by varying secular trends. Trends (for example, in mortality rates) should ideally be observed in both the intervention and reference regions over several years before starting an intervention to obtain an impression of the grade of congruence of the matched communities.

Efforts to detect weak intervention effects

Unexpected or unknown inequalities between the communities can be responsible for different variances and trends in the outcome parameters. These circumstances, together with the limited population size of the units, make it difficult to draw conclusions and to detect the real intervention effects. As shown by the preliminary results of the Kilkenny Health Project it might happen that in the reference community significantly better trends in risk factors are observed than in the intervention community (see Table 12.1; Shelly *et al.* 1991). It is not very likely that the intervention efforts had a negative influence on the health behaviour in the intervention population, but rather unknown effects may be responsible for these results.

The three major community intervention trials in the USA, the Stanford Five City Project (Farquhar *et al.* 1990), the Minnesota Heart Health Program (Luepker *et al.* 1994), and the Pawtucket Heart Health Study (Carleton *et al.* 1995) did not observe homogeneous and substantial net reductions of risk factors (see Table 12.1), although for single risk factors in selected sex or age groups significant changes occurred. The change in total cardiovascular risk score did not differ significantly between the intervention and reference populations in these trials. A final evaluation on the basis of changes in mortality rates has still to be performed.

The researchers of these three United States intervention trials concluded that the influence of intervention might have been too weak to change behaviour. This conclusion might be true. Contrary to the findings mentioned above, however, the Stanford trial shows favourable net reductions for most of the risk factors, although significant changes could not be ascertained. Perhaps the sample sizes were too small to ascertain the weak net changes that could be achieved in the Stanford study and in several other studies (see Table 12.1). However, even weak risk factor reductions conducted in large populations are likely to contribute substantially to community health.

Evaluation of changes

The complexity of community intervention trials requires evaluation instruments which can measure the various dimensions of possible influences. Changes in health knowledge, health attitudes and health behaviour, means and prevalences of risk factors, and physical symptoms and signs should be followed in the intervention versus reference populations. Specific morbidity as well as the prevalence of pain and life quality are outcomes of interest, which should be evaluated. Finally, the overall impact of intervention has to be evaluated by following specific and total mortality rates. For assessment and explanation of these changes, data on the social environment and economic conditions in communities have to be gathered as well (societal evaluation). The evaluation instruments and methods used in community intervention trials are discussed in the following subsection.

Interview instruments

The main instrument for measuring health knowledge, health attitudes, and individual health behaviour, as well as subjective levels of symptoms, signs, diseases, and quality of life in population samples is the questionnaire. Widely used and validated scales and question blocks from epidemiologic and social science research are available for intervention trials. Self-instructing or interviewer-instructed questionnaires are useful in measuring the following issues and many others in a standardized, reliable, and valid way.

Nowadays, interactive computer questionnaires with integrated quality, plausibility, and validity checks are often used.

The following parameters are assessable through questionnaire:

1. smoking;

2. drinking (including alcohol consumption);

3. food consumption and eating behaviour (with food frequency lists, food protocol, 24-hour recall, and diet history questionnaires);

4. sport and physical activity;

5. prevalence of chronic diseases, symptoms, signs, and pain;

6. medication use;

7. subjective health status and life quality;

8. frequency of visiting physicians, and health institutions;

9. occupation and social status.

Analytic procedures

Physical and biochemical parameters can be measured with high precision and accuracy. Following the principles of good laboratory practice, analytical procedures or measurements will normally result in methodological errors in the range of 2 to 5 per cent. Changes achieved through intervention programmes thus can be determined in representative population samples. The expected changes should be pinpointed at the beginning of the trial. These expected differences should be used for calculating a sample size sufficient to confirm the statistical significance of these differences.

The physical measurements should be performed under the highest quality standards for preanalytical and analytical procedures. Specially trained persons should perform the sampling, storage, and transport of blood and other materials in order to minimize method differences. Altering procedures of blood sampling (such as using the sitting versus the lying position), for example, would lead to unacceptable variances. Since considerable seasonal differences of risk factor levels and behaviour (for example, cholesterol level, nutrition, and physical activity) can occur, the intervention and reference should be sampled during the same time of the year. Clinical analyses should be performed in a central laboratory with internal and external quality controls. In this way methodological differences between laboratories are reduced. A person could systematically measure too high blood pressure values due to his personality ('Rosenthal' effect), so this should be checked and interviewers should be rotated regularly from the intervention to reference samples.

Morbidity and mortality estimates

Despite the generally large populations in intervention studies, objective and complete assessment of disease events by standardized medical examinations is hard to achieve. Only frequently occurring and strictly defined diseases like ischaemic heart disease can be assessed sufficiently well. A continuous registration might be the ideal way to measure morbidity rates. This has, however, not been done in community trials. Morbidity data can also be gathered from practising physicians or from hospitals in the communities. This has to be done with careful monitoring of completeness and comparability of the data.

During morbidity and mortality evaluation, it is also important to ensure that availability of medical services and medical treatment do not differ between intervention and reference populations. Although the impact of curative measures like bypass surgery, programs for early detection of certain cancers (breast, cervix, colon) on morbidity and mortality rates is controversial, it seems likely that improved medical treatment has a positive influence on morbidity and mortality.

Mortality evaluation

Every intervention trial should evaluate disease specific mortality and total mortality rates. Since deaths from certain diseases and even from all causes are rare events, long observation times and large communities are necessary. As with risk factor changes, the expected reduction in mortality by intervention has to be pin-pointed at study start to estimate the necessary community size. In most intervention trials, the total number of mortality cases in the intervention and reference populations are counted and cumulative mortality rates during the study time (extended with a certain period after intervention) are compared. Causes of death can be ascertained from death certificates, hospital records and interviews with relatives. In the GCP the official national and regional (age adjusted) mortality rates from the Federal Statistical Office will be used.

As can be seen from Table 12.1, for most of the major community intervention trials on cardiovascular disease, the mortality evaluation has still to be done. For those who already performed a mortality evaluation (North Karelia Project; Five City Project), no convincing intervention effect could be observed. This may be due to insufficient influence on risk factors and health behaviour by intervention activities as well as uncontrolled secular trends. Problems in evaluating mortality rates can also arise by different developments in the population structure between intervention and reference regions. Thus, not only the mortality cases but also the drop-out and drop-in rates have to be considered. The denominator, which means the living part of population in communities and their movements has to be estimated carefully.

Statistical procedures

The mean levels (or prevalence rates) of outcome variables of the independently drawn samples represent the initial and final health status in the intervention and reference population. In intervention trials with more than two surveys, the additional measurements during intervention time can give insight in the process of intervention induced changes.

The statistical analysis procedures normally derive their statistical power from the number of individuals within the survey samples. The community is the unit of intervention, but changes in response to the intervention programme can only be measured by looking at individuals. This apparently paradoxical situation for the evaluation process limits the use of usual statistical procedures to

measure the changes. Furthermore, the evaluator has to correct for the initial differences between the intervention and reference groups.

The classical way to measure intervention effects is by the use of simple formulas for net changes. Figure 12.4 shows the imaginary risk factor level in the intervention community (I_0) and in the reference (R_0). At the end of the intervention period, the level was changed in the intervention community (I_1) and reference (R_1). In this example a reduction in the intervention community ($I_1 - I_0$) was achieved whereas the level increased in the reference ($R_1 - R_0$). The net change is often expressed as the percentage change in the intervention community minus the percentage change in the reference (formula (a)) which can be rewritten as a substraction of ratios ($I_1/I_0 - R_1/R_0$). Variations of this formula have been used in literature ((b) and (c)) to measure net changes. The second formula has the advantage that it allows a direct estimation of confidence intervals because it is defined as a ratio of ratios. The third formula gives the relative change divided by the baseline level in the reference which is assumed to be the baseline for the total population.

The general procedures used to calculate the net changes in intervention communities assume that baseline differences are still the same at the final measurement in the absence of an intervention programme (see Fig. 12.4). This assumption, however, is not very realistic and will be the exception in health changes within communities. Initial differences between community levels can cause complications for the evaluation. If initially measured levels differ between the observed communities, this can be partly due to chance and it is likely that trends similar to a 'regression to the mean' will occur: strong differences due to chance at a first measurement are likely to become smaller at the second measurement. Moreover, an initially high risk factor level could motivate individuals within the community to change their lifestyle independently of the intervention programme.

In addition, the possible occurrence of a 'ceiling effect' has to be considered: individuals (or parts of communities) with high risk factor levels may have reached their upper limits. A rising secular trend for this group will stagnate. The evaluation analyses would then over- or underestimate the potential of an intervention measure depending on the occurrence of such an effect in the intervention or reference community. In Fig. 12.5 a possible ceiling effect is presented graphically. The level of a certain risk factor at baseline in the reference (R_0) rises further during the intervention period and reaches its biologic upper limit (R_1). The observed net changes ($I_1 - I_0$ versus $R_1 - R_0$) give an underestimation of the 'true' intervention effect which would be observed when no ceiling effect occurred. A larger effect would be measured if, for instance, the reference were to start at a lower baseline level. Of course one can argue that such an effect is a part of nature and an intervention should be successful in altering such 'natural' trends. However, this example illustrates how difficult it may be to detect intervention-based changes in reality. On the contrary, a very healthy population can hardly be improved in their risk factor levels due to a similar effect. Multiple samples between the start and endpoint of intervention and the use of multivariate statistical models can be used to correct for such effects.

An example of a multivariate model to estimate the effect of intervention on various risk factor changes is given in Fig. 12.6.

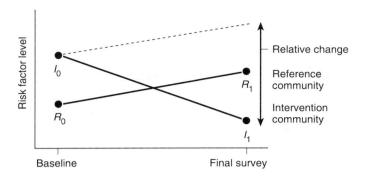

(a) Net change $= \dfrac{I_1 - I_0}{I_0} - \dfrac{R_1 - R_0}{R_0}$ (percentage change in intervention minus percentage change in reference)

$$\Rightarrow \left[\dfrac{I_1}{I_0} - 1 \right] - \left[\dfrac{R_1}{R_0} - 1 \right] \Rightarrow \dfrac{I_1}{I_0} - \dfrac{R_1}{R_0}$$

Multiplicative proposal[1]

(b) Net change $= \dfrac{(I_1 / I_0)}{(R_1 / R_0)} - 1 \Rightarrow \dfrac{I_1 \times R_0}{I_0 \times R_1} - 1$

note: (a) can be written as $\dfrac{1}{R_0} \times \dfrac{I_1 (R_0 - I_0) R_1}{I_0}$

(b) can be written as $\dfrac{1}{R_1} \times \dfrac{I_1 (R_0 - I_0) R_1}{I_0}$; so (a) $= \dfrac{R_1}{R_0}$ (b)

Proposal where reference serves as base level

(c) Net change $= \dfrac{(I_1 - I_0) - (R_1 - R_0)}{R_0} \Rightarrow \dfrac{(I_1 - I_0 - R_1)}{R_0} + 1$

[1]The addition of '−1' makes the direction of the net changes comparable to the other formulas.

Fig. 12.4. Formulas to calculate net changes on the basis of community levels.

Such a model allows correction for different time trends and omits variance problems. Additional corrections for within-community correlations have been proposed by Murray *et al.* (1994). Significant changes in the GCP (using the model in Fig. 12.5) were so evident that no further refinement was considered necessary. Further community intervention research should, however, con-

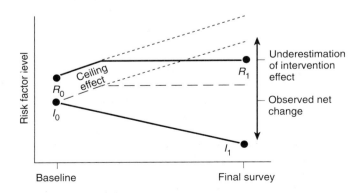

Fig. 12.5. Biased estimate of intervention net change due to 'ceiling effect'.

centrate on stronger methods to improve health behaviour and to reduce risk factor levels in large populations rather than to refine the statistical handling to detect weak effects.

Summary

Various concepts to influence a populations' health behaviour and risk have been developed and are now available. The effectiveness of such strategies for primary prevention in large populations can be tested with community intervention trials. The outcome of important community intervention trials is described and discussed with respect to their design. Such trials raise specific design problems (such as choice of intervention and reference, sampling, and secular trends), because the intervention is conducted and changes are measured at a community level and not at an individual level.

The success of prevention programmes can be measured from changes in health behaviour, risk factor levels, morbidity and mortality of specific diseases (diseases of interest), and total mortality. Process evaluation can give information about how such changes were achieved. For the final evaluation of intervention effects specific statistical methods are available.

$$Y = \text{age} + \text{community} + \text{time}_1 + \text{time}_2 + (\text{community} \times \text{time}_1) + (\text{community} \times \text{time}_2)$$

where

$Y =$	in linear regression: continuous risk factor like systolic BP, cholesterol
	in logistic regression: dichotomous (like smoking, hypertension)
age $=$	age of individual in years at time of observation
community $=$	intervention or reference
$\text{time}_1 =$	sample at midtime or other sample
$\text{time}_2 =$	final sample (after intervention) or other

The interaction terms (multiplicative terms of community $\times$ time$_1$ and community $\times$ time$_2$) represent the intervention effect at midtime and after the intervention period.

Fig. 12.6. Multivariate regression model to estimate intervention effects (Hoffmeister *et al.* 1996).

References

Ajzen, I. and Madden, T.J. (1986). Prediction of goal directed behaviour, attitudes, intentions and perceived behavioural control. *Journal of Experimental Social Psychology*, **22**, 414–53.

Bandura, A. (1986). *Social foundation of thought and action*. Prentice Hall, Englewood Cliffs, NJ.

Carleton, R.A., Lasater, T.M., Assaf, A.R., Feldman, H.A., and McKinlay, S. (1995). The Pawtucket Heart Health Program: community changes in cardiovascular risk factors and projected disease risk. *American Journal of Public Health*, **85/6**, 777–85.

Cox, D.R. and Oakes, D. (1984). *Analysis of survival data*. Chapman & Hall, New York.

Egger, G., Fitzgerald, W., Frape, G. *et al.* (1983). Results of a large scale media antismoking campaign: North Coast "Quit for Life" Programme. *British Medical Journal*, **286**, 1125–8.

Farquhar, J.W., Fortmann, S.P., Flora, J.A., Barr Taylor, C.B., Haskell, W.L., Williams, P.T., *et al.* (1990). Effects of communitywide education on cardiovascular disease risk factors, The Stanford Five-City Project. *Journal of the American Medical Association*, **264/3**, 359–65.

Feruglio, G.A., Vanuzzo, D., Pilotto, L., and Zuliani, A. (1988). The Martignacco Project. In *Comprehensive cardiovascular community control programmes in Europe. EURO Reports and Studies 106*, (ed. P. Puska). pp. 52–8. WHO Regional Office for Europe, Copenhagen.

Giampaoli S., Urbinati G.C., Menotti A., and Ricci G., with the technical assistance of Pasquali, M. and the Research Group of the DISCO Project (1991). Short term changes in cardiovascular risk factors in the DI.S.CO. Intervention Project. *European Journal of Epidemiology*, **7/4**, 372–9.

Green, L. and Kreuter, M. (1991). *Health promotion planning: an educational and environmental approach* 2nd edn. Mayfield Publishing, Palo Alto, Ca.

Gutzwiller, F., Junod, B., and Schweizer, W. (ed.) (1985). *Wirksamkeit der gemeindeorientierten Prävention kardiovaskulärer Krankheiten: Ergebnisse des Nationalen Forschungsprogrammes 1 A – Prävention von Herz-Kreislauf-Krankheiten in der Schweiz*. Verlag Hans Huber, Bern, Stuttgart, Toronto.

Hoffmeister, H., Mensink, G.B.M., Stolzenberg, H., Hoeltz, J., Kreuter, H.,

Laaser, U. *et al.* (1996). Reduction of coronary heart disease risk factors in the German Cardiovascular Prevention Study. *Preventive Medicine*, **25**, 135–45.

Kotler, P. and Clarke, R.N. (1987). *Marketing for health care organizations*. Prentice Hall, Englewood Cliffs NJ.

Luepker, R.V., Murray, D.M., Jacobs, D.R., Mittelmark, M.B., Bracht, N., Carlaw, R. *et al.* (1994). Community education for cardiovascular disease prevention: risk factor changes in the Minnesota Heart Health Program. *American Journal of Public Health*, **84/9**, 1383–93.

McGuire, W.J. (1984). Public communication as a strategy for inducing health promotion behavioural change. *Preventive Medicine*, **13**, 299–319.

Murray, D.M., Hannan, P.J., Jacobs, D.R., McGovern, P.J., Schmid, L, Baker, W.L., and Gray, C. (1994). Assessing intervention effects in the Minnesota Heart Health Program. *American Journal of Epidemiology*, **139/1**, 91–103.

Nüssel, E. (1985). Community-based prevention: the Eberbach-Wiesloch Study. In *Primary and secondary prevention of coronary heart disease*, (ed. H. Hofmann), pp. 50–9. Springer, New York.

Rossouw, J.E., Jooste, P.L., Chalton, D.O., Jordaan, E.R., Langenhoven, M.L., Jordaan, P.C.J. *et al.* (1993). Community-based intervention: the Coronary Risk Factor Study (CORIS). *International Journal of Epidemiology*, **22**, 428–38.

Schechter, C., Stunkard, A.J., and Stolley, P. (1982). The Pennsylvania County Health Improvement Program. *Pennsylvania Medicine*, **85/4**, 18–20.

Shea, S., Basch, C.E., Lantigua, R., and Wechsler, H. (1992). The Washington Heights-Inwood Healthy Heart Program. *Preventive Medicine*, **21/2**, 203–17.

Shelley E., Daly L., Collins, C., *et al.* (1995). Cardiovascular risk factor changes in the Kilkenny Health Project. *European Heart Journal*, **16**, 752–60.

Vartiainen, E., Puska, P., Jousilahti, P., Korhonen, H.J., Tuomilehto, J., and Nissinen, A. (1994). Twenty-year trends in coronary risk factors in North Karelia and in other areas of Finland. *International Journal of Epidemiology*, **23**, 495–504.

World Health Organization European Collaborative Group (1983). Multifactorial trial in the prevention of coronary heart disease: 3. Incidence and mortality results. *European Heart Journal*, **4**, 141–7.

13 Methodology of intervention trials in individuals

Julie E. Buring and Charles H. Hennekens

The intervention study, or clinical trial, is the epidemiological design strategy that, if well designed and conducted, can provide data most closely resembling the controlled experiments performed by basic science researchers (Hennekens and Buring 1987). As in a cohort study, individuals are enrolled on the basis of their exposure status; however, the distinguishing characteristic of an intervention study is that the investigators themselves allocate the exposure. The primary advantage of this feature is that, if the treatments are allocated at random in a sample of sufficiently large size, intervention studies have the potential to provide a degree of assurance about the validity of a result that is simply not possible with any observational design option.

Rarely is the introduction of a new treatment or procedure accompanied by benefits as striking and unequivocal as those that followed the introduction of the antibiotic penicillin or pharmacological treatment of malignant hypertension. A randomized trial of these drugs seemed neither necessary nor, for ethical reasons, desirable, in part because the benefits were so large and immediate that they seemed clearly due to the drugs themselves. Most often, however, the effects of the therapeutic or preventive measures of interest are small to moderate, of the order of 10, 20, or 30 per cent differences in disease outcomes. Such differences can be extremely important from a clinical or public health standpoint, particularly when the outcome of interest relates to a common disease. However, these small to moderate differences are very difficult to establish reliably from observational studies, since the effects of uncontrolled and uncontrollable confounding are likely to be as large as the magnitudes of the postulated effects of the treatment or procedure. In these circumstances a randomized trial will yield the strongest and most direct epidemiological evidence on which to base a judgement of whether an observed association is one of cause and effect.

Types of intervention studies

Intervention studies can generally be considered either therapeutic or preventive. Therapeutic (or secondary prevention) trials are conducted among patients with a particular disease to determine the ability of an agent or procedure to diminish symptoms, prevent recurrence, or decrease risk of death from that disease. For example, to test the therapeutic effects of aspirin, the Aspirin Myocardial Infarction Study (AMIS) randomized 4524 men and women with a history of at least one prior myocardial infarction to either 1g of aspirin daily or placebo and looked at subsequent

occurrence of total mortality and non-fatal reinfarction (AMIS Research Group 1980).

A preventive (or primary prevention) trial involves the evaluation of whether an agent or procedure reduces the risk of developing disease among those free from that condition at enrolment. Primary prevention trials can be conducted among healthy individuals at usual risk or those already recognized to be at increased risk of developing a disease because of the presence of certain factors. An example of the former is the Women's Health Study, a randomized placebo-controlled trial testing the anti-oxidant vitamin vitamin E as well as low-dose aspirin in the primary prevention of cancer and cardiovascular disease among 40 000 apparently healthy American women (Buring and Hennekens 1992). With respect to trials enrolling high-risk participants, the Alpha Tocopherol, Beta Carotene Cancer Prevention Study randomized 29 133 middle-aged male cigarette smokers, who are at high risk of lung cancer, in order to test whether supplements of alpha-tocopherol and beta-carotene reduce the risk of lung cancer (Alpha-Tocopherol, Beta Carotene Cancer Prevention Study Group 1994).

While therapeutic trials are almost always conducted among individuals, primary prevention measures can be studied among either individuals or entire populations. One example of the latter, also termed a community trial, is the Newburgh–Kingston dental caries study, in which one entire community (Newburgh) was allocated at random to receive sodium fluoride added to the water supply, while the other (Kingston) continued to receive water without supplementation (Ast et al. 1950). In this chapter we focus on intervention trials among individuals; trials in which populations are the unit of randomization are the focus of Chapter 12 (Volume 2).

Unique problems of intervention studies

While the investigator is merely a passive observer in observational analytical study designs, there is active assignment of participants to a particular treatment or procedure in the intervention study. Consequently, for reasons of both ethics and feasibility, the timing of a randomized trial is crucial in that there must be sufficient belief in an agent's potential to justify exposing half the trial population to it, and at the same time there must be sufficient doubt about a treatment's efficacy to justify withholding it from the remaining half of the study population. Ethical considerations preclude the evaluation of some treatments or procedures in an intervention study. Certainly, practices or substances already known to be harmful cannot be allocated by an investigator, although such agents can be tested indirectly in trials of their removal, such as the effects of smoking cessation programmes on subsequent morbidity and mortality. Similarly, therapies that have been clearly demonstrated to be beneficial, such as medical treatment of severe hypertension, cannot be withheld from an affected individual. In many instances, however, there is insufficient evidence in either direction. In these circumstances, the question then becomes not whether it is ethical to conduct a trial, but whether it is ethical *not* to proceed with a randomized intervention in order to answer the question definitively.

The widespread adoption of measures by either the medical community or the general public before demonstration of efficacy and safety can cause insurmountable problems of feasibility. It may become difficult to find a sufficiently large population of individuals willing to forgo a treatment or practice believed to be beneficial for the duration of a trial, even if there is no sound evidence to support this view. For example, in recent years there has been growing public awareness concerning the possibility that antioxidant vitamins may reduce risks of developing cancer, cardiovascular disease, or other chronic conditions (Hennekens *et al.* 1994). To date, the scientific evidence for a benefit of antioxidant vitamins is far from conclusive. None the less, from 1988 to 1993 sales of beta-carotene supplements in the United State rose steeply from $7 million to $82 million per year, while sales of vitamin E rose from $260 million to $338 million (*Newsweek* 7 June 1993). If randomized trials testing the possible health benefits of antioxidants are not conducted over the next few years, vitamin consumption may become so generally widespread a practice that it might no longer be feasible to conduct the trials. Reliable evidence on this issue is essential, for if antioxidant vitamins do not reduce disease risk, the proportion of the United States public using them may be too high, while if there is substantial benefit, those not using them may wish to consider doing so. Thus, for reasons of ethics and feasibility, it is best to conduct a randomized trial as soon as there is sufficient evidence to suggest a possible benefit of an agent or procedure, rather than after it gains widespread acceptance and becomes considered standard practice.

Issues in the design and conduct of clinical trials

There are a number of issues to consider in the design and conduct of clinical trials. These include the selection of the study population, allocation of the treatment regimens, maintenance and assessment of compliance, and achieving high and uniform rates of ascertainment of outcomes (Hennekens and Buring 1987).

Selection of a study population

The groups of individuals among whom an intervention study is conducted are derived from a number of interrelated populations, which can be considered as a population hierarchy (Fig. 13.1). The reference population is the general group to whom the investigators expect the results of the particular trial to be applicable. It may include all people if it seems likely that the study findings are universally applicable, or it may be restricted by age, sex, or a

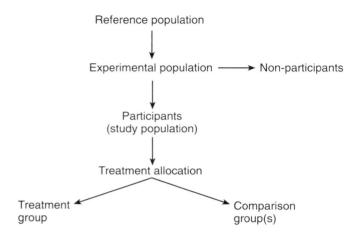

Fig. 13.1 Population hierarchy in an intervention study.

medical characteristic that is thought to modify the existence or magnitude of the effects seen in the trial. Thus the reference population represents the scope of the public health impact of the intervention. For example, the Physicians' Health Study (Steering Committee 1989) is a randomized trial of low-dose aspirin in the reduction of cardiovascular disease and beta-carotene in decreasing cancer incidence which has been ongoing since 1982 among 22 071 male American physicians, aged 40–84 years at baseline. There seems to be no reason to believe that the effects of either aspirin or beta-carotene on cardiovascular disease and cancer would be inherently different among male physicians who participated in the trial than in a comparable group of males who are not physicians or among men who do not live in the United States. Therefore, the reference population of this trial was reasonably felt to include all men 40 years of age and older. However, while some consider the reference population to be as broad as all people over 40 years of age, others have hesitated to make an automatic generalization of the findings of this trial to women. Thus the reference population is related to the issue of generalizability, which involves a judgement about an intervention based on considerations beyond the data from an individual trial.

The experimental population is the actual group in which the trial is conducted. While, in general, it is preferable that this group should not differ from the reference population in such a way that generalizability to the latter is not possible, the primary consideration in the design of the trial should always be to obtain a valid result. The selection of the experimental population is crucial to achieving that aim and involves consideration of several important issues. First, it is essential to determine whether the proposed experimental population is sufficiently large to achieve the necessary sample size for the trial. For example, in considering design features for a trial comparing the relative benefits and risks of the three principal thrombolytic drugs used to treat acute myocardial infarction—streptokinase, tissue plasminogen activator, and anisoylated plasminogen-streptokinase activator complex—a single hospital would certainly not enrol the requisite number of participants to detect the most plausible treatment differences among these drugs, even over a study period of several years. Therefore, to carry out such a trial, more than 900 hospitals in 17 different countries were recruited into an international multicentre trial that randomized more than 41 000 acute myocardial infarction patients (ISIS–3 Collaborative Group 1992).

Analogously, it is essential to choose an experimental population that will experience a sufficient number of the end-points or outcomes of interest to permit meaningful comparisons among various treatments or procedures within a reasonable period of time. For example, the Physicians' Health Study randomized 22 071 male physicians, aged 40–84, in order to assess the primary prevention effects of aspirin on cardiovascular disease. In contrast, the Women's Health Study, a similar primary prevention trial of aspirin among women, needed to randomize approximately 40 000 women, aged 45 or older, to achieve the same aim, since age-specific cardiovascular disease rates in women are lower than those in men (Buring and Hennekens 1994).

A third major concern is the likelihood of obtaining complete and accurate follow-up information for the duration of the trial. A long-term trial conducted among a highly mobile group such as college students or a study requiring frequent clinic visits among a group of infirm elderly subjects might result in low follow-up rates, which would render the findings uninterpretable.

Once the experimental population has been defined, subjects must be invited to participate after being fully informed as to the purposes of the trial, the study procedures, and the possible risks and benefits. The actual study population of a trial is often not only relatively small but also a select subgroup of the experimental population. It is well recognized that those who participate in an intervention study are very likely to differ from non-participants in many ways that may affect the rate of development of the end-points under investigation (Friedman et al. 1985). Among all who are eligible, those willing to participate in clinical trials tend to experience lower morbidity and mortality rates than those who do not, regardless not only of the hypothesis under study but of the actual treatment to which they are assigned (Wilhelmsen et al. 1976). Volunteerism is likely to be associated with age, sex, socioeconomic status, education, and other less well-defined correlates of health consciousness that might significantly influence subsequent morbidity and mortality. Whether the subgroup of participants is representative of the entire experimental population will not affect the validity of the results of a trial conducted among that group. However, it may affect the ability to generalize those results to either the experimental or the reference populations.

If it is possible to obtain baseline data and/or to ascertain outcomes for subjects who are eligible but unwilling to participate, such information is extremely valuable for assessing the presence and extent of differences between participants and non-participants in a particular trial. This will aid in judging to which reference population the results among trial participants are generalizable.

Allocation of study regimens

Since participants and non-participants may differ in important ways related to the outcome under study, allocation to the various treatment groups should take place only after subjects have been determined to be eligible and have agreed to participate. The effects of a treatment, procedure, or programme can be compared with those of one or more of a variety of groups, such as another dosage of the same drug, another therapy or programme, standard medical practice, or a placebo. To maximize the probability that the groups receiving these differing interventions will be comparable,

assignment to a study group should be random. Random assignment implies that each individual has the same chance of receiving each of the possible treatments and that the probability that a given subject will receive a particular allocation is independent of the probability that any other subject will receive the same treatment assignment. This is usually achieved through the use of a table of random numbers or a computer-generated randomization list. When the outcome under study is anticipated to vary appreciably in frequency among subgroups of the study population (for instance between men and women, or by age, or when response is likely to differ markedly between subjects such as those with different severity of disease at entry), the efficiency of the study may be increased by ensuring that treatment groups are approximately equal or balanced with respect to such characteristics. This can be accomplished by a somewhat more complex form of randomization, called blocking, in which every participant is classified with respect to each such variable before allocation and then randomized within the subgroup. Since randomization of large samples virtually guarantees comparability of treatment groups, blocking has particular relevance when the study size is limited (Peto et al. 1976, 1977).

Randomization has many unique advantages when compared with other methods of allocation. First, if randomization is performed properly, nobody either involved in deciding whether a patient is eligible to enter into a trial or responsible for the allocation procedure will know what the assigned treatment group will be. Thus the potential for bias in allocation to study groups is removed and investigators can be confident that observed differences are not due to the selection of particular patients to receive a given therapy. Whenever a system can be predicted, as with the use of other procedures to allocate treatment, there is the potential for manipulation. For example, alternative assignment to study and comparison groups is often used but is always liable to potential bias. Specifically, if two willing and eligible subjects presented at the same time with different prognoses, a physician might, consciously or not, enter them into the study in the order that would allow the more seriously ill patient, for example, to receive the treatment that the physician already believed to be more (or perhaps even less) promising in terms of efficacy or to have fewer side-effects. If a large proportion of subjects were entered in this way, there would be a serious imbalance in the treatment groups with respect to baseline factors that would probably affect the outcome under study. In fact, a truly more promising treatment could appear less effective than the alternative, simply because it was administered to a group less likely to benefit from any form of therapy than the individuals who were systematically assigned to the alternative being studied. Similarly, allocation on the basis of the day of the week is also subject to the potential for systematic bias, particularly for patients presenting at or near midnight.

Another unique advantage of randomization is that, on average, the study groups will tend to be comparable with respect to all factors except for the interventions being studied. 'On average' implies that the larger the sample size, the more successful the randomization process will be in distributing these factors equally among the groups. This feature of randomization is important because all baseline characteristics that differ between the treatment groups and independently affect risk of the outcome under study could potentially confound the relationship between the intervention under study and the disease. However, an even more crucial implication is that, on average, not only will all known confounding variables be equally distributed, but so will all potential confounders that are unknown or unmeasured by the investigator at the time that the trial is initiated. Variables that are not identifiable cannot be dealt with by any analytical procedures. Consequently, the only possible way of achieving control for the influence of unknown variables is through randomization. When the sample size is sufficiently large, both known and unknown confounding factors are distributed equally among treatment groups. Thus randomization can provide a degree of assurance about the comparability of the study groups that is simply not possible in any observational study design.

Finally, a significant advantage of randomization is the deservedly favourable impression that this strategy has on those reading the published results of a trial. When exposure is assigned by a method other than randomization, the burden of proof is on the investigator to show that none of the possible biases in the allocation of patients to a study group or the confounding effects of known or unknown factors that may differ between the study groups account for the observed result. Thus there is an inherent confidence in the results of a well-designed and conducted randomized trial that cannot be achieved with any alternative allocation scheme (Friedman et al. 1985).

A type of non-randomized intervention study that is sometimes seen in the literature is one in which the comparison group is historical. In this instance, the experience of a group of patients allocated to a new agent or procedure is compared with that of other patients who experienced the previous standard form of treatment. In general, such observational comparisons can provide reliable evidence when there is a relatively large effect of the new treatment compared with previous standard therapy. For example, the efficacy of treatment of malignant hypertension was demonstrated by observing a far lower mortality experience among newly treated patients than among those previously untreated (Dustan et al. 1958). However, in the more common circumstance, where the effects of a new intervention are small to moderate in size, it is difficult to distinguish reliably such differences between the study groups. Since data on the new treatment and the standard therapy are collected during two different time periods, there may have been changes in the patient population admitted to the hospital, other advances in diagnostic or treatment methods, or even general modifications of health behaviour. Any or all of these factors may result in changes in the frequency of the disease that are totally unrelated to the intervention being tested.

Maintenance and assessment of compliance

By definition, an intervention study requires the active participation and co-operation of the study subjects. After agreeing to participate, subjects in a trial of medical therapy may deviate from the protocol for a variety of reasons, including developing side-effects, forgetting to take their medication, or simply withdrawing their consent after randomization. Analogously, in a trial of surgical versus medical therapy, those who were randomized to one group may choose to obtain the alternative treatment on their own initiative. In addition, there will be instances where participants cannot comply, such as when the condition of a randomized patient rapidly worsens to the point where surgical therapy becomes

indicated. Consequently, the problem of achieving and maintaining high compliance is an issue in the design and conduct of all clinical trials.

The extent of non-compliance in any trial is related to the length of time that participants are expected to adhere to the intervention, as well as to the complexity of the study protocol. There are a number of possible strategies that can be adopted to try to enhance compliance among the participants in a trial. Selection of a population of individuals who are at increased risk of developing the outcome can enhance compliance rates, since such individuals in general have a much stronger motivation to comply with a study regimen than those at usual risk. Other ways of attempting to increase compliance include frequent contact with participants by home or clinic visits, telephone, or mail; the use of calendar packs of study medication, in which each pill is labelled with the day it is to be taken; and the use of incentives such as the provision of detailed medical information not ordinarily available from their usual source of health care.

Monitoring compliance is important because non-compliance will decrease the statistical power of a trial to detect any true effect of the study treatment. To the extent that participants in the alternative treatment group receive the intervention under study or those in the intervention group do not actually adhere to their assigned regimen, the two groups will become more similar in terms of exposure. Consequently, any true magnitude of effect of the intervention may be obscured. For example, in the Multiple Risk Factor Intervention Trial (MRFIT), 12 866 healthy men, aged 35–57 years, who were at high risk of developing coronary heart disease on the basis of current cigarette smoking, elevated blood pressure, and high blood cholesterol were randomized either to a special intervention programme designed to promote the reduction of these three risk factors or to their usual sources of health care in the community (MRFIT Research Group 1982). After 7 years of follow-up, there was a non-significant 7 per cent decrease in deaths from coronary heart disease in the special intervention group compared with those allocated to usual medical care. The confidence interval for this reduction in risk was very wide and in fact, was compatible with the magnitude of the postulated benefits. One factor that contributed to the inability of the study to detect a significant effect of the special intervention group, despite sizeable reductions in the levels of all three risk factors, was that a large proportion of individuals in the usual care group also stopped smoking, received antihypertensive medication, and lowered their serum cholesterol through weight loss or dietary changes, in large part due to an increasing awareness among the general public of the adverse effects of these risk factors.

The higher the degree of compliance with the offered programme, the greater is the extent to which observed differences between those allocated to alternative therapies reflect real differences in the effects of the treatments themselves. Thus compliance levels must be measured, which is generally not easy. All the measures available to estimate compliance have inherent limitations. The simplest measure is self-report. In fact, for some interventions, such as exercise programmes or behavioural modification, this may be the only practical way to assess compliance. Pill counts, where participants bring unused medication to each clinic visit or return it to the investigators at specified intervals, have been used in trials of pharmacological agents. Although this method may eliminate inaccuracies due to poor memory, it assumes that the subject has ingested all medication that has not been returned to the clinic. A more objective means of assessing compliance, which is also expensive and logistically difficult, is the use of biochemical parameters to validate self-report. Laboratory determinations on either blood or urine can frequently detect the presence of active drugs or metabolites. In cases where drugs or metabolites are difficult to measure, or for subjects taking an inert placebo, a safe biochemical marker such as trace amounts of riboflavin can be added to the treatment. However, laboratory determinations are limited in that usually they can only reflect whether medication was taken in the preceding day or two and thus cannot be used as a reliable measure for long-term compliance.

Inevitably, some proportion of participants in a trial will become non-compliant despite all reasonable efforts. In such instances, maintaining any level of compliance is preferable to complete non-compliance. Moreover, as will be discussed, every randomized subject should be included in the primary analysis of any intervention study, so that it is essential to obtain as complete follow-up information as possible on those who have discontinued the treatment programme. Investigators should pursue follow-up data on outcome for such individuals for the duration of the trial in a manner identical to that for subjects who continue to comply.

Uniform and high rates of ascertainment of outcome

Another crucial issue to be considered in the design and conduct of an intervention study is the ascertainment of the outcome(s) of interest. The primary objective is to ensure that results are not biased by the collection of more complete or accurate information from one or another of the study groups. In addition to the need for uniform ascertainment of outcome, complete follow-up of study participants over the duration of the trial is required. Ascertainment of the outcome of some research questions, such as a study of in-hospital mortality after treatment of acute myocardial infarction or a trial assessing the acute toxicity following administration of a new chemotherapeutic agent, may require only a short follow-up period. In these circumstances, it is often relatively easy to maintain contact with all participants during the entire study period. Often, however, many years of follow-up will be needed, particularly for trials of treatments or other interventions that affect the risk of developing or dying from chronic diseases. As the period of time over which subjects must be followed increases, maintaining complete ascertainment of outcomes becomes more difficult. When outcomes for a small proportion of study subjects are not identified and that proportion is similar for all treatment groups, the magnitude of any potential bias from loss to follow-up is likely to be small. However, if the proportion of outcomes that are not ascertained is large or differs among the study groups, the observed results could be an underestimate, an overestimate, or reflect the true effect simply by chance. To avoid a situation where it is not possible to know the magnitude or direction of the bias, it is crucial to keep the number of individuals lost to follow-up to an absolute minimum. For studies with mortality as an end-point, the availability of the United States National Death Index has enabled researchers, at the very least, to assess the vital status on virtually every individual entered into a trial (Stampfer et al. 1985).

The potential for observation bias in ascertainment of outcome can exist in an intervention trial since knowledge of a participant's treatment status might, consciously or not, influence the identification or reporting of a relevant event. The likelihood of such bias is directly related to the subjectivity of the outcomes under study. If the end-point being considered is total mortality, observation bias is unlikely, since the fact of death is objective and indisputable and cannot be affected by knowledge of a patient's treatment regimen. In contrast, ascertainment of a specific cause of death may be less clear cut and thus may be influenced by a clinician's knowledge of treatment assignment. Moreover, there are trials in which the end-points of interest may include subjective outcomes such as severity of illness, frequency of side effects, increased mobility, or decreased pain. In all these circumstances, it is particularly important to utilize methods to minimize the likelihood of any systematic difference in the ascertainment of outcomes between study groups.

One such approach is to keep the study participants and/or the investigators blinded as far as possible to the identity of the interventions until data collection has been completed. In a double-blind design, neither the participants nor the investigators responsible for assessment of outcomes know to which treatment group an individual has been assigned. The ability to conduct a double-blind trial is dependent on having almost identical treatment and comparison programmes. Consequently, in many trials, particularly of drug therapies, the comparison group is assigned to receiving a placebo, which is an inert agent indistinguishable from the active treatment. By making it extremely difficult, if not impossible, to differentiate between the treatment and comparison groups, the use of a placebo will minimize bias in the ascertainment of both subjective disease outcomes and side-effects.

One problem in the evaluation of subjective end-points is the well-documented potential for individuals to report a favourable response to any therapy regardless of the physiological efficacy of what they receive. This phenomenon is referred to as the placebo effect. If a study does not use placebo control, it is impossible to tell whether subjective outcomes are due to the actual trial treatments, to the extra attention that participants receive, or merely to their belief that the treatment will help. For example, Wangensteen et al. (1962) introduced a new technique for the treatment of duodenal ulcer, gastric 'freezing', in which a coolant was administered by nasogastric tube to suppress secretions. All of their case series of 31 patients reported marked or complete relief of pain following this procedure. Despite the fact that the data were descriptive and therefore could not test the hypothesis, gastric freezing began to be used in many clinical centres. Subsequent concern about the efficacy and safety of this treatment led to the initiation of a randomized trial (Ruffin et al. 1969). In this trial of 137 patients with duodenal ulcer, 69 were assigned at random to gastric freezing and 68 received a placebo treatment in which the nasogastric tube was inserted but coolant was applied only as far as the upper oesophagus. Using these procedures, all patients were aware of the presence of the coolant, but no direct effect on gastric secretions was possible in the placebo group. The trial showed similar proportions of marked or complete relief of pain, suppression of secretions, and frequency and severity of recurrence between those who received the actual freezing procedure and those who did not. These results suggested that the relief of symptoms reported by all subjects in the case series may have been due to the psychological effect of the procedure rather than any true physiological benefits.

However, persons taking a drug or undergoing a medical procedure may be sensitized to their physical condition and tend to ascribe every symptom or unusual occurrence to their treatment. For example, in the Veterans Administration Cooperative Study of Antihypertensive Agents, 186 men were randomized to a combination of hydrochlorothiazide, reserpine, and hydralazine, and 194 were assigned to placebo (Veterans Administration Cooperative Study Group on Antihypertensive Agents 1972). One of the anticipated side-effects of these agents was impotence, and 29 per cent of the active treatment group reported this outcome at some time during the study period. However, a similar proportion reported these symptoms in the placebo group (28 per cent). Thus the true rate of impotence attributable to hypertensives is the difference between these two rates. Similarly, in the Aspirin Myocardial Infarction Study, 23.7 per cent of subjects randomized to receiving 1 g of aspirin daily reported symptoms suggestive of peptic ulcer, gastritis, or erosion of gastric mucosa, whereas 14.9 per cent of those receiving placebo reported similar symptoms (AMIS Research Group 1980). If the trial had not used placebo control, an erroneously high rate of gastrointestinal side-effects would have been attributed to aspirin, whereas the actual rate was 8.8 per cent (23.7 - 14.9 per cent). Thus the use of a placebo will ensure that all aspects of the programme offered to participants are identical except for the actual experimental treatment. Consequently, by comparing the proportions of individuals in the active treatment and placebo groups who report a particular symptom or outcome, the true incidence of subjective treatment-related effects can be determined.

Thus the primary strength of a double-blind design is to minimize the potential for observation bias. Of course, a concomitant limitation is that such trials are usually more complex and difficult to conduct. Procedures must be established for immediate 'unblinding' in the event of serious side-effects or other clinical emergencies in which this information seems essential. Moreover, in some circumstances, it is not possible to blind both the participants and the investigators to the allocated treatment regimen. For example, it is very difficult to design a double-blind trial for the evaluation of programmes involving substantial changes in life-style (such as exercise, cigarette smoking, or diet), surgical procedures, or drugs with characteristic side-effects. In these circumstances, a single-blind or unblinded trial may be necessary. In a single-blind design the investigator alone is aware of which intervention a subject is receiving, while in an unblinded or open trial both the subject and the investigator know to which study group the individual has been assigned.

Single-blind or unblinded trials are simpler to execute than double-blind studies and may be more acceptable to both physicians randomizing their patients and the participants themselves. Of course, these designs also have special problems. For example, subjects aware that they are not on the new or experimental programme may become dissatisfied and drop out of the trial, thus resulting in differential compliance or loss to follow-up. Moreover, as discussed earlier, knowledge of the intervention to which the participant has been assigned raises the potential for observation bias in the reporting of side-effects or assessment of outcomes. Thus, when a double-blind design is not possible, it is imperative

that special precautions be taken to reduce the potential for observation bias. Objective criteria should be used for measurement of both side-effects and end-points, and outcomes should be assessed by independent examiners who are unaware of the subjects' treatment status.

Sample-size considerations: statistical power

Although sample size must be addressed early in the planning stage of any analytical epidemiological investigation, it has particular importance in an intervention study. Observational analytical study designs can most reliably study large effects, so that the sample may be moderate in size. In contrast, a trial must have a sufficient sample size to have adequate statistical power to detect reliably the small to moderate but clinically important differences between treatment groups that are most likely to occur. Even if an investigator feels confident that a new intervention will have a large benefit (i.e. a 50 per cent or greater reduction in the primary end-point), it is far more preferable to design a trial to test the more likely small to moderate benefits (i.e. 20–30 per cent) and stop the trial early than to anticipate a larger effect and have no ability to detect smaller but none the less clinically important differences.

In designing a clinical trial, investigators often devote much time and effort to increasing the total number of participants enrolled. However, the statistical power of a trial to detect a postulated difference between treatment groups, if one truly exists, is dependent not simply on the sample size but more specifically on two factors: (1) the total number of end-points experienced by the study population and (2) the difference in compliance between the treatment groups (Hennekens and Buring 1987).

Accumulation of adequate end-points

To accumulate sufficient numbers of end-points, two major strategies may be considered: (1) selecting a high-risk population for study, and (2) ensuring an adequate duration of follow-up.

Selection of a high-risk population

A primary strategy to ensure the accumulation of an adequate number of end-points is to select individuals at increased risk of developing the outcomes of interest. With respect to the general population, a simple but important criterion for this selection is age, since the frequency of most outcomes rises markedly with increasing age. Other risk factors on which selection of a study population might be based include gender, occupation, geographic area, or one or more medical or life-style variables. For example, as described earlier, the Alpha-Tocopherol, Beta Carotene Cancer Prevention Study enrolled 29 133 middle-aged male cigarette smokers in Finland in order to test whether supplements of vitamin E and beta-carotene reduce the risk of lung cancer (Alpha-Tocopherol, Beta Carotene Cancer Prevention Study Group 1994). To evaluate this same question in a general population group at usual risk of lung cancer would require a substantially greater sample size since the baseline rate of lung cancer is lower in this group.

The collection of baseline data can be planned to increase the sensitivity of the trial to detect an effect of a treatment, if one is truly present, by identifying particular subgroups whose members might experience different effects of an intervention. For example, in the Physicians' Health Study, if the true reduction in cancer incidence due to beta-carotene supplementation is 30 per cent or greater, there is excellent power to detect that difference among the 22 071 randomized physicians. In contrast, if the overall reduction in risk is only 10 per cent, it would not be possible to detect such an effect with great assurance. However, a 10 per cent overall reduction could result from a much larger effect confined exclusively to a particular subgroup, in this case, those with the lowest levels of beta-carotene or vitamin A at baseline. This finding could easily be detected if participants were stratified by baseline levels of these parameters. For this reason, pre-randomization blood specimens were collected by mail from 14 916 of the participating physicians and will be analysed for baseline levels of retinol, carotene, retinol-binding protein, as well as other relevant parameters. The availability of these pre-randomization blood specimens will increase the sensitivity of the trial to identify which particular subgroup of participants, if any, stands to benefit most from beta-carotene (Hennekens and Buring 1989). If there is a benefit confined to those with low baseline levels, future public health interventions could be aimed at that target population. Conversely, if there is no true effect of beta-carotene supplementation on cancer incidence, this strategy would in fact produce a more convincing and truly informative null result, for then it could be stated that not only was there no significant overall effect observed but, in addition, no effect of supplementation with this agent was apparent regardless of initial blood levels. Despite the fact that such hypotheses are formulated before data collection, it remains important to keep in mind that such subgroup comparisons are not strictly randomized.

Length of the follow-up period

The planned length of follow-up for any trial should take into account the likelihood that the actual rate of accrual of end-points will be less than projected. This situation is not unusual in clinical trials and may occur for reasons beyond the control of the investigators. First, as discussed earlier, those who volunteer to participate are a self-selected group who also tend to experience generally lower morbidity and mortality rates than those who do not take part, regardless of the hypothesis under study or the treatment allocated at random (Wilhelmsen et al. 1976). They may also tend to adopt healthier practices irrespective of the specific intervention being studied (Kuller 1985). Moreover, there may be secular changes in disease rates during the course of the trial, sometimes as great as that postulated as attributable to the intervention being studied.

In cancer prevention trials, a particularly important consideration in determining the duration of treatment and follow-up is the postulated mechanism by which the intervention exerts its effects as well as the latency period for the cancer outcome of interest. For example, observational studies of cessation of smoking and risk of lung cancer indicate that eight to ten years are required before the benefit becomes optimal, at which time the lung cancer risk for ex-smokers decreases to a level about mid-way between that of never-smokers and current smokers (Doll and Peto 1978). An analogy with this model suggests that interventions such as micronutrient supplements are likely to require at least several years of treatment before any decrease in risk begins to become apparent, and perhaps a decade or more before the effect becomes

maximal. For example, a randomized trial of beta-carotene among 1805 patients with a recent non-melanoma skin cancer found similar rates of subsequent skin cancer among those receiving daily beta-carotene supplements (50 mg) and placebo (Greenberg et al. 1990). However, the five-year duration of treatment and follow-up in this trial may simply have been inadequate to yield a clearly detectable reduction in skin cancer, which is a multistage process that often proceeds over many years. Therefore, the findings do not preclude the possibility that a benefit of beta-carotene might emerge with longer duration of treatment.

Every effort should be made during the planning phase to choose the appropriate length of follow-up to answer the scientific question definitively. Nonetheless, the emergence of new evidence on mechanisms, changes in rates of disease within the general population, and even, on occasion, the failure to achieve a sufficient sample size or to accrue sufficient end-points within the trial itself may raise the question of increasing the duration of the study beyond the planned period of follow-up. Any such decision should be made as early in the trial as possible to maintain scientific credibility and avoid any implication that the change in design was based on last-minute efforts to achieve statistical significance (Friedman et al. 1985).

The effect of compliance

In addition to the number of end-points accrued, the second major factor influencing the power of the study to detect a true difference between treatment groups is compliance. With an intention-to-treat analysis, all study participants randomized to treatment A are compared with those randomized to treatment B, regardless of actual compliance. Thus the effect of any non-compliance will be to make the intervention and comparison groups more alike, with the result of decreasing the power of the trial to detect any true differences between the treatment groups.

One strategy to maximize compliance that is being used more frequently in clinical trials is the implementation of a run-in period prior to actual randomization. During this period, all participants experience, to the extent possible, the requirements and procedures employed in the actual trial. This permits potentially eligible participants who have difficulty adhering to the intervention programme or those perceiving adverse effects to withdraw or be withdrawn by the investigators before randomization. Such a strategy is particularly logistically feasible in trials where it is not necessary for an intervention to begin during or immediately following an acute event.

The Physicians' Health Study utilized a pre-randomization run-in period by sending all 33 223 initially willing and eligible participants calendar packs containing active aspirin and beta-carotene placebo. Since the postulated beneficial effects of aspirin are acute and side-effects are relatively common, it was decided to expose all willing and eligible subjects to active aspirin during the run-in period. However, the possible beneficial effects of beta-carotene are cumulative and the side-effects are minimal, so that it was optimal to use carotene placebo. After 18 weeks, participants were mailed a brief follow-up questionnaire, and those who reported apparent side-effects to aspirin or who reported taking less than two-thirds of their pills were deemed ineligible to be randomized. Following this run-in period, 22 071 physicians were randomized into the actual trial. Therefore, although the sample size of the study, was reduced by about one-third, a study population of 22 071 that remains compliant with the regimen for the duration of the trial will, in fact, have greater statistical power to answer the scientific questions posed than the larger group of 33 000, one-third of whom become non-compliant during the trial (Lang *et al.* 1991).

One possible limitation of a run-in is that when a trial is restricted to a group of proven good compliers, the study subjects may differ from the general population with respect to a number of factors that might affect the development of the outcomes of interest. Of course, to the extent that the non-compliers who were eliminated during the run-in can be followed, this question can be evaluated directly. However, from a more theoretical perspective, this issue relates solely to the generalizability of the study findings to the total experimental or reference populations. In this regard, the primary goal in the design of a trial must be to ensure that the results obtained are valid. Consequently, any procedure that maximizes compliance, thus increasing the validity of the study results, will positively affect the ability to generalize that finding to other populations. The good compliers proven in a run-in period who contribute to a valid result are a far greater asset to the generalizability of the trial results than would be a more representative study population whose members were unable to maintain adequate compliance for the duration of the study.

Issues in analysis and interpretation

In the analysis of an intervention study, the fundamental comparison is between the rate of the outcome of interest in the treated group(s) and the corresponding rate in the comparison group(s). As for any analytical epidemiological study, the roles of chance, bias, and confounding must be evaluated as possible alternative explanations for the findings. However, the unique design features of clinical trials have special implications for their analysis and interpretation.

With respect to confounding, the unique strength of randomization is that it tends to distribute both known and unknown confounders evenly among the treatment groups. If the sample size is large, this comparability is virtually guaranteed. However, with a small sample size or even, in rare instances, as a result of the play of chance in a large sample, randomization may not always result in groups that are alike with respect to baseline characteristics that might affect the outcomes under study. Consequently, one important early step in the analysis of any clinical trial is to compare the relevant characteristics of the randomized treatment and comparison groups to ensure that balance was achieved. This comparison should be presented as one of the first tables in the report of the study findings. If such a comparison indicates that randomization was not effective and that there were imbalances between the study groups with respect to known confounding factors, such discrepancies can be controlled in the analysis using a variety of statistical techniques (Hennekens and Buring 1987). However, this can only be done for variables that are known and measured, and the strength of randomization to control other confounders is no longer present.

A second important issue that often arises in clinical trials is the question of which subjects to include in the analysis. Some investigators remove from the analysis subjects who were determined to be ineligible after randomization or who did not comply with the study protocol. However, the exclusion of any randomized patients from the analysis can lead to biased results. First, perfect compliers represent only a fraction of the total study population in most trials. As with losses to follow-up, non-compliance may be related to factors that also affect the risk of the outcome under study, and failure to analyse data on all randomized participants could introduce bias. For example, in the Coronary Drug Project, a trial testing clofibrate in the reduction of mortality following myocardial infarction, the five-year total mortality rates in the treatment and placebo groups were very similar when all randomized subjects were included in the major analysis (18.0 versus 19.5 per cent) (Coronary Drug Project Research Group 1980, 1981). Since a number of individuals had been non-compliant with the clofibrate regimen, the investigators then analysed the mortality experience within the clofibrate group and found that those whose compliance was at least 80 per cent had a mortality rate of 15.0 per cent compared with 24.6 per cent among those who were poor compliers. Such a finding might be erroneously interpreted to indicate that clofibrate is effective in reducing mortality. However, a similar analysis within the placebo group found a comparable disparity in mortality among compliers and non-compliers, with rates of 15.1 per cent and 28.2 per cent, respectively. These data indicate that in both the active and placebo groups, compliers are different from non-compliers in ways that affect their prognosis. Even after controlling for 40 known possible confounders, there was still a difference in the mortality rates in the placebo group between good (16.4 per cent) and poor (25.8 per cent) compliers. Thus there must be additional but unknown variables associated with both compliance and mortality in this trial.

A second limitation in evaluating data on only those subjects who comply with the study regimen is that such an analysis does not address the actual research question being posed in an intervention study—whether the offering of a treatment programme is of benefit. While we wish to study the actual effect of the treatment, we are, in fact, randomizing only on the basis of the offering of treatment, so that we must analyse the data on this basis to preserve the power of randomization. Only the entire groups allocated by randomization are truly comparable. Once participants are randomized to a treatment group, their subsequent health experience must be assessed and analysed along with all others in that group, regardless of whether they comply with their assigned regimen. This methodological issue emphasizes the need to maintain high compliance with their assigned regimen among all study participants. It is also important to keep in mind that if a particular regimen is so difficult and uncomfortable that it is likely to be accepted and used by only a small proportion of the reference population, it may not be practical to recommend its use, no matter how effective the actual treatment may be.

Thus, in all circumstances, the most valid comparison to estimate the true benefit to be obtained from the intervention programme is to analyse by intention to treat—in other words, 'once randomized, always analysed.' For this reason, it is imperative to maintain high levels of compliance, to keep losses to follow-up at a minimum, and to collect complete information on all randomized subjects. Those who are no longer complying with the study regimen should continue to provide all follow-up information whenever possible or, at the very least, their vital status should be ascertained. Subsequent analyses can certainly be performed based on that subgroup of participants who actually received their assigned treatment. However, if this is done, it is impossible to regain the control of unknown confounders that had been achieved originally through randomization, despite the ability to perform analyses that achieve balance in the distribution of known confounders.

The need to perform randomized comparison in the analyses of data from a trial is equally important when subgroups are identified on the basis of other characteristics besides compliance. Investigators are often tempted to examine differences in treatment effects among those with various baseline characteristics such as age, prognostic factors, or previous medical history. For example, a Multiple Risk Factor Intervention Trial subgroup analysis by presence or absence of resting electrocardiogram abnormalities suggested that, among men with such abnormalities at baseline, those receiving the special intervention programme actually had an increased risk of death from coronary heart disease relative to those in the group allocated to usual medical care (MRFIT Research Group 1985). This finding led to a further exploration of the effects of the intervention among those with various levels of hypertension. However, the investigators noted that 'subgroup analyses must be interpreted with caution' and added that 'these findings pose hypotheses for investigation by other researchers in systemic hypertension' (MRFIT Research Group 1985).

In general, the caveats needed to compare subgroups defined a priori by baseline characteristics are far less than those required when comparisons are made on the basis of variables chosen after randomization, such as compliance. With regard to the former, a minor concern involves a loss of statistical power because only subgroups of the total number of randomized subjects are being compared. However, a greater concern is to ensure adequate control of variables that may no longer be distributed at random among the subgroups. With respect to analyses of subgroups defined a posteriori on the basis of information accumulated after randomization, in general they can only raise data-derived hypotheses, not test particular research questions.

Stopping rules: decision for early termination of a trial

In the design phase of a trial, there is a need to develop guidelines for deciding whether a trial should be modified or terminated before it was originally scheduled to end. To ensure that the welfare of the participants is protected, the unblinded data should be monitored by a group that is independent of the investigators conducting the trial. If the data indicate a clear and extreme benefit on the primary end-point due to the intervention, or if a treatment is clearly harmful, the modification or early termination of the trial must be considered.

A decision to terminate a study early is based on a number of complex issues and must be made with a great deal of caution. It is critical that a trial is not stopped prematurely solely on the basis of trends emerging from a small number of patients, since such findings might well be only transient and disappear or even reverse after data have accumulated from a larger sample. As a general rule, the first requirement for even considering modification or early termination of an ongoing trial is the observation of a sustained statistical association that is so extreme, and therefore so highly

statistically significant, that it is virtually impossible that it arose by chance alone. The observed association must then be considered in the context of the totality of evidence. While a number of specific guidelines have been used in various studies, the aim is to achieve an equitable balance between protection of randomized participants against real harm and minimizing the risks of mistakenly modifying or stopping the trial prematurely.

It must be clearly kept in mind that whenever a trial is ended prematurely because of findings related to one end-point, there may be a resultant loss of ability to answer other, often equally important questions that are of interest. For example, the Physicians' Health Study among 22 071 male American physicians was designed to evaluate two primary prevention hypotheses: whether low-dose aspirin reduces cardiovascular mortality, and whether beta-carotene decreases cancer incidence. In early 1988, the Data Monitoring Board of the trial terminated the aspirin component prematurely (Steering Committee 1989). This decision was based on all available evidence, including three major considerations: the presence of a statistically significant ($p < 0.00001$) reduction in the risk of total myocardial infarction among those in the aspirin group; the fact that no effect of aspirin on cardiovascular mortality could be detected in the trial until the year 2000 or later, because of the exceptionally low cardiovascular death rates among the participating physicians; and the fact that aspirin was prescribed for more than 85 per cent of the participants who experienced a non-fatal myocardial infarction, which would render any subsequent findings about cardiovascular mortality particularly difficult to interpret. However, two other significant outcomes of interest in relation to aspirin were stroke and overall cardiovascular death, both of which occurred less frequently than myocardial infarction. As a result of the early termination of the aspirin component, there were inadequate numbers of strokes and cardiovascular deaths to permit a reliable assessment of aspirin's effect. There was an apparent increased risk for stroke—primarily in the subgroup of haemorrhagic strokes—but this was not statistically significant. With respect to cardiovascular mortality, no reduction in risk was associated with aspirin, but the confidence interval was wide and consistent with the postulated benefit. While a number of explanations for the lack of benefit on cardiovascular death have been proposed, the primary consideration must be that the number of cardiovascular deaths in this trial at the time of the termination of the aspirin component was simply too small to evaluate the end-point reliably. Thus two major pieces of the 'benefit to risk' equation for the use of aspirin in the primary prevention of heart disease could not be determined owing to the ethical and practical considerations that prompted the early termination of the aspirin component of the trial.

Meta-analysis or statistical overview

As discussed earlier, the sample size of a trial and its resultant statistical power determine the extent to which the play of chance may have influenced the study findings. If a study is of inadequate sample size, then a finding of no statistically significant association between intervention and outcome (a so-called null result) may well be uninformative, since a true lack of association will be difficult or impossible to distinguish from a true association that simply cannot be detected statistically because of inadequate power.

The ambiguity of results from individual trials of small sample size provides a strong rationale for the conduct of much larger trials that can detect reliably modest treatment effects. Some investigators have argued that small trials should be pursued first, with larger investigations undertaken only if shown necessary. However, null results from small trials that are uninformative may erroneously suggest no effect. For this reason, it would appear far preferable to mount a large trial once there is sufficient belief in a treatment's potential. If the effect is far greater than anticipated, a large trial can always be terminated earlier than scheduled.

A single well-designed and well-conducted trial of sufficient sample size to detect the true effects of an intervention is always best. However, in the absence of a definitive study, statistical overviews or meta-analyses that consider, in aggregate, the data from several smaller trials can provide useful information by minimizing the role of chance as an explanation for the findings. This does not mean that meta-analysis can overcome any effects of bias or confounding present in the individual trial results. Moreover, since randomization works 'on average' to distribute confounding factors evenly between treatment groups, a major concern in combining the results from several small trials is that residual confounding may very likely be affecting the magnitude of the effect observed in any one small trial.

Perhaps, then, the chief utility of such meta-analysis is not to answer the question definitively but to provide a reliable estimate of the most likely effect of an intervention which can be used in planning a future trial with adequate power to detect such an effect if it truly exists. With respect to estimating the size of any risk reduction, results from a pilot study or even a single small trial are likely to be quite unstable owing to sampling variability. In contrast, the unique strength of meta-analysis of data from all randomized trials is to minimize the variability of the overall estimate obtained from each individual study. Thus risk estimates from meta-analysis are the most reliable that can be obtained in the absence of a single trial of adequate statistical power.

The pitfalls of estimating the probable effects of an intervention from a single small trial instead of an overview can be illustrated by a comparison of two trials testing the effects of beta-blocker drugs given in the acute phase of myocardial infarction: the Metoprolol in Acute Myocardial Infarction (MIAMI) trial and the First International Study of Infarct Survival (ISIS–1). Before the initiation of the MIAMI trial, the investigators conducted a pilot study among approximately 1400 participants. Based on an observed 36 per cent reduction in total mortality, approximately 6000 individuals were enrolled in the full-scale trial. In contrast, the sample size for ISIS–1 was calculated from an overview of 21 previous trials of beta-blocker therapy, which indicated an approximate 10 per cent reduction in total mortality. On the basis of this estimate, over 16 000 patients were enrolled in ISIS–1. When the two trials were completed, the estimates of the effects of treatment were similar, with reductions in vascular mortality of approximately 13 per cent in MIAMI and 15 per cent in ISIS–1. However, the results from the MIAMI trial did not achieve statistical significance, whereas the results from ISIS–1 did (MIAMI Trial Research Group 1985; ISIS–1 Collaborative Group 1986). This clearly reflects the effect of inadequate sample size on the power of the MIAMI trial to detect an effect of this magnitude.

Thus, the use of a statistical overview or meta-analysis provides a quantitative method of obtaining an overall estimate of effect. However, the quality and usefulness of any overview is entirely dependent on the quality of the component studies. Not only must they be free from the effects of uncontrolled bias or confounding, but the studies combined should be similar with respect to the disease and the exposure or intervention being studied, and the characteristics of the subjects must be sufficiently similar to make combining the results of such studies reasonable. In addition, the magnitude of the effect of each of the studies must be sufficiently similar that their combination will not provide a distorted estimate. To the extent that there is substantial heterogeneity, the information provided by a single overall estimate of effect will decrease.

Conclusion

The ultimate aim of any intervention study is to provide either a definitive positive result on which public policy can be based or a reliable and informative null finding that can then safely permit the redistribution of resources to other important areas of research. Intervention studies can certainly be more difficult to design and conduct than observational epidemiological studies owing to their unique problems of ethics, feasibility, and costs. However, trials that are sufficiently large, randomized, and carefully designed, conducted, and analysed can provide the strongest and most direct epidemiological evidence on which to make a judgement about the existence of a cause–effect relationship.

References

Alpha-Tocopherol, Beta Carotene Cancer Prevention Study Group (1994). The effect of vitamin E and beta carotene on the incidence of lung cancer and other cancers in male smokers. *New England Journal of Medicine*, **330**, 1029–35.

AMIS (Aspirin Myocardial Infarction Study) Research Group (1980). A randomized, controlled trial of aspirin in persons recovered from myocardial infarction. *Journal of the American Medical Association*, **243**, 661–9.

Ast, D.B., Finn, S.B., and McCaffrey, I. (1950). The Newburgh–Kingston Caries Fluorine Study. I. Dental findings after three years of water fluoridation. *American Journal of Public Health*, **40**, 716–24.

Buring, J.E. and Hennekens, C.H. (1992). The Women's Health Study: summary of the study design. *Journal of Myocardial Ischemia*, **4**, 27–9.

Buring, J.E. and Hennekens, C.H. (1994). Randomized trials of primary prevention of cardiovascular disease in women: an investigator's view. *Annals of Epidemiology*, **4**, 111–4.

Coronary Drug Project Research Group (1980). Influence of adherence to treatment and response of cholesterol on mortality in the Coronary Drug Project. *New England Journal of Medicine*, **303**, 1038–41.

Coronary Drug Project Research Group (1981). Practical aspects of decision making in clinical trials: the Coronary Drug Project as a case study. *Controlled Clinical Trials*, **1**, 363–76.

Doll, R. and Peto, R. (1978). Cigarette smoking and bronchial carcinoma: dose and time relationships among regular smokers and lifelong non-smokers. *Journal of Epidemiology and Community Health*, **32**, 303–13.

Dustan, H.P., Schneckloth, R.E., Corcoran A.S., *et al.* (1958). The effectiveness of long-term treatment of malignant hypertension. *Circulation*, **18**, 644–51.

Friedman, L.M., Furberg, C.D., and DeMets, D.L. (1985). *Fundamentals of clinical trials*, (2nd edn). PSG, Littleton, MA.

Greenberg, E.R., Baron, J.A., Stukel, T.A., *et al.* (1990). A clinical trial of beta carotene to prevent basal-cell and squamous-cell cancers of the skin. *New England Journal of Medicine*, **323**, 789–95.

Hennekens, C.H. and Buring, J.E. (1987). *Epidemiology in medicine*. Little, Brown, Boston, MA.

Hennekens, C.H. and Buring, J.E. (1989). Methodologic considerations in the design and conduct of randomized trials: the US Physicians' Health Study. *Controlled Clinical Trials*, **10** (Suppl.), 142–50S.

Hennekens, C.H., Buring, J.E., and Peto, R. (1994). Antioxidant vitamins—benefits not yet proved. *New England Journal of Medicine*, **330**, 1080–1.

ISIS–1 Collaborative Group (1986). ISIS–1: a randomized trial of intravenous atenolol among 16 027 cases of suspected acute myocardial infarction. *Lancet*, **ii**, 57–66.

ISIS–3 Collaborative Group (1992). ISIS–3: a randomised trial comparing SK vs tPA vs APSAC and comparing aspirin plus heparin vs aspirin alone among 41 299 suspected acute myocardial infarction. *Lancet*, **339**, 1–18.

Kuller, L.H. (1985). Pilot studies. In *Chemoprevention clinical trials: problems and solutions, 1984*, (ed. M. A. Sestili and J. G. Dell). NIH Publication No. 85–2715, US Department of Health and Human Services, Hyattsville, MD.

Lang, J.M., Buring, J.E., Rosner, B., *et al.* (1991). Estimating the effect of the run-in on the power of the Physicians' Health Study. *Statistics in Medicine*, **10**, 1585–93.

MIAMI Trial Research Group (1985). Metoprolol in Acute Myocardial Infarction (MIAMI): a randomized placebo-controlled international trial. *European Heart Journal*, **6**, 199–226.

MRFIT (Multiple Risk Factor Intervention Trial) Research Group (1982). Multiple Risk Factor Intervention Trial: risk factor changes and morbidity results. *Journal of the American Medical Association*, **248**, 1465–77.

MRFIT (Multiple Risk Factor Intervention Trial) Research Group (1985). Baseline resting electrocardiographic abnormalities, antihypertensive treatment, and mortality in the Multiple Risk Factor Intervention Trial. *American Journal of Cardiology*, **55**, 1–15.

Peto, R., Pike, M.C., Armitage, P., *et al.* (1976). Design and analysis of randomized clinical trials requiring prolonged observation of each patient: I. Introduction and design. *British Journal of Cancer*, **34**, 585–612.

Peto, R., Pike, M.C., Armitage, P., *et al.* (1977). Design and analysis of randomized clinical trials requiring prolonged observation of each patient: II. Analyses and examples. *British Journal of Cancer*, **35**, 1–39.

Ruffin, J.M., Grizzle, J.E., Hightower, N.C., *et al.* (1969). A cooperative double-blind evaluation of gastric 'freezing' in the treatment of duodenal ulcer. *New England Journal of Medicine*, **281**, 16–19.

Stampfer, M., Buring, J.E., Willett, W., *et al.* (1985). The 2 × 2 factorial design: its application to a randomized trial of aspirin and carotene in US physicians. *Statistics in Medicine*, **4**, 111–16.

Steering Committee of the Physicians' Health Study Research Group (1989). Final report on the aspirin component of the ongoing Physicians' Health Study. *New England Journal of Medicine*, **321**, 129–35.

Veterans Administration Cooperative Study Group on Antihypertensive Agents (1972). Effect of treatment on morbidity in hypertension: III. Influence of age, diastolic pressure, and prior cardiovascular disease; further analysis of side effects. *Circulation*, **45**, 991–1004.

Wangensteen, O.H., Peter, E.T., Bernstein, E.F., *et al.* (1962). Can physiological gastrectomy be achieved by gastric freezing? *Annals of Surgery*, **156**, 579–91.

Wilhelmsen, L., Ljungberg, S., Wedel, H., *et al.* (1976). A comparison between participants and non-participants in a primary preventive trial. *Journal of Chronic Diseases*, **29**, 331–9.

14 Concepts of validity in epidemiological research

Sander Greenland

Some of the major validity concepts in epidemiological research are outlined in this chapter. The contents are organized around three main sections: validity in prediction problems, validity in casual inference, and special validity problems in case–control and retrospective cohort studies. Familiarity with the basics of epidemiological study design and a number of terms of epidemiological theory, among them risk, competing risk, average risk, population at risk, and rate, are assumed.

A number of textbooks provide more background and depth than can be given here. Among them, Schlesselman (1982), Kelsey et al. (1986), Rothman (1986), Checkoway et al. (1989), and Walker (1991) provide practical epidemiological treatments, while Breslow and Day (1980, 1987), Kleinbaum et al. (1982), Miettinen (1985), and Clayton and Hills (1993) focus on statistical and theoretical details.

Despite broad parallels there is considerable diversity and conflict among the classification schemes and terminologies employed in the various textbooks. This diversity reflects the fact that there is no unique way of classifying the various validity conditions, biases, and measures that have been described in the literature. In particular, the classification schemes employed here and elsewhere should not be regarded as anything more than convenient frameworks for organizing discussions of study validity and epidemiological inference.

Several important study designs, including prevalence studies and ecological studies, are not discussed in this chapter. Such studies require consideration of the above validity conditions and also require special considerations of their own. Further details of these and other designs can be found in the general textbooks cited above. For a review of the special problems of ecological studies, see Greenland and Robins (1994). Meta-analytic methods are reviewed and discussed by Greenland (1987b, 1994).

Also not covered are a number of central problems of epidemiological inference, including choice of effect measures and interpretation of statistics. Critical discussions of effect measures are given by Greenland (1987a), Greenland and Robins (1988), and Greenland et al. (1986, 1991). Oakes (1990) presents an extensive introduction to competing schools of statistical inference. He emphasizes the shortcomings of the prevailing approaches to statistics and critically discusses alternative approaches as well; see also Berger and Berry (1988) and Goodman and Royall (1988). Rubin (1991) contrasts different statistical approaches to causal inference. Finally, Miettinen (1985), Rothman (1986), Poole (1987a,b), Goodman (1992, 1993), and Greenland (1990, 1993b) discuss the use and misuse of statistical inference in epidemiological research.

Inference and validity

Epidemiological inference is the process of drawing inferences from epidemiological data, such as prediction of disease patterns or identification of causes of diseases or epidemics. These inferences must often be made without the benefits of direct experimental evidence or established theory about disease aetiology. Consider the problem of predicting the risk and incubation (induction) time for acquired immunodeficiency syndrome (AIDS) among persons infected with type 1 human immunodeficiency virus (HIV-1). Unlike an experiment, in which the exposure is administered by the investigator, the date of HIV-1 infection cannot be accurately estimated in most cases; furthermore, the mechanism by which 'silent' HIV-1 infection progresses to AIDS is not known with certainty. Nevertheless, some prediction must be made from the available data if one is to prepare effectively for future health care needs.

As another example, consider the problem of estimating how much excess risk of coronary heart disease (if any) is produced by coffee drinking. Unlike an experimental exposure, coffee drinking is self-selected; it appears that persons who use coffee are more likely to smoke than non-users and probably tend to differ in many other behaviours as well (Greenland 1987b). As a result, even if coffee use if harmless, we should not expect to observe the same pattern of heart disease in users and non-users. Thus small coffee effects should be very difficult to disentangle from the effects of other behaviours. Nevertheless, because of the high prevalence of coffee use and the high incidence of heart disease, determination of the effect of coffee on heart disease risk may be of considerable public health importance.

In both these examples, and in general, inferences will depend on evaluating the **validity** of the available studies, i.e. the degree to which the studies meet basic logical criteria for absence of bias. In each section of this chapter major concepts of validity in epidemiological research as applied in three settings—prediction from one population to another, causal inference from cohort studies, and causal inference from case–control and retrospective cohort studies —are outlined and illustrated. Parallel aspects of each application will be emphasized. In particular, each problem requires consideration of comparison validity, follow-up validity, specification validity, and measurement validity. Case–control studies require the additional consideration of case- and control-selection validity, and are often subject to additional sources of measurement error beyond those occurring in prospective cohort studies. Similar problems arise in retrospective cohort studies.

Validity in prediction problems

The following prediction problem will be used to illustrate the basic concepts of validity in epidemiological inference.

A health clinic for homosexual men is about to begin enrolling HIV-1-negative men in an unrestricted programme that will involve re-testing each participant for HIV-1 antibodies at six-month intervals. We can expect that, in the course of the programme, many participants will seroconvert to positive HIV-1 status. Such participants will invariably ask difficult questions, such as: What are my chances of developing AIDS over the next five years? How many years do I have before I develop AIDS? In attempting to answer these questions, it will be convenient to refer to such participants (i.e. those who seroconvert) as the **target cohort**. Even though membership of this cohort is not determined in advance, it will be the target of our predictions. It will also be convenient to refer to the time from HIV-1 infection until the onset of clinical AIDS as the **AIDS incubation time**. We could provide reasonable answers to a participant's questions if we could accurately predict AIDS incubation times, although we would also have to estimate the time elapsed between infection and the first positive test.

There might be someone who responds to the questions posed above with the following anecdote: 'I've known several men just like the ones in this cohort, and they all developed AIDS within five years after a positive HIV-1 test'. No trained scientist would conclude from this anecdote that all or most of the target cohort will develop AIDS within five years of seroconversion. Of course, one reason is that the men in the anecdote cannot be 'just like' men in our cohort in every respect: they may have been older or younger when they were infected; they may have experienced a greater degree of stress following their infection; they may have been heavier smokers, drinkers, or drug users, etc. In other words, we know that the anecdotal men and their post-infection life events could not have been exactly the same as the men in our target cohort with respect to all factors that affect AIDS incubation time, including measured, unmeasured, and unknown factors. Furthermore, it may be that some or all of the men referred to in the anecdote had been infected long before they were first tested, so that (unlike men in our target cohort) the time from their first positive test to AIDS onset was much shorter than the time from seroconversion to AIDS onset.

Any reasonable predictions must be based on observing the distribution of AIDS incubation times in another cohort. Suppose that we obtain data from a study of homosexual men who underwent regular HIV-1 testing, and we then assemble from these data a study cohort of men who were observed to seroconvert. Suppose also that most of these men were followed for at least five years after seroconversion. We cannot expect any member of this study to be 'just like' any member of our target cohort in every respect. Nevertheless, if we could identify no differences between the two cohorts with respect to factors that affect incubation time, we might argue that the study cohort could serve as a point of

reference for predicting incubation times in the target cohort. Thus we shall henceforth refer to the study cohort as our **reference cohort**. Note that our reference and target cohorts may have originated from different populations; for example, the clinic generating the target cohort could be in New York, but the study that generated the reference cohort may have been in San Francisco. Of course, for both the target and reference cohorts, the actual times of HIV-1 infection will have to be imputed, based on the dates of the last negative and the first positive tests.

Suppose that our statistical analysis of data from the reference cohort produces estimates of 0.05, 0.25, and 0.45 for the average risk of contracting AIDS within two, five, and eight years of HIV-1 infection. What conditions would be sufficient to guarantee the validity of these figures as estimates or predictions of the proportion of the target cohort that would develop AIDS within two, five, and eight years of infection? If by 'valid' we mean that any discrepancy between our predictions and the true target proportions is purely random (unpredictable in principle), the following conditions would be sufficient.

(C) *Comparison validity* The distribution of incubation times in the target cohort will be approximately the same as the distribution in the reference cohort.

(F) *Follow-up validity* Within the reference cohort, the risk of censoring (i.e. follow-up ended by an event other than AIDS) is not associated with risk of AIDS.

(Sp) *Specification validity* The distribution of incubation times in the reference cohort can be closely approximated by the statistical model used to compute the estimates. For example, if one employs a lognormal distribution to model the distribution of incubation times in the reference cohort, this model should be approximately correct.

(M) *Measurement validity* All measurements of variables used in the analysis closely approximate the true values of the variables. In particular, each imputed time of HIV-1 infection closely approximates the true infection time, and each reported time of AIDS onset closely approximates a clinical event defined as AIDS onset.

The first condition concerns the external validity of making predictions about the target cohort based on the reference cohort. The remaining conditions concern the internal validity of the predictions as estimates of average risk in the reference cohort. The following sections will explore the meaning of these conditions in prediction problems.

Comparison validity

Comparison validity is probably the easiest condition to describe, although it is difficult to evaluate. Intuitively, it simply means that the distribution of incubation times in the target cohort could be almost perfectly predicted from the distribution of incubation times in the reference cohort, if the incubation times were observed without error and there was no loss to follow-up. Other ways of stating this condition are that the two cohorts are **comparable** (Miettinen 1985) or **exchangeable** (Greenland and Robins 1986) with respect to incubation times, or that the AIDS experience of the target cohort can be predicted from the experience of the reference cohort.

Confounding

If the two cohorts are not comparable, some or all of our risk estimates for the target cohort based on the reference cohort will be biased* as a result. This bias is sometimes called **comparison bias** or **confounding**. There has been much research on methods for identifying and adjusting for such bias (see the textbooks cited earlier for overviews of such methods).

To evaluate comparison validity, we must investigate whether the two cohorts differ on any factors that influence incubation time. If so, we cannot reasonably expect the incubation time distributions of the two cohorts to be comparable. A factor responsible for some or all of the confounding in an estimate is called a **confounder** or **confounding variable**, the estimate is said to be **confounded** by the factor, and the factor is said to **confound** the estimate.

To illustrate these concepts, suppose that men infected at younger ages tend to have longer incubation times and that the members of the reference cohort are on average younger than members of the target cohort. If there were no other differences to counterbalance this age difference, we should then expect that members of the reference cohort will on average have longer incubation times than members of the target cohort. Consequently, unadjusted predictions of risk for the target cohort derived from the reference cohort would be biased (confounded) by age in a downward direction. In other words, age would be a confounder for estimating risk in the target cohort, and confounding by age would result in underestimation of the proportion of men in the target cohort who will develop AIDS within five years.

Now suppose that we can compute the age at infection of men in the reference cohort, and that within one-year strata of age, for instance, the target and reference cohorts had virtually identical distributions of incubation times. The age-specific estimates of risk derived from the reference cohort would then be free of age confounding and so could be used as unconfounded estimates of age-specific risk for men in the target cohort. Also, if we wished to construct unconfounded estimates of average risk in the entire target cohort, we could do so via the technique of **age standardization**.

To illustrate, let P_x denote our estimate of the average risk of AIDS within five years of infection among members of the reference cohort who become infected at age x. Let W_x denote the proportion of men in the target cohort who are infected at age x. Then the estimated average risk of AIDS within five years of infection, standardized to the target cohort's age distribution, is simply the average of the age-specific reference estimates P_x weighted by the age distribution (at infection) of the target cohort; algebraically, this average is the sum of the products W_xP_x over all ages and is denoted by $\Sigma_xW_xP_x$. Considered as an estimate of the overall proportion of the target cohort that will contract AIDS within five years of HIV-1 infection, the standardized proportion $\Sigma_xW_xP_x$ will be free of age confounding.

The preceding illustration brings forth an important and often overlooked point: when one employs standardization to adjust for potential biases, the choice of standard distribution should never be considered arbitrary. In fact, the standard distribution should always be taken from the target cohort or the population about which inferences will be made. If inferences are to be made about several different groups, it may be necessary to compute several different standardized estimates.

Methods for removing bias in estimates by taking account of variables responsible for some or all of the bias are known as **adjustment** or **covariate control** methods. Standardization is perhaps the oldest and simplest example of such a method; methods based on multivariate models, which are discussed below, are more complex.

Unmeasured confounders

If all confounders were measured accurately, comparison validity could be achieved simply by adjusting for these confounders (although various technical problems might arise when attempting to do so). Nevertheless, in any non-randomized study we would ordinarily be able to think of a number of possible confounders that had not been measured or had been measured only in a very poor fashion. In such cases, it may still be possible to predict the direction of uncontrolled confounding by examining the manner in which persons were selected into the target and reference cohorts from the population at large. If the cohorts are derived from populations with different distributions of predictors of the outcome, or the predictors themselves are associated with admission differentially across the cohorts, these predictors will become confounders in the analysis.

To illustrate this approach, suppose that HIV-1 infection via an intravenous route (e.g. through needle sharing) leads to shorter incubation times than HIV-1 infection through sexual activity. Suppose also that the reference cohort had excluded all or most intravenous drug users, whereas the target cohort was non-selective in this regard. Then incubation times in the target cohort will on average be shorter than times in the reference cohort owing to the presence of intravenously infected persons in the target cohort. Thus we should expect the results from the reference cohort to underestimate average risks of AIDS onset in the target cohort.

Random sampling and confounding

Suppose, for the moment, that our reference cohort had been formed by taking a random sample of the target cohort. Can predictions about the target made from such a random sample still be confounded? With the above definition of confounding, the answer is yes. To see this, note for example that by chance alone men in our sample reference cohort could be younger on average than the total target; this age difference would in turn downwardly bias the unadjusted risk predictions if men had longer incubation times at younger ages.

Nevertheless, random sampling can help to ensure that the distribution of the reference cohort is not too far from the distributing of the target cohort. In essence, the probability of severe confounding can be made as small as necessary by increasing the sample size. Furthermore, if random sampling is used, any confounding left after adjustment will be accounted for by the standard errors of the estimates, provided that the correct statistical model is used to compute the estimates and standard errors. We shall examine the latter condition under the section on specification validity.

---

* Readers with some background in mathematical statistics may substitute inconsistent for biased throughout this chapter.

Follow-up validity

In any cohort study covering an extended period of risk, subjects will be followed for different lengths of time. Some subjects will be lost to follow-up before the study ends. Others will be removed from the study by an event that precludes AIDS onset, which in this setting is death before AIDS onset from fatal accidents, fatal myocardial infarctions, etc. Because subjects come under study at different times, those who are not lost to follow-up or who die before developing AIDS will still have had different lengths of follow-up when the study ends; traditionally, a subject still under follow-up at study end is said to have been 'withdrawn from study' at the time of study end.

Suppose that we wish to estimate the average risk of AIDS onset within five years of infection. The data from a member of the reference cohort who is not observed to develop AIDS but is also not followed for the full five years from infection are said to be **censored** for the outcome of interest (AIDS within five years of infection). Consider, for example, a subject killed in a car crash two years after infection but before contracting AIDS: the incubation time of this subject was censored at two years of follow-up.

Follow-up validity means that over any span of follow-up time, risk of censoring is unassociated with risk of the outcome of interest. In our example, follow-up validity means that over any span of time following infection, risk of censoring (loss, withdrawal, or death before AIDS) is unassociated with risk of AIDS. All common methods for estimating risk from situations in which censoring occurs (e.g. person-years, life table, and Kaplan–Meier methods) are based on the assumption of follow-up validity. Given follow-up validity, we can expect that, at any time t after infection, the distribution of incubation times will be the same for subjects lost or withdrawn at t and subjects whose follow-up continues beyond t.

Violations of follow-up validity can result in biased estimates of risk; such violations are referred to as **follow-up bias** or **biased censoring**. To illustrate, suppose that younger reference subjects tend to have longer incubation times (i.e. lower risks) and are lost to follow-up at a higher rate than older reference subjects. In other words, lower-risk subjects are lost at a higher rate than higher-risk subjects. Then, after enough time, the average risk of AIDS in the observed portion of the reference cohort will tend to be overestimated, i.e. higher than the average risk occurring in the full reference cohort (as the latter includes both censored and uncensored subject experience).

The follow-up bias in the last illustration would not affect the age-specific estimates of risk (where age refers to age at infection). Consequently, the age bias in follow-up would not produce bias in age-standardized estimates of risk. More generally, if follow-up bias can be traced to a particular variable that is a predictor of both the outcome of interest and censoring, bias in the estimates can be removed by adjusting for that variable. Thus, some forms of follow-up bias can be dealt with in the same manner as confounding.

Specification validity

All statistical techniques, including so-called 'distribution-free' or 'non-parametric' methods as well as basic contingency table methods, are derived by assuming the validity of a **sampling** model or **error distribution**. A common example is the binomial model, which is discussed in all the textbooks cited in the introduction. For parametric methods, the sampling model is a mathematical formula that expresses the probability of observing the various possible data patterns as a function of certain (possibly unknown) constants or *parameters*. Although the parameters of this model may be unknown, the mathematical form of this model incorporates only known or purely random aspects of the data-generation process; unknown systematic aspects of this process (such as most follow-up and selection biases) will not be accounted for by the model.

All parametric statistical techniques also assume a **structural model**, which is a mathematical formula that expresses the parameters of the sampling model as a function of study variables. A common example is the logistic model (Breslow and Day 1980; Schlesselman 1982; Kelsey *et al.* 1986; Checkoway *et al.* 1989). The structural model is most often incorporated into the sampling model, and the combination is referred to as the statistical model. An estimate can be said to have specification validity if it is derived using a statistical model that is correct or nearly so.

If either the sampling model or the structural model used for analysis is incorrect, the resulting estimates may be biased. Such bias is sometimes called **specification bias**, while the use of an incorrect model is known as **model misspecification** or **specification error**. Even when misspecification does not lead to bias, it can lead to invalidity of statistical tests and confidence intervals.

The true structural relation among the study variables is almost never known in studies of human disease. Furthermore, in the absence of random sampling and randomization, the true sampling process (i.e. the exact process leading people to enter and stay in the study groups) will also be unknown. It follows that we should ordinarily expect some degree of specification error in an epidemiological analysis. Minimizing such error largely consists of contrasting the statistical model against the data and against any available information about the processes that generated the data (Greenland 1989; McCullagh and Nelder 1989), such as prior information on demographic patterns of incidence.

Many statistical techniques in epidemiology are based on assuming some type of logistic model. Examples include all the popular adjusted odds ratios, such as the Woolf, maximum-likelihood, and Mantel–Haenszel estimates, as well as tests for odds ratio heterogeneity. Classical 'indirect' adjustment of rates and other comparisons of standardized morbidity ratios depend on similar multiplicative models for their validity (Breslow and Day 1987).

The degree of bias in traditional epidemiologic analysis methods when the model assumptions fail has not been extensively studied. Fortunately, a few traditional methods, such as directly standardized comparisons and the Mantel–Haenszel test, remain valid under a wide variety of structural models. In addition, risk regression has been extended to situations involving more general models than assumed in classical theory (Breslow and Day 1987; Hastie and Tibshirani 1990). Leamer (1978) and White (1993) give more details on the effects of specification error in multiple regression problems.

Measurement validity

An estimate from a study can be said to have measurement validity if it suffers from no bias due to errors in measuring the study variables. Unfortunately there are sources of measurement error in nearly all studies, and nearly all sources of measurement error will contribute to bias in estimates. Thus evaluation of measurement validity primarily focuses on identifying sources of measurement error and attempting to deduce the direction and magnitude of bias produced by these sources.

To aid in the task of identifying sources of measurement error, it may be useful to classify such errors according to their source. Errors from specific sources can then be further classified according to characteristics that are predictive of the direction of the bias they produce. One classification scheme divides errors into three major categories, according to their source.

1. *Procedural error*: arising from mistakes or defects in measurement procedures.

2. *Proxy-variable error*: arising from using a 'proxy' variable as a substitute for an actual variable of interest.

3. *Construct error*: arising from ambiguities in the definition of the variables.

Regardless of their source, errors can be divided into two basic types, differential and non-differential, according to whether the direction or magnitude of error depends on the true values of the study variables. Two different sources of error may be classified as dependent or independent, according to whether or not the direction or magnitude of the error from one source depends on the direction or magnitude of the error from the other source. Finally, errors in continuous measurements can be factored into systematic and random components. As described in the following sections, these classifications have important implications for bias.

Procedural error

Procedural error is the most straightforward to imagine. It includes errors in recall when variables are measured through retrospective interview (for example, mistakes in remembering all medications taken during pregnancy). It also includes coding errors, errors in calibration of instruments, and all other errors in which the target of measurement is well defined and the attempts at measurement are direct but the method of measurement is faulty. In our example, one target of measurement is HIV-1 antibody presence in blood. All available tests for antibody presence are subject to error (false negatives and false positives), and these errors can be considered to be procedural errors of measurement.

Proxy-variable error

Proxy-variable error is distinguished from procedural error in that use of proxies necessitates imputation and hence virtually guarantees that there will be measurement error. In our example, we must impute the time of HIV-1 infection. For instance, we might take as a proxy the infection time computed as six weeks before the midpoint between the last negative test and the first positive test for HIV-1 antibodies. Even if our HIV-1 tests are perfect, this measurement incorporates error if (as is certainly the case) time of infection does not always occur six weeks before the midpoint between the last negative and first positive tests.

Construct error

Construct error is often overlooked, although it may be a major source of error. Consider our example in which the ultimate target of measurement is the time between HIV-1 infection and onset of AIDS. Before attempting to measure this time span, we must unambiguously define the events that mark the beginning and end of the span. While it may be reasonable to think of HIV-1 infection as a point event, the same cannot be said of AIDS onset. Various symptoms and signs may gradually accumulate, and then it is only by convention that some point in time is declared the start of the disease. If this convention cannot be translated into reasonably precise clinical criteria for diagnosing the onset of AIDS, the construct of incubation time (the time span between infection and AIDS onset) will not be well defined let alone accurately measurable. In such situations it may be left to various clinicians to improvise answers to the question of time of AIDS onset, and this will introduce another source of extraneous variation into the final 'measurement' of incubation time.

Differential and non-differential error

Errors in measuring a variable are said to be **differential** when the direction or magnitude of the errors tend to vary across the true values of other variables. Suppose, for example, that recall of drug use during pregnancy is enhanced among mothers of children with birth defects. Then a retrospective interview about drug use during pregnancy will yield results with differential error, since false-negative error will occur more frequently among mothers whose children have no birth defects.

Another type of differential error occurs in the measurement of continuous variables when the distribution of errors varies with the true value of the variable. Suppose, for example, that women more accurately recall the date of a recent cervical smear test (Papanicolaou (Pap) test) than the date of a more distant test. Then a retrospective interview to determine length of time since a woman's last cervical smear test would tend to suffer from larger errors when measuring longer times.

Errors in measuring a variable are said to be **non-differential** with respect to another variable if the magnitudes of errors do not tend to vary with the true values of the other variable. Measurements are usually assumed to be non-differential if neither the subject nor the person taking the measurement knows the values of other variables. For example, if drug use during pregnancy is measured by examining prepartum prescription records for the mother, it would ordinarily be assumed that the error will be non-differential with respect to birth defects discovered postnatally. Nevertheless, such 'blind' assessments will not guarantee non-differential error if the measurement scale is not as fine as the scale of the original variable (Flegal *et al.* 1991; Wacholder *et al.* 1991) or if there is a third uncontrolled variable that affects both the measurement and the other study variables.

Dependent and independent error

Errors in measuring two variables are said to be **dependent** if the direction or magnitude of the errors made in measuring one of the variables is associated with the direction or magnitude of the errors made in measuring the other variable. If there is no association of errors, the errors are said to be **independent**.

In our example, errors in measuring age at HIV-1 infection and AIDS incubation time are dependent. Our measure of incubation time is equal to our measure of age at AIDS onset minus our measure of age at infection; hence overestimation of age at infection will contribute to underestimation of incubation time, and underestimation of age at infection will contribute to overestimation of incubation time. In contrast, in the same example it is plausible that the errors in measuring age at infection and age at onset are independent.

Misclassification and bias toward the null

Measurement of a binary (dichotomous) variable is called better than random if, regardless of the true value, the probability that the measurement yields the true value is higher than the probability that it does not. In other words, the measurement is better than random if it is more likely to be correct than incorrect, no matter what the true value is. Given two binary variables, better-than-random measurements with independent non-differential errors cannot inflate or reverse the association observed between the variables. In other words, any bias produced by independent non-differential error in better-than-random measurements can only be towards the null value of the association (which is one for a relative-risk measure) and not beyond.

If either variable has more than two levels, then (contrary to assertions in most pre-1990 literature) the preceding conditions are not sufficient to guarantee that the resulting bias will only be towards the null and not beyond (Dosemeci *et al.* 1990). Despite this insufficiency, knowing that errors are independent and non-differential can increase the plausibility that any resulting bias is towards the null. For further discussions of sufficient conditions for error to produce bias toward the null, see the correspondence in the *American Journal of Epidemiology*, 15 August 1991, as well as articles by Flegal *et al.* (1991), Wacholder *et al.* (1991), and Weinberg *et al.* (1993).

There is one important situation in which the assumption of independent non-differential measurement error and hence bias towards the null have particularly high plausibility: in a double-blind clinical trial with a dichotomous treatment and outcome, successful blinding of treatment status during outcome evaluation should lead to independence and non-differentiality of treatment and outcome measurement errors. Successful blinding thus helps to ensure (although it does not guarantee) that any bias produced by measurement error contributes to underestimation of treatment differences (conservative bias).

Systematic and random components of error

For well-defined measurement procedures on continuous variables, measurement errors can be subdivided into systematic and random components. The systematic component (sometimes called the bias of the measurement) measures the degree to which the procedure tends to underestimate or overestimate the true value on repeated application. The random component is the residual error left after subtracting the systematic component from the total error.

To illustrate, suppose that in our study HIV-1 infection time was unrelated to time of antibody testing and that the average time of HIV-1 seroconversion was eight weeks after infection. Then, even if one used a perfect HIV-1 test, a procedure that estimated infection time as six weeks before the midpoint between the last negative and first positive test would on average yield an estimated infection time that was two weeks later than the true time. Thus the systematic component of the error of this procedure would be +2 weeks. Since AIDS incubation time is AIDS onset time minus HIV-1 infection time, use of this procedure would add −2 weeks (i.e. a two-week underestimation) to the systematic component of error in estimating incubation time.

Each of the components of an error, systematic and random, may be differential (i.e. may vary with other variable values) or non-differential, and may or may not be independent of the error components in other variables. We shall not explore the consequences of the numerous possibilities. However, one important (but semantically confusing) fact is that, for certain quantities, independent and non-differential systematic components of error will not harm measurement validity in that they will produce no bias in estimation.

To illustrate, suppose that in our example we wish to estimate the degree to which AIDS incubation time depends on age at HIV-1 infection. Suppose also that the systematic components of the measurements of incubation time and age of infection are −2 weeks and +2 weeks (as above), and do not vary with true incubation time or age at measurement (i.e. the systematic components are non-differential). Then the systematic components, being equal, will cancel out when we compute differences in incubation time and differences in age at infection. Since only these differences are used to estimate the association, the observed dependence of incubation time on age at infection will not be affected by the systematic components of error (although it may be biased by the random components of error).

Summary of example

The example of this section provides an illustration of the most common threats to the validity of predictions. The unadjusted estimates of AIDS risk may be confounded if the target and reference cohorts differ in composition, and may also be biased by losses to follow-up or use of an incorrect statistical model. Finally, our predictions are likely to be compromised by errors in measurements. These sources of error should be borne in mind in attempts to predict AIDS incidence in populations newly infected by HIV-1.

Validity in causal inference

Concepts of valid prediction are applicable in evaluating studies of causation; comparison validity, follow-up validity, specification validity, and measurement validity must each be considered. In fact, as we shall see, problems of causal inference can be viewed as a special type of prediction problem, namely prediction of what would happen (or what would have happened) to a population if certain characteristics of the population were (or had been) altered.

To illustrate validity issues in causal inference, we shall consider the hypothesis that coffee drinking causes acute myocardial infarction. This hypothesis can be operationally interpreted in a number of ways, such as the following.

1. There are people for whom the consumption of coffee results in their experiencing a myocardial infarction sooner than they might have, had they avoided coffee.

While this hypothesis is appealingly precise, it offers little practical guidance to an epidemiological researcher. The problem lies in our inability to recognize an individual whose myocardial infarction was caused by coffee drinking. It is quite possible that myocardial infarctions precipitated by coffee use are clinically and pathologically indistinguishable from myocardial infarctions due to other causes. If so, the prospect of finding convincing physiological evidence concerning the hypothesis is not good.

We could overcome this impasse by examining a related epidemiologic hypothesis, i.e. a hypothesis that refers to the distribution of disease in populations. One of many such hypotheses is given next.

2. Among five-cup-a-day coffee drinkers, cessation of coffee use will lower the frequency of myocardial infarction.

This form not only involves a population (five-cup-a-day coffee drinkers) but also asserts that a mass action (coffee cessation) will reduce the frequency of the study disease. Thus the form of the hypothesis immediately suggests a strong test of the hypothesis: conduct a randomized intervention trial to examine the impact of coffee cessation on myocardial infarction frequency. This solution has some profound practical limitations, not least of which would be persuading anyone to give up or take up coffee drinking to test a speculative hypothesis.

Having ruled out intervention, we might consider an observational cohort study. In this case our epidemiological hypothesis should refer to natural conditions, rather than intervention. One such hypothesis is as follows.

3. Among five-cup-a-day coffee drinkers, coffee use has elevated the frequency of myocardial infarction.

In fact there have been a number of conflicting cohort and case–control studies of coffee and myocardial infarction. The present discussion will be confined to the issues arising in the analysis of a single study. For a review of issues arising in the analysis of multiple studies (meta-analysis) using the coffee–myocardial infarction literature as an example, see Greenland (1987*b*, 1994). Additional references to the coffee-myocardial infarction literature are given by Greenland (1993*a*).

Consider a cohort study of coffee and first myocardial infarction. At baseline, a cohort of people with no history of myocardial infarction is assembled and classified into subcohorts according to coffee use (for example never-drinkers, ex-drinkers, occasional drinkers, one-cup-a-day drinkers, two-cup-a-day drinkers, etc.). Other variables are measured as well: age, sex, smoking habits, blood pressure, and serum cholesterol. Suppose that at the end of ten years of monitoring this cohort for myocardial infarction events, we compare the five-cup-a-day and never-drinker subcohorts, and obtain an unadjusted estimate of 1.22 for the ratio of the person-time incidence rates of first myocardial infarction among five-cup-a-day drinkers and never-drinkers (with 95 per cent confidence limits of 1.00 and 1.49). In other words, it appears that the rate of first myocardial infarction among five-cup-a-day drinkers was 1.22 times higher than the rate among never-drinkers. (Hereafter, myocardial infarction means first myocardial infarction, risk means average risk, and rate means person-time incidence rate.)

The estimated rate ratio of 1.22 may not seem large. Nevertheless, if it accurately reflects the impact of coffee use on the five-cup-a-day subcohort, this estimate implies that persons drinking five cups a day at baseline suffered a 22 per cent increase in their myocardial infarction rate as a result of their coffee use. Given the high frequency of both coffee use and myocardial infarction in many populations, this could represent a substantial health impact.

Therefore we should want to perform a careful evaluation of the validity of the estimate.

As in the previous AIDS example, we can proceed by examining a series of conditions sufficient for validity of the estimate as a measure of coffee effect.

(C) *Comparison validity*   If the members of the five-cup-a-day subcohort had instead never drunk coffee, their distribution of myocardial infarction events over time would have been approximately the same as the distribution among the never-drinkers.

(F) *Follow-up validity*   Within each subcohort, the risk of censoring (i.e. follow-up ended by an event other than myocardial infarction) is not associated with the risk of myocardial infarction.

(Sp) *Specification validity*   The distribution of myocardial infarction events over time in the subcohorts can be closely approximated by the statistical model on which the estimates are based.

(M) *Measurement validity*   All measurements of variables used in the analysis closely approximate the true values of the variables.

These four conditions are sometimes called internal validity conditions because they pertain only to estimating effects within the study cohort rather than to generalizing results to other cohorts. They are sufficient but not necessary for validity, in that certain violations of the conditions will not produce bias in the effect estimate (although most violations will produce some bias). The meaning of these conditions for an observational cohort study of a causal hypothesis is explored in the following sections. An important phenomenon known as effect modification, which is relevant to both internal validity and generalizability, is also discussed.

Comparison validity

In our example, comparison validity simply means that the distribution of myocardial infarctions among never-drinkers accurately predicts what would have happened in the coffee-drinking groups had the members of these groups never drunk coffee. Another way of stating condition **C** is that the five-cup-a-day and never-drinker subcohorts would be comparable or exchangeable with respect to myocardial infarction times if no one had ever drunk coffee.

Despite its simplicity, note that the comparison validity condition depends on the hypothesis of interest in a very precise way. In particular, the research hypothesis (hypothesis 3 above) is a statement about the impact of coffee among five-cup-a-day drinkers. Thus this subcohort is the target cohort, while never-drinkers serve as the reference cohort for making predictions about this target.

To illustrate further the correspondence between comparison validity and the hypothesis at issue, suppose for the moment that our research hypothesis was as follows.

4. Among never-drinkers, five-cup-a-day coffee use would elevate the frequency of myocardial infarction.

In examining this hypothesis, the never-drinkers would be the target cohort and the coffee drinkers would be the reference cohort. Thus the comparison validity condition would have to be replaced by a condition such as the following.

> **(C')** If the never-drinkers had drunk five cups of coffee per day, their distribution of myocardial infarctions would have been approximately the same as the distribution among five-cup-a-day drinkers.

Other ways of stating condition **C'** are that the five-cup-a-day and never-drinker subcohorts would be comparable or exchangeable with respect to myocardial infarction times if everyone had been five-cup-a-day drinkers, and that the myocardial infarction experience of five-cup-a-day drinkers accurately predicts what would have happened to the never-drinkers if the latter had drunk five cups a day.

Confounding

Failure to meet condition **C** results in a biased estimate of the effect of five-cup-a-day coffee drinking on five-cup-a-day drinkers, a condition sometimes referred to as confounding of the estimate. Similarly, failure to meet condition **C'** results in a biased estimate of the effect that five-cup-a-day drinking would have had on never-drinkers.

To evaluate comparison validity, we must check whether the subcohorts differed at baseline on any factors that influence myocardial infarction time. If so, we could not reasonably expect the myocardial infarction distributions of the subcohorts to be comparable, even if the subcohorts had the same level of coffee use. In other words, we could not expect condition **C** (or **C'**) to hold, and so we should expect our estimates to suffer from confounding.

In our example, we should note that several studies have found a positive association between cigarette smoking (an established risk factor for myocardial infarction) and coffee use (Greenland 1987*b*). It also seems a priori sensible that a person habituated to a stimulant such as nicotine would be attracted to coffee use as well. Thus we should expect to see a higher prevalence of smoking among coffee users in our study.

Suppose then that, in our cohort, smoking is more prevalent among five-cup-a-day subjects than never-drinkers. This elevated smoking prevalence should have led to elevated myocardial infarction rates among five-cup-a-day drinkers, even if coffee had no effect. More generally, we should expect the myocardial infarction rate among never-drinkers to underestimate the myocardial infarction rate that five-cup-a-day drinkers would have had if they had never drunk coffee. The result would be an inflated estimate of the impact of coffee on the myocardial infarction rate of five-cup-a-day drinkers. Similarly, we should expect the myocardial infarction rate among five-cup-a-day drinkers to overestimate the myocardial infarction rate that never-drinkers would have had if they had drunk five cups a day.

Adjustment for measured confounders

As in the prediction problem, we can stratify the data on potential confounders with the objective of creating strata within which confounding is minimal or absent. We can also employ standardization to remove confounding from estimates of overall effect. Again, some care in the selection of the standard is required.

To illustrate, let R_{xz} denote the estimated rate of myocardial infarction among cohort members who drank x cups of coffee per day and smoked z cigarettes per day at baseline, with R_{0z} denoting the estimated rate among never-drinkers. Let W_{xz} denote the proportion of person-time among x-cup-per-day drinkers that was contributed by z-cigarette-per-day smokers. Finally, let R_{xc} be the crude (unadjusted) rate observed among cohort members who drank x cups per day at baseline, with R_{0c} denoting the estimated crude rate among never-drinkers.

Suppose for the moment that any change in coffee-use patterns would have negligible impact on the longitudinal smoking distribution of the cohort. The predicted (i.e. expected) rate among five-cup-per-day drinkers had they never drunk coffee, adjusted for confounding by smoking, is the average of the smoking-specific estimates from the never-drinker (reference) subcohort weighted by the smoking distribution of the five-cup-per-day (target) cohort. Algebraically, this average is the following sum (over z):

$$\Sigma_z W_{5z} R_{0z}.$$

This sum is commonly termed the rate in the never-drinkers standardized to the distribution of smoking among five-cup-a-day drinkers. Such terminology obscures the fact that the sum is a prediction about the five-cup-a-day drinkers, not the never-drinkers.

Given the last computation, a smoking-standardized estimate of the increase in myocardial infarction rate produced by coffee drinking among five-cup-per-day drinkers is the rate ratio standardized to the five-cup-per-day smoking distribution:

$$\Sigma_z W_{5z} R_{5z} / \Sigma_z W_{5z} R_{0z}.$$

This formula reveals a property common to (and essential for) any standardized rate ratio: the same weights W_{xz} must be used in the numerator and denominator sums. Some insight into this formula can be obtained by noting that the crude rate R_{5c} among the five-cup-a-day drinkers is equal to

$$\Sigma_z W_{5z} R_{5z},$$

so that the standardized rate ratio can be rewritten as

$$R_{5c} / \Sigma_z W_{5z} R_{0z}.$$

This version shows that the ratio is a classical observed (crude) over expected ratio, or standardized morbidity ration (SMR). Another standardized rate ratio is

$$\Sigma_z W_{0z} R_{5z} / \Sigma_z W_{0z} R_{0z}.$$

This differs from the previous standardized ratio in that the weights are taken from the never drinkers (W_{0z}) instead of five-cup-a-day drinkers (W_{5z}). Insight into this formula can be obtained by noting that the numerator sum is simply a prediction (expectation) of what would have happened to the never-drinkers if they had been five-cup-a-day drinkers, while the denominator sum is equal to the crude rate R_{0c}, among never-drinkers. Thus the last standardized ratio is a smoking-standardized estimate of the increase in the myocardial infarction rate that five-cup-a-day drinking would have produced among the never-drinkers.

Standardization is appealingly simple in both justification and computation. Unfortunately, if the number of cases occurring within the confounder categories tends to be small (under five or so), the technique will be subject to various technical problems including possible bias. These problems can be avoided by broadening confounder categories or by not adjusting for some of the measured confounders. Unfortunately, both these strategies are likely to result in incomplete control of confounding. To avoid having to adopt these strategies, many researchers attempt to control confounding by using a multivariate model. This remedy has problems of its own, some of which we shall address in the section on specification validity.

Another problem is that standardized procedures (as well as typical modelling procedures) take no account of potential exposure effects on the adjustment variables or their distribution. Thus, in the above example, to justify use of the fixed weights W_{xz} we had to invoke the dubious assumption that changes in coffee use would only negligibly affect the smoking distribution. We shall briefly discuss this issue in the section on intermediate variables.

Unmeasured confounders
Among the possible confounders not measured in our hypothetical study are diet and exercise. Suppose that 'health conscious' subjects who exercise regularly and eat low-fat diets also avoid coffee. The result will be a concentration of these lower-risk subjects among coffee non-users and a consequent overestimation of coffee's effect on risk.

Confounding by unmeasured confounders can sometimes be minimized by controlling variables along pathways of the confounders' effect. For example, if exercise and low-fat diet lowered myocardial infarction risk only by lowering serum cholesterol and blood pressure, control of serum cholesterol and blood pressure would remove confounding by exercise and dietary fat. Unfortunately, such control may also generate bias if the controlled variables are intermediates between our study variable and our outcome variable.

If external information is available to indicate the relationship in our study between an unmeasured confounder and the study variables, we can attempt to use an indirect method to adjust for the confounder (Schlesselman 1978; Flanders and Khoury 1990). If external information is unreliable or unavailable, we can still examine the sensitivity of our results to unmeasured confounding (Cornfield et al. 1959; Rosenbaum 1995; Flanders and Khoury 1990).

Randomization and confounding
Suppose, for the moment, that the level of coffee use in our cohort had been assigned by randomization and that the participants diligently consumed only their assigned amount of coffee. Could our estimates of coffee effects from such a randomized trial still be confounded? By our earlier definition of confounding, the answer is yes. To see this, note for example that by chance alone the five-cup-a-day drinkers could be older on average than the never-drinkers; this difference would in turn result in an upward bias in the unadjusted estimate of the effect of five cups a day, since age is an important risk factor for myocardial infarction.

Nevertheless, randomization can help to ensure that the distributions of confounders in the different exposure groups are not too far apart. In essence, the probability of severe confounding can be made as small as necessary by increasing the size of the randomized groups. Furthermore, if randomization is used and subjects comply with their assigned treatments, any confounding left after adjustment will be accounted for by the standard errors of the estimates, provided that the correct statistical model is used to compute the effect estimates and their standard errors (Robins 1988; Greenland 1990).

Intermediate variables
In effect estimation, we must take care to distinguish intermediate variables from confounding variables. Intermediate variables represent steps in the causal pathway from the study exposure to the outcome event. The distinction is essential, for control of intermediate variables can increase the bias of estimates.

To illustrate, suppose that coffee use affects serum cholesterol levels (as suggested by the results of Curb et al. (1986)). Then, given that serum cholesterol affects myocardial infarction risk, serum cholesterol is an intermediate variable for the study of coffee effects on this risk. Now suppose that we stratify our cohort data on serum cholesterol levels. Some coffee drinkers will be in elevated cholesterol categories because of coffee use and so will be at elevated myocardial infarction risk because of coffee effects, yet these subjects will be compared with never-drinkers in the same stratum who are also at elevated risk due to their elevated cholesterol. Therefore the effect of coffee on myocardial infarction risk via the cholesterol pathway will not be apparent within the cholesterol strata, and so cholesterol adjustment will contribute to underestimation of the coffee effect on myocardial infarction risk. Analogously, if coffee affected myocardial infarction risk by elevating blood pressure, blood-pressure adjustment will contribute to underestimation of the coffee effect. Such underestimation can be termed overadjustment bias.

Intermediate variables may also be confounders and thus present the investigator with a severe dilemma. Consider that most of the variation in serum cholesterol levels is not due to coffee use and that much (perhaps most) of the association between coffee use and cholesterol is not due to coffee effects, but rather to factors associated with both coffee and cholesterol (such as exercise and dietary fat). This means that serum cholesterol may also be viewed as a confounder for the coffee–myocardial infarction study, and that estimates unadjusted for serum cholesterol will be biased unless they are also adjusted for the factors contributing to the coffee–cholesterol association.

Suppose that a variable is both an intermediate and a confounder. It will usually be impossible to determine how much of the change in the effect estimate produced by adjusting for the variable is due to introduction of overadjustment bias and how much is due to removal of confounding. Nevertheless, a qualitative assessment may be possible in some situations. For example, if we know that the effects of coffee on serum cholesterol are weak and that most of the association between coffee and serum colesterol is due to confouding of this association by uncontrolled factors (such as exercise and diet), we can conclude that the cholesterol-adjusted estimate is the less biased of the two. Alternatively, if we have accurately measured all the factors that confound the coffee–cholesterol association, we can control these factors instead of cholesterol to obtain an estimate free of both overadjustment bias and confounding by cholesterol. Finally, if we have multiple measurements of coffee use and cholesterol over time, techniques are available that adjust for the confounding effects of cholesterol but do not introduce overadjustment (Robins 1989; Robins and Greenland 1994).

Direct and indirect effects

Often, one may wish to estimate how much of the effect under study is indirect relative to an intermediate variable (in the sense of being transmitted through the intermediate), or how much of the effect is direct relative to the intermediate (i.e. not mediated by the intermediate). For example, we might wish to estimate how much of coffee's effect on myocardial infarction risk is due to its effect on serum cholesterol, or how much is due to coffee effects on cardiovascular variables other than cholesterol.

One common approach to this problem is to adjust the coffee–myocardial infarction association for serum cholesterol level via ordinary stratification or regression methods and then use the resulting estimate as the estimate of the direct coffee effect. This procedure is potentially biased as it may introduce new confounding by determinants of serum cholesterol, even if these determinants did not confound the total (unadjusted) association (Robins and Greenland 1992). However, given sufficient data, it is possible to obtain separate estimates for direct and indirect effects using special stratification or modelling techniques (Robins and Greenland 1994).

Follow-up validity

In our example, follow-up validity means that follow-up is valid within every subcohort being compared. In other words, over any span of time during follow-up, myocardial infarction risk within a subcohort is unassociated with censoring risk in the subcohort. Given follow-up validity, we can expect that, at any follow-up time t, the myocardial infarction rates in a subcohort will be the same for subjects lost or withdrawn at t and subjects whose follow-up continues beyond t.

In fact, we should expect follow-up to be biased by cigarette smoking: smoking is associated with mortality from myocardial infarction and from many other causes; the association of smoking with socio-economic status might also produce an association between smoking and loss to follow-up. The result would be elevated censoring among high-risk (smoking) subjects. As a consequence, unadjusted estimates of myocardial infarction risks will underestimate those risks in the complete subcohorts (as the latter includes both censored and uncensored subject experience). If the degree of underestimation varies across subcohorots, bias in the relative-risk estimates will result.

In fact, the degree of underestimation should vary in this example because of the variation in smoking prevalence across subcohorts. Nevertheless, variation in smoking prevalence is not necessary for smoking-related censoring to produce biased estimates of absolute effect. For example, if smoking-related censoring produced a uniform 15 per cent underestimation of the myocardial infarction rate in each subcohort, all rate differences would also be underestimated by 15 per cent.

Analogous to control of confounding, any bias produced by smoking's association with myocardial infarction and censoring can be removed by smoking adjustment. As before, if adjustment is by standardization, the standard distribution should be chosen from the target subcohort.

Because the same correction methods can sometimes be applied, some authors (e.g. Miettinen 1985) classify follow-up bias as a form of confounding. Nevertheless, the two phenomena are reversed with respect to the causal ordering of the third variable responsible for the bias: confounding arises from an association of the study exposure (coffee use) with other exposures (such as smoking) that affect outcome risk; in contrast, follow-up bias arises from an association between the risk of the study outcome (myocardial infarction) and risks of other endpoints (such as other-cause mortality or loss to follow-up) that are affected by exposure. Furthermore, certain forms of follow-up bias cannot be removed by adjustment. These problems are discussed in the statistics literature under the heading dependent competing risks; see Kalbfleisch and Prentice (1980) and Slud and Byar (1988) for discussions of this issue.

Some authors (e.g. Kelsey *et al.* 1986) classify follow-up bias as a form of selection bias. Here, we reserve the latter term for a special problem of case–control studies (discussed below).

Specification validity

As noted earlier, the use of a statistical method based on an incorrect model (specification error) can lead to bias in estimates and improper performance of statistical tests and interval estimates. All statistical techniques, including non-parametric methods, must assume some sort of model for the process generating the data; however, in the absence of randomization or random sampling, it will rarely be possible to identify a 'correct' sampling model. In addition, structural assumptions are rarely (if ever) exactly satisfied. Thus some specification error should be expected. As before, minimization of specification error must rely on checking the model against the data and against background information about the processes generating the data.

Recall that the unadjusted rate ratio estimate for five-cup-a-day versus never-drinkers is 1.22 in the present example, with 95 per cent confidence limits of 1.00 and 1.49, and a p value of 0.05. Suppose that these figures were obtained by the person-time methods given in epidemiological textbooks such as Kleinbaum *et al.* (1982, pp. 285–8) or Rothman (1986, pp. 153–6). These methods are based on a binomial sampling model for the number of cases who drank five cups a day at baseline, given the combined total number of cases among five-cup-a-day and never-drinkers. In our example, the validity of this model depends on the assumption that the myocardial infarction rate remains constant within subcohorts over the follow-up period. It follows that the model (and hence the statistics given earlier) cannot be valid in our example; the subcohort members grow older over the follow-up period, and hence the myocardial infarction rates must increase with follow-up time.

The invalidity just noted can be rectified by stratifying either on follow-up time or the variable responsible for the change in rates over follow-up time (here, age). The stratification need only be fine enough to ensure that the myocardial infarction rate change within strata is negligible over follow-up. As we noted earlier, however, we must also adjust for smoking and perhaps other factors responsible for confounding or follow-up bias. If we stratify finely enough to remove all the bias from these sources, the resulting estimates would be undefined or so unstable that they would tell us nothing about the association of coffee and myocardial infarction.

The standard solution to such problems is to compute adjusted estimates using regression models. These are structural models representing a set of assumptions (usually rather strong ones) about the joint effects of the study variables. Such models allow estimates and tests to be extracted from what would otherwise be hopelessly sparse data. Of course, the cost is a greater risk of bias arising from violations of the assumptions underlying the models (Robins and Greenland 1986). An overview of the problem of finding a reasonably correct model is provided elsewhere (Greenland 1989). For further details of cohort modelling, see Kleinbaum *et al.* (1982), Kelsey *et al.* (1986), Breslow and Day (1987), Checkoway *et al.* (1989), Hosmer and Lemeshow (1989), or Clayton and Hills (1993).

Measurement validity

Unlike sex, the continuous variables of coffee use, cigarette use, blood pressure, cholesterol, and age are time-dependent covariates. With the exception of age (whose value at any time can be computed from birth date), this fact adds considerable complexity to measuring these variables and estimating their effects.

Consider that we cannot reasonably expect a single baseline measurement, no matter how accurate, to summarize adequately a subject's entire history of coffee drinking, smoking, blood pressure, or cholesterol. Even if the effect of a subject's history could be largely captured by using a single summary number (for example total number of cigarettes smoked), the baseline measurement may well be a poor proxy for this ideal and unknown summary. For these reasons, we should expect proxy-variable errors to be very large in our example.

Proxy-variable error in the study variables

The degree of proxy-variable error in measuring the study variables depends on the exact definitions of the variables that we wish to study. In turn, this definition should reflect the hypothesized effect that we wish to study. To illustrate, consider the following acute effect hypothesis.

Drinking a cup of coffee produces an immediate rise in short-term myocardial infarction risk. In other words, coffee consumption is an acute risk factor.

Note that this hypothesis does not exclude the possibility that coffee use also elevates long-term risk of myocardial infarction, perhaps through some other mechanism; it simply does not address the issue of chronic effects.

One way of examining the hypothesis would be to compare the myocardial infarction rates among person-days in which one, two, three, etc. cups were drunk with the rate among person-days in which no coffee was drunk (adjusting, of course, for confounding and follow-up bias). However, if we had only baseline data, baseline daily consumption would have to serve as the proxy for consumption on every day of follow-up. This would probably be a poor proxy for daily consumption at later follow-up times where more outcome events occur. It turns out that a 'standard' analysis, which simply examines the association of baseline coffee use with myocardial infarction rates, is equivalent to an analysis that uses baseline consumption as a proxy for consumption on all later days. Thus, estimates from a standard analysis would suffer large bias if considered as estimates of acute coffee effect.

Note that the proxy-variable error in the last example could easily be differential with respect to the outcome: person-days accumulate more rapidly in early follow-up, where the error from using baseline consumption as the proxy is relatively low; in contrast, myocardial infarction events accumulate more rapidly in later follow-up, where the error is probably higher. This illustrates an important general point: errors in variables can be differential, even if the variables are measured before the outcome event. Such phenomena occur when errors are associated with risk factors for the outcome; in our example, the error is associated with follow-up time and hence age. In turn, such associations are likely to occur when measurements are based on proxy variables.

Suppose now that we examine the following chronic effect hypothesis.

Each cup of coffee drunk eventually results in a long-term elevation of myocardial infarction risk.

This hypothesis was suggested by reports that coffee drinking produces a rise in serum lipid levels (Curb *et al.* 1986). Note that it does not address the issue of acute effects. One way to examine the hypothesis would be to compare the myocardial infarction rates among person-months with different cumulative doses of coffee (perhaps using a lag period in calculating dose; for example, one might ignore the most recent month of consumption). If we had only baseline data, however, baseline daily consumption would have to be used to construct a proxy for cumulative consumption at every month of follow-up. This could be done in several different ways. For example, we could estimate subjects' cumulative doses up to a particular date by multiplying their baseline daily consumption by the number of days that they had lived between age 18 and the date in question. This estimate assumes that coffee drinking began at age 18 and the baseline daily consumption is the average daily consumption since that age. We should expect considerable error in such a crude measure of cumulative consumption.

The degree of bias in estimating chronic effects could be quite different from the degree of bias in estimating acute effects. Furthermore, as discussed below, the errors in each proxy will make it virtually impossible to discriminate between acute and chronic effects.

Measurement error and confounding

If a variable is measured with error, estimates adjusted for the variable as measured will still be somewhat confounded by the variable. This residual confounding arises because measurement error prevents construction of strata that are internally homogeneous with respect to the true confounding variable (Greenland 1980).

To illustrate, consider baseline daily cigarette consumption. This variable can be considered a proxy for consumption on each day of follow-up or can be used to construct an estimate of cumulative consumption (analogous to the cumulative coffee variable discussed above).

Suppose that we stratify the data on a cumulative smoking index constructed from the baseline smoking measurement. Within any stratum of the index, there would remain a broad range of cumulative cigarette consumption. For example, two subjects who were age 40 and smoked one pack a day at baseline would receive the same value for the smoking index and so end up in the same stratum. However, if one of them stopped smoking immediately after baseline, while the other continued to smoke a pack a day, after 10 years of follow-up the former subject would have ten less pack-years of cigarette consumption than the continuing smoker.

Suppose now that cumulative cigarette consumption is positively associated with cumulative coffee consumption. Then, even within strata of the smoking index, we should expect subjects with high coffee consumption to exhibit elevated myocardial infarction rates simply by virtue of having higher levels of cigarette consumption. As a consequence, the estimate of coffee effect adjusted for the smoking index would still be confounded by cumulative cigarette consumption.

In some cases a study variable may appear to have an effect (or no effect) only because of poor measurement of an apparently unimportant confounder. This can occur, for example, when an important confounding variable is measured with a large amount of non-differential error. Such an error would ordinarily reduce the apparent association of the variable with the exposure, and would also make the variable appear to be a weak risk factor, perhaps weaker than the study exposure. This in turn would make the variable appear to be only weakly confounding, in that adjustment for the variable as measured would produce little change in the result. However, this appearance would be deceptive because adjustment for the variable as measured would eliminate little of the actual confounding by the variable.

To illustrate this phenomenon, suppose that coronary proneness of personality was measured only by the baseline yes–no question: Do you consider yourself a hard-driving person? Such a crude measure of the original construct would be unlikely to show more than a weak association with either coffee use or myocardial infarction, and adjusting for it would produce little change in our estimate of coffee effect. Suppose, however, that coronary-prone personalities have an elevated preference for coffee. Such a phenomenon would lead to a concentration of coronary-prone persons (and hence a spuriously elevated myocardial infarction rate) among coffee drinkers, even after stratification on response to the above question.

One would ordinarily expect adjustment for a non-differentially misclassified confounder to produce an estimate lying somewhere between the crude (unadjusted) estimate and the estimate adjusted for the true values of the confounder (Greenland 1980). Unfortunately, if the true confounder has more than two levels, it is possible for adjustment by the misclassified confounder to be more biased than the crude estimate (Brenner 1993). It is also possible for adjustment by factors that affect misclassification to worsen bias (Greenland and Robins 1985).

Measurement error and separation of effects
Because of their impact on the effectiveness of adjustment procedures, measurement errors can severely reduce our ability to separate different effects of the study variable. Suppose in our example that we wished to estimate the relative strength of acute and chronic coffee effects. To do so we must take account of the fact that acute and chronic effects will be confounded. When examining acute effects, person-days with high coffee consumption will occur most frequently among persons with high cumulative coffee consumption. As a consequence, if cumulative coffee consumption

is a risk factor, it will be a confounder for estimating the acute effects of coffee consumption. By similar arguments, if coffee consumption has acute effects, these will confound estimates of the chronic effects of cumulative consumption.

Unfortunately, both cumulative and daily consumption are measured with considerable error. As a result, any effect observed for one may be wholly or partially due to the other, even if the other has little or no apparent effect.

Repeated measures
One costly but effective method for reducing the degree of proxy-variable error in measuring time-dependent variables is to take repeated (serial) measurements over the follow-up period and ask subjects to report their pre-baseline history of such variables at the baseline interview. In our example, subjects could be asked about their age at first use and level of consumption at different ages for coffee and cigarettes; they could then be recontacted every year or two to assess their current consumption. Of course, not all subjects may be willing to co-operate with such active follow-up, but the penalties of some extra loss may be far outweighed by the benefit of improved measurement accuracy.

Errors in assessing incidence
A particularly important form of measurement error in assessing incidence is misdiagnosis of the outcome event. In the AIDS example, a false-positive diagnosis of AIDS would result in underestimation of incubation time, while a false-negative diagnosis would result in overestimation. In the present example, false-positive errors would result in overestimation of myocardial infarction rates, while false-negative errors would result in underestimation. These errors will be of particular concern when the study depends on existing surveillance systems or records for detection of outcome events. However, there are some special cases in which the errors will induce little or no bias in estimates (Poole 1985).

If the only form of misdiagnosis is false-negative error, if the proportion of outcome events missed in this fashion is the same across cohorts, and if there is no follow-up bias, then the relative-risk estimates will not be distorted by the underdiagnosis. Suppose in our example that all recorded myocardial infarction events are true myocardial infarctions, but that in each subcohort 10 per cent of myocardial infarctions are missed. The myocardial infarction rates in each subcohort will then be underestimated by 10 per cent; nevertheless, if we consider any two of these rates, say R_0 and R_5, the observed rate ratio will be

$$\frac{0.9R_5}{0.9R_0} = \frac{R_5}{R_0}$$

which is undistorted by the underdiagnosis of myocardial infarction. However, if coffee primarily induced 'silent' myocardial infarctions and these were the most frequently undiagnosed events, the coffee effect would be underestimated.

In an analogous fashion, if the only form of misdiagnosis is false-positive error, if the rate of false positives is the same across cohorts, and if there is no follow-up bias, then rate differences will not be distorted by the overdiagnosis. Suppose that the rate of false positives in our example is R_f in all subcohorts; then if we consider any two true rates, say R_0 and R_5, the observed rate difference will be

$$(R_5 + R_f) - (R_0 + R_f) = R_5 - R_0$$

which is undistorted by the overdiagnosis of myocardial infarction. However, if there is non-differential underdiagnosis of myocardial infarction, as is probably the case in our example, the rate difference will be underestimated.

Effect modification (heterogeneity of effect)

Estimation of effects usually requires consideration of effect-measure modification, which is also known as effect modification, effect variation, or heterogeneity of effect. As an example, suppose that drinking five cups of coffee a day elevated the myocardial infarction rate of men in our cohort by a factor of 1.40 (i.e. a 40 per cent increase), but elevated the myocardial infarction rate of women by a factor of only 1.10 (i.e. a 10 per cent increase). This situation would be termed modification (or variation or heterogeneity) of the rate ratio by sex, and sex would be called a modifier of the coffee–myocardial infarction rate ratio.

As another example, suppose that drinking five cups of coffee a day elevated the myocardial infarction rate in men in our cohort by a factor of 400 cases per 100 000 person-years but elevated the rate in women by a factor of only 40 cases per 100 000 person-years. This situation would be termed modification of the rate difference by sex, and sex would be called a modifier of the coffee–myocardial infarction rate difference.

As a final example, suppose that drinking five cups of coffee per day elevated the myocardial infarction rate in our cohort by a factor of 1.22 in both men and women. This situation would be termed homogeneity of the rate ratios across sex.

Note that effect modification and homogeneity are not absolute properties of an effect but instead are properties of the way that the effect is measured. For example, suppose that drinking five cups of coffee per day elevated the myocardial infarction rate in men from 1000 cases per 100 000 person-years to 1220 cases per 100 000 person-years, but elevated the rate in women from 400 cases per 100 000 person-years to 488 cases per 100 000 person-years. Then the sex-specific rate ratios would both be 1.22, homogeneous across sex. In contrast, the sex-specific rate differences would be 220 cases per 100 000 person-years for males and 88 cases per 100 000 person-years for females, and so are heterogeneous or 'modified' by sex. Examples such as this show that one should not equate effect modification with biological concepts of interaction such as synergy or antagonism. Further discussions of this point can be found in Kleinbaum *et al.* (1982) and Rothman (1986).

Effect modification can be analysed by stratifying the data on the potential effect modifier under study, estimating the effect within each stratum, and comparing the estimates across strata. There are several potential problems with this approach. The number of subjects in each stratum may be too small to produce stable estimates of stratum-specific effects, particularly after adjustment for confounder effects. Estimates may fluctuate wildly from stratum to stratum owing to random error. A related problem is that statistical tests for heterogeneity in stratified data have extremely low power in many situations, and therefore are likely to miss much if not most of the heterogeneity when used with conventional significance levels (such as 0.05). Finally, the amount of bias from confounding, measurement error, etc. may vary from stratum to stratum, in which case the observed pattern of modification will be biased.

Effect modification and generalizability

Suppose that we succeed in obtaining approximately unbiased estimates from our study. We can then confront issues of generalizability (external validity) of our results. For example, we can ask whether they accurately reflect the effect of coffee on myocardial infarction rates in a new target cohort. We can view such a question as a prediction problem in which the objective is to predict the strength of coffee effects in the new target cohort. From this perspective, generalizability of an effect estimate involves just one validity issue in addition to those discussed so far, namely confounding of the predicted effect by effect modifiers.

Suppose that the rate increase (in cases per 100 000 person-years) produced by coffee use is 400 for males and 40 for females among five-cup-a-day drinkers in both our study cohort and the new target. If our study cohort is 70 per cent male while the new target is only 30 per cent male, the average increase among five-cup-a-day drinkers in our study cohort would be $0.7 \times 400 + 0.3 \times 40 = 292$, whereas the average increase in the new target would be only $0.3 \times 400 + 0.7 \times 40 = 148$. Thus any valid estimate of the average increase in our study cohort will tend to overestimate greatly the average increase in the new target. In other words, modification of coffee's effect by sex confounds the prediction of its effect in the new target. This bias can be avoided by making only sex-specific predictions of effect or by standardizing the study results to the sex distribution of the new target population.

Summary of example

The example used in this section provides an illustration of the most common threats to the validity of effect estimates from cohort studies. The unadjusted estimates of coffee effect on myocardial infarction will be confounded by many variables (such as smoking), and there will be follow-up bias. As a result, the number of variables that must be controlled is too large to allow adequate control using only stratification. The true functional dependence of myocardial infarction rates on coffee and the confounder is unknown, so that estimates based on multivariate models are likely to be biased. Even if this bias is unimportant, our estimates will remain confounded because of our inability to measure the key confounders accurately. Finally, our inability to summarize coffee consumption accurately would further bias our estimates, making it impossible to separate acute and chronic effects of coffee use reliably.

Given that there are several sources of bias of unknown magnitude and different directions, it would appear that no conclusions about coffee effect could be drawn from a study like the one described above, other than that coffee does not appear to have a large effect. This type of result—inconclusive, other than to rule out very large effects—is common in thorough epidemiological analyses of observational data. In particular, inconclusive results are common when the data being analysed were collected for purposes other than to address the hypothesis at issue, for such data often lack accurate measurements of key variables.

Validity in case–control and retrospective cohort studies

Case–control studies

The practical difficulties of cohort studies have led to extensive development of case–control study designs. The distinguishing feature of such designs is that sampling is intentionally based on the outcome of individuals.

In a population-based or population-initiated case–control study, one first identifies a population at risk of the outcome of interest, which is to be studied over a specified period of time or risk period. As in a cohort study, one attempts to ascertain outcome events in the population at risk. Nevertheless, unlike a cohort study, one selects persons experiencing the outcome event (cases) and a 'control' sample of the entire population at risk for ascertainment of exposure and covariate status.

In a case-initiated case–control study, one starts by identifying a source of study cases (for example a hospital emergency room is a source of myocardial infarction cases). One then attempts to identify a population at risk such that the source of cases provides a random or complete sample of all cases occurring in this population. Study cases recruited from the source occur over a risk period; controls are selected in order to ascertain the distribution of exposure in the population at risk over that period.

Case–control studies may also begin with an existing series of controls (Greenland 1985). Regardless of how a case–control study is initiated, evaluation of validity must ultimately refer to a population at risk that represents the target of inference for the study.

Relative-risk estimation in case–control studies

The control sample may or may not be selected in a manner that excludes cases. If persons who become cases over the risk period are ineligible for inclusion in the control group (as in traditional case–control designs), a 'rare-disease' assumption may be needed to estimate relative risks from the case–control data. However, if persons who become cases over the risk period are also eligible for inclusion in the control group (as in newer case–control designs), the rare-disease assumption can be discarded. These points are discussed in detail in the textbooks cited at the beginning of this chapter.

The basics of case–control estimation will be illustrated with the following example. We wish to study the effect of coffee drinking on rates of first myocardial infarction and we have selected a population for study (for example, all residents aged 40–64 in a particular town) over a one-year risk period. At any point during the risk period, the population at risk comprises persons in this selected population who have not yet had a myocardial infarction.

Suppose that the average number of never-drinkers in the population at risk was 20 000 over the risk period, the average number of five-cup-a-day drinkers was 10 000, there were 120 first myocardial infarctions among never-drinkers, and there were 90 first myocardial infarctions among five-cup-a-day drinkers. Then, if one observed the entire population without error, the estimated rates among never-drinkers and five-cup-a-day drinkers would be

$$\frac{120}{20\,000 \text{ person-years}} \quad \text{and} \quad \frac{90}{10\,000 \text{ person-years}}$$

Thus, if we observed the entire population, the estimated rate ratio would be

$$\frac{90/10\,000 \text{ person-years}}{120/20\,000 \text{ person-years}} = \frac{90/120}{10\,000/20\,000} = 1.50.$$

This estimate depends on only two figures: the relative prevalence of five-cup-a-day versus never-drinkers among cases (90/120), and the same relative prevalence in the person-years at risk (10 000/ 20 000). These two relative prevalences are often called the **case exposure odds** and the **population exposure odds**.

The first relative prevalence (numerator) could be estimated by interviewing an unbiased sample of all the new myocardial infarction cases that occur over the risk period, and the second relative prevalence (denominator) could be estimated by interviewing an unbiased sample of the population at risk over the risk period. The ratio of relative prevalences from the case- and control-sample interviews would then be an unbiased estimate of the population rate ratio of 1.50. This estimate is called the **sample odds ratio**.

Three points about the preceding argument should be carefully noted. First, no rare-disease assumption was made. Second, the control sample of the population at risk was accumulated over the entire risk period (rather than at the end of the risk period); such sampling is called density sampling (Kleinbaum *et al.* 1982) or risk-set sampling (Breslow and Day 1987). Third, because of the density sampling, someone may be selected for the control sample, and yet have a myocardial infarction later in the risk period and become part of the case sample as well. Specific methods for carrying out density sampling can be found in the textbooks cited at the beginning of this chapter.

Validity conditions in case–control studies

The primary advantages of case–control studies are their short time frame and the large reduction in the number of subjects needed to achieve the same statistical power as a cohort study. The primary disadvantage is that more conditions must be met to ensure their validity (in addition to the four listed in the cohort study example).

Suppose that our case–control study data yield an unadjusted rate-ratio estimate (odds ratio) of 1.50, with 95 per cent confidence limits of 1.00 and 2.25. The following series of conditions would be sufficient for the validity of this figure as an estimate of the effect of drinking five cups of coffee a day (versus none) on the myocardial infarction rate.

(C) *Comparison validity*   If five-cup-a-day drinkers in the population at risk had instead drunk no coffee, their distribution of myocardial infarction events over time would have been approximately the same as the distribution among never-drinkers.

(F) *Follow-up validity*   Within each subpopulation defined by coffee use, censoring risk (i.e. population membership ended by an event other than myocardial infarction, such as emigration or death from another cause) is not associated with myocardial infarction risk.

(Sp) *Specification validity*   The distribution of myocardial infarction events over time in the subpopulations can be closely approximated by the statistical model on which the estimates are based.

(M) *Measurement validity*   All measurements of variables used in the analysis closely approximate the true values of the variables.

(Se) *Selection validity*   This has two components.

  1. *Case-selection validity*   If one studies only a subset of the myocardial infarction cases occurring in the population over the risk period (for example, because of failure to detect all cases), this subset provides unbiased estimates of the prevalence of different levels of coffee use among all cases occurring in the population over the risk period.

  2. *Control-selection validity*   The control sample provides unbiased estimates of the prevalences of different levels of coffee use in the population at risk over the risk period.

Issues of comparison validity, follow-up validity, specification validity, effect modification, and generalizability in case–control studies parallel those in follow-up studies, and so will not be discussed here. Case–control studies are vulnerable to certain problems of measurement error that are less severe or do not exist in prospective cohort studies. We shall discuss these problems first, and then examine selection validity and modelling. Finally, we shall briefly discuss analogous issues in retrospective cohort studies.

Retrospective ascertainment

A special class of measurement errors arises from **retrospective ascertainment** of time-dependent variables, i.e. attempting to measure past values of the variables. Retrospective ascertainment must be based on individual memories, existing records of past values, or some combination of the two. Therefore such ascertainment usually suffers from faulty recall, missing or mistaken records, or lack of direct measurements in existing records.

Retrospective ascertainment may be an important component of a cohort study. For example, the cohort study of coffee and myocardial infarction discussed above could have been improved by asking subjects about their coffee use and smoking prior to the start of follow-up. This information would allow one to construct better cumulative indices than could be constructed from baseline consumption alone, although the resulting indices would still incorporate error due to faulty recall.

Unless records of past measurements are available for all subjects, measurements on cases and controls must be made after the time period under study since subjects are not selected for study until after that period. Thus, unlike cohort studies, most case–control studies of time-dependent variables depend on retrospective ascertainment. Considering our example, there may be much more error in determining daily coffee consumption ten years before interview than one month before interview. Given this, one might then expect case–control studies to be more accurate for studying acute effects than for studying chronic effects. However, if acute and chronic effects are heavily confounded, the elevated inaccuracies of long-term recall will make it impossible to disentangle short-term from long-term effects. As illustrated earlier, this confounding can arise in a cohort study. Nevertheless, in a cohort study such confounding can be minimized by taking repeated measurements. In contrast, such confounding would be unavoidable in a case–control study based on recall, even if detailed longitudinal histories were requested from the subjects.

The preceding observations should be tempered by noting that some case–control studies have access to exposure measurements of the same quality as found in cohort studies and that the exposure measurements in some cohort studies may be no better than those used in some case–control studies. For example, a cohort study in which measurements are derived by abstracting routine medical records would suffer from no less measurement error than a case–control study in which measurements are derived by abstracting the same records.

Outcome-affected measurements

One common potential problem in case–control studies is **outcome-affected recall**, often termed **recall bias**. These terms refer to the differential measurement error that originates when the outcome event affects recall of past events. Examples arise in case–control studies of birth defects, for instance. If the trauma of having an affected child either enhances recall of prenatal exposures among case mothers or increases the frequency of false-positive reports among case mothers, estimates of relative risk will be upwardly biased by effects of the outcome on case recall (although this bias may be counterbalanced by other biases, such as recall bias among controls (Drews and Greenland 1990)).

One method commonly proposed for preventing bias due to outcome-affected recall is to restrict controls to a group believed to have recall similar to the cases. Unfortunately, one usually cannot tell to what degree this restricted selection corrects the bias from outcome-affected recall. Even more unfortunately, one usually cannot tell if the selection bias produced by such restriction is worse than the recall bias one is attempting to correct (Swan *et al.* 1992; Drews *et al.* 1993).

A problem similar to outcome-affected recall can occur when the outcome event affects a psychological or physiological measurement. This is of particular concern in case–control studies of nutrient levels and chronic disease. For example, if colon cancer leads to a drop in serum retinol levels, the relative risk for the effect of serum retinol will be underestimated if serum retinol is measured after the cancer develops. Errors of this type can be viewed as proxy-variable errors in which the post-outcome value is a poor proxy for the pre-outcome value of interest.

Selection validity

Selection validity is straightforward to understand but can be extraordinarily difficult to verify. A violation of the selection validity conditions is known as **selection bias**. Many case–control designs and field methods are devoted to avoiding such bias (Schlesselman 1982).

In some instances it may be possible to identify a factor or factors that affect chance of selection into the study. If in such instances we have accurate measurements of one of these factors, we can stratify on (or otherwise adjust for) the factor and thereby remove the selection bias due to the factor. Because of this possibility, some authors classify selection bias as a form of confounding. Nevertheless, there are some forms of selection bias that cannot be removed by adjustment. These points will be illustrated in the following subsections.

Case-selection validity

Unbiased selection of a case series can be best assured if one can identify every case that occurs in the population at risk over the risk period. This requires a surveillance system for the outcome of interest, such as a population-based disease registry. In our coffee–myocardial infarction example, we would probably have to construct a myocardial infarction surveillance system from existing resources, such as emergency room admission records, ambulance service records, and paramedic records.

Even if all cases of interest can be identified, selection bias may arise from failure to obtain information on all the cases. In our example, many cases would be dead before interview was possible. For such cases, there are only two alternatives: attempt to obtain information from some other source, such as next of kin or co-workers, or exclude such cases from the study. The first alternative increases measurement error in the study. The second alternative will introduce bias if coffee affects risk of fatal and non-fatal myocardial infarction differently, or if coffee affects risk of myocardial infarction survivorship. To illustrate, suppose that coffee drinking reduced one's chance of reaching the hospital alive when a myocardial infarction occurred. Then the prevalence of coffee use among myocardial infarction survivors would under-represent the prevalence among all myocardial infarction cases. Underestimation of the rate ratio would result if fatal myocardial infarction cases were excluded from the study.

Note that, in the previous example, we could remove the case selection bias by redefining the study outcome as non-fatal myocardial infarction. Unfortunately, this does not remove the bias but only leads to its reclassification as a bias due to differential censoring (here classified as a form of follow-up bias). In a study of non-fatal myocardial infarction, fatal myocardial infarction is a censoring event associated with risk of non-fatal myocardial infarction; if fatal myocardial infarction is also associated with coffee use, the result will be underestimation of the rate ratio for non-fatal myocardial infarction. More generally, it is usually not possible to remove bias by placing restrictions on admissible outcomes.

Unfortunately, exclusion is the only alternative for cases that refuse to participate or cannot be located. In our example, if such cases tend to be heavier coffee users than others, underestimation of the rate ratio would result. However, suppose that, within levels of cigarette use, such cases were no different from other cases with respect to coffee use. Then adjustment for smoking would remove the selection bias induced by refusals and failures to locate cases. (Of course, such adjustment would require accurate smoking measurement, which is a problem in itself.)

Bias that arises from failure to detect certain cases is sometimes called *detection bias*. If our surveillance system used only hospital admissions, many out-of-hospital myocardial infarction deaths would be excluded, and a detection bias of the sort described above could result.

Control-selection validity

Unbiased selection of a control group can best be assured if one can potentially identify every member of the population at risk at every time during the risk period. In such a situation one could select controls with one of many available probability sampling techniques, using the entire population at risk as the sampling frame. Unfortunately, such situations are exceptional.

Many studies attempt to approximate the ideal sampling situation through use of existing population lists. An example is control selection by random digit dialling; here, the list (of residential telephone numbers) is not used directly but nevertheless serves as a partial enumeration of the population at risk. This list excludes people without telephone numbers. In our example, if people without telephones drink less coffee than people with telephones, a control group selected by random digit dialling would over-represent coffee use in the population at risk. The result would be underestimation of the rate ratio.

Note that one could redefine the population at risk in the previous example so that the telephone-related selection bias did not exist by restricting the study to persons with telephones. This would require excluding persons without telephones from the case series. The resulting relative risk estimate would suffer no selection bias. The only important penalty from this restriction is that the resulting estimate might apply only to the population of persons with telephones; however, this is a problem of generalizability rather than a problem of selection validity. More generally, it is often possible to prevent confounding or selection bias by placing restrictions on the population at risk (and hence the control group). In such instances, however, one must take care to apply the same restrictions to the case series and avoid using restrictions based on events that occur after exposure.

Even if all members of the population at risk can be identified, selection bias may arise from failure to obtain information on all people selected as controls. The implications are the reverse of those for case-selection bias. In our example, if controls who refuse to participate or cannot be located tend to be heavier coffee users than other controls, overestimation of the rate ratio would result. This should be contrasted with the underestimation that results from the same tendency among cases.

More generally, we might expect an association of selection probabilities with the study variable to be in the same direction for both cases and controls. If so, the resulting case-selection and control-selection biases would be in opposite directions and so, to some extent, they would cancel one another out, although not completely. To illustrate, suppose that among cases the proportions who refuse to participate are 0.05 for five-cup-a-day drinkers and 0.02 for never-drinkers, and among controls the analogous proportions are 0.20 and 0.10. These refusals will result in the odds of five-cup-a-day versus never-drinkers among cases being underestimated by a factor of $0.95/0.98 = 0.97$; this in turn results in a 3 per cent underestimation of the rate ratio. Among controls, the odds will be underestimated by a factor of $0.80/0.90 = 0.89$; this results in a $1/0.89 = 1.12$, or a 12 per cent overestimation of the rate ratio. The net selection bias in the rate-ratio estimate will then be $0.97/0.89 = 1.09$, or 9 per cent overestimation.

For further discussions of control-selection validity, see the textbooks cited in the beginning of this chapter, particularly

Schlesselman (1982), and the papers by Savitz and Pearce (1988), Swan *et al.* (1992), and Wacholder *et al.* (1992).

Case–control matching

In cohort studies, **matching** refers to selection of exposure subcohorts in a manner that forces the matched factors to have similar distributions across the subcohorts. If the matched factors are accurately measured and the proportion lost to follow-up does not depend on the matched factors, cohort matching can prevent confounding by the matched factors, although there are statistical reasons to control the matched factors in the analysis (Kleinbaum *et al.* 1982).

In case–control studies, matching refers to selection of subjects in a manner that forces the distribution of certain factors to be similar in cases and controls. Because the population at risk is not changed by case–control matching, such matching does not prevent confounding by the matched factors. In fact, it is now widely recognized that case–control matching is a form of selection bias that can be removed by adjusting for the matching factor; to the extent the factor has been closely matched and accurately measured, this adjustment also controls for confounding by the factor. These points are discussed further by Kleinbaum *et al.* (1982), Miettinen (1985), and Rothman (1986).

As an example, suppose that our population at risk is half male, that the men tend to drink less coffee than the women, and that about 75 per cent of our cases are men. Unbiased control selection should yield about 50 per cent men in the control group. However, if we matched controls to cases on sex, about 75 per cent of our controls would be men. Since men drink less coffee than women and men would be over-represented in the matched control group, the matched control group would under-represent coffee use in the population at risk. Note, however, that matching does not affect the sex-specific prevalence of coffee use among controls, and so the sex-specific and sex-adjusted estimates would be unaffected by matching. In other words, the selection bias produced by matching could be removed by adjustment for the matching factor.

The conclusion to be drawn is that matching can necessitate control of the matching factors. Thus, in order to avoid increasing the number of factors requiring control unnecessarily, one should limit matching to factors for which control would probably be necessary anyway. In particular, matching is usually best limited to known strong confounders, such as age and sex in the above example (Schlesselman 1982).

More generally, the primary theoretical value of matching is that it can sometimes reduce the variance of adjusted estimators (see Kleinbaum *et al.* (1982) and Miettinen (1985) for discussions of this point). However, there are circumstances in which matching can facilitate control selection and so is justified on practical grounds. For example, neighbourhood controls may be far easier to obtain than unmatched general population controls. In addition, although neighbourhood matching would necessitate use of a matched analysis method, the neighbourhood-matched results would incorporate some control of confounding by factors associated with neighbourhood (such as socio-economic status and air pollution).

Special control groups

It is not unusual for investigators to select a special control group that is clearly not representative of the population at risk if they can argue that (1) the group will adequately reflect the distribution of the study factor in the population at risk or (2) that the selection bias in the control group is of the same magnitude of (and so will cancel with) the selection bias in the case group. The first rationale is common in case-control studies of mortality, in which persons dying of other selected causes of death are used as controls; in such studies, selection validity can be assured only if the control causes of death are unrelated to the study factor. The second rationale is common in studies using hospital cases and controls; in particular, selection validity can be assured in such studies if the control conditions are unrelated to the study factor, and the study disease and the control conditions have proportional exposure-specific rates of hospital admission (Kleinbaum *et al.* 1982).

Selection into a special control group usually requires membership in a small and highly select subset of the population at risk. Thus use of a special control group requires careful scrutiny for mechanisms by which the study factor may influence entry into the subset. See Schlesselman (1982) and Kelsey *et al.* (1986) for discussions of practical issues in evaluating special control groups, and Miettinen (1985) and Rothman (1986) for validity principles in mortality case–control studies (so-called proportionate mortality studies).

Case–control modelling

The most popular model for case–control analysis is the logistic model. Details of logistic modelling for case–control analysis are covered in many textbooks, including Breslow and Day (1980), Kleinbaum *et al.* (1982), Schlesselman (1982), Kelsey *et al.* (1986), Hosmer and Lemeshow (1989), and Clayton and Hills (1993).

One important aspect of case–control modelling is that matched factors require special treatment. For example, suppose that matching is done on age in five-year categories and age is associated with the study exposure. To control for the selection bias produced by matching, one must either employ conditional logistic regression with age as a stratifying factor, or else enter indicator variables for each age-matching category into an ordinary logistic regression (the latter strategy has the drawback of requiring about ten or more subjects per age stratum to produce valid estimates). Simply entering age into the model as a continuous variable may not adequately control for the matching-induced bias.

Summary of example

The example in this section provides an illustration of the most common threats to validity in case–control studies (beyond those already discussed for cohort studies). After adjustments for possible confounding and follow-up bias (along the lines described for the cohort study), there may still be irremediable selection bias, especially if we use only select case groups (for example myocardial infarction survivors) or control groups (for example hospital controls). In addition, retrospective ascertainment will lead to greater measurement error than prospective ascertainment, and some of this additional error may be differential.

Given the even greater number of potential biases of unknown magnitude and different directions, it would appear that (as in the cohort example) no conclusions about coffee effect could be drawn from a study like the one described above, other than that coffee does not have a large effect. Again, this is a common result in thorough epidemiological analyses of observational data.

Retrospective cohort studies

Two major types of cohort studies can be distinguished depending on whether members of the study cohort are identified before or after the follow-up period under study. Studies in which all members are identified before their follow-up period are called concurrent or **prospective** cohort studies, while studies in which all members are identified after their follow-up period are called historical or **retrospective** cohort studies. Like case–control studies, retrospective cohort studies often require special consideration of retrospective ascertainment and selection validity.

In particular, retrospective cohort studies that obtain exposure or covariate histories from post-event reconstructions are vulnerable to bias from outcome-affected measurements. Suppose, for example, that a study of cancer incidence at an industrial facility had to rely on company personnel to determine the location and nature of various exposures in the plant during the relevant exposure periods. If these personnel were aware of the locations at which cases worked (as when a publicized 'cluster' of cases has occurred), biased exposure assessment could result. Of course, such problems can also occur in a prospective cohort study if exposure or covariate histories are based on post-event reconstructions.

Retrospective cohort studies can also suffer from selection biases analogous to those found in case–control studies. Suppose, for example, that a retrospective cohort study relied on company records to identify members of the cohort of plant employees. If retention of an employee's records (and hence identification of the employee as a cohort member) were associated with both the exposure and outcome status of the employee, the exposure–outcome association observed in the incomplete study cohort could poorly represent the exposure–outcome association in the complete cohort of plant employees.

Conclusion

Uncertainty about validity conditions is responsible for most of the inconclusiveness inherent in epidemiological studies. This inconclusiveness can be partially overcome when multiple complementary studies are conducted, i.e. when new studies are conducted under conditions that effectively limit bias from one or more of the sources present in earlier studies. Ideally, after enough complementary studies have been conducted, each known or suspected source of bias will have been rendered unimportant in at least one study. If at this point all the study results appear consistent with one another (which is not the case for coffee and myocardial infarction, although the studies of smoking and lung cancer provide a good example), the epidemiological community may reach some consensus about the existence and strength of an effect.

Even in such ideal situations, however, one should bear in mind that consistency is not validity. For example, there may be some unsuspected source of bias present in all the studies, so that they are all consistently biased in the same direction. Alternatively, all the known sources of bias may be in the same direction, so that all the studies remain biased in the same direction if no one study eliminates all known sources of bias. For these and other reasons, many authors warn that all causal inferences should be considered

tentative, at least if drawn from observational epidemiological data alone. The reader is referred to Schlesselman (1982) and Rothman (1986, 1988) for further discussion and references on this point.

Acknowledgement

The author wishes to thank Irva Hertz-Picciotto, Philip Kass, Jennifer Kelsey, George Maldonado, Staffan Norrell, James Schlesselman, and Alexander Walker for their helpful comments on this chapter.

References

Berger, J.O. and Berry, D.A. (1988). Statistical analysis and the illusion of objectivity. *American Scientist*, **76**, 159–65.

Brenner, H. (1993). Bias due to nondifferential misclassification of a polytomous confounder. *Journal of Clinical Epidemiology*, **46**, 57–63.

Breslow, N.E. and Day, N.E. (1980). *Statistical methods in cancer research*. I: *The analysis of case–control studies*. IARC, Lyon.

Breslow, N.E. and Day, N.E. (1987). *Statistical methods in cancer research*. II: *The analysis of cohort data*. IARC, Lyon.

Checkoway H., Pearce N., and Crawford-Brown, D. (1989). *Research methods in occupational epidemiology*. Oxford University Press, New York.

Clayton, D. and Hills, M. (1993). *Statistical models in epidemiology*. Oxford University Press, New York.

Cornfield, J., Haenszel, W.H., Hammond, E.C., *et al.* (1959). Smoking and lung cancer: recent evidence and a discussion of some questions. *Journal of the National Cancer Institute*, **22**, 173–203, Appendix A.

Curb, J.D., Reed, D.M., Kautz, J.A., *et al.* (1986). Coffee, caffeine, and serum cholesterol in Japanese men in Hawaii. *American Journal of Epidemiology*, **123**, 648–55.

Dosemeci, M., Wacholder, S., and Lubin, J.H. (1990). Does nondifferential misclassification of exposure always bias a true effect towards the null value? *American Journal of Epidemiology*, **132**, 746–8.

Drews, C.D. and Greenland, S. (1990). The impact of differential recall on the results of case–control studies. *International Journal of Epidemiology*, **19**, 1107–12.

Drews, C., Greenland, S., and Flanders, W.D. (1993). The use of restricted controls to prevent recall bias in case–control studies of reproductive outcomes. *Annals of Epidemiology*, **3**, 86–92.

Flanders, W.D. and Khoury, M.J. (1990). Indirect assessment of confounding: graphic description and limits on effects of adjusting for covariates. *Epidemiology*, **1**, 239–46.

Flegal, K.M., Keyl, P.M., and Nieto, F.J. (1991). Differential misclassification arising from nondifferential errors in exposure measurement. *American Journal of Epidemiology*, **134**, 1233–44.

Goodman, S.N. (1992). A comment on replication, *p*-values and evidence. *Statistics in Medicine*, **11**, 875–9.

Goodman, S.N. (1993). *P*-values, hypothesis tests, and likelihood: implications for epidemiology of a neglected historical debate. *American Journal of Epidemiology*, **137**, 485–96.

Goodman, S.N. and Royall, R.M. (1988). Evidence and scientific research. *American Journal of Public Health*, **78**, 1568–74.

Greenland, S. (1980). The effect of misclassification in the presence of covariates. *American Journal of Epidemiology*, **112**, 564–9.

Greenland, S. (1985). Control initiated case–control studies. *International Journal of Epidemiology*, **14**, 130–4.

Greenland, S. (1987a). Interpretation and choice of effect measures in epidemiologic analyses. *American Journal of Epidemiology*, **125**, 761–8.

Greenland, S. (1987b). Quantitative methods in the review of epidemiologic literature. *Epidemiologic Reviews*, **9**, 1–30.

Greenland, S. (1989). Modelling and variable selection in epidemiologic analysis. *American Journal of Public Health*, **79**, 340–9.

Greenland, S. (1990). Randomization, statistics, and causal inference. *Epidemiology*, **1**, 421–9.

Greenland, S. (1993a). A meta-analysis of coffee, myocardial infarction, and coronary death. *Epidemiology*, **4**, 366–74.

Greenland, S. (1993b). Summarization, smoothing, and inference. *Scandinavian Journal of Social Medicine*, **21**, 421–9.

Greenland, S. (1994). A critical look at some popular meta-analytic methods. *American Journal of Epidemiology*, **140**, 290–6.

Greenland, S. and Robins, J.M. (1985). Confounding and misclassification. *American Journal of Epidemiology*, **122**, 495–506.

Greenland, S. and Robins, J.M. (1986). Identifiability, exchangeability, and epidemiological confounding. *International Journal of Epidemiology*, **15**, 413–19.

Greenland, S. and Robins, J.M. (1988). Conceptual problems in the definition and interpretation of attributable fractions. *American Journal of Epidemiology*, **128**, 1185–97.

Greenland, S. and Robins, J.M. (1994). Ecologic studies: biases, misconceptions, and counterexamples. *American Journal of Epidemiology*, **139**, 747–60.

Greenland, S., Schlesselman, J.J., and Criqui, M.H. (1986). The fallacy of employing standardized regression coefficients and correlations as measures of effect. *American Journal of Epidemiology*, **123**, 203–8.

Greenland, S., Maclure, M., Schlesselman, J.J., *et al.* (1991). Standardized coefficients: a further critique and a review of alternatives. *Epidemiology*, **2**, 387–92.

Hastie, T. and Tibshirani, R. (1990). *Generalized additive models*. Chapman and Hall, New York.

Hosmer, D.W. and Lemeshow, S. (1989). *Applied logistic regression*. Wiley, New York.

Kalbfleisch, J.D. and Prentice, R.L. (1980). *The statistical analysis of failure-time data*. Wiley, New York.

Kelsey, J.L., Thompson, W.D., and Evans, A.S. (1986). *Methods in observational epidemiology*. Oxford University Press, New York.

Kleinbaum, D.G., Kupper, L.L., and Morgenstern, H. (1982). *Epidemiologic research: principles and quantitative methods*. Lifetime Learning, Belmont, CA.

Leamer, E.E. (1978). *Specification searches*. Wiley, New York.

McCullagh, P. and Nelder, J.A. (1989). *Generalized linear models* (2nd edn.), Chapman and Hall, New York.

Miettinen, O.S. (1985). *Theoretical epidemiology*. Wiley, New York.

Oakes, M. (1990). *Statistical inference*. Epidemiology Resources, Chestnut Hill, MA.

Poole, C. (1985). Exceptions to the rule about nondifferential misclassification (abstract). *American Journal of Epidemiology*, **122**, 508.

Poole, C. (1987a). Beyond the confidence interval. *American Journal of Public Health*, **77**, 197–9.

Poole, C. (1987b). Confidence intervals exclude nothing. *American Journal of Public Health*, **77**, 492–3.

Robins, J.M. (1988). Confidence intervals for causal parameters. *Statistics in Medicine*, **7**, 773–85.

Robins, J.M. (1989). The control of confounding by intermediate variables. *Statistics in Medicine*, **8**, 679–701.

Robins, J.M. and Greenland, S. (1986). The role of model selection in causal inference from nonexperimental data. *American Journal of Epidemiology*, **123**, 392–402.

Robins, J.M. and Greenland, S. (1992). Identifiability and exchangeability for direct and indirect effects. *Epidemiology*, **3**, 143–55.

Robins, J.M., and Greenland, S. (1994). Adjusting for differential rates of prophylaxis theraphy for PCP in high- versus low-dose AZT treatment arms in an AIDS randomized trial. *Journal of the American Statistical Association*, **90**, 737–49.

Rosenbaum, P.R. (1995). *Observational studies*. Springer-Verlag, New York.

Rothman, K.J. (1986). *Modern epidemiology*. Little, Brown, Boston, MA.

Rothman, K.J. (1988). *Causal inference*. Epidemiology Resources, Chestnut Hill, MA.

Rubin, D.R. (1991). Practical implications of modes of statistical inference for causal effects, and the critical role of the assignment mechanism. *Biometrics*, **47**, 1213–34.

Savitz, D.A. and Pearce, N. (1988). Control selection with incomplete case ascertainment. *American Journal of Epidemiology*, **127**, 1109–17.

Schlesselman, J.J. (1978). Assessing the effects of confounding variables. *American Journal of Epidemiology*, **108**, 3–8.

Schlesselman J.J. (1982). *Case–control studies: design, conduct, analysis*. Oxford University Press, New York.

Slud E. and Byar D. (1988). How dependent causes of death can make risk factors appear protective. *Biometrics*, **44**, 265–70.

Swan, S.H., Shaw, G.R., and Schulman, J. (1992). Reporting and selection bias in case–control studies of congenital malformations. *Epidemiology*, **3**, 356–63.

Wacholder, S., Dosemeci, M., and Lubin, J.H. (1991). Blind assignment of exposure does not always prevent differential misclassification. *American Journal of Epidemiology*, **134**, 433–7.

Wacholder, S., McLaughlin, J.K., Silverman, D.T., and Mandel, J.S. (1992). Selection of controls in case-control studies. *American Journal of Epidemiology*, **135**, 1019–50.

Walker, A.M. (1991). *Observation and inference: an introduction to the methods of epidemiology*. Epidemiology Resources, Chestnut Hill, MA.

Weinberg, C.R., Umbach, D., and Greenland, S. (1994). When will non-differential misclassification preserve the direction of the trend? *American Journal of Epidemiology*, **140**, 565–71.

White, H. (1993). *Estimation, inference, and specification analysis*. Cambridge University Press, New York.

15 Causation and causal inference

Kenneth J. Rothman and Sander Greenland

In *The magic years*, Fraiberg (1959) characterized every toddler as a scientist, busily fulfilling an earnest mission to develop a logical structure for the strange objects and events that make up the world that he or she inhabits. To survive successfully requires a useful theoretical scheme to relate the myriad events that are encountered. As a youngster, each person develops and tests an inventory of causal explanations that brings meaning to the events that are perceived and ultimately leads to increasing power to control those events.

Parents can attest to the delight that children take in forming causal hypotheses and then meticulously testing them, often through exasperating repetitions that are motivated mainly by the joy of understanding. At a certain age, a child will, when entering a new room, search for a wall switch to operate the electric light. Upon finding one, the child will switch it on and off repeatedly to test the discovery beyond any reasonable doubt. Experiments such as those designed to examine the effect of gravity on free-falling liquids are usually conducted with careful attention, varying the initial conditions in subtle ways and reducing extraneous influences whenever possible by conducting the experiments safely removed from parental interference. The fruit of such scientific labours is a working knowledge of the essential system of causal relations that enables each of us to navigate our complex world.

A general model of causation

If everyone begins life as a scientist, creating his or her own inventory of causal explanations for the empirical world, everyone also begins life as a pragmatic philosopher, developing a general causal theory that some events or states of nature are causes with specific effects or effects with specific causes. Without a general theory of causation, there would be no skeleton on which to hang the substance of the many specific causal theories that one needs to survive. Unfortunately, the concepts of causation that are established early in life are too rudimentary to serve well as the basis for scientific theories. We need to develop a more refined set of concepts that can serve as a common starting point in discussions of causal theories.

Concept of sufficient cause and component causes

To begin, we need to define cause. We can define a cause of a specific disease event as an antecedent event, condition, or characteristic that was necessary for the occurrence of the disease at the moment it occurred, given that other conditions are fixed. In other words, a cause of a disease event is an event, condition, or characteristic that preceded the disease event and without which the disease event would not have occurred at all or until some later time. In this definition it may be that no specific event, condition, or characteristic is sufficient by itself to produce disease. This definition, then, does not define a complete causal mechanism, but only a component of it.

A common characteristic of the concept of causation that we develop early in life is the assumption of a one-to-one correspondence between the observed cause and effect. Each cause is seen as necessary and sufficient in itself to produce the effect. Thus, the flick of a light switch appears to be the singular cause that makes the lights go on. There are less evident causes, however, that also operate to produce the effect: the need for an unspent bulb in the light fixture, wiring from the switch to the bulb, and voltage to produce a current when the circuit is closed. To achieve the effect of turning on the light, each of these is equally as important as moving the switch, because absence of any of these components of the causal constellation will prevent the effect.

For many people, the roots of early causal thinking persist and become manifest in attempts to find single causes as explanations for observed phenomena. However, experience and reflection should easily persuade us that the cause of any effect must consist of a constellation of components that act in concert (Mill 1862). A 'sufficient cause', which means a complete causal mechanism, can be defined as a set of minimal conditions and events that inevitably produce disease; 'minimal' implies that all of the conditions or events are necessary. In disease aetiology, the completion of a sufficient cause may be considered equivalent to the onset of disease. (Onset here refers to the onset of the earliest stage of the disease process, rather than the onset of signs or symptoms.) For biologic effects, most and sometimes all of the components of a sufficient cause are unknown (Rothman 1976).

For example, smoking is a cause of lung cancer, but by itself it is not a sufficient cause. First, the term smoking is too imprecise to be used in a causal description. One must specify the type of smoke, whether it is filtered or unfiltered, the manner and frequency of inhalation, and the onset and duration of smoking. More important, smoking, even defined explicitly, will not cause cancer in everyone. So who are those who are 'susceptible' to the effects of smoking? Or, to put it in other terms, what are the other components of the causal constellation that act with smoking to produce lung cancer?

When causal components remain unknown, we are inclined to assign an equal risk to all individuals whose causal status for some components is known and identical. Thus, men who are heavy

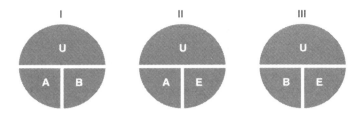

Fig. 15.1 Three sufficient causes of a disease.

Table 15.1 Exposure frequencies for three component causes in two hypothetical populations according to the possible combinations of the component causes

Exposures			Response	Frequency of exposure pattern	
A	B	E	(outcome)	Population 1	Population 2
1	1	1	1	100	900
1	1	0	1	100	900
1	0	1	1	900	100
1	0	0	0	900	100
0	1	1	1	900	100
0	1	0	0	900	100
0	0	1	0	100	900
0	0	0	0	100	900

cigarette smokers are said to have approximately a 10 per cent lifetime risk of developing lung cancer. Some interpret this statement to mean that all men would be subject to a 10 per cent probability of lung cancer if they were to become heavy smokers, as if the outcome, aside from smoking, were purely a matter of chance. In contrast, we view the assignment of equal risks as reflecting nothing more than assigning to everyone within a specific category, in this case male heavy smokers, the average of the individual risks for people in that category. In the classical view, these risks are either 1 or 0, according to whether or not the individual will or will not get lung cancer.

We cannot measure the individual risks and assigning the average value to everyone in the category reflects nothing more than our ignorance about the determinants of lung cancer that interact with cigarette smoke. It is apparent from epidemiologic data that some people can engage in chain smoking for many decades without developing lung cancer. Others are or will become 'primed' by unknown circumstances and need only to add cigarette smoke to the nearly sufficient constellation of causes to initiate lung cancer. In our ignorance of these hidden causal components, the best we can do in assessing risk is to classify people according to measured causal risk indicators and then assign the average risk observed within a class to persons within the class. As knowledge expands, the risk estimates assigned to people will depart from the average according to the presence or absence of other factors that affect the risk.

For example, we now know that smokers with substantial asbestos exposure are at higher risk of lung cancer than those who lack asbestos exposure. Consequently, with adequate data we could assign different risks to heavy smokers based on their asbestos exposure. Within categories of asbestos exposure, the average risks would be assigned to all heavy smokers until other risk factors are identified.

Figure 15.1 provides a schematic diagram of sufficient causes in a hypothetical individual. Each constellation of component causes represented in Fig. 15.1 is minimally sufficient to produce the disease, that is there are no redundant or extraneous component causes—each one is a necessary part of that specific causal mechanism. Component causes may play a role in one, two, or all three of the causal mechanisms pictured.

Figure 15.1 does not depict aspects of the causal process such as prevention, sequence of action, dose, and other complexities. These aspects of the causal process can be accommodated in the model by an appropriate definition of each causal component. Thus, if the outcome is lung cancer and factor E represents cigarette smoking, it could be defined more explicitly as smoking at least two packs a day of unfiltered cigarettes for at least 20 years. If the outcome is smallpox, which is completely prevented by immunization, factor

U could represent 'unimmunized'. More generally, the preventive effects of a factor C can be represented by placing its complement 'no C' within sufficient causes.

Strength of causes

The causal model exemplified by Fig. 15.1 can facilitate an understanding of some key concepts such as 'strength of effect' and 'interaction.' As an illustration of strength of effect, Table 15.1 displays the frequency of the eight possible patterns for exposure to A, B, and E in two hypothetical populations. Suppose that U is always present (ubiquitous) and Fig. 15.1 represents all the sufficient causes capable of acting for each individual in each population. Here and throughout the book we will assume that 'disease' refers to a non-recurrent event, such as death or first occurrence of a disease. Under these assumptions, the response of each individual under the exposure pattern in a given row can be found under the response column.

The proportion acquiring a disease in any subpopulation (the incidence proportion) can be found simply by multiplying the number at each exposure pattern by the response for that pattern, summing these products to get the total number of disease cases in the subpopulation, and dividing this total by the population size. If exposure A is unmeasured, the pattern of these incidence proportions in population 1 would be those in Table 15.2.

As an example of how the proportions in Table 15.2 were calculated, let us review how the incidence proportion among persons with B present, but E absent was calculated: There were 100 persons with A present, B present and E absent, all of whom became cases, because A and B are sufficient to produce the disease in combination with the background causes. There were 900 persons with A absent, B present, and E absent, none of whom

Table 15.2 Pattern of incidence proportions for component causes B and E in hypothetical population 1 assuming that component cause A is unmeasured

	B = 1, E = 1	B = 1, E = 0	B = 0, E = 1	B = 0, E = 0
Cases	1000	100	900	0
Total	1000	1000	1000	1000
Proportion	1.00	0.10	0.90	0.00

Table 15.3 Pattern of incidence proportions for component causes B and E in hypothetical population 2 assuming that component cause A is unmeasured

	B = 1, E = 1	B = 1, E = 0	B = 0, E = 1	B = 0, E = 0
Cases	1000	900	100	0
Total	1000	1000	1000	1000
Proportion	1.00	0.90	0.10	0.00

became cases, because they did not have a sufficient cause. Thus, among all 1000 people with B present and E absent, there were 100 cases, for a proportion of 0.10.

It is evident from Table 15.2 that for population 1, E is a much stronger determinant of incidence than B. This difference is reflected in the fact that the presence of E increases the incidence by 0.9, whereas the presence of B increases incidence by only 0.1.

Table 15.3 shows the analogous results for population 2. Although the members of this population have exactly the same causal mechanisms operating within them as do the members of population 1, the relative strengths of E and B are reversed: B is now a much stronger determinant of incidence than E. This is so despite the fact that the crude proportions of members with A, B, and E are exactly 50 per cent in both populations and even though within each population, A, B, and E have no association with one another.

One key difference between populations 1 and 2 is that the conditions under which E acts as a necessary and sufficient cause—the presence of A or B, but not both—is common in population 1 but rare in population 2. In population 1, 3600 people or 90 per cent of the total have A or B but not both and the incidence proportion for E merely reflects this percentage. In contrast, only 400 people or 10 per cent of the total in population 2 have A or B but not both. This difference in the frequency of necessary and sufficient conditions for E to act explains the difference in the strength of the effect of E for the two populations. A similar explanation applies to the different strength of effect for factor B in the two populations.

We will call the set of conditions necessary and sufficient for a factor to produce disease the causal complement of the factor. Thus, the condition '(A and U) or (B and U)' is the causal complement of E in the above example. This example shows that the strength of a factor's effect on a population depends on the relative prevalence of its causal complement. This dependence of the effects of a specific component cause on the prevalence of its causal complement has nothing to do with the biologic mechanism of the component's action, since the component is an equal partner in each mechanism in which it appears. Nevertheless, a factor is a strong cause if its causal complement is common. Conversely, a factor with a rare causal complement will appear to be a weak cause.

The strength of a cause may have tremendous public health significance, but it may have little biological significance. The reason is that given a specific causal mechanism, any of the component causes can be either strong or weak. The actual identity of the constituent components of the cause amount to the biology

of causation, whereas the strength of a cause is a relative phenomenon that depends on the time- and place-specific distribution of component causes in a population. Over a span of time, the strength of individual causal risk factors within a specific causal mechanism for a given disease may change, because the prevalence of specific component causes in various mechanisms may also change. The causal mechanisms in which these components act could remain unchanged, however.

The preceding discussion has focused on the absolute increase in incidence (often referred to as 'risk difference') as the measure of the strength of effect. More commonly, a ratio measure is used. The arguments we have just given also apply to ratio measures. The magnitude of such measures depends profoundly on the prevalence of complements to the factor under study. In addition, however, ratio measures depend on the prevalences of components of sufficient causes in which the factor does not participate. Thus, in the above example, the prevalence of A will affect the apparent strength of E, as measured by the ratio of incidence proportions, not only though completion of sufficient cause II (in which A is complementary to E), but also through completion of sufficient cause I (in which E does not participate). The net impact can be observed by comparing the incidence ratios for E when B = 1: in population 1 this ratio is 0.90/0.10 = 9, whereas in population 2 this ratio is only 1.00/0.90 = 1.1.

Interactions between causes

Two component causes acting in the same sufficient cause may be thought of as interacting biologically to produce disease. Indeed, one may define biological interaction as the participation of two component causes in the same sufficient cause. Such interaction is also known as causal co-action or joint action. The joint action of the two component causes does not have to be simultaneous action: one component cause could act many years before the other, but it would have to leave some effect that interacts with the later component.

For example, suppose a traumatic injury to the head leads to a permanent disturbance in equilibrium. Many years later, the faulty equilibrium may lead to a fall while walking on an icy path, causing a broken hip. The causal mechanism for the broken hip includes the traumatic injury to the head as a component cause, along with its consequence of a disturbed equilibrium. The causal mechanism also includes the walk along the icy path. These two component causes have interacted with one another, although their time of action is many years apart. They also would interact with the other component causes, such as the type of footwear, the absence of a handhold, and any other conditions that were necessary to the causal mechanism of the fall and the broken hip that resulted.

The degree of observable interaction between two specific component causes depends on how many different sufficient causes produce disease and the proportion of cases that occur through sufficient causes in which the two component causes both play some role. For example, in Fig. 15.2, suppose that G were only a hypothetical substance that did not actually exist. Consequently, no disease would occur from sufficient cause II, because it depends on an action by G and factors B and F would act only through the distinct mechanisms represented by sufficient causes I and III. Thus, B and F would be biologically independent. Now suppose that C is completely replaced by G. Factors B and F will then act

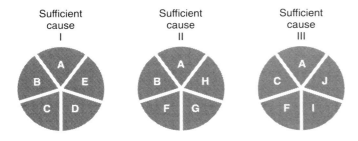

Fig. 15.2 Three sufficient causes of a disease.

together in the mechanism represented by sufficient cause II and, thus, will be found to interact biologically. Thus, the extent of biological interaction between two factors is dependent on the relative prevalence of other factors.

Proportion of disease due to specific causes

In Fig. 15.1, assuming that the three sufficient causes in the diagram are the only ones operating, what fraction of disease is caused by U? The answer is all of it; without U, there is no disease. U is considered a 'necessary cause'. What fraction is due to E? E causes disease through two mechanisms, I and II and all disease arising through either of these two mechanisms is due to E. This is not to say that all disease is due to U alone or that a fraction of disease is due to E alone; no component cause acts alone. It is understood that these factors interact with others in producing disease.

A widely discussed but unpublished paper from the 1970s, written by scientists at the National Institutes of Health, proposed that as much as 40 per cent of cancer is attributable to occupational exposures. Many scientists thought that this fraction was unacceptably high and argued against this claim (Higginson 1980; Ephron 1984). One of the arguments used in rebuttal was as follows: x per cent of cancer is caused by smoking, y per cent by diet, z per cent by alcohol, and so on; when all these percentages are added up, only a small percentage, much less than 40 per cent, is left for occupational causes. This rebuttal is fallacious, because it is based on the naive view that every case of disease has a single cause. In fact, since diet and smoking and asbestos and other factors interact with one another and with genetic factors to cause cancer, each case of cancer could be attributed to many separate component causes.

There is a tendency to think that the sum of the fractions of disease attributable to each of the causes of the disease should be 100 per cent. For example, in their widely cited work, *The causes of cancer*, Doll and Peto (1981) created a table (Table 20) giving their estimates of the fraction of all cancers caused by various agents; the total for the fractions was nearly 100 per cent. Although they acknowledged that any case could be caused by more than one agent, which would mean that the attributable fractions would not sum to 100 per cent, they referred to this situation as a 'difficulty' and an 'anomaly'. It is, however, neither a difficulty nor an anomaly, but simply a consequence of allowing for the fact that no event has a single agent as the cause. The fraction of disease that can be attributed to each of the causes of disease in all the causal mechanisms actually has no upper limit: for cancer or any disease, the total of the fraction of disease attributable to all the component

causes of all the causal mechanisms that produce it is not 100 per cent but infinity. Only the fraction of disease attributable to a single component cause cannot exceed 100 per cent.

A single cause or category of causes that is present in every sufficient cause of disease will have an attributable fraction of 100 per cent. Much publicity attended the pronouncement in 1960 that as much as 90 per cent of cancer is environmentally caused (Higginson 1960). Since 'environment' can be thought of as an all-embracing category that represents non-genetic causes, which must be present to some extent in every sufficient cause, it is clear on *a priori* grounds that 100 per cent of any disease is environmentally caused. Thus, Higginson's (1960) estimate of 90 per cent was an underestimate.

Similarly, one can show that 100 per cent of any disease is inherited. MacMahon (1968) cited the example given by Hogben (1933) of yellow shanks, a trait occurring in certain genetic strains of fowl fed on yellow corn. Both the right set of genes and the yellow corn diet are necessary to produce yellow shanks. A farmer with several strains of fowl, feeding them all only yellow corn, would consider yellow shanks to be a genetic condition, since only one strain would acquire yellow shanks, despite all strains having the same diet. A different farmer, who owned only the strain liable to get yellow shanks, but who fed some of the birds yellow corn and others white corn, would consider yellow shanks to be an environmentally determined condition because it depends on diet. In reality, yellow shanks is determined by both genes and the environment; there is no reasonable way to allocate a portion of the causation to either genes or the environment. Similarly, every case of every disease has some environmental and some genetic component causes and, therefore, every case can be attributed both to genes and to the environment. No paradox exists as long as it is understood that the fractions of disease attributable to genes and to the environment overlap with one another.

Many researchers have spent considerable effort in developing heritability indices, which are supposed to measure the fraction of disease that is inherited. Unfortunately, these indices only assess the relative role of environmental and genetic causes of disease in a particular setting. For example, some genetic causes may be necessary components of every causal mechanism. If everyone in a population has an identical set of the genes that cause disease, however, their effect is not included in heritability indices, despite the fact that having these genes is a cause of the disease. The two farmers in the example above would offer very different values for the heritability of yellow shanks, despite the fact that the condition is always 100 per cent dependent on having certain genes.

If all genetic factors that determine disease are taken into account, whether or not they vary within populations, then 100 per cent of disease can be said to be inherited. Analogously, 100 per cent of any disease is environmentally caused, even those diseases that we often consider purely genetic. Phenylketonuria (**PKU**), for example, is considered by many to be purely genetic. None the less, the mental retardation that it may cause can be successfully prevented by appropriate dietary intervention.

The treatment for PKU illustrates the interaction of genes and the environment to cause a disease commonly thought to be purely genetic. What about an apparently purely environmental disease such as 'killed in an automobile accident'? It is easy to conceive of genetic traits that lead to psychiatric problems such as alcoholism, which in turn lead to drunk driving and consequent fatality. Consider another more extreme environmental example, 'killed by lightning'. Again, partially heritable psychiatric conditions can influence whether someone will take shelter during a lightning storm. The argument may be stretched on this example, but the point that every case of disease has both genetic and environmental causes is theoretically defensible and has important implications for research.

Induction period

The diagram of causes in Fig. 15.2 also provides a model for conceptualizing the induction period, which may be defined as the period of time from causal action until disease initiation. If, in sufficient cause I, the sequence of action of the causes is A, B, C, D, and E and we are studying the effect of B, which, let us assume, acts at a narrowly defined point in time, we do not observe the occurrence of disease immediately after B acts. Disease occurs only after the sequence is completed, so there will be a delay while C, D, and, finally, E act. When E acts, disease occurs. The interval between the action of B and the disease occurrence is the induction time for the effect of B.

In the example given earlier of an equilibrium disorder leading to a later fall and hip injury, the induction time between the occurrence of the equilibrium disorder and the later hip injury might be very long. In an individual instance, we would not know the exact length of an induction period, since we cannot be sure of the causal mechanism that produces disease in an individual instance, nor when all the relevant component causes acted. We can characterize the induction period relating the action of a component cause to the occurrence of disease in general, however, by accumulating data for many individuals. A clear example of a lengthy induction time is the cause–effect relation between exposure of a female fetus to diethylstilboestrol (**DES**) and the subsequent development of adenocarcinoma of the vagina. The cancer occurs generally between the ages of 15 and 30 years. Since exposure to DES occurs before birth, there is an induction time of 15 to 30 years for the carcinogenic action of DES. During this time, other causes presumably are operating; some evidence suggests that hormonal action during adolescence may be part of the mechanism (Rothman 1981).

It is incorrect to characterize a disease itself as having a lengthy or brief induction time. The induction time can be conceptualized only in relation to a specific component cause. Thus, we say that the induction time relating DES to clear cell carcinoma of the vagina is 15 to 30 years, but we cannot say that 15 to 30 years is the induction time for clear cell carcinoma in general. Since each component cause in any causal mechanism can act at a time different from the other component causes, each can have its own induction time. For the component cause that acts last, the induction time equals zero. If another component cause of clear cell carcinoma of the vagina that acts during adolescence were identified, it would have a much shorter induction time for its carcinogenic action than DES. Thus, induction time characterizes a specific cause–effect pair rather than just the effect.

In carcinogenesis, the terms initiator and promotor have been used to refer to component causes of cancer that act early and late, respectively, in the causal mechanism. Cancer itself has often been characterized as a disease process with a long induction time. This

characterization is a misconception, however, because any late-acting component in the causal process, such as a promotor, will have a short induction time. Indeed, by definition the induction time will always be 0 for at least one component cause, the last to act.

Disease, once initiated, will not necessarily be apparent. The time interval between disease occurrence and detection has been termed the latent period (Rothman 1981), although others have used this term interchangeably with induction period. The latent period can be reduced by improved methods of disease detection. The induction period, on the other hand, cannot be reduced by early detection of disease, since disease occurrence marks the end of the induction period. Earlier detection of disease, however, may reduce the apparent induction period (the time between causal action and disease detection), since the time when disease is detected, as a practical matter, is usually used to mark the time of disease occurrence. Thus, diseases such as slow-growing cancers may appear to have long induction periods with respect to many causes because they have long latent periods. The latent period, unlike the induction period, is a characteristic of the disease and the detection effort applied to the person with the disease.

Although it is not possible to reduce the induction period proper by earlier detection of disease, it may be possible to observe intermediate stages of a causal mechanism. The increased interest in biomarkers, such as DNA adducts, is an example of attempting to focus on causes more proximal to the disease occurrence. Biomarkers reflect the effects of earlier-acting agents on the organism.

Some agents may have a causal action by shortening the induction time of other agents. Suppose that exposure to factor A leads to epilepsy after an interval of 10 years, on average. It may be that exposure to a drug, B, would shorten this interval to 2 years. Is B acting as a catalyst or as a cause of epilepsy? The answer is both: a catalyst is a cause. Without B the occurrence of epilepsy comes 8 years later than it comes with B, so we can say that B causes the onset of the early epilepsy. It is not sufficient to argue that the epilepsy would have occurred anyway. First, it would not have occurred at that time and the time of occurrence is part of our definition of an event. Second, epilepsy will occur later only if the individual survives an additional 8 years, which is not certain. Agent B not only determines when the epilepsy occurs, it can determine whether it occurs. Thus, we should call any agent that acts as a catalyst of a causal mechanism, speeding up an induction period for other agents, as a cause in its own right. Similarly, any agent that postpones the onset of an event, drawing out the induction period for another agent, is a preventive. It should not be too surprising to equate postponement to prevention: we routinely use such an equation when we employ the euphemism that we prevent death, which actually can only be postponed. What we prevent is death at a given time, in favour of death at a later time.

Generality of the model

The main utility of this model of sufficient causes and their components lies in its ability to provide a general but practical conceptual framework for causal problems. The attempt to make the proportion of disease attributable to various component causes add to 100 per cent is an example of a fallacy that is exposed by the model: the model makes it clear that, because of interactions, there is no upper limit to the sum of these proportions. The epidemiological evaluation of interactions themselves can be clarified with the help of the model.

How could the model accommodate varying doses of a component cause? Since the model appears to deal qualitatively with the action of component causes, it might seem that dose variability cannot be taken into account. But this view is overly pessimistic. To account for dose variability, one need only to postulate a set of sufficient causes, each of which contains as a component a different dose of the agent in question. Small doses might require a larger or rarer set of complementary causes to complete a sufficient cause than that required by large doses (Rothman 1976). In this way the model could account for the phenomenon of a shorter induction period accompanying larger doses of exposure, because there would be a smaller set of complementary components needed to complete the sufficient cause.

Those who believe that chance must play a role in any complex mechanism might object to the intricacy of this deterministic model. A probabilistic (stochastic) model could be invoked to describe a dose–response relation, for example, without the need for a multitude of different causal mechanisms; the model would simply relate the dose of the exposure to the probability of the effect occurring. For those who believe that virtually all events contain some element of chance, deterministic causal models may seem to misrepresent reality. Nevertheless, the deterministic model presented here can accommodate classical 'chance', but it does so by reinterpreting chance as deterministic events beyond the current limits of knowledge or observability.

For example, the outcome of a flip of a coin is usually considered a chance event. In classical physics, however, the outcome can in theory be determined completely by the application of physical laws and a sufficient description of the starting conditions. To put it in terms more familiar to epidemiologists, consider the explanation for why an individual acquires lung cancer. One hundred years ago, when little was known about the aetiology of lung cancer, a scientist might have said that it was a matter of chance. Nowadays we might say that the risk depends on how much the individual smokes, how much asbestos and radon the individual has been exposed to, and so on. One might then ask, for an individual who has smoked a specific amount and has a specified amount of exposure to all the other known risk factors, what determines if this individual will get lung cancer. Today's answer might well be that it is a matter of chance. We can explain much more of the variability in lung cancer occurrence nowadays than we formerly could, by taking into account specific factors known to cause it, but at the limits of our knowledge we ascribe the remaining variability to what we call chance. In this view, chance is seen as a catch-all term for our ignorance about causal explanations.

We have so far ignored more subtle considerations of sources of unpredictability in events, such as transcomputably complex deterministic behaviour, chaotic behaviour (in which even the slightest uncertainty about initial conditions leads to vast uncertainty about outcomes), and quantum-mechanical uncertainty. In each of these situations, a random (stochastic) model component may be essential for any useful modeling effort. Such components can be introduced in the above conceptual model by treating unmeasured component causes in the model as random events, so that the causal model based on components of sufficient causes can have a random element.

Philosophy of scientific inference

Causal inference may be viewed as a special case of the more general process of scientific reasoning. The literature on this topic is too vast for us to review, but we will provide a brief overview of certain points relevant to epidemiology, at the risk of some over-simplification.

Modern science began to emerge around the sixteenth and seventeenth centuries, when the knowledge demands of emerging technologies (such as artillery and transoceanic navigation) stimulated inquiry into the origins of knowledge. An early codification of the scientific method was Bacon's *Novum organum* (1620), which presented an inductivist view of science. In this philosophy, scientific reasoning is said to depend on making generalizations or inductions from observations to general laws of nature; the observations are said to induce the formulation of a natural law in the mind of the scientist. Thus, an inductivist would have said that Jenner's observation of a lack of smallpox among milkmaids induced in his mind the theory that cowpox (common among milkmaids) conferred immunity to smallpox. Inductivist philosophy reached a pinnacle of sorts in the canons of John Stuart Mill (1843), which evolved into inferential criteria that are still in use today.

Inductivist philosophy was a great step forward from the medieval scholasticism that preceded it, for at least it demanded that a scientist make careful observations of people and nature, rather than appeal to faith, ancient texts, or authorities. None the less, by the eighteenth century, the Scottish philosopher David Hume (1739) had described a disturbing deficiency in inductivism: an inductive argument carried no logical force; instead, such an argument represented nothing more than an assumption that certain events would in the future follow in the same pattern as they had in the past. Thus, to argue that cowpox caused immunity to smallpox because no one got smallpox after having cowpox corresponded to an unjustified assumption that the pattern observed so far (no smallpox after cowpox) will continue into the future. Hume (1739) pointed out that, even for the most reasonable sounding of such assumptions, there was no logic or force of necessity behind the inductive argument.

Of central concern to Hume (1739) was the issue of causal inference and failure of induction to provide a foundation for it.

Thus not only our reason fails us in the discovery of the *ultimate connexion* of causes and effects, but even after experience has inform'd us of their *constant conjunction*, 'tis impossible for us to satisfy ourselves by our reason, why we shou'd extend that experience beyond those particular instances, which have fallen under our observation. We suppose, but are never able to prove, that there must be a resemblance betwixt those objects, of which we have had experience, and those which lie beyond the reach of our discovery (Hume 1739).

In other words, no number of repetitions of a particular sequence of events, such as the appearance of a light after flipping a switch, can establish a causal connection between the action of the switch and the turning on of the light. No matter how many times the light comes on after the switch has been pressed, the possibility of coincidental occurrence cannot be ruled out. Hume (1739) pointed out that observers cannot perceive causal connections, but only a series of events. Russell (1945) illustrated this point with the example of two accurate clocks that perpetually chime on the hour, with one keeping time slightly ahead of the other; although one invariably chimes before the other, there is no causal connection from one to the other. Thus, assigning a causal interpretation to the pattern of events cannot be a logical extension of our observations, since the events might be occurring together only by coincidence or because of a shared earlier cause.

Causal inference based on mere coincidence of events constitute a logical fallacy known as *post hoc ergo propter hoc* (Latin for 'after this therefore on-account-of this'). This fallacy is exemplified by the inference that the crowing of a rooster is necessary for the sun to rise because sunrise is always preceded by the crowing.

The *post hoc* fallacy is a special case of a more general logical fallacy known as the 'fallacy of affirming the consequent'. This fallacy of confirmation takes the following general form: 'We know that if H is true, B must be true and we know that B is true; therefore H must be true.' This fallacy is used routinely by scientists in interpreting data. It is used, for example, when one argues as follows: 'if sewer service causes heart disease, then heart disease rates should be highest where sewer service is available; heart disease rates are indeed highest where sewer service is available; therefore, sewer service causes heart disease'. There, H is the hypothesis 'sewer service causes heart disease' and B is the observation 'heart disease rates are highest where sewer service is available'. The argument is of course logically unsound, as demonstrated by the fact that we can imagine many ways in which the premises could be true but the conclusion false, for example economic development could lead to both sewer service and elevated heart disease rates, without any effect of the latter on the former.

Russell (1939) summarized the fallacy this way:

'If p, then q; now q is true; therefore p is true.' E.g., 'If pigs have wings, then some winged animals are good to eat; now some winged animals are good to eat; therefore pigs have wings.' This form of inference is called 'scientific method.'

Russell was not alone in his lament of the illogicality of scientific reasoning as ordinarily practised. Many philosophers and scientists from Hume's time forward attempted to set out a firm logical basis for scientific reasoning. Perhaps none has attracted more attention from epidemiologists than the philosopher Karl Popper.

Popper addressed Hume's problem by asserting that scientific hypotheses can never be proven or established as true in any logical sense. Instead, Popper observed that scientific statements can simply be found to be consistent with observation. Since it is possible for an observation to be consistent with several hypotheses that themselves may be mutually inconsistent, consistency between a hypothesis and observation is no proof of the hypothesis. In contrast, a valid observation that is inconsistent with a hypothesis implies that the hypothesis as stated is false and so refutes the hypothesis. If you wring the rooster's neck before it crows and the sun still rises, you have disproved that the rooster's crowing is a necessary cause of sunrise. Or consider a hypothetical research programme to ascertain the boiling point of water (Magee 1985). A scientist who boils water in an open flask and repeatedly measures the boiling point at 100°C will never, no matter how many confirmatory repetitions are involved, prove that 100°C is always the boiling point. On the other hand, merely one attempt to boil the water in a closed flask or at high altitude will refute the proposition that water always boils at 100°C.

According to Popper (1968), science advances by a process of elimination that he called conjecture and refutation. Scientists form hypotheses based on intuition, conjecture, and previous experience. Good scientists use deductive logic to infer predictions from the hypothesis, and then compare observations with the predictions. Hypotheses whose predictions agree with observations are confirmed only in the sense that they can continue to be used as explanations of natural phenomena. At any time, however, they may be refuted by further observations and replaced by other hypotheses that better explain the observations. This view of scientific inference is sometimes called refutationism or falsificationism.

Refutationists consider induction to be a psychological crutch: repeated observations did not in fact induce the formulation of a natural law, but only the belief that such a law has been found. For a refutationist, only the psychological comfort that induction provides explains why it still has its advocates.

One way to rescue the concept of induction from the stigma of pure delusion is to resurrect it as a psychological phenomenon, as Hume (1739) and Popper (1968) claimed it was, but one that plays a legitimate role in hypothesis formation. The philosophy of conjecture and refutation places no constraints on the origin of conjectures. Even delusions are permitted as hypotheses and, therefore, inductively inspired hypotheses, however psychological, are valid starting points for scientific evaluation. This concession does not admit a logical role for induction in confirming scientific hypotheses, but it allows the process of induction to play a part, along with imagination, in the scientific cycle of conjecture and refutation.

The philosophy of conjecture and refutation has profound implications for the methodology of science. The popular concept of a scientist doggedly assembling evidence to support a favourite thesis is objectionable from the standpoint of refutationist philosophy, because it encourages scientists to consider their own pet theories as their intellectual property, to be confirmed, proven, and, when all the evidence is in, cast in stone and defended as natural law. Such attitudes hinder critical evaluation, interchange, and progress. The approach of conjecture and refutation, in contrast, encourages scientists to consider multiple hypotheses and to seek crucial tests that decide between competing hypotheses by falsifying one of them. Since falsification of one or more theories is the goal, there is incentive to depersonalize the theories. Criticism levelled at a theory need not be seen as criticism of its proposer. It has been suggested that the reason why certain fields of science advance rapidly while others languish is that the rapidly advancing fields are propelled by scientists who are busy constructing and testing competing hypotheses; the other fields, in contrast, 'are sick by comparison, because they have forgotten the necessity for alternative hypotheses and disproof' (Platt 1964).

Some twentieth century philosophers of science, most notably Kuhn, have emphasized the role of the scientific community in determining the validity of scientific theories. These critics of the conjecture and refutation model have suggested that the refutation of a theory involves making a choice. Every observation is itself dependent on theories. For example, observing the moons of Jupiter through a telescope seems to us like a direct observation, but only because the theory of optics on which the telescope is based is so well accepted. When confronted with a refuting observation, a scientist faces the choice of rejecting either the validity of the theory being tested or the validity of the scientific infrastructure of the theories on which the refuting observation is based. Observations that are falsifying instances of theories may at times be treated as 'anomalies', tolerated without falsifying the theory in the hope that the anomalies may eventually be explained. An epidemiological example is the observation that shallow-inhaling smokers had higher lung cancer rates than deep-inhaling smokers. This anomaly was eventually explained when it was noted that smoking-associated lung tumours tend to occur high in the lung, where shallowly inhaled smoke tars tend to be deposited (Wald 1985).

In other instances, anomalies may eventually lead to the over-throw of current scientific doctrine, just as Newtonian mechanics was discarded (remaining only as a first order approximation) in favour of relativity theory. Kuhn (1962) claimed that in every branch of science the prevailing scientific viewpoint, which he termed 'normal science', occasionally undergoes major shifts that amount to scientific revolutions. These revolutions signal a decision of the scientific community to discard the scientific infrastructure rather than to falsify a new hypothesis that cannot be easily grafted onto it. Kuhn (1962) and others have argued that the consensus of the scientific community determines what is considered accepted and what is considered refuted.

Kuhn's critics characterized this description of science as one of an irrational process, 'a matter for mob psychology' (Lakatos 1970). Those who cling to a belief in a rational structure for science consider Kuhn's vision to be a regrettably real description of much of what passes for scientific activity, but not prescriptive for any good science. The philosophical debate about Kuhn's description of science hinges on whether he meant to describe only what has happened historically in science or instead meant to describe what ought to happen, an issue about which he has not been completely clear:

Are Kuhn's remarks about scientific development . . . to be read as descriptions or prescriptions? The answer, of course, is that they should be read in both ways at once. If I have a theory of how and why science works, it must necessarily have implications for the way in which scientists should behave if their enterprise is to flourish (Kuhn 1970).

The idea that science is a sociological process, whether considered descriptive or normative, is an interesting thesis. Regardless of the answer, we suspect that most epidemiologists (and most scientists) will continue to function as if the following classical view of the goal of science is correct: the ultimate goal of scientific inference is to capture some objective truths and any theory of inference should ideally be evaluated by how well it leads us to these truths.

Those holding the objective view of scientific truth nevertheless concede that our knowledge of these truths will always be tentative. For refutationists this tentativeness has an asymmetric quality: we may know a theory is false because it consistently fails the tests we put it through, but we cannot know that it is true, even if it passes every test we can devise, for it may fail a test as yet undevised. With this view, any theory of inference should ideally be evaluated by how well it leads us to detect errors in our hypotheses and observations.

There is another philosophy of inference that, like refutation-ism, holds an objective view of scientific truth and a view of knowledge as tentative or uncertain, but which focuses on an evaluation of knowledge rather than truth. Like refutationism, the modern form of this philosophy evolved from the writings of eighteenth century British philosophers, but the focal arguments first appeared in a pivotal essay by Thomas Bayes (1763) and, hence, the philosophy is usually referred to as Bayesianism (Howson and Urbach 1989). Like refutationism, it did not reach a complete expression until after the First World War, most notably in the writings of Ramsey (1931) and DeFinetti (1937) and, like refutationism, it did not begin to appear in epidemiology until the 1970s (see, for example, Cornfield 1976).

The central problem addressed by Bayesianism is the following. In classical logic, a deductive argument can provide you no information about a scientific hypothesis unless you can be 100 per cent certain about the truth of the premises of the argument. Consider the centerpiece of refutationism, the logical argument called *modus tollens*: 'If H implies B and B is false, then H must be false.' This argument is logically valid, but it does the scientist little of the good claimed by refutationists, because the conclusion follows only on the assumptions that the premises 'H implies B' and 'B is false' are true statements. If these premises are statements about the physical world, we cannot possibly know them to be correct with 100 per cent certainty, since all observations are subject to error. Furthermore, the claim that 'H implies B' will often depend on its own chain of deductions, each with its own premises of which we cannot be certain.

For example, if H is 'television viewing causes homicides' and B is 'homicide rates are highest where televisions are most common', the first premise used in *modus tollens* to test the hypothesis that television viewing causes homicides will be 'if television viewing causes homicides, homicide rates are highest where televisions are most common'. The validity of this premise is doubtful—after all, even if television does cause homicides, homicide rates may be low where televisions are common because of socio-economic advantages in those areas.

Continuing to reason in this fashion, we could arrive at a more pessimistic state than even Hume imagined: not only is induction without logical foundation, but *deduction* has no scientific utility because we cannot insure the validity of all the premises. The Bayesian answer to this problem is partial, in that it makes a severe demand on the scientist and puts a severe limitation on the results. It says roughly this. If you can assign a degree of certainty or personal probability to the premises of your valid argument, you may use any and all the rules of probability theory to derive a certainty for the conclusion and this certainty will be a logically valid consequence of your original certainties. The catch is that your concluding certainty, or posterior probability may depend heavily on what you used as initial certainties or prior probabilities. And, if those initial certainties are not those of a colleague, that colleague may very well assign a different certainty to the conclu-sion than you derived.

Because the posterior probabilities emanating from a Bayesian inference depend on the person supplying the initial certainties and, thus, may vary across individuals, the inferences are said to be subjective. This subjectivity of Bayesian inference is often mistaken for a subjective treatment of truth. Not only is such a view of Bayesianism incorrect, but it is diametrically opposed to Bayesian philosophy. The Bayesian approach represents a constructive attempt to deal with the dilemma that scientific laws and facts should not be treated as known with certainty, yet classical deductive logic yields conclusions only when some law, fact, or connection between is asserted with 100 per cent certainty.

A common criticism of Bayesian philosophy is that it diverts attention away from the classical goals of science, such as the discovery of how the world works, towards psychological states of mind called 'certainties', 'subjective probabilities', or 'degrees of belief' (Popper 1968). This criticism fails, however, to recognize the importance of the scientist's state of mind in determining what theories to test and what tests to apply.

In any research context there will be an unlimited number of hypotheses that could explain an observed phenomenon. Some argue that progress is best aided by severely testing (empirically challenging) those explanations that seem most probable in light of past research, so that shortcomings of currently 'received' theories can be most rapidly discovered. Indeed, much research in certain fields takes this form, as when theoretical predictions of particle mass are put to ever-more precise tests in physics experiments. This process does not involve a mere improved repetition of past studies. Rather, it involves tests of previously untested but important predictions of the theory.

Probabilities of auxiliary hypotheses are also important in study design and interpretation. Failure of a theory to pass a test can lead to rejection of the theory more rapidly when the auxiliary hypotheses upon which the test depends possess high probability. This observation provides a rationale for preferring population-based to hospital-based case–control studies, because the former has a higher probability of unbiased subject selection.

Even if one disputes the above arguments, most epidemiologists desire some interval estimate or evaluation of the likely range for an effect in light of available data. This estimate must inevitably be derived in the face of considerable uncertainty about methodologic details and various events that led to the available data and can be extremely sensitive to the reasoning used in its derivation. Psychological investigations have found that most people, including scientists, reason poorly in general and especially poorly in the face of uncertainty (Kahnemann et al. 1982). Bayesian philosophy provides a methodology for such reasoning and, in particular, provides many warnings against being overly certain about one's conclusions.

Such warnings are echoed in refutationist philosophy. As Medawar (1979) put it, 'I cannot give any scientist of any age better advice than this: the intensity of the conviction that a hypothesis is true has no bearing on whether it is true or not.'

We would only add that the intensity of a conviction that a hypothesis is false has no bearing on whether it is false or not.

Vigorous debate is a characteristic of modern scientific philosophy, no less in epidemiology than in other areas (Rothman 1988). Perhaps the most important common thread that emerges from the debated philosophies is Hume's legacy that proof is impossible in empirical science. This simple fact is particularly important to epidemiologists, who often face the criticism that proof is impossible in epidemiology, with the implication that it is possible in other scientific disciplines. Such criticism may stem from a belief by some that an experiment can somehow provide proof, whereas the non-experimental nature of much epidemiological work precludes definitive proof. Others hold the view that 'statistical' relations are only suggestive and believe that detailed study of mechanisms within single individuals can reveal cause–effect rela-

tions with certainty. Both of these views unfairly devalue epidemiological work.

Regarding the first view, the non-experimental nature of a science does not preclude impressive scientific understanding; presumably geologists and astronomers do not lose sleep over their inability to conduct double-blind randomized trials. Even when they are possible, randomized trials do not provide anything approaching proof—many have only fuelled controversies (Rothman 1985). As for the second view, it overlooks the fact that all relations are suggestive in exactly the manner discussed by Hume: even the most careful and detailed mechanistic dissection of individual events cannot provide more than associations, albeit at a finer level.

All of the fruits of scientific work, in epidemiology or other disciplines, are, at best, only tentative formulations of a description of nature, even when the work itself is carried out without mistakes. The tentativeness of our knowledge does not prevent practical applications, but it should keep us sceptical and critical, not only of everyone else's work, but our own as well.

Causal inference in epidemiology

Biological knowledge about epidemiological hypotheses is often scant, making the hypotheses themselves at times little more than vague statements of causal association between exposure and disease. These vague hypotheses have only vague consequences that can be tested, apart from a simple iteration of the observation. To cope with this vagueness, epidemiologists usually focus on testing the negation of the causal hypothesis, that is, the null hypothesis that the exposure does not have a causal relation to disease. Then, any observed association can potentially refute the hypothesis, subject to the assumption (auxiliary hypothesis) that biases are absent.

None the less, if the causal mechanism is stated specifically enough, epidemiologic observations can provide crucial tests of competing non-null causal hypotheses. For example, when toxic shock syndrome was first studied, there were two competing hypotheses about the origin of the toxin. Under one hypothesis, the toxin was a chemical in the tampon, so that women using tampons were exposed to the toxin directly from the tampon. Under the other hypothesis, the tampon acted as a culture medium for staphylococci that produced the toxin. Both hypotheses explained the relation of toxic shock occurrence to tampon use. The two hypotheses, however, lead to opposite predictions about the relation between the frequency of changing tampons and the risk of toxic shock. Under the hypothesis of a chemical intoxication, more frequent changing of the tampon would lead to more exposure to the toxin and possible absorption of a greater overall dose. This hypothesis predicted that women who changed tampons more frequently would have a higher risk than women who changed tampons infrequently. The culture-medium hypothesis predicts that the women who change tampons frequently would have a lower risk than those who leave the tampon in for longer periods, because a short duration of use for each tampon would prevent the staphylococci from multiplying enough to produce a damaging dose of toxin. Thus, epidemiological research examining how the risk of toxic shock relates to the frequency of tampon changing was able to refute one of these theories (the chemical theory was refuted).

Another example of a theory easily tested by epidemiological data related to the finding that women who took replacement oestrogen therapy were at a considerably higher risk of endometrial cancer. Horwitz and Feinstein (1978) conjectured a competing theory to explain the association: they proposed that women taking oestrogen experienced symptoms such as bleeding that induced them to consult a physician. The resulting diagnostic work-up led to the detection of endometrial cancer in these women. Many epidemiological observations could have been and were used to evaluate these competing hypotheses. The causal theory predicted that the risk of endometrial cancer would tend to increase with increasing use (dose, frequency, and duration) of oestrogens, as for other carcinogenic exposures. The detection bias theory, on the other hand, predicted that women who had used oestrogens only for a short while would have the greatest risk, since the symptoms related to oestrogen use that led to the medical consultation tend to appear soon after use begins. Because the association of recent oestrogen use and endometrial cancer was the same in both long-term and short-term oestrogen users, the detection bias theory was refuted as an explanation for all but a small fraction of endometrial cancer cases occurring after oestrogen use. (Refutation of the detection bias theory also depended on many other observations. Particularly important was the theory's implication that there must be a large reservoir of undetected endometrial cancer in the typical population of women to account for the much greater rate observed in oestrogen users.)

The endometrial cancer example illustrates a critical point in understanding the process of causal inference in epidemiological studies: many of the hypotheses being evaluated in the interpretation of epidemiologic studies are non-causal hypotheses, in the sense of involving no causal connection between the study exposure and the disease. For example, hypotheses that amount to explanations of how specific types of bias could have led to an association between exposure and disease are the usual alternatives to the primary study hypothesis that the epidemiologist needs to consider in drawing inferences. Much of the interpretation of epidemiological studies amounts to the testing of such non-causal explanations for observed associations.

Causal criteria

In practice, how do epidemiologists separate out the causal from the non-causal explanations? Despite philosophical criticisms of inductive inference, inductively oriented causal criteria have commonly been used to make such inferences. If a set of necessary and sufficient causal criteria could be used to distinguish causal from non-causal relations in epidemiologic studies, the job of the scientist would be eased considerably. With such criteria, all the concerns about the logic or lack thereof in causal inference could be forgotten: it would only be necessary to consult the check-list of criteria to see if a relation were causal. We know from philosophy that such a set of criteria does not exist. Nevertheless, lists of causal criteria have become popular, possibly because they seem to provide a road map through complicated territory.

A commonly used set of criteria was proposed by Hill (1965); it was an expansion of a set of criteria offered previously in the landmark Surgeon General's report on smoking and health (US Department of Health, Education and Welfare 1964), which in turn were inspired by the inductive canons of Mill (1862). Hill sug-

gested that the following aspects of an association be considered in attempting to distinguish causal from non-causal associations: strength, consistency, specificity, temporality, biologic gradient, plausibility, coherence, experimental evidence, and analogy. The popular view that these criteria should be used for causal inference makes it necessary to examine them in detail.

1. Strength

For Hill and others, the strength of association refers to the magnitude of the ratio of incidence ('relative risk') or some analogous ratio measure. Hill's argument was essentially that strong associations are more likely to be causal than weak associations because, if they could be explained by some other factor, the effect of that factor would have to be even stronger than the observed association and therefore would have become evident. Weak associations, on the other hand, are more likely to be explained by undetected biases. To some extent this is a reasonable argument, but, as Hill himself acknowledged, the fact that an association is weak does not rule out a causal connection. A commonly cited counter-example is the relation between cigarette smoking and cardiovascular disease: one explanation for this relation being weak is that cardiovascular disease is common, making any ratio measure of effect comparatively small compared with ratio measures for diseases that are less common (Rothman and Poole 1988). Nevertheless, cigarette smoking is not seriously doubted as a cause of cardiovascular disease. Another example would be passive smoking and lung cancer, a weak association that few consider to be non-causal.

Counter-examples of strong but non-causal associations are also not hard to find; any study with strong confounding illustrates the phenomenon. For example, consider the strong but non-causal relation between Down's syndrome and birth rank, which is confounded by the relation between Down's syndrome and maternal age. Of course, once the confounding factor is identified, the association is diminished by adjustment for the factor. These examples remind us that a large association is neither necessary nor sufficient for causality, nor is weakness necessary nor sufficient for the absence of causality. In addition to these counter-examples, we have to remember that neither relative risk nor any other measure of association is a biologically consistent feature of an association; rather it is a characteristic of a study population that depends on the relative prevalence of other causes. A strong association serves only to rule out hypotheses that the association is due to some weak unmeasured confounder or some other modest source of bias.

2. Consistency

Consistency refers to the repeated observation of an association in different populations under different circumstances. Lack of consistency, however, does not rule out a causal association, because some effects are produced by their causes only under unusual circumstances. More precisely, the effect of a causal agent cannot occur unless the complementary component causes act or have already acted to complete a sufficient cause. These conditions will not always be met. Thus, transfusions can cause HIV infection but they do not always do so: the virus must also be present. Tampon use can cause toxic shock syndrome, but only rarely when certain other, perhaps unknown, conditions are met. Consistency is apparent only after all the relevant details of a causal mechanism are understood, which is to say very seldom. Furthermore, even studies of exactly the same phenomena can be expected to differ in their results simply because they differ in their methodologies. Consistency serves only to rule out hypotheses that the association is attributable to some factor that varies across studies.

3. Specificity

The criterion of specificity requires that a cause lead to a single effect, not multiple effects. This argument has often been advanced to refute causal interpretations of exposures that appear to relate to myriad effects, in particular by those seeking to exonerate smoking as a cause of lung cancer. Unfortunately, the criterion is wholly invalid. Causes of a given effect cannot be expected to lack other effects on any logical grounds. In fact, everyday experience teaches us repeatedly that single events or conditions may have many effects. Smoking is an excellent example: it leads to many effects in the smoker. The existence of one effect does not detract from the possibility that another effect exists.

Furthermore, specific effects are as liable to be confounded as non-specific effects. Therefore, specificity for an exposure does not result in greater validity for any causal inference regarding the exposure. Hill's discussion of this criterion for inference is replete with reservations, but, even so, the criterion is useless and misleading.

4. Temporality

Temporality refers to the necessity that the cause precede the effect in time. This criterion is inarguable, in so far as any claimed observation of causation must involve the putative cause C preceding the putative effect D. It does not, however, follow that a reverse time order is evidence against the hypothesis that C can cause D. Rather, observations in which C followed D merely shows that C could not have caused D in these instances; they provide no evidence for or against the hypothesis that C can cause D in those instances in which it precedes D.

5. Biologic gradient

Biologic gradient refers to the presence of a monotonic (unidirectional) dose–response curve. We often expect such a monotonic relation to exist. For example, more smoking means more carcinogen exposure and more tissue damage and, hence, more opportunity for carcinogenesis. Some causal associations, however, show a single jump (threshold) rather than a monotonic trend; an example is the association between DES and adenocarcinoma of the vagina. A possible explanation is that the doses of DES that were administered were all sufficiently great to produce the maximum effect from DES. Under this hypothesis, for all those exposed to DES, the development of disease would depend entirely on other component causes.

The somewhat controversial topic of alcohol consumption and mortality is another example. Death rates are higher among non-drinkers than among moderate drinkers, but ascend to the highest levels for heavy drinkers. There is considerable debate about which parts of the J-shaped dose–response curve are causally related to alcohol consumption and which parts are non-causal artifacts stemming from confounding or other biases. Some studies appear to find only an increasing relation between alcohol consumption and mortality, possibly because the categories of alcohol consumption are too broad to distinguish different rates among moderate drinkers and non-drinkers.

Associations that do show a monotonic trend are not necessarily causal; confounding can result in a gradual relation between a non–causal risk factor and disease if the confounding factor itself demonstrates a biologic gradient in its relation with disease. The non-causal relation between birth rank and Down's syndrome mentioned above shows a biological gradient that merely reflects the progressive relation between maternal age and Down's syndrome occurrence.

These issues imply that the existence of a monotonic association is neither necessary nor sufficient for a causal relation. A non-monotonic relation only refutes those causal hypotheses specific enough to predict a monotonic dose–response curve.

6. Plausibility

Plausibility refers to the biological plausibility of the hypothesis, an important concern but one that may be difficult to judge. Sartwell (1960), emphasizing this point, cited the remarks of Cheever (1861), who was commenting on the aetiology of typhus before its mode of transmission (via body lice) was known.

It could be no more ridiculous for the stranger who passed the night in the steerage of an emigrant ship to ascribe the typhus, which he there contracted, to the vermin with which bodies of the sick might be infested. An adequate cause, one reasonable in itself, must correct the coincidences of simple experience.

The point is that what was to Cheever (1861) an implausible explanation turned out to be the correct explanation, since it was indeed the vermin that caused the typhus infection. Such is the problem with plausibility: it is too often not based on logic or data, but only on prior beliefs.

The Bayesian approach to inference attempts to deal with this problem by requiring that one quantify, on a probability (0 to 1) scale, the certainty that one has in those prior beliefs, as well as in new hypotheses. This quantification displays the dogmatism or open-mindedness of the analyst in a public fashion, with certainty values near 1 or 0 betraying a strong commitment of the analyst for or against a hypothesis. It can also provide a means of testing those quantified beliefs against new evidence (Howson and Urbach 1989). Nevertheless, the Bayesian approach cannot transform plausibility into an objective causal criterion.

7. Coherence

Taken from the Surgeon General's report on smoking and health (US Department of Health, Education and Welfare 1964), the term coherence implies that a cause and effect interpretation for an association does not conflict with what is known of the natural history and biology of the disease. The examples Hill (1965) gave for coherence, such as the histopathological effect of smoking on the bronchial epithelium (in reference to the association between smoking and lung cancer) or the difference in lung cancer incidence by sex, could reasonably be considered examples of plausibility as well as coherence; the distinction appears to be a fine one. Hill emphasized that the absence of coherent information, as distinguished, apparently, from the presence of conflicting information, should not be taken as evidence against an association being considered causal. Consequently, at least according to Hill, coherence should not be a criterion for causal inference. On the other hand, the presence of conflicting information may indeed refute a hypothesis, but one must always remember that the conflicting information may be mistaken or misinterpreted (Wald 1985).

8. Experimental evidence

It is not clear what Hill meant by experimental evidence. It might have referred to evidence from laboratory experiments on animals or to evidence from human experiments. Evidence from human experiments, however, is seldom available for most epidemiological research questions and animal evidence relates to different species and usually to levels of exposure very different from those experienced by humans. From Hill's examples, it seems that what he had in mind for experimental evidence was the result of removal of some harmful exposure in an intervention or prevention programme, rather than the results of formal experiments (Susser 1991). The lack of availability of such evidence would at least be a pragmatic difficulty in making this a criterion for inference. Logically, however, experimental evidence is not a criterion but a test of the causal hypothesis, a test that is simply unavailable in most circumstances. It is also not as decisive as often thought. For example, the hypothesis that malaria is caused by swamp gas can be tested by draining swamps to see if the malaria rates in local residents goes down. Indeed, the rates will drop, but not because swamp gas causes malaria.

9. Analogy

Whatever insight might be derived from analogy is handicapped by the inventive imagination of scientists who can find analogies everywhere. At best, analogy provides a source of more elaborate hypotheses about the associations under study; the absence of such analogies only reflects lack of imagination or experience, not the falsity of the hypothesis.

Conclusion

As is evident, these standards of epidemiological evidence offered by Hill to judge whether an association is causal are saddled with reservations and exceptions. Hill himself was ambivalent about the utility of these 'standards' (he did not use the word criteria in the paper). On the one hand he asked 'in what circumstances can we pass from this observed *association* to a verdict of *causation*?' (Hill 1965, emphasis in original) Yet, despite speaking of verdicts on causation, he disagreed that any 'hard-and-fast rules of evidence' existed by which to judge causation: 'None of my nine viewpoints [criteria] can bring indisputable evidence for or against the cause-and-effect hypothesis and none can be required as a *sine qua non*' (Hill 1965).

Actually, the fourth viewpoint, temporality, is a *sine qua non* for causality: if the putative cause did not precede the effect, that indeed is indisputable evidence that the observed association is not causal (although this evidence does not rule out causality in other situations, for in other situations the putative cause may precede the effect). Other than this one condition, however, which may be viewed as part of the definition of causation, there is no necessary or sufficient criterion for determining whether an observed association is causal.

This conclusion accords with the views of Hume, Popper, and others that causal inferences cannot attain the certainty of logical deductions. Although some scientists continue to promulgate causal criteria as aids to inference (Susser 1991), others argue that it is actually detrimental to cloud the inferential process by

considering check-list criteria (Lanes and Poole 1984). An intermediate refutationist approach seeks to alter the criteria into deductive tests of causal hypotheses (Maclure 1985; Weed 1986).

References

Bayes, T. (1763). An essay towards solving a problem in the doctrine of chances. *Philosophical Transactions of the Royal Society*, **53**, 370–418.

Cornfield, J. (1976). Recent methodological contributions to clinical trials. *American Journal of Epidemiology*, **104**, 408–24.

DeFinetti, B. (1937). Foresight: its logical laws, its subjective sources. Reprinted in *Studies in subjective probability* (ed. H.E. Kyburg and H.E. Smokler. Wiley, New York.

Doll, R. and Peto, R. (1981). *The causes of cancer.* Oxford University Press, New York.

Ephron, E. (1984). *The apocalyptics. Cancer and the big lie.* Simon and Schuster, New York.

Fraiberg, S. (1959). *The magic years.* Scribner's, New York.

Higginson, J. (1960). Population studies in cancer. *Acta Union Internationale Contra Cancrum*, **16**, 1667–70.

Higginson, J. (1980). Proportion of cancer due to occupation. *Preventive Medicine*, **9**, 180–8.

Hill, A.B. (1965). The environment and disease: association or causation? *Proceedings of the Royal Society of Medicine*, **58**, 295–300.

Hogben, L. (1933). *Nature and nurture.* Williams and Norgate, London.

Horwitz, R.I. and Feinstein, A.R. (1978). Alternative analytic methods for case–control studies of estrogens and endometrial cancer. *New England Journal of Medicine*, **299**, 1089–94.

Howson, C. and Urbach, P. (1989). *Scientific reasoning. The Bayesian approach.* Open Court, LaSalle, Ill.

Hume D. (1739). *A treatise of human nature.* Oxford University Press edition, with an Analytical Index by L.A. Selby-Bigge, published 1888. Second edition with text revised and notes by P.H. Nidditch, 1978.

Kahnemann, D., Slovic, P., and Tversky, A. (1982). *Judgment under uncertainty; heuristics and biases.* Cambridge University Press, New York.

Kuhn, T.S. (1962). *The structure of scientific revolutions* (2nd edn). University of Chicago Press, Chicago.

Kuhn, T.S. (1970). Reflections on my critics. In *Criticism and the growth of knowledge* (ed. I. Lakatos and A. Musgrave) Cambridge University Press.

Lakatos, I. (1970). Falsification and the methodology of scientific research programmes. In *Criticism and the growth of knowledge* (ed. I. Lakatos and A. Musgrave). Cambridge University Press.

Lanes, S.F. and Poole, C. (1984). 'Truth in packaging?' The unwrapping of epidemiologic research. *Journal of Occupational Medicine*, **26**, 571–4.

Maclure, M. (1985). Popperian refutation in epidemiology. *American Journal of Epidemiology*, **121**, 343–50.

MacMahon, B. (1986). Gene–environment interaction in human disease. *Journal of Psychiatric Research*, **6**, 393–402.

Medawar, P.B. (1979). *Advice to a young scientist.* Basic Books, New York.

Magee, B. (1985) *Philosophy and the real world. An introduction to Karl Popper.* Open Court, La Salle, Ill.

Mill, J.S. (1862). *A system of logic, ratiocinative and inductive* (5th edn). Parker, Son and Bowin, London. Cited in D.W. Clark and B. MacMahon (ed.) (1981). *Preventive and community medicine* (2nd edn). Little, Brown, Boston.

Platt, J.R. (1984). Strong inference. *Science*, **146**, 347–53.

Popper, K.R. (1957). Probability magic or knowledge out of ignorance. *Dialectica*, **11**, 354–74.

Popper, K.R. (1968). *The logic of scientific discovery.* Harper & Row, New York.

Ramsey, F.P. (1931). *Truth and probability.* Reprinted in Kyburg, H.E. and Smokler, H.E. (ed.) (1964). *Studies in subjective probability.* Wiley, New York.

Reichenbach, H. (1951). *The rise of scientific philosophy.* University of California Press, Berkeley.

Rothman, K.J. (1976). Causes. *American Journal of Epidemiology*, **104**, 587–92.

Rothman, K.J. (1981). Induction and latent periods. *American Journal of Epidemiology*, **114**, 253–9.

Rothman, K.J. (1985). Sleuthing in hospitals. *New England Journal of Medicine*, **313**, 258–60.

Rothman, K.J. (ed.) (1988). *Causal inference*. Epidemiology Resources, Inc., Boston.

Rothman, K.J. and Poole, C. (1985). Science and policy making. *American Journal of Public Health*, **75**, 340–1.

Rothman K.J. and Poole C. (1988). A strengthening programme for weak associations. *International Journal of Epidemiology*, 17 (Suppl.), 955–9.

Russell, B. (1945). Dewey's new 'Logic'. (1939). In *The philosophy of John Dewey*. (ed. P.A. Schlipp). Tudor, New York. Reprinted in Egner, R.E. and Denonn, L.E., eds. (1961). *The Basic Writings of Bertrand Russell*. Simon and Schuster, New York.

Sartwell, P. (1960). On the methodology of investigations of etiologic factors in chronic diseases—further comments. *Journal of Chronic Diseases*, **11**, 61–3.

Susser, M. (1988). Falsification, verification and causal inference in epidemiology: reconsiderations in the light of Sir Karl Popper's philosophy. In *Causal inference*, (ed. K.J. Rothman). Epidemiology Resources, Inc., Boston.

Susser, M. (1991). What is a cause and how do we know one? A grammar for pragmatic epidemiology. *American Journal of Epidemiology*, **133**, 635–48.

US Department of Health, Education and Welfare (1964). *Smoking and health: report of the Advisory Committee to the Surgeon General of the Public Health Service*. Government Printing Office, Washington, DC.

Wald, N.A. (1985). Smoking. In *Cancer risks and prevention* (ed. M.P. Vessey and M. Gray). New York.

Weed, D. (1986). On the logic of causal inference. American Journal of Epidemiology, **123**, 965–79.

16 Meta-analysis and data synthesis in medical research

G. Davey Smith, Matthias Egger, and Andrew N. Phillips

Introduction

The volume of data which needs to be considered by medical researchers in any particular field is constantly expanding. In many areas it is impossible for the individual worker to read, critically evaluate and synthesize the state of current knowledge, let alone keep updating this on a regular basis. Furthermore, with regard to summaries of empirical research, different authorities will often disagree in their interpretations, even when the research findings they are reviewing are essentially the same. It is difficult for third parties to determine the basis for such disagreements and have any sound basis for deciding which reading of the data is correct. In response to this situation there has, in recent years, been an increasing focus on formal methods of combining data from studies, to produce explicitly formulated, quantitative, summary measures of effects. This process has been called 'meta-analysis' and its growing popularity is reflected in the sharp increase in the number of papers concerning meta-analysis published between 1983 and 1993 (Fig. 16.1).

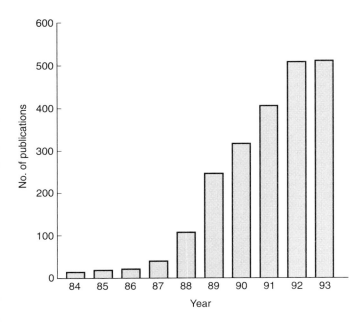

Fig.16.1 Number of publications concerning meta-analysis, 1984 to 1993. Results from MEDLINE search using text word and medical subject heading 'meta-analysis'.

Meta-analysis in medical research has been best developed with respect to the findings of randomized controlled trials (**RCTs**). While there are several problems which can lead to misleading results of such meta-analyses, restricting the admissible evidence to that produced from RCTs means that the central potential problem of observational studies—the exposed and unexposed groups differ systematically in other ways than their exposure status—is avoided (Davey Smith *et al.* 1992*a*). Meta-analysis has been extended to observational studies—within the fields of both aetiologic epidemiology and the evaluation of medical interventions. Here the reception has been more mixed (Shapiro 1994), since interpretation of the causal importance of the associations under study is more problematic. Methods to combine experimental and non-experimental data—for example, the results of RCTs of mammography with the findings of case–control studies and databases (Eddy *et al.* 1988)—are currently being developed. Such an analysis strategy—sometimes referred to as 'cross-design synthesis' (General Accounting Office 1992)—is intended to take advantage of the totality of data available, whether it be experimental or observational. While this seems an attractive proposition, the technique has not gone uncriticized (Anonymous 1992).

Despite its widespread use, meta-analysis thus continues to be a controversial technique. While some exponents feel that 'meta-analyses should replace traditional review articles of single topic issues whenever possible' (Chalmers *et al.* 1990) others think of it as 'a new *bête noire*' which represents 'the unacceptable face of statisticism' and should 'be stifled at birth' (Oakes 1986, p. xii). Davis (1992) wrote that

Meta-analysis begins with scientific studies, usually performed by academics or government agencies, and sometimes incomplete or disputed. The data from the studies are then run through computer models of bewildering complexity, which produce results of implausible precision. (p. 1)

This mixed reception is not surprising. The pooling of results from a particular set of studies may be inappropriate from a clinical point of view, producing a population 'average' effect, while clinicians want to know how to best treat their particular patients. Additional problems arise in meta-analysis of observational studies and in cross-design synthesis. While systematic overviews which include meta-analyses have clear advantages over conventional reviews, meta-analysis is not an infallible tool, and its potentials and limitations, summarized in Table 16.1, must be considered carefully.

Table 16.1 Potentials and limitations of meta-analytic research

Potentials	Limitations
More objective appraisal of the evidence than in traditional narrative reviews	Results of meta-analyses, albeit precise, may be misleading. Bias is difficult to exclude when combining observational studies
Enhanced precision of pooled estimate, leading to reduced probability of false-negative results	Selection bias: inclusion or exchange of a few studies may change results. For example, inclusion of published studies only may give misleading results (publication bias)
Resolution of uncertainty when original research, reviews, and editorials disagree	Equal weight is given to studies of high quality and to more doubtful studies
Heterogeneity in study results may be deciphered in additional analyses	Statistical procedures alone cannot resolve the issue of heterogeneity between study results
Testing hypotheses not posed at the start of individual trials, e.g. regarding subgroups of patients who are likely to respond particularly well (or the reverse) to an intervention	Extensive data-dredging results in subgroup findings which are likely to be spurious even though they may achieve statistical significance
Generation of promising research questions to be addressed in future studies	Important further research may be prevented if meta-analyses are falsely perceived as providing definite answers
Accurate calculation of the sample sizes needed in future studies	The clinical interpretation of meta-analyses is often problematic

We will focus our exposition of the principles of data synthesis in medical science on the case of meta-analysis of RCTs. In this exposition we will deal in detail with the problems which can distort the results of such quantitative data syntheses. It should be remembered that all these apply to meta-analyses of observational data and to exercises in cross-design synthesis, but that these latter studies are also subject to the additional potential biases which apply only to observational research.

History

Efforts to pool results from a number of separate studies are not new. In his account on the preventive effect of serum inoculations against enteric fever, the statistician Pearson (1904), was probably the first researcher to report the use of formal techniques to combine data from different samples. The rationale put forward by Pearson (1904) for pooling studies is still one of the main reasons for undertaking meta-analysis today: 'Many of the groups . . . are far too small to allow of any definite opinion being formed at all, having regard to the size of the probable error involved.' Noticeably, Pearson's authority as a statistician did not prevent his conclusions going unchallenged and the heated correspondence in the *British Medical Journal* that followed his publication was critical of the data synthesis exercise which he carried out (Susser 1977). Meta-analysis has, of course, continued to attract controversy since Pearson's time.

The first meta-analysis assessing the effect of a therapeutic intervention was published in 1955. Interestingly the therapy being evaluated was the placebo (Beecher 1955). A simple average was calculated of the effectiveness of placebos in such diverse conditions as post operative wound pain, cough and angina pectoris: the placebo was apparently effective in 35 per cent of patients. The development of more sophisticated statistical techniques took place in the social sciences, in particular in education research, in the 1970s. The term meta-analysis was coined in 1976 by the psychologist Glass (1976), with meta-analysis in the social and psychological sciences generally being applied to the combination of results from observational or quasi-experimental studies. Meta-analysis was rediscovered by medical researchers to be used mainly in randomized clinical trial research, particularly in the fields of cardiovascular disease (Yusuf *et al.* (1985), oncology (Early Breast Cancer Trialists Collaborative Group 1988), and perinatal care (Chalmers *et al.* 1989).

In 1982 a meta-analysis of the trials of the use of streptokinase therapy after myocardial infarction was published (Stampfer *et al.* 1982), which demonstrated a large, statistically highly significant benefit of such therapy, which could not be seen in the small individual trials the results of which were being combined. The use of such therapy remained relatively uncommon (Collins and Julian 1991), however, but very large RCTs have since established its effectiveness (Gruppo Italiano per lo Studio della Streptochinasi nell' Infarto Miocardico 1986; ISIS-2 Collaborative Group 1988). Many deaths which could have been delayed were thus allowed to occur earlier than necessary because of inadequate understanding and implementation of research which had already been carried out. In order to minimize future similar occurrences, a network of centres for the systematic meta-analysis of RCTs, named after a pioneer in the field of evaluation of medical interventions, Archie Cochrane, was created (Chalmers *et al.* 1992). This, it is hoped, will share resources, reduce duplication of effort, and facilitate dissemination of the results of meta-analyses. The logo of the Cochrane Collaboration, discussed in more detail below, is shown in Fig. 16.2.

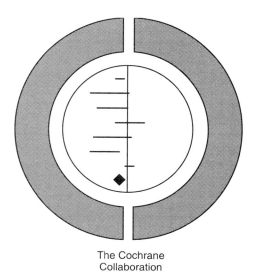

The Cochrane Collaboration

Fig. 16.2 The logo of the Cochrane Collaboration.

Terminology

There is debate about what the process of combining and analysing data from separate studies should be called (Dickersin *et al.* 1990). Apart from 'meta-analysis', the terms 'overview', 'pooling', and 'quantitative synthesis' have been used synonymously. There is clearly a need for an agreed term in order to improve communication and to help in the identification of relevant literature. We believe the term for the mathematical process of producing an overall effect estimate should be meta-analysis, for the following reasons. First, the term makes sense. Meta stands for something occurring later, which is more comprehensive and the word is often used to name a new but related discipline designated to deal critically with the original one. The alternative terms are less specific. Overview, for example, is also used for traditional, narrative reviews. Pooling incorrectly implies that the source data are actually merged together. Finally, the keyword meta-analysis has recently been included as a Medical Subject Heading (MeSH) within the MEDLINE indexing system of the National Library of Medicine (Dickersin *et al.* 1990). The term 'systematic review' has been proposed to denote a comprehensive review in which explicit methods have been used to reduce bias and, if possible and appropriate, imprecision (Chalmers *et al.* 1993). Systematic reviews can include formal meta-analyses, together with critical assessments of single trials and reviews of other sources of evidence. Therefore meta-analysis is a useful term for describing a component of systematic reviews—the production of summary effect estimates—and distinguishing between the two terms can contribute to methodological clarity.

Problems with traditional reviews

Traditional narrative reviews have a number of disadvantages which meta-analyses may overcome. First, the classical review is subjective and therefore prone to bias and error (Teagarden 1989). Without guidance by formal rules, reviewers can disagree about issues as basic as what types of studies it is appropriate to include and how to balance the quantitative evidence they provide. Selective inclusion of studies which support the author's view is common. This is illustrated by the observation that the frequency of citation of clinical trials is related to their outcome, with studies supporting the prevailing opinion being quoted more frequently than unsupportive studies (Ravnskov 1992). Once a set of studies has been assembled a common way to review the results is to count the number of studies supporting various sides of an issue and to choose the view receiving the most votes. This procedure is clearly unsound, since it ignores sample size, effect size, and research design. It is thus hardly surprising that reviewers using traditional methods often reach opposite conclusions (Mulrow 1987) and miss small but potentially important effects (Cooper and Rosenthal 1980). Reviews have often been commissioned to end an argument and help reach a consensus. However, it has been shown that in controversial areas the conclusions drawn from a given body of evidence may be associated more with the specialty of the reviewer than with the available data (Chalmers *et al.* 1990). By integrating the actual evidence, meta-analysis allows for a more objective appraisal, which can help to resolve uncertainties when the original research, classical reviews, and editorial comments disagree.

Potentials of meta-analysis

A single study can often not detect or exclude with certainty a modest, albeit clinically relevant, difference in the effects of two therapies. A trial may thus show no statistically significant treatment effect when in reality such an effect exists—it may produce a false–negative result. In this case we are dealing with a type II error, whose probability of occurrence (β) can be calculated for the particular circumstances of the study in question. Generally better recognized is the type I error—when a trial produces a statistically significant difference due to chance—whose probability, α, corresponds to the significance level. An examination of clinical trials which reported no statistically significant differences between experimental and control therapy has shown that type II errors in clinical research are common: for a clinically relevant difference in outcome, β (that is the *a priori* probability of missing this effect given the trial size) was greater than 20 per cent in 115 of the 136 trials examined (Freiman *et al.* 1992). The number of patients included in clinical trials is thus often inadequate, a situation which has changed little over recent years. In some cases, however, the required sample size may be difficult to achieve. A drug which reduces the risk of death from myocardial infarction by 10 per cent could, for example, delay many thousands of deaths each year in the United Kingdom. In order to detect such an effect at an $\alpha = 0.05$ with 90 per cent certainty or, in other words, with a type II error of no more than 10 per cent, over 10 000 patients in each treatment group would be needed (Collins *et al.* 1992).

The meta-analytic approach appears to be an attractive alternative to such a large, expensive and logistically problematic study. Data from patients in trials evaluating the same or a similar drug in a number of smaller but comparable studies are considered. In this way the necessary number of patients may be reached and relatively small effects can be detected or excluded with confidence.

Meta-analysis can also contribute to considerations regarding the generalizability of study results. The findings of a particular study may only be valid for a population of patients with the same characteristics as those investigated in the trial. If many trials exist in different groups of patients, with similar results being seen in the various trials, then it can be concluded that the effect of the intervention under study has some generality.

By putting together all available data meta-analyses are also better placed than individual trials to answer questions regarding whether an overall study result varies between subgroups, for example between men and women, older and younger patients, or subjects with different degrees of severity of disease. New hypotheses which were not posed in the single studies can thus be tested in meta-analyses. Meta-analyses lead to the identification of the most promising or the most urgent research question and may permit a more accurate calculation of the sample sizes needed in future studies. This is illustrated by an early meta-analysis of four trials that compared different methods of monitoring the fetus during labour (Chalmers 1979). The meta-analysis led to the hypothesis that, compared with intermittent auscultation, continuous fetal heart monitoring and acid–base assessment when indicated reduced the risk of neonatal seizures. This hypothesis was subsequently confirmed in a single RCT of almost seven times the size of the four previous studies combined (MacDonald *et al.* 1985).

Meta-analysis renders an important part of the review process transparent. In traditional narrative reviews it is often not clear how the conclusions follow from the data examined. In an adequately presented meta-analysis it should be possible for readers to replicate the quantitative component of the argument.

The increased openness required by meta-analysis leads to the replacement of unhelpful descriptors such as 'no relationship', 'some evidence of a trend', 'a weak relationship' and 'a strong relationship', with numerical, clearly defined values (Rosenthal 1990). Furthermore, performing a meta-analysis may lead to reviewers moving beyond the conclusions authors present in the abstracts of papers, to a thorough examination of the actual data.

Steps in carrying out meta-analysis

The performance of a meta-analysis should be viewed as an observational study of the evidence which has accrued on issues such as the relative merits and disadvantages of medical interventions (Sacks et al. 1987). The steps involved are indeed similar to any other research undertaking: formulation of the problem to be addressed, collection and analysis of the data, and reporting of the results. Likewise, a detailed research protocol which clearly states the objectives, the hypotheses to be tested, the subgroups of interest and the statistical methods to be employed should be written in advance. If the process is not clearly defined at the outset, variations of the procedures can introduce biases which may reduce the validity of the findings. Departures from the predefined plan, together with the reasons for such deviations, should be reported (Hedges 1991).

Eligibility criteria and literature search

As with patient inclusion and exclusion criteria in well-designed clinical studies, eligibility criteria have to be defined for the data to be included in a meta-analysis. They relate to the quality of trials and to the combinability of treatments, patients, outcomes, and lengths of follow-up. The quality and design features of a study can influence the results. For example, trials using a historical control group tend to show greater treatment effects than RCTs (Sacks et al. 1982). Ideally, only controlled trials with proper patient randomization, which report on all follow-up data on all initially included patients (analysis according to the intention to treat principle) and with an objective, preferably blinded, outcome assessment would be considered for inclusion (Prendiville et al. 1988). Evaluating the quality of a study can be a subjective process, however, in particular since the information reported is often inadequate for the purposes of reaching such a decision. It is therefore preferable to define only basic inclusion criteria and to test the robustness of the findings of the meta-analysis to any changes in criteria in a thorough sensitivity analysis.

The search strategies for the identification of the relevant studies should be clearly delineated. In particular, it has to be decided whether the search will be extended to include unpublished studies, as their results may systematically differ from published trials. As discussed below, a meta-analysis which is restricted to published evidence may produce distorted results due to such publication bias. For locating published studies, electronic databases such as MEDLINE are useful, but, on their own may miss a substantial proportion of relevant studies (Dickersin et al. 1985). Current Contents, citation indices and the bibliographies of review articles, monographs, and the located studies should be scrutinized as well. Registers of clinical trials and experts in the field may be useful sources to identify unpublished trials.

Data collection

Data collection consists of the detailed scrutiny of candidate studies with respect to the study design, treatment regimens, patient characteristics and outcome measures. A standardized record form for abstracting the data from published studies is useful for this purpose. Records should be kept about all trials considered for inclusion in the meta-analysis, with details being recorded for the reasons for the exclusion of certain studies.

It is useful if two independent observers extract the data from original papers, so errors can be avoided. At this stage, observers may also rate the quality of the studies, using one of the several scales which have been developed for this purpose (Chalmers et al. 1981; Prendiville et al. 1988). It is unclear to what extent blinding of observers to the names of the authors, institutions, and journals is of importance. Some authorities recommend separating data extraction and quality rating, so that the observers who are rating the quality of studies can also be blinded to the results of the studies. Blinding involves such strategies as photocopying papers and cutting out title pages and methods sections (Chalmers 1991) or scanning the text of papers into a computer and preparing standardized formats. Ongoing research will help decide whether these extra efforts actually improve the validity of the findings.

Standardized outcome measure

Once a complete set of studies which fulfil the eligibility criteria is identified, analysis can start. First, it is necessary to bring the results of each individual trial into a standardized format to allow for a comparison between the studies. If the endpoint is continuous (for example, blood pressure) the mean difference between the treatment and control groups is often used as a measure of effect. A mean difference of zero indicates no difference in efficacy between the groups. The size of a difference, however, is influenced by the underlying population value. For example, an antihypertensive drug is likely to have a greater absolute effect in overtly hypertensive patients than in borderline hypertensive patients. Differences are therefore often presented in standard deviation units. If the endpoint is binary (for example, disease versus no disease or dead versus alive) then odds ratios are often calculated. The advantage of the odds ratio lies in its convenient mathematical properties, which allow for ease in the combination of data from all studies and the testing of the overall effect for statistical significance. However, other indices can be used with binary endpoints, for example the difference in the proportion of patients in the treatment and control group who are alive at the end of the trial. The statistical methods required for the combining of such outcomes have been implemented in dedicated computer software, making the choice of outcome measure less dependent upon ease of calculation (Eddy et al. 1992; EGRET 1993).

Graphical display of individual results

Odds ratios can usefully be graphically displayed, together with their confidence intervals. The results of each study are influenced by random variability, the degree of which will be inversely related to the size of the study. The 95 per cent confidence intervals

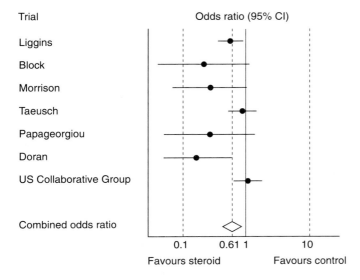

Fig. 16.3 Meta-analysis of seven trials of a short course of a corticosteroid in women expected to give birth prematurely. The evidence indicates that steroids reduce the odds of the baby dying from immaturity by 39 per cent. This is the meta-analysis depicted in the logo of the Cochrane Collaboration (see Fig. 16.2).

calculated for each trial will contain the true underlying odds ratio in 95 per cent of the occasions such trials are performed. If the confidence interval for the odds ratio includes 1, then the difference in the effect of experimental and control therapy will not be statistically significant at conventional levels, in other words, the p-value is greater than 0.05 ($p > 0.05$).

Figure 16.3 illustrates a meta-analysis of seven RCTs of a short corticosteroid course in women expected to give birth prematurely which had appeared in the decade from 1972 to 1981 (Crowley 1994). The outcome considered is whether the baby died or not from the complications of immaturity. The 95 per cent confidence intervals of five out of the seven studies include 1—no statistically significant ($p > 0.05$) effect was thus found in these studies. For two trials (Liggins and Doran) the confidence intervals exclude 1. The beneficial effect was thus significant at $p < 0.05$. The diamond shows the overall odds ratio with 95 per cent confidence intervals. It indicates a reduction in the odds of death when treated with corticosteroids of 39 per cent (combined odds ratio 0.61, 95 per cent confidence interval of 0.46 to 0.81, $p < 0.001$). The overlapping confidence intervals demonstrate that the combined odds ratio is compatible with the findings from the individual trials. This meta-analysis is depicted in the logo of the Cochrane Collaboration (see Fig. 16.2). Since 1981, the beneficial effect of corticosteroids has been confirmed in seven further trials.

The graphical display gives a visual indication of the consistency of the findings and of the uncertainty attached to the results of each trial. The display of all study results in this manner together with the overall effect makes an important contribution to the interpretation of the evidence.

Statistical methods for calculation of the overall effect

The last step consists of the calculation of the overall effect by combining the data. A simple arithmetic average of all the trial results would give misleading results. The results from small studies contributing few events are more subject to the play of chance and should, therefore, be given less weight. Methods used for meta-analysis employ a weighted average of the results in which the larger trials have more influence than the smaller ones. There are a variety of statistical techniques available for this purpose, which can be broadly classified into two models (Berlin et al. 1989). The difference consists of the way the variability of the results between the studies is treated. The so-called 'fixed effects' model considers this variability as exclusively due to random variation, on the assumption that there is a single underlying effect of therapy (Yusuf et al. 1985). The main alternative, the 'random effects' model, assumes that a different underlying therapy effect is acting in each study and, therefore, takes this into consideration as an additional source of variation in results between individual studies (DerSimonian and Laird 1986). It leads to somewhat wider confidence intervals than the fixed effects model. However, only if the results of the individual studies are markedly heterogeneous, that is if the between study variability is large, will a substantial difference in the overall average effect calculated by the fixed and random effects models be seen (Berlin et al. 1989).

The fixed effects model, often unreasonably, makes the assumption that all the studies try to give fundamentally the same answer, within the constraints of sampling variation. Therefore, if all the studies were infinitely large they would give identical answers. The random effects model, on the other hand, assumes that each study reflects a different treatment effect. Therefore, even if the individual studies were infinitely large, they would still give treatment effects of differing magnitudes. These are assumed to be normally distributed. The central point of this distribution is then the focus of the combined effect estimate. Neither of the two statistical approaches can be said to be the 'correct' method and the issue regarding why and when one is more appropriate than the other is the subject of ongoing debate.

Testing for heterogeneity between study results

If the individual study results are very different then it must be considered whether it is legitimate to pool the results to give a single, overall, effect estimate. One common approach is to examine statistically the degree of similarity in the study outcomes, in other words, to test for heterogeneity across studies. In such procedures, whether the individual study results reflect a single underlying effect, as opposed to a distribution of effects, is assessed. If this test indicates homogeneous results, then it is assumed that the trials are randomly distributed around a single underlying effect and the differences between individual studies are a consequence of sampling variation. A fixed effects model is then regarded as appropriate. If, on the contrary, the test indicates that significant heterogeneity among study results exists, a random effects model may be advocated. A major limitation with this approach is that the statistical tests lack power—they often fail to reject the null hypothesis of homogeneous results even if substantial inter-study differences exist.

Heterogeneity between study results should not only be seen as a problem for meta-analysis, since it also provides an opportunity for examining why treatment effects differ in different circumstances. The approach to heterogeneity should be to scrutinize—and attempt to explain—it, rather than simply to ignore it after applying some statistical test (Bailey 1987). There is no statistical solution to this issue, which is one reason why some uncertainty must remain with meta-analyses, as with other forms of research (Fleiss 1987).

Sensitivity analyses

As there will often be diverging opinions on the correct method for performing a particular meta-analysis, the robustness of the findings to different assumptions should be examined in a thorough sensitivity analysis. Such sensitivity analyses should include the calculation of effect sizes and confidence intervals using both fixed effects and random effects methods. An attempt should be made to determine the quality of the individual studies and the effect of excluding studies perceived as of lower quality should then be investigated. As discussed below, the possible impact of publication bias should also be considered. This can be done by excluding smaller studies, whose publication is more likely to be dependent on the statistical significance and direction of the results. If it is demonstrated that all such analyses lead to similar overall effects and conclusions, this stability of the results lends credence to the findings. If different assumptions lead to different results and conclusions, however, this fact should be made known. Thus a good meta-analysis is not complete without a good sensitivity analysis.

An example: β-blockers after myocardial infarction

An early influential meta-analysis which concerned the role of β-blockers in myocardial infarction was published in 1985 (Yusuf *et al.* 1985). In total over 60 RCTs were analysed. One component concerned the use of β-blockers following myocardial infarction. By combining data from 15 trials it could be shown that oral β-blockade starting a few days to a few weeks after the acute infarction reduces subsequent mortality by an estimated 23 per cent (combined odds ratio of 0.77, 95 per cent confidence intervals of 0.69 to 0.86, $p < 0.0001$ by the fixed effects model). We have updated this meta-analysis for the present example. A MEDLINE search was conducted and reviews and meta-analyses were scrutinized for relevant studies. Two additional studies were identified. One study showed no effect (Lopressor Intervention Trial Research Grove 1987), but the confidence intervals included the effect size demonstrated earlier. The other study (Boissel *et al.* 1990) showed a statistically significant ($p = 0.027$) beneficial effect of β-blockade. The same fixed effects model was used for combining the 17 studies. The odds ratios from the individual trials and the overall odds ratio, together with the 95 per cent confidence intervals, are shown in Fig. 16.4. The combined odds ratio of 0.78 (95 per cent confidence interval of 0.71 to 0.87) is close to the one obtained in 1985.

How robust are the findings of this meta-analysis? This was examined in the sensitivity analysis presented in Fig. 16.5. First, the overall effect was calculated by different statistical methods, using both a fixed and a random effects model. It is evident from the figure that the overall estimate is virtually identical and that the confidence intervals are only slightly wider when using the random effects model.

The methodological quality was assessed in terms of how study

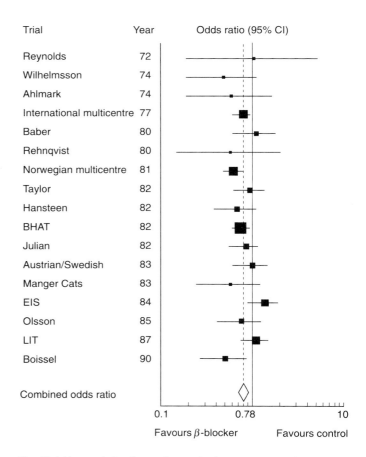

Fig. 16.4 Meta-analysis of mortality results from 17 trials of β-blockade in secondary prevention after acute myocardial infarction.

patients were allocated to active treatment or control groups, how outcome was assessed, and how the data were analysed (Prendiville *et al.* 1988). For each criteria and study, one to three points was assigned and a summary score was calculated. The maximum credit of nine points was given if the patient allocation was truly random, if the assessment of vital status was independent of the treatment group, and if the data from all patients initially included were analysed according to the intention to treat principle. Conversely, only one point was given if there was potential bias in the treatment allocation (for example, alternate allocation), assessment of outcome (no blinding of observers to treatment group), and analysis (selective exclusion of patients). Trials which earned eight or nine points were considered to be of good quality. Trials which received less were classified as of doubtful quality. The figure shows that the three low-quality studies indicated more benefit than the high-quality trials, although the confidence intervals are wide. Exclusion of these three studies, however, leaves the overall effect and the confidence intervals practically unchanged.

Statistically significant results are more likely to get published than non-significant findings (Easterbrook *et al.* 1991; Dickersin *et al.* 1992) and this can distort the findings of meta-analyses. As discussed in detail below, whether such publication bias is present can be examined in different ways. One approach is to stratify the analysis by study size. Smaller effects can be statistically significant in larger studies. If publication bias is present, it is expected that of published studies, the larger ones will report the smaller effects.

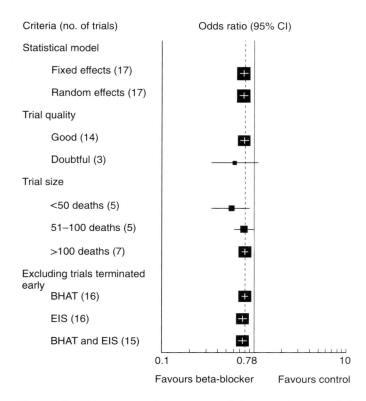

Criteria (no. of trials)   Odds ratio (95% CI)

Statistical model
    Fixed effects (17)
    Random effects (17)
Trial quality
    Good (14)
    Doubtful (3)
Trial size
    <50 deaths (5)
    51–100 deaths (5)
    >100 deaths (7)
Excluding trials terminated early
    BHAT (16)
    EIS (16)
    BHAT and EIS (15)

0.1   0.78   10

Favours beta-blocker   Favours control

Fig. 16.5 Sensitivity analyses relating to meta-analysis of mortality results of 17 trials of β-blockade after myocardial infarction (see text).

The figure clearly shows that in the present example this is indeed the case with the smallest trials (50 deaths or less) showing the largest effect. However, exclusion of the smaller studies has little effect on the overall estimate.

Finally, two studies, the BHAT and European Infarction Study (EIS) trials, were terminated earlier than anticipated on the grounds of the results from interim analyses. Estimates of treatment effects from trials which were stopped early because of a significant treatment difference are liable to be biased away from the null value. Bias may thus be introduced in a meta-analysis which includes such trials (Green *et al.* 1987). Exclusion of these trials, however, again affects the overall estimate only marginally (Fig. 16.5).

Based on these sensitivity analyses it can thus be concluded that the results from this meta-analysis are robust to the choice of the statistical method and to the exclusion of trials of lesser quality or of studies terminated early and that publication bias is unlikely to have distorted its findings.

Limitations of meta-analysis

That there are limitations to this technique is illustrated by the fact that meta-analyses of the same issue have reached opposite conclusions. Examples include assessments of low molecular weight heparin in the prevention of perioperative thrombosis (Leizorovicz *et al.* 1992*b*; Nurmohamed *et al.* 1992); and second-line anti-rheumatic drugs in the treatment of rheumatoid arthritis (Felson *et al.* 1990; Gøtzsche *et al.* 1992). In the following subsections the problems pertinent to meta-analysis are discussed in some detail.

The most important problem clearly relates to including different sets of studies in the meta-analysis.

Publication bias

The most obvious problem with regard to the inclusion of studies is brought about by the fact that some studies may never get published. If the reasons why studies remain unpublished are associated with their outcome, then the results of a meta-analysis could be seriously biased. Hypothetically, with a putative therapy which has no actual effect on a disease, it is possible that studies which suggested a beneficial treatment effect would end up being published, while an equal mass of data pointing the other way would remain unpublished. In this situation, a meta-analysis of the published trials would identify a spurious beneficial treatment effect.

Such publication bias has been investigated by following up research proposals approved by ethics committees or institutional review boards. Of the studies approved by a research ethics committee in Oxford between 1984 and 1987 which had been analysed by 1990, those with statistically significant ($p < 0.05$) results were more likely to have been published than those with non-significant results (Easterbrook *et al.* 1991). Studies with statistically significant results were also more likely to generate multiple publications and presentations. Pharmaceutical industry-sponsored studies were less likely to be published than those supported by the government or by a charity, with investigators citing the data management by these companies as a reason for non-publication. This is in agreement with a review of publications of clinical trials which separated them into those which were sponsored by the pharmaceutical industry and those supported by other means (Davidson 1986). The results of 89 per cent of published industry-supported trials favoured the new therapy, as compared to 61 per cent of the other trials. Similar results have been reported from an overview of non-steroidal anti-inflammatory drug trials (Rochon *et al.* 1994). The implication is that after funding trials the pharmaceutical industry discourages the publication of negative studies.

A study based on institutional review boards at The Johns Hopkins Health Institutions reported similar findings to the Oxford investigation (Dickersin *et al.* 1992). Both studies identified selective submission of papers as a more important contributor to publication bias than selective acceptance of papers by journals. However, that the latter does occur is illustrated by the 'instructions to authors' section of one major diabetes journal, which states that reports of studies with negative results were not desired (Anonymous 1984). Many authors will not submit negative studies in anticipation of rejection.

Another approach to examining for publication bias is to compare the results from a meta-analysis of trials identified in a literature search with a meta-analysis of trials contained in an international trials registry (Easterbrook 1992). Registration of trials generally takes place before completion of the study, so the inclusion of a study in a trials registry can therefore be assumed not to be influenced by its results. The studies enlisted in a registry thus constitute a more representative sample of all the studies which have been performed in a given area than a sample of published studies. This has been examined for trials of different cancer chemotherapies, using the International Cancer Research

Table 16.2 Meta-analysis of published and registered trials comparing combination chemotherapy to alkylating agent monotherapy in patients with advanced ovarian cancer: an illustration of publication bias

	Published trials	Registered trials
Survival ratio	1.16	1.06
95% confidence intervals	1.06–1.27	0.97–1.15
p-value	0.004	0.17

Adapted from Simes (1987).

Data Bank (Simes 1981). As shown in Table 16.2 for advanced ovarian cancer the analysis of published RCTs indicated better survival with combination chemotherapy as compared to alkylating agent monotherapy. However, an analysis of the registered trials failed to confirm this.

The possibility of publication bias should be considered in any meta-analysis. Different methods have been proposed for this purpose. In funnel plots, the estimates of effect size obtained in the studies are plotted against the sample size. In the absence of publication bias, the plot should resemble a symmetrical inverted funnel with the results of smaller studies being more widely scattered than those of the larger studies. If the plot shows an asymmetrical shape, publication bias may be present. This usually takes the form of a gap in the wide part of the funnel which indicates the absence of negative small studies. The funnel plot for the meta-analysis of 17 trials assessing β-blockers in myocardial infarction which we discussed earlier is shown in Fig. 16.6. The somewhat asymmetrical shape of the funnel does indicate that there was selective non-publication of a few smaller trials which showed less sizeable benefit. However, it is clear from the sensitivity analyses presented in Fig. 16.5 that inclusion of the biased sample of small studies has little effect on the overall estimate.

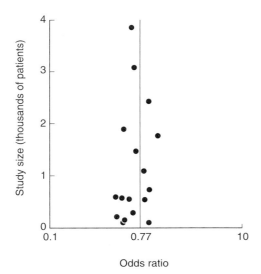

Fig. 16.6 Funnel plot relating mortality reduction to study size: trials of β-blockade in secondary prevention after myocardial infarction.

Another approach to publication bias is to calculate the number of unpublished negative studies which would be necessary to invalidate the results obtained in a meta-analysis: the so-called fail-safe N (Rosenthal 1979). If this number is very large then it is unlikely that the conclusions drawn from the sample of studies included in the analysis are offset by publication bias. The fail-safe N can be calculated both assuming that the unpublished studies show, on average, no effect or an opposite effect (Oakes 1993). In the β-blocker example, 159 studies showing no effect would need to exist to render the combined result of the 17 original studies non-significant ($p > 0.05$). This hypothetical number is reduced when it is assumed that the unpublished studies show an adverse effect of β-blocker therapy, but is still large enough to make publication bias an improbable explanation for the findings of this meta-analysis.

The most effective way of minimizing the risk of publication bias and related biases is to establish registers of clinical trials (Easterbrook 1992), with new studies being documented at the time they are established. In addition, the process of ethical committees approving studies could be linked to a requirement that reports of results are submitted to the ethical committee within a certain time period (Levy 1992). The registers of ethical committees and the reports could be kept centrally and requests for unpublished reports sent to this body. At present, however, it requires much effort to ensure that the set of studies located for a meta-analysis is not a biased sample of all existing studies and it is improbable that this will change in the near future.

Other biases in location of data

While publication bias has long been recognized (Sterling 1959) and much discussed (Dickersin *et al.* 1987; Begg and Berlin 1989), other factors can contribute to biased inclusion of studies in meta-analyses. Incomplete search bias can occur when inadequate efforts have been made to locate reports of studies. In this regard it is important to note that even experienced users of electronic literature databases such as MEDLINE fail to locate a substantial proportion of eligible studies (Dickersin *et al.* 1985; Bernstein 1988). This appears to be due both to inadequate indexing of studies in the databases and suboptimal search strategies.

In locating studies, searches of computerized databases are supplemented by contacting experts in the field and checking the reference lists of other studies and reviews. In this process citation bias could play an important role. In the field of cholesterol lowering, it has been shown that trials which are supportive of a beneficial effect are cited more frequently than unsupportive trials, regardless of the size and quality of the studies involved (Ravnskov 1992). Thus, the use of reference lists would be more likely to locate supportive than unsupportive studies, which could clearly bias the findings of a meta-analysis.

Which journals papers are published in could also influence the ease of their location and their inclusion in meta-analyses. One influential cholesterol-lowering trial was originally planned as a study with primary prevention and secondary prevention arms (Manninen 1983). The results of the primary prevention component were interpreted as being favourable by the investigators and the results were published in the *New England Journal of Medicine* in 1987 (Frick *et al.* 1987). The secondary prevention arm finished at the same time, but in this case the results were unfavourable (Frick *et al.* 1993). The trial was not reported until

1993, when a paper was finally published in the *Annals of Medicine* (Frick *et al.* 1993). The primary prevention trial has received nearly 1000 citations since 1987; even an important paper in a journal with limited circulation such as the *Annals of Medicine* would be unlikely to receive more than a handful of citations in this time.

The production of multiple publications from single studies can lead to bias in two ways. First, studies with significant results are more likely to lead to multiple publications and presentations (Easterbrook *et al.* 1991), which makes it more likely that they will be located and included in a meta-analysis. Second, it may not always be obvious that multiple publications come from a single study and one set of study participants may be included in an analysis twice. In a meta-analyses of low molecular weight heparin (Nurmohamed *et al.* 1992), for example, it appears that combined data from a multicentre trial were included, together with a subset of the same data which had also been reported separately by the individual centres which contributed to the trial (Leizorovicz *et al.* 1992*a*). Indeed it may not always be easy for investigators to determine whether two papers represent duplicate publications of one trial or two separate trials, since examples exist where two articles reporting the same trial do not share a single common author (Felson 1992).

Once an exhaustive search has been carried out it may prove difficult to obtain data for inclusion into a meta-analysis for the unpublished trials. Many factors could influence the willingness of investigators to make their data available, but one element could be the direction of the results. Such provision of data bias could also occur in the case of publications of trials which do not provide adequate data breakdown for inclusion into a meta-analysis and for which requests have to be made to the investigators to provide further details.

Biases in selecting studies for inclusion in a meta-analysis

Once studies have been located and data obtained, there are still potential biases involved in setting the inclusion criteria for a meta-analysis. If, as is usual, the inclusion criteria are developed by an investigator familiar with the area under study, they can be influenced by knowledge of the results of the set of potential studies. Manipulating the inclusion criteria could lead to selective inclusion of positive studies and exclusion of negative studies. For example, some meta-analyses of trials of cholesterol lowering therapy (Peto *et al.* 1985; MacMahon 1992) have excluded certain studies on the grounds that the treatments used appear to have had an adverse effect which is independent of cholesterol lowering itself. These meta-analyses have, however, included trials of treatments which are likely to influence the risk of coronary heart disease favourably, independently of cholesterol lowering. Clearly such an asymmetrical approach introduces the possibility of selection bias, with the criteria for inclusion into the meta-analysis being derived from the results of the studies. The most appropriate way of handling the problems associated with the selection of studies to be included in a meta-analysis is to include all studies which meet very basic entry criteria, then perform sensitivity analyses with regard to the different possible entry criteria. Any conclusions from a meta-analysis which are highly sensitive to altering the entry criteria should be treated with caution.

Application to clinical practice

The main aim of a meta-analysis of RCTs is to produce an estimate of the average effect seen in trials of a particular treatment modality. The direction and magnitude of this average effect is intended to help guide decisions about clinical practice for a wide range of patients. In some sense the clinician is being asked to treat his or her patients as though they were well represented by the patients in the clinical trials included in the meta-analysis. Furthermore, he or she is also encouraged to make clinical decisions for individual patients based upon the assumption that they can all be treated like an 'average' patient. This runs against the concerns physicians have for using the specific characteristics of a particular patient to tailor management accordingly (Wittes 1987).

The problem with identifying those who benefit most

It is clearly implausible to assume that the effect of a given treatment is identical across different groups of patients, for example the young versus the elderly and those with mild versus those with severe disease. It therefore seems reasonable to base treatment decisions upon the results of those trials which have included participants with similar characteristics to the particular patient under consideration, rather than on the totality of the evidence as furnished by meta-analysis.

Although seemingly sound, decisions based on subgroup analyses are often misleading. Consider, for example, a physician in Germany being confronted by the meta-analysis of long-term β-blockade following myocardial infarction, as presented earlier in this chapter. Whilst there is a robust beneficial effect seen in the overall analysis, in the only trial recruiting a substantial proportion of German patients, the European Infarction Study (EIS) Group (1984), there was, if anything, a detrimental effect of using β-blockers (Fig. 16.4). Should the physician give β-blockers to their German post infarct patients? In this case, it would seem sensible to believe that the poor outcome in the EIS represents the play of chance and to base treatment decisions for German patients upon the evidence coming from trials originating in other countries. Common sense would suggest that being German does not prevent a patient obtaining benefit from β-blockade. Thus, the best estimate of the outcome for German patients may actually come through, essentially, discounting the trial carried out in these patients. This may seem paradoxical; indeed a statistical expression of this phenomenon is known as Stein's paradox (Efron and Morris 1977).

Making decisions such as this is not just a problem created by meta-analysis; it also applies to the interpretation of individual clinical trials (Oxman and Guyatt 1992). Authors of trial reports often spend more time discussing the results within subgroups of the patients included in the trial than on the overall results. Yet frequently the findings of these subgroup analyses, upon which much attention is focused, fail to be confirmed by later research. For example, the various individual trials of β-blockade after myocardial infarction yielded several subgroup findings with apparent clinical significance (Yusuf *et al.* 1991). Treatment was said to be beneficial in patients under 65 years and harmful in those older than this or only beneficial in patients with anterior myocardial infarction, for example. When examined in subsequent studies or in a formal pooling project (The Beta-blocker Pooling Project Research Group 1988), these findings received no support (Yusuf *et al.* 1991). This situation is not unique to the case of trials of β-blockade following myocardial infarction—rather, it is a general phenomenon. It can be shown that if a treatment effect overall is statistically significant at the 5 per cent level ($p < 0.05$) and the patients are divided at random into two similarly sized groups, then there is a one in three chance that the treatment effect will be large and statistically significant in one group but irrelevant and non-significant in the other (Peto 1982). The subgroup that 'clearly' benefits from an intervention thus largely varies at random—inundating the literature with contradictory findings from subgroup analyses (Buyse 1989). Sufficient care is not always taken in the interpretation of such findings. For example, in the GISSI–1 study of streptokinase in acute myocardial infarction, results from subgroup analyses were interpreted as indicating that patients with infarcts affecting less than four leads in the electrocardiogram would not benefit from the intervention (Mauri *et al.* 1989). This report may have induced clinicians not to use streptokinase in patients with electrocardiographically less extensive infarctions—despite the fact that it was based on a subgroup finding from a single trial which was not confirmed in subsequent trials and meta-analyses (Fibrinolytic Therapy Trialist's (FTT) Collaborative Group 1994).

Meta-analyses of large numbers of trials clearly offer a sounder basis for subgroup analyses—however, they are not exempt from producing misleading findings. One of the explanations put forward for the disappointing result seen in the aforementioned β-blocker trial in German post infarct patients was that the agent used, Oxprenolol, had intrinsic sympathomimetic activity (**ISA**) (Schroeder 1985). It seemed plausible that agents with ISA would be less effective as the beneficial effect was assumed to be entirely mediated by blockade of the β-1 receptor. This interpretation received support from a meta-analytic subgroup analysis which showed less benefit in patients treated with ISA agents (Yusuf *et al.* 1985). The difference between the two classes of β-blockers was statistically significant ($p < 0.01$). Since then, however, a trial was published which showed a particularly strong beneficial effect of acebutolol, an agent with ISA (Boissel *et al.* 1990), while another trial using metoprolol, a β-blocker without ISA, was negative (Lopressor Intervention Trial Research Group 1987). Adding the results from these two trials renders the difference between the two classes of β-blockers non-significant (Peto 1987).

Examining for gradients in treatment effects

A more powerful way of assessing differences in treatment effects is to relate the outcome to some underlying patient characteristic on a continuous or ordered scale. In other words, the aim is to examine whether the effect of a given treatment depends in a graded way on the level of some other factor. In trials of cholesterol reduction, for example, the degree of cholesterol lowering attained differs markedly between studies, and the reduction in coronary heart disease mortality is greater in the trials in which larger reductions in cholesterol are achieved (Davey Smith *et al.* 1993). Many other interventions in which the outcome in terms of morbid or mortal events is dependent upon changes in a mediating factor can be examined in this way. Such graded associations are not limited to situations where greater benefits would be expected consequent on

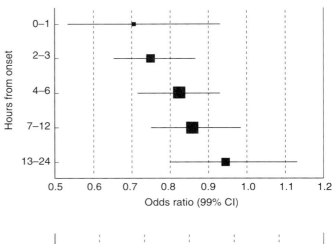

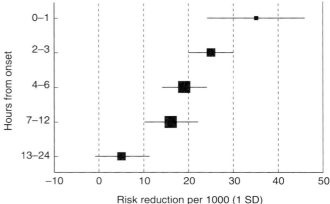

Fig. 16.7 Relative and absolute reductions in mortality from thrombolytic therapy in myocardial infarction according to the delay from symptom onset. Results from the Fibrinolytic Therapy Trialist's Collaborative Group's meta-analysis. Adapted from Fibrinolytic Therapy Trialist's (FTT) Collabarative Group (1994).

greater changes in a risk factor. In the case of thrombolytic therapy after acute myocardial infarction, for example, the greater the delay before therapy is given, the smaller the benefit consequent on thrombolysis (Zelen 1983; EMERAS Collaborative Group 1993; Fibrinolytic Therapy Trialist's (FTT) Collaborative Group 1994). This is illustrated with respect to both relative and absolute benefit in Fig. 16.7. In such cases, there is a graded association between the outcome seen in a trial and a characteristic of the treatment which is used. This allows for a more powerful examination of differences in outcomes, since a statistical test for trend can be performed, rather than the less powerful test for evidence of global heterogeneity. Other attributes of study groups—such as age and length of follow-up—can readily be analysed in this way.

A factor which is often related to a given treatment effect is the underlying risk of occurrence of the event the treatment aims to prevent. It makes intuitive sense that patients at high-risk are more likely to benefit than low-risk patients. In the case of trials of cholesterol lowering, for example, the patient groups have ranged from heart attack survivors with gross hypercholesterolaemia, to groups of healthy asymptomatic individuals with moderately elevated cholesterol levels. The coronary heart disease death rates of the former group have been up to 100 times higher than the death rates of the latter groups. The outcome of treatment in terms of all-cause mortality has been considerably more favourable in the trials recruiting participants at high risk than in the trials involving relatively low-risk individuals. This is demonstrated in Fig. 16.8, in which all-cause mortality outcomes of the trials of pharmacological cholesterol lowering are presented, stratified into three groups according to the coronary heart disease (**CHD**) death rate in the control group of each trial (Davey Smith *et al.* 1993). There are two factors contributing to this. First, among the high-risk participants, the great majority of deaths will be from CHD, the risk of which is reduced by cholesterol reduction. A 30 per cent reduction in CHD mortality therefore translates into a near-equivalent reduction in total mortality. In the low-risk participants, on the other hand, a much smaller proportion—around 40 per cent—of deaths will be from CHD. In this case a 30 per cent reduction in CHD mortality would translate into a much smaller—around 10 per cent—reduction in all-cause mortality. Second, if there is any detrimental effect of treatment, it may easily outweigh the benefits of cholesterol reduction in the low risk group, whereas in high-risk patients among whom a substantial benefit is achieved from cholesterol reduction, this will not be the case.

A similar association between the level of risk and benefit obtained can be seen in meta-analyses carried out for other types of medical treatment (Davey Smith and Egger 1994). Thus, the use of antiplatelet agents such as aspirin after an acute myocardial infarction produces a 23 per cent reduction in all-cause mortality, whereas in the primary prevention setting there is only a (non-significant) 5 per cent reduction in mortality (Antiplatelet Trialist's Collaboration 1994). This may reflect a small increase in the risk of haemorrhagic stroke consequent on the use of antiplatelet agents which counterbalances the beneficial effects among low-risk individuals, but not among those at higher risk. In the case of the treatment of HIV infection with zidovudine, a large reduction in the risk of death was seen in the single placebo controlled RCT of Zidovudine monotherapy which has been reported among patients with AIDS (Fischl *et al.* 1987). However, in a meta-analysis of seven trials it was seen that the use of zidovudine early in the course of HIV-infection was not associated with any long-term survival benefit (Egger *et al.* 1994) Fig. 16.9.

In situations where outcomes are very different in groups at different levels of risk, it is inappropriate to perform a meta-analysis in which an overall estimate of the effect of treatment is calculated. In the case of the zidovudine trials, for example, an

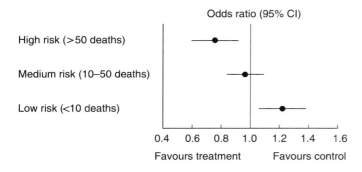

Fig. 16.8 Effect of cholesterol lowering treatment on total mortality stratified by number of deaths from coronary heart disease per 1000 person-years in control subjects. Meta-analysis of 35 trials. Adapted from Davey Smith *et al.* (1993).

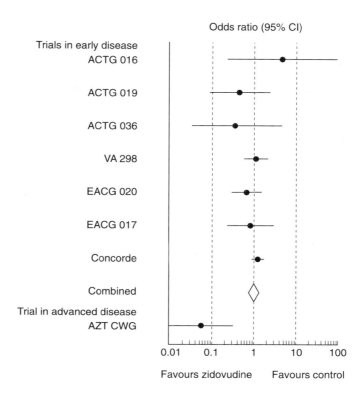

Fig. 16.9 Meta-analysis of mortality results of seven trials of zidovudine in asymptomatic or early symptomatic HIV infection. The results are in stark contrast to the beneficial effect seen in the only trial in high-risk patients (Azidothymidine Collaborative Working Group (AZT CWG) trial. Adapted from Egger *et al.* (1994).

overall effect estimate from all the eight trials (odds ratio of 0.96, 95 per cent confidence interval of 0.75 to 1.22) is very different from that seen in the only trial among patients with AIDS (odds ratio of 0.04, 95 per cent confidence interval of 0.006 to 0.33). If there had been more trials among patients with AIDS the overall effect would appear highly beneficial. Conversely, if there had been more large trials among asymptomatic patients there would apparently be no benefit from treatment and, indeed, the confidence intervals around the overall effect estimate would exclude any useful benefit, which would be misleading if applied to patients with AIDS.

When there have been many trials conducted in a particular field, it is possible to perform risk stratification at the level of individual trials. This was carried out in the case of cholesterol lowering (Davey Smith *et al.* 1993), using the CHD mortality rate in the control arm of the trials as the stratification variable (Fig. 16.8). This stratification is of clinical use, since this is the risk of CHD death of patients without treatment—that is the risk level which the clinician would want to use for deciding whether or not patients will benefit from therapeutic cholesterol lowering. The analysis can also be performed using control group CHD mortality risk as a continuous variable, through the examination of the interaction between treatment effect and risk in a logistic regression analysis. A significant statistical test for interaction suggests that there is a real difference in outcome at different levels of risk.

In many cases there are simply too few trials or the range of risk across control groups of the trials is too small to be able to perform a stratified analysis at the level of the individual trials. In these cases it may be possible to consider risk strata within the trials, which may be included in published reports. However it will often be necessary to obtain additional analyses or the complete original data from the authors for this purpose.

Several collaborative groups have now gone beyond obtaining summary data from individual trials to the collection of data on each participant within the separate trials. This greatly increases flexibility for defining common subgroups within the different trials for subgroup analyses and also allows for the use of exact time to event data for each participant, rather than the less precise data regarding grouped outcomes, such as deaths at 2 years. Thus the Fibrinolytic Therapy Trialist's Collaborative Group (1994) could investigate the effect of thrombolytic therapy after myocardial infarction according to the electrocardiographic abnormalities of patients at study entry, to the time from symptom onset at which treatment was received (Fig. 16.7), to the age and sex of the patients, and to presence or absence of various co-morbid conditions. This allows for comparisons which retain the advantage of the original randomization, with the proviso that the separate trials did not necessarily employ stratified randomization according to these characteristics.

Cumulative meta-analysis

Cumulative meta-analysis is defined as the repeated performance of meta-analysis whenever a new relevant trial becomes available for inclusion. Such cumulative meta-analysis has allowed the retrospective identification of the point in time when a treatment effect first reached conventional levels of statistical significance. For example, in cumulative meta-analysis of the trials of intravenous streptokinase in acute myocardial infarction, a statistically significant ($p < 0.05$) difference in total mortality became evident by 1971 (Lau *et al.* 1992). At that time, 962 patients had been randomized in four small trials. The results of the subsequent 29 studies which included the large GISSI–1 (1986) and International Study of Infarct Survival–2 (ISIS–2) (1988) trials and enrolled a total of 36 012 additional patients reduced the significance level to $p < 0.001$ in 1977 and to $p < 0.0001$ in 1986, narrowing the confidence intervals around an essentially unchanged estimate of 25 per cent reduction in the risk of death. A similar picture is apparent in the case of β-blockade in the secondary prevention of myocardial infarction, with a statistically significant beneficial effect ($p < 0.05$) being evident by 1977 (Fig. 16.10). Again, subsequent trials in a further 16 616 patients only confirmed this result. This situation has been taken to suggest that further studies in large numbers of patients may be at best superfluous and costly if not unethical (Murphy *et al.* 1994), once a statistically significant treatment effect is evident from meta-analysis of the existing smaller trials.

In this context, the disappointing results of the very large ISIS–4 multicentre study must be considered (ISIS–4 Collaborative Group 1995). Among other treatments, ISIS–4 tested the effect of intravenous magnesium in over 58 000 patients with acute myocardial infarction and showed a statistically non-significant adverse effect of magnesium. This result from a mega-trial is in stark contrast to an earlier meta-analysis of seven small trials published between 1984 and 1990 (Teo *et al.* 1991). This meta-

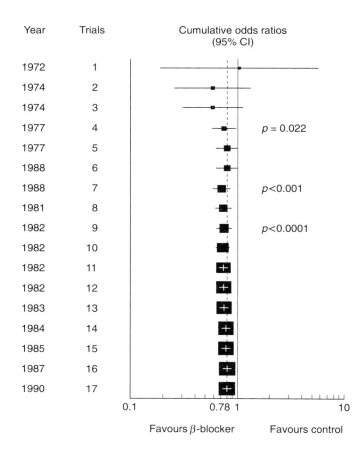

Fig. 16.10 Cumulative meta-analysis of mortality results from 17 trials of β-blockade in secondary prevention after acute myocardial infarction (see text).

analysis concluded that substantial benefit was associated with the use of magnesium, the results indicating a 50 per cent reduction of the risk of death ($p = 0.0007$). Three further trials appeared up to 1992, including the larger Leicester Intravenous Magnesium Intervention Trial–2 (LIMIT–2) trial (Woods *et al.* 1992). The updated meta-analysis continued to indicate a substantial beneficial effect which was now highly statistically significant ($p < 0.0001$) (Teo *et al.* 1993). There was discussion in the ISIS–4 data monitoring committee whether it would be ethical to continue to randomize ISIS–4 participants to groups not receiving magnesium (Peto *et al.* 1995). A similar situation arose with regard to the role of intravenous nitrates in acute myocardial infarction. Again, meta-analysis of small trials indicated a statistically significant beneficial effect (Yusuf *et al.* 1988) which was not confirmed by ISIS–4.

Retrospectively, it is easy to see that it was correct to continue with ISIS–4 as planned. But what can be learnt from the discrepancies of results between early meta-analyses and later large trials? Table 16.3 shows a comparison of two meta-analyses of treatment trials in acute myocardial infarction: intravenous magnesium and intravenous streptokinase. All trials were cumulatively included, until the treatment effect became significant at $p < 0.001$. For magnesium, seven small trials appearing in the 1980s were sufficient to establish the effect. Although trials tended to be larger in the case of fibrinolytic therapy, twice as many studies and two decades were necessary to reach the same level of statistical

Table 16.3 Comparison of two meta-analyses refuted and confirmed by subsequent large randomized controlled trials: intravenous magnesium and streptokinase for acute myocardial infarction

	Refuted by mega-trials[a]: magnesium	Confirmed by mega-trial[b]: streptokinase
Year of first publication	1984	1959
Year of $p < 0.001$ achieved	1990	1977
Estimated mortality reduction (%)	55	23
Number of trials	7	15
Total number of deaths per patients	78/1301	926/4314
Size of trials		
10– 99	3	4
100–199	1	3
200–499	3	4
500–999	–	4
Average number of patients per trial	186	288

[a] By ISIS–4 Collaborative Group (1995).
[b] By Gruppo Italiano per lo Studio del le Streptochinasi nell'Infarto Miocardico (GISSSI) (1986) and ISIS–2 Collaborative Group (1988). Trials were cumulatively included until $p < 0.001$.

significance. The funnel plots for the magnesium and streptokinase trials which appeared prior to the relevant mega-trials are shown in Fig. 16.11, with mega-trials added. The plot for the streptokinase trials is symmetrical and the pooled estimate in line with the results from GISSI–1 (1986) and ISIS–2 (1988). This is clearly not the case for magnesium. The pooled estimate is at odds with ISIS–4 and there is a gap in the bottom right of the funnel which indicates the absence of negative small studies. Selective non-publication of negative trials thus appears to be a likely explanation for the false-positive findings of the magnesium meta-analysis (Egger *et al.* 1995). The situation regarding magnesium indicates that the results from meta-analyses of a small number of relatively small trials should be treated with great caution—even if the combined odds ratio indicates a statistically highly significant effect—and it highlights the importance of careful sensitivity analysis.

A further application of cumulative meta-analysis has been to correlate the accruing evidence with the recommendations made by experts in review articles and textbooks. Antman *et al.* (1992) showed for thrombolytic drugs that recommendations for routine use first appeared in 1987, 14 years after a statistically significant ($p < 0.01$) beneficial effect became evident in cumulative meta-analysis. Conversely, the prophylactic use of lidocaine continued to be recommended for routine use in myocardial infarction despite the lack of evidence for any beneficial effect and the possibility of a harmful effect being evident in cumulative meta-analysis. In this context it is noteworthy that the publication of single large studies appear to have a stronger effect on recommendations than meta-analyses. In the light of the meta-analyses mentioned which were subsequently contradicted by large randomized trials, this may be seen as a wise response by the medical community. However, more research is clearly needed into the factors associated with false-positive (or false-negative) meta-analyses (Egger *et al.* 1995).

Meta-analysis of observational studies: false precision?

A clear distinction should be made between meta-analysis of RCTs and meta-analysis of observational epidemiological studies. Statistically combining RCTs is based on the assumption that each trial provides an unbiased estimate of the effect of an experimental treatment as compared to some control intervention. Clearly, before calculating an overall estimate the meta-analyst must examine the set of RCTs with regard to their 'combinability'. As discussed earlier, this concerns the various differences between trials, for example with regard to the patient populations studied, the exact mode of treatment, or the length of follow-up. It follows that the overall effect calculated from a group of sensibly combined RCTs provides an unbiased estimate of the treatment effect whose precision is enhanced.

A different situation arises in the case of observational studies. The findings from such studies are potentially biased—principally because those exposed to the factor under investigation may differ in a number of other aspects which are relevant to the risk of developing the disease in question.

Even if adjustments for such confounding factors are made in the analysis, residual confounding remains a potentially serious problem in observational research. Residual confounding arises whenever a confounding factor cannot be measured with sufficient precision—a situation which often occurs in epidemiological studies (Phillips and Davey Smith 1991). This is illustrated by the case of smoking and the risk of cervical cancer. Observational studies, most of them case–control studies, have generally shown a positive association between smoking and the risk of cervical cancer (Winkelstein 1990). In most studies, cervical cancer was also associated with sexual behaviour—reflecting the role of a viral sexually transmitted agent, the human papilloma virus (**HPV**) in the aetiology of cervical cancer (Gissmann and Schneider 1980). In industrialized societies, smoking in turn is associated with sexual behaviours which lead to an increased risk of exposure to HPV. Therefore, when adjustment for markers of exposure to HPV was made in these studies—for the number of lifetime sexual partners or for age at first intercourse—then the odds ratio associated with smoking was reduced. For example, in one study the crude odds ratio associated with current smoking was 10.1 (95 per cent confidence interval of 7.0 to 14.7) which was reduced to 3.4 (95 per cent confidence interval of 2.1 to 5.6) after adjustment in a multivariate model (Slattery *et al.* 1989). Meta-analyses of case––control studies, combining the adjusted figures, have resulted in overall odds ratios of around 1.6, with narrow confidence intervals indicating a statistically highly significant ($p < 0.0001$) association (Licciardone *et al.* 1990; Sood 1991). Based on these results, it was concluded that a causal relationship between smoking and the risk of cervical cancer was highly probable. However, asking for the number of sexual partners or for age at first intercourse is clearly an imprecise surrogate measure for actual exposure to HPV. Residual confounding may easily explain odds ratios of this magnitude (Phillips and Davey Smith 1991). Indeed, a number of more recent studies using the polymerase chain reaction (**PCR**) for direct assessment of the presence of HPV support this hypothesis (Bosch *et al.* 1994). When considering HPV-positive women only—thus removing HPV as a confounding factor—no association between

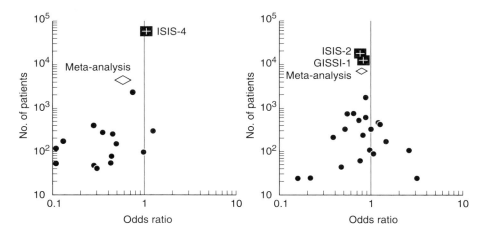

Fig. 16.11 Funnel plots for meta-analyses refuted and confirmed by subsequent mega-trials: intravenous magnesium (left panel) and streptokinase (right panel) in acute myocardial infarction. Points indicate odds ratios from small and medium-sized trials, diamonds show combined odds ratios with 95 per cent confidence intervals from meta-analysis of these trials and squares odds ratios with 95 per cent confidence intervals from mega-trials. Adapted from Egger and Davey Smith (1995).

smoking and cervical cancer was evident (Bosch *et al.* 1994). Statistically combining the results from observational studies would, in this situation, lead to a very precise, but spurious result. Indeed, consideration of the heterogeneity between observational study results will provide many more insights than the mechanistic calculation of an overall measure of effect. In the case of smoking and cervical cancer, it may be of particular interest to examine the strength of the association in settings where smoking may have different cultural associations and therefore different relationships with HPV infection. Much could be gained by establishing whether the strength of the association between smoking and cervical cancer depends upon or is independent of the strength and direction of the association between smoking and sexual behaviour in a given cultural setting (Davey Smith and Phillips 1990). The meta-analysis of the results of observational studies may, therefore, be highly misleading and calls have been made for this practice to be abandoned (Shapiro 1994). Such analyses may simply pool a series of equally spurious results.

Interestingly, one of the first meta-analyses of observational epidemiological data concerned case–control studies of smoking and lung cancer, (Comfield 1956) all of which showed the now well-established, strong association. While tabulating the studies and demonstrating their consistency was useful, it is unlikely that the mathematical synthesis of the results convinced people to take an already clear association (Davey Smith *et al.* 1995) more seriously. Today, on the other hand, if a meta-analysis of prospective studies of the association between smoking and suicide were to be performed, including the studies which have (generally parenthetically) reported on this, then the fact that smokers are more likely to commit suicide would be clear (Davey Smith *et al.* 1992a; Tverdal *et al.* 1993; Doll *et al.* 1994). It is unlikely, however, that such a meta-analysis would convince the reader that a causal association between smoking and suicide exists.

The data included in meta-analyses of observational studies are likely to contain associations which are due, to differing degrees, to bias and confounding. It is easy for analysts to come up with hypotheses for factors underlying the discrepancies or similarities in the results they find. Thus, a meta-analysis of the association

between blood cholesterol levels and the development of cancer suggested that the increased cancer risk among participants with low blood cholesterol levels was only seen in cohorts recruiting from poor socioeconomic strata (Law and Thompson 1991). The hypothesis was changed in a further meta-analysis by the same team (Law *et al.* 1994), to agree with the suggestion (Davey Smith *et al.* 1992b) that the inverse associations were only seen in general population samples, which unlike cohorts of working people contained sizeable numbers of sick individuals. Clearly meta-analysis in this situation can be a moveable feast, with little appearance of objectivity.

Statistically combining the results from observational studies may thus lead to very precise, albeit equally biased results. This is not to say that findings from different observational studies should not be compared on a common scale. Indeed, thoughtful examination of the heterogeneity between observational study results has much to contribute to the interpretation of the observed associations. For example, the bringing together of the data from the various large prospective observational studies of circulating cholesterol and mortality (Jacobs *et al.* 1992) allowed informative comparisons to be made between the associations of blood cholesterol and particular causes of death in different situations. However, the pooling of these associations into common effect estimates was probably combining common non-causal phenomena (Davey Smith 1994), which has led to these being widely misinterpreted, but with the added and spurious authority of 'meta-analysis'.

Cross-design synthesis

RCTs provide the most robust evidence regarding both the effectiveness of interventions aimed at improving health and the causal nature of associations between exposures and disease. Therefore, the meta-analysis of data from such trials, if taking into account the potential problems discussed above, is a powerful methodology. There are, however, limitations to the scope of RCTs which can make it difficult to apply their results to clinical practice. Patients unfortunately fail to conform to the characteristics of participants in RCTs. Unjustified assumptions are required when applying, for example, the results of trials of treatment for acute myocardial infarction—mainly carried out on middle-aged men—to women and the elderly (Gurwitz et al. 1992). Many other less obvious, but probably equally important, differences exist between trial participants and patients presenting in the surgery. Interventions carried out in randomized controlled trial settings are also probably implemented in different—and often more favourable—circumstances, compared to routine practice. RCTs are taken to measure the efficacy of interventions—whether they work in ideal circumstances—while what health service planners want to know is their effectiveness—how well they work in field settings.

Conversely, various factors can lead to RCTs underestimating the benefits of interventions. First, dilution can occur if some trial participants in the active arm of an RCT fail to take the treatment under study. Second, contamination of the control group—by participants who though randomized to this arm take the active treatment outwith the RCT protocol. Examples of both of these can be seen in the Multiple Risk Factor Intervention Trial Research Group (1982), in which middle-aged men were randomized to lifestyle counselling aimed at lowering blood cholesterol and blood pressure and stopping smoking or to usual care. Some of the men in the special intervention group would reject all advice, while some in the usual care group would take up the advice—received through other sources and perhaps stimulated by the knowledge that they were in this trial. Thus the difference in exposure to the treatment between the special intervention and usual care groups would be attenuated, leading to reduced estimates of the efficacy of risk factor modification. Similar considerations apply to drug trials, in which some of the participants randomized to receive treatment fail to comply and some of the control participants obtain prescribed treatment by their non-trial physician. Abandoning the intention to treat analysis and analysing trial participants according to whether they actually take the treatment, leads to serious bias and therefore is no solution to this problem (Coronary Drug Project Research Group 1980).

Failing RCTs with 100 per cent treatment adherence carried out in every conceivable patient subgroup, are there reliable methods of research which could guide therapeutic decisions? This is the question which various research groups have recently addressed (Eddy et al. 1992; General Accounting Office 1992), answering with a form of data analysis sometimes referred to as cross-design synthesis. The recommended strategy in essence consists of combining the results of RCTs with findings from the analysis of databases of patient records. These databases link details of patient characteristics, the treatments received, and outcomes, from which estimates of the ostensible effectiveness of treatments are made (Anonymous 1989). The advantage of database analyses is that they look at patients in settings which may be substantially different than the academic medical centres participating in trials (Hartz et al. 1992). The findings of these analyses may, it is therefore argued, be more generalizable to clinical practice.

When trying to make decisions regarding the effectiveness of treatments, however, this increased generalizability is bought at a potentially high cost. Database analyses suffer from the problem of non-comparability of treatment groups (Green and Byar 1984). Without randomization treatment decisions will depend upon patient characteristics, producing groups which differ in ways which will be related to the treatment they receive. This makes it difficult to attribute differences in outcomes to treatment itself.

The apparent solution to this problem is statistical adjustment for the factors which differ between the treatment groups. In a series of papers (Hlatky et al. 1988; Califf et al. 1989; Hlatky 1991), the Duke University Medical Centre Cardiovascular Disease Database has been analysed in just this manner, in order to compare the outcomes for patients receiving coronary artery bypass surgery (**CABG**) with those of patients under medical treatment for angina. Patients undergoing CABG generally do better than patients under medical therapy, with the differences observed between the treatments being in the main similar to those seen in the RCTs (Hlatky et al. 1988). Once the predictions of the database analyses have been shown to be comparable to the results of RCTs, statistical models based on the observational data can be used to predict outcomes for particular patient groups, even ones not included in the trials. Such 'projecting to empty strata' is one of the central features of the effectiveness research strategy advocated by a US governmental agency report (General Accounting Office 1992).

While this methodology appears attractive, it could produce seriously misleading results. In the Duke database, the medically and surgically treated groups were markedly different in some respects, with approximately half of the latter and two-thirds of the former having suffered a myocardial infarction (Califf et al. 1989). Previous myocardial infarction is, of course, an important factor indicating poor prognosis, thus favouring the surgically treated group. As with all observational findings, statistical adjustments for unmeasured or inadequately characterized confounding factors could produce strong associations which are nevertheless completely spurious (Petitti et al. 1986; Davey Smith et al. 1992a).

Perhaps the most well-developed approach in this area has been that of the 'confidence profile method', put forward by Eddy et al. (1992). This strategy involves adjusting the results of studies of different designs for the biases they are considered to be susceptible to, then combining the estimates. Thus, RCTs are susceptible to dilution and contamination and the treatment effects they produce are adjusted—generally towards improved benefit—for this. Case-control studies and databases, relating outcomes to patient treatment histories, are susceptible to patient selection biases—which are adjusted for—but not to dilution and contamination. Other data sources can be similarly adjusted. The adjusted estimates are then, in essence, meta-analysed—with the production of confidence intervals on effect estimates and the performance of sensitivity analysis—to produce a summary of the available evidence on a particular issue.

This approach appears attractive and has the advantage of making decisions about the weighting of evidence explicit. However, it is likely that in many cases the effect of biases cannot be adequately known, but the 'adjustments' which are performed can lead to a spurious sense that they are under control. Therefore in an early confidence profile analysis relating to the use of mammography, the findings of RCTs, case–control studies, and simple observation were brought together, it being concluded that mammography would reduce mortality for women under 50 years (Eddy et al. 1988). Evidence from randomized trials accruing since publication of this analysis seriously challenges its conclusions, however (Miller et al. 1992).

Even cross-design synthesis analyses in which some RCT data are included can be misleading. In many cases data synthesis exercises contain less robust data. The various database analyses which suggested that transurethral resection for prostatic hyper-trophy (**TURP**) resulted in higher postoperative mortality than open prostatectomy (Roos *et al.* 1989; Anderson *et al.* 1990), have been called into question by a recent study suggesting that sicker patients are assigned to TURP and that more complete adjustment for co-morbidity eliminates the apparent excess mortality risk associated with this operation (Concato *et al.* 1992). Therefore, while the database analyses have questioned the prevailing practice regarding the management of prostatic hypertrophy and indicate the need for an RCT, they do not of themselves provide the urologist with the information he or she requires to make the best decision for their current patients.

Patient databases are required for various reasons and analyses of such data can suggest important areas of medical practice which require further scrutiny. The danger is that the type of data which are collected, often for administrative reasons, can dictate the questions about therapeutic effectiveness which are asked. One researcher happily wrote that 'I utilize data that is available. I do not start out with "what is the problem, what is the outcome?" I say "Given this data, what can I do with it?"' (Blumberg 1991). Observational data are unable to provide definitive answers to questions regarding therapeutic effectiveness, but the difficulties in applying the results of meta-analyses of RCTs to individual patients remain (Kassirer 1992) and these difficulties sometimes appear to be under appreciated. While in an ideal world therapies would be evaluated separately in all the different potential patient groups and such evaluation would be repeated each time the regime changes, there is no sign that this is going to happen. Treatment decisions will continue to be made, patients will continue to be treated, and useful information can be derived by finding out what happens to the patients after treatment and comparing this to expectations from other available data sources, including RCTs. The risk with cross-design synthesis is that the more expensive, time-consuming but also more reliable component, RCTs, will come to be replaced by database analyses. Formal methods of combining results from different study modalities can confuse rather than clarify the issues and should not substitute for the informed interpretation of all the available evidence.

Conclusions

Meta-analysis should be seen as structuring the processes through which a thorough review of previous research is carried out—it is clearly superior to the narrative approach to reviewing medical research. In addition to providing a precise estimate of the overall treatment effect in some instances, appropriate examination of heterogeneity across individual studies can produce clinically useful information. The inappropriate pooling of data from obser-vational studies and the unconsidered synthesis of disparate results from randomized controlled trials threaten to damage the reputa-tion of meta-analysis. Some of the shortcomings of meta-analysis are, however, a consequence of a more general failing with respect to the dissemination of research findings. At present, this process is highly dependent on the publication of aggregated data in peer-reviewed journals. This can result in a selected portion of all the evidence becoming accessible. Registers of clinical trials are the only solution to this problem; however, current levels of support are insufficient to get such registers widely established.

References

Andersen, T.F., Bronnum-Hansen, H., Sejr, T., and Roepstorff, C. (1990). Elevated mortality following transurethral resection of the prostate for benign hypertrophy! But why? *Medical Care*, **28**, 870–9.

Anonymous. (1984). Manuscript guideline. *Diabetologia*, **25**, 4A.

Anonymous. (1989). Databases for health care outcomes. *Lancet*, ii, 195–6.

Anonymous. (1992). Cross design synthesis: a new strategy for studying medical outcomes?. *Lancet*, **340**, 944–6.

Antiplatelet Trialist's Collaboration. (1994). Collaborative overview of rando-mised trials of antiplatelet therapy—I: prevention of death, myocardial infarction, and stroke by prolonged antiplatelet therapy in various categories of patients. *British Medical Journal*, **308**, 81–106.

Antman, E.M., Lau, J., Kupelnick, B., Mosteller, F., and Chalmers, T.C. (1992). A comparison of results of meta-analyses of randomized control trials and recommendations of clinical experts. *Journal of the American Medical Association*, **268**, 240–8.

Bailey, K.R. (1987). Inter-study differences: how should they influence the interpretation and analysis of results?. *Statistics in Medicine*, **6**, 351–8.

Begg, C.B. and Berlin, J.A. (1989). Publication bias and dissemination of clinical research. *Journal of the National Cancer Institute*, **81**, 107–15.

Berlin, J.A., Laird, N.M., Sacks, H.S., and Chalmers, T.C. (1989). A compar-ison of statistical methods for combining event rates from clinical trials. *Statistics in Medicine*, **8**, 141–51.

Bernstein, F. (1988). The retrieval of randomized clinical trials in liver diseases from the medical literature: manual versus MEDLARS searches. *Contribu-tions to Clinical Trials*, **9**, 23–31.

Beecher, H.K. (1955). The powerful placebo. *Journal of the American Medical Association*, **159**, 1602–6.

Beta-Blocker Pooling Project Research Group. (1988). The Beta-Blocker Pooling Project (BBPP): subgroup findings from randomized trials in post infarction patients. *European Heart Journal*, **9**, 8–16.

Blumberg, M.S. (1991). Potentials and limitations of database research illus-trated by the QMMP AMI Medicare mortality study. *Statistics in Medicine*, **10**, 637–46.

Boissel, J.P., Leizorovicz, A., Picolet, H., and Peyrieux, J.C. (1990). Secondary prevention after high-risk acute myocardial infarction with low-dose acebu-tolol. *American Journal of Cardiology*, **66**, 251–60.

Bosch, F.X., De Sanjos, S., and Munñoz, N. (1994). Cigarette smoking and cervical cancer. *International Journal of Epidemiology*, **23**, 1100–1.

Buyse, M.E. (1989). Analysis of clinical trial outcomes: some comments on subgroup analyses. *Contributions to Clinical Trials*, **10**, 187S–194S.

Califf, R.M., Harrell, F.E., Lee, K.L., *et al.* (1989). The evolution of medical and surgical therapy for coronary artery disease: a 15–year perspective. *Journal of the American Medical Association*, **261**, 2077–86.

Chalmers, I. (1979). Randomised controlled trials of fetal monitoring 1973–1977. In *Perinatal Medicine* (ed. O. Thalhammer, K. Baumgarten, and A. Pollak) p.260. Thieme, Stuttgart.

Chalmers, I., Enkin, M., and Keirse, M.J.N.C. (1989). *Effective care during pregnancy and childbirth.* Oxford University Press, New York.

Chalmers, I., Dickersin, K., and Chalmers, T.C. (1992). Getting to grips with Archie Cochrane's agenda. *British Medical Journal*, **305**, 786–8.

Chalmers, I., Enkin, M., and Keirse, M.J.N.C. (1993). Systematic reviews of randomized controlled trials. *Millbank Quarterly*, **71**, 411–37.

Chalmers, T.C., Smith, H., Blackburn, B., *et al.* (1981). A method for assessing the quality of a randomized control trial. *Contributions to Clinical Trials*, **2**, 31–49.

Chalmers, T.C. (1991). Problems induced by meta-analyses. *Statistics in Medicine*, **10**, 971–80.

Chalmers, T.C., Frank, C.S., and Reitman, D. (1990). Minimizing the three stages of publication bias. *Journal of the American Medical Association*, **263**, 1392–5.

Collins, R. and Julian, D. (1991). British Heart Foundation surveys (1987 and 1989) of United Kingdom treatment policies for acute myocardial infarction. *British Heart Journal*, **66**, 250–5.

Collins, R., Keech, A., Peto, R.,*et al.* (1992). Cholesterol and total mortality: need for larger trials. *British Medical Journal*, **304**, 1689.

Concato, J., Horwitz, R.I., Feinstein, A.R., Elmore, J.G., and Schiff, S.F. (1992). Problems of comorbidity in mortality after prostatectomy. *Journal of the American Medical Association*, **267**, 1077–82.

Cooper, H.M. and Rosenthal, R. (1980). Statistical versus traditional procedures for summarising research findings. *Psychological Bulletin*, **87**, 442–9.

Cornfield, J. (1956). A statistical problem arising from retrospective studies. *Proceedings of the 3rd Berkley Symposium on Mathematical Statistics*, **4**, 135–48.

Coronary Drug Project Research Group. (1980). Influence of adherence to treatment and response of cholesterol on mortality in the CDP. *New England Journal of Medicine*, **303**, 1038–41.

Crowley, P. (1994). Corticosteroids prior to preterm delivery. In *Pregnancy and Childbirth Module* (ed. M.W. Enkin, M.J.M.C. Keirse, M.J. Renfrew, and J.P. Neilson) p.2955. Update Software, Oxford.

Davey Smith, G. (1994). Blood cholesterol level and non-coronary mortality. *Coronary Artery Disease*, **4**, 860–6.

Davey Smith, G. and Phillips, A.N. (1990). Declaring independence: why we should be cautious. *Journal of Epidemiology and Community Health*, **44**, 257–8.

Davey Smith, G. and Egger, M. (1994). Who benefits from medical interventions? Treating low risk patients can be a high risk strategy. *British Medical Journal*, **308**, 72–4.

Davey Smith, G., Phillips, A.N., and Neaton, J.D. (1992a). Smoking as "independent" risk factor for suicide: illustration of an artifact from observational epidemiology. *Lancet*, **340**, 709–11.

Davey Smith, G., Shipley, M., Marmot, M.G., and Rose, G. (1992b). Plasma cholesterol concentration and mortality: The Whitehall Study. *Journal of the American Medical Association*, **267**, 70–6.

Davey Smith, G., Song, F., and Sheldon, T.A. (1993). Cholesterol lowering and mortality: the importance of considering initial level of risk. *British Medical Journal*, **306**, 1367–73.

Davey Smith, G, Ströbele, S., and Egger, M. (1995). Smoking and death. *British Medical Journal*, **310**, 369.

Davidson, R.A. (1986). Source of funding and outcome of clinical trials. *Journal of General and Internal Medicine*, **1**, 155–8.

Davis, B. (1992). What price safety? Risk analysis measures need for regulation, but it's no science. *Wall Street Journal*, **August 6**, 1.

DerSimonian, R. and Laird, N. (1986). Meta-analysis in clinical trials. *Contributions to Clinical Trials*, **7**, 177–88.

Dickersin, K., Hewitt, P., Mutch, L., Chalmers, I., and Chalmers, T.C. (1985). Perusing the literature: comparison of Medline searching with a perinatal clinical trial data base. *Contributions to Clinical Trials*, **6**, 306–17.

Dickersin, K., Chan, S., Chalmers, T.C., Sacks, H.S., and Smith, H. (1987). Publication bias in clinical trials. *Contributions to Clinical Trials*, **8**, 343–53.

Dickersin, K., Higgins, K., and Meinert, C.L. (1990). Indentification of meta-analyses. The need for standard terminology. *Contributions to Clinical Trials*, **11**, 52–66.

Dickersin, K., Yuan-I, M., and Meinert, C.L. (1992). Factors influencing publication of research results. Follow-up of applications submitted to two institutional review boards. *Journal of the American Medical Association*, **267**, 374–8.

Doll, R., Peto, R., Wheatley, K., Gray, R., and Sutherland, I. (1994). Mortality in relation to smoking: 40 years' observation on male British doctors. *British Medical Journal*, **309**, 901–11.

Early Breast Cancer Trialists' Collaborative Group. (1988). Effects of adjuvant tamoxifen and of cytotoxic therapy on mortality in early breast cancer. An overview of 61 randomized trials among 28,896 women. *New England Journal of Medicine*, 319, 1681–1892.

Easterbrook, P.J. (1992). Directory of registries of clinical trials. *Statistics in Medicine*, **11**, 345–423.

Easterbrook, P.J., Berlin, J.A., Gopalan, R., and Matthews, D.R. (1991). Publication bias in clinical research. *Lancet*, **337**, 867–72.

Eddy, D.M., Hasselblad, V., McGivney, W., and Hendee, W. (1988). The value of mammographic screening in women under age 50 years. *Journal of the American Medical Association*, **259**, 1512–19.

Eddy, D.M., Hasselblad, V., and Shachter, R. (1992). *Meta-analysis by the confidence profile method. The statistical synthesis of evidence.* Academic Press, Boston.

Efron, B. and Morris, C. (1977). Stein's paradox in statistics. *Scientific American*, **236**, 119–27.

Egger, M. and Davey Smith, G. (1995). Misleading meta-analysis. Lessons from "an effective, safe, simple" intervention that wasn't. *British Medical Journal*, **310**, 752–4.

Egger, M., Neaton, J.D., Phillips, A.N., and Davey Smith, G. (1994). Concorde trial of immediate versus deferred zidovudine. *Lancet*, **343**, 1355.

EGRET. (1993). Seattle: Statistics and Epidemiology Research Corporation.

EMERAS (Estudio Multicentrico Estreptoquinasa Republicas de América del Sur) Collaborative Group. (1993). Randomised trial of late thrombolysis in patients with suspected acute myocardial infarction. *Lancet*, **342**, 767–72.

European Infarction Study Group. (1984). European Infarction Study (E.I.S). A secondary prevention study with slow release oxprenolol after myocardial infarction: morbidity and mortality. *European Heart Journal*, **5**, 189–202.

Felson, D.T. (1992). Bias in meta-analytic research. *Journal of Clinical Epidemiology*, **45**, 885–92.

Felson, D.T., Anderson, J.J., and Meenan, R.F. (1990). The comparative efficacy and toxicity of second-line drugs in rheumatoid arthritis. *Arthritis and Rheumatism*, **33**, 1449–61.

Fibrinolytic Therapy Trialists' (FTT) Collaborative Group. (1994). Indications for fibrinolytic therapy in suspected acute myocardial infarction: collaborative overview of early mortality and major morbidity results from all randomised trials of more than 1000 patients. *Lancet*, **343**, 311–22.

Fischl, M.A., Richman, D.D., Griego, M.H., *et al.* (1987). The efficacy of azidothymidine (AZT) in the treatment of patients with AIDS and AIDS-related complex. A double-blind, placebo-controlled trial. *New England Journal of Medicine*, **317**, 185–91.

Fleiss, J. (1987). Discussion. *Statistics in Medicine*, **6**, 359–60.

Freiman, J.A., Chalmers, T.C., Smith, H.,and Kuebler, R.R. (1992). The importance of beta, the type II error, and sample size in the design and interpretation of the randomized controlled trial. In *Medical uses of statistics*. (ed. J.C. Bailar and F. Mosteller), p.357. NEJM Books, Boston, MA.

Frick, M.H., Elo, O., Haapa, K., *et al.* (1987). Helsinki Heart Study: primary prevention trial with gemfibrozil in middle aged men with dyslipidaemia. *New England Journal of Medicine*, **317**, 1237–45.

Frick, M.H., Heinonen, O.P., Huttunen, J.K., Koskinen, P., Manttari, M., and Manninen, V. (1993). Efficacy of gemfibrozil in dyslipidaemic subjects with suspected heart disease. An ancillary study in the Helsinki Heart Study frame population. *Annals of Medicine*, **25**, 41–5.

General Accounting Office. (1992). *Cross design synthesis: a new strategy for medical effectiveness research.* G.O.A., Washington DC.

Gissmann, L. and Schneider, A. (1986). The role of human papillomaviruses in genital cancer. In *Herpes and papilloma viruses. Their role in the carcinogenesis of the lower genital tract* (ed. G. De Palo, F. Rilke, and H. zur Hausen) p.15. Raven Press, New York.

Glass, G.V. (1976). Primary, secondary and meta-analysis of research. *Education Research*, **5**, 3–8.

Gøtzsche, P.C., Podenphant, J., Olesen, M., and Halberg, P. (1992). Meta-analysis of second-line antirheumatic drugs: sample size bias and uncertain benefit. *Journal of Clinical Epidemiology*, **45**, 587–94.

Green, S.B. and Byar, D.P. (1984). Using observational data from registries to compare treatments: the fallacy of omnimetrics. *Statistics in Medicine*, **3**, 361–70.

Green, S., Fleming, T.R., and Emerson, S. (1987). Effects on overviews of early stopping rules for clinical trials. *Statistics in Medicine*, **6**, 361–7.

Gruppo Italiano per lo Studio della Streptochinasi nell'Infarto Miocardico (GISSI). (1986) Effectiveness of intravenous thrombolytic treatment in acute myocardial infarction. *Lancet*, **397**, 402.

Gurwitz, J.H., Col, N.F., and Avorn, J. (1992). The exclusion of the elderly and women from clinical trials in acute myocardial infarction. *Journal of the American Medical Association*, **268**, 1417–22.

Hartz, A.J., Kuhn, E.M., Pryor, D.B., *et al.* (1992). Mortality after coronary angioplasty and coronary artery bypass surgery (The National Medicare Experience). *American Journal of Cardiology*, **70**, 179–85.

Hedges, L.V. (1990). Directions for future methodology. In *The future of meta-analysis* (ed. K.W. Wachter and M.L. Straf). p.11. Russel Sage Foundation, New York.

Hlatky, M.A., Califf, R.M., Harrell, F.E., Lee, K.L., Mark, D.B., and Pryor, D.B. (1988). Comparison of predictions based on observational data with the results of randomised controlled clinical trials of coronary artery bypass surgery. *Journal of the American College of Cardiology*, **11**, 237–45.

Hlatky, M.A. (1991). Using databases to evaluate therapy. *Statistics in Medicine*, **10**, 647–52.

ISIS–2 Collaborative Group. (1988). Randomised trial of intravenous streptokinase, oral aspirin, both, or neither among 17187 cases of suspected acute myocardial infarction: ISIS–2. *Lancet*, ii, 349–60.

ISIS–4 Collaborative Group. (1995). ISIS–4: A randomised factorial trial assessing early oral captopril, oral mononitrate, and intravenous magnesium sulphate in 58,050 patients with suspected acute myocardial infarction. *Lancet*, **345**, 669–87.

Jacobs, D., Blackburn, H., Higgins,M., *et al.* (1992). Report of the Conference on Low Blood Cholesterol: mortality associations. *Circulation*, **86**, 1046–60.

Kassirer, J.P. (1992). Clinical trials and meta-analysis: what do they do for us?. *New England Journal of Medicine*, **327**, 273–4.

Lau, J., Antman, E.M., Jimenez-Silva, J., Kupelnick, B., Mosteller, F., and Chalmers, T.C. (1992). Cumulative meta-analysis of therapeutic trials for myocardial infarction. *New England Journal of Medicine*, **327**, 248–54.

Law, M.R. and Thompson, S.G. (1991). Low serum cholesterol and the risk of cancer: an analysis of the published prospective studies. *Cancer Causes and Control*, **2**, 253–61.

Law, M.R., Thompson, S.G., and Wald, N.J. (1994). Assessing possible hazards of reducing serum cholesterol. *British Medical Journal*, **308**, 373–9.

Leizorovicz, A., Haugh, M.C., and Boissel, J.P. (1992a). Meta-analysis and multiple publications of clinical trial reports. *Lancet*, **340**, 1102–3.

Leizorovicz, A., Haugh, M.C., Chapuis, F.-R., Samama, M.M., and Boissel, J.-P. (1992b). Low molecular weight heparin in prevention of perioperative thrombosis. *British Medical Journal*, **305**, 913–20.

Levy, G. (1992). Publication bias: its implications for clinical pharmacology. *Clinical and Pharmacological Therapy*, **52**, 115–19.

Licciardone, J.C., Brownson, R.C., Chang, J.C., and Wilkins, J.R. (1990). Uterine cervical cancer risk in cigarette smokers: a meta-analytic study. *American Journal of Preventive Medicine*, **6**, 274–81.

Lopressor Intervention Trial Research Group. (1987). The Lopressor Intervention Trial: multicentre study of metoprolol in survivors of acute myocardial infarction. *European Heart Journal*, **8**, 1056–64.

MacDonald, D., Grant, A., Sheridan-Pereira, M., Boylan, P., and Chalmers, I. (1985). The Dublin randomised controlled trial of intrapartum fetal heart rate monitoring. *American Journal of Obstetrics and Gynecology*, **152**, 524–39.

MacMahon, S. (1992). Lowering cholesterol: effects on trauma death, cancer death and total mortality. *Australian and New Zealand Journal of Medicine*, **22**, 580–2.

Manninen, V. (1983). Clinical results with gemfibrozil and background to the Helsinki Heart Study. *American Journal of Cardiology*, **52**, 35B–38B.

Mauri, F., Gasparini, M., Barbonaglia, L., *et al.* Prognostic significance of the extent of myocardial injury in acute myocardial infarction treated by streptokinase (the GISSI trial). *American Journal of Cardiology*, **63**, 1291–5.

Miller, A.B., Baines, C.J., To, T., and Wall, C. (1992). Canadian National Breast Screening Study: 1. Breast cancer detection and death rates among women aged 40 to 49 years. *Canadian Medical Association Journal*, **147**, 1459–76.

Mulrow, C.D. (1987). The medical review article: state of the science. *Annals of Internal Medicine*, **106**, 485–8.

Multiple Risk Factor Intervention Trial Research Group. (1982). Multiple Risk Factor Intervention Trial. Risk factor changes and mortality results. *Journal of the American Medical Association*, **248**, 1465–77.

Murphy, D.J., Povar, G.J., and Pawlson, L.G. (1994). Setting limits in clinical medicine. *Archives of Internal Medicine*, **154**, 505–12.

Nurmohamed, M.T., Rosendaal, F.R., Bueller, H.R., *et al.* (1992). Low-

molecular-weight heparin versus standard heparin in general and orthopaedic surgery: a meta-analysis. *Lancet*, **340**, 152–6.

Oakes, M. (1986). *Statistical inference: a commmentary for the social and behavioural sciences*. John Wiley & Sons, Chichester.

Oakes, M. (1993). The logic and role of meta-analysis in clinical research. *Statistical Methods in Medical Research*, **2**, 147–60.

Oxman, A.D. and Guyatt, G.H. (1992). A consumer's guide to subgroup analyses. *Annals of Internal Medicine*, **116**, 78–84.

Pearson,K. (1904). Report on certain enteric fever inoculation statistics. *British Medical Journal*, **3**, 1243–6.

Peto, R. (1982). Statistical aspects of cancer trials. In *Treatment of cancer* (ed. K.E. Halnan). Chapman and Hall, London.

Peto, R. (1987). Why do we need systematic overviews of randomized trials. *Statistics in Medicine*, **6**, 233–40.

Peto, R., Yusuf, S., and Collins, R. (1985). Cholesterol-lowering trial results in their epidemiologic context. *Circulation*, **72** (suppl. 3), 451.

Peto, R., Collins, R., and Gray, R. (1995). Large, simple trials and overviews of trials. *Journal of Clinical Epidemiology*, **48**, 23–40.

Petitti, D.B., Perlman, J.A., and Sidney, S. (1986). Postmenopausal estrogen use and heart disease. *New England Journal of Medicine*, **315**, 131–2.

Phillips, A.N. and Davey Smith, G. (1991). How independent are "independent" effects? Relative risk estimation when correlated exposures are measured imprecisely. *Journal of Clinical Epidemiology*, **44**, 1223–31.

Prendiville, W., Elbourne, D., and Chalmers, I. (1988). The effects of routine oxytocin administration in the management of the third stage of labour: an overview of the evidence from controlled trials. *British Journal of Obstetrics and Gynaecology*, **95**, 3–16.

Ravnskov, U. (1992). Cholesterol lowering trials in coronary heart disease: frequency of citation and outcome. *British Medical Journal*, **305**, 15–19.

Rochon, P.A., Gurwitz, J.H., Simms, R.W., *et al.* (1994). A study of manufacturer-supported trials of nonsteroidal anti-inflammatory drugs in the treatment of arthritis. *Archives of Internal Medicine*, **154**, 157–63.

Roos, N.P., Wennberg, J.E., Malenka, D.J., *et al.* (1989). Mortality and reoperation after open and transurethral resection of the prostate for benign prostatic hyperplasia. *New England Journal of Medicine*, **320**, 1120–4.

Rosenthal, R. (1979). The 'file drawer problem' and tolerance for null results. *Psychological Bulletin*, **86**, 638–41.

Rosenthal, R. (1990). An evaluation of procedures and results. In *The future of meta-analysis* (ed. K.W. Wachter and M.L. Straf ML) p.123. Russel Sage Foundation, New York.

Sacks, H., Chalmers, T.C., and Smith, H.Jr. (1982). Randomized versus historical controls for clinical trials. *American Journal of Medicine*, **72**, 233–40.

Sacks, H.S., Berrier, J., Reitman, D., Ancona-Berk, V.A., and Chalmers, T.C. (1987). Meta-analyses of randomized controlled trials. *New England Journal of Medicine*, **316**, 450–5.

Schroeder, R. (1985). Oxprenolol in myocardial infarction survivors: brief review of the European Infarction Study results in the light of other beta-blocker post infarction trials. *Zeitschrift für Kardiologie*, **74** (suppl. 6), 165–72.

Shapiro, S. (1994) Meta-analysis/Shmeta-analysis. *American Journal of Epidemiology*, **140**, 771–8.

Simes, R.J. (1987). Confronting publication bias: a cohort design for meta-analysis. *Statistics in Medicine*, **6**, 11–29.

Slattery, M.L., Robison, L.M., Schuman, K.L., *et al.* (1989). Cigarette smoking and exposure to passive smoke are risk factors for cervical cancer. *Journal of the American Medical Association*, **261**, 1593–8.

Sood, A.K. (1991). Cigarette smoking and cervical cancer: meta-analysis and critical review of recent studies. *American Journal of Preventive Medicine*, **7**, 208–13.

Stampfer, M.J., Goldhaber, S.Z., Yusuf, S., Peto, R., and Hennekens, C.H. (1982). Effect of intravenous streptokinase on acute myocardial infarction. Pooled results from randomized trials. *New England Journal of Medicine*, **307**, 1180–2.

Sterling, T.D. (1959). Publication decisions and their possible effects on inferences drawn from tests of significance—or vice versa. *Journal of the American Statistics Association*, **54**, 30–4.

Susser, M. (1977). Judgment and causal inference: criteria in epidemiologic studies. *American Journal of Epidemiology*, **105**, 1–15.

Teagarden, J.R. (1989). Meta-analysis: whither narrative review?. *Pharmacotherapy*, **9**, 274–84.

Teo, K.K. and Yusuf, S. (1993). Role of magnesium in reducing mortality in acute myocardial infarction. A review of the evidence. *Drugs*, **46**, 347–59.

Teo, K.K., Yusuf, S., Collins, R., Held, P.H., and Peto, R. (1991). Effects of intravenous magnesium in suspected acute myocardial infarction: overview of randomised trials. *British Medical Journal*, **303**, 1499–503.

Tverdal, A., Thelle, D., Stensvold, I., Leren, P., and Bjartveit, K. (1993). Mortality in relation to smoking history: 13 years follow-up of 68000 Norwegian men and women 35–49 years. *Journal of Clinical Epidemiology*, **46**, 475–87.

Winkelstein, W. (1990). Smoking and cervical cancer—current status: a review. *American Journal of Epidemiology*, **131**, 945–57.

Wittes, R.E. (1987). Problems in the medical interpretation of overviews. *Statistics in Medicine*, **6**, 269–76.

Woods, K.L., Fletcher, S., Roffe, C., and Haider, Y. (1992). Intravenous magnesium sulphate in suspected acute myocardial infarction: results of the second Leicester Intravenous Magnesium Intervention Trial (LIMIT–2). *Lancet*, **339**, 1553–8.

Yusuf, S., Peto, R., Lewis, J., Collins, R., and Sleight, P. (1985). Beta blockade during and after myocardial infarction: an overview of the randomized trials. *Progress in Cardiovascular Disease*, **17**, 335–71.

Yusuf, S., Collins, R., MacMahon, S., and Peto, R. (1988). Effect of intravenous nitrates on mortality in acute myocardial infarction: an overview of the randomised trials. *Lancet*, **i**, 1088–92.

Yusuf, S., Wittes, J., Probstfield, J., and Tyroler, H.A. (1991). Analysis and interpretation of treatment effects in subgroups of patients in randomized clinical trials. *Journal of the American Medical Association*, **266**, 93–8.

Zelen, M. (1983). Intravenous streptokinase for acute myocardial infarction. *New England Journal of Medicine*, **308**, 593.

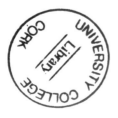

17 Statistical methods

A.V. Swan

Introduction

Statistical methods are required whenever groups of individuals, not entirely predictable in their characteristics or behaviour, need to be described or compared. A wide range of techniques has been developed, and this text cannot cover them all. The most useful are known as regression techniques. In this chapter we concentrate on statistical methods commonly used in epidemiology and public health research and service work. The material on case–control studies is dealt with more fully in a separate chapter.

The chapter is divided into six sections, which can be regarded as a course in three parts. The first two sections after this introduction, 'Design and sampling' and 'Practical questions from a statistical point of view', provide a general survey of statistical ideas and practical problems. These are followed by a more advanced discussion of the underlying principles of statistical reasoning under the heading 'Basic concepts'. The final part, 'Types of analyses', discusses, in some detail, the application of the statistical methods appropriate to the problems presented in the 'Practical questions' section.

The aim of the chapter as a whole is to give a clear picture of the range of problems that can be handled by statistical methods, with a general appreciation of the methods and the underlying statistical concepts necessary for analyses using computer packages such as Minitab (Ryan *et al.* 1985), SPSS (SPSS Inc. 1990), GLIM (Francis *et al.* 1993), and Stata (Stata Corporation 1993). In addition, more comprehensive details are provided for the special cases where the problem can be simplified sufficiently for the analysis to be performed by hand.

Design and sampling

The statistical design of an investigation is determined by the form of analysis appropriate to answering the question of interest, the precision required, and the assumptions that appear justified. The practical question should indicate quite clearly what analyses are necessary. The design is then determined by what is necessary to make these analyses possible and sufficiently precise.

Circumstances and ethics may mean that an **observational** study, i.e. a study where subjects exposed to a variety of influences are simply observed, must be used. In such cases sampling is restricted to a process of choosing who enters the study. If the investigation is using previously collected data, for example cardio-vascular mortality figures from areas of differing water hardness, no sampling is involved. If an experiment or clinical trial involving intervention by the investigator is possible, the sampling process also includes allocation to the groups to be compared. A compre-hensive discussion of this and other aspects of clinical trials is given by Pocock (1983). Because it is often important to determine the most effective treatment as quickly as possible and to minimize the number of patients receiving the other treatments, what are known as sequential trials with special allocation rules may be very useful. The subject is well covered by Armitage (1960) and Whitehead (1992).

In general, sampling does not need to be complicated. Although it may be awkward in an administrative sense, the process is straightforward in principle. The first necessity is to decide on the population of interest and to identify that part of the population that is accessible in practice. The sampling process is then applied to that subgroup of the population with due regard to the possibility that it is not properly representative of the whole. For the sampling process, it is usually sufficient in both selection and allocation to use what is known as simple random sampling. This means the use of any technique, such as 'tossing coins', 'drawing names from a hat', 'taking every tenth name on a list assumed to be in random order', etc., that gives every subject an equal chance of selection.

In practice, the problem tends to be that of obtaining a list, called a sampling frame, of all the candidates for inclusion. In community health surveys in the United Kingdom, a commonly used sampling frame is the electoral register.

For complex sampling problems, it may be necessary to use random sampling numbers which are included in most sets of statistical tables (Lindley and Miller 1964). They usually consist of sequences of two–digit numbers (for example, 87, 31, 47, 55, 56, . . .) generated in such a way that in any reasonably long sequence, the number of 0s, 1s, 2s, . . . , 9s and, consequently, 00s, 01s, . . . , 99s are the same. On average, each single digit will occur once in every ten digits and each double-digit combination will occur once in every hundred pairs. For example, to allocate subjects to three groups in a trial, a sequence of digits, ignoring the zeros, would be assigned, one at a time, to each of the subjects. Then allocation is determined by taking the digits 1, 2, and 3 to represent group 1, the digits 4, 5, and 6 to represent group 2, and the digits 7, 8, and 9 to represent group 3. Sometimes particular subgroups (essentially subpopulations) of individuals are of specific interest, for example sex or age groups. In that case it may be appropriate to identify the individuals belonging to the groups, known as strata, and to sample separately within each. This is known as stratified random sampling. This process can also be performed using 'pseudo-random' numbers generated with a computer.

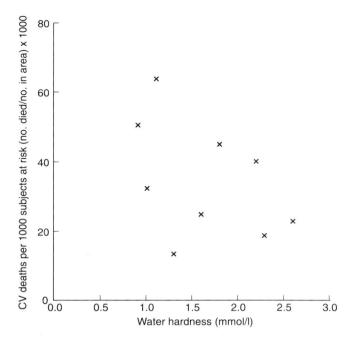

Fig. 17.1 Cardiovascular (CV) mortality by water hardness. *Source*: Pocock *et al.* 1980.

Practical questions from a statistical point of view

Trends—routinely collected grouped data

It has been suggested that the 'hardness' of drinking water may affect the risk of an individual developing heart disease. The cardiovascular death rates and some measure of the water 'hardness' in each of a number of geographic areas (for a particular year) might give a picture as shown in Fig. 17.1, which is known as a scatter diagram.

The question is: Does the risk of cardiovascular disease change according to the 'hardness' of the water you drink? In terms of the pattern in the diagram, the question becomes: What is the trend in this sample of points and does it reflect a real trend in all the points from the other subjects, other years, and other areas that these points represent?

The 'truth', were it possible to see it, might be as in Fig. 17.2(a) or 17.2(b). The analysis is a process of determining which is the most likely 'truth'.

Trends—individuals in an observational study

In an investigation of blood pressure and salt intake, the question could be: Does an increase in salt intake increase systolic blood pressure?

If it were possible to determine salt intake for a sample of individuals, a plot of each individual might give a scatter diagram such as that shown in Fig. 17.3. As before, the question becomes: Is there a trend in these points consistent enough to suggest a real trend in the large population of points that this sample is taken to represent?

If data were available from men and women (Fig. 17.4), the question would be more complicated. The relationship between

systolic blood pressure and salt intake could differ between the sexes. The initial question becomes several separate questions: (i) Are the trends in the populations of men and women represented by these samples different? (ii) If they are different, are either of them non-horizontal? (iii) What are the trends?

There is also information with which to answer the following questions:

(a) At a given salt intake, do the male and female populations differ on the systolic blood pressure scale? That is, at a given salt intake, are the population points for the males higher or lower, on average, than those of the females?

(b) Do the male and female populations differ with respect to salt intake? Or, in the population, are the male and female points positioned differently on the salt intake scale?

Simply introducing another factor, sex, has considerably complicated the problem.

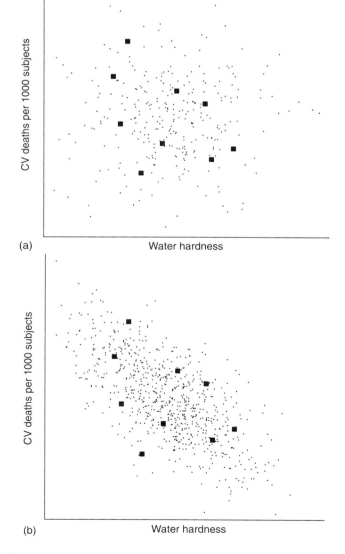

Fig. 17.2 Possible population patterns for cardiovascular (CV) death rates with water hardness: (a) no trend; (b) a negative trend.

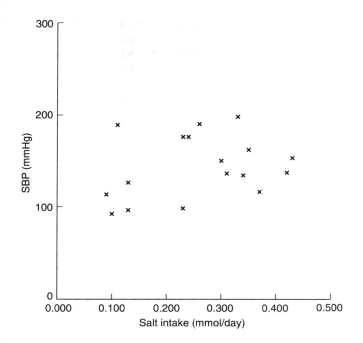

Fig. 17.3 Systolic blood pressure (SBP) versus salt intake (simulated data).

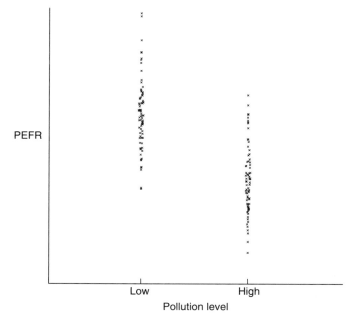

Fig. 17.5 Peak expiratory flow rate (PEFR) in children versus air pollution levels (simulated data).

In practice it may be necessary to consider weight, exercise, age, and possibly other factors related to systolic blood pressure, in which case the complications multiply rapidly.

Comparing groups of individuals

Investigations of air pollution and respiratory health encounter considerable problems in determining an individual's exposure. Often the design has to be a simple two-group comparison of

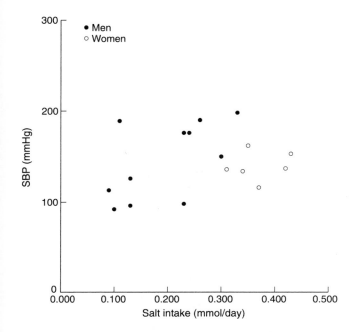

Fig. 17.4 Systolic blood pressure (SBP) versus salt intake in men and women (simulated data).

individuals living in an area of high pollution with those living in one of low pollution. Such a study might produce peak expiratory flow rate values from children in high and low pollution areas as shown in Fig. 17.5.

The question is: Does air pollution affect lung function in children? With some assumptions, this can be rephrased as: Do children in areas with different pollution levels have different lung function values on average? On the plot this becomes: Do the heights of these two samples of points differ enough to suggest a difference between the populations they represent?

Proportions from two categories of outcome

Frequently an all-or-nothing response, such as the presence or absence of a symptom, will be the outcome measure of interest. The appropriate response scale is the proportion with the symptom (i.e. the prevalence of the symptom). An investigation of pollution as above may be interested in the prevalence of morning cough in children from areas with different levels of pollution.

The question is: Does exposure to pollution increase the risk of a child developing morning cough? A plot of the prevalences against pollution level with the points joined by straight lines will generally give a line with a number of bends in it (Fig. 17.6). The question becomes: Do these sample proportions differ enough to suggest that differences would be seen if the populations of all such children exposed to these pollution levels could be observed? In other words, is the equivalent population line horizontal?

Information on parents' smoking habits will give a plot of two lines (Fig. 17.7). There are now several questions:

(i) Are the differences between the pollution level groups in the population the same in the two parental smoking groups? That is, are the population lines parallel to each other?

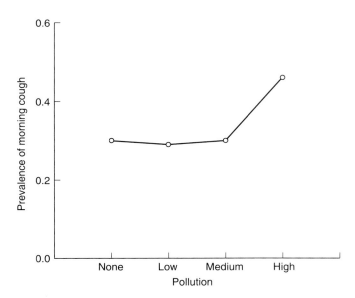

Fig. 17.6 Prevalence of morning cough in children versus pollution level (simulated data).

(ii) Are the population differences between the pollution groups non-zero in either parental smoking group? That is, is either population line non-horizontal?

(iii) At a fixed pollution level is there a difference between the parental smoking groups in the population? That is, is there a vertical separation between the population lines?

Proportions: case–control studies

In a study of sudden infant death syndrome, various information was collected on all the infants dying this way in a particular area and period of time—these were the cases. The same information was collected for the same number of randomly selected control children born in the same period and still alive. Such studies are known as case–control or retrospective studies. The latter name

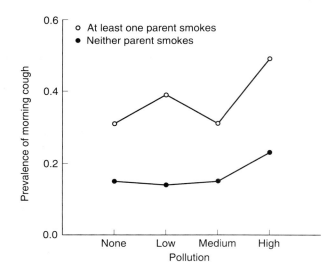

Fig. 17.7 Prevalence of morning cough in children versus pollution level by parents' cigarette smoking habits (simulated data).

Table 17.1 Cases of sudden infant death and controls by mother's age

	Mother's age (years)			
	<20	29 –	25 –	30+
Cases	17	22	17	5
Controls	9	23	16	13
Cases and controls	26	45	33	18
P	0.65	0.49	0.52	0.28

arises because the study starts after the event of interest and consists of looking back in time at what preceded the event. These data are given in Table 17.1.

The question here is: Does the risk of sudden infant death change with the age of the mother? It is not possible to obtain a direct estimate of this risk, which is that of an infant becoming a case (risk = number of cases/number at risk), because the number at risk is not known. However, with some assumptions, mainly that the sampling fraction for the controls (the proportion the sample is of the population) is the same for all the age groups, it is possible to manage without it. A proxy measure, the proportion P = cases/(cases + controls), is constructed and used to investigate the patterns in the data. These proportions are given in the last row of Table 17.1. When they are plotted against the mid-point of the mother's age group (Fig. 17.8), they show a slightly negative trend with increasing mother's age.

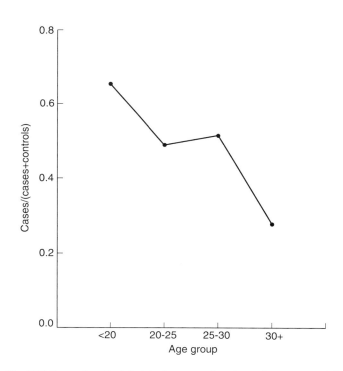

Fig. 17.8 Cases of sudden infant death as proportions (cases/(cases + controls)) versus mother's age group.

If the controls were known to be 1 per cent of all possible controls, i.e. a sampling fraction of 0.01, then the usual estimates of risk would be

$$\frac{17}{17 + 900} \qquad \frac{22}{22 + 2300} \qquad \frac{17}{17 + 1600} \qquad \frac{5}{5 + 1300}$$

or

$$0.0185 \qquad 0.0095 \qquad 0.0105 \qquad 0.0038.$$

These are much smaller than the proportions but, when plotted, give a line with practically the same shape. The question then becomes: Does the line deviate from the horizontal more than could easily arise by chance if the equivalent population line is horizontal?

Three or more categories of outcome

A study of illness behaviour in women used the number of positive responses to questions on 'loss of appetite', 'nerves', 'depression or irritability', 'sleeplessness', and 'undue tiredness' as a measure of depression.

The numbers in the various depression categories and their marital states are given in Table 17.2. The question is: Does the pattern of depression in women differ according to their marital status?

Statistically, as a deduction from the sample to the population, the question becomes: Is the proportional distribution among the depression categories in the population of all such women the same for each marital status? That is, are the 38 single women distributed among the depression categories in the same proportions, apart from differences that could arise from sampling variation, as the 88 married and the 60 widowed or divorced women? The proportional allocation can be seen more easily if the frequencies are expressed as percentages of the total in that particular marital status group (Table 17.2).

Figure 17.9 gives a plot of the percentage frequencies as a separate line for each marital status group. If the proportional allocation to the depression categories were the same, these lines would fall on top of one another.

Therefore the question becomes: Are these lines, obtained from a sample, more different than could easily arise by chance if the three equivalent population lines are really identical?

Survival data

This general title is used to cover data that arise when the interest is in the risk of some event occurring. The event may be death, but

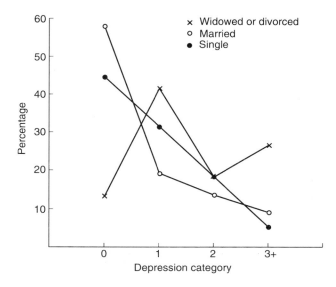

Fig. 17.9 Percentage of women in each marital status group plotted against depression category.

it need not be; survival data techniques are appropriate for comparing the chances of remission for patients on different treatments and other such events.

The first example considered annual mortality in relatively large groups of people. The usual analyses for data of that type assume that all subjects were at risk of the event for the whole of a specified period. However, if someone is lost to observation half-way through the year, they have been at risk, as far as the study is concerned, for only half a year. With large numbers and small risks, the numbers observed for only part of a period are small, and ignoring the problem does little harm. When the numbers in the groups to be compared are relatively small, the times at risk must be taken into account.

If it can be assumed that, within each group of subjects to be compared, each individual is running the same risk throughout the chosen time period, this is relatively straightforward. The periods of time that each individual was observed are summed over all the individuals in the group. If the period of time is a year and the times at risk are expressed as fractions of a year, this gives the number of 'person years at risk' (obviously, at other times it may be necessary to use 'woman years at risk', 'patient weeks at risk', and so on).

Then the estimate of the annual risk of death (or other event) is simply the ratio of the number of deaths to the number of person years at risk.

In an occupational health study of cancer, groups of current and ex-workers in two industrial environments were observed for a number of years. The overall mortality is as given in Table 17.3. The initial question is: Is the risk of death from any cause different in the two environments?

The estimated risks per person per year are given in Table 17.3, and Fig. 17.10 shows the estimated risks plotted against age. The question becomes: Are these lines surprisingly far apart if the equivalent lines in the population represented by this sample of individuals are identical?

The techniques for answering this question are essentially the same as those for the previous examples.

Table 17.2 Classification of women by marital status and answers to questions related to depression

Marital status	No. of positive responses (%)				
	0	1	2	3 or 4	Total
Single	17(45)	12(32)	7(18)	2(5)	38(100)
Married	51(58)	17(19)	12(14)	8(9)	88(100)
Widowed or divorced	8(13)	25(42)	11(18)	16(27)	60(100)

Table 17.3 Mortality from all causes and estimated risk of death from any cause per person per year by age group and factory

Age at start of study (years)	Factory 1			Factory 2		
	Numbers dying	Person years at risk	Estimated risk of death	Numbers dying	Person years at risk	Estimated risk of death
50–59.9	7	4045	0.0017	7	3701	0.0019
60–69.9	27	3571	0.0076	37	3702	0.0100
70–79.9	30	1771	0.0169	35	1818	0.0193
80–89.9	8	381	0.0210	9	350	0.0257

When risks are changing during the period of observation, techniques assuming one overall risk are inappropriate. To illustrate data of this sort, survival curves are used. These are plots of the percentage in a group still surviving against time elapsed since some defined starting point, such as date of entry to the study.

Data of this type arose from a clinical trial comparing radiotherapy with hormone treatment for cancer of the prostate. The question was: Which is the better treatment?

This is not at all a simple question. The treatment giving the greater chance of survival at five years, say, is not necessarily the treatment that gives the longest life expectancy. It is necessary to look at the relative shapes of the survival curves. During the trial, 44 patients received radiotherapy and 48 received hormone treatment. The survival curves for the two groups are shown in Fig. 17.11.

There is some divergence of the curves and the primary question becomes: Do the curves for the population represented by these samples differ? In other words, are these sample curves too different to have easily arisen by chance sampling from populations with identical survival curves?

Basic concepts

Because individuals subject to biological variation are to some extent unpredictable in their characteristics and behaviour, factual statements concerning them take the form:

> Individuals like **this**
> treated like **this**
> tend to respond like **this**.

The **individuals** are the items being observed. They may be patients, tissue samples, rats, or geographic areas. They may even be the same patient observed at different times (for example when a sequence of separate blood samples is taken or results are obtained from a repeatedly administered psychiatric test).

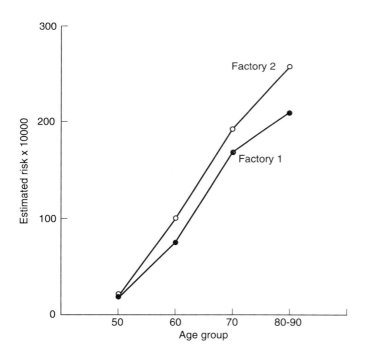

Fig. 17.10 Estimated risks of death versus age for each factory.

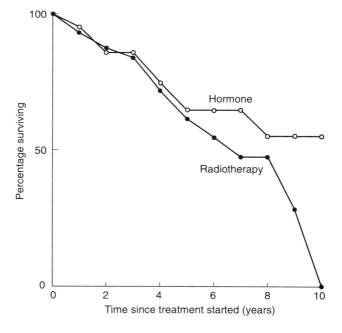

Fig. 17.11 Survival curves for patients with cancer of the prostate receiving radiotherapy or hormone treatment.

The **individuals like this** make up the **population** in the statistical sense (i.e. any strictly defined group of individuals).

The human population of a country may be the statistical population of interest, but it will usually be a sample of the general population of all such humans who might exist now or in the future. Researchers in London, England, will want to be able to generalize their findings beyond Londoners and generally will wish to conclude that the results apply to all such patients in the United Kingdom now and possibly in the future.

The population should be defined before the study begins, and the sample to represent it chosen accordingly. However, practical circumstances can have a considerable effect on the sampling. This makes it necessary for the researcher to indicate how, and with what qualifications, results from a sample apply to a particular population. In addition, most studies will involve individuals from identifiable subpopulations. For example, studies involving physical characteristics such as lung function, which may differ systematically between the sexes, require that results are obtained separately for the two samples representing the male and female subpopulation. If that is not done, and the findings in the two samples not shown to be consistent, it is not safe to combine all the data to arrive at a general conclusion.

This implies that if there are two subpopulations that may differ in respects important to the study in question, data must be collected to identify from which subpopulation each individual arose. These subpopulation-defining characteristics or variables, such as sex, age, social class, and so on, are often a nuisance. For example, it is not usually necessary to study how the sexes differ—this is mostly known. It is necessary only in order to confirm that the effects of interest are consistently found in all the subpopulations. If this can be assumed at the beginning, studies can be simplified by restricting them to one sex or one age group, for example, a simplifying option that is always worth considering at the design stage. Generally, however, data must be collected on individuals from a number of subpopulations.

Clinical trials are studies of subjects who have been treated in some way that must be defined and possibly measured, for example as a dose. In most trials two or more groups receiving different treatments will be compared, and so the treatment, type, or dosage may vary from one individual to another. Therefore the treatment is a variable and will be represented in the data collected during the trial by numerical values identifying the type of treatment and/or the dosage.

Observational studies of naturally occurring 'experiments' may be concerned with assessing the effect on individuals of some experience or exposure to some aspect of the environment. As for a treatment, it is necessary to define and measure the experience or exposure. Again, it must be represented by a variable with numerical values.

To assess the manner in which individuals treated in some way or undergoing some experience tend to respond, a variable is required to measure or classify the response. This is the response or outcome variable. Furthermore, because they will vary in a random way even among individuals from a homogeneous population in which all are treated in the same way, these variables are known as random variables. The way in which they vary is described by the distribution of their values in the sample and by inference in the populations.

Types of variables

Which analytical approach to use largely depends on the nature of the response variable. There are two main categories: quantitative and qualitative.

Quantitative variables have an obvious associated scale on which distances have a clear interpretation. They can arise in two forms, continuous or discrete. Continuous variables are generally measurements, and every value within some sensible range is possible (for example serum cholesterol or peak expiratory flow rate). Discrete variables are generally counts where only certain values on the scale are possible (such as number of previous heart attacks or number of schistosome eggs in a stool sample).

Qualitative variables are those associated with a set of categories. The categories may have a natural ordering as in severity of a condition, category of remission, social class, and so on. These are known as ordinal variables and, although they have to be treated as categories, they are usually interpretable as sections of an underlying scale. Categories such as blood group and type of health services contact do not have an order and are termed nominal variables.

Functions of variables

The function of response variables is clear. They provide the 'yardstick' by which the effects of treatment or experience are measured. However, variables are also used to identify the subpopulation to which an individual belongs so that an analysis can assess and allow for differences between subpopulations. They are also used to measure or classify treatment or experience.

There is no obvious general term for these last two classes of variable. They are sometimes called 'predictor' variables because studies are often concerned with how well they predict outcome or response. They may also be referred to as independent or explanatory variables because the analysis is essentially assessing how variations in response or outcome depend or can be explained by differences in their values. The response variable is often referred to as the dependent variable.

Perhaps the simplest terminology of all follows mathematical convention. The treatment, exposure, and subpopulation variables, all of which tend to appear on the horizontal axis of graphical plots, are classed as x variables. The response variables generally appear on the vertical axis of such plots and are known as y variables.

Describing data patterns—models

A model, in the statistical sense, is simply an algebraic formula for describing some pattern or structure in variable data.

Consider the relationship between forced expiratory volume in 1 second FEV_1 and height in a sample of students (Fig. 17.12). There is a tendency for the taller individuals to have larger FEV values. If the individuals are grouped on the height scale (for example all individuals with heights between 62 and 64 inches are treated as if they were 63 inches, those between 65 and 67 as if they were 66 inches, and so on), the plot becomes a set of separate groups of points (Fig. 17.13).

For each height group there is an array or distribution of FEV values. These are known as conditional distributions. They are the distributions of FEV values conditional on the concerned individuals all having the same height (or, in this case, being in the same height group). It can now be seen that the trend in FEV values is

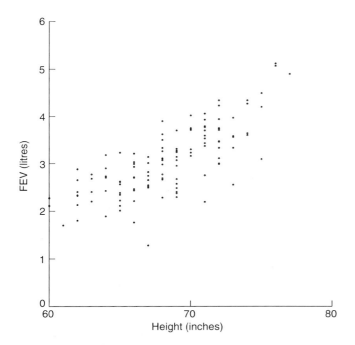

Fig. 17.12 Forced expiratory volume FEV (litres/minute) in young adults versus height in inches.

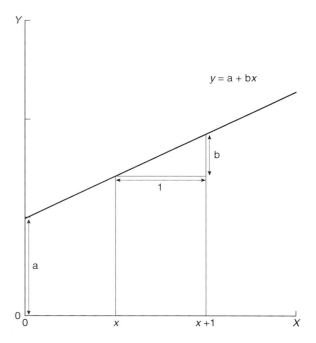

Fig. 17.14 Diagrammatic representation of the straight-line regression model $y = a + bx$.

a systematic tendency for these conditional distributions to move up as height increases. The distributions overlap, but their centres are located at a generally higher position in the taller height groups. It is not easy to describe the behaviour of the individual points, but it is possible to be reasonably precise about the relative positioning or location of the conditional distributions.

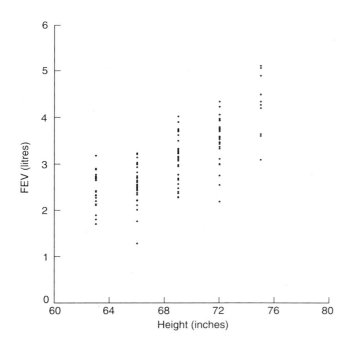

Fig. 17.13 Forced expiratory volume FEV (litres/minute) in young adults versus height groups.

The models to describe this sort of pattern have the form:

location of distribution = reference value + horizontal position effect.

The behaviour of individual points has to be described in terms of the location of their particular distribution and the way in which they are dispersed or spread about the location. In Fig. 17.13 the data were grouped to show the conditional distributions, but this is wasteful of information. Some method is needed to describe the trend in the raw data.

The simplest model is a straight-line trend. This model assumes that the height (x variable) effect is a steady increase (or decrease) in the FEV (y variable) distribution locations, usually represented by the arithmetic mean defined below. That is to say, for each unit change in height, there is the same change in mean FEV at all points on the height axis. The model for this is

mean FEV = reference value + change/unit height × height

This is known as a regression line model. In more general terms it becomes

$$y = a + bx$$

which is the equation representing a straight line on a plot of y against x (in this case FEV against height). This is shown diagrammatically in Fig. 17.14, where a (the height of the line when $x = 0$) is known as the intercept and b (the slope of the line) is called the regression coefficient. FEV at zero height makes no practical sense, but it makes the algebra simpler to represent the regression line by

$$FEV = intercept + b \times height.$$

Finding the 'best' straight line to describe a trend means estimating the appropriate intercept and slope; this is known as fitting the regression line. In theory, any values of a and b are possible and so the possibilities are infinite. The problem is to define the 'best' line to describe a set of data and then to deduce the values of *a* and *b* that give this 'best' line as functions of the data values.

In practice, the 'best' fitting line is defined by the **principle of least squares**. This principle can be illustrated by considering a general line on a scatter diagram with *a* and *b* unspecified (Fig. 17.15). Each point deviates from the line (in the *y* direction) by some amount. The principle of least squares states that the 'best' line is the one that makes the 'sum of all the deviations squared' as small as possible. This means that *a* and *b* must be chosen to make the sum of all the d^2 a minimum. Using this principle, it is possible to deduce mathematically standard formulae with which the appropriate values of *a* and *b* can be calculated for any set of data.

Before further discussion of how models are defined and used, it is necessary to consider how to define and measure the important characteristics of the distributions whose relative positioning they are used to describe and test.

The characteristics of distributions

The characteristics of the distributions represented by the arrays of points in Fig. 17.13 are not at all clear. Their location can be judged to some extent, but how the individuals are dispersed about the central location cannot be seen so easily. Single distributions are better displayed as histograms.

To represent a sample as a histogram, the scale is divided into intervals of equal length and the points within an interval are drawn on top of one another as shown in Fig. 17.16. Points falling where two intervals join could be placed in either, but this does not really matter for graphic techniques. Usually they are allocated to the higher interval.

The shape is rather 'ragged', but one can see, in addition to its location and spread, that the distribution is rather asymmetrical. There is a longer 'tail' on the high-value or positive side. Such

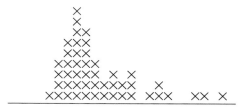

Fig. 17.16 Representation of a sample of values as a histogram.

distributions are called skew, and since skewness can affect the analysis, some method is needed to detect and measure it. There are specific measures of skewness, but they are rarely necessary in practice. Graphic techniques are usually adequate to detect whether it is present to an extent that matters. However, location and dispersion require precise measures, and, on occasion, a complete numerical specification of the distribution is required, for which centiles (sometimes referred to as percentiles) are used.

Measures of location

There are three commonly used measures of location.

The **arithmetic mean** is the sum of all the values in a distribution or a sample divided by the number of values. It is by far the most useful measure of location and is usually referred to simply as the mean. For a sample it is

mean = sum of all values/number of values.

The **median** is the variable value such that half of the values in a distribution are above it and half are below. It is easy to find and useful for simple descriptions of asymmetrical distributions. However, it is not very easy to handle in more complex analyses.

The **mode** is the value in a distribution that occurs most frequently. It is of occasional use for describing single distributions.

Measures of dispersion

There are a multitude of measures of dispersion in the literature, but only a few are commonly used.

The **range** is the distance, on the scale of measurement, between the highest and lowest values. It is occasionally used for describing the spread of small samples. Obviously, as sample sizes increase, the range will automatically increase and, since it depends on the least characteristic pair of individuals in the sample, its usefulness is limited.

The **variance** is a direct measure of spread about the arithmetic mean. For a sample it is defined as

sum for all values of (value − mean value)²/(number of values − 1)

Notice that 'squaring' the deviations of values from their mean ensures that negative deviations from low values do not cancel out with those from high values. The variance cannot be calculated in this way for a population (usually defined so generally that the size is infinite). In this case it is defined as the value approached by the calculated value as the sample size increases indefinitely.

Because the variance is an average squared deviation, it is not in the original units of the variable in question. For this reason its square root, the **standard deviation** (SD), is frequently more useful. This gives quite an accurate measure of how far from the mean individuals are likely to occur in a given distribution. Unless

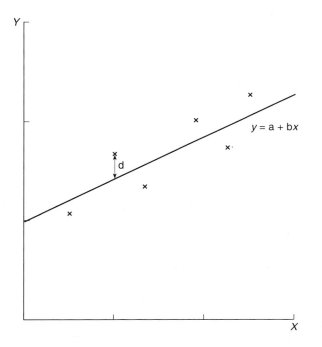

Fig. 17.15 Deviations of data points from the model *y* = a + b*x*.

Table 17.4 Frequency distribution of a sample of ten adult males according to their systolic blood pressures

Systolic blood pressure (mmHg)	Frequency of values	Cumulative total
From 100 to just under 110	1	1
From 110 to just under 120	2	3
From 120 to just under 130	4	7
From 130 to just under 140	2	9
From 140 to just under 150	0	9
From 150 to just under 160	1	10

a distribution is very asymmetrical, individuals more than three SDs from the mean will occur only very rarely and most individuals (approximately 95 per cent) will fall within two SDs of the mean.

Centiles

Centiles are points on the variable scale that exceed a specified percentage of the distribution. Consider a sample of ten systolic blood pressure values with the distribution shown in Table 17.4. Ten per cent (one value) of the sample is below 110 mmHg, and therefore that is the 10th centile. Seven values (70 per cent) are below 130 mmHg so that is the 70th centile, and so on. However, this approach only gives the centiles that occur at the ends of the intervals. Considering the sample as a representative of a much larger population, it is possible to go a little further by plotting the cumulative frequency, as a percentage, against the upper ends of the intervals (Fig. 17.17). It is far from smooth, but various centiles can be deduced by estimating where the 'curve' reaches the equivalent

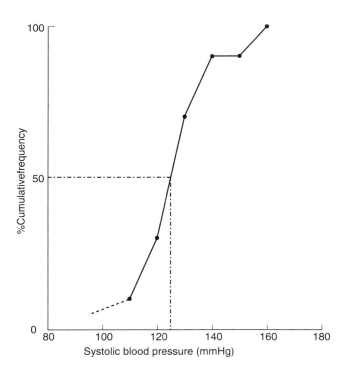

Fig. 17.17 Cumulative frequency plot of a sample of systolic blood pressure values.

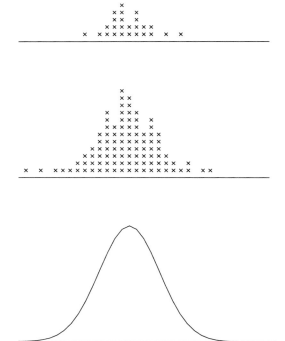

Fig. 17.18 Histograms from samples of increasing size approaching a smooth population curve.

height on the per cent cumulative frequency scale. This method estimates the 50th centile, which is the median, as 125 mmHg. For more precise estimates, a smooth curve could be drawn through the points. Alternatively, assumptions about the shape of the population curve can be made and the appropriate estimates deduced mathematically. To understand this process, it is necessary to consider in detail how sample distributions and their characteristics relate to those of the population.

Inferring the truth—sample to population
Distributions

Consider a sequence of histograms obtained from larger and larger samples of an infinite population (Fig. 17.18). As the sample size increases, the distribution becomes smoother with a more clearly defined shape. As the sample size is increased indefinitely (with the vertical scale reduced appropriately), the shape tends to a smooth curve. For many biological variables this will be close to the symmetrical 'bell-shaped' distribution known as the normal distribution, which can be defined in precise mathematical terms.

Probabilities

In the sample of ten systolic blood pressures (Table 17.4), two out of ten were in the range 110–120 mmHg. Therefore the proportion

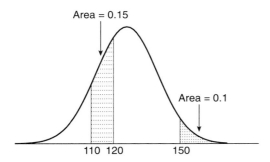

Fig. 17.19 Areas of the population distribution as probabilities.

of the sample between 110 and 120 mmHg is $2/10 = 0.2$. If the names of the ten individuals were written on pieces of paper, mixed up in a hat, and then one was picked at random, the probability that it was an individual in the range 110–120 would be 2/10 (0.2). There are two of the sort required and ten in total.

The probability of selecting an individual with a systolic blood pressure less than 100 mmHg from this hat is 0/10, i.e. zero or impossible. The probability of selecting an individual with a pressure less than 180 is 10/10, i.e. 1.0 or certain. Notice that 120 is the 30th centile and the probability of an individual below 120 is 0.3 or 30 per cent. The probability of an individual below the 15th centile is 0.15 or 15 per cent, and so on.

From the probability of selecting an individual below a particular point, it is possible to deduce the probability of an individual on or above that point. Three of the ten individuals are below 120, which gives the probability of such an individual as 0.3. Seven of the ten are equal to or greater than 120, i.e. a probability of 0.7. Thus probability (value ≥ 120) is

$$\frac{No. \geq 120}{Total \ no.} = \frac{10 \ - No. < 120}{Total \ no.} = \frac{10 \ - \ 3}{10}$$

$$= 7/10 \ or \ (10 \ - \ 3)/10.$$

The probability that an individual will be greater than or equal to some value is 1 minus the probability of being less than that value:

$$p \ (value \geq 120) = 1 - p \ (value < 120).$$

For example

$$p \ (< 110) = 1/10 = 0.1,$$

$$p \ (\geq 110) = 9/10 = 1 - p \ (< 110) = 0.9,$$

and so on.

As sample sizes increase and the histogram approaches the smooth population curve, the numbers become indefinitely large. However, the area above an interval and beneath the curve is in the same ratio to the total areas as the number in that interval to the total number. In practice, population distributions are scaled so that the curve encloses an area exactly equal to unity. This means that the area above any interval is the proportion of individuals with values in that interval. This in turn is the probability that an individual picked at random has a value in that particular interval. For example, if the area of the population distribution between two values, 110 and 120, is 0.15, the population having a systolic blood pressure between 110 and 120 is 0.15 (Fig. 17.19).

The probability that an individual selected at random has a value greater than 150 is the area A under the curve from 150 upward. Since $A = 0.1$, this means that 10 per cent of the population will have systolic blood pressures of 150 or above.

The area below 150 is $1 - A$, so that the probability of an individual below 150 is $1 - A = 0.9$. This means that the remaining 90 per cent of individuals have systolic blood pressures below 150. Consequently, 150 is the 90th centile of the population distribution.

The centiles of the population can be obtained as long as there is some way of obtaining the areas under the population distribution curve. If we represent the 10th centile of the variable y as $y_{0.1}$, the area below $y_{0.1}$ is 0.1, the area below $y_{0.2}$ is 0.2, and so on.

The normal distribution

For various reasons random variables that appear to follow a normal distribution are common in nature—for example human height, haemoglobin levels, systolic blood pressure, and so on. Others can be made to follow a normal distribution by a transformation of their scale. Possibly even more important is the fact that, for all but the smallest samples, averages are themselves random variables from approximately normal distributions whatever the distributions of the original values. Because of this and its amiable mathematical nature, the normal distribution holds a central place in statistical theory and practice.

The theoretical normal distribution is completely specified by its mean and variance. The distribution is symmetrical about the mean, and areas beneath the curve can be obtained mathematically. For example it is known that if the variable is y, the 2.5th centile is

$$y_{0.025} = \text{mean} - 1.96 \ \text{SD}.$$

This implies that in a normal distribution only 2.5 per cent of the individuals will be more than 1.96 SDs below the mean. Similarly, only 2.5 per cent will be more than 1.96 SDs above it. Combining these, it further implies that the range of values

$$\text{mean} - 1.96 \ \text{SD to mean} + 1.96 \ \text{SD}$$

will include 95 per cent of individuals in the population and exclude only 5 per cent.

The normal distribution is so useful that the percentage cumulative frequencies for the standard distribution, which has a mean of zero and a variance of unity, have been widely tabulated (Lindley and Miller 1964) and are easily calculated with most statistical software (e.g. Minitab, Stata, GLIM). The equivalent values for a normal variable with any mean and variance can be deduced from these.

The tabulated values are the areas under the mathematically defined population distribution curve below the given values of the standard normal variable u, say, as in Fig. 17.20. The area P_0 in Fig. 17.20 is the percentage cumulative frequency at u_0, which is the probability of a value below u_0, i.e.

$$p \ (value < u_0) = P_0.$$

The probability of a value at or above u_0 is

$$p \ (value < u_0) = 1 - P_0$$

and the probability of a value between u_0 and u_1 is

$$p \ (u_0 < value < u_1) = P_1 - P_0$$

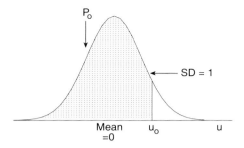

Fig. 17.20 Probabilities and the standardized normal distribution curve.

where P_1 is the area under the curve below u_1.

The variable u is effectively the number of SDs that a value is from the mean. Equivalent probabilities for variables with a different mean and variance are deduced by calculating how many SDs each value is from its mean and treating these as values of u. For example, suppose that the systolic blood pressure in adult males is normally distributed with mean 130 and SD 15. To calculate the probability of an individual value less than 160 mmHg, note that it is 30 mmHg above the mean (i.e. two SDs). This implies that

$$p \text{ (value} < 160) = p \text{ } (u < 2)$$

and since from tables

$$p \text{ } (u < 2) = 0.977$$

it can be deduced that

$$p \text{ (value} < 160) = 0.977$$

and the required probability is 97.7 per cent.

If the population distribution is known, these techniques allow the probabilities of individual sample values to be deduced.

However, the problem is really in the opposite direction. The need is to deduce the population characteristics from the sample values. A method is required to assess the closeness of sample values such as the mean to the unknown population equivalents. This is done by considering how the values of a sample estimate might vary if further samples were taken from the same population. Each sample will differ and estimates from them will vary.

Estimation and sampling distributions

It is simplest to start by considering how the sample mean varies in a sequence of samples all taken from the same population in the same way. The result can be generalized to any estimate (for example a regression coefficient, a difference between means, and so forth) calculated from a sample. Suppose that a sequence of samples of four values ($n = 4$) is taken from the systolic blood pressure (SBP) distribution, and the mean is calculated for each. These sample means will themselves have a distribution which, because it can only arise as a result of repeated sampling, is known as a **sampling distribution**. In this distribution of means, samples with all values at one extreme of the population distribution will be rare. As a result the sample means will be more tightly clustered about the population mean than are the individual observations. In addition, as long as the sampling was properly random, the mean of the sampling distribution will be the same as the population mean. Because of this, the sample mean is said to be an unbiased estimate of the population mean. It can be shown that if the sampling is

repeated indefinitely, the sampling distribution of the mean will tend to a smooth curve with the same mean as the population of individual values but a smaller standard deviation. In fact, it can be shown mathematically that this standard deviation of the mean is

$$SD \text{ (mean SBP)} = SD \text{ (SBP)}/\sqrt{} \text{ (sample size } n).$$

Therefore, for samples of size 4 and SD = 15,

$$SD \text{ (mean SBP)} = 15 / \sqrt{4} = 15 / 2 = 7.5$$

and the spread of the sampling distribution for this mean is half the spread of the population distribution of the individual SBP values.

It should be remembered that the complete sampling distribution exists only in theory. In practice there is only a single sample mean which is one observation from the distribution. The narrower the spread of this distribution, the nearer the single value available is likely to be to the truth. This spread, represented by the standard deviation of the sampling distribution, indicates how precise a single sample mean is as an estimate. It indicates the likely error in the estimate. Largely because of this, the standard deviations of sampling distributions are almost universally referred to as standard errors (SEs):

$$SE \text{ (mean)} = SD \text{ (mean)} = SD \text{ (original variable)}/\sqrt{n}$$

Thus the standard error of a mean (or of any other estimate) indicates its precision as an estimate. For samples of 100 values ($n = 100$), the sample means would have had a standard deviation of $15/10 = 1.5$, which is a very small spread. The estimate can be made as precise as required by increasing the sample size.

Therefore the standard error of a sample mean is

$$SE \text{ (mean)} = SD \text{ (original variable)}/\sqrt{(sample\ size)}$$
$$= SD/\sqrt{n} \qquad (17.1)$$

which can be deduced mathematically by the application of some fairly general rules. The same techniques can be used to deduce the standard errors of regression coefficients, differences between means, and so on. In fact, appropriate standard errors can be obtained for any value calculated from a sample.

Confidence intervals

Although the estimate is chosen as the 'best guess' at the population value, usually it will not be exactly right. In practice, the standard error and the estimate are used to obtain a range of values defining an interval on the original variable scale which will contain the unknown population value with some chosen probability.

Fortunately, for reasonably large samples ($n > 30$) and some fairly mild assumptions, the sampling distributions of many common estimates are close to normal. This means, for example, that the sample value will only fall outside the range

true value $-$ 1.96 SEs to true value $+$ 1.96 SEs

for 5 per cent of such samples. With some algebra it follows that the interval

estimate $-$ 1.96 SEs to estimate $+$ 1.96 SEs

will include the true population value in 95 per cent of such samples. This means that one can be 95 per cent confident that an interval calculated in this way will include the true population value. Other confidence intervals, such as 99 per cent, are obtained by taking the appropriate centile of the standard normal distribution instead of 1.96.

These calculations require the population standard deviation of the original variable. Since this is rarely known, it is necessary to use the sample value as an estimate. This does not matter very much for large samples, but it may if the sample size falls below about $n = 30$. As a result, the standard normal distribution cannot be used for small samples. It is necessary to use what is known as the t distribution. The centiles of the normal distribution, such as $u_{0.975} = 1.96$, have to be replaced by the equivalent centiles of the t distribution appropriate to the sample size. None the less, the appropriate 97.5 centiles are all close to 2. These centiles are commonly denoted by $t_{f, 0.975}$, where f is known as the number of degrees of freedom and represents the amount of information available to estimate the population standard deviation used in the calculation of the standard error. The degrees of freedom are invariably the total sample size minus the number of values estimated from the sample. It can be seen from tables (e.g. Lindley and Miller (1964) or statistical programs such as GLIM) that

$$t_{20, \ 0.975} = 2.09$$

$$t_{30, \ 0.975} = 2.04$$

$$t_{40, \ 0.975} = 2.02$$

$$t_{60, \ 0.975} = 2.00$$

and, only when the number of degrees of freedom approaches 500 do the 97.5 centiles of the two distributions become the same to two decimal places:

$$t_{473, \ 0.975} = 1.96 = u_{0.975}.$$

However, for most practical purposes, once there are more than 60 degrees of freedom, the t distribution can be assumed to be the same as the normal distribution.

Sample sizes for estimation

The sample size for an estimation is determined by the precision required. The usual approach to defining precision is to stipulate that there should be a high probability (often 95 per cent) that the estimate is close to the true value. Close is usually defined as within some small percentage, such as 5 per cent, of the correct value. Clearly, this means that the approximate size of the value being estimated must be known.

Consider the problem of estimating a population mean from a sample. Ninety-five per cent of means from unbiased samples will be within 1.96 SEs of the true value. This implies that if $1.96 \times SE$ is less than 5 per cent of the true value, then the precision will be as specified.

If M represents the value to be estimated, then the sample will be large enough if

$$1.96 \times SD / \sqrt{n} \leq 0.05 \times M,$$

i.e. if

$$n \geq (1.96)^2 \times SD^2 / (0.05 \times M)^2 \qquad (17.2)$$

With this sample size one can be 95 per cent confident that the estimate will be within 5 per cent of the true value.

Example

To estimate the mean systolic blood pressure for men between 30 and 60 years old to within 5 per cent with 95 per cent confidence.

From previous work it is known that the true value M is about 150 mmHg and the standard deviation is about 15. Using eqn (17.2), this means that the sample size needs to be

$$n \geq (1.96 \times 15)^2 / (0.05 \times 150)^2 = 16.$$

This is very small, so that 5 per cent is not a very stringent requirement in this context. Requiring a higher degree of precision (for example that the estimate must be accurate to 1 per cent) implies a sample size of

$$n \geq (1.96 \times 15)^2 / (0.01 \times 150)^2 = 385.$$

Significance tests

The probability that a sample 95 per cent confidence interval will not contain the true population value is less than or equal to 5 per cent. This means that, for any hypothetical population value, it is possible to judge whether the sample estimate is surprisingly far from it by seeing whether it falls outside the 95 per cent confidence interval. If a value hypothesized for the population falls outside the interval, then the probability of the sample giving this interval and hence the estimate, assuming that the hypothesized population value is correct, is less than 5 per cent. Therefore

$$p \ (\text{estimate} \mid \text{population value}) \leq 0.05$$

or, as it is frequently written, ($p < 0.05$).

Assuming that the hypothesis to be tested is true, a significance test is a procedure that can be used to calculate the probability p of sample values occurring as far or further from those expected as those actually observed. Some value, called a test statistic, that has a known sampling distribution is calculated from the sample. This is frequently the number of standard errors that an estimate is from the population value expected from the hypothesis. The p value can then be obtained from the sampling distribution of the test statistic. If the p value is less than 5 per cent, then the sample value is taken as evidence significant at the 5 per cent level that the hypothesis is untrue.

In 5 per cent of tests using a 5 per cent significance level, surprising values of the test statistic will occur even though the hypothesis is correct. This error—concluding that a hypothesis is not true when it is—is known as a type 1 error. Therefore, if a test uses a 5 per cent level of significance, there will be a 5 per cent risk when using the test that a type I error will occur. Notice that the risk may be set as required in a test by altering the level of significance to be used. Finally, there is a risk that even when the hypothesis is false, samples may be obtained that produce unsurprising values of the test statistic. This leads to the error of accepting as true a hypothesis that is actually false; this is a type II error. The size of sample needed to give a reliable test of some hypothesis must take both types of error into account. Sample size calculations for significance testing are discussed in a later section.

There is a close relationship between confidence interval calculations and significance tests. Any hypothesis that predicts a population value can be tested by inspecting whether the value falls inside the appropriate confidence interval. Using the 99 per cent confidence interval, this is equivalent to $p < 0.01$.

Suppose that a study is estimating the population mean systolic blood pressure for adult males. For a moderately large sample ($n > 30$) with mean 120 mmHg and standard error 2.0, the 95 per cent confidence interval is

$$120 \pm 1.96 \times 2.0 \quad \text{or} \quad 116.1–123.9$$

If the true value is 130, the probability of results as extreme as 120 is less than 5 per cent since 130 is well outside the interval. The estimated 120 mmHg is significantly different from 130 mmHg at the 5 per cent level because it is surprisingly far from the population value of 130 ($p < 0.05$). It is reasonably clear that the sample is from a population with a lower mean value than 130 mmHg. However, it must be remembered that, by definition, 5 per cent of the confidence intervals will exclude the true value. This is the type I error above. If this system is used in making decisions, they will be wrong 5 per cent of the time.

Although the use of confidence intervals is quite sufficient, it is common to calculate the p values directly. As implied above, this is most frequently done by calculating, as a test statistic, how many standard errors separate the estimate and the hypothetical value:

$$\frac{\text{estimate} - \text{hypothetical value}}{\text{SE of the estimate}}.$$

What centile this is of the t or standard normal distribution is then determined from tables which, for a given value of the variable, give the probability of values below it, say P.

The probability of values equal to or above that obtained is $1 - P$, which is the probability of surprisingly high values. Surprisingly low values will also be possible, so that the probability of values as surprising as that observed will be twice $1 - P$ or

$$p = 2(1 - P).$$

These are the basic concepts of statistics. It is now necessary to consider how these techniques are used to answer practical questions from real data.

Types of analyses
Measured outcomes
Simple regression
Figure 17.21 shows some data on chromosome abnormalities and blood lead levels from female workers in a battery factory. The research question was: Does lead exposure damage chromosomes?

If it is assumed that current lead levels in the blood reflect overall exposure, the question can be expressed as follows. In the population of all such subjects as these, is the number of chromosome abnormalities higher, on average, in those with high blood lead levels than it is in those with low levels?

This is the same as asking: Is the trend in these points sufficiently non-horizontal to indicate a real trend in the population?

To answer the question it is necessary to fit the least-squares regression line and test whether the sample regression coefficient is consistent with a true value of zero. Alternatively, it is simply necessary to show that a non-zero trend model fits the data

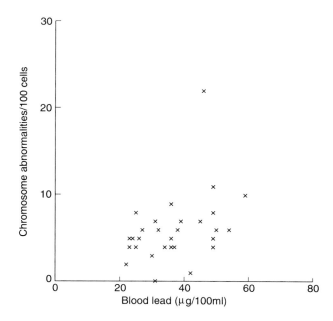

Fig. 17.21 Chromosome abnormalities per 100 cells and blood lead levels. *Source*: Forni and Sciame 1975.

significantly better than a horizontal line model to demonstrate that the apparent trend is unlikely to be due to chance.

To demonstrate how a regression line is fitted, a number of algebraic definitions are needed. The variance of a set of values has already been introduced as

sum for all values (value − mean value)^2/(number of values − 1)

which, for values of a variable y, becomes

$$\text{sum } (y - \bar{y})^2/(n - 1) \tag{17.3}$$

where $\bar{y}$ (pronounced y bar) is the conventional abbreviation for the mean of a sample of y values. The sum of squared deviations construction is so common in statistical calculations that it is convenient to have a special notation. In this chapter we shall use

$$Syy = \text{sum } (y - \bar{y})^2 \tag{17.4}$$

Although it will not be used here, many statistical texts use Σ to denote summation. In that notation, the above becomes:

$$Syy = \Sigma(y - \bar{y})^2$$

For an x variable, the equivalent is

$$Sxx = \text{sum } (x - \bar{x})^2 \tag{17.5}$$

and finally

$$Sxy = \text{sum } (y - \bar{y})(x - \bar{x}). \tag{17.6}$$

The sum of squared deviations minimized when we fit a regression line is essentially Sdd, but it is more often called the residual sum of squares (RSS) or Sr.

In general

$$Sr = \text{sum } (y - \text{value predicted by the model})^2$$

which, for a simple regression line, becomes

$$Sr = \text{sum } (y - \text{height of line})^2.$$

Now, to fit a regression line of the form

$$y = a + bx$$

to describe the trend in chromosome abnormalities as blood lead increases means choosing the most appropriate values for a and b. The principle of least squares means that a and b are required to make the sum of the squared deviations Sr a minimum. For this line the residual sum of squares is

$$Sr = \text{sum } (y - a - bx)^2. \qquad (17.7)$$

It can be shown mathematically that this is a minimum when

$$b = Sxy/Sxx \qquad (17.8)$$

and

$$a = \bar{y} - b\bar{x}. \qquad (17.9)$$

The minimum value of Sr when a and b take these values is

$$Sr = Syy - Sxy^2/Sxx. \qquad (17.10)$$

The residual sum of squares is the basic measure of how well a model, in this case $y = a + bx$, fits the data. If points are widely scattered about the line, Sr will be large, indicating a bad fit. If the points fall more or less on a straight line, Sr will be small, indicating that a straight-line model fits the data well.

The variance of the deviations about the line is called the residual variance and is denoted by

$$s^2 = Sr/(n - 2) \qquad (17.11)$$

where $n - 2$ is the number of degrees of freedom and is the amount of information available to estimate the residual variance. This is the number of observations (or points on the plot) minus the number of parameters in the model that need to be estimated. Here it was necessary to estimate two parameters, the intercept and the slope.

The residual variance can be used to calculate the standard error of b which is

$$SE(b) = \sqrt{(s^2/Sxx)}. \qquad (17.12)$$

For the data on women battery factory workers, where y is the number of chromosome abnormalities per 100 cells and x is the blood lead level in μg/100 ml, the values required in the analysis to fit a simple regression line are

$$n = 30 \qquad \bar{y} = 5.97 \qquad \bar{x} = 36.37$$

with

$$Syy = 432.97 \qquad Sxx = 3302.96 \qquad Sxy = 460.37$$

Therefore the estimates of a and b are

$$b = Sxy/Sxx = 460.37/3302.96 = 0.14$$

$$a = \bar{y} - b\bar{x} = 5.97 - 0.14 \times 36.37 = 0.90.$$

From eqn (17.10)

$$Sr = 432.97 - 460.37^2/3302.96 = 368.80$$

so that

$$s^2 = Sr/(n - 2) = 368.80/28 = 13.17$$

and

$$SE\ (b) = \sqrt{(s^2/Sxx)} = 0.06.$$

Therefore the line giving the 'best' representation of the apparent trend in the least-squares sense is

$$ABS = 0.90 + 0.14 \times BL$$

where ABS denotes chromosome abnormalities and BL denotes blood lead levels. If it is assumed that the sampling distribution of b is sufficiently near normal, the 95 per cent confidence interval for the 'true' value of the slope is

$$0.14 - 1.96\ (0.06) \quad \text{to} \quad 0.14 + 1.96\ (0.06)$$

or

$$0.02 \text{ to } 0.16.$$

Since this does not include zero, it is a reasonably strong indication that the population trend is not zero (i.e. the observed trend is significantly different from a population value of zero at the 5 per cent level). A sample regression slope could not easily occur this far from zero by chance ($p < 0.05$).

The significance test of the zero-slope hypothesis is performed by calculating how many standard errors the slope 0.14 is from the expected zero, i.e.

$$\frac{\text{observed slope} - \text{expected slope}}{SE\ (\text{slope})} = \frac{0.14 - 0}{0.06} = 2.33$$

which is well above 1.96, as the confidence interval also showed. Therefore there is strong evidence of a trend in the population represented by this sample. Higher numbers of chromosome abnormalities will be found in those individuals who have the higher blood lead levels.

There was one 'outlying' individual with 22 abnormalities on the plot. If the results had been less conclusive, then it might have been wise to repeat the analysis excluding this individual. Her effect on the analysis could then be assessed and the interpretation modified appropriately, but it is not really necessary here. Note that the t distribution should be used for samples this size. The t distribution centile equivalent to the standard normal 1.96 for 28 DF is 2.05 (about 5 per cent higher); however, even if the t value is used, the conclusions are exactly the same.

It is still unclear whether these results really mean that lead in the blood damages chromosomes. Partly for this reason it is customary to describe significant trends as indicating only a real 'association' between the variables, in order to make it clear that the existence of a trend in the population in no way proves a 'causal relationship'. This single finding must be added to the whole body of knowledge on the subject before conclusions can be carried that far.

Apart from tests of the assumptions that the population line is straight and not a curve, that there is a similar residual variance at all x values, and that the underlying distribution is normal, this analysis is complete.

In fact, since any trend is indicative of the relationship—in this case between lead exposure and chromosome abnormalities, whether or not it is straight hardly matters. Whether the residuals have a normal distribution is more crucial since inferences from confidence intervals and significance tests all assume that they do. How to test these assumptions will be discussed later. Meanwhile it is useful to consider how this analysis can be approached in a more general way applicable to most common problems. In some circumstances the question cannot be phrased so that it becomes a test of a single parameter. In those cases the question has to be expressed as a comparison of different models.

In the lead data example the equivalent model comparison is between a model of the form

$$y = a + bx$$

which is a sloping straight line and the model

$$y = a$$

which represents a horizontal line.

If there is a significant trend, then the second model will fit the data significantly worse than the first. How well a model describes data is measured by the residual sum of squares—the smaller Sr, the better the fit. Comparisons of the fits of two models are made by comparing their residual sums of squares.

As should be clear from this example, the more parameters there are in a model, the smaller the residual sum of squares Sr can be made. Choosing the intercept and the slope, two parameters for a sloping line, makes it possible to fit the model closer to the data points than when the fitting process is restricted to choosing one parameter (e.g. the intercept for a horizontal line). For the model

$$y = a + bx$$

the residual sum of squares is

$$Sr = 368.75$$

and the residual variance is

$$s^2 = 13.17.$$

For the horizontal-line model when the intercept (height of the line) is simply the mean of y, the residual sum of squares is

$$Sr = 433.0,$$

i.e. an increase of 64.25.

The increase has one degree of freedom associated with it since one parameter has been dropped from the more complicated model. On the hypothesis that the trend is a chance event in this particular sample, 64.25 is a further estimate of the residual variance. This means that, if the hypothesis is true, $64.25/s^2$ should be about 1.0 since it is the ratio of two estimates of the same variance; the value in this example is $64.25/13.17$ or 4.88.

The numerator, which is the increase in Sr resulting from simplifying the model, has one degree of freedom. The denominator, which is the residual variance from the most complicated model, has $n - 2 = 28$ degrees of freedom. If the 'no-trend' hypothesis is true, then this variance ratio can be shown to have a sampling distribution with a particular mathematical form called the F distribution (in this case with 1 and 28 degrees of freedom). By giving what is known as an F test, this can be used to assess how surprising an observed variance ratio is.

The F distribution of 1 and 28 degrees of freedom is illustrated in Fig. 17.22. The 95th centile of the F distribution is 4.20, and less than 5 per cent of F values calculated from a sample in this way should occur this far above 1.0. This implies that the value of 4.88 is surprisingly large ($p < 0.05$) if the population has no trend. It suggests that the horizontal-line model is incorrect. Surprisingly

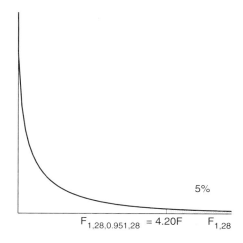

Fig. 17.22 *F* distribution with one and 28 degrees of freedom.

low values can occur, but they have little meaning. If anything, they imply that the model fits the data surprisingly well given the amount of variation present. Generally, they are treated as insignificant.

The interpretation of this analysis is that it is either necessary to assume a freak sample or that the non-zero trend model was necessary to describe this data. In practice it would be taken as reasonably strong evidence that there was a trend in the population. The estimated regression coefficient with a confidence interval should then be obtained to demonstrate the magnitude of the effect.

This model comparison approach to the analysis is best presented in tabular form, giving what is known as an 'analysis of variance' (although it is actually an analysis of residual sums of squares). The analysis is given in Table 17.5 where the residual sum of squares from model 1 is S_1 and the mean square MS is the sum of squares divided by the number of degrees of freedom for a model.

To construct such analysis of variance tables it is only necessary to obtain the residual sum of squares for the two models. A test of the parameters omitted when model 1 is changed to the simpler model 2 is then immediately available as

$$F_{1,28} = (S_2 - S_1)/s^2. \tag{17.13}$$

Since all that is needed for this approach is the residual sum of squares for each model, it is not even necessary to fit them. In practice they are fitted because it is necessary to know the likely magnitudes of the effects, not just whether they do or do not exist.

Non-linear regression

In a given analysis a straight-line trend may well be inadequate; a curved-line trend might fit the data better. To test this a model representing a curved trend is fitted, and the fit is compared with that of a straight-line model. The simplest model for a curved trend is known as a quadratic and takes the form

$$y = a + bx + cx^2$$

In the lead data example, this is equivalent to

$$ABS = intercept + bBL + cBL^2$$

Model		SS	DF	MS	F
1.	Intercept and trend on BL: sloping line	$S_1 = 368.75$	28	$s^2 = 13.17$	
2.	Incercept, but no trend: horizontal line	$S_2 = 433.00$	29		
(2 − 1)	Due to trend	64.25	1	64.25	$F_{1,28} = 64.25/13.17$ $= 4.88$

Table 17.5 Analysis of variance to test for a linear trend in chromosome abnormalities by blood lead (BL) levels

SS, sum of squares; DF, degrees of freedom; MS, mean sum of squares.

where ABS and BL denote chromosome abnormalities and blood lead levels respectively. The model is fitted exactly as before with a, b, and c chosen so that the residual sum of squares is minimized.

The formulae are rather more complicated than for the straight-line model; therefore, although this model can be fitted by hand, it is tedious. It is very easy with a professionally produced package program on a computer, and it is not necessary to know the formulae in detail.

The hypothesis that there is no curvature in the population can be tested very easily by calculating

$$t = \frac{c - \text{expected } c}{\text{SE}(c)} = \frac{c - 0}{\text{SE}(c)}$$

and, since we have fitted three parameters, this has $n - 3$ degrees of freedom where n is the number of data points. The fitted model for the lead data gives

intercept	$a = 2.77$
linear coefficient	$b = 0.03$
quadratic coefficient	$c = 0.0014$ with $\text{SE}(c) = 0.0066$.

Therefore, for the t test of curvature,

$$t = \frac{0.0014 - 0}{0.0066} = 0.2 \text{ with 27 degrees of freedom.}$$

This is very far from the value needed for significance, which is a little above 2.0 ($t_{0.975} = 2.05$ on 27 degrees of freedom). Obviously there is little evidence that the population trend is not a straight line.

Comparing two groups

The above analysis of the lead study data looked at the association between chromosome abnormalities and blood lead levels. However, the current blood lead level may not reflect long-term

exposure. Figure 17.23 compares the individuals from lead-free areas in the factory with those exposed to lead in their work. The values for the exposed individuals appear to be slightly higher with a wider spread. To investigate this more precisely, it is necessary to calculate the mean and standard deviations for the two groups (Table 17.6).

The question becomes: Are the means surprisingly different? This is tested by fitting a model of the form

mean ABS = reference value + group effect.

Taking the 'reference value' as the mean for group 1 (not exposed), the group effect is zero for that group and equal to the difference between the two means for the second group.

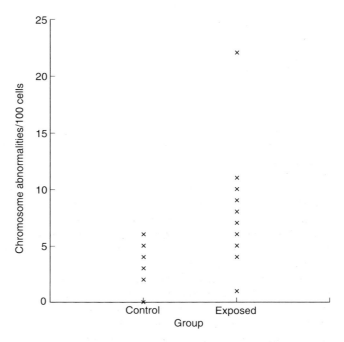

Fig. 17.23 Chromosome abnormalities and exposure group.

Table 17.6 Chromosome abnormalities (ABS) in female battery factory workers by exposure group

	Not exposed	Exposed	All
Number	12 (12)	18 (17)	30 (29)
Mean	4.00 (4.00)	7.28 (6.41)	5.97 (5.41)
SD	1.71 (1.71)	4.36 (2.43)	3.87 (2.44)

The findings when one woman with ABS = 22 was excluded are shown in parentheses.

Fitting this model by least squares is exactly the same as allowing each group to have its own mean:

$$\text{mean ABS} = 4.00 + 0 \qquad \text{for group 1}$$

$$\text{mean ABS} = 4.00 + (7.28 - 4.00) \quad \text{for group 2.}$$

Each mean minimizes the sum of squared deviations within its own group, S_{yy1} and S_{yy2} say, so that the total residual sum of squares $S_r = S_{yy1} + S_{yy2}$ is a minimum.

The variances for the groups separately are calculated as $S_{yy1}/(n_1 - 1)$ for group 1 and $S_{yy2}/(n_2 - 1)$ for group 2. To compare the group means, it is necessary to assume one underlying residual variance. On this assumption, both samples contain information on the residual variance, and the information is pooled as the overall residual sum of squares S_r to estimate it. Therefore the pooled estimate of variance is S_r divided by its degrees of freedom.

The number of degrees of freedom for the above model is $n_1 + n_2 - 2$ because there are $n_1 + n_2$ values in total and two parameters (the two means) have been estimated. Now

$$S_{yy1} = 32.00 \qquad S_{yy2} = 323.61.$$

Therefore

$$S_r = S_{yy1} + S_{yy2} = 355.6$$

and, since $n_1 = 12$ and $n_2 = 18$,

$$s^2 = S_r/(n_1 + n_2 - 2) = 355.6/28 = 12.7. \qquad (17.14)$$

The difference between the means, which is the group 2 effect since the reference value is the group 1 mean, is

$$\text{difference} = 7.28 - 4.00 = 3.28$$

which has the standard error

$$\text{SE (difference)} = \sqrt{[s^2(1/n_1 + 1/n_2)]} \qquad (17.15)$$

$$= \sqrt{[12.7(1/12 + 1/18)]} = 1.33.$$

A significance test of the hypothesis that the population difference is zero is obtained as

$$t = \frac{\text{difference} - \text{hypothesized difference}}{\text{SE (difference)}}$$

$$= \frac{3.28 - 0}{1.33} = 2.47$$

and the probability of values as far from zero as 2.47 occurring by chance, obtained from tables of the t distribution with 28 degrees of freedom, is about 0.02 ($p < 0.05$). The difference is significant at the 5 per cent level ($p < 0.05$) on the assumption that the two samples came from populations with identical variances.

However, the two groups actually have very different SDs and therefore different variances (Table 17.6), and so the assumption should be tested. This is done using a form of the F test. If the population variances are the same, the variances from the two groups are estimating the same thing. In that case their ratio will be an observation from an F distribution and should have a value close to unity. If the hypothesis of equal population variances is false, then the variance ratio will deviate from unity. Whether this gives large or small values depends on which way the variance ratio is calculated: large/small or small/large. Since this is arbitrary, surprisingly small values are just as interesting, in this context, as surprisingly large values.

It is usual to calculate the ratio with the larger variance as the numerator. The probability of F values as high as the calculated ratio is then obtained from tables and doubled to give p, the probability of variances as different as those observed occurring by chance. This means that the probability of values as high as the ratio calculated must be less than 0.025 in order for the probability that variances this different were obtained by chance to be less than 0.05.

The standard deviations of the two groups were 1.71 and 4.36, so that the variance ratio (large/small) is

$$F = (4.36/1.71)^2 = 6.50$$

with $18 - 1 = 17$ and $12 - 1 = 11$ degrees of freedom. The tables show that only 2.5 per cent of values from the $F_{17, 11}$ distribution should occur above 3.33. This implies that our variances are significantly different at the 5 per cent level ($p < 0.05$). The assumption of equal variances is clearly unsafe and some corrective action is required.

In these data the difference between the variances is largely due to one very high value of ABS (22) from an individual in the exposed group. If she is removed (Table 17.6), although the standard deviations are still different, the F value

$$F_{16, 11} = (2.43/1.71)^2 = 2.02$$

is less than the 95th centile of $F_{16, 11}$, which is 2.37. Thus the probability of variances this different by chance is at least 2×0.05 or 0.10. There is now no real evidence of unequal variances and no reason not to perform the standard analysis. The residual sum of squares reduces to 126.12 with 27 degrees of freedom, so that the residual variance becomes 4.67.

The difference between the means is $6.41 - 4.00 = 2.41$, and the standard error of this difference is now

$$\text{SE (difference)} = \sqrt{[4.67(1/12 + 1/17)]} = 0.81.$$

The t test becomes $t = 2.41/0.81 = 2.98$, which is even more significant than before; removing the extreme point has reduced the standard error more than it has the difference.

The above analysis in which a single model is fitted is possible and sufficient because the question of interest can be reduced to a test of a single parameter. However, when several groups have to be compared this is not really possible and the model comparison approach is required.

In a model comparison analysis of these data there are two models. The first is the one assuming that the population means are different:

$$(1) \quad \text{mean ABS} = \text{reference value} + \text{group effect}$$

Table 17.7 Analysis of variance for comparing the mean number of chromosome abnormalities in two groups

Model	RSS	DF	MS	Variance ratio F
1. Groups different	126.12	27	4.67	
2. Groups same	167.03	28		
(2 − 1) Due to difference	40.91	1	40.91	$F_{1,27} = 40.91/4.67 = 8.76$

where the reference value is the group 1 mean. As before, the residual sum of squares for this model is Syy for group 1 plus Syy for group 2. Calling this S_1, we have

$$S_1 = 126.12$$

(omitting the individual with ABS = 22). The residual variance from this model is $s^2 = 4.67$.

The second model, assuming no difference, is

(2) mean ABS = reference value

where the reference value is the overall mean of the two groups estimating the supposedly constant population mean. The residual sum of squares for this model is the value of Syy calculated from both groups combined into one sample. Calling this S_2, we have

$$S_2 = 167.03$$

and the analysis of variance table is as given in Table 17.7. Since $F_{1, 27, 0.99} = 7.68$, this gives a probability of a difference of this magnitude—given the hypothesis of no difference between the populations—of $p < 0.01$. This is the same p value as for $t = 2.98$, which was obtained using the alternative t test of the relevant parameter in a single fitted model. In fact, they are the same test in two different forms.

Comparing three or more groups

Consider data from an Italian study designed to assess the effects of well-publicized hypertension clinics on blood pressure levels in the community (Forni and Sciame 1975). There is some evidence that systolic blood pressure increases with age in a non-linear way. For this reason, the analyses were performed using age groups rather than exact ages. At the beginning of the study, the mean systolic blood pressure (SBP) for males in the control district that had no clinic was as shown in Table 17.8.

There is a tendency for the mean value to increase with age (Fig. 17.24). The SDs are all about the same, and so an assumption of equal variances is reasonable. The appropriate model is

(1) mean SBP = reference value + group effect.

Because it simplifies the interpretation of the fitted parameters, the group 1 mean (men aged 20–29 years) is taken as the 'reference value'. The 'group effects' are then the differences between the mean of that particular group and the group 1 mean (i.e. the reference value). The model then has five parameters:

the reference value (mean for group 1)

the group 2 effect G_2 (mean for group 2 − reference value)

the group 3 effect G_3 (mean for group 3 − reference value)

the group 4 effect G_4 (mean for group 4 − reference value)

the group 5 effect G_5 (mean for group 5 − reference value).

To fit the model, estimates for these five parameters must be obtained as the means and differences implied above with the residual sum of squares Sr and hence the SEs of the parameter estimates. Since the model essentially allows each group to have its own mean, Sr is the sum of the values of Syy obtained separately from each of the groups. Calling this S_1 and its degrees of freedom f_1, where

$$f_1 = (\text{total number of values} - \text{the number of parameters})$$

gives

$$S_1 = 685\,211 \quad \text{with} \quad f_1 = (1440 - 5) = 1435$$

Thus the residual variance is

$$s^2 = 685\,211/1435 = 477.5$$

Table 17.8 Mean systolic blood pressure by age in males from a study of the effect of hypertension clinics

	Age group (years)					
	20–29.9	30–39.9	40–49.9	50–59.9	60+	All
Number	340	303	302	207	288	1440
Mean	141.9	146.0	150.1	149.2	156.9	148.5
SD	20.4	19.9	22.7	21.4	24.7	22.4

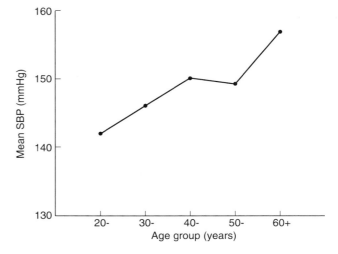

Fig. 17.24 Mean systolic blood pressure (SBP) by age in males, from a study of hypertension clinics.

Table 17.9 Analysis of variance comparing mean systolic blood pressures in five age groups

Model	SS	DF	MS	F
1. Groups different	S_1 = 685 211	1435	s^2 = 477.5	
2. One overall mean	S_2 = 723 110	1439		
(2 – 1) Due to group differences	$S_2 - S_1$ = 37 899	4	9475	19.8

The simpler model, where differences are assumed to be chance, is simply one overall mean:

$$(2) \text{ mean SBP} = \text{reference value.}$$

with the overall mean as the reference value that represents a single horizontal line. How well this fits the data is measured by the residual sum of squares about the overall mean. This is simply S_{yy} from all 1440 individuals treated as one sample, which is S_2 = 723 110. The analysis of variance is given in Table 17.9.

F values of 19.8 with 4 and 1435 degrees of freedom are extremely unlikely to occur by chance ($p \ll 0.01$). The sample sizes are so large that the small but consistent changes in SBP are highly significant. A linear trend model

$$(3) \text{ mean SBP} = \text{intercept} + b \text{ age,}$$

taking individuals in the same group as having the same age, gives a test of whether the population trend is curved in any way.

When the data are treated as one large sample and a simple regression line is fitted, the residual sum of squares from eqn (17.10) is

$$S_3 = S_{yy} - S_{xy}^2/S_{xx}$$

and

$$S_3 = 688\ 123$$

for these data. Since two parameters have been fitted, the number of degrees of freedom is

$$1440 - 2 = 1438.$$

The analysis of variance is given in Table 17.10. Since F with 3 and 1435 degrees needs to exceed 2.60 for significance at the 5 per cent level, there is little evidence that a linear trend is not an adequate representation. The estimated slope is

$$b = S_{xy}/S_{xx} = 0.68 \text{ mmHg/year}$$

Table 17.10 Analysis of variance testing whether mean systolic blood pressure follows a linear trend over five age groups.

Model	SS	DF	MS	F
1. Groups different (any trend)	685 211	1435	s^2 = 477.5	
3. Linear trend	688 123	1438		
(3 – 1) Due to non-linearity	2912	3	970.7	203

and, from eqn (17.12),

$$\text{SE}(b) = 0.08.$$

The analysis shows that the means differ significantly and that the way that they differ is adequately represented by a linear trend. This implies that the slope of the linear trend is significantly non-zero and the direct test is

$$t = 0.68/0.08 = 8.5 \ (p < 0.01).$$

Comparing groups allowing for trends

Consider the problem of comparing lung function, in particular FEV, in smokers and non-smokers. The underlying question is: Does smoking affect lung function?

It appears that the study simply requires samples of smokers and non-smokers to test whether their respective populations differ. However, for an efficient analysis, the samples need to be as similar as possible in other respects so that, for example, a preponderance of males in the smokers will not bias the comparison. It is possible to avoid this bias by restricting the study to one sex. Unfortunately this approach cannot be used to avoid bias due to such variables as height. Some height differences will inevitably occur. It is possible to ensure that the groups have the same range of heights, which avoids the problem of systematic bias. None the less the variation in lung function is increased as a result of height differences. This decreases the sensitivity with which group differences can be detected.

Quantitative variables that interfere with group comparisons in this way are known as covariates, and analyses involving them are known as analyses of covariance. The analysis of covariance uses regression techniques to deduce from the data in this example (i) whether FEV changes with height in the same way for both groups, and, if it does, (ii) what FEV differences would be seen between smokers and non-smokers if they all had the same height. Four main circumstances can arise, as illustrated in Fig. 17.25.

The biases illustrated in Fig. 17.25 can be avoided by designing the study to keep the height distributions of the groups similar. In practice it is more important to remove the variation due to covariate differences in order to increase the sensitivity with which the analysis estimates and tests the group differences.

If the trend lines in two groups are parallel, the groups differ by the same amount at all heights. As long as both groups have the same range of height, it is possible to predict how they will differ without specifying a height. To investigate this it is necessary to compare the fit of parallel and non-parallel models. Assuming straight-line trends, an assumption that would need testing in practice, the models are:

1. Non-parallel

   mean FEV = group intercept + group slope × height

(i.e. each group has its own slope and intercept)

2. Parallel

   mean FEV = group intercept + common slope × height

(i.e. each group has its own intercept, but the same slope).

If there are $n = n_1 + N_2$ points in total, the residual sum of squares for model 1 is

$$S_1 = \text{sum for both groups of } (S_{yy} - S_{xy}^2/S_{xx})$$

with $n - 4$ degrees of freedom since four parameters have been

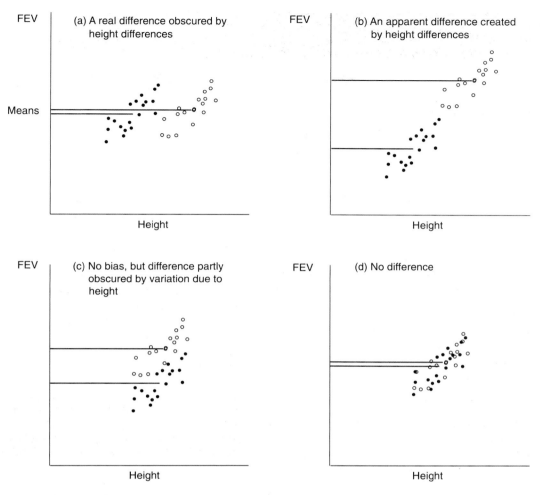

Fig. 17.25 Two-group scatter diagrams to illustrate the ways in which a covariate may influence a group comparison.

fitted (two slopes and two intercepts). The residual variance about this model is $s^2 = S_1/(n - 4)$.

The residual sum of squares from model 2 is

$$S_2 = \text{sum } Syy - (\text{sum } Sxy)^2/\text{sum } Sxx$$

where 'sum' implies that the Syy, Sxx, and Sxy are calculated for each group separately and then summed. S_2 has $n - 3$ degrees of freedom since in this model only three parameters are required (two intercepts and one slope). The test of parallelism, from eqn (17.13), is

$$F_{1,\ n-4} = (S_2 - S_1)/s^2$$

which is compared with the appropriate F distribution centile.

If it seems reasonable to accept that the population trends are parallel, the estimated slope is, from eqn (17.8),

$$b = \text{sum } Sxy/\text{sum } Sxx$$

and, from eqn (17.12),

$$SE(b) = \sqrt{(s^2/\text{sum } Sxx)}.$$

The group difference allowing for height is then constant for all heights and most easily calculated as the difference between the intercepts, i.e.

mean FEV difference $-$ slope $\times$ mean height difference.

Although the algebra is beyond the scope of this text, it can be shown that the variance of this is

$$\text{var(diff)} = s^2[1/n_1 + 1/n_2 + (\text{mean height difference}^2/\text{sum } Sxx)]$$

from which we can obtain

$$SE(\text{diff}) = \sqrt{(\text{var(diff)})}$$

which gives us a t test of the group difference allowing for height.

For more complex situations with several groups and possibly more than one covariate, the group differences are more easily tested by model comparison. Considering the single covariate case to avoid excessive complications, a third model is fitted assuming that all intercepts and slopes are the same in the population. This means that only one intercept and one slope need to be estimated. To fit them the groups are ignored and all the data combined as one. The model is

3. Coincident trend lines

mean FEV = intercept + slope $\times$ height.

Table 17.11 Construction of analysis of covariance table for comparing groups allowing for the interfering effect of a covariate

Model	SS	DF	MS	F
1. Non-parallel	S_1	$n-4$	$s^2 = S_1(n-4)$	
2. Parallel	S_2	$n-3$		
(2 – 1) Due to non-parellelism	$S_2 - S_1$	1		$F_{1,n-4} = (S_2 - S_1)/s^2$
3. Same intercept and slope	S_3	$n-2$		
(3 – 2) Due to group differences	$S_3 - S_2$	1		$F_{1,n-4} = (S_3 - S_2)/s^2$

The residual sum of squares from this model is

$$S_3 = \mathrm{S}yy \text{ all data} - (\mathrm{S}xy \text{ all data})^2/\mathrm{S}xx \text{ all data}$$

with $n-2$ degrees of freedom. The test for group differences is again an F test performed by obtaining the difference between the Sr for the two models and dividing by the residual variance obtained from the most complex model, in this case model 1 as in eqn (17.13):

$$F_{1, n-4} = (S_3 - S_2)/s^2.$$

When this is expressed as an analysis of variance (Table 17.11), it is easier to see how this approach can be generalized to more than two groups.

Example Mean FEV values were obtained for 50 males of whom five were regular smokers (Table 17.12). The smokers have slightly lower FEV values than the non-smokers, but the comparison makes no allowance for differences in height. In fact the mean heights are different, with the smokers being slightly shorter on average. The analysis is given in Table 17.13.

Since F values will exceed unity for surprising values, and both these F values are less than unity, there is no evidence that the trends have different slopes or that the smokers and non–smokers in general differ on the FEV scale.

Groups in a cross-classification

The effects of intervention in an Italian hypertension study (Forni and Sciame 1975) were assessed at the end of a five-year period. Samples of males and females were obtained from the control and intervention areas. The mean systolic blood pressure values for those aged 60 years and over are given in Table 17.14. This is a 2×2 classification because the table has two rows and two columns. The groups are defined by the categorical variables sex in one direction and treatment in the other. For historic reasons variables used to classify individuals are known as factors and their values, the actual categories, are known as levels.

To assess the effects of intervention, it is necessary to determine whether the difference between the intervention and control areas is the same in both sexes. If it is, an overall estimate of the effect using data from both sexes is required. This must then be tested against zero to assess whether the hypothetical population of such individuals treated in this way would show a non–zero effect. If the effects are different for the two sexes, they have to be estimated and tested for each sex separately.

Figure 17.26 shows that the intervention means are well below

Table 17.13 Analysis of covariance comparing FEV in cigarette smokers and non-smokers allowing for height differences

Model	MS	DF	SS	F
1. Non-parallel trends with height	12.91	46	$s^2 = 0.28$	
2. Parallel trends	12.99	47		
(2 – 1) Due to non-parallelism	0.08	1	0.08	$F<1$
3. Same intercept	13.03	48		
(3 – 2) Due to group differences	0.04	1	0.04	$F<1$

Table 17.12 Mean FEV values for 50 males by smoking behaviour together with mean height in inches

	Non-smokers	Smokers
Number	45	5
Mean	3.34	3.23
SD	2.33	2.83
Mean height	70.6	69.0

Table 17.14 Mean systolic blood pressures by sex and intervention group of subjects in a hypertension study

	Area	
	Control	Intervention
Male		
Number	200	223
Mean	158.5	150.1
SD	24.2	21.0
Female		
Number	191	283
Mean	167.4	154.7
SD	27.5	21.5

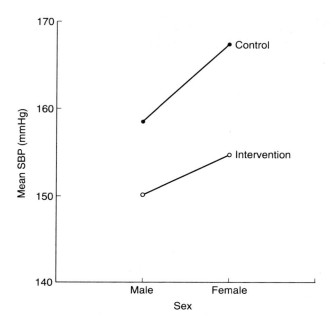

Fig. 17.26 Mean systolic blood pressure (SBP) versus sex and treatment group from a study of hypertension.

those of the equivalent control groups. The females have consistently higher values than the males, and there is a slight suggestion that the difference between intervention and control groups is greater in females. This makes the lines joining the sample means non-parallel.

Two models must be fitted to test this non-parallelism or interaction between the effects of treatment and sex. These are a non-parallel model, where each group has it own mean, and a model where the population means are constrained to fall on parallel lines.

In Fig. 17.26 the parameter representing the deviation from parallelism is the difference between the control–intervention interval for the females and that for the males. Consequently if T is the treatment effect in the males (i.e. the control mean − the intervention group mean) and $T + I$ is the equivalent effect in the females, then I is the deviation from parallelism. Because it represents an influence of the factor sex on the treatment effect (cf. synergy and antagonism in pharmacology), it is often referred to as an interaction. The sex effect (S say) is taken as the difference between the sexes in the intervention group. The model is

(1) mean SBP = reference value + sex effect + treatment effect

which represent four equations for the four sex–treatment combinations:

male intervention	mean	=	rv
male control	mean	=	$rv + T$
female intervention	mean	=	$rv + S$
female control	mean	=	$rv + S + T + I$

The estimate of the interaction can be calculated using

$\hat{I}$ = (control mean − intervention mean) females
    − (control mean − intervention mean) males

which, when the data are substituted, gives

$$(167.4 - 154.7) - (158.5 - 150.1) = 12.7 - 8.4 = 4.3$$

The Sr from this model is

$$S_1 = \text{sum of } Syy \text{ from the four groups} = 488\ 486.2$$

with $n - 4$ degrees of freedom where n is the total number of subjects in all four groups and 4 is subtracted since four parameters need to be estimated. Therefore the residual variance is

$$s^2 = S_1/(n - 4) = 488\ 486.2/893 = 547.0$$

which can be used to obtain a standard error for $\hat{I}$:

$$\text{SE}(\hat{I}) = \sqrt{[s^2(1/n_1 + 1/n_2 + 1/n_3 + 1/n_4)]} = 3.16.$$

Therefore, a test of the hypothesis that the true deviation from parallelism is zero is

$$t = (\hat{I} - 0)/\text{SE}(\hat{I}) = 4.3/3.16 = 1.36.$$

Since there are 893 degrees of freedom, the t distribution is almost the same as the standard normal distribution (Fig. 17.20). This means that the value would have to exceed 1.96 for significance at the 5 per cent level. Since it does not, there is little evidence of an interaction. The effect of intervention, if any, is the same for both sexes.

The parallel-line model is

(2) mean SBP = reference value + sex effect + treatment effect.

Unfortunately there is no simple formula for Sr from this model, and the analysis cannot easily be performed without a statistical package on a computer. When there are only two treatment groups, a technique due to Yates (described very thoroughly by Snedecor and Cochran (1967)) using averages of the mean differences weighted according to the group sizes can be used. However, it is laborious and not very general. The Sr from this model, S_2 say, will have $n - 3$ degrees of freedom. The three fitted parameters will be the reference mean, the average difference between the sexes, and one treatment effect averaged over both sexes. The effects can be tested using

$$t = \text{estimate}/\text{SE(estimate)}$$

or, for the generality required for comparing several groups, by fitting models without them. To test the treatment effect it is necessary to fit

(3) mean SBP = rv + sex effect

with S$r = S_3$ and $n - 2$ degrees pf freedom. The F test for the treatment effect is then

$$F_{1, n - 4} = (S_3 - S_2)/s^2.$$

Exactly the same procedure can be used to test the sex effect. The full analysis of variance is given in Table 17.15.

Example The actual analysis for the Italian systolic blood pressure data is given in Table 17.16. Since the 95th centile $F_{1,\ 893}$ is 3.84, there is no evidence of interaction. The other two F values are highly significant, indicating that the differences between both the treatment groups and the sexes are highly significant ($p < 0.001$).

The treatment effect was estimated using model 2 and was found to be 10.6 with SE 1.58. This means that, all else being equal, individuals receiving the second treatment (the intervention)

Table 17.15 Analysis of variance comparing means in a two-way classification

Model	SS	DF	MS	F
1. With interaction	S_1	$n - 4$	$s^2 = S_1/(n - 4)$	
2. No interaction	S_2	$n - 3$		
(2 – 1) Due to interaction	$S_2 - S_1$	1	$S_2 - S_1$	$F_{1,n-4} = (S_2 - S_1)/s^2$
3. No treatment effect	S_3	$n - 2$		
(3 – 2) Due to treatment	$S_3 - S_2$	1	$S_3 - S_2$	$F_{1,n-4} = (S_3 - S_2)/s^2$
4. No sex effect	S_4	$n - 2$		
(4 – 2) Due to sex	$S_4 - S_2$	1	$S_4 - S_2$	$F_{1,n-4} = (S_4 - S_2)/s^2$

will be on average 10.6 mmHg below the control group. The approximate 95 per cent confidence interval for the 'true' effect of intervention is estimate ± 2 SEs, which gives −13.76 to −7.44. The 'true' difference between the sexes is estimated in a similar way, showing females to be higher on average by 6.5 mmHg with an approximate 95 per cent confidence interval of 6.5 ± 1.57 mmHg.

The general principles of the above analyses apply to much more complicated situations. A study design may lead to cross-classifications with many more than two factors. Any of the factors may have more than two levels. As well as a cross-classification, it may be necessary to allow for one or more covariates in the analysis. Even so the pattern of the analysis is more or less the same. A computer can be used to obtain the appropriate residual sums of squares together with estimated parameters representing the group differences of interest and their standard errors.

Repeated or paired measurements

Repeated observations are made on the same subjects when changes over time are of interest. In addition, subjects may be matched in pairs or larger groups to increase the precision of an investigation.

An important reason for performing analyses using covariates or interfering factors is to explain and remove some of the variation observed in the response variable and thus increase the precision of the analysis. In comparisons of a treatment with a control, the main source of variation is between the individuals within the groups. There may be a clear difference between the means of the control and treatment groups, but the degree of overlap among individual values may well mean that the observed difference cannot be distinguished from possible chance effects.

In certain circumstances it is possible to use each individual as his or her own control or, as in studies of twins, there may be a very well-defined pairing. This means that the part of the response unique to the individual (or the pair) appears in both the control and the treatment measurement and cancels out when the difference is calculated. As Fig. 17.27 shows, the consistent way in which the lines joining paired points slope upward gives a much stronger impression of a genuine treatment effect than the points alone.

The questions dictating which models need to be fitted and compared are as follows.

(i) Is the effect of treatment the same for all subjects? That is, are the population lines parallel?

(ii) Assuming the effect is the same for all, is it non-zero? That is, are the population lines non-horizontal?

The first question cannot be answered if, as is usual, there is only one measurement for each subject within a group. In a non-

Table 17.16 Analysis of variance comparing mean systolic blood pressure in groups classified by sex and treatment

Model	SS	DF	MS	F
1. With interaction	488 486.2	893	$s^2 = 547.0$	
2. No interaction	489 499.2	894		
(2 – 1) Due to interaction	1013.0	1	1013.0	$F_{1,893} = 1.85$
3. No treatment	514 316.2	895		
(3 – 2) Due to treatment	24 817.0	1	24 817.0	$F_{1,893} = 45.4$
4. No sex	498 866.2	895		
(4 – 2) Due to sex	9367.0	1	9367.0	$F_{1,893} = 17.1$

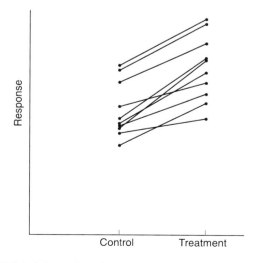

Fig. 17.27 Paired observations plotted against treatment category.

Table 17.17 Analysis of variance for paired measurements

Model	SS	DF	MS	F
1. Parallel lines	S_1	$n-1$	s^2	
2. Horizontal lines	S_2	n		
(2 – 1) Due to non-parallelism	$S_2 - S_1$	1	$S_2 - S_1$	$F_{1, n-1} = (S_2 - S_1)/s^2$

parallel-line model every pair of points has its own line, which fits them exactly, and there are no deviations. This means that there is no information about the underlying variation and therefore inferences cannot be made about the population. To address this particular question, it is necessary to replicate some of the measurements.

To answer the second question it is necessary to fit a set of parallel lines to the pairs of points. The model is

(1) mean $Y = rv$ + subject effect + treatment effect

where the 'treatment effect' is actually the mean of the differences between treatment and control. The subject effects represent the heights of the lines in Fig. 17.27. It is not necessary to estimate these effects since they are included in the model to keep them out of the residual sum of squares and hence reduce the residual variance. There are $2n$ points from n subjects; the model requires n parameters for the subjects and one parameter for the treatment group difference. Thus the residual sum of squares S_1 has $2n - (n + 1) = n - 1$ degrees of freedom.

The model appropriate to the hypothesis that the treatment has no effect is

(2) mean $Y = rv$ + subject effect

which is simply a set of horizontal lines. The model requires one parameter for each subject, so the residual sum of squares S_2 has $2n - n = n$ degrees of freedom. The analysis of variance is given in Table 17.17.

This is a very simple example. In practice, there may well be subpopulations such as sex represented in the sample, and it will be necessary to check that effects are the same in each. There will frequently be more than two treatment groups.

The model comparison approach can be extended quite simply to handle both situations. However, it does need quite sophisticated computing facilities.

In this simplest of cases, the test of the treatment effect can be expressed as what is known as the paired t test. Denoting the treatment–control difference for each subject by d, we have

treatment effect = mean d

and the test of the estimate against zero is

$$t = \text{mean } d \bigg/ \sqrt{(s_d^2 / n)}$$

where s_d is the standard deviation of the n differences.

Example In an investigation of the accuracy of blood pressure measurements, two measurements of systolic blood pressure were taken about 5 minutes apart. These replicated readings ought to differ in a purely random way unless the process of measurement affects the value. The comparison here is not between two treatments, but between the first and second readings. The mean values are given in Table 17.18. If these are treated as two independent groups, the apparent decrease is far from significant.

Table 17.19 gives the analysis of variance obtained by fitting the models with subject parameters to take account of the pairing. The F value on 1 and 9 degrees of freedom for testing the effect is 4.55. The 95th centile of this F distribution is $F_{1, 9, 0.95} = 5.12$ and the 90th centile is 3.35; hence it can be deduced that $0.05 < p \leqslant 0.10$. The model incorporating a reading effect fits better but not startlingly so. The evidence is ambiguous. It is probably necessary to repeat the investigation with a larger sample before coming to a conclusion as to the existence or otherwise of a reading effect.

Treating the analysis as a straight paired t test, the mean difference is

$$d = 5.55 \ (\text{1st} - \text{2nd reading})$$

and the residual sum of squares of the differences about their mean is

$$S_{dd} = 598.6$$

with 9 degrees of freedom. Therefore the variance of the differences is

$$S_d^2 = 598.6/9 = 66.5$$

Table 17.18 Means of paired blood pressure readings

	First reading	Second reading
Number	10	10
Mean	157.6	152.1
SD	17.0	17.0

Table 17.19 Analysis of variance to test for a change over time in duplicate systolic blood pressure readings

Model	SS	DF	MS	F
1. Reading effect	299.3	9	33.25	
2. No reading effect	450.5	10		
(2 – 1) Due to reading effect	151.2	1	151.2	$F_{1,9} = 4.55$

and

$$t = d \Big/ \mathrm{SE}(d) = 5.5 \Big/ \sqrt{(66.5/10)} = 2.13.$$

This must be compared with the 97.5th centile of the t distribution with nine degrees of freedom, which is 2.26. Thus, as for the F test, p obtained in this way is greater than 0.05. In fact this t value is the square root of the above F value $(2.26^2 = 5.12)$, illustrating that in this case F and t are effectively the same test and will always produce the same answer.

Sample size calculations for comparing means

Sample sizes for significance tests of means are calculated in much the same way as they are for estimation (see the section on sample sizes for estimation) with one extra complication. The probability of accepting an incorrect hypothesis, i.e. a type II error, must be taken into account. Since the standard error of the test statistic is a function of the sample size n and the residual variance, which must be known or estimated, the calculation amounts to solving for n

$$\frac{\text{smallest interesting value of test statistic—value expected if hypothesis is true}}{\text{standard error of test statistic.}} \geq Za + Zb$$

The values Za and Zb are centiles of the standard normal distribution and are determined by the size of the type I and type II errors considered acceptable. The t distribution might be more appropriate. However, since the t distribution centiles can be determined only if the degrees of freedom, and hence the sample size, are known, the argument becomes circular. It is simpler to use the normal distribution and remember that the calculated sample sizes may be slightly smaller than is necessary.

Za will usually be 1.96 for a type I error of 5 per cent. Demanding an 80 per cent chance of detecting when the hypothesis is false, which implies a type II error of 20 per cent, means that Zb must be taken as 0.84, the 80th centile of the standard normal distribution.

For a paired t test, as above, the expected difference (given the usual hypothesis of no effect) is zero. If the smallest interesting difference is D, a 5 per cent significance level must be used ($Za = 1.96$), and if an 80 per cent chance of detecting a real difference as large as D is required ($Zb = 0.84$), the sample size n (the number of pairs) must satisfy

$$(D - 0) \Big/ s_d / \sqrt{n} \geq 1.96 + 0.84.$$

Note that D is assumed positive, which makes no difference and simplifies the calculations. This requires that

$$n \geq (1.96 + 0.84)^2 \times 2s_d^2/D^2.$$

Example Suppose that it is important to detect a difference of 5 mmHg between paired blood pressure measurements. With type I and type II errors of 5 per cent and 20 per cent respectively, this requires a sample size of

$$n \geq (1.96 + 0.84)^2 \times 66.5/25 = 20.9.$$

Thus at least 21 pairs of measurements are required.

If two independent groups are to be compared, the calculations are similar except that the form of the standard error becomes that given in eqn (17.14). If D is the smallest interesting difference, the sample size is obtained by solving

$$(D - 0) \Big/ \sqrt{[s^2 (1 / n_1 + 1 / n_2)]} \geq Za + Zb.$$

for n_1 and n_2. Since analyses are most efficient if the sample sizes are equal, if we assume $n_1 = n_2 = n$ the number in each group must satisfy

$$n \geq (Za + Zb)^2 \, 2s^2/D^2.$$

Example In a study to assess the effect of jogging on systolic blood pressure, two independent groups, one consisting of joggers and one of non-joggers, are compared. The appropriate test statistic is the difference between the means. This is known as a two-group t test. If D is set at 5 mmHg, the error levels I and II are taken as 5 per cent and 20 per cent respectively, and the residual variance taken from previous studies is 225, the number in each group must be

$$n \geq (1.96 + 0.84)^2 \times 2 \times 225/25 = 141.1,$$

i.e. 142 subjects are required in each group.

The analyses in the preceding sections cover most of the situations that arise in practice when responses are measured.

Qualitative responses—two-category outcomes
Maximum likelihood estimation

Exactly the same questions arise for qualitative as for quantitative responses, and the same general approach is used as described above. However, there are a few essential differences which must be discussed.

Typically two-category outcomes arise when the effects of some treatment or experience are judged according to whether an individual responds or not, has a symptom or not, and so on. The outcome variables are responses with the values **no** or **yes**. It is conventional to represent such variables numerically as 0 and 1. Clearly, such variables cannot have normal distributions and the principle of least squares cannot be used; however, apart from this, the conceptual approach to the analysis is identical with that for measured outcome variables.

In general, the underlying distribution is taken as binomial, and, instead of mean values, it is the proportions of individuals in each category that are of interest. In the population these proportions are the probabilities or 'risks' of individuals picked at random belonging to the specified category. An algebraic model is needed to describe how the 'risk' of an individual being in category 1 (responding, having a symptom, etc.) changes from one group to another or according to values of some measured x variable or covariate.

To fit these models (i.e., to estimate the parameters) the 'maximum likelihood principle' is used instead of least squares. Essentially this means assuming not only that the sample obtained is not unusual, but also that it is the most likely sample to occur. Once the form of the conditional distributions is determined—in this case binomial—the probability of the sample can be calculated for any algebraic model describing the pattern in the population 'risks', for example

population risk = some function of $(a + bx) = g(a + bx)$.

The likelihood or probability of the sample is then a more complex function involving $g(a + bx)$ and the data values. The values of the parameters a and b are then chosen to maximize this probability or likelihood. Apart from this difference, the process follows much the same lines as the least-squares approach.

To illustrate the analysis of this type of data, consider several groups of similar men exposed to differing levels of pollution and classified according to whether they have a persistent cough or not. If there is a positive relationship, the proportion with cough will start close to some minimum (it cannot go below zero) for low pollution levels, begin to rise at some point, and then level off as it approaches some upper limit (it cannot exceed 1.0) for high levels of pollution. This produces an S-shaped or sigmoid curve, which is characteristic of data where the response variable is constrained between two limits, in this case 0 and 1. From a sample it may appear that there is some sort of relationship even when there is none. The curve may be a chance deviation from a horizontal line. A test is needed to assess whether there really is an effect of exposure on the risk of response. This is obtained by using an algebraic model to describe the curve. The parameters representing how increasing the dose affects response can then be estimated and tested.

If subpopulations are represented in the sample, it will be necessary to compare two or more such dose–response curves. For example, the effect of pollution on respiratory symptoms might have to be assessed using a sample containing smokers and non-smokers. Smokers might well have a consistently higher risk. It is necessary to allow for this when assessing the apparent dose–response relationship. There will be two sigmoid curves representing how risk changes with pollution, one for each of the smoking effects while assessing the effect of pollution. At the tails of such curves the risks are very close to 0 or 1. Small changes in these may be, proportionally, very important. It is necessary to take into account that a change in risk from 0.01 to 0.02 (1 to 2 per cent) is a doubling of the risk, while the same absolute change in the middle of the curve, say 0.50 to 0.51 (50 to 51 per cent), is a relatively trivial proportional change in risk.

In practice this is allowed for by converting the values to the 'logistic' or log(odds) scale. Using the variable y, values for the proportion with cough, i.e. p (cough), are calculated as

$$y = \log\{p(\text{cough})/[1 - p(\text{cough})]\}$$

where the logarithmic function is the natural logarithm to the base e, and the function $p/(1 - p)$ is known as the odds. Therefore

if $p(\text{cough}) = 0.01$, then $y = \log(0.01/0.99) = -4.6$

if $p(\text{cough}) = 0.50$, then $y = \log(0.5/0.5) = 0.0$

if $p(\text{cough}) = 0.99$, then $y = \log(0.99/0.01) = +4.6$.

This pulls the lower tail of the curve down and pushes the upper tail up with an overall effect of straightening the sigmoid curves.

The order of points on the curve is unchanged by moving from the p to the y scale. An increase on the logistic scale automatically implies an increase on the risk scale.

Transforming proportions to the logistic scale

$$y = \log[p/(1 - p)]$$

turns a sigmoid curve into a straight line. The reverse transformation, which is

$$p = 1/[1 - \exp(-y)]$$

turns a straight line into a sigmoid curve. The exponential function is the antilogarithm for logarithms to the base e. This means that trends in proportions can be assessed and compared by fitting straight-line models

$$y = a + bx$$

on the logistic scale. Specific risks can be estimated or compared using the reverse transformation.

All the analyses of the section on measured outcomes can be applied to proportions using this approach. Any proportion can be considered as a point on a sigmoid curve and the same approach can be used for comparing two or more groups, possibly in some cross-classification, at the same time as allowing for the effects of covariates.

However, because maximum likelihood and not least squares is used to fit the models, the residual sum of squares cannot be used to indicate how well a model fits the data. It is necessary to use what Nelder and Wedderburn (1972) have called the 'deviance' which is defined as

$$\text{deviance} = -2 \times \log (\text{likelihood})$$

where the 'likelihood' is the probability of the sample for the given model.

The analysis of variance to compare two models produces a ratio that is an observation from an F distribution if the two models fit the data equally well. In the analysis of deviance for qualitative response variables, the difference between two deviances is, approximately, an observation from a distribution known as the χ^2 distribution. This distribution is widely used, and so values from it can be calculated in most general statistical software packages and tables (Lindley and Miller 1964) are available from which centiles and p values can be obtained.

Unfortunately, most practical problems involving proportions can be handled only with the aid of a computer and a good statistical package. The analysis can only be performed by hand if the problem is greatly simplified. The following sections cover the general approaches first and then indicate how simpler analyses can be performed at the cost of a few assumptions.

Comparing two groups allowing for a covariate

Table 17.20 gives some simulated data on the prevalence of cough in children exposed to different levels in pollution. The proportions increase steadily with increasing pollution, and they may well arise from the tails of sigmoid curves.

The questions are as follows.

1. Is the effect of pollution the same in both groups? That is, are the equivalent population lines parallel on the logistic scale?

If parallelism can be assumed:

Table 17.20 Prevalence (number at risk) of children with cough by pollution level and smoking in the home (simulated data).

	SO$_2$ pollution level		
	Low (100 µg/m^3)	**Medium** (200 µg/m^3)	**High** (300 µg/m^3)
Smoking in the home			
No	0.05 (37)	0.20 (25)	0.33 (12)
Yes	0.09 (32)	0.29 (28)	0.53 (17)

2. Is there an effect of pollution? That is, are the equivalent population lines non-horizontal?

3. Is there an effect of exposure to smoking? That is, are the equivalent population lines separated vertically?

For this analysis it is necessary to fit the following models.

1. **Non-parallel**—a different pollution effect in each smoking group:

$y = rv$ + smoking effect + smoking group pollution effect

where rv is the reference value that is the predicted proportion for the low pollution/non-smoking reference group transformed to a value on the logistic scale.

2. **Parallel**:

$y = rv$ + smoking effect + pollution effect.

3. **Horizontal**—no pollution effect:

$y = rv$ + smoking effect.

4. **Coincident lines**—no smoking effect:

$y = rv$ + pollution effect.

The analysis was performed using a computer and the statistical package GLIM (Francis *et al*. 1993). Other packages such as BMD-P (Dixon 1981), Stata (Stata Corporation 1993), and Egret (Statis-tics and Epidemiology Research Corporation 1992) can be used to perform the same analyses, but, in many cases, not as easily. GLIM requires as input the numbers at risk and the numbers responding (i.e. those with symptoms) for each cell of the two-way table (Table 17.20) to fit the models and obtain their deviances. From these, the analyses of deviance in Table 17.21 can be constructed.

From line (2–1), there is no evidence of non-parallelism. The difference between the two deviances gives a χ^2 value of 0.04, which is trivial compared with the 95th centile of the χ^2 distribution with one degree of freedom, which is 3.84. Whatever the association, it is the same whether or not the child is exposed to cigarette smoking in the home.

From line (3–2), omitting the pollution effect from the parallel-line model gives a much worse fitting model. Values as large as the χ^2 value testing the slope of the pollution trend against zero (i.e. 17.2) should occur by chance in less than 0.1 per cent of such investigations. The 99.9th centile of the χ^2 distribution on one degree of freedom is only 10.83. These simulated data indicate very strongly that there is an association at these levels between increasing pollution levels and increasing risk of having a symptom.

The effect of smoking in the home is not so clear. The smoking effect (i.e. the separation of the two lines) appears to be no more than could easily occur by chance. The χ^2 value of 1.94 on one degree of freedom is well below the value of 3.84 required for significance.

The parallel-line model (2) is adequate to describe these data,

Table 17.21 Analysis of deviance for comparing prevalences of respiratory symptoms in children classified by exposure to air pollution and cigarette smoking

Model	Deviance	DF	Approximate χ^2
1. Different pollution effects non-parallel	0.40	2	
2. Identical effects parallel	0.44	3	
(2 – 1) Due to different effects	0.04	1	0.04 (cf. $\chi^2_{1,0.95} = 3.84$)
3. No pollution effect horizontal	17.64	4	
(3 – 2) Due to pollution effect	17.20	1	17.20 ($p < 0.01$)
4. No smoking effect coincident lines	2.38	4	
(4 – 2) Due to smoking effects	1.94	1	1.94 (not significant)

and it provides estimates of the effects. On the logistic scale the model is,

$$y = a + smk + b \times \text{pollution}$$

where a is the intercept for the non-smoking group, the smoking effect smk is the vertical separation of the lines, and b is the slope or regression coefficient of the pollution trends. The computed analysis gives estimates with the following approximate standard errors:

$$a = -3.87 \quad \text{with SE } (a) = 0.69$$
$$smk = 0.61 \quad \quad \text{SE } (smk) = 0.44$$
$$b = 0.0113 \quad \quad \text{SE } (b) = 0.0029.$$

The pollution effect can be tested by comparing b with zero using the standardized normal distribution

$$u = 0.0113/0.0029 = 3.90 \text{ (cf. 1.96)}$$

This gives an equally significant result to that of the χ^2 test. They are essentially two ways of doing the same thing using different assumptions.

The test of the smoking effect, $0.61/0.44 = 1.39$, is consistent with this χ^2 result, i.e. well below 1.96. The confidence interval, which therefore includes zero, is

$$0.61 \pm 1.96 \times 0.44 \quad \text{or} \quad -0.25 \text{ to } 1.47$$

This shows that the data are consistent with quite large values, up to 1.47. In such circumstances it is wise to investigate what the effects on the logistic scale mean in terms of estimated risks.

Taking pollution as $100 \ \mu g/m^3$, the low category on the logistic scale, the model predicts that for the non-smoking group (ns)

$$y_{ns} = -3.87 + 0.0113 \times 100 = -2.74$$

and for the smoking group (s)

$$y_s = -8.87 + 0.61 = 0.0113 \times 100 = -2.13.$$

If $y = \log[p/(1-p)]$, then the value of p is

$$p = 1/[1 + \exp(-y)]$$

so that

$$p_{ns} = 1/[1 + \exp(+2.74)] = 0.061$$

and

$$p_s = 1/[1 + \exp(+2.13)] = 0.106.$$

This means that the estimated risks of having the symptom 'cough' are 6.1 per cent and 10.6 per cent respectively. Although it does not reach significance in this data set, the effect of exposure to smoking is estimated as an increase in risk of 4.5 per cent. The risk of 6.1 per cent has nearly doubled on going from children not exposed to smoking to those who are. If this were to represent a real effect, obviously it would be important.

The ratio of the two risks is known as the relative risk, i.e. the risk of those exposed relative to the risk of those not exposed. This is calculated as

relative risk $= 0.106/0.061 = 1.74$

which is nearly 2, indicating that the risk is nearly doubled by exposure to pollution.

An approximation of the relative risk is provided by the odds ratio, which, for the smoking factor, is

$$p_s / (1 - p_s) \Big/ p_{ns} / (1 - p_{ns}).$$

Because the analysis uses the logistic scale, this is in fact

$$\exp(smk) = \exp(0.61) = 1.84$$

which is rather larger than the relative risk. None the less for small risks (about 5 per cent or less), the odds ratio is a good approximation to the relative risk.

There are a number of tests specifically designed for comparing such estimates of relative risk with the value expected (1.0) if the true risks are identical. (For further discussion of this topic, see Volume 2, Chapter 10). Apart from slightly differing assumptions, they are effectively the same as the test derived from the model comparison in the analysis of deviance. In addition, fitting and comparing models has allowed the use of all the data from several pollution groups. The model comparison approach is much more general. It can be extended to cover very complicated data sets, and it allows estimates of all the various effects to be obtained in a relatively straightforward way.

Approximate confidence intervals for the estimates of risk and relative risk can be obtained from the parallel-line model. However, this can be done only indirectly by first calculating the confidence limits on the logistic scale as

estimate ± 1.96 SE (estimate)

and then converting the limits of the confidence interval back to the risk scale. The predicted y value for the smoking group is

$$y = a + b \times 100.$$

The standard error of y, SE(y), which is the square root of the sampling variance of y, is a function of the sampling variances of a and b with what is known as their covariance. The interdependence of estimates has not been discussed, but this must be taken into account when standard errors of functions of estimates are required. A full discussion is given by Armitage and Berry (1987). All that is needed are the covariances of the estimates, and these are readily obtained during computer analysis. For $y = a + bx$, the variance of y [var(y)] is then calculated by

$$\text{var}(y) = \text{var}(a) + 2x \times \text{covariance } (a,b) + x^2 \times \text{var}(b).$$

For this analysis, the computer produced the values

$$\text{var}(y) = 0.48$$
$$\text{var}(b) = 8.3 \times 10^{-6}$$
$$\text{cov}(a,b) = -0.0017.$$

Therefore

$$\text{var}(y) = 0.48 + 200 \, (-0.0017) + 100^2 \times 10^{-6} \times 8.30$$
$$= 0.22$$

Table 17.22 Numbers of children with cough classified by exposure to smoking in the home and the numbers expected if there was no association between exposure and risk of cough (in parentheses)

Cough	Smoking in the home		
	No	Yes	Total
Yes	4(5.4)	9(7.6)	13
No	8(6.6)	8(9.4)	16
Total	12	17	29

and

$$\text{SE} (y) = \sqrt{[\text{var}(y)]} = 0.47.$$

Therefore the 95 per cent confidence interval for y in the non-smoking group is

$$-2.74 \pm 1.96 \times 0.47 \qquad \text{or} \qquad -3.66 \text{ to } -1.82.$$

Converting back to the risk scale, the equivalent confidence interval for the risk in this group is 0.025–0.139. In the group exposed to smoking, the equivalent figures are 10.6 per cent for the best estimate of risk with a confidence interval of 5.0 to 21.3 per cent. This gives an estimated relative risk of 10.6/6.1 = 1.75.

It is not simple to obtain a confidence interval for the true relative risk, but it is quite straightforward for the odds ratio. On the logistic scale, the effect of smoking is $0.61 \pm 1.96 \times 0.44$ or -0.25 to 1.47. The odds ratio is estimated as exp(0.61), and exp(−0.25) to exp(1.47) (i.e. 0.77 to 4.35) are the approximate confidence limits.

The data are reasonably consistent with a true odds ratio as low as 0.77 (i.e. the non-smoking group having a lower risk than the smoking group) or as high as 4.35 (i.e. the group exposed to smoking having a risk of more than four times that of those not exposed). Since this range includes 1, it means that the odds ratio is not significantly different from 1.

The conclusions from these simulated data are as follows. First there is strong evidence of a pollution effect—going from low to medium to high pollution in these individuals at least doubles and then trebles the risk in both the smoking and non-smoking groups. Second, there is some suggestion that a larger study might identify an important effect of exposure to smoking, since these results are not inconsistent with a fourfold increase in risk of cough in those exposed to smoking compared with those not so exposed.

Comparing two proportions

If data are available only for the high pollution group, as in Table 17.22, the problem reduces to comparing two proportions. The prevalence of cough is 4/12 or 33.3 per cent in the non-smoking homes and 9/17 or 52.9 per cent in the smoking homes. The question is: Are these two proportions more different than could easily occur by chance?

The hypothesis to test is that there is a single 'true' risk, which is the same for both groups, and that the differences arose by chance. This single risk, assuming that the hypothesis is true, is best estimated using all the data, i.e. by 13/29 = 44.8 per cent.

This means that, in studies like this, on average 44.8 per cent of each group would be expected to fall in the cough category. On this basis the expected numbers can be calculated for each cell of the table: 5.4 is 44.8 per cent of 12, 7.6 is 44.8 per cent of 17, and so on. The problem becomes one of assessing whether the cell frequencies are surprisingly far from those expected. For each cell the measure of how far apart the observed and expected frequencies are is taken as

$$\frac{(\text{observed frequency} - \text{expected frequency})^2}{\text{expected frequency}}$$

or, more simply, using an abbreviated notation:

$$(O - E)^2/E.$$

The summation of this over all the cells in the table gives a measure of how the table as a whole deviates from what should be expected if the hypothesis were true, i.e. sum for all cells of $(O - E)^2/E$, which can be shown to have a χ^2 distribution on one degree of freedom. This is because the analysis is essentially comparing a model with two different proportions or parameters with a model with one proportion or parameter. Measures of the difference between these two models have one degree of freedom. In this case

$$\chi^2 = \frac{(4 - 5.4)^2}{5.4} + \frac{(9 - 7.6)^2}{7.6} + \frac{(8 - 6.6)^2}{6.6} + \frac{(8 - 9.4)^2}{9.4}$$
$$= 1.09$$

which is a long way from significance at the 5 per cent level (cf. 3.84).

Practical problems rarely reduce to the comparison of two proportions without gross simplification. None the less, a number of alternatives to this test have been developed over the years. There is also much discussion as to which is right. Fortunately, it rarely matters. Yates (1934) pointed out that sum $(O - E)^2/E$ was more nearly a χ^2 variable if the test was slightly modified by subtracting 0.5 from the frequencies on the diagonal with the largest product (in this case, the 8,9 diagonal). This is probably the most sensible test to use in this context. When only small numbers are available, a test known as Fisher's exact test is more precise.

Fisher's test calculates the exact probability of this or more surprising tables occurring given the marginal totals and the hypothesis. Therefore it gives p values directly. Those requiring the algebraic details should consult Armitage and Berry (1987). A number of statistical packages (for example EpiInfo (Dean et al. 1994) and StatXact (Mehta and Patel 1992)) provide a facility for performing Fisher's exact test for 2×2 tables.

Sample sizes for comparing proportions

The exact solution to this problem leads to a very complicated formula, which can be found in a paper by Casagrande et al. (1978). This has been implemented in the menu-driven sample-size calculation system Sample (Andrews and Swan 1994) using the macro-facility in GLIM (Francis *et al.* 1993). However, for most practical purposes it will be sufficient to use a calculation analogous to that for comparing means. The sample sizes obtained will be slightly smaller than optimum, but this can be regarded as an increase in the risk of a type II error. If this matters, the risk can be set lower and the calculations repeated. The calculations are based on expressing the χ^2 test above in the form

$$\frac{\text{estimate} - \text{expected value}}{\text{SE (estimate)}}$$

where the estimate is the difference between two proportions; The expected value is usually zero. The test statistic is

$$(r_1/n_1 - r_2/n_2)\sqrt{[p(1 - p)(1/n_1 + 1/n_2)]}$$

where $p = (r_1 + r_2)/(n_1 + n_2)$. This has a sampling distribution close to normal even for quite small proportions and values of n_1 and n_2. This means that the statistic can be tested against 1.96 for a 5 per cent significance level. As for comparing means, it is efficient to keep the groups the same size. The number in each group must then satisfy

$$D\Big/\sqrt{[p\,(1 - p)\,2/n]} \geq Za + Zb$$

where D is the smallest difference of interest, and Za and Zb are centiles of the standard normal distribution determined by the choice of what risks of type I and type II errors are acceptable. In this calculation p is taken as the average of the two proportions expected if the hypothesis is false. The number must satisfy

$$n \geq (Za + Zb)^2 \times 2\,p(1 - p)/D^2$$

Example What sample size is needed to detect a difference in the prevalence of respiratory symptoms between children in two towns with differing air pollution levels?

If the prevalence is about 20 per cent and the smallest interesting difference is 5 per cent, then $p = 0.20 + 0.05/2 = 0.225$. If the acceptable risks of type I and type II errors are 5 per cent and 20 per cent respectively, the number in each group must satisfy

$$n \geq (1.96 + 0.84)^2 \times 2 \times 0.225\,(1 - 0.225)/(0.05)^2$$

which gives $n \geq 1093.7$. Thus 1094 subjects are needed in each group and 2188 in total.

This and the earlier section on sample size for comparing means give a simplified guide to sample size calculations. Lachin (1981) gives a very comprehensive guide, and the Sample system (Andrews and Swan 1994) provides a conveniently automated approach for most practical problems.

Repeated observations

An individual can be classified as having or not having a symptom several times during a course of treatment. This produces an analysis problem analogous to that of repeated measurements. Using a subject parameter in the model allows it to be analysed in much the same way, employing an analysis of deviance instead of the analysis of variance. Odds ratio estimates for risks before and after some treatment or exposure can then be obtained as the square root of the equivalent estimate as in the section above on comparing two groups allowing for a covariate. In practice, a modified form of

Table 17.23 Distribution of subjects according to errors made in their drug regimen before and after provision of a patient-held treatment record

| | After record | |
	Errors	No errors
Before record		
Errors	4	4
No errors	0	2

model fitting is used for this type of data, which also arises in the matched case–control studies discussed below and in Volume 2, Chapter 10. A comprehensive discussion of the model-fitting approach in this context is given by Breslow and Day (1980), and the method of analysis with the computer package GLIM is fully described in the *GLIM4 manual* (Francis *et al.* 1993).

In the simplest case analogous to the paired t test problem, a technique known as McNemar's test can be used.

Example using McNemar's test Geriatric patients in the community often have complex drug regimens to follow. Table 17.23 gives some data from a study to assess whether a specially designed, patient-held treatment record affects the error rate when the patients are questioned on their regimen.

It is possible to analyse these data using a model-fitting approach, but in this simple case it is not necessary. On the hypothesis that the subjects are equally likely to make errors before and after, as many should improve as become worse. This means that those who changed should be equally divided between the two types of change possible.

In these data four changed—they all became better at identifying their drug dosages. The probability of a result as surprising as this if there was only a 50 per cent chance of improving is required. This is exactly the same as the probability of getting 'heads' in all four tosses of a coin, which is $0.5 \times 0.5 \times 0.5 \times 0.5 = 0.0625$. An equally surprising result would have been all four becoming worse—the equivalent of four 'tails'. Since this also has probability $p = 0.0625$, the probability of a result this surprising is $p = 0.0625 \times 2 = 0.125$. Therefore, although the result seems interesting, the probability of such extreme results is certainly not less than 0.05. If the effect was genuinely of this magnitude, then a larger sample would be needed to show it as significant.

Comparing proportions from separate samples—case–control or retrospective studies

If cases with a particular disease or condition and controls are not matched to have the same values of potentially interfering factors (such as age and sex), the data from case–control studies are analysed in exactly the same way, using the model-fitting approach, as any other set of proportions, taking the ratio of cases to (cases + controls) as the proportions. Odds ratios, assessing the effects on risk of factors in the model, are obtained from the fitted model as described earlier.

If the cases and controls have been matched in some way according to factors that might be related to the risk of becoming a case, then the correct analysis is more complicated. Further

Table 17.24 Distribution of Hodgkin's disease patients by treatment and remission category (treatment group percentages in parentheses)

Treatment	Remission category			Total
	1. None/died	2. Partial remission	3. Complete remission	
A	16 (40)	9 (23)	15 (37)	40 (100)
B	11 (24)	4 (9)	31 (67)	46 (100)

discussion can be found in Breslow and Day (1980), Schlesselman (1982), Greenberg and Ibrahim (1991), and Francis *et al.* (1993).

More than two categories of outcome

Categorical outcomes arise when individuals can respond to treatment or experience in several ways that are not easily measured. For example, a treatment for Hodgkin's disease can be assessed according to whether the patients 'died', 'became worse', 'stayed the same', or 'showed signs of remission'. In this case the clinician's overall classification is preferred to a single measure of well-being, such as white cell count.

It is always possible to combine some of the categories so that there are only two, for example 'no remission' and 'remission'. This permits the response to be treated as a proportion and allows the use of the methods in the previous section. In practice this is often the most sensible thing to do, although it wastes information. Alternatively, some way must be found for describing responses in many categories by models.

Consider data from a trial comparing two treatments (A and B) for Hodgkin's disease. The outcomes, assessed after a fixed period of treatment, were 'no response or died', 'partial remission', and 'complete remission'. The results are given in Table 17.24.

It is necessary to compare how the two treatment groups are distributed among the response categories. This is best done by plotting the frequencies against the remission category for each of the treatment groups. Joining the points within each treatment group makes the diagram easier to interpret (Fig. 17.28). The true responses are represented on the horizontal axis. However, if the frequencies on the y axis are considered as the response variable, the pattern to be described by an algebraic model has exactly the same form as discussed in previous sections on means and proportions. In this context the y variable is a 'count' or frequency. It is usual to assume that these arise from a theoretical distribution called the Poisson distribution.

For proportions obtained from counts in two categories of response, it was necessary to use the logistic scale to fit the models. It is necessary to use another scale for frequencies, and the most useful and appropriate is the logarithmic scale. This is logical because changes in frequencies seen when moving to groups at higher risk are likely to be proportional. On the frequency scale, distances representing the same proportional difference will change with the frequency. On the log (frequency) scale, these distances will stay constant, which means that constant proportional effects will give parallel-line models. For this reason this analysis has come to be known as 'log linear modelling'.

Notice that if there had been many more subjects in treatment

group A, the frequencies would all be larger. The A line would have been much higher than the B line, even if the treatments were equally effective. Because of this it is the parallelism of the lines that is of most interest, not their separation.

To test whether there are significant differences in the shapes of the distributions, it is necessary to compare models with and without interaction parameters. Because the height of the lines does not matter, it is not necessary to treat it as a random variable and waste information estimating some 'true' height. This is avoided by forcing the model-fitting process to choose estimates for the 'height' parameters so that the model fits or predicts the observed total frequencies exactly.

Apart from the use of the log scale, since the constraints on the models and the interaction are the model parameters of prime interest, the analysis is much the same as for proportions. Maximum likelihood and the analysis of deviance are used to produce approximate χ^2 tests of the interaction parameters quantifying the hypothesis of interest.

Comparing two groups with three outcomes

The models to be compared are as follows.

1. **Non-parallel lines:**

   $y = rv$ + treatment effect + remission category effect
   + treatment × remission category interaction.

2. **Parallel lines:**

   $y = rv$ + treatment effect + remission category effect.

Model 1 requires six parameters. Since there are only six points, it will fit the data exactly and there are no degrees of freedom and no deviance. A computer analysis gave the deviance from the parallel-line model as 8.17 on two degrees of freedom, and so the analysis of deviance is as in Table 17.25.

Since the 95th centile of the χ^2 distribution with two degrees of freedom is 5.99, the outcome distributions of the two treatment

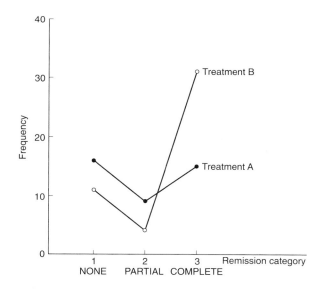

Fig. 17.28 Frequency of Hodgkin's disease patients versus remission category by treatment group. *Source*: British National Lymphoma Investigation 1975.

Table 17.25 Analysis of deviance comparing the frequency distribution of Hodgkin's disease patients among three remission categories for two treatment groups

Model		Deviance	DF	χ^2
1.	Non-parallel	0	0	
2.	Parallel	8.17	2	
(2 – 1) Due to non-parallelism		8.17	2	8.17

groups are significantly different ($p < 0.05$). It only remains to make quantitative statements about how the 'relative risk' of ending up in the various remission categories varies according to treatment using the estimated frequencies from the non-parallel model and the treatment group totals. In this simple case, this gives estimates of risk equal to the percentages given in Table 17.24.

This approach easily extends to more complex problems, for example if initial severity subgroups had to be taken into account.

Comparing frequencies in a two-way classification

If the data are as simple as in the above example, the frequencies can be compared directly with a χ^2 test using expected frequencies calculated on the assumption that the hypothesis to be tested is true (Table 17.26).

On the hypothesis that the treatments are equally effective, 31.4, 15.1, and 53.5 per cent of individuals would be expected to fall into the three response categories whatever the treatment (Table 17.26). This means that 31.4 per cent of the 40 patients receiving treatment A are expected to fall into response category 1:

$$\frac{31.4}{100} \times 40 = \frac{27}{86} \times 40 = 12.6$$

in category 2, 15.1 per cent of 40 = 6, and so on.

As when comparing two proportions, the test of whether the frequencies are surprisingly far from those expected on the hypothesis of equally effective treatments is

$$\chi^2 = \text{sum } (O - E)^2/E = 8.03.$$

Table 17.26 Distribution of Hodgkin's disease patients by treatments and remission category

	Response*			
	Category 1	Category 2	Category 3	Total
A	16 (12.6)	9 (6.0)	15 (21.4)	40
B	11 (14.4)	4 (7.0)	31 (24.6)	46
Total	27	13	46	86
Percentage	31.4	15.1	53.5	100

* Frequencies expected assuming equally effective treatments are given in parentheses.

This is not quite the same as the analysis of deviance χ^2 value because slightly different assumptions are made in the analyses. However, the conclusion is much the same, and unless 5 per cent is inappropriately regarded as a 'magic' cut-off point these two approaches will usually lead to the same conclusions.

Survival or event data

These data arise when individuals observed over time are at risk of some event. The event may be death, menarche, coronary heart attack, and so on. After death or menarche, the individual is no longer at risk—the event cannot occur again. In fact, a coronary heart attack could be the first of many, but if observation of the subject is discontinued after the event, it can be treated as terminal and standard analyses can be used.

If the data consist of numbers of people dying in a cohort that is observed for a fixed period, then the analysis is simply a comparison of proportions. The techniques of the earlier section on qualitative two-category responses will usually suffice. Annual mortality rates from different geographic areas can be analysed in this way, treating them as proportions, but there may be complications as discussed by Pocock *et al.* (1981). None the less, the analysis of mortality data of this sort by a model-fitting approach avoids the use of standardizing techniques, which traditionally adjusted mortality figures for age and sex effects before group comparisons were made, notably using standardized mortality ratios. Such adjustments make possibly unwarranted and certainly untested assumptions about the effects of age and sex being the same in all the groups to be compared and, for that reason, must be used with care. Standardization methods are well covered by Armitage and Berry (1987).

When the individuals are at risk of the event for varying periods of time, the problem cannot easily be considered as an analysis of proportions. There are two main types of problems. In the first it is assumed that the risk is constant over time within the groups to be compared. In the second case the risk changes with time. The remaining discussion will be restricted to these two types of survival data.

Constant risks

From the number experiencing the event in a group of individuals observed for varying lengths of time, the risk per unit time for an individual in the group can be estimated by dividing the number of deaths by the accumulated time at risk. The modelling approach to analysing such data requires that the number of deaths in each group is taken as the response variable and the accumulated time at risk is used as a covariate.

In the occupational health study data given in Table 17.27, the deaths were classified according to factory and age at the start of the observation period. The table also gives the total person years at risk (PYR) within each group. Since the response variable is a count, the appropriate analysis requires using the number of deaths as a Poisson response variable and fitting the models on the logarithmic scale.

The question to be answered is: Is the effect of age the same in both factories? If it is: Are the risks, allowing for age, different in the two factories? The models required to answer these are as follows.

Table 17.27 Number of deaths by age group and factory from a study of occupational mortality

Age at start of study (years)	Number of deaths*	
	Factory 1	Factory 2
50–59.9	7 (4045)	7 (3701)
60–69.9	27 (3571)	37 (3702)
70–79.9	30 (1777)	35 (1818)
80–89.9	8 (381)	9 (350)

* Person years at risk in parentheses.

1. **Non-parallel age trends**:

$$y = \log (\text{PYR}) + rv + \text{factory effect} + \text{factory specific slope} \times \text{age}.$$

If straight-line age trends are assumed, the models are as follows.

2. **Parallel age trends**:

$$y = \log (\text{PYR}) + rv + \text{factory effect} + \text{slope} \times \text{age}.$$

3. **No factory effect**:

$$y = \log (\text{PYR}) + rv + \text{slope} \times \text{age}.$$

4. **No age effect** (for completeness):

$$y = \log (\text{PYR}) + rv + \text{factory effect}.$$

When these models are fitted, the analysis of deviance in Table 17.28 is obtained.

The 95th centile of the χ^2 distribution with one degree of freedom is 3.84, and values less than this could well occur by chance. Obviously the age effect producing a χ^2 value of 89.19 is very marked and real. The factory effect gives a χ^2 value of 1.73, which does not appear to indicate much. However, the initial deviance of 12.70 on four degrees of freedom indicates that the first model is a long way from the data points. The linear age trends do not fit the data well, and so the subsequent analysis must be treated with caution. In fact fitting an age-squared term to allow for curvature gives a much smaller deviance. The following model with such a term, but assuming a zero difference between the two factories,

Table 17.28 Analysis of deviance comparing mortality in two factories allowing for different age structures

Model		Deviance	DF	χ^2
1.	Non-parallel linear age trends	12.70	4	
2.	Parallel trends	12.71	5	
(2 – 1)	Due to non-parallelism	0.01	1	0.01
3.	No factory effect	14.44	6	
(3 – 2)	Due to factory effect	1.73	1	1.73
4.	No age effect	101.90	6	
(4 – 2)	Due to age effect	89.19	1	89.19

5. $y = \log (\text{PYR}) + rv + b \times \text{age} + c \times \text{age}^2$

fits the data well with a deviance of 2.09 on five degrees of freedom. Therefore there is very little evidence of a factory effect.

Observed and expected deaths

In simple cases a hypothesis can be used to deduce the number of deaths expected, and these can then be used to calculate $(O - E)^2/E$ for appropriate groups. This is used to obtain a simple χ^2 test.

In the above example, the hypothesis to be tested was that the risks were equal in the two factories. The risk for each age group per person year is calculated as

sum of deaths/sum of PYRs.

The expected deaths in each factory are obtained from this value multiplied by the appropriate PYR. For the 50-year-olds in factory 1, this gives

$$\text{expected deaths} = 4045 \times \frac{7 + 7}{4045 + 3701}$$
$$= 4045 \times 0.0018 = 7.3.$$

Similarly, for factory 2

$$\text{expected deaths} = 3701 \times 0.0018 = 6.7$$

and so on for all age groups.

The overall χ^2 value to test the hypothesis of no factory effect on risk is the sum of the eight $(O - E)^2/E$ values:

$$(7 - 7.3)^2/7.3 + (7 - 6.7)^2/6.7$$
$$+ \quad (27 - 31.4)^2/31.4 + (37 - 32.6)^2/32.6$$
$$+ \quad (30 - 32.1)^2/32.1 + (35 - 32.9)^2/32.9$$
$$+ \quad (8 - 8.9)^2/8.9 + (9 - 8.1)^2/8.1$$
$$= 1.70.$$

This has four degrees of freedom because there were eight observations and it was necessary to estimate four parameters (the risks for the four age groups) to calculate the χ^2 value. The conclusions are the same, but this approach is impossibly tedious if there are many more than two groups to compare. The modelling approach is almost inevitable for a thorough analysis that estimates the magnitude of the various effects.

Changing risks—survival curves

For each individual, data of this type will consist of the length of time observed and the reason he or she was lost to observation. The period of observation may start at birth, diagnosis, start of treatment, or some other appropriate point in time. An individual who dies, has some other terminal event, or drops out during the course of the study is then lost to observation. When a study is concluded, observation stops on the survivors.

Life-table survival curves are used to investigate survival in a group of individuals observed for differing periods of time. The survival curve is a plot of the individuals surviving against time elapsed from diagnosis, or other appropriate points. The life-table calculations to obtain these percentages from individuals observed for varying lengths of time are fairly simple, but not obvious.

Consider a number of subjects entering and leaving a trial at

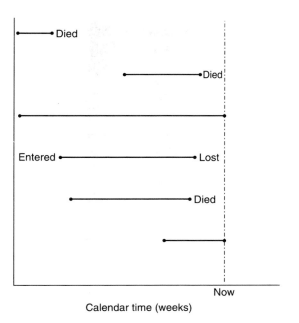

Fig. 17.29 Observation periods of subjects in a trial.

different times as shown in Fig. 17.29. Using time since entry as the horizontal scale gives a modified plot (Fig. 17.30) from which the number of subjects at risk and the number dying in each week since entry can be seen. In the first week after entry six subjects were at risk and one had died. This gives an estimated death rate of 0.17 and hence a survival rate of 0.83. In the second week there were four at risk all the time, one for half a week, and one died, giving a death rate of $1/4.5 = 0.22$ and a survival rate for individuals reaching the second week of 0.78.

The chance of an individual surviving the second week, which requires that he or she survives both the first and the second weeks,

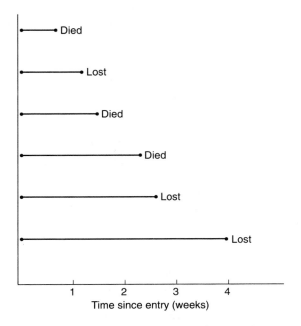

Fig. 17.30 Observation periods of subjects in a trial from time of entry.

is $0.83 \times 0.78 = 0.65$. This is the estimated cumulative survival rate. Plotting it against time from treatment gives the survival curve. Conventionally, individuals lost in any interval are treated as having been at risk for half the interval.

The life-table for patients with prostate cancer in the radiotherapy group of a trial comparing radiotherapy and hormone treatments is given in Table 17.29. The adjusted number at risk is the number entering the interval minus half the number lost to observation during it. Plotting the percentage surviving S against the upper end of the time intervals gives the survival curve shown in Fig. 17.31. It is not appropriate to draw a smooth curve through the points since such curves give a spurious impression of accuracy.

Comparisons of a small number of survival curves can be made by hand using what is known as the 'log rank' test. On the hypothesis of no difference between two curves, the number of deaths expected in each group can be calculated. By calculating $(O - E)^2/E$ for each group, a χ^2 test on one degree of freedom comparing the curves can be obtained. The method can be used to compare survival curves within a cross-classification of treatment or other groups, but it is not simple. The method is described in detail by Peto *et al.* (1977).

At the cost of a few testable and often reasonable assumptions, a full modelling approach can be used that is analogous to those discussed in earlier sections. This approach was introduced by Cox (1972) and is discussed by Anderson *et al.* (1980) and Kalbfleisch and Prentice (1980). Although these texts are rather mathematical, computer programs are now available that make it possible to fit sequences of models to survival data with relative ease (GLIM, Egret, Stata, BMDP, etc.). This approach provides quantitative estimates with standard errors, thus aiding considerably the interpretation and presentation aspects of the analysis.

Quantitative reviews—meta-analysis

Quantitative reviews or overviews are exercises combining the results from different studies of the same problem using formal statistical techniques. Strictly speaking, they are an application of statistical methods rather than a statistical method in themselves. However, they have become increasingly important in making the best use of the results from several clinical trials assessing the same treatment and for combining observational studies investigating factors associated with a particular outcome. Consequently, it would be remiss of a discussion on statistical methods in public health to neglect them. A good discussion of the role and use of meta-analysis is given by Pocock and Thompson (1991*a*), and the same authors give a clear account of the methods and assumptions involved in a paper entitled 'Can meta-analysis be trusted?' (Pocock and Thompson 1991*b*). (Also see Chapter 16, Volume 2.)

Effectively, the statistical methods involved are the same as those discussed earlier using the study, i.e. the study from which each part of the overall data set was obtained, as a factor. If differences between exposed and unexposed, or treated and untreated, are not systematically different from one study (or category of studies) to the next, then it will be appropriate to obtain a single combined estimate of the effect of interest. This is done by calculating an overall pooled estimate of the effect of exposure or treatment using the results from the separate studies weighted appropriately to take

Table 17.29 Life-table for patients with cancer of the prostate in the radiotherapy group of a clinical trial

Time since entry (years)	No. died	No. at risk	No. lost	Adjusted no. at risk	Estimated probability of		Estimated proportion of surviviors at end of interval
					Death	Survival	
0–1	3	44	3	42.5	0.071	0.929	0.929
1–2	2	38	10	33.0	0.061	0.939	0.873
2–3	1	26	3	24.5	0.041	0.959	0.837
3–4	3	22	3	20.5	0.146	0.854	0.715
4–5	2	16	4	14.0	0.143	0.857	0.613
5–6	1	10	1	9.5	0.105	0.895	0.548
6–7	1	8	1	7.5	0.133	0.867	0.475
7–8	0	6	3	4.5	0.000	1.000	0.475
8–9	1	3	1	2.5	0.400	0.600	0.085
9–10	1	1	0	1.0	1.000	0.000	0.000

their size into account. This will give a more precise estimate of the true effect. If the raw data can be obtained, such weighting is done automatically in a routine regression analysis. If the data are in the form of means, explicit weighting is required according to the numbers of observations involved. Data in the form of proportions or 2 × 2 tables can be combined using logistic regression or, in the simpler cases, a procedure known as the Mantel–Haenszel test can be used (described fully by Schlesselman (1982)).

A good example of an overview meta-analysis of the benefits of diuretics in pregnancy is given by Collins *et al.* (1985).

Design, data management, and data analysis

Although surveys and other epidemiological studies may appear simple, it is easy to perform them ineffectively. The design stage needs the aims and objectives of the study specified in a detailed

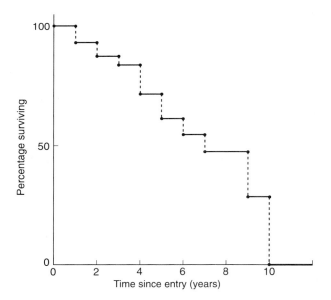

Fig. 17.31 Life-table survival curve for the radiotherapy group in a trial of treatments for cancer of the prostate.

protocol. Even in a pilot study these need to be expressed in quantitative terms so that it is clear how the success of the study will be measured. For example, the study might be a pilot study of doctors in general practice to assess whether a good enough response rate can be obtained for a major study. The aims must specify the minimum acceptable response rate and the pilot study must be large enough to demonstrate reasonably conclusively whether such a response rate will be achievable in the larger study. This will involve testing an observed response rate against the minimum response rate considered acceptable for the main study. The test can be used, as described earlier, to infer the sample size needed for the pilot study, and the calculations should also be part of the protocol. The protocol must also include the data collection documents (for example questionnaires, specification of computer screens to be used, and so on) in sufficient detail to make it clear that all the data required to meet the aims and objectives will be collected accurately and unambiguously. These must be constrained to give as simple a data structure as possible; further, they must be restricted to the data needed to meet the aims and objectives. If extra data are collected for any reason, this may, by increasing the effort required, reduce the care with which the important information is recorded and may complicate the data management system required by absorbing time and resources. The data will be wasted if they are not analysed, and, if analysed, they will effectively reduce the confidence that can be put in all positive findings. The last disadvantage arises because the more analyses that are performed, the greater is the chance that a type I error (i.e. a false-positive finding) will occur. These are more important points than they might seem because most studies suffer from collecting too much data; indeed, very few suffer from collecting insufficient data. Finally, the protocol should have a section clarifying the analysis strategy and methodology to be used so that the needs of the analysis, in terms of data content and structure, and its appropriateness are given careful thought early in the design stage.

Data management can range from the relatively trivial (for example a survey where a single questionnaire is completed by an easily accessible sample of individuals and entered into the computer in a format immediately readable by the statistical packages to be used in the analysis) to the potentially very complex systems required for multicentre longitudinal studies which follow subjects recruited continuously and for long periods. However, even in the simplest case, entry into the computer may introduce errors in the data, and systems of checking and verifying the process (for example double-entry verification) need to be employed. It is tempting to use routine commercial database packages for storing data from epidemiological studies, but there are dangers in this. Unless the package is similar to EpiInfo (Dean *et al.* 1994), which was specifically designed for such studies, it will be unlikely to include good data entry checking facilities. By tempting the user into using the 'electronic filing cabinet' facilities, it may also lead to the collection of data in a form quite inappropriate for statistical analysis (for example free-text responses, alphabetic variables potentially misspelt, individual subject data spread over an unpredictable number of separate records, etc.). There may be circumstances where all of these may be necessary, but they complicate the data management and analysis considerably and, where possible, they should be avoided. Statistical packages generally require what are known as 'flat' files where there is a fixed (i.e. constant) number of variable values for each individual study unit and which variable each value represents is deducible from its position in the individual record. For example, the third value in every record may be a 1 or 2, indicating an individual's gender (1 for male, 2 for female), the 15th value could indicate their systolic blood pressure on entry to the study, and so on. Any system of data collection and storage must be designed so that the data can be converted into this form or the statistical analysis will become extremely difficult to organize and very time consuming.

The analysis will vary considerably according to the nature of the study. However, there are a few general principles that should guide the analysis strategy so that a process starting with, possibly, hundreds of variable values for each subject converges to a few appropriate and justifiable conclusions relevant to the aims and objectives of the study. Most analyses will be concerned with assessing whether some outcome (for example death, recovery, etc.) is systematically affected by some explanatory variable (for example exposure, treatment, etc.). This will generally require an analysis involving the comparison of regression models. A strategy is needed for deciding how to handle both outcome and explanatory variables in the analysis. The study protocol should have identified the outcome variable or variables to be studied in order to meet the aims. However, when several outcomes have been identified, as is often the case, it is necessary to identify which is of primary importance and how to deal with them overall. In most cases the best strategy is to identify the primary outcome variable and pursue the analysis right through with that. Other outcome variables should then be analysed on the same lines and the results of those analyses used in support of the conclusions that emerged from the main analysis. In this way the type I and type II errors can be considered as confined largely to the tests and decisions involved in the main analysis.

The explanatory variables frequently generate an even larger problem. In many studies, even when experienced statisticians have been thoroughly involved in the design, information is collected on very large numbers of potential explanatory or x variables. Some of these will be of primary importance to the aims of the study (for

example the treatment in a clinical trial or the exposure of interest in an observational study). Others will be variables known to have an effect on the outcome of interest, such as age and sex in a study of blood pressure. In addition, there will probably be a number of variables which it was thought might affect outcome and hence have effects that could, by confounding, bias the estimation of the effects of interest. Estimating these confounding effects may even be a subsidiary part of the aims and objectives of the study.

A strategy that is usually effective for coping with large numbers of explanatory variables is to group them into three categories. The first includes such essential variables as all those that must be present in the final analysis—the intervention, exposure variables implied by the study aims, and the confounding variables generally agreed to have an effect on the outcome under consideration whose effects cannot safely be assumed zero. The second category should contain the possibly interesting x variables whose effects could be assumed to be zero, in this study at least, if an analysis including the first category variables showed them to be unable to contribute any further explanatory effect on variation in the outcome variable. The third category, which in good studies would generally be empty, is for the variables on which information was collected just in case they might have an effect or because they seemed interesting and the marginal cost of collecting them had appeared very small to the questionnaire designer. Once collected, these variables should be included in the analysis or their collection will have been futile.

The overall strategy is first to assess, possibly in groups, whether variables from the third category contribute anything to explaining variation in the outcome variable after all variables in the first category, and possibly those in the second, have been taken into account. Only those third-category variables with a clear association with outcome in these analyses should be considered further. The remainder can be ignored in subsequent analyses and the finding reported as evidence that they appear not to have independent effects on outcome. Secondly, the effects of second-category variables need to be investigated systematically to assess which of them contribute anything to explain variation beyond that contributed by the category-one variables and any from category three that could not be ignored.

By this stage a modelling analysis should have focused on a manageable set of x variables whose independent effects, separately and combined, can be assessed from a single model. At this point, if not earlier, consideration should be given to investigating the possibility of interactions, or effect modifications as they are termed in the epidemiological literature. Until they have been assessed and shown negligible, any inferences concerning individual effects are based on an untested assumption that all interactions are zero. If significant interactions are found, the situation becomes quite complicated. For example, if the effect of treatment, say, is different in males to that found in females, this needs to be allowed for in all further analyses. The efficient way is to keep that interaction term in the model. In more complex situations with several interactions involving gender it may be easier, particularly in the interpretation and presentation, to perform separate analyses for males and females. Comparing the results, identifying where they are similar and where different, is then a relatively clear way of presenting the results of a complex analysis of a complex data set.

If it is assumed that interactions can be ignored or are taken into account appropriately, the remainder of the analysis is a process of testing the main effects of interest and obtaining their estimates and confidence limits for a clear presentation identifying the nature and import of the findings, focusing clearly on those of most importance for the aims of the study.

In practice, it is usually a good idea to develop the analysis system, i.e. stored sequences of commands for the chosen statistical package, on a part of the data following the above strategy from beginning to end. In this way all the unforeseen pitfalls in the computing and analysis sequence are identified early enough for solutions to be found before the full data set is ready for analysis. The final analysis can then be completed quickly and efficiently as soon as the data set is complete and results can be obtained while the data are young.

Conclusion

Obviously special problems which require special techniques which cannot be discussed here. None the less, the range of problems discussed and the appropriate analytical approaches cover the major part of statistical activity in public health research and epidemiology. With reasonable computing facilities, most practical problems that are likely to be met can be tackled using these methods. More detailed texts covering most of the material presented here from a more traditional point of view are Armitage and Berry (1987), Bland (1987), and Altman (1991). In addition, Clayton and Hills (1993) cover most of the methodology in this chapter and more from a slightly different, and helpful, perspective in their excellent text *Statistical models in epidemiology*.

References

Altman, D.G. (1991). *Practical statistics for medical research*. Chapman and Hall, London.

Anderson, S., Auquier, A., Hanck, W., *et al.* (1980). *Statistical methods for comparative studies*. Wiley, New York.

Andrews, N.J. and Swan, A.V. (1994). A sample size investigation system using GLIM4. *GLIM Newsletter*, **23**, 4–11.

Armitage, P. (1960). *Sequential medical trials*. Blackwell Scientific, Oxford.

Armitage, P. and Berry, G. (1987). *Statistical methods in medical research*. Blackwell Scientific, Oxford.

Bland, M. (1987). *An introduction to medical statistics*. Oxford University Press.

Breslow, N.E. and Day, N.E. (1980). *Statistical methods in cancer research*. Vol. 1, *The analysis of case–control studies*. IARC Scientific Publications No. 32, International Agency for Research on Cancer, Lyon.

British National Lymphoma Investigation (1975). Value of prednisone in combination chemotherapy of stage IV Hodgkin's disease. *British Medical Journal*, iii, 413.

Casagrande, J.T., Pike, M.C., and Smith, P.G. (1978). An improved approximate formula for calculating sample sizes for comparing two binomial distributions. *Biometrics*, **34**, 483.

Clayton, D. and Hills, M. (1993). *Statistical models in epidemiology*. Oxford University Press.

Collins, R., Yusuf, S., and Peto, R. (1985). Overview of randomised trials in pregnancy. *British Medical Journal*, **290**, 17–22.

Cox, D.R. (1972). Regression models and life tables (with discussion). *Journal of the Royal Statistical Society B*, **34**, 187.

Dean, A.G., Dean, J.A., Coulombier, D., *et al.* (1994). *Epi Info, Version 6*. US Centers for Disease Control and Prevention, Atlanta, GA.

Dixon, W.J. (ed.) (1981). *BMDP statistical software*. University of California Press, Berkeley, CA.

Forni, A. and Sciame, A. (1975). Chromosome and biochemical studies in women occupationally exposed to lead. *Archives of Environmental Health*, **35**, 139.

Francis, B., Green, M., and Payne, C. (ed.) (1993). *The GLIM system release 4 manual*. Oxford University Press.

Greenberg, R.S. and Ibrahim, M.A. (1991). The case–control study. In *Oxford Textbook of Public Health* (ed. W. W. Holland, R. Detals, and G. Knox), 2nd edn. pp. 121–44. Oxford University Press, Oxford, UK.

Kalbfleisch, J. and Prentice, R.L. (1980). *The statistical analysis of failure time data*. Wiley, New York.

Lachin, J.M. (1981). Introduction to sample size determination and power analysis for clinical trials. *Clinical Trials*, **1**, 93.

Lindley, D.V. and Miller, J.C.P. (1964). *Cambridge elementary statistical tables*. Cambridge University Press.

Mehta, C. and Patel, N. (1992). *StatXact*. Cambridge University Press.

Nelder, J.A. and Wedderburn, R.W.M. (1972). Generalised linear models. *Journal of the Royal Statistical Society A*, **135**, 370.

Peto, R., Pike, M.C., Armitage, P., *et al.* (1977). Design and analysis of randomised clinical trials requiring prolonged observation of each patient: II. Analysis and examples. *British Journal of Cancer*, **35**, 1.

Pocock, S.J. (1983). *Clinical trials—a practical approach*. John Wiley & Sons, Chichester.

Pocock, S.J. and Thompson, S.G. (1991a). The role of meta-analyses in clinical and epidemiological research. In *Coronary heart disease epidemiology; from aetiology to public health* (ed. M. Marmot and P. Elliott) Oxford University Press, Oxford.

Pocock, S.J. and Thompson, S.G. (1991b). Can meta-analysis be trusted? *Lancet* **338**, 1127–30.

Pocock, S.J., Shaper, A.G., Cook, D.G., *et al.* (1980). British regional heart study—geographical variation in cardiovascular mortality and the role of water quality. *British Medical Journal*, **280**, 1243.

Pocock, S.J., Cook, D.G., and Beresford, S.A.A. (1981). Regression of area mortality rates on explanatory variables: what weighting is appropriate. *Journal of Applied Statistics*, **30**, 286.

Ryan, B.F., Joiner, B.L., and Ryan, Jr., T.A. (1985). *Minitab Handbook*. 2nd ed. Duxbury Press, Boston.

Schlesselman, J.J. (1982). *Case–control studies—design, conduct, analysis*. Oxford University Press.

Snedecor, G.W. and Cochran, W.G. (1967). *Statistical methods* (6th edn). Iowa State University Press, Ames, IA.

SPSS Inc. (1990). *SPSS*. Chicago, IL.

Stata Corporation (1993). *Stata reference manual: release 3.1*. (6th edn). Stata Corporation, College Station, TX.

Statistics and Epidemiology Research Corporation and Cytel Software Corporation (1992). *Egret*. Statistics and Epidemiology Research Corporation, Seattle, WA.

Whitehead, J. (1992). *The design and analysis of sequential clinical trials*. Ellis Horwood, Chichester.

Yates, F. (1934). Contingency tables involving smaller numbers and the chi-squared test. *Journal of the Royal Statistical Society*, **1** (suppl.), 217.

18 Mathematical models of transmission and control

Roy Anderson and D. James Nokes

Introduction

The aim of this chapter is to show how simple mathematical models of the transmission of infectious agents within human communities can help to aid the interpretation of observed epidemiological trends, to guide the collection of data towards further understanding, and to help in the design of programmes for the control of infection and disease. A central theme is to improve understanding of the interplay between the variables that determine the typical course of infection within an individual and the variables that control the pattern of infection and disease within communities of people. This theme hinges on an understanding of the basic similarities and differences between different infections in terms of the number of population variables (and consequent equations) needed for a sensible characterization of the system, the typical relations between the various rate parameters (such as birth, death, recovery, and transmission rates), and the form of expression that captures the essence of the transmission process.

Model construction, whether mathematical, verbal, or diagrammatic, is in principle the conceptual reduction of a complex biological or population-based process into a more simple idealized and easily understandable sequence of events. Consequently, the use of mathematical modelling as a descriptive and interpretative tool is a very common exercise in scientific study. Its use, therefore, in epidemiological study should not be viewed as intrinsically difficult or beyond the comprehension of those trained in medical or biological disciplines. The reductionist approach, inherent to model construction, which helps to define processes clearly and identify the most important components of a system, is employed in many areas of public health research and practice. The following situations, for example, are all likely to involve, at the very least, the implicit use of models to simplify and aid understanding: the assessment of the cause and severity of sporadic epidemics of *Salmonella* or hepatitis A virus (HAV) food poisoning or legionnaires' disease, the cost–effectiveness analysis of various measures used to combat an infection within a hospital, within a community, countrywide, or globally, or the identification of the factors that control the maintenance of an endemic infection within a community.

Most epidemiological problems, by definition, are concerned with the study of populations and so involve quantitative scores of, for example, abundances and rates of spread. Thus, it is invariably necessary to convert any descriptive model of process into a more formal mathematical framework so that we work with numbers and not words. The use of a more formal structure enables us to incorporate quantitative estimates of abundances or rates, derived from experiment or field observations, into the model and to make predictions of the likely behaviour of the system under varying conditions, particularly when we are concerned with the introduction or alteration of measures to control infection or disease.

It is the step of translation from verbal or diagrammatic description, into a formal mathematical framework, that arouses the deepest suspicions amongst medical or public health workers. Quite naturally this response is in part a consequence of the use of, what is to many, a strange symbolism to describe familiar verbal or conceptual identities. It must be remembered, however, that mathematics is the most precise language we have available for scientific study and once a problem is formulated in mathematical terms many techniques are available to pursue the logical consequences of the stated assumptions. The clear and unambiguous statement of assumptions is of course a particular attribute of mathematical, as opposed to verbal, description. Excessive use of symbolism or formal methods of analysis can confuse as opposed to clarify and it must be admitted that some sections of the mathematical epidemiological literature have drifted from their original moorings and sail free from the constraints of data or relevance. But to jump from this observation to the belief that mathematical models have nothing to contribute in practice to the design of public health programmes is a mistake. Sensibly used, mathematical models are no more and no less than tools for thinking about things in a precise way.

The second area of suspicion, aside from symbolism, concerns simplification. A frequent criticism of mathematical work in epidemiology is that model formulation involves too many simplifying assumptions despite known biological complexity. This is often true, and needs to be remedied, but it is in part a consequence of the infancy of the discipline and, in some cases, a result of inadequate quantitative understanding of a particular problem. There are, however, two important counter-arguments to the criticism of simplification. First and most importantly, it is often the case in biological study that a few processes dominate the generation of observed pattern despite the fact that many more can, to a lesser degree, influence the outcome. The identification of the dominant processes is an important facet of model construction and, what is termed, sensitivity analysis. The second point concerns scientific method. The process of understanding the consequences of a series of simple assumptions and building upon this by slowly adding complexity is directly analogous to the laboratory scientist's approach of carefully controlling most variables and allowing a few to vary in a planned design. Carefully building complexity on a simple framework can greatly facilitate our understanding of the major factors that influence or control a particular process or pattern.

The chapter is organized as follows. The second section following this introduction provides a brief review of the historical development of mathematical epidemiology and outlines the types of infection that will be considered in latter sections. The third section addresses the problems of model construction, design, and application. The fourth section examines the major concepts in quantitative epidemiology that have been derived from mathematical study, such as threshold host densities for the persistence of an infection, the basic reproductive rate, and herd immunity. In the fifth section methods are explored by which to obtain some of the basic epidemiological parameters from empirical observation. The sixth section turns to applied problems and considers the use of models in the design of control strategies for infection and disease, and the final section is reserved for concluding thoughts. Throughout, mathematical details are kept to a bare minimum and the reader interested in technical details of model construction and analysis is referred to papers in specialist journals.

Historical perspective

The application of mathematics to the study of infectious disease appears to have been initiated by Daniel Bernoulli in 1760 when he used a mathematical method to evaluate the effectiveness of the techniques of variolation against smallpox (Bernoulli 1760). Further interest did not occur until the middle of the nineteenth century when, in 1840, William Farr effectively fitted a normal curve to smoothed quarterly data on deaths from smallpox in England and Wales over the period 1837 to 1839 (Farr 1840). This empirical approach was further developed by John Brownlee (1906) who considered in detail the 'geometry' of epidemic curves. The origins of modern mathematical epidemiology owe much to the work of Hamer, Ross, Soper, Kermack, and McKendrick who, in different ways, began to formulate specific theories about the transmission of infectious disease in simple but precise mathematical statements and to investigate the properties of the resulting models (e.g. Ross, 1911; Kermack and McKendrick, 1927; Soper, 1929). The work of Hamer (1906), Ross (1911), Soper (1929), and Kermack and McKendrick (1927) led to one of the cornerstones of modern mathematical epidemiology via the hypothesis that the course of an epidemic depends on the rate of contact between susceptible and infectious individuals. This led to the so-called 'mass-action' principle in which the net rate of spread of infection is assumed to be proportional to the density of susceptible people multiplied by the density of infectious individuals. In turn this principle generated the celebrated threshold theory according to which the introduction of a few infectious individuals into a community of susceptibles will not give rise to an epidemic outbreak unless the density or number of susceptibles is above a certain critical value (see the review by Fine (1993)).

Since these early beginnings the growth in the literature has been very rapid and recent reviews have been published by Bailey (1975), Becker (1979), Anderson and May (1985c, 1991), Dietz (1987), and Scott and Smith (1994). In recent work there has been an emphasis on the application of control theory to epidemic models (Wickwire 1977), the study of the spatial spread of the disease (Cliff et al. 1993), the investigation of the mechanisms underlying recurrent epidemic behaviour (Anderson and May 1982), the importance of heterogeneity in transmission (Anderson and May 1985a), the formulation of stochastic (=probabilistic) models (Ball 1983), the formulation of models for indirectly transmitted infections with complex lifecycles (Anderson and May 1985b; Rogers 1988), the study of sexually transmitted infections such as gonorrhoea and the human immunodeficiency virus (HIV) (Hethcote and Yorke, 1984; Anderson et al. 1986; May and Anderson 1987), and the development of models for infectious agent transmission in developing countries with positive net human population growth rates (Anderson et al. 1988; McLean and Anderson 1988a, b). Such theoretical work is beginning to play a role in the formulation of public health policy (Babad et al. 1995) and the design of control programmes (Nokes and Anderson 1991) but there is a need in future work for greater emphasis on data-oriented studies that link theory with observation.

In the following sections we attempt to give a flavour of recent work and to distil the major conclusions that have emerged in particular areas. We have deliberately chosen to concentrate on directly transmitted viral and bacterial infections that constitute the major infectious diseases of children in developed countries and, as a consequence of the recent pandemic of the acquired immuno-deficiency syndrome (AIDS), sexually transmitted infections. Our reasons are simply that the mathematical models are more highly developed in these fields by comparison with others (for example, vector-borne infections), that theory has close contact with empirical epidemiological data in these areas, and that model structure is somewhat simpler than for other infections such as metazoan parasites.

Model construction

Definition of terms

Epidemiology

Epidemiology as a subject is concerned with the study of the 'behaviour' of an infection or disease within a population or populations of hosts (=humans). 'Behaviour' refers to observed patterns such as the incidence (the rate at which new cases arise or are reported) of infection or disease. Examples of 'behaviour' are epidemics (a rise and subsequent fall in incidence) and endemicity (the stable maintenance of infection within the human community). The aim of the discipline is to determine the underlying processes and understand the interactions between them, that generate observed patterns, (for example, the rate of spread of infection and the pattern of susceptibility to infection). Epidemiology is a quantitative discipline that draws on statistical techniques for parameter estimation and mathematical methods for delineating the dynamic changes that occur through time, across age classes, or over different spatial locations. The discipline also make use of modern molecular (for example, DNA probes and polymerase chain reaction (PCR)) and immunological (measures of the abundances of antibodies specific to an infectious agent's antigens) techniques for the detection and quantification of current and past infection or disease.

Table 18.1 Epidemiological classification of infectious diseases of public health importance in developed countries

Mode of transmission	Type of parasite	Examples (diseases or agents)
VERTICAL*	Micro†	
	Viruses	Rubella, hepatitis B, cytomegalovirus, retroviruses
	Protozoa	*Toxoplasma gondii*
HORIZONTAL		
Direct		
Close contact	Micro	
	Viruses	Measles, mumps, rubella, Epstein–Barr virus, herpes simplex-1, respiratory syncytical virus, influenza-2, varicella, common cold
	Bacteria	Diphtheria, pertussis, bacterial meningitis
	Macro‡	
	Nematodes	*Enterobius vermicularis* (pinworm)
Environmental	Micro	
	Viruses	Hepatitis A, polio, Coxsackie
	Bacteria	Tetanus, shigella, salmonella. typhoid, cholera, legionnaires' disease
	Protozoa	*Giardia intestinalis*, amoebiasis
	Macro	
	Nematodes	Pinworm
Sexual	Micro	
	Viruses	Hepatitis B, human immunodeficiency virus, herpes simplex-2, cytomegalovirus
	Bacteria	*Neisseria gonorrhoeae*, syphilis
	Protozoa	*Trichomonas vaginalis*
Not direct		
Via other host species (zoonoses)	Micro	
	Virus	Rabies
	Protozoa	*Toxoplasma gondii*
	Macro	
	Nematodes	*Toxocara species*
	Cestodes	*Taenia solium, T. saginata, Echinococcus granulosus* (hydatid)
Vector-borne§	Mirco	
	Viruses	Hepatitis B, human immunodeficiency virus
	Bacteria	*Yersinia* species (plague)
	Protozoa	*Plasmodium* species (malaria)

* Inclusive of transplacental and perinatal infection.

† Microparasites are those that multiply directly within the host individual, usually resulting in acute infections and subsequent durable immunity to reinfection.

‡ Macroparasites are larger parasites whose reproductive stages pass out of the host. Infection intensity is thus a process of accumulation, and can be measured as worm burden.

§ Needle transmission is included.

Populations

The definition and description of the host and parasite populations is of obvious importance in epidemiological studies. A population is an assemblage of organisms of the same species (or genetic type, and so on) which occupy a defined point or points in the plane created by the dimensions of space and time. The basic unit of such populations is the individual organism (that is, parasite or human host). Populations may be divided (=stratified) into a series of categories or classes, the members of which possess a unifying character or characters such as age, sex, or their stage of development. Such subdivisions may be made on spatial or temporal criteria to distinguish a local population from a larger assemblage. The boundaries in space, time, and genetic constitution between different populations are often vague, but it is important to define what constitutes the 'study population' as clearly as possible.

The natural history of infection

Mathematical models are often used to depict the rate of spread or transmission of an infectious agent through a defined human community. For their formulation three broad classes of information are required:

1. The modes and rates of transmission of the agent.

2. The typical course of events within an individual following infection.

3. The demographic and social characteristics of the human community.

The mode of transmission (that is direct, indirect, horizontal, vertical, and so on) is of obvious importance (see Table 18.1), but

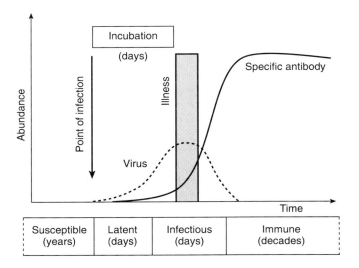

Fig. 18.1 Schematic representation of the typical time-course of an acute viral or bacterial infection in a host individual and the corresponding progression through infection classes (note the different time durations within each of these classes) (Source: Nokes and Anderson 1988, with permission from the editors of *Epidemiology and Infection*.)

if there is more than one route the relative efficiency of each in determining overall transmission must be understood. When considering microparasitic infections (for example, viruses, bacteria, and protozoa that multiply directly within the host) it is generally not possible to measure the pathogen abundance within the host (that is, the burden or intensity of infection). However, following invasion it is important to obtain quantitative information on the typical durations of the latent and infectious periods of the infection and the incubation period of the disease it induces. As depicted in Fig. 18.1, the latent period is defined as the average period of time from the point of infection to the point when an individual becomes infectious to others, the infectious period denotes the average period over which an infected person is infectious to others, and the incubation period defines the average period from infection to the appearance of symptoms of disease. In practice all these periods are variable between individuals, depending on factors such as the size of the inoculum of the infectious agent that initiates infection, the genetic background of host and parasite, past experience of infections, and the nutritional status of the host. The use of an average is an economy of thought and where knowledge permits models should be based on distributed latent and infectious periods. In some instances the infectious period may be influenced by patient management practices such as the confinement of an infected person once symptoms of infection are diagnosed (for example, measles and tuberculosis).

There are instances in the case of viral and bacterial infections when a knowledge of pathogen abundance within blood, excretions, secretions, and other tissues or organs of the host can be of importance in determining the infectivity of an infected person to susceptible contacts. A good example is provided by HIV-1. Current evidence suggests that the infectiousness of an infected person varies greatly over the long and variable incubation period of the disease AIDS that the virus induces (Fig. 18.2). It is believed on the basis of recorded fluctuations in HIV antigenaemia that a short period of high infectiousness occurs shortly after infection,

followed by a long period of low to negligible infectiousness (perhaps many years) before infectiousness again increases as the infected patient develops symptoms of AIDS-related complex (**ARC**) and AIDS (Anderson and May 1988). In these cases rather complex models are required to mirror the natural history of infection (Anderson 1988).

The human immune response to infection, its ability to confer protection against reinfection, and the duration of this protection have important implications for model construction. For the majority of childhood viral infections the assumption of lifelong immunity following recovery appears to be correct. However, as one moves up a scale of parasite structural (antigenic) complexity from viruses to bacteria to protozoa in general the duration of acquired immunity decreases. For certain infections, such as gonorrhoea, acquired immunity is absent while for many protozoan infections it is of short duration (for example, *Plasmodium* sp.). The inability to develop effective immunity is often related to the genetic diversity of the infectious agent population (antigenic diversity) such that infection with one genetic strain fails to protect against invasions by another (for example, *Neisseria gonorrhoea*, *Neisseria menigitidis*, and influenza viruses). The question of immunity can be complicated by a degree of cross-immunity (non-specific in character) resulting from infection by dissimilar organisms (for example, many bacterial infections of the respiratory tract).

Demographic and behavioural characteristics of the human community are usually important in the study of transmission dynamics. For infections that confer lifelong immunity on host recovery the rate of input by births of new susceptibles will influence the overall pattern of infection in a community. Similarly, the rate of transmission of 'close contact' infections (see Table 18.1) will depend upon the degree of mixing between individuals and the density and age distribution of susceptibles and those infected. Heterogeneity in behaviour within a community is of particular importance in the study of sexually transmitted infections since rates of sexual partner change vary greatly between individuals (Johnson *et al.* 1992, 1994). More generally heterogeneity in any

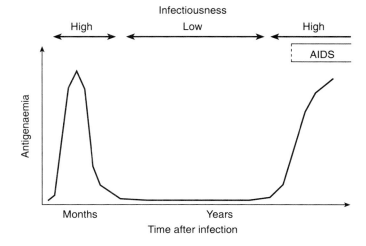

Fig. 18.2 Possible changes in human immunodeficiency virus 1 concentration in the blood of an infected individual (antigenaemia) and in the associated degree of infectiousness during the long incubation period of acquired immune deficiency syndrome (AIDS).

behaviour, whether sexual or social mixing, must be captured in model formulation.

It will be clear from the preceding comments that much quantitative detail about the natural history of infection must be understood for accurate model formulation. In many instances such detail is not available, but model formulation can greatly facilitate our knowledge of what needs to be understood to define the transmission dynamics of a given infection. With respect to many childhood viral and bacterial infections, such as measles, rubella, mumps, pertussis, and diphtheria, a great deal is understood about the natural history and, hence, much of the work on mathematical models has focused on those infections. Their direct route of transmission, their tendency to induce lifelong immunity plus, in most cases, the availability of serological or virological techniques to detect past or current infection facilitates the acquisition of quantitative data.

Units of measurement

The unit of measurement employed in epidemiological study depends on the type of infection. The most basic unit is that of the individual parasite. As already discussed, in most cases this unit is not a practicable option for microparasitic organisms due to difficulties in detection and quantification (advances in molecular biology and biochemistry, however, are generating new techniques which may be of value in the near future). As such, the most useful unit is that of the infected host which allows the human community to be stratified on the basis of whether individuals are susceptible, infected but not yet infectious (=latent or pre-patent), infectious, and recovered (=immune in the case of many viral infections). Infection may be detected directly (for example, DNA probes, virus, or bacterial culture) or indirectly by the presence of antibodies specific to pathogen antigens (serological and salivary tests). Seropositivity does not necessarily discriminate between infected and recovered individuals, but for many viral and bacterial infections serological surveys of a population, perhaps stratified by age, sex, and other variables carried out longitudinally (through time via cohort monitoring) or horizontally (across age classes) provide a key measure of transmission and the broad epidemiological characteristics of the infection.

What models describe

At any point in time a population may be classified by the density or number of susceptible, infected, and immune individuals. With the passing of time and concomitantly as individuals age, people may move from one infection class to the next. As such, with the recruitment of new susceptibles by birth and, in some cases, the loss of immunity, the population structure is a dynamic process with individuals flowing from one class to the next. Mathematical models of transmission attempt to capture the dynamic nature of these changes in the form of difference (discrete time steps) or differential (continuous time) equations (Scott and Smith (1994) give a simple introduction). With respect to microparasitic infections where the population is stratified or compartmentalized by infection status, the resulting models are often referred to as compartmental models. The types and numbers of compartments will depend upon the type of infectious agent and the details of its natural or life history. A number of examples are recorded in

Fig. 18.3 in the form of flow diagrams. These diagrams form a useful intermediary step between biological comprehension and mathematical formulation.

Population rates of flow

Following the introduction of an infection into a stable population the number or density of individuals within the various infection compartments will depend on the rates of flow between compartments such as infection and recovery rates. The size of a population in a specific compartment will depend on the magnitude of those rates that determine the entry and duration of stay. In general, the shorter the duration of stay (the higher the rate of leaving) in a particular compartment the smaller the size of the population in that category (the inverse relationship between 'standing crop' and 'rate of turnover'). If the infection attains a stable endemic equilibrium in the human community, the net input into each compartment will exactly balance the net output. The relative numbers in each compartment will be directly related to the duration of stay. Thus, for example, in the case of endemic measles in a developed country where immunity is lifelong (many decades), individuals remain in the susceptible class for an average of 4 to 5 years and in the latent and infectious classes for a few days (say 7 days on average in each). As such, most people are in the immune class, followed by the susceptible class, and few individuals at any point in time are in the latent and infectious classes. Figure 18.4 provides a diagrammatic representation of this point.

A formal demonstration of the influence of rates of flow (or durations of stay) on the proportion of susceptibles, those infected, and immunes in a population is made possible by the translation of the flow diagram of movement between compartments (see Fig. 18.3) into a set of coupled differential equations. Typically, these describe the rates of change with respect to time (or age or both) of the densities of infants with maternally derived immunity (due to maternal antibodies), susceptibles, infecteds not yet infectious, infectious individuals, and immunes, denoted respectively by $M(t)$, $X(t)$, $H(t)$, $Y(t)$ and $Z(t)$ at time t (see Fig. 18.3(e)). In writing down these equations we need to define the rates of flow between compartments by a series of symbols. For example, in common notation δ (delta) defines the loss of maternally derived immunity. That is, the average per person rate of loss of passive protection. The absolute rate of loss from or movement out of class M (Fig. 18.3) requires that the per capita rate (that is, /person/unit of time) be multiplied by the size of the M subpopulation, that is δM (which has units of persons/unit of time). If δ is the per capita rate of movement out of class M then the average duration of maternally derived immunity is $1/\delta$. These principles apply to the other rate terms shown in Fig. 18.3(e). Hence, using conventional symbols, β (Beta) is the transmission coefficient that defines the probability of contact and infection transfer between a susceptible and infectious person, σ (sigma) defines the per capita rate of leaving the latent class (average latent period $1/\sigma$), γ (gamma) the per capita rate of leaving the infectious class (average infectious period $1/\gamma$), and μ (mu) the natural per capita mortality rate ($1/\mu$ is average life expectancy). For developed countries it is commonly assumed that population size is approximately constant such that net births exactly balance net deaths. Therefore the net death rate, μN (where N is the total population size = $M + X + H + Y + Z$) is equated

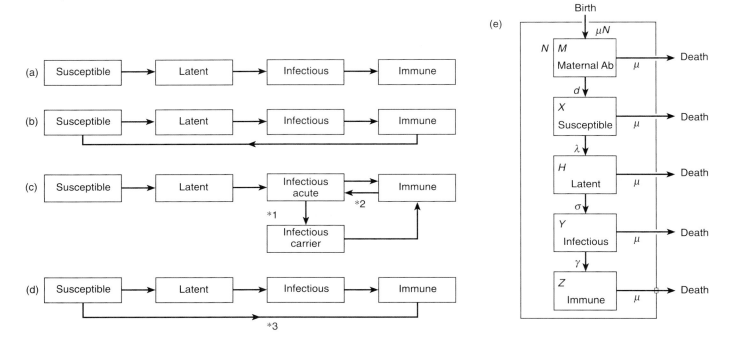

Fig. 18.3 Flow diagrams used to describe the movement of individuals within populations compartmentalized according to infection status to particular parasitic agents. (a) Simple model for infections inducing lasting immunity (e.g. measles, mumps, rubella, yellow fever, and poliomyelitis) or (b) in which immunity is transient and individuals subsequently return to the susceptible pool (e.g. *Neisseria gonorrhoea*, typhoid, cholera, *Trichomonas vaginalis*). (c) Many infections persist within the host for long periods of time, during which the infected individual may remain infectious (*1), as is the case for carriers of hepatitis B virus, gonorrhoea, *Salmonella typhi*, and *Treponema pallidum* (syphilis), chronic tuberculosis patients, or during recrudescence of herpes viruses and malaria. The epidemiological importance of this characteristic is that it enables the perpetuation of such infections in low density communities (see discussion of the mass-action principle in text). For other infections immunity is defence against disease but not asymptomatic reinfection (*2) from which new infectious individuals arise (e.g. *Haemophilis influenzae* and *Neisseria meningitidis*). (d) Vaccination (*3) has the effect of transferring individuals directly from the susceptible to the immune class. (e) More detailed description of the transmission dynamics of an acute microparasitic infection which explicitly accounts for births and deaths in the population. All neonates are born possessing maternally derived protective antibody. The net birth-rate is assumed to equal the sum of the net death-rates for each subpopulation (compartment), i.e. births = μN, where $N = M + X + H + Y + Z$ = constant population size. The *per capita* rates defining movement between infection classes are described in the text.

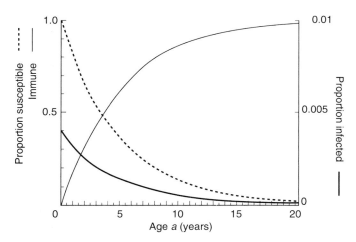

Fig. 18.4 The proportions of a population who are in the susceptible, infected (either latent or infectious), and immune classes for a typical childhood viral infection. In this example, which is based on measles, the force of infection, $\lambda = 0.2$ per year (corresponding to an average age at infection of 5 years) and the rate of movement from the latent class, σ, and recovery from infectiousness, γ, is 52 per year (corresponding to an average duration of stay in each of these infected classes of 1 week). Note that the proportion of the population in the infected classes is always much less than that in the susceptible or the immune classes (Fig 18.1). (Source: May 1986.)

by births (hence the term μN for births in Fig. 18.3(e)). Additionally, it is assumed that infection does not induce an extra case mortality rate over and above natural mortality. With this notation we can define the equations for M, X, H, Y, and Z as

$$dM/dt = \mu N - (\delta + \mu)\, M \qquad (1)$$
$$dX/dt = \delta M - (\beta Y + \mu)\, X \qquad (2)$$
$$dH/dt = \beta XY - (\sigma + \mu)\, H \qquad (3)$$
$$dY/dt = \sigma H - (\gamma + \mu)\, Y \qquad (4)$$
$$dZ/dt = \gamma Y - \mu Z \qquad (5)$$

In these equations, which constitute a simple model of infection transmission, $d\square/dt$ simply refers to the rate of change of the number or density of individuals in a class (M, X, H, Y, or Z) with respect to (over) time. The right-hand side of each of these equations then expresses precisely what the rate of change is. For a simple introduction to the definition, manipulation, and interpretation of such differential equations in the epidemiological context, the reader is referred to Scott and Smith (1994). The major assumptions incorporated in the above equations are that the net rate of infection βXY is proportional to the density of susceptibles multiplied by the density of infectious individuals, that individuals leave each compartment at a constant per capita rate (other than for the susceptible class, X; see below) because it is assumed that the per person rates δ, μ, σ, and γ, do not change over time, and that net births exactly balance net deaths (reasonably accurate for developed countries). To explore what these assumptions imply in terms of the dynamics of transmission and the numbers or proportions of individuals in each class we need to solve these equations either analytically to obtain explicitly expressions for $M(t)$, $X(t)$, $H(t)$, $Y(t)$, and $Z(t)$ in terms of the rate parameters and the variable time (t) or numerically to generate projections of changes in the numbers in each compartment through time (Scott and Smith 1994). In the case of simple models we can often obtain exact analytical solutions as is the case for the equation for $M(t)$ in the model defined by eqns 1 to 5. The solution gives us the number of infants with maternally derived protection at time t, $M(t)$, that is

$$M(t) = \{(\mu N)/(\mu+\delta) \ [1-e^{-(\mu+\delta)t}]\} + M(0)e^{-(\mu+\delta)t} \qquad (6)$$

where $M(0)$ is the number protected at time $t = 0$.

More generally, the complexity of the life histories of many infections makes analytical solution difficult or impossible and numerical methods are required. Modern computers make light work of very complex systems of equations describing disease transmission and many software packages are available for the solution of sets of differential equations and now for model making. Nevertheless, in these cases some general analytical insights can be obtained by examining the equilibrium properties of the model which is done by setting the time derivatives (that is, the $d\square/dt$) equal to zero, that is such that there are assumed to be no further changes in the number of individuals within each infection class because the flows into and out of any one category are equal. These equations can then be solved to determine the numbers at equilibrium (that is at stable endemicity) in each class (referred to as M^*, X^*, H^*, Y^*, and Z^*). For example, in the simple model of eqns (1) to (5) by simple algebraic manipulations we obtain

$$M^* = \mu N/(\delta+\mu) \qquad (7)$$
$$X^* = (\sigma+\mu)(\gamma+\mu)/(\beta\sigma) \qquad (8)$$
$$H^* = (\gamma+\mu)Y^*/\sigma \qquad (9)$$
$$Y^* = (\delta M^*-\mu X^*)/\beta X^* \qquad (10)$$
$$Z^* = \gamma Y^*/\mu \qquad (11)$$

where N is the constant representing the total population size. These equilibrium solutions illustrate how the various rate parameters that determine flow between compartments influence the numbers of individuals in each compartment when the infection is at an endemic steady state. For example, based upon the assumptions in our model for an acute childhood infection, eqns (1) to (5), we can suggest that at endemic equilibrium the number or density of individuals in the maternal antibody class, M^*, is directly dependent upon the net rate of births (where births equal deaths, μN) and inversely related to the rate of loss from the class, $(\delta+\mu)$ (where $1/(\delta+\mu)$ is the average duration in the maternal antibody protected class).

Parameter estimation

The preceding section provided a clear illustration of the numerous parameters that are necessary to define even the simplest model of direct transmission within a human community. To make the best use of a model it is desirable to have available estimates for each of the parameters for a given infection. Some, such as the demographic rates of birth and mortality and total population size, can

be easily obtained via national census databases (usually finely stratified by age and sex in developed countries). Others, such as the average latent and infectious periods, must be determined either by clinical studies of the course of infection in individual patients (for example, measures of change in viral abundance during the course of infection) or by detailed household studies of case to case transmission. Statistical methodology plays an important role in this instance since, as noted earlier, latent, infectious, and incubation periods are rarely constant from one individual to the next. Statistical estimation procedures have been developed to help derive summary statistics of these distributions (for example, means and variances) (Bailey 1975).

Invariably, the most difficult parameter to estimate is the transmission coefficient β (see eqn 2), which is a measure of the rate of contact between members of a population plus the likelihood of infection resulting from contact. In some cases, such as certain sexually transmitted infections (for example, gonorrhoea), direct estimates can be obtained via contact tracing methods (see Hethcote and Yorke 1984). More commonly, indirect methods must be employed, often themselves based on model formulation and analysis. A simple example employs the model defined in the previous section by eqns (1) to (5). We may define the component βY of the transmission term as the per capita rate at which susceptibles (X) acquire infection. This rate is commonly referred to as the 'force of infection' and denoted by the symbol λ (lambda). Analysis of the model reveals that the average age at which an individual typically acquires infection, A, is approximately related to the force of infection by the expression

$$A \cong 1/\lambda \qquad (12)$$

Hence if we can estimate A from an age-stratified serological profile or from age-defined case-notification records (see Box 18.1) we can, via eqn (12) estimate λ. More generally, this rate often varies with age and more complex methods of estimation must be employed given good age-stratified serological data (see (Grenfell and Anderson 1985)). Put in simple terms, if the proportion susceptible at age $a + 1$ is $x(a + 1)$ then the force of infection over the age interval $a \rightarrow a + 1$ (defined per unit of age) is simply

$$\lambda = -\ln[x(a+1)/x(a)] \qquad (13)$$

Box 18.1 Surveillance profiles

Two infections (i) and (ii), are at endemic equilibrium (i.e. roughly constant incidence in time) in a stationary host population (i.e. births are equal to deaths). The changes, with time or increasing age, in the proportion of the population that has experienced each infection may be estimated from longitudinal cohort or horizontal cross-sectional surveys (serological or case notifications) of individuals from birth to life expectancy, L, as shown on next page.

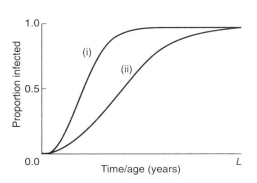

The steeper profile of (i) compared with (ii) is an indication that the basic reproductive potential R_0, of infection (i) exceeds that for infection (ii) such that:

$$R_0(i) > R_0(ii)$$

Assume that each infection induces lifelong immunity, then, from the above profiles, changes with age/time in the proportion susceptible, x, to each infection are:

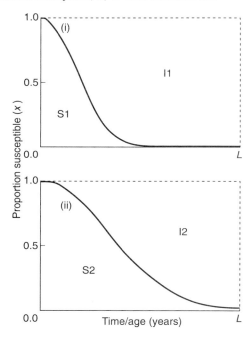

The (equilibrium) proportion of the total population susceptible to infection (i) is:

$$x^*(i) = \text{area S1}/(\text{area S1} + \text{area I1})$$

and infection (ii):

$$x^*(ii) = \text{area S2}/(\text{area S2} + \text{area I2})$$

Note that the equilibrium proportion susceptible to infection (i) (with the higher reproductive rate) is smaller than that for infection (ii) (with a lower rate of reproduction) i.e.:

$$x^*(i) < x^*(ii)$$

and the relationship between these two epidemiological parameters may be usefully expressed as:

$$R_0(i) = 1/x^*(i)$$

and

$$R_0(ii) = 1/x^*(ii)$$

Summing the proportion susceptible, $x(a)$, in the above graphs for each age class from age 0 years (time 0) to L years, we can determine the average age at infection, A, thus:

$$x(a) = x(0) + x(1) + x(2) + \ldots + x(L) = A = S$$

from which it can be seen:

$$A(i) < A(ii)$$

Note also that:

$$R_0(i) = L/A(i) = L/S1$$

and

$$R_0(ii) = L/A(ii) = L/S2$$

(See also eqns 12 and 13, and Anderson and May (1983), for estimation of the force of infection from surveillance profiles.)

Summary examples

Assume infection (i) is measles and (ii) is rubella in the United Kingdom with average life-span, L, of 75 years. If S1 = 5 and S2 = 10, then $A(i) = 5$ years and $A(ii) = 10$ years, and:

$$x^*(i) = 5/75 = 0.066'$$
$$x^*(ii) = 10/75 = 0.133'.$$

Therefore:

$$R_0(i) = 1/0.066' = 15$$
or
$$= 75/5 = 15$$

and

$$R_0(iI) = 1/0.133' = 7.5$$
or
$$= 75/10 = 7.5$$

The implications of this difference in the basic reproductive rate of infection to the proportion of the population that must be vaccinated in order to eradicate each infection can be seen in Fig. 18.11.

With serological data finely stratified by age, under the assumption that the infection confers lifelong immunity upon recovery, eqn (13) can be used to estimate how λ changes with age in a given community. For most childhood viral and bacterial infections λ is a function of age changing from low values in infant classes to high in child to young teenage classes back to low in adult age classes (Fig. 18.5). This is thought to reflect patterns of intimate contact via attendance at school and play activities.

Further complications may arise if rates of contact or transmission vary through time, perhaps due to seasonal factors such as the aggregation and dispersal of children at term and school holiday periods (Yorke et al. 1979; Anderson 1982; Bolker and Grenfell 1993). The problems of parameter estimation are considered in more detail in a later section.

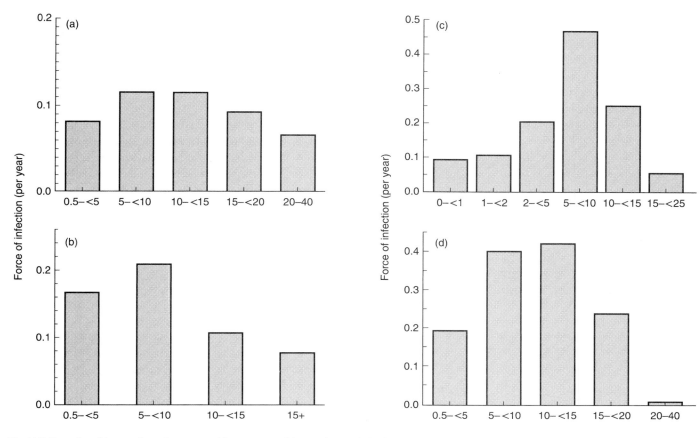

Fig. 18.5 Examples of the age-dependent nature of the per susceptible rate of transmission for common childhood viral and bacterial infections. Graphs (a) and (b) derive from horizontal cross-sectional serological surveys in the United Kingdom, of rubella (Nokes *et al.* 1986) and mumps (Anderson *et al.* 1987), respectively. Graphs (c) and (d) provide estimates based on case-notification data for England and Wales, for whooping cough (Anderson and May 1985*b*) and measles (Grenfell and Anderson 1985), respectively.

Concepts in quantitative epidemiology

The incidence of infection and disease

Transmission by direct contact and the law of mass action

When close contact between infectious and susceptible individuals is necessary for transmission, the number of new cases in a population which arise in a unit of time (that is, incidence of infection) is often assumed to be approximately given by the density (or number) of susceptibles, X, multiplied by the density (or number) of infectious persons, Y, multiplied by the probability of an effective (infectious) contact between an infectious person and a susceptible, β (that is, βXY). This relationship is commonly referred to as the 'law of mass action' by analogy with particles colliding within an ideal gas system (see Box 18.2). The basic assumption implicit in this concept is that the population mixes in a random manner (often referred to as homogeneous mixing). The term βXY which describes net transmission is the major non-linear expression in most compartmental models of directly transmitted viral and bacterial infections. It is, of course, a crude approximation of what actually occurs in human communities and more realistic refinements of this assumption are discussed in later sections. However, it provides a convenient point of departure for model construction and analysis.

Box 18.2 The law of mass action and the incidence of infection

Imagine susceptible and infectious individuals behaving as ideal gas particles within a closed system with no immigration or emigration and occupying a defined space, where: X = number of particles of one gas (i.e. susceptibles); Y = number of particles of a second gas (i.e. infectious people); and β = collision coefficient for the formation of molecules of a new gas from one molecule each of the original gases (i.e. new cases of infection) (a).

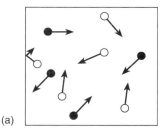

(a)

Gas particles (individuals) are mixing in a homogeneous manner such that collisions (contacts) occur at random. The law of mass action states that the net rate of production of new molecules (i.e. cases), I, is simply:

$$I = \beta X Y$$

The coefficient β is a measure of (i) the rate at which collisions (contacts) occur and (ii) the probability that the repellent forces of the gas particles can be overcome to produce new molecules, or, in the case of infection, the likelihood that a contact between a susceptible and an infectious person results in the transmission of infection. Under these assumptions, the incidence of infection will be increased by larger numbers (or densities) of infectious and susceptible persons and/or high probabilities (β) of transmission (b).

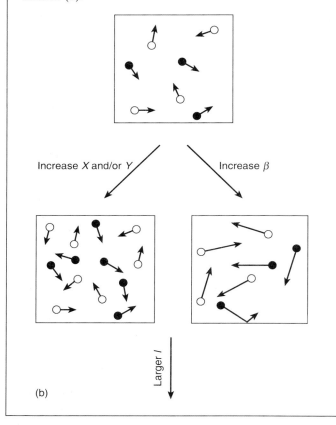

(b)

The transmission coefficient, β

The probability of transmission, β, is made up of two components, namely, the rate at which contacts occur between susceptible and infectious persons and the likelihood that transmission will result from a contact. Consequently β is dependent on sociological and behavioural factors within the host population (that is rate of mixing) and the biological properties that determine the infectiousness of an infected person and the susceptibility of an uninfected individual. These biological properties involve factors such as the virulence of the infectious agent and the genetic background plus the nutritional status of the human host.

Incidence estimates

The incidence of infection, I, can be measured by direct observation of new cases, such as notifications of measles or pertussis.

Unfortunately, however, measures of incidence tell us nothing about the respective densities of susceptibles or infectious people, nor the magnitude of the transmission coefficient β. It is common practice in epidemiology for I to be expressed as the number of cases per unit of population (usually 100 000 people in a defined class (for example, age or sex)) over a defined period of time such as 1 year (for example, 5/100 000 per annum). Such measures are often referred to as attack rates (**ARs**). However, they are a rather poor measure of the intensity of transmission within a population since they take no account of the proportion of the community (or age or sex class) that is susceptible to infection (see Box 18.3). A better measure of the rate at which susceptibles acquire infection is provided by a parameter termed 'the force of infection' commonly denoted by the symbol λ. It simply defines the probability that a susceptible individual will acquire infection over a short period of time (that is, a per susceptible (= per capita) rate of infection) and, in the terminology of the mass-action principle, is defined as $\lambda = \beta Y$. Here β might be thought of as the force of infection for one infectious person in a community. Estimates of this rate λ can be derived from age-stratified serological profiles or case notifications (Anderson and May 1983, 1991; Grenfell and Anderson 1985) (see Fig. 18.5).

Box 18.3 Interpreting attack rates

Care should be exercised when interpreting attack rates in the absence of information on the proportion of individuals within the population who are immune as a result of previous infection (assuming we are considering an infection such as measles that induces lasting immunity on recovery). A simple illustrative example is given below based on case notification for measles.

Age (years)	Attack rate per head of population in that age class	Percentage immune in the age class	Modified attack rate based on infection per head of the susceptible population
2	180/100 000	10	180/90 000
10	20/100 000	90	180/90 000

At a first glance at column two, the attack rate suggests that infants aged 2 years have a much greater chance of acquiring infection than children aged 10 years. However, if we adjust the denominator of the attack rate from per head of population in that age class to per head of susceptible population in the age class, we see from the fourth column that the rate of infection is identical in both age classes.

Validity of the mass-action principle

Despite the simplicity of the notion of homogeneous mixing implicit in the mass-action principle of transmission, the predic-

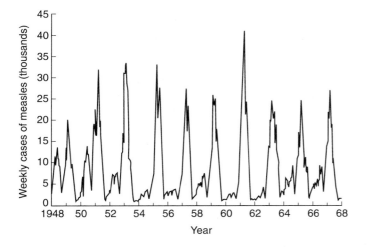

Fig. 18.6 The number of cases of measles reported each week in England and Wales between 1948 and 1968. (Source: Office of Population Censuses and Surveys, London.)

tions of simple compartmental models based on this assumption often mirror observed epidemiological patterns surprisingly well (Anderson and May, 1982). In part, this is a consequence of increased travel, movement, and mixing within many societies in developed countries. Measles epidemics, for example, are often synchronous in England and Wales, with a clear distinction in all parts of these regions between years of high incidence and years of low incidence (Fig. 18.6). However, the less able an infection to spread through a particular population (lower R_0, see below) then the more important are slight deviations from homogeneous mixing, resulting in a lower degree of synchrony of epidemics in a country (Fig. 18.7). The assumption is most appropriate for infections which are spread by close contact between individuals such as respiratory infections transmitted by contaminated droplets and nasopharyngeal secretions. In such cases, the survival of the infectious agent in the external environment is of very short duration (that is, minutes). As such, there is no significant reservoir

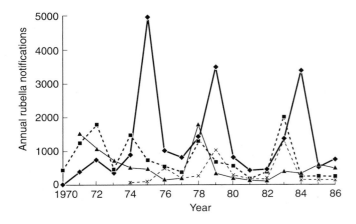

Fig. 18.7 Annual rubella case notifications reported by four city health authorities in England: Leeds (◆), Bristol (■), Manchester (▲), and Newcastle (X). The dominant interepidemic period is roughly 4–5 years with peak incidence often slightly out of phase between cities (compare with Fig. 18.6). (Source: Communicable Disease Surveillance Centre, London.)

of infectious stages to maintain transmission in the absence of infectious persons.

Many kinds of heterogeneities can invalidate the mass-action principle and much attention in recent years has been devoted to their inclusion in compartmental models. The major sources are heterogeneities arising from age-related factors, that determine contact and mixing patterns (that is, 'who mixes with whom') and spatial factors such as differences in population densities in urban and rural areas of a country (Anderson and May 1984, 1991; May and Anderson 1984). Such sources of heterogeneity are very important in the design of control policies based, for example, on mass vaccination and models have been developed to assess their impact.

Heterogeneity in behaviour is of particular importance in the study of sexually transmitted infections such as gonorrhoea and HIV. One of the major determinants of the rate of spread of such infections is the distribution of the rate of sexual-partner change within a defined community (Fig. 18.8). These distributions are typically highly heterogeneous in character (that is the variance in the rate of partner change is much greater in value than the mean rate of partner change) where most people have few different sexual partners in a lifetime (or over a defined period of time) and a few have very many. The activities of individuals in the 'tail' of the distribution (the highly sexually active) are clearly important for the persistence and spread of infection since those with many partners are both more likely to acquire infection and more likely to transmit it to others.

Simple theory based on compartmental models of the transmission of infections such as gonorrhoea and HIV assumes that the net rate at which infection is spread in, for example, a male homosexual community, is determined by the proportion of infectious persons (Y/N where N is the total size of the sexually active population) multiplied by the density of susceptibles (X) multiplied by a transmission coefficient β. This coefficient is defined as the probability that a sexual contact (per partner) results in transmission, B, multiplied by the effective rate of sexual-partner change, c (which determines contacts). If the population mixed homogeneously, this effective rate would simply be the mean rate of sexual-partner change, m. When great heterogeneity in rates of partner change is present within a population the effective rate must be defined in terms of this variability as well as the mean rate of activity. If we assume that the population is divided into classes with different rates of partner change and that partners are chosen (from any class) in proportion to their representation in the population multiplied by the rate of partner change in each group (an assumption of 'proportional mixing', see Anderson *et al.*, 1986; May and Anderson 1987; Garnett *et al.* 1992; Gupta and Anderson 1992), then the effective rate of partner change, c, is given by

$$c = m + (s^2/m) \qquad (14)$$

where m is the mean rate of partner change and s^2 is the variance in the rate. The importance of variability in contact is clear from this simple equation. For example, suppose the mean rate per year is unity but the variance is five times greater. If we assumed that homogeneous mixing occurred our estimate of the effective rate would be 1, but if we take account of heterogeneity the effective rate is six times as large. The influence of the small proportion of

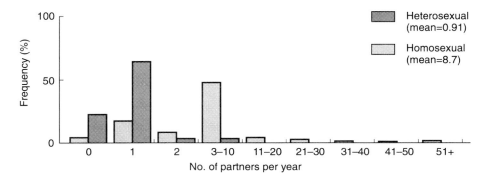

Fig. 18.8 Variation in the numbers of different sexual partners per year revealed from surveys of the male homosexual and the heterosexual communities in the United Kingdom, 1986 (Anderson 1988). The skewed distribution observed in each instance (an indication that although the majority of individuals have few partners, a few have very many), and the mean rate of sexual-partner change (indicated), are both of significance to the perpetuation and rate of spread of sexually transmitted diseases in the community.

highly sexually active individuals on the overall transmission rate is very significant.

Transmission thresholds and the basic reproductive rate of infection

The basic reproductive rate of infection R_0
A key measure of the transmissibility of an infectious agent is provided by a parameter termed the basic reproductive rate (or, also in the literature, basic reproduction number or ratio) and denoted by the symbol R_0. It measures the average number of secondary cases of infection generated by one primary case in a susceptible population. Its value is defined by the number of susceptibles present with which the primary case can come into contact (X) multiplied by the length of time the primary case is infectious to others, D, multiplied by the transmission coefficient, β (rate of effective mixing):

$$R_0 = \beta XD \quad (15)$$

Note that R_0 is a dimensionless quantity (that is, the units of measurement cancel out) that defines the potential to produce secondary cases (in a totally susceptible population) per generation time (that is the average duration of the infection).

The basic reproductive rate is of major epidemiological significance since the condition $R_0 = 1$ defines a transmission threshold below which the generation of secondary cases is insufficient to maintain the infection within the human community. For values above unity the infection will trigger an epidemic and, with a continual input of susceptibles, will result in endemic persistence. A further quantity of interest is the effective reproductive rate R which defines the generation of secondary cases in a population which contains susceptibles and immunes (as opposed to just susceptible individuals). If the prevalence or incidence of infection is stable through time, the effective reproductive rate R must equal unity in value; a situation in which each primary case gives rise, on average, to a single secondary infectious individual.

Factors that influence R_0
The simple expression $R_0 = \beta XD$ (appropriate for directly transmitted infections under the mass-action assumption) provides a framework for assessing how different epidemiological factors influence transmission success. Clearly high transmission coeffi-

cients, long periods of infectiousness, and high densities of susceptibles enhance the generation of secondary cases. Note that its value depends not only on the properties that define the course of infection in an individual (that is, the duration of infectiousness, D), but also on attributes of the host population such as the density of susceptibles, X and the component of β that determines the rate of contact or mixing. A good example of the influence of population level characteristics is provided by the rate of transmission of the measles virus in urban centres in developed and developing countries. The more rapid rise in the proportion of children who have experienced infection, with age, in developing countries by comparison with developed regions is in part a consequence of higher population densities and poorer living conditions (McLean and Anderson 1988a).

Principles of control
The threshold condition for persistence of an infection, defined by $R_0 = 1$, captures the essence of the problem of control. To eradicate an infection we must reduce the value of the basic reproductive rate below unity. Similarly, to reduce incidence the value of R_0 must be reduced below the level that pertains prior to the introduction of control measures. Reductions can be achieved by reducing the infectious period, D, by, for example, the isolation of infectious persons (perhaps recognized by clinical symptoms of disease), reducing the number or density of susceptibles, usually by immunization, and by altering the social and behavioural factors that determine transmission such as improving living conditions to reduce overcrowding (in the case of sexually transmitted infections, education can serve to reduce rates of sexual-partner change or promote the use of condoms to lower the probability of transmission).

The threshold density of susceptibles
It is clear from the definition of R_0 given above that to maintain the value of the basic reproductive rate above unity the density of susceptibles in the population must exceed a critical value. More precisely, this critical level, X_T, is (for the mass-action assumption) obtained by setting $R_0 = 1$ in eqn (15) and rearranging thus:

$$X_T = 1/(\beta D). \quad (16)$$

The aim of mass vaccination, aside from protecting the individual, is to lower the density of susceptible people in the population. If

Table 18.2 Island community size and endemic persistence of measles

Island	Population size (units of 100 000)	Percentage of months in which no cases were reported
Hawaii	5.50	0
Fiji	3.46	36
Iceland	1.60	39
Samoa	1.18	72
Solomon	1.10	68
Fr. Polynesia	0.75	92
New Caledonia	0.68	68
Guam	0.63	20
Tonga	0.57	88
New Hebrides	0.52	70
Gilbert and Ellice	0.40	85
Greenland	0.28	76
Bermuda	0.41	49
Faroe	0.34	68
Cook	0.16	94
Niue	0.05	95
Nauru	0.03	95
St Helena	0.05	96
Falkland	0.02	100

Source: Anderson (1982b).

eradication is the aim of control then the density of susceptibles must be reduced to less than X_T in value.

Critical community size

The magnitude of R_0 and, concomitantly, the size of the threshold density of susceptibles determines whether or not an epidemic of an infection will occur when introduced into a given community. In practice, however, for infections that induce lasting immunity in those who recover, the long-term endemic persistence of infection will depend on the renewal of the supply of susceptibles by new births or, to a lesser extent, by immigration. As such, the net birth rate in a community, which is itself dependent on the total population size (or density), will influence the likelihood of persistence. There is, therefore, a critical community size for the endemic persistence of a given infection. In certain island communities, immigration of susceptibles and infectious individuals may also play a role in the long-term persistence of a given infection (Black 1966; Anderson and May 1986, 1991). These factors are of growing significance as rates of population movement increase as a result of, for example, improved air transport services. Table 18.2 provides an example of the relationship between community size and the likelihood of the endemic persistence of the measles virus.

The concepts of a threshold density of susceptibles and a critical community size are most relevant for directly transmitted viral and bacterial infections that induce lasting (=lifelong) immunity. The production of long-lived infective stages or the use of vectors (such as mosquitoes) lessen the importance of the human population density for the persistence of an infection. In the case of sexually transmitted infections, simple models suggest that there is no

critical density of susceptibles for persistence since the magnitude of R_0 can be approximately given by

$$R_0 = BcD \tag{17}$$

where c is the effective rate of sexual-partner change, D is the average duration of infectiousness, and B is the transmission probability per partner contact (Anderson et al. 1986). This is simple to arrive at theoretically. If, as stated earlier, the incidence of cases of a sexually transmitted disease (**STD**) is defined as

$$I = BcXY/N \tag{18}$$

then following the introduction of a single infectious person ($Y = 1$), infectious over a period D, into a totally susceptible population ($N = X$), the number of secondary cases will be represented by eqn (17).

The dependence upon the number of susceptibles is lost. Biologically this is more difficult to grasp, but it does seem reasonable that the rate of sexual-partner change should be more important to the potential for spread of a STD than the number of susceptibles in the population.

Regulation of infection within human communities

The regulation (that is, modulation or control) of the incidence or prevalence of a particular infection within a human community is largely determined by the level of herd immunity (that is, the proportion of the population immune to infection) and the net rate of input of new susceptible individuals. A simple example serves to illustrate this point. Consider a closed population with no inflow or outflow of susceptible, infected, or immune individuals. If the densities of susceptibles, infecteds, and immunes at time t are defined by $X(t)$, $Y(t)$, and $Z(t)$, respectively, then under the mass-action assumption of transmission the rates of change in the densities with respect to time can be captured by three coupled differential equations:

$$dX / dt = -\beta XY \tag{19}$$
$$dY / dt = \beta XY - \gamma Y \tag{20}$$
$$dZ / dt = \gamma Y \tag{21}$$

It is here assumed that there is no latent period of infection (individuals are infectious once infected), that the average duration of infectiousness, D, is given by $D = 1/\gamma$ where γ is the rate of recovery from infection, that immunity is lifelong, and that no losses occur due to mortality. If we start with a totally susceptible population and introduce a few infecteds, the occurrence of an epidemic will depend upon the magnitude of the basic reproductive rate R_0 ($R_0 = \beta XD$) and, concomitantly, whether or not the density of susceptibles exceeds the critical threshold value X_T ($X_T = 1/\beta D$) (Fig. 18.9). Assuming that R_0 is greater than unity then an epidemic will occur, but as time progresses the density of susceptibles will decline ($X \rightarrow Y \rightarrow Z$) until the effective reproductive rate R is less than unity (that is, susceptible numbers fall below the threshold X_T) and the infection dies out.

For the persistence of the infection one of two things must happen. First, suppose susceptibles are continually introduced into the population at a net rate bN where b is the per capita birth rate and that natural mortalities occur in each class at a per capita rate μ. For simplicity we further assume that net births exactly balance net deaths ($bN = \mu N$) to maintain the total population at a constant

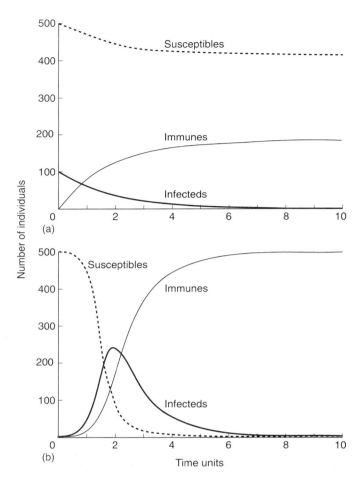

(a)

(b)

Time units

Fig. 18.9 Conditions for an epidemic. (a) Host density (susceptibles) below the threshold level (at time 0, $X = 500$, $Y = 100$, $Z = 0$, $\beta = 0.0001$, $\gamma = 1$, $R_0 = 0.005$, $X_T = 10000$). (b) Host density above the threshold level (at time 0, $X = 500$, $Y = 1$, $Z = 0$, $\beta = 0.01$, $\gamma = 1$, $R_0 = 5$, $X_T = 100$).

size. With these assumptions and provided $R_0 \geq 1$, we find that the infection persists in the population (see Fig. 18.10(a)) with an endemic equilibrium density of susceptibles again equal to X_T and equilibrium densities of infecteds, Y^* and immunes, Z^*, given by

$$Y^* = [\mu/(\mu + \gamma)]\,(N - X_T) \tag{22}$$
$$Z^* = (\gamma/\mu)\,Y^* \tag{23}$$

Second, suppose there are no new births and no mortality but that immunity is of short duration such that individuals leave the immune class Z to regain the susceptible class X at a per capita rate α (alpha) where $1/\alpha$ is the average duration of immunity. We again find that the infection can persist (Fig. 18.10(b)) (provided $R_0 \geq 1$) with equilibrium densities of infecteds and immunes of

$$Y^* = [\alpha \,/\, (\alpha + \gamma)]\,(N - X_T) \tag{24}$$

$$Z^* = (\gamma \,/\, \alpha)\,Y^* \tag{25}$$

Note that the faster the loss of immunity (α large) the higher the equilibrium density of infecteds and the lower Z^*.

These two examples show how the net input of susceptibles and the degree of herd immunity (as controlled by the duration of

immunity to reinfection following recovery) influence the likelihood that an infection will persist endemically after the initial epidemic has swept through a susceptible population following the introduction of an infection. In these simple models of the transmission of direct-contact infections, the density of infecteds tends to exhibit oscillatory behaviour after the introduction of infection due to the rise and fall in the density of susceptibles taking the effective reproductive rate above and below unity in value. These oscillations are seen to damp down, settling to the equilibrium values given analytically (for example eqns 22 to 25). This propensity to exhibit oscillatory behaviour is more apparent if the infection is of short duration such that infection prevalence is sensitive to the availability of susceptibles and induces long-lasting immunity since it takes some time, under these circumstances, for new births or loss of immunity to replenish the supply of susceptibles such that R is again above unity in value. Maintenance of these oscillations over

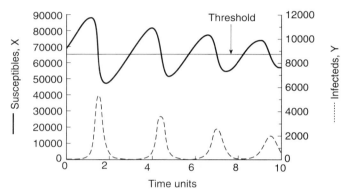

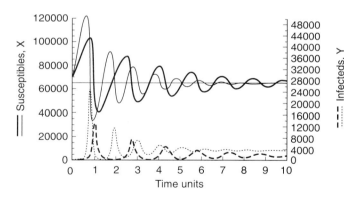

Fig. 18.10 Conditions for the persistence of an infection in a community. In each case solid curves represent susceptible numbers and dashed lines are infected. (a) Renewal of susceptibles by births (initial conditions: $X = 70\,000$, $Y = 1$, $Z = 930\,000$, $\beta = 0.0004$, $\gamma = 26$, $\mu = 0.02$, $\alpha = 0$, $R_0 = \beta N/(\mu + \gamma) \cong 15$, $X = 65\,050$). Notice that the numbers of susceptibles oscillates above and below the threshold susceptible number, X_T (marked) and that each epidemic starts when susceptible numbers exceed the threshold, X_T and subsequently decays as susceptibles fall below the threshold, X_T. Oscillations of X and Y (and Z, not shown) gradually damp over time towards the predicted equilibrium values, X^*, Y^*, and Z^* (see text). (b) Renewal of susceptibles through waning immunity, at rate $\alpha = 0.05$ (thick lines) or 0.1 (thin lines) (corresponding average durations of immunity being 20 and 10 units of time, respectively) (other initial settings as for (a) above except for no mortality, that is $\mu = 0$). Notice that for the two different rates of loss of immunity the equilibrium susceptible numbers are the same ($X^* = X_T$) since waning immunity has no impact on R_0; a higher rate of loss of immunity does, however, result in an increase in numbers of infecteds at equilibrium, Y^*.

the longer period would require a force to be applied periodically—in reality this might derive from seasonal changes in mixing rates as a result of school opening and closing. In Fig. 18.10(a) and (b) it should be noted that the numbers infected, Y, are always increasing when susceptibles, X, exceed the threshold X_T (thus $R > 1$) and are always on the decrease when $X < X_T$ (when $R < 1$). Hence, infection is being driven by the availability of susceptibles.

Other factors that can promote long-term persistence include the production of infective stages that are able to survive for long periods in the external environment, sexual transmission, vertical transmission, from mother to unborn offspring, vector transmission, and the carrier state in which some individuals (for genetic or other reasons) atypically harbour the infection for long periods of time (see Table 18.1 and Fig. 18.3 for examples).

Herd immunity and mass vaccination

When an infection is persisting endemically in a community such that the net rate at which new cases of infection arise is approximately equal to the net rate at which individuals recover and acquire immunity, the effective reproductive rate R is equal to unity in value. This is known as endemic equilibrium. In practice, for many common viral and bacterial infections the incidence of infection fluctuates both on seasonal and longer-term cycles. The effective reproductive rate therefore fluctuates below and above unity in value as the incidence and density of susceptibles change (see Figs. 18.6 and 18.10). However, the average value over a series of incidence cycles (both seasonal and longer term) will be approximately equal to unity in the absence of control intervention or changing social and demographic patterns. The effective reproductive rate is reduced below the basic reproductive rate in relation to the fraction of contacts that are with susceptible individuals $x = X/N$, that is, by the simple equation

$$R = R_0 x. \tag{26}$$

At equilibrium when R is on average unity, the proportion susceptible represents a threshold, x^*, below which infection rates would decline (see Fig. 18.10(a) and (b)). Thus from eqn (26) we see that at equilibrium this proportion susceptible x^* is equal to the reciprocal of the basic reproductive rate R_0 (that is $R_0 \approx 1/x^*$). The magnitude of x^* (and therefore R_0) can be determined from cross-sectional serological surveys given data on the age structure of the population. If x_i is the proportion susceptible in age class i and p_i is the proportion of the population in the same age class then

$$x^* = \sum_{i=1}^{n} x_i p_i$$

in a population with n age classes. This assumes that the serological profile is unchanging over time (see Box 18.1).

To block transmission and eliminate an infection it is necessary to raise the level of herd immunity by mass vaccination such that the magnitude of the effective reproductive rate is less than unity in value. If x^* is the threshold susceptible proportion then $1-x^*$, which we call p_c, represents the herd immunity threshold. Vaccinating a proportion of the population $p > p_c$ will lead to elimination of the infection. This quantity is therefore a critical level for mass vaccination and since from eqn (26) $x^* = 1/R_0$, p_c may be related to the basic reproductive rate in the following way:

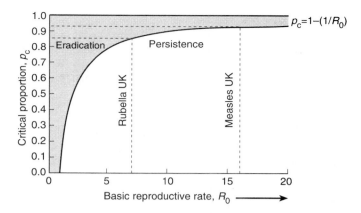

Fig. 18.11 Relationship between the proportion of the population vaccinated at or near birth and the likelihood of an infection persisting or, alternatively, being eliminated. Infectious agents with high basic reproductive rates in defined communities will be more difficult to control by mass vaccination as illustrated by the example of measles and rubella in the United Kingdom. (Source: Nokes and Anderson 1988.)

$$p_c = 1 - 1 / R_0. \tag{28}$$

The relationship between p_c and R_0 is depicted diagrammatically in (Fig. 18.11); the larger the magnitude of the infection's transmission potential (as measured by R_0) the greater the proportion of the population that must be immunized to block transmission. Note that it is not necessary to vaccinate everyone in the community to prevent the spread of infection. The principle of herd immunity implies the indirect protection of the individual conferred by the protection (= vaccination) of the population. The mechanism underlying this concept is that of the critical density of susceptibles required to maintain the magnitude of the reproductive rate above unity in value.

Age at vaccination

In general, immunization programmes are introduced by focusing on cohorts of children such that the level of immunization coverage is built up over many years of routine vaccination, that is as children pass some age gateway. In these circumstances, p_c of eqn (28) must be interpreted as the proportion of each cohort vaccinated as soon after birth as is practically feasible, taking account of the need to immunize after the decay in maternally derived specific antibody. For most viral infections the average duration of protection against infection provided by maternal antibodies is approximately 6 months. It will clearly take many years of cohort immunization to achieve the desired level of artificially induced herd immunity. A further complication is that it is often the case that the average age at vaccination is higher than what is epidemiologically ideal, resulting from the desire to link vaccination with a delivery opportunity (such as first attendance at school) or variation in the age of delivery resulting perhaps from inefficiency in the coordination system or motivation of the population. In this case, simple mathematical models suggest that the level of vaccination coverage required to eradicate the infection under a policy which vaccinates (with a vaccine with 100 per cent efficacy) at an average age of V years is

$$p > [1+(V/L)]/[1+(A/L)] \tag{29}$$

EPIDEMIOLOGICAL APPROACHES

Here L is human life expectancy and A is the average age at which the infection was acquired prior to the introduction of vaccination (Anderson and May 1983). It is clear from this expression that transmission cannot be interrupted unless the average age at vaccination, V, is less than the average age at infection, A, prior to control.

Imperfect vaccines

Various forms of vaccine failure can be specified. At the time of delivery only a proportion of individuals may respond by generating protective immunity postimmunization. This has been called vaccine 'take' (McLean and Blower 1993). In addition, a proportion of those who initially 'take' still may not be able to fend off an infection if exposed. This might be thought of as an exposure –dose-dependent phenomenon and a vaccine exhibiting this effect might be said to provide only a 'degree' of protection. Finally, vaccine-induced immunity may wane with the passing of time such that a previously protected individual once again becomes susceptible. A vaccine therefore may only confer protection for a particular duration.

The impact of these three vaccine failings is to reduce the effectiveness or impact of a specified level of vaccination coverage and therefore increase the level of coverage required to achieve elimination of the infection. This new required vaccination proportion, $p^\wedge$, of an imperfect vaccine, may be related to the critical proportion that needs to be effectively vaccinated for elimination, p_c, in the form

$$P^\wedge = P_c/\phi \qquad (30)$$

where ϕ is the effective vaccine efficacy defined as

$$\phi = \omega_1 \omega_2 [\mu/(\mu + \omega_3)] \qquad (31)$$

(McLean and Blower 1993). Here ω_1 is 'take', ω_2 is 'degree', $1/\omega_3$ is 'duration' (that is ω_3 is the rate of waning vaccine-induced immunity), and μ is the death rate. The effects of 'take' and 'degree' are clearly going to be in direct proportion to their magnitude. For example, if a vaccine is being used to interrupt transmission of an infection with an R_0 value of 10 (for which, from eqn (28), the critical proportion to be effectively immunized, p_c, is 0.9) but only 90 per cent of those vaccinated respond (that is $\omega_1 = 0.9$), then the new proportion needing to be vaccinated is $0.9/0.9 = 1.0$, that is 100 per cent coverage. The effect of a vaccine waning over time is less obvious but may be seen from Fig. 18.12. Here vaccine impact ϕ due to the waning immunity effect (for a vaccine which has perfect 'take' and 'degree') is related to the rate of loss of vaccine-induced immunity, expressed as the time taken for 10 per cent of those vaccinated to lose protection. We can see from this graph that even a slight waning of immunity may cause a very significant reduction in the impact of a vaccine, for example if 10 per cent of those effectively vaccinated at birth lose their immunity by age 30 years vaccine impact is reduced by 20 per cent (that is, $\phi = 0.8$ from Fig. 18.12) and in our above example of an infection with $R_0 = 10$, 100 per cent vaccination in infants would not be sufficient to eliminate transmission.

As a final note of caution, the components that make up the term vaccine impact, ϕ, have a compounding effect since they are multiplied by one another. Thus even if each individually is of little significance, the compounded effect on impact may still be very significant.

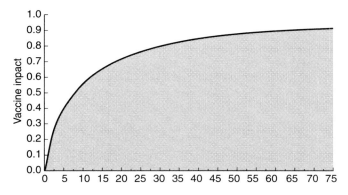

Time taken for 10% to lose immunity (years)

Fig. 18.12 The impact of an imperfect vaccine. The time taken for 10 per cent, of individuals to lose their immunity after vaccination is related to the impact of a vaccine, $\phi = \mu/(\mu + \omega)$ (the vaccine is assumed to have perfect 'take' and 'degree'). Here, the proportion whose immunity has waned in τ years, p_τ, is related to the rate of loss of immunity by the expression $p_\tau = \exp(-\omega\tau)$.

The prevalence of infection and the basic reproductive rate

A further epidemiological feature arising from the existence of a critical density of susceptibles to maintain infection concerns the relationship between the magnitude of the basic reproductive rate and the prevalence of infection in a population in which the infectious agent persists endemically. As depicted in Fig. 18.13 simple models predict that the relationship is non-linear such that a marked reduction in the endemic prevalence or incidence will only occur as the transmission potential is reduced to an extent where it approaches the threshold level $R_0 = 1$. The practical implication is that we should not expect the decline in the incidence of infection induced by mass vaccination to be directly proportional

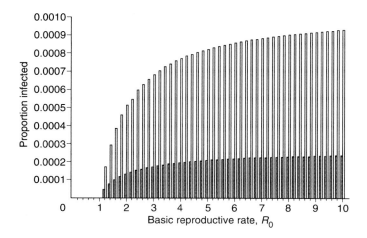

Basic reproductive rate, R_0

Fig. 18.13 Predicted changes in the equilibrium proportion of a population infected (i.e. the stable endemic prevalence of an infection) as the transmission potential of the microparasitic agent varies. For infections where there is no loss of immunity, the level of the plateau of prevalence is dependent upon the rate of input of new susceptibles (i.e. the birth rate, b) and the duration of infectiousness, $1/\gamma$. In the figure, $b = 1/75$ per year and $\gamma = 52$ per year (i.e. a 1-week infectious period) (closed bars) or $\gamma = 13$ per year (i.e. a 4-week period) (open bars). An important point to observe is that the greatest changes in the proportion infected occur over the first few increments of R_0 (irrespective of the magnitude of b or γ.)

to the level of vaccination coverage. The greatest changes are predicted to occur when coverage attains high levels.

Interepidemic period, T

Many viral and bacterial infections that induce lasting immunity to reinfection and which have high transmission potentials (R_0 large) tend to exhibit oscillatory fluctuations in incidence. A good example is that of measles which in the United Kingdom prior to mass vaccination oscillated on a seasonal basis (due to the aggregation and desegregation of children for school term and holiday periods) and a longer-term 2 year cycle with years of high incidence separated by years of low incidence (Anderson et al. 1984) (see Fig. 18.6). Time-series analyses reveal that these longer-term cycles for infection such as measles, mumps, rubella, and pertussis, are not due to chance fluctuations but arise as a result of the dynamic interaction between the net rates of acquisition of infection and immunity on recovery.

Simple models based on the mass-action assumption suggest that the interepidemic period, T, of the longer-term cycles is determined by the generation time of the infection, k, defined as the sum of the latent and infectious periods and the transmission potential of the infection inversely measured by the average age at infection, A, where

$$T = 2\pi(AK)^{\frac{1}{2}}. \tag{32}$$

This simple prediction well matches the observation for a variety of common childhood infections prior to mass vaccination (that is the 2-year cycles of measles, the 3-year cycles of mumps, the 4- to 5-year cycles of rubella, and the 3- to 4-year cycles of pertussis). Non-seasonal oscillation arises as a consequence of the exhaustion of a supply of susceptibles, as an epidemic passes through a population, plus the time lag that arises before new births replenish the pool to trigger the next epidemic. As such the interepidemic period is also influenced by the birth rate of the community (which influences the average age of infection, A, in eqn 32). For example, in developing countries such as Kenya with high birth rates, measles tends to cycle on a 1-year time scale in urban centres as opposed to the 2-year cycle in the United Kingdom prior to control (McLean and Anderson 1988b).

Parameter estimation

Survey data

Survey data on the incidence or prevalence of infection (past or current) can be obtained in a variety of ways. Longitudinal (= through time) data can be acquired by monitoring a cohort of people through time and recording infection as it occurs. Horizontal (= one point in time) –cross-sectional (= across age and sex classes) can be acquired by a survey at one point in time or over a short interval of time, by the examination of different age classes within the population. Such surveys are of most use when based on serological examinations to determine the proportion of individuals in a given age class who have antibodies specific to the antigens of a particular infectious agent. These cross-sectional serological profiles reflect the proportion in each age class who have, at some time in the past, experienced infection. Case-notification data stratified by age and sex and recorded over a set interval of time such as 1 year, can be accumulated to indicate what proportion of the cases occurs by any given age. This may then be used to infer changes in the proportion who experience infection as a function of age. Such data are clearly less reliable than serological information since they are dependent on a lack of bias in reporting efficiency by age class. Bias is to be expected if the seriousness of the disease induced by infection changes with age (for example, rubella in women and mumps in men) or where the incidence of subclinical (that is, undetectable) infections is age dependent.

An alternative to the use of serum for the detection of specific antibodies to infectious agents is saliva. More specifically, when looking for systemic antibodies (for example, IgG and IgM) the fluid which collects around the gums and under the tongue (as distinct from salivary gland secretions) is rich in serum antibodies. This is known as gingivocrevicular exudate or secretion. The disadvantage of using salivary fluid for antibody detection is the low concentration of immunoglobulin it contains relative to serum. IgG in whole saliva is approximately 1000-fold less concentrated than in serum, although in crevicular fluid it may only be 5-fold more dilute (Mortimer and Parry 1991). In recent years highly sensitive assays have been developed to overcome the dilution problems and, accompanied by developments in devices for the collection of crevicular fluid samples, have now been successfully employed in the detection of antibodies to a variety of infections, including measles, rubella, and mumps (Perry et al. 1993; Brown et al. 1994) human parvovirus, and hepatitis B virus (core antibodies) (Parry et al. 1989), and HIV (Van Den Akker et al. 1992; Holmstrom et al. 1990; Behets et al. 1991).

The advantages of using saliva over serum are numerous and associated largely with the collection procedure. For example, sampling is non-invasive and is more acceptable which will assist in response level, the collection process is easier, and may be carried out by non-technical personnel and there is lower risk to both subject and investigator (Mortimer and Parry 1991). Surveys based on saliva collection offer great potential in the fields of epidemiology and surveillance, including the measurement of population immunity in the evaluation of the impact of vaccination programmes of infection prevalence in assessing the rate of spread of infections, such as HIV, through communities. The opportunity for longitudinal surveillance will be beneficial to studies of spatial and temporal patterns of disease spread and salivary diagnosis will become increasingly useful in outbreak investigation and control.

When conducting surveys a number of points should be borne in mind. First, sample sizes should be as large as practically possible, finely stratified by age (preferably infants to elderly people). How large will depend upon what we wish the accuracy or power (see Sokal and Rohlf 1981) of subsequent analyses to be, but 25 to 50 per yearly age class is a rough working estimate. Second, the incidence of infection may oscillate on a seasonal or longer-term basis. As such, it is good practice to carry out surveys that span epidemic and interepidemic years. Third, systematic changes through time may occur in a given population due to social, behavioural, economic, or other changes. Examples include the observed reduction in the incidence of hepatitis A in northern European countries over the past few decades due to improved standards of hygiene and the rise in the incidence of gonorrhoea in certain developed countries during the 1960s and 1970s due to changes in sexual behaviour (for example, increased rates of sexual-partner change). Basic reproductive rates and rates of infection may

Table 18.3 Epidemiological parameters for a variety of childhood infections in developed countries in the absence of mass vaccination. Parameter definitions given in text (data from a variety of sources)

Infection	Average age at infection, A (years)	Location and date	Data type	Life expectancy, L	$R_0{}^*$	p_c (%)
Measles	5.0	England and Wales, 1948–68	Case notifications	70	15.6	94
	5.5	US, large families, 1957	Serology	70	14.0	93
	8.0	US, small families, 1957	Serology	70	9.3	89
Whooping cough	4.5	England and Wales, 1944–78†	Case notifications	70	17.5	94
	4.9	US, urban, 1908–17	Case notifications	60	13.6	93
	6.5	US, rural, 1908–17	Case notifications	60	10.0	90
Chickenpox	8.6	US, urban, 1913–17	Case notifications	60	7.4	86
	6.8	US, urban, 1943	Case notifications	70	11.1	91
Mumps	7.0	UK, urban, 1977	Serology	75	11.5	91
	5.7	Netherlands, urban, 1980	Serology	75	14.4	93
	9.9	US, urban, 1943	Case notifications	70	7.4	86
Diphtheria	10.4	US, 1912–28	Case notifications	60	6.1	84
Rubella	10.8	England, urban, 1980–84‡	Serology	75	7.3	86
	10.2	GDR, 1972	Serology	70	7.2	86
Scarlet fever	8.0	US, urban, 1908–17	Case notifications	60	8.0	88
	12.3	US, rural, 1918–19	Case notifications	60	5.1	80

* $R_0 = L/(A - F)$ where F is duration of maternally derived protection, assumed to last for 6 months in all cases. Note that no consideration of age-dependent forces of infection is given (see text).

† Encroaches on to vaccination era.

‡ Male serology—only females vaccinated under selective immunization policy.

therefore change through time irrespective of the impact of control measures.

The basic reproductive rate of infection

Estimating individually the component parameters that determine the magnitude of the basic reproductive rate, R_0, is fraught with many problems. In the case of directly transmitted viral and bacterial infections, we require a knowledge of the transmission coefficient, β, the density of susceptibles, X, and the average duration of infectiousness. In practice it is often easier to use indirect methods to arrive at estimates of R_0 employing serological data finely stratified by age. As discussed earlier, the rate of decay with age in the proportion susceptible to infection provides measures of the age-dependent forces of infection (the $\lambda(a)$). These in turn can be used to obtain an estimate of the average age, A, at which an individual typically acquires infection. Mathematical models can be used to define a relationship between the magnitude of R_0 and the average age at infection. In the simplest case the relationship is of the form

$$R_0 = Q / A \tag{33}$$

where Q denotes the reciprocal of the net birth rate of the community. In developed countries where net births are approximately equal to net deaths the quality Q is equal to the average life expectancy (from birth), L (Anderson and May 1985a). More generally, if maternally derived antibodies provide protection for an average of F years R_0 is related to A by the expression

$$R_0 = Q / (A - F) \tag{34}$$

A simple example of the use of this equation is provided by the transmission of the measles virus in the United Kingdom prior to the introduction of mass vaccination. In this case the values of A, L, and F, respectively, were 5, 75, and 0.5 years leading to an R_0 estimate of between 16 and 17. The inverse relationship between R_0 and A makes good intuitive sense; infections with high transmission potentials will tend to have low average ages at infection and vice versa. These notions are depicted diagrammatically in Box 18.1, and Table 18.3 lists some estimates of R_0, A, L and the critical level of vaccination coverage to block transmission, p_c, for a variety of common infectious agents in defined localities.

An alternative method to that outlined above is based on the prediction of simple models that the magnitude of R_0 is related to the fraction of the population susceptible to infection, x^* when the infection has attained its endemic equilibrium. The relationship is simply

$$R_0 = 1 / x^* \tag{35}$$

and arises from the fact that at equilibrium the effective reproductive rate is equal to unity in value (see eqn 26). Note that eqns (33) and (35) imply that the average age at infection, A, is inversely related to the equilibrium fraction of susceptibles in a population, x^* required to ensure each primary case gives rise on average to at least one secondary case (see Box 18.1). In general, however, the method based on estimating the average age at infection is the better one given good age-stratified serological data.

Latent and infectious periods

Two sources of data are available to estimate latent and infectious periods. The first derives from clinical, virological, and immuno-

Table 18.4 Average duration of infection classes for a variety of microparasites

Infectious disease	Latent period, $1/\sigma$ (days)	Infectious period, $1/\gamma$ (days)	Incubation period (time to appearance of symptoms; days)
Measles	6–9	6–7	11–14
Chickenpox	8–12	10–11	13–17
Rubella	7–14	11–12	16–20
Hepatitis A	13–17	19–22	30–37
Mumps	12–18	4–8	12–26
Polio	1–3	14–20	7–12
Smallpox	8–11	2–3	10–12
Influenza	1–3	2–3	1–3
Scarlet fever	1–2	14–21	2–3
Whooping cough	6–7	21–23	7–10
Diphtheria	2–5	14–21	2–5

Source: Anderson (1982b).

logical studies of the course of infection in individual patients. For some common microparasitic infections, the presence of the infectious agent in host tissues, excretions, and secretions can be directly assessed. Durations of antigenaemia in body fluids and secretions or of infective particles in specific cells will, in many instances, reflect the period over which an infected person is infectious to others (although this is, of course, not always the case as, for example, with the latent herpesviruses).

Alternatively, statistical methods can be employed in the study of transmission within small groups of individuals. The classic data on measles, collected by Hope Simpson (1952) in the Cirencester area of England during the years 1946 to 1952, record the distribution of the observed time interval between two cases of measles in 219 families with two children under the age of 15 years. The bulk of these observations represent case-to-case transmissions within a family. However, in a small number of families, where the observed interval is only a few days it may be assumed that these cases are double primaries, both children having been simultaneously infected from some outside source. Statistical methods, based on chain binomial models, can be used to derive estimates of the latent, infectious, and incubation periods (see Bailey 1973). A rough guide to these periods for various common viral and bacterial infections is presented in Table 18.4. Some of these estimates are based on detailed analyses of case to case data while others are more speculative.

Sexually transmitted infections

Rather different problems in parameter estimation, to those outlined above, are presented by sexually transmitted infections. By way of an illustration and given the topicality of the infection, we focus on the human immunodeficiency virus (**HIV**).

The characteristics of most sexually-transmitted diseases (STDs) cause their epidemiology to differ from that of common childhood viral and bacterial infections. First, the rate at which new infections are produced does not appear to be closely correlated with population density. Second, the carrier phenomenon in which certain individuals harbour asymptomatic infection is often important. Third, many STDs induce little or no acquired immunity on recovery and, fourth, net transmission depends on the degree of heterogeneity in sexual activity prevailing in the population and the degree to which individuals in one sexual activity class (perhaps

defined in terms of the rate of sexual-partner change) mix with those in the same and in different classes (that is 'who has sex with whom').

The basic reproductive rate, R_0, in its simplest form is determined by the transmission probability, B, multiplied by the effective rate of sexual-partner change, c, multiplied by the average duration of infectiousness, D. Heterogeneity in sexual activity is a major influence on the magnitude of transmission success. Recent national surveys of sexual attitudes and lifestyles suggest that most people have few different sexual partners and a few have many (Anderson and May 1988; ACSF 1992; Johnson *et al.* 1994). The distributions of reported numbers of sex partners per defined period of time therefore tend to be skewed with a long right-hand tail where a few individuals report many partners (Fig. 18.14). As we pointed out earlier, under these circumstances the variance in partner numbers, s^2, is much greater in value than the mean, m and the effective rate of sexual partner change, c, is defined as $c = m + (s^2/m)$ (as in eqn 14). It follows that those with high rates of sexual partner change play a disproportionate role (relative to their proportional representation in a community) in the spread of infection. In the case of HIV each component of R_0 is difficult to measure due to the sensitivity and the practical difficulties associated with the study of sexual behaviour and the long and variable incubation period of the disease AIDS induced by the infection. Over the long incubation period infectiousness appears to vary widely for an individual and between individuals.

As a consequence some indirect measure of transmission potential is required. Mathematical models of transmission suggest that the doubling time, t_d (the average time over which the number of cases of infection doubles), of an epidemic of HIV in a defined risk group (for example, male homosexuals), during the early stages of the epidemic, is related to the magnitude of R_0 by the equation

$$t_d = D\ln(2)/(R_0 - 1) \qquad (36)$$

where D denotes the average duration of infectiousness. Current estimates of the incubation period of AIDS suggest a mean period of approximately 8 years. It is probable that the average infectious period is much shorter perhaps of the order of 2 years or so (however, this is uncertain at present; see Anderson and May 1988). If we assume the value of D lies between 2 and 6 years eqn (32)

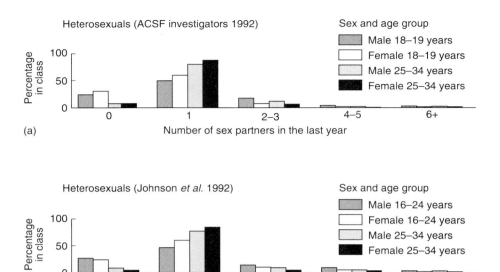

Fig. 18.14 Frequency distributions of the reported number of different sexual partners over the past year in two surveys (in France (a) and Britain (b)) of sexual attitudes and lifestyles (ACSF 1992; Johnson *et al.* 1992) stratified by age and sex. The similarities in the results of the two surveys are striking.

gives estimates of R_0 in the range of 2.7 to 6, given an observed doubling time of around 10 months in male homosexual communities in the United States during the early 1980s (May and Anderson 1987). Of course, this method of estimation is very crude, but it provides a rough guide to the degree to which sexual habits must change in order to reduce the magnitude of R_0 below unity in value (that is by a factor of 3 to 6).

More generally, certain of the parameters that determine the magnitude of R_0 may vary between the sexes. This is certainly the case for gonorrhoea (see Hethcote and Yorke 1984) and it may be true for HIV. In these circumstances, when considering transmission via heterosexual contact, the basic reproductive rate adopts the form

$$R_0 = (B_1 B_2 c_1 c_2 D_1 D_2) \qquad (37)$$

where the subscripts 1 and 2 denote males and females, respectively.

Further complications arise in the definition of the case reproductive number, R_0, when we take into account the pattern of mixing between different strata of the sexually active population. For example, in light of the data presented in Fig. 18.14 concerning heterogeneity in reported rates of sexual partner acquisition per year in France and Britain, it seems sensible to stratify the population by the rate of sexual partner change into low-, medium-, and high- 'activity' classes. The magnitude of any epidemics of an STD and the endemic level of infection in a community will depend on the degree to which the small number of people with high rates of sexual-partner change mix with the medium- and low-activity classes. If mixing is random across activity classes the infection will be widely disseminated in the community. However, if mixing is highly assortative (that is, like with like) the infection will tend to be restricted to the small proportion of individuals in the high-activity class (the so-called 'core' group) with a few cases in the other classes. The prevailing pattern of mixing is therefore of great importance in determining the prevalence of an STD and the

degree to which it is disseminated in a defined community. Recent studies of mixing patterns based on contact tracing via STD clinics suggest that mixing is more assortative than random in character (Garnett and Anderson 1993). Once mixing is taken into account it is necessary to redefine transmission success in terms of the number of secondary cases of infection in group i generated by contact with infectives in group j, R_{0ij}, where

$$R_{0ij} = p_{ij} B c D. \qquad (38)$$

Here p_{ij} is the probability that a susceptible in group i has a sexual contact with someone in group j.

Again, more generally, the population is structured by other variables such as age, ethnicity, area of residence, and educational attainment. Here again, behavioural studies suggest a degree of assortative mixing with respect to the choice of sexual partner —except in contact with commercial sex workers.

Models and the design of control programmes

Mathematical models can be of help in defining the targets for a control programme, in interpreting observed epidemiological changes under the impact of control, and in discriminating between different approaches (Nokes and Anderson 1987, 1988, 1991, 1992, 1993; Garnett *et al.* 1992; Gupta and Anderson 1992). In this section we consider two themes, namely, the design of mass vaccination programmes to control childhood viral and bacterial infections and education to induce changes in sexual behaviour to control STDs.

Impact of mass vaccination

In practical terms, the level of vaccination coverage in a given community or country is determined by a variety of economic and logistic factors (developing countries) or motivational and legislative issues (industrialized countries). However, models can define the ideal goal of a given programme. We have already outlined the relationship between the critical level of vaccination coverage required to block transmission, p_c and various epidemiological (R_0), demographic (net birth rate and life expectancy, Q and L), and logistical (V, the average age at vaccination) parameters (see eqns 28 and 29 and Table 18.3) and vaccine properties (see eqns 30 and 31). In many instances, the high transmission potentials of common childhood viral and bacterial infections imply very high levels of infant vaccination coverage if transmission is to be interrupted. If vaccine efficacy is less than 100 per cent (for example, the current pertussis vaccines) then problems may arise in attaining these targets even if legislation enforces vaccination of all children before entry to school (as in the United States). Models emphasize the point that to obtain the best effects very high levels of coverage should be aimed at with vaccination at as young an age as is practically feasible given the complications presented by the presence of maternally derived antibodies in infants.

Aside from defining targets for vaccination coverage, models can assist in interpreting the impact of a given programme on epidemiological parameters such as the incidence of infection, the average age at infection and the interepidemic period. In a later part of this section we consider the principles underlying an alternative approach to mass vaccine intervention, that of pulsed immunization across age cohorts, which has recently met with such success in controlling polio and measles in Central and South America.

Incidence of infection

Immunization has the direct effect of reducing the number of cases of infection as a result of the protection of the vaccinated individuals ($X - > Z$, see Fig. 18.3(d)). Since this reduces the number of infectious persons in the vaccinated population, an indirect effect is a reduction in the net rate of transmission of the virus or bacterium. This is the principle of herd immunity, where susceptibles gain protection from the vaccinated proportion of the population. Provided the infection is able to persist endemically (that is, the level of coverage is less than that required for eradication), models suggest that the equilibrium proportion of susceptibles in the population will remain constant irrespective of the level of coverage below the critical point for eradication. This prediction is illustrated diagrammatically in Fig. 18.15. The level of coverage simply reduces the proportion of seropositive individuals who have acquired immunity via infection as opposed to via vaccination. As mentioned earlier (see Fig. 18.13) the manner in which the incidence declines as the level of coverage rises is non-linear in form with the most dramatic reductions occurring as the proportion vaccinated approaches the critical point for the interruption of transmission. As the level of coverage approaches the critical point the proportion of immune persons who possess vaccine-induced immunity approaches unity.

The average age at infection

As a direct result of reducing the net rate of transmission, vaccination acts to increase the average age at which susceptibles acquire infection over that pertaining prior to control (that is, by reducing the probability of coming into contact with an infectious person). Observation now bears out the expectation of an increased average age of susceptibles and of infection as a result of mass vaccination programmes. The example shown in Fig. 18.16, shows

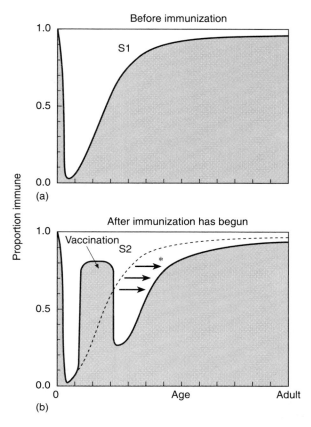

Fig. 18.15 Diagrammatic representation of the predicted impact of mass immunization (against a typical childhood viral or bacterial infection) on the age distribution of susceptibility in a population. Before immunization (a) there is a 'valley' of susceptibles (S1) in the young age classes. Attempts to fill in this valley by vaccination (b) reduces the rate of transmission of the infection thus lowering the probability of unvaccinated individuals being infected. As a consequence there is an upward shift in the ages of susceptibles (*) from that pertaining before vaccination (dotted line). Two points are important: (i) the number or proportion of susceptibles after immunization has begun (area S2) is roughly unchanged from that which existed before immunization (area S1); and (ii) the average age of susceptibles increases. (Source: Nokes and Anderson 1988, with permission from the editors of *Epidemiology and Infection*.)

the prevaccination (1982) serological profile (or distribution of susceptibles by age) for rubella in Finland (Fig. 18.16(a)) and the profile (for males only) in 1986 4 years after mass infant MMR (measles, mumps and rubella) vaccine was introduced (Fig. 18.16(b)) (Ukkonen and Von Bonsdorf 1988). The similarity with Fig. 18.15. is striking. Also shown in Fig. 18.16 is the changing distribution of diagnosed rubella cases, with a marked increase in the average age. Later we discuss how this change in the age distribution of the incidence of infection can influence the incidence of disease arising from infection if older people differ in their vulnerability to complications and concomitant morbidity when compared with younger people.

Interepidemic period

Simple models also predicted that a reduction in the transmission rate in a vaccinated population will act to lengthen the interepidemic period over that pertaining prior to control (Anderson and May 1983). This may be shown easily using our model in Fig. 18.10 if a proportion of all individuals entering the population are

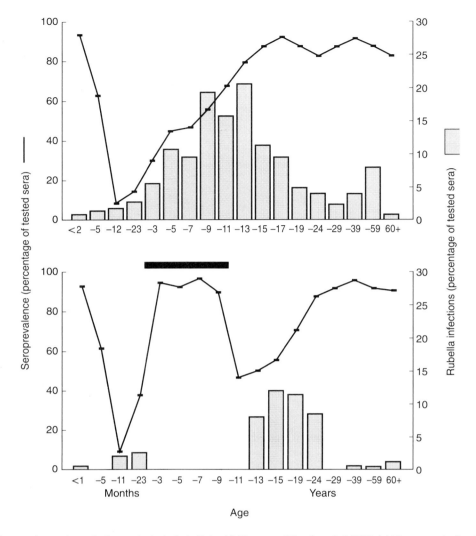

Fig. 18.16 The observed impact of mass immunization against rubella in Finland (Ukkonen and Von Bonsdorf 1988). (a) The prevaccination (1982) age seroprevalence of specific rubella antibodies (line) with the age distribution of diagnosed cases (bars). (b) Four years after mass infant MMR vaccination was introduced with the age range affected shown by the solid bar (data for males only) (other details as for (a)) (Nokes and Anderson 1993). Reproduced with kind permission of the editors of *Reviews in Medical Microbiololology.*

vaccinated at the time of birth (starting from time unit 5 onwards), resulting in an increase in the time taken for susceptibles to build up to threshold numbers and, hence, an increase in the interval between epidemics (Fig. 18.17). This pattern has been observed in various vaccinated communities (for example, Fig. 18.18).

Cautionary notes

The changes in epidemiological patterns of infection induced by vaccination are not always beneficial. An increased interepidemic period, for example, can induce complacency in the community with respect to the need to maintain high levels of vaccination coverage. Motivating parents to ensure that their children are vaccinated during long periods of low incidence (the troughs in the epidemic cycle) can be problematic particularly if there is some small but measurable risk associated with vaccination. At the start of a mass immunization programme the probability of serious disease arising from vaccination is usually orders of magnitude smaller than the risk of serious disease arising from natural

infection. As the point of eradication is approached, the relative magnitude of these two probabilities must inevitably be reversed.

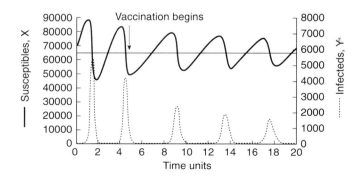

Fig. 18.17 Predicted impact of vaccination on the interepidemic period. Vaccination of 50 per cent of all births was introduced at time 5 into the model given in Fig. 18.10. (with the same initial settings).

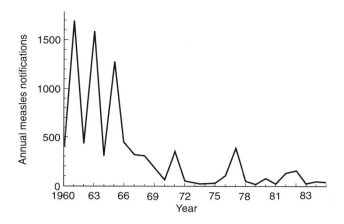

Fig. 18.18 Annual measles notifications for the city of Oxford, England, for the period 1960–85. The introduction of measles vaccination in 1966 has resulted in a significant increase in the period between epidemics. (Source: Office of Population Censuses and Surveys, London.)

The optimum strategy for the individual (not to be vaccinated) therefore becomes at odds with the needs of society (to maintain her immunity) (Nokes and Anderson 1991). This issue—which was central to the decline in the uptake of pertussis vaccine in the United Kingdom during the mid- to late-1970s—can be overcome by legislation to enforce vaccination (as in the United States), but its final resolution is only achieved by global eradication of the disease agent so that routine vaccination can cease.

Other problems concern doubts over the role played by exposure to natural infection in boosting vaccine-induced immunity and, in some cases, worries over the duration of protection provided by vaccination. If enough is understood about these problems mathematical models could be used to decide whether or not to revaccinate a proportion of the immunized population and, if so, what is the best age to revaccinate. Similarly, recent evidence for measles suggests that passive immunity in infants of mothers whose own protection was vaccine derived wanes more rapidly than in infants whose mothers were naturally infected (Markowitz *et al.* 1995). The consequences of this are that, on the one hand, infants become susceptible to infection at an earlier age than was previously the case, but, on the other hand, it may allow for the lowering of the age of vaccine delivery. The merits of this latter issue could well be addressed using mathematical models.

Variation in vaccine uptake

Ideally, vaccination coverage should be high and constant both through time and in different regions of a country. In practice, however, this is rarely the case. With respect to time, once incidence is reduced to a low level, problems can arise in stimulating public health workers to maintain coverage at high levels. More importantly, after introduction, most immunization programmes show a slow increase in rates of coverage. This obviously results in a delay in experiencing the full benefits and must be recognized in assessing the impact of a given policy. It takes many decades before the full benefits of a cohort immunization programme are manifest. Model simulations of the impact of such programmes on the incidence of infection and disease clearly illustrate this point (Anderson and May 1983, 1985*a*,*c*). Of greater concern, however, is

the variation in vaccine uptake in different regions of a country. Levels of vaccine coverage for sentinel antigens (measles, diphtheria 3, and pertussis 3) in the United Kingdom, for example, varied widely between different regions in the late 1980s (Fig. 18.19), a problem which has been greatly diminished as a result of improved vaccine programme coordination. To block transmission country-wide effectively it is necessary to ensure that the targets laid out in Table 18.3 are attained in each area. Otherwise, pockets of infection in regions of low uptake will continue to trigger small epidemics in other areas. The upsurge of mumps in certain states in the United States in the late 1980s (Wharton *et al.* 1988) is an example of the potential hazards of spatial variation in vaccine uptake.

Non-uniformity in human population density

Non-uniformity in the spatial distribution of humans, with some people living in dense aggregates and others living in isolated or small groups, can lead to heterogeneity in transmission rates. Models suggest that this can result in the transmission potential of an infection (R_0) being greater on average than suggested by estimation procedures which assume spatial homogeneity (Anderson and May 1984; May and Anderson 1984). Under these circumstances, theory suggests that the optimal solution appears to involve 'targeting' vaccination coverage in relation to group size with dense groups receiving the highest levels of coverage. The optimal programme is defined as that minimizing the total, communitywide number of immunizations needed for elimination or for a defined level of control. This strategy reduces the overall proportion that must be vaccinated to block transmission, compared with that estimated on the assumption of spatial homogeneity. This conclusion has practical significance for the control of infections such as measles and pertussis in some developing countries, where rural–urban differences in population density tend to be much more marked than in developed countries (Anderson and May 1991). It is probable that in many regions of Africa and Asia, diseases such as measles cannot persist endemically in rural areas without frequent movement of people between low-density (rural) and high-density (urban) populations. Under these circumstances, transmission might be blocked in both regions by high levels of mass immunization in the urban centres alone.

Age-dependent factors

Analyses of case-notification records and serological profiles suggest that, for many common infections (measles, rubella, and pertussis), the per capita rate of infection ($\lambda(a)$) depends on the ages of susceptible individuals, changing from a low level in the 0 to 5-year age classes, via a high level in the 5 to 15-year age classes back to a lower level in the adult age classes (Fig. 18.5). This is of interest both because it reflects behavioural attributes of human communities and because of its impact on the predicted level of vaccination required to eliminate transmission. The high levels of the force of infection in the 5 to 15-year-old classes are thought to arise as a consequence of frequent and intimate contacts within school environments (Anderson and May 1985*c*; Nokes *et al.* 1986; Anderson *et al.* 1987). Theoretical studies which take account of age dependence in the force of infection predict somewhat lower rates of vaccination than those arrived at under the simple mass-action assumption (see Table 18.3). However, it should be emphasized that the values listed in Table 18.3 provide a good first

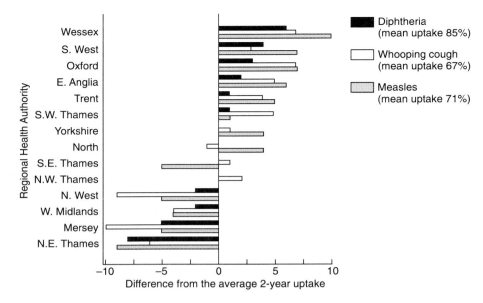

Fig. 18.19 Regional variation in immunization uptake for sentinel agents in England, 1986. (Source: Nokes and Anderson 1988, with permission from the editors of *Epidemiology and Infection*.)

approximation of the targets to be obtained in a vaccination programme. The reason why the observed age-related changes in the force of infection influence the predicted level of coverage relates to the tendency for mass vaccination to shift the age distribution of susceptibility (Figs. 18.15 and 18.16). Susceptibles who avoid infection and vaccination may move from an age class with a high force of infection into an older class with a lower rate.

Does mass vaccination always reduce disease incidence?

The risk of complications arising from infection is often dependent upon the age at which exposure occurs. The newborn are particularly vulnerable due to their immunological immaturity and are therefore more likely to suffer morbidity and even mortality (Fig. 18.20). Protection by maternally derived antibody moderates the risk during this time of great vulnerability but, in developing countries, factors such as malnutrition and high incidences of secondary 'opportunist' infections can result in high mortality rates as a result of infant and childhood viral and bacterial infection. In general where the risk of serious disease is higher in the young than old people, mass vaccination will always act to reduce the incidence of disease.

In developed countries case fatalities are much less common and the greatest problem is morbidity and the risk of serious disease. Of particular concern are infections where the risk of severe complications increases with age (Fig. 18.21). Whether this trend is important depends on the quantitative details of such factors as how risk changes with age, the average age at which the vaccine is administered, the average age at infection, and how the rate (or force) of infection changes with age prior to the introduction of immunization (Knox 1980; Anderson and May 1983, 1985*a*; Anderson *et al.* 1987; Nokes and Anderson 1991) (see Fig. 18.21).

Rubella and mumps are clear examples because of the risk of

congenital rubella syndrome (**CRS**) in infants born to mothers who contracted rubella in their first trimester of pregnancy and the occurrence of orchitis and the associated risk of sterility in post-pubertal males plus infection of the central nervous system following mumps infection. The crux of the problem relates to how mass vaccination changes the age profile of the incidence of infection. Any level of coverage will reduce the incidence of infection but by increasing the average age at which those still susceptible acquire infection certain levels of coverage may increase the incidence of disease. The important question is whether the increase in the proportion of cases in older people will result in an increase in the absolute numbers of cases of serious disease.

This problem has resulted in the adoption of different vaccina-

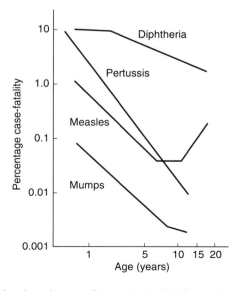

Fig. 18.20 Age-dependent mortality associated with infection from a variety of childhood viruses and bacteria. (Source: MIMS 1987.)

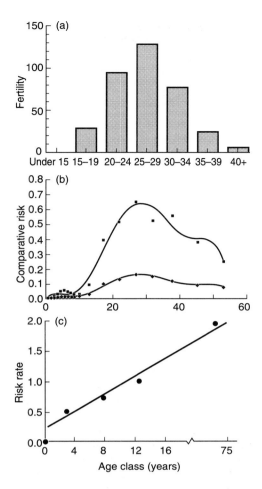

Fig. 18.21 Age-dependent risk of complications from infection: (a) the likelihood of fetal transmission of rubella virus with concomitant risk of congenital rubella syndrome is directly related to age-specific fertility of women (data for England and Wales, 1985; source OPCS Monitor FMI 86/2); (b) changes in the risk of complications from mumps infection in the United Kingdom relative to age and sex. In addition to meningitis and encephalitis, males (■) may suffer orchitis. (Source: Anderson *et al.* 1987). Note here that the term comparative risk, refers to the risk compared to other age classes; (c) measles encephalitis per 100 000 cases in the United States. (Source: Anderson and May 1983.)

tion programmes against rubella (to control CRS) in different countries (Table 18.5). Until the introduction of MMR vaccine in the United Kingdom in 1988, girls only were vaccinated at an average age of around 12 years, so as to allow rubella virus to circulate in males and young females and create naturally acquired immunity in the early years. By contrast, it has always been the case in the United States for both boys and girls to be vaccinated at around 2 years of age, with the aim of blocking rubella virus transmission. Mathematical models predict that the United States policy is best if very high levels of vaccination (80 to 85 per cent of each yearly cohort) can be achieved at a young age, while the United Kingdom policy is better if this cannot be guaranteed (see Fig. 18.22). A mixed policy is predicted to be of additional benefit over the selective policy alone if moderate to high levels of vaccine uptake among boys and girls can be achieved at a young age (>60 per cent) (Anderson and Grenfell 1986).

The process of using mathematical models to evaluate the impact of a particular mass vaccination policy in a community is

detailed in Box 18.4, in this case for mumps. At the time of the introduction of MMR infant vaccination in the United Kingdom in November 1988 such studies as these suggested that provided moderate to high levels of coverage (60 to 65 per cent) could be achieved then the change in policy was unlikely to increase the incidence of serious disease (Anderson *et al.* 1987). Following the implementation of the MMR vaccine, coverage rose from the level of uptake for measles vaccine at the time of around 70 per cent by age 2 years (the level of update for measles vaccine at the time) to 90 per cent within the space of 2 years. Thoughts have now turned to the required strategy for elimination of these three infections and use is being made of mathematical models to explore the possible options, such as a two-dose schedule (Babad *et al.* 1995). For rubella and specifically the issue of when to remove the selective arm of the vaccination strategy, we now have the example from the Scandinavian countries to guide our policy. Data from Finland, for example, clearly show the need to continue schoolgirl vaccination until the cohorts with high-level immunity through infant vaccination span the entire high-fertility age groups. Note that this concurs with predictions made prior to the observations becoming available (Nokes and Anderson 1987).

Box 18.4 Epidemiology and control of mumps virus infection.

Incidence of infection

Mumps is typical of the childhood viral infections with peak incidence in the young age classes and relatively few cases occurring in adulthood (a).

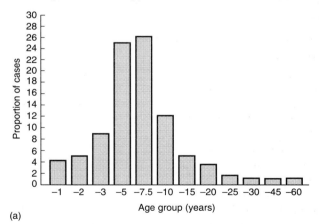

(a)

Information of this sort, obtained from age-specific case notification data or age-serological profiles, is used to derive age-dependent rates of transmission as shown in Fig. 18.5(b) in the main text.

Incidence of disease

Various types of complications are associated with mumps virus infection (b). In the prevaccination era mumps was the most common cause of viral meningitis in the United Kingdom, and is also a significant cause of encephalitis and, in post-pubertal males, of orchitis.

(continued on next page)

Table 18.5 Strategies of rubella immunization

	Selective	Mass cohort
Aim	Eliminate congenital rubella, not rubella infection	Eliminate rubella infection, and so congenital rubella
Age at vaccination	Pre-pubertal girls (10–15 years)	Boys and girls of 1–2 years
Philosophy	(i) Build upon levels of herd immunity attained through childhood (ii) Reduce the proportion of susceptible women of childbearing age (ii) Allow continued circulation of virus in male and young female segments of the population	(i) Reduce circulation of wild virus in community, especially children (ii) Lower the probability of susceptible women catching infection via the action of herd immunity
Overall incidence of infection	Very little impact at any level of coverage	(i) Reduction in cases in a non-linear manner as vaccine level increases (see Fig. 18.13) (ii) Increase in average age at infection
Other concerns	(i) Cannot eradicate congenital rubella unless 100 per cent of women 'at risk' are immune (via infection in childhhod or immunization) (ii) Herd immunity largely natural with continued re-exposure to infection and boosting of antibody response	(i) Proportion of remaining cases increases in older age classes, hence possible to increase congenital rubella at certain levels of immunization (ii) Herd immunity ultimately all vaccine induced. Less solid? No boosting of immunity by re-exposure to virus
Which policy?	Sutiable for lower levels of vaccination coverage (see Fig. 18.22)	Sutiable if high levels of uptake can be achieved (see Fig. 18.22)
Country (as example)	UK	US

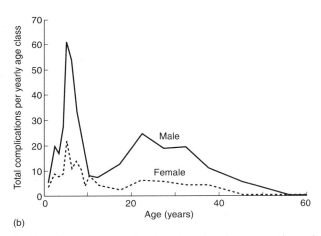

(b)

Scaling these age-complication data by the proportion of cases of *infection* in the corresponding age classes (shown above), it is possible to drive the relative risk of complications from infection, as shown in Fig. 18.21(b) in the main text. What becomes apparent from these data analyses is that although fewest cases of infection occur in the older age classes, there remain substantial numbers of cases of complications, such that infection in older persons runs a considerably greater risk of resulting in complications when compared with infection in the young.

Mass vaccination and the incidence of infection

The figure below shows the predicted numbers of cases of mumps infection across a wide range of age classes, through time, before and after the introduction of a programme of mass cohort immunization (60 per cent of 2 year olds).

The force of infection is assumed to remain constant with age at 0.15 per year (corresponding to an average age at infection before immunization of 6.7 years). The epidemic peaks in the prevaccine period show the majority of cases occurring in the youngest age classes. Subsequent to the initiation of immunization two changes should be noted: (a) the obvious and expected decline in infection incidence (particularly in the young); and (b) an increase in the age at which the remaining cases occur, indicated by the wave of infections migrating, in time, into the older age classes. The implications of this shift in the age distribution of cases on the incidence of disease are addressed on the next page.

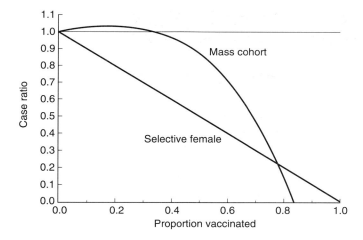

Fig. 18.22 Effectiveness of different rubella immunization programmes. Changes in the predicted case ratio (i.e. the average number of rubella infections in pregnant women after the introduction of immunization divided by average prevaccination number) under increasing levels of coverage for two types of policy, namely, selective immunization of girls of average age 12 years or mass vaccination of children (aged 2 years). Low to medium levels of uptake favour adoption of a selective immunization programme compared with mass vaccination which has the undesirable effect of increasing the average age at infection.

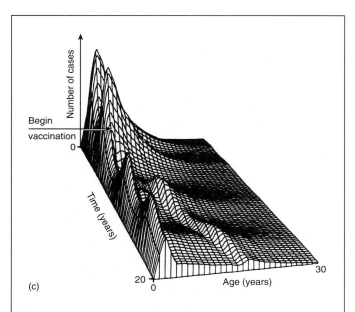

Mass vaccination and the incidence of disease

The effect of a rise in the proportion of cases in the older age classes (predicted above) on the incidence of complications is dependent upon two things: (a) the level of cohort immunization that can be attained; and (b) the age-dependent nature of the risk of complications seen in Fig. 18.21. Simulations that help to unravel this problem are shown in figure (d) (adapted from Anderson *et al.* 1987), recording the change in the predicted risk ratio (i.e. the average number of complications after immunization has begun divided by the average number of complications occurring before) over various levels of childhood immunization (note that the risk ratio is unity for no benefit from immunization).

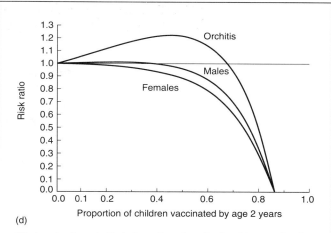

Obviously there is little benefit to be obtained by vaccination at less than 60 per cent, and indeed vaccination at anything less than 70 per cent is potentially hazardous when considering orchitis alone. Such a phenomenon is a direct result of the combination of increased average age at infection and of the risk of complications with age.

The strategy of pulse vaccination

The use of the alternative strategy of pulse vaccination as a method of control of childhood vaccine-preventable diseases has gained prominence in the early 1990s largely as a result of success in the Americas against polio and measles (De Quadros *et al.* 1991). Pulse vaccination may be defined as the repeated application of vaccine across a wide age range (Agur *et al.* 1993; Nokes and Swinton 1995) and usually takes the form of vaccination days or campaigns repeated once or twice yearly in which all children under a specified age, for example 15 years, are offered vaccine (usually irrespective of vaccination history). Repeated vaccination days or weeks in central and South America have seen the elimination of polio from the region since 1991 and very marked reductions in measles incidence. Although a basic understanding of the rationale underlying pulse vaccination guided its use in the Latin American context, there is good reason to seek greater quantitative insight into the underlying mechanism of action prior to advocating more widespread use in other regions with different social patterns and health infrastructure.

Remember that it is the presence of a threshold density or proportion of susceptibles in a population which enables endemic persistence of acute vaccine-preventable infections (that is infections requiring close contact to effect transmission and which develop lasting immunity following recovery). Vaccination of a fraction of an endemic proportion susceptible lowers the effective reproductive rate below unity and incidence declines (this may be quite a considerable reduction if a pulse is administered across a wide age range). Lowering the number of infectious persons in the population results in a lowering of the force of infection acting upon susceptibles. In turn fewer infections leads to a build up once more in susceptible numbers to the threshold level. The principle behind pulse vaccination rests upon these simple conditions. The aim of repeatedly pulsing is to maintain susceptible numbers below the threshold density or fraction and thereby maintain a continual decline in incidence (that is, by maintaining $R < 1$). In practical quantitative terms we are interested in the timing of successive pulses to achieve this objective.

The interpulse interval depends upon three factors: what fraction of the population are susceptible at endemic equilibrium, how much of this susceptible population is immunized as a result of the campaign, and how rapidly are susceptibles replenished after a campaign. Translating these into epidemiological terms, we note that the proportion of the susceptible population vaccinated in a single pulse is $p'x^*$ where p' is the vaccination coverage and x^* is the endemic fraction susceptible (related to the basic reproductive rate in the form $x^* = 1/R_0$). In addition, if the total population is approximately constant in size, then, ignoring any further infection, the rate of replenishment of susceptibles by births is equal to the death rate, $\mu = 1/L$ (where L is life expectancy at birth). Therefore, the minimum time taken after pulsing to recover the equilibrium fraction, that is the interpulse period, T_v, is

$$T_v = p'x^*L \qquad (39)$$

and since, $x^* = 1/R_0 = A/L$, we obtain

$$T_v = p'A \qquad (40)$$

(Agur *et al.* 1993). This gives the common-sense result that if all susceptibles were to be immunized by a pulse of vaccine, that is $p' = 1.0$, then the time taken to recover the threshold fraction would be equivalent to the average age at infection. The higher the average age at infection, that is the lower the transmission potential of the infection, the higher the endemic fraction susceptible and the consequent increase in the permitted interval between pulses. An observation from this analysis is that it is possible to eliminate an infection using a pulse vaccination proportion, p', which is less than the critical level of coverage predicted to be required for a continuous immunization process. The reason for this is that by vaccinating repeatedly across an age range, some individuals will receive multiple opportunities to receive the vaccine and there is therefore a build-up of vaccine-induced immunity with increasing age.

One complication that ought to be considered is the effect of combining a routine vaccination programme with a pulse regime (Nokes and Swinton 1995). Clearly, if a fraction of susceptibles are being vaccinated at or near to birth, then the rate of replenishment of susceptibles following a pulse will be lowered. It may be shown that, providing the vast majority of individuals acquire immunity some time during their lives, then the interpulse period in the presence of a routine vaccination programme in which a proportion p are vaccinated, is

$$T_v = p'\,A/(1-p). \qquad (41)$$

In other words the pulse interval is lengthened in direct relation to the new fraction of births which are susceptible, $(1-p)$.

Major simplifying assumptions underlie these simple relationships for the interpulse period. It is assumed that a proportion p' of susceptibles of any age are vaccinated and that on successive occasions each individual in a population has the same likelihood of being vaccinated. Such assumptions entail that the expressions given provide simple guidelines to aid understanding. Models of greater complexity are required which expand upon these ideas to give more practical guidelines (Nokes and Swinton 1995).

Monitoring the impact of control programmes

There is an ever-growing need to establish a coordinated surveillance programme to monitor the impact of control programmes against microparasitic infections (Nokes and Cutts 1993). The needs include the following.

1. To establish the impact of a specified control programme on a particular outcome variable, such as incidence of infection. This is of increasing importance as control programmes near their goals of elimination, where indicators of process, such as vaccination coverage, simply do not relate well enough to outcome;

2. To establish the accuracy of outcome indicators, such as notifications of infectious disease, the efficiency of which commonly fall off dramatically as incidence declines. This is crucial to the identification of outbreaks (and perhaps areas of low vaccine uptake) and to the validation of elimination targets, for example surveillance of acute flaccid paralysis as a marker for poliomyelitis

3. To monitor the appearance of wild-type variants, either introduced from other countries, or which have gained selective advantage over persisting strains in the presence of high selective pressure of vaccination or chemotherapy.

Various modern tools are now at our disposal to assist in this process. For example, saliva antibody assays which are being used to confirm clinical diagnoses and may be useful in establishing longitudinal surveillance systems and molecular probes by which to identify the origins of strains in infection outbreaks and the arrival of variants able to circulate in the presence of high-level, vaccine-associated immunity.

Mathematical models have a role to play in this area of epidemiology also. They facilitate the assessment of the impact of mass vaccination programmes through their predictive capability, where suitable outcome indicators may not be available (for example, infections with poor differential diagnosis) or may only be measurable many years after a programme has begun (for example, hepatitis B virus (HBV) and the occurrence of hepatic disorders). In addition, models can be used to explore the potential (and the time course) for strain variants to establish themselves in highly vaccinated populations, where they would otherwise normally be out-competed by a dominant (higher R_0) strain, for which immunity through vaccination is more solid.

Changes in sexual behaviour and the transmission of sexually transmitted infections

The current pandemic of AIDS and the absence of effective drugs and a vaccine to combat infection, has focused much attention in recent years on how to induce changes in sexual behaviour via education and media publicity campaigns to slow the spread of infection. The most important behaviour relevant to the rate of spread is the distribution of the rates of acquiring new sexual partners within a defined population (see Fig. 18.8). A major characteristic of this behaviour is the heterogeneity between individuals within a given community. A central question in this problem is whether it is best to aim health educational programmes at the whole population, with the aim of reducing average rates of sexual-partner change or whether it is best to target education at high-risk groups such as those with very high rates of sexual-partner change (in either male homosexual or heterosexual communities). This is a complicated question and its resolution depends, in part, on a detailed quantitative knowledge of the pattern of sexual behaviour within a given population. However, simple mathematical models can help to provide some clues to the resolution of this issue. Of particular importance in understanding the dynamics of transmission of HIV is determining how sexual behaviour influences the magnitude of the basic reproductive rate, R_0. As discussed earlier, for an STD such as HIV, the magnitude of R_0 is (in simple terms) defined by the probability of transmission per partner contact, B, multiplied by the effective rate of sexual-partner change, c, multiplied by the average duration of infectiousness, D, of an infected person. As noted earlier the variance in the rate of sexual-partner acquisition is typically much larger in value than the mean and, hence, those with high rates of partner change play a disproportionate role (relative to their proportional representation within a sexually active population) in the spread of infection (Fig. 18.14). This simple theoretical result suggests that greater benefit is to be gained (in terms of reducing R_0) by targeting education at those with higher than average rates of sexual-partner change. In practice the identification of such individuals is problematic in the absence of detailed survey data that relate this behaviour to other characteristics. The surveys of sexual behaviour that have been completed to date show a strong age dependency (with young adults having the highest rates of sexual-partner change) but little else of help in identifying correlates (ACSF 1992; Johnson *et al.* 1992). However, attendees at STD clinics are an important target group, since STDs other than HIV are more frequently present among those with high rates of partner change. Small changes in behaviour in the highly sexually active are likely to have a major impact on the prevalence of STDs in a community.

Conclusions

We have glossed over much detail and ignored many complications in model formulation and analysis in this chapter. The interested reader is therefore urged to consult the source references. Our aim has been to define, as simply as possible, the central concepts underpinning the study of the transmission dynamics of infectious diseases and the major conclusions that have emerged from the development and analysis of mathematical models of transmission and control.

The recent convergence of mathematical theory and observation in epidemiology has created a powerful set of tools for the study of the population biology of infectious disease agents. At present the potential value of these techniques is not widely appreciated by public health scientists and medical personnel. Many people have rightly criticized models that pursue the mathematics for its own sake, making only perfunctory attempts to relate the findings to epidemiological data. But there is a converse danger which is less widely understood. The complexities of the course of infection within an individual and its spread between people are such that years of clinical experience and the most refined intuition will not always yield reliable insights into the factors that control the transmission dynamics of a given infectious agent and how these are influenced by perturbations introduced by control measures. Moreover, insensitive use of a computer will not always help in understanding these problems, for if a computer is given inappropriate instruction it will usually give inappropriate answers. What is needed, in our view, is increased collaboration between epidemiologists and mathematicians, with the models being founded on data (and with their predictions being tested against available facts) and with verbal hypotheses being founded on clear mathematical statements of the assumptions. We hope that the contents of this chapter stimulate interest in this goal.

References

ACSF (1992). AIDS and sexual behaviour in France. *Nature*, **360**, 407–9.

Agur, Z., Cojocaru, L., Mazor, G., Anderson, R.M., and Danon, Y.L. (1993). Pulse mass measles vaccination across age cohorts. *Proceedings of the National Academy of Sciences USA*, **90**, 11698–702.

Anderson, R.M. (1982). Directly transmitted viral and bacterial infections of man. In *Population dynamics of infectious diseases—theory and applications* (ed. R.M. Anderson) Ch 1, pp. 1–37. Chapman & Hall, London.

Anderson, R.M. (1988). Epidemiology of HIV infection: variable incubation plus infectious periods and heterogeneity in sexual activity. *Journal of the Royal Statistical Society, Series A*, **151**, 66–93.

Anderson, R.M. and Grenfell, B.T. (1986). Quantitative investigation of different vaccination policies for the control of congenital rubella syndrome (CRS) in the U.K. *Journal of Hygiene (Cambridge)*, **96**, 305–33.

Anderson, R.M. and May, R.M. (1983). Vaccination against rubella and measles: quantitative investigations of different policies. *Journal of Hygiene (Cambridge)*, **90**, 259–325.

Anderson, R.M. and May, R.M. (1984). Spatial, temporal and genetic heteogeneity in host populations and the design of immunization programmes. *IMA Journal of Mathematics Applied in Medicine and Biology*, **1**, 233–66.

Anderson, R.M. and May, R.M. (1985a). Age-related changes in the rate of disease transmission: implications for the design of vaccination programmes. *Journal of Hygiene (Cambridge)*, **94**, 365–436.

Anderson, R.M. and May, R.M. (1985b). Herd immunity to helminth infection and implications for parasite control. *Nature (London)*, **315**, 493–6.

Anderson, R.M. and May, R.M. (1985c). Vaccination and herd immunity to infectious diseases. *Nature*, **318(6044)**, 323–9.

Anderson, R.M. and May, R.M. (1986). The invasion, persistence and spread of infectious diseases within animal and plant communities. *Philosophical Transactions of the Royal Society of London*, **314**, 533–70.

Anderson, R.M. and May, R.M. (1988). Epidemiological parameters of HIV transmission. *Nature (London)*, **333**, 514–22.

Anderson, R.M. and May, R.M. (1991). *Infectious diseases of humans: dynamics and control*. Oxford University Press, Oxford.

Anderson, R.M. and May, R.M. (1982). Directly transmitted infectious diseases: control by vaccination. *Science*, **215**, 1053–60.

Anderson, R.M., Grenfell, B.T., and May, R.M. (1984). Oscillatory fluctuations in the incidence of infectious disease and the impact of vaccination: time series analysis. *Journal of Hygiene (Cambridge)*, **93**, 587–608.

Anderson, R.M., Medley, G.F., May, R.M., and Johnson, A.M. (1986). A preliminary study of the transmission dynamics of the human immunodeficiency virus (HIV), the causative agent of AIDS. *IMA Journal of Mathematics Applied in Medicine and Biology*, **3**, 229–63.

Anderson, R.M., Crombie, J.A., and Grenfell, B.T. (1987). The epidemiology of mumps in the UK: a preliminary study of virus transmission, herd immunity and the potential effect of immunization. *Epidemiology and Infection*, **99**, 65–84.

Anderson, R.M., May, R.M., and McLean, A.R. (1988). Possible demographic consequences of AIDS in developing countries. *Nature*, **332**, 228–34.

Babad, H.R., Nokes, D.J., Gay, N.J., Miller, E., Morgan-Capner, P., and Anderson, R.M. (1995). Predicting the impact of measles vaccination in

England and Wales: model validation and analysis of policy options. *Epidemiology and Infection*, **114**, 319–44.

Bailey, N.T.J. (1973). Estimation of parameters from epidemic models. In *Mathematical theory of the dynamics of biological populations* (ed. M.S. Bartlett and R.W. Hiorns), p. 253. Academic Press, London.

Bailey, N.T.J. (1975). *The mathematical theory of infectious diseases and its implications*. Griffin, London.

Ball, F. (1983). The threshold behaviour of epidemic models. *Journal of Applied Probability*, **20**, 227–41.

Becker, N. (1978). The uses of epidemic models. *Biometrics*, **35**, 295–305.

Behets, F.M., Edidi, B., Quinn, T.C., Atikala, L., Bishagara, K., Nzila, N. *et al.* (1991). Detection of salivary HIV-1-specific IgG antibodies in high risk populations in Zaire. *Journal of Acquired Immune Deficiency Syndromes*, **4(2)**, 183–7.

Bernoulli, D. (1760). Essai d'une nouvelle analyze de la mortalite causee pour la verole et des avantages de l'incubation pour la prevenir. *Mem. Math. Phys. Acad. Roy. Sci (Paris)*, **1**, 1–45.

Black, F.L. (1966). Measles endemicity in insular populations: critical community size and its evolutionary implications. *Journal of Theoretical Biology*, **II**, 207–11.

Bolker, B.M. and Grenfell, B.T. (1993). Chaos and biological complexity in measles dynamics. *Philosophical Transactions of the Royal Society of London B Biological Sciences*, **251**, 75–81.

Brown, D.W.G., Ramsay, M.E.B., Richards, A.F., and Miller, E. (1994). Salivary diagnosis of measles: a study of notified cases in the UK, 1991–3. *British Medical Journal*, **308**, 1015–17.

Brownlee, J. (1906). Statistical studies in immunity: the theory of an epidemic. *Proceedings of the Royal Society (Edinburgh)*, **26**, 484–521.

Cliff, A., Haggett, P., and Smallman-Raynor, M. (1993). *Measles an historical geography* (1st edn). Blackwell, Oxford.

De Quadros, C.A., Andrus, J.K., Olive, J.-M., Da Silveira, C.M., Eikhof, R.M., Carrasco, P. *et al.* (1991). Eradication of poliomyelitis: progress in the Americas. *The Pediatric Infectious Disease Journal*, **10(3)**, 222–9.

Dietz, K. (1987). Mathematical models for the control of malaria. In *Malaria* (ed. W.H. Wensdorfe and J.A. MacGregor), p. 1087. Churchill Livingstone, Edinburgh.

Farr, W. (1840). Progress of epidemics. *Second Report of the Registrar General of England and Wales*, HMSO pp. 91–8.

Fine, P.E.M. (1993). Herd immunity: history, theory, practice. *Epidemiologic Reviews*, **15(2)**, 265–302.

Garnett, G.P. and Anderson, R.M. (1993). Contact tracing and the estimation of sexual mixing patterns: the epidemiology of Gonococcal infections. *Sexually Transmitted Diseases*, **20**, 181–91.

Garnett, G.P., Swinton, J., Brunham, R.C., and Anderson, R.M. (1992). Gonococcal infection, infertility and population growth: II. The influence of heterogeneity in sexual behaviour. *IMA Journal of Mathematics Applied in Medicine and Biology*, **9**, 127–44.

Grenfell, B.T. and Anderson, R.M. (1985). The estimation of age-related rates of infection from case notifications and serological data. *Journal of Hygiene*, **95**, 419–36.

Gupta, S. and Anderson, R.M. (1992). Sex, AIDS and mathematics. *New Scientist*, **12 September**, 34–8.

Hamer, W.H. (1906). Epidemic disease in England. *The Lancet*, **1**, 733–9.

Hethcote, H.W. and Yorke, J.A. (1984). Gonorrhoea: transmission dynamics and control. *Lecture Notes in Biomathematics*, **56**, 1–105.

Holmstrom, P., Syrjanen, S., Laine, P., Valle, S.-L., and Suni, J. (1990). HIV antibodies in whole saliva detected by ELISA and Western blot assays. *Journal of Medical Virology*, **30(4)**, 245–8.

Hope Simpson, R.E. (1952). Infectiousness of communicable diseases in the household. *The Lancet*, **I**, 1145–55.

Johnson, A.M., Wadsworth, J., Wellings, K., Bradshaw, S., and Field, J. (1992). Sexual lifestyles and HIV risk. *Nature*, **360**, 410–12.

Johnson, A.M., Wadsworth, J., Wellings, K., Field, J., and Bradshaw, S. (1994). *Sexual attitudes and lifestyles*. Blackwell Scientific Publications, Oxford.

Kermack, W.O. and McKendrick, A.G. (1927). A contribution to the mathematical theory of epidemics. *Proceedings of the Royal Society of London, Series A*, **115**, 700–21.

Knox, E.G. (1980). Strategy for rubella vaccination. *International Journal of Epidemiology*, **9(1)**, 13–23.

McLean, A.R. and Anderson, R.M. (1988a). Measles in developing countries. Part II. The predicted impact of mass vaccination. *Epidemiology and Infection*, **100**, 419–42.

McLean, A.R. and Anderson, R.M. (1988b). Measles in developing countries. Part I. Epidemiological parameters and patterns. *Epidemiology and Infection*, **100**, 111–33.

McLean, A.R. and Blower, S. (1993). Impefect vaccines and herd immunity to HIV. *Proceedings of the Royal Society London B*, **253**, 9–13.

Markowitz, L.E., Albrecht, P., Rhodes, P., Demonteverde, R., Swint, E., Maes, E.F. *et al.* (1996). Changing levels of measles antibody titers in women and children in the United States: impact on response to vaccination. *Paediatrics*, **97**, 1061–5.

May, R.M. and Anderson, R.M. (1984). Spatial heterogeneity and the design of immunization programs. *Mathematical Biosciences*, **72**, 83–111.

May, R.M. and Anderson, R.M. (1987). The transmission dynamics of HIV infection. *Nature (London)*, **326**, 137–42.

Mortimer, P.P. and Parry, J.V. (1991). Non-invasive virological diagnosis: are saliva and urine specimens adequate substitutes for blood? *Reviews in Medical Virology*, **1**, 73–8.

Nokes, D.J. and Anderson, R.M. (1987). Rubella vaccination policy: a note of caution. *The Lancet*, **I**, 1441–2.

Nokes, D.J. and Anderson, R.M. (1988). The use of mathematical models in the epidemiological study of infectious diseases and in the design of mass immunization programmes. *Epidemiology and Infection*, **101**, 1–20.

Nokes, D.J. and Anderson, R.M. (1991). Vaccine safety versus vaccine efficacy in mass immunization programmmes. *The Lancet*, **338**, 1309–12.

Nokes, D.J. and Anderson, R.M. (1992). Mathematical models of infectious agent transmission and the impact of mass vaccination. *Reviews in Medical Microbiology*, **3**, 187–95.

Nokes, D.J. and Anderson, R.M. (1993). Application of mathematical models to the design of immunization strategies. *Reviews in Medical Microbiology*, **4**, 1–7.

Nokes, D.J. and Cutts, F.T. (1993). Immunizations in the developing world: strategic challenges. *Transactions of the Royal Society of Tropical Medicine and Hygiene*, **87**, 353–4, 398.

Nokes, D.J. and Swinton, J. (1995). The control of childhood infection by pulse vaccination: an epidemiological approach. *IMA Journal of Mathematics Applied in Medicine & Biology*, **12**, 29–53.

Nokes, D.J., Anderson, R.M. and Anderson, M.J. (1986). Rubella epidemiology in south-east England. *Journal of Hygiene, (Cambridge)*, **96**, 291–304.

Parry, J.V., Perry, K.R., Panday, S., and Mortimer, P.P. (1989). Diagnosis of hepatitis A and B by testing saliva. *Journal of Medical Virology*, **28(4)**, 255–60.

Perry, K.R., Brown, D.W.G., Parry, J. V., Panday, S., Pipkin, C., and Richards, A. (1993). Detection of measles, mumps and rubella antibodies in saliva using antibody capture radioimmunoassay. *Journal of Medical Virology*, **40**, 235–40.

Rogers, D.J. (1988). A general model for the African trypanosomiases. *Parasitology*, **97**, 193.

Ross, R. (1911). *The prevention of malaria* (2nd edn). Murray, London.

Scott, M.E. and Smith, G. (ed.) (1994). *Parasitic and infectious diseases epidemiology and ecology* (1st edn). Academic Press, London.

Sokal, R.R. and Rohlf, F.J. (1981). *Biometry* (2nd edn). W.H. Freeman & Company, San Francisco, CA.

Soper, M.A. (1929). Interpretation of periodicity in disease prevalence. *Journal of the Royal Statistical Society A*, **92**, 34–61.

Ukkonen, P. and Von Bonsdorf, C.-H. (1988). Rubella immunity and morbidity: effects of vaccination in Finland. *Scandinavian Journal of Infectious Diseases*, **20**, 255–9.

Van Den Akker, R., Van Den Hoek, J.A.R., Van Den Akker, W.M.R., Kooy, H., Vijge, E., Roosendaal, G., Coutinho, R.A., and Van Loon, A.M. (1992).

Detection of HIV antibodies in saliva as a tool for epidemiological studies. AIDS, **6(9)**, 953– 957.

Wharton, M., Cochi, S.L., Hutcheson, R. H., Bistowish, J.M., and Shaffner, W. (1988). A large outbreak of mumps in the post vaccine era. *The Journal of Infectious Diseases*, **158(6)**, 1253–60.

Wickwire, K. (1977). Mathematical models for the control of pests and infectious diseases: a survey. *Theoretical Population Biology*, **11**, 182–238.

Yorke, J.A., Nathanson, N., Pianigiani, G., and Martin, J. (1979). Seasonality and the requirements for perpetuation and eradication of viruses in populations. *American Journal of Epidemiology*, **109(2)**, 103–23.

19 Microcomputers and epidemiology

Ralph R. Frerichs and Beatrice J. Selwyn

Introduction

The microcomputer has empowered epidemiologists around the world to serve the interests of science and society in many ways. Of course, different disease patterns prevail in every country. Heart disease, cancer, and stroke are of primary importance in the more developed countries, while infectious conditions such as malaria, tuberculosis, and onchocerciasis prevail in less developed regions. Yet the methods necessary to unravel the local determinants of these diseases are the same. As Rothman (1986) has stated, 'Although some specialized methods have been developed solely to study the spread of infectious illness, whatever distinctions exist between traditional and modern areas of epidemiology are certainly less important than the broad base of concepts that are shared.' The microcomputer both permits and encourages these methods to be used throughout the world by epidemiologists who are interested in unravelling the complexity of disease occurrence in society.

In the following sections of this chapter, we shall first describe the microcomputer hardware and software that has fostered the process of empowerment for epidemiologists. Next, we shall present seven applications of microcomputer use in epidemiology: medical record studies, rapid surveys, vaccine effectiveness, use of available data, surveillance, telecommunications, and distance learning. Other applications, including the use of microcomputers for conducting case–control studies, cohort studies, and understanding misclassification, were presented in an earlier edition of this book (Frerichs and Selwyn 1991). We conclude with a view of the future.

Microcomputer hardware and software

The components necessary for a functioning microcomputer are often divided into two groups, hardware and software. Hardware is a term used to describe the parts of a computer that have a physical presence, such as microcomputers, monitors, memory boards, and printers. Software, however, describes the programs or instructions that tell a computer what to do. In this section we shall first describe the typical microcomputer hardware. The following section focuses on several categories of software currently being used by epidemiologists.

Categories of hardware

Microcomputers are categorized as portable and desktop computers. Portable computers are further divided by weight into four categories: laptop computers, notebook computers, subnotebook computers, and personal digital assistants (PDAs). Desktop machines are typically less expensive per unit of computing power

than portable units, much larger and heavier, and composed of a separate central processing unit, monitor, and keyboard. Portable microcomputers, with all the components joined in a single unit, tend to be much more rugged than desktop machines and, in many ways, are ideal for field use or for general use in developing countries. Although a PDA resembles a calculator, it is actually a very small computer with a greatly reduced keyboard and viewing screen.

Central processing unit

The microcomputer's brain resides in the central processing unit (CPU). Here a series of small silicon chips are mounted on a motherboard on the floor of the unit. These chips are microprocessors, which understand and process a series of binary numbers, the basic units of a computer known as **bits**, with values of either 1 or 0. All communication with the microcomputer has to be translated into bits before the computer can work with the information. Bits are combined to create numeric, alphabetic, and graphic characters termed **bytes**. An example of a byte is the letter Q, which is written as 10101001. Typically, eight bits are needed by the computer to create one character or byte. Most computers can process more than one byte at a time; this ability defines the speed of the computer. Thus a 32-bit computer processes four characters simultaneously while a 64-bit computer can process eight characters at a time.

There are various ways of communicating with the computer. The message can be written in binary code, often termed **machine language**, which speaks directly to the computer. Alternatively, a programming language that translates alphabetic or numeric terms common to human communication into bits or machine language can be employed. Both these approaches require the help of computer programmers who have specialized knowledge of the respective languages. The third mode of communication, which relies on words, sentences, or symbols to instruct the computer, has helped to revolutionize the way computers are being used by epidemiologist and other scientists. This special software translates binary code to words that non-programmers can readily understand and use. Thus the epidemiologist is able to interact directly with the microcomputer to perform a wide variety of tasks.

As well as the microprocessor, the CPU also contains the computer memory. Memory is measured in kilobytes (approximately one thousand bytes) or megabytes (approximately one million bytes), denoted by the symbols K and MB respectively. There are actually two kinds of memory internal to the microcomputer, both of which are maintained in small chips attached to the motherboard. The first is random-access memory or RAM.

This memory can be filled with words or data entered either by typing on the keyboard or from disks or other modes of storage. This information can easily be altered or erased, depending on the wishes of the computer operator. Once the machine is turned off, however, all information in the RAM is usually cleared. Thus it must first be stored on disks or some other storage device. Some computers are equipped with special RAM chips, which use very little power, known as complementary metal oxide semiconductor (CMOS) chips. A small battery in the microcomputer maintains just enough power for the CMOS chips to ensure that the information is retained in the RAM even when the machine is turned off.

The size of the microcomputer's RAM is a major determinant of how fast information can be analysed. If all the data reside in the internal memory of the machine, the computer can quickly fulfill the requests of the operator. Conversely, the computer can only process a portion of a large data set at one time if the RAM is too small and must constantly go back and forth to the disk where the complete data set is stored. While the software program also takes up internal memory, a microcomputer with 16 MB of RAM can easily hold in its memory a data set comprising of 5000 subjects, 400 variables per subject, and five to six characters per variable.

As well as the RAM, the microcomputer also has read-only memory (ROM). This second form of memory contains instructions written in machine language which cannot be erased or altered by the operator. The ROM often contains a set of instructions that allow the computer to use words when interacting with the operator. ROM chips may also hold a programming language. Finally, various forms of ROM are available that contain favourite software programs or reference data sets, such as a dictionary or a thesaurus, that do not need to be changed.

Although not part of the CPU, fixed or hard disks that store specialized instructions, software, and data are housed internally in most microcomputers. Typically, such hard disks hold 200–1000 MB (1 gigabyte (GB)) of information. Owing to their need for extensive storage space, many software programs now require a hard disk to operate.

Input devices

The most common microcomputer input device is the keyboard, which is often equipped with a separate set of numeric keys off to one side for entering numbers. Information can also be entered with voice recognition devices, enabling memoranda or letters to be dictated rather than typed into the machine. Another common input device is known as a mouse. These small devices control a cursor or arrow on the computer screen, which either points to and activates an instruction statement or is used to draw graphs or other symbols. A pen-like stylus, related to a mouse, is commonly used with PDAs because of their small size.

A useful input mechanism for epidemiologists is the optical scanner. For instance, questionnaire responses made with a special pencil can be read directly into the computer using this device rather than relying on someone to enter the data. Scanners can also read both text and graphs from reports, manuscripts, or other non-copyrighted documents for entry into the microcomputer. When used with magnetic tapes or other forms of data storage, the investigator can save appropriate written material and create an extensive reference library of non-published work requiring very

little physical space. More important, the epidemiologist can use simple search statements to access specific text, graphs, or topics in his or her personal reference library.

A source of extensive data is the CD–ROM or read-only compact disc, the same kind of disc on which stereo music is recorded. Note that this disc is spelled with a *c* (referring to the round disc-shaped object) rather than the *k* used to spell magnetic disks (abbreviation for diskette). Compact discs hold 600–1400 MB of information and therefore are ideal for storing and providing access to large data sets from health surveys or population censuses, reference material such as dictionaries or encyclopedias, and book chapters and journal articles. Recently, sound and pictures have been added to CD–ROM discs, creating further opportunities for disseminating information in a variety of forms.

Disk drives, also discussed in the next section, serve as both input and output devices. They often use small magnetic disks, the main information storage mechanism for microcomputers. Since magnetic disks are easily transported, they are used to send both programs and data from one investigator to another. Commercial software is usually distributed on magnetic disks. In addition, magnetic tapes, which hold up to 300 MB of data, are frequently used to back up the internal hard disks in microcomputers. They also serve as an inexpensive means of data storage since information can be both retrieved from and written onto them.

Local networks link together multiple computers at one site (either through local cables or telephone lines), enabling them to share information, common programs, and data sets. Information from computers in other cities or locations within a city can also be shared using a modem, which serves as both an input and an output device. The words or data arrive over a telephone line in the form of sounds generated by the transmitting computer, and the modem converts the sound signals to the binary machine language used by the microcomputer.

Output devices

The four main microcomputer output devices are the monitor, the printer, magnetic disks or tapes (serving as both input and output devices), and a network or modem link.

The monitor is by far the most important output device for most epidemiologists using microcomputers. Since much time is spent reading text or viewing graphs on the screen, the monitor must be of a high quality. Contributing to the sharpness of the screen image (displayed in either colour or black and white) is the number of dots or pixels that appear on the screen. Quality monitors display 1024×768 pixels, while high-resolution monitors can display several thousand pixels on each axis of the screen. Most monitors resemble a television set and use a cathode-ray tube (CRT). Low-energy monitors with a flat liquid-crystal display (LCD) are often found on portable computers. Typically, laptop, notebook, and some subnotebook computers have colour LCDs, while PDAs use monochrome displays.

For epidemiologists and other scientists, the written word remains the most common form of communication. Therefore reports, memoranda, letters, or manuscripts (often including figures) all require output to a printer of sufficient quality to produce both text and graphs. The highest print quality is produced by laser printers, which are output devices employing technology similar to some photocopying machines. Ink jet printers, which spray a jet of ink on to a page through small pin-holes, and dot matrix printers, which use small pins to produce dots in various patterns on the paper, are also in widespread use.

A third output device is the magnetic disk or tape. Although information can be stored on 'hard' or fixed disks, 'floppy' disks are most commonly used. This name refers to the original disk construction, which had thin external covers that were easy to bend. Floppy disks are now encased in a non-bendable plastic cover with a small spring-loaded door that opens when the disk is inserted into the computer. They hold up to 2 MB of information and serve as inexpensive storage and software distribution mechanisms. The most common form of magnetic tape typically holds 300 MB of information, but tapes capable of storing several gigabytes are becoming readily available.

The recordable CD will become popular in the future since each disk is capable of storing 600–700 MB of text, graphics, and sound information. Although recordable disks are inexpensive today, the recordable CD drives are not. Until their price is reduced, it is likely that CD recorders will only be used by specialty groups who create CD–ROM packages for general use. Such groups include government agencies (including census bureaux), news media, and publishers of magazines and professional journals.

Finally, electronic linkage to a modem or to networks can transmit information to one or more microcomputers in the same office or facility or to computers in another region or even another country. Transmission may occur through telephone lines using a modem at each site, by direct-line connection using a dedicated cable and special boards that fit into the computer, or through higher-frequency airways (similar to radio and television signals) which require local transmitters and receivers. Infrared linkage, which sends information through the air in a manner similar in concept to a short-distance cellular telephone, is commonly used for communicating with small PDAs.

Categories of software

Without commercial software, most epidemiologists would find computers to be nothing more than complicated machines. Software allows the operator to dictate what the microcomputer should do. We have included descriptions in general terms of several common categories of software, which may or may not be sold as separate packages, since software programs are constantly changing.

Word processing

One of the most common applications of microcomputers for epidemiologists is likely to be word processing. Whether designing questionnaires, preparing lecture notes, writing reports, or drafting manuscripts, microcomputers greatly reduce the amount of time necessary to complete each task. Word-processing programs enable the user to type, edit, and change documents when they appear on the screen and then store the revised document on the computer's hard drive or on a magnetic disk. One possible use is to create individualized form letters for sending messages to field staff or colleagues in other agencies. Text and figures or graphs can be printed in many formats with various type styles, depending on the printer's capabilities. These programs offer many editing and proof-reading functions which utilize electronic dictionaries, thesauri, and grammar guides. Some programs will also translate text from one language to another. Once completed, the text can be sent via a network connection to local colleagues or by modem and telephone lines to the microcomputers of collaborators in other cities or countries. Researchers can use word-processing software in battery-powered portable computers to abstract reference material while visiting a library or other facility.

Database management

Database management programs have been developed for the rapid transformation of raw data collected by epidemiologists into useful information for unravelling disease aetiology, assisting administrators, or formulating public policy. McNichols and Rushinek (1988) have described seven data management functions that, historically, have been carried out manually but are now more efficiently performed by this category of program: (1) recording, (2) storing, (3) retrieving, (4) selecting or classifying, (5) sorting, (6) computing, and (7) displaying. **Recording** consists of capturing individual facts in a form that allows later reference, either from questionnaires, interview, or examination forms, or by direct entry into the microcomputer. **Storing** is the transfer of data to floppy or hard disks or laser disks for later retrieval. **Retrieving** is quickly extracting specific information from the computer (such as the person's name or disease status). **Selecting or classifying** is separating information into different categories (such as never smoked, current smoker, or ex-smoker) for subsequent retrieval. **Sorting** is arranging data in numerical or alphabetical order. **Computing** is summarizing, transforming, or cross-tabulating data. **Displaying** is showing the results in an interpretable form in tables or possibly graphs. Most database management programs allow the user to request particular kinds of information using written or verbal commands. The user can then set up the format in which the information will be presented on the display screen.

Statistical

Statistical software has become essential to most practising epidemiologists for two kinds of statistical analyses: descriptive and inferential. Descriptive analysis summarizes common data properties, such as the mean value of a given variable and the frequency of various responses. In contrast, inferential statistics determines whether study findings are based on fact or are the result of chance. Typical functions performed by statistical software packages are data handling, contingency tables, non-parametric tests, T tests, correlation, regression, analysis of variance, log-linear models, survival analysis, cluster analysis, and time series analysis. However, functions or tests favoured by epidemiologists, such as direct and indirect standardization, Mantel–Haenszel adjusted risk and odds ratios, or logistic regression, are not always included in every statistical software package, nor can all of them be used for the analysis of population surveys that typically measure groups of persons in villages, neighbourhoods, and households. The variability of observations is typically greater when measuring people in groups rather than as independent individuals. By not recognizing groups or clusters, most statistical packages underestimate the variance of survey data and thus imply more precise results than are actually measured. Fortunately, version 6 (or later) of the Epi Info program used by many epidemiologists (see section on medical records studies) has a statistical module designed specifically for cluster surveys.

Spreadsheet

Spreadsheet programs are among the most useful for epidemiologists. The concept was originated on the microcomputer, although spreadsheet programs are now available for use in mainframe computers as well. The terms 'spreadsheet' originates from the practice of accountants who spread large sheets of paper on a table to examine columns and rows of financial data. These programs divide the computer screen into a series of columns and rows with individual cells containing data, text, or formulae relating one cell to another. When a cell entry is changed, it may affect the numerical or text values in many other cells, depending on how the variables are related. This procedure is often referred to as doing a 'what if' or 'sensitivity' analysis. Spreadsheet programs are most frequently used for organizing, calculating, and presenting financial, statistical, and other numerical data that serve as the basis for decision-making. Spreadsheets are also used to model disease processes and to understand the consequences in studies of factors such as selection and misclassification bias (Frerichs and Selwyn 1991).

Graphics

Graphics software programs permit epidemiologists and others to visualize quickly relationships that may not be as apparent when viewing information organized in a table format. In the past epidemiologists have been notoriously dull in their graphic presentations, almost exclusively using histograms and plain-line graphs to describe their findings. Selwyn's findings, based on a one-year review of the graphics contents of a leading epidemiology journal (Selwyn 1985), are typical: 98 per cent of 121 graphs were either histograms or line graphs. Only 2 per cent were pie charts and none were three-dimensional graphs, which is an ideal method of representation for illustrating the modifying or intervening effect of a third variable when considering the association between a risk factor and disease. For example, the relationship between the number of antenatal care vists and neonatal mortality might differ by birth weight. This could be visualized easily in a graph with the number of antenatal care vists on the horizontal or x axis, neonatal mortality on the vertical or y axis, and birth-weight categories on the third axis.

Many database management, statistics, and spreadsheet programs include graphics of acceptable quality. However, special graphics software can create a wide variety of graphs, including three-dimensional bar and line graphs, pie charts with separable slices, graphs with superimposed symbols, detailed geographic maps, and word charts. The graphs can be printed on paper or transparencies or can be converted to slides. Alternatively, the graphic images can be shown as they appear on the computer monitor using a real-time overhead display. These displays are flat panels containing a transparent LCD, the same monitor as found on many portable computers. The display is placed on an overhead projector, which projects the image onto a wall or screen as the text, graph, or figure is created by the microcomputer. Using the display panels and current graphics or presentation programs, epidemiologists can create a set of electronic slides, arrange them in the desired order, and show them directly to an audience. If a colour printer and colour photocopy machine are available, the graphs can easily be made into colourful transparencies for use with an overhead projector. Alternatively, computer-generated graphics can

be transferred to 35 mm slide film through the use of a slide-maker attached to the microcomputer's parallel port. Finally, computer graphic files can be sent directly to private companies that make individual slides.

Communications

Communications programs use telephone lines to link one microcomputer with either another microcomputer or a mainframe computer. Modems, which convert the machine language to sound and back to machine language again, and their associated software, which instructs the computer when to send and receive the data, are required at both the transmitting and receiving computers. Most communications programs will work with a variety of modems and hardware configurations. Standard features are auto-dialling, auto-answering, and the maintenance of a directory with telephone numbers and other relevant information. The transfer of data or text from one computer to another is often referred to as electronic mail (or e-mail). This form of communication is almost instantaneous and may be less expensive than conventional mail, depending on the telephone charges.

Software is also available for epidemiologists and others who need to communicate with information services using mainframe computers. Typically, these are electronic encyclopaedias, newspaper and magazine articles, and abstracting services, such as the Medical Literature Analysis and Retrieval System (MEDLARS) maintained by the United States National Library of Medicine. Finally, programs can also be purchased to connect microcomputers as networks for sharing files or for linking computers both nationally and internationally to a wide variety of databases or users. Included in this category is Internet, a set of computer networks that allow worldwide written or graphic communication with those linked into the system (Nicoll 1994a).

Project management

Performing an epidemiological study usually requires careful balancing of time, money, and resources. Project management software allows investigators to separate the proposed study into various components and to estimate both the order of completion and the time and resources necessary for completion of the individual components. Such items as unexpected sick days, reductions in funds, or the availability of extra interviewers can quickly be entered into the program to determine what is the most efficient course to take. Reporting and monitoring features of this category of software can also be used for progress reports required by funding agencies.

Special interest

Some software cannot be easily categorized. Various groups are constantly developing programs of special interest to epidemiologists or others interested in population-based research. Notable among these are two programs developed at the United States Centers for Disease Control in Atlanta, Georgia: Epi Info and Epi Map. Epi Info is intended for outbreak investigations or other epidemiological studies and consists of a series of computer programs used to create and analyse questionnaires for various types of epidemiological studies, including cluster surveys, design interview or examination schedules, and other common epidemiological tasks (Dean et al. 1991; Editor 1993). Epi Map is a computer mapping program for microcomputers, which produces maps from geographic boundary files and data values entered directly from the keyboard or supplied by Epi Info or another database management program (Epidemiology Program Office 1994). Data values for the maps may be counts, rates, or other numerical values, which can be represented as shading or colour patterns for each geographic entity. They can also be depicted as dot maps, with dots proportional in number to the values placed in each geographic area. Finally, the program can produce cartograms in which the size of an area is increased or decreased depending on the number of events or persons in the area.

Applications

Microcomputers are being used by epidemiologists to perform a wide variety of activities. Seven examples with relevance to epidemiologists in many different settings are presented in this section. These applications were selected to demonstrate this variety as well as for their use of different types of software and hardware.

Medical record studies

One of the most common sources of information in epidemiological research is the medical record. Abstracting relevant data that is of 'research quality' is definitely enhanced by the use of microcomputers. Even though most medical records departments lack space, the modern portable microcomputer is generally welcomed. Microcomputers are now small enough (laptop, notebook, or subnotebook size) to use in a space no larger than a piece of paper. Microcomputers do not need much electrical power and often have enough battery power to use without an external electrical source. Most portable microcomputers weigh 3–7 pounds (1.4–3.2 kg), so that field workers do not protest about having to carry them to the site of data collection. A less powerful (and therefore less expensive) microcomputer is very suitable for this activity. Since data abstraction from a medical record moves slowly, speed in the microcomputer is less important than its size, cost, and weight.

Software designed with epidemiologists in mind, such as Epi Info, performs very well for this data abstraction activity. As an example of this application of portable microcomputers to epidemiological research, we shall feature a study that assessed factors associated with preterm birth in which the required information was abstracted from medical records in several different hospitals.

Data entry

The Epi Info software program is installed on the microcomputer and modified for this specific use. Data collectors are trained in its use as well as in the protocol for using the data collection record, including the necessity of making two back-up diskettes of the files that they create each day. In order to facilitate data entry, the data collection record on the microcomputer monitor is prepared to look just as it would on paper. Using programmed instructions to assist with coding and other decision-making, the person entering the data rarely needs to look up guidelines during record abstraction. Places where data are to be entered are marked according to the requirements of the software program. An example of such a data entry screen is shown in Fig. 19.1.

The computer monitor screen contains the study variables in the first column (enclosed for program identification with {}

PRETERM BIRTH PREVENTION EVALUATION LABOUR DATA ABSTRACTION INSTRUMENT		
ITEM	DESCRIPTION	CODE
1. [Schedule] ID	3. Schedule D Preintervention	#
2. [Clinic] Name	1. South East	#
	2. North Side	
	4. Lyons	
	5. Humble	
	6. La Porte	
3. [Study] Number	0001 – 9999	####
4. Gestation age when seen [OB]	01 – 45 Weeks	##
5. [Date] admitted to labour	01/01/89 – 05/31/90	<mm/dd/yy>
	11/11/11 = Not admitted	
	12/12/12 = Not recorded	
6. Screening used: [Hydration]	1. Yes	#
	2. No	
7. [Time] placed on monitor	8. Not applicable	
	9. Not recorded	
	00:00 – 23:59	####
	88:88 = Not applicable	
	99:99 = Not recorded	
8. [Contr]actions on monitor	1. Yes, regular	#
	2. Yes, irregular	
	3. Yes, but quit	
	4. None	
	8. Not applicable	
	9. Not recorded	

Note: Data are entered in the areas to the right, marked with ## marks or date codes, i.e.,<mm/dd/yy>. During data entry the user has access to these parts of the screen only. All other parts appear on the screen, but are not available to the user.

Fig. 19.1 Example of a data entry screen prepared for direct entry from medical records.

brackets), a list of choices to be coded in the second column, and the format for entering the data in the third column. Epi Info uses # to indicate a single-digit number, ## for a two–digit number, and so forth. Dates are entered as three sets of two–digit numbers indicating month (mm), day (dd), and year (yy).

Range and logical checks

Effective software allows data checking at the time of data entry. Epi Info is equipped with checks for the range of codes allowable for each item of information. This range check prevents the entry of data that might result from inadvertently hitting the wrong number key or attempting to use the wrong data entry line. It calls the problem to the attention of the date abstractor with a sound cue.

Another useful feature of data entry software is the ability to check for logical inconsistencies that might occur in abstraction. This feature is also applied during the data abstraction process. For example, suppose that the study requires information on the date of childbirth as well as the date of the first prenatal visit, but the abstractor enters one of the dates incorrectly. The microcomputer can be programmed to check these dates for the amount of time that has passed between them and then to alert the abstractor of a possible error. If the two dates are more than 45 weeks apart, for

COMMAND IN THE COMPUTER	INTERPRETATION
	For Questions 1 and Questions 2
SCHEDUL1	The item code name.
Repeated	Tells computer to repeat the same code for all the following records
MustEnter	Tells computer not to allow a blank entry
Range 3 3	Specifies the range: minimum is 3, maximum is 3
END CLINIC2	Tells computer that this question instruction is finished
Repeated	Tells computer to repeat the same code for all the following records
MustEnter	Tells computer not to allow a blank entry
KEY	Tells the computer that this is an identifier for the case
Range 1 6	Specifies the range: minimum is 1, maximum is 6
END	Tells computer that this question instruction is finished
	For Question 6: Screening used: hydration
HYDRAT6	
MustEnter	Tells computer not to allow a blank entry
Range 1 2	Specifies the range: minimum is 1, maximum is 2
Legal 8 9	States codes 8 and 9 are legal, even though outside the accepted range
END	Tells computer that this question instruction is finished
IF DATLAB5='11/11/11' ANDHYDRAT6 < > 8	
THEN	Checking for inconsistency #1
HELP 'Possible error. Check Ques 5 with Ques 6.'	
ENDIF	Tells computer to end the IF statement
END	Tells computer that this question instruction is finished

NOTE:
#1: The logical check says: IF Question 5 (the date admitted to labour) is coded 'not admitted'(11/11/11), and Question 6 (screening with hydration therapy) is not coded as 'not applicable'(code 8), THEN place a HELP message on the screen that says 'Possible error. Check Ques 5 with Ques 6. Press ESC.' The message shows on the screen only when a logical inconsistency is detected.

Fig. 19.2 Example of the range and logical checking used when abstracting medical record data directly into the microcomputer (corresponds to Fig. 1 data collection record).

example, there is an error somewhere since pregnancy rarely lasts longer than this. The specific instructions for range and logical checking used in the abstraction of medical records in the preterm birth study are shown in Fig. 19.2. They were programmed for selected variables that both limit the range of entries and check for inconsistencies in the entries.

Verification and reabstraction

Another useful feature of the Epi Info software is its verify function, which checks for consistency of answers. Data from collection records are entered twice; the verify function then checks for inconsistent entries and flags any that are found. This is the most rigorous data entry protocol, and prevents many data entry errors from creeping into the final data set. However, verification by double entry is often not feasible when collecting data directly since it may take 30–45 minutes to read each medical record for the desired data. As a result, data entry proceeds so slowly that errors rarely occur while keying in the answer. However, errors do occur

in interpreting the medical records, locating the correct information to be entered as data, and using standardized definitions. To address such problems, a sample of records must be reabstracted from the original sources and the data entered a second time. Reabstraction differs from verification, which catches errors in data entry, since it monitors the general reliability of the entire abstraction process. With the use of such a sampling scheme, inconsistencies in abstraction are detected shortly after initial collection and the overall error rate can be determined. If the problem is very troublesome, it can be corrected by total reabstraction of the specific data collected since the last reabstraction occurred. Corrective measures can be discussed with staff to prevent future occurrences. Thus the skill of abstractors is regularly monitored. Ultimately, this approach saves time for the study.

Using portable microcomputers for direct data entry has several advantages over the past method of using paper for medical record abstraction. The two methods of data collection are compared in Table 19.1. The major advantages of using portable microcomputers is in quality of data and time of acquisition of data. Problems are corrected on site before the medical record is returned to the hospital files. This is particularly important when dealing with busy hospital staff who have no connection with the study. When the day's abstraction is finished, the microcomputer-based system provides edited data which are more valid than would result from the use of a paper record for the initial collection. Finally, use of paper for record abstraction is more time consuming since the abstractor must first write the information on a sheet of paper and then enter the data into a computer located at another site. With large epidemiological studies, excess time per single record soon becomes a major cost item in salary expenses. The data entry process takes longer and thus increases the cost of data acquisition.

Rapid surveys

Decision-makers often ask epidemiologists about the burden at the community level that illness places on people and how resources are being allocated to address various health problems. While the questions are easy to ask, the answers are often hard to acquire. One solution is to rely more extensively on rapid epidemiological assessment methods (Selwyn et al. 1989; Smith 1989), including health surveys (US CDC 1992). Trained interviewers or examiners, using correct methods, can sample populations and obtain standardized data of high quality. Until recently, however, the processing and analysis of most survey data has been so cumbersome and has taken so long that the information is old and often irrelevant before it is available for dissemination. The increased affordability of portable computers is helping to address this problem, particularly when combined with new software such as the Csample module in version 6 of Epi Info, which is designed specifically for the statistical analysis of cluster surveys. In addition, Ariawan and Frerichs (1994) have recently created the Csurvey module for Epi Info which (1) selects clusters to be sampled with probability proportionate to size, (2) derives the necessary sample size for both clusters and persons per cluster, and (3) creates a random number table for selecting the random start household or persons within a household.

Surveys can now be performed very quickly, as happened in Florida and Louisiana after Hurricane Andrew, using existing

Table 19.1 Comparison of data collection activities from medical records using paper versus microcomputer

Paper medium	Microcomputer medium
1. Design data collection record in word processor and print to paper	1. Design data collection record in word processor
2. Abstract medical record on paper	2. Abstract medical record to microcomputer
3. Perform a reliability check on a sample of medical records; this means reabstracting onto paper and checking the second abstract against the first	3. Check the range and logical inconsistencies of the computerized data at the same time as abstraction is occurring.
4. Carry out any corrective actions	4. Fix problems
5. Enter information from paper record into the microcomputer	5. Perform a reliability check on a sample of medical records in the microcomputer
6. Verify data entry by entering the information from the paper record a second time	6. Carry out any corrective action
7. Correct any data entry errors	
8. Check the range and logical inconsistencies of the computerized data; note any problems	
9. Check where the error is; if the error is in the abstracted data, return to the medical record and correct the error	

software and hardware (US CDC 1992). Such rapid gathering, processing, and analysis of survey data occur in even the poorest countries (Frerichs 1989; Frerichs and Tar 1989; Bennett et al. 1991). For example, health department staff in rural Myanmar (formerly Burma) were able to gather appropriate survey data, complete an analysis, prepare simple tables and graphs, and present survey findings to the local medical official and his staff in less than five days. Another five days later, they presented a 50-page report, written with a word-processing program, to the Director of Public Health in Yangon (formerly Rangoon). Thus, within ten days of going into the field, the Myanmar health department staff were able to provide detailed information necessary for decision-making at both the local and national levels.

Rapid surveys are commonly planned for measuring vaccination coverage, as advocated by the World Health Organization (WHO) (Lemeshow and Robinson 1985). Current practice focuses on data collection by maternal interview. Actual immunization status confirmed by serum antibody titre is rarely known since serological surveys are considered to be inappropriate in most societies owing to the cost of medically trained personnel, the need for cooling equipment, and the resistance of parents and children to giving blood. However, antibodies to common childhood diseases can also be detected in saliva (Perry et al. 1993; Brown et al. 1994). Thus future rapid surveys will probably use the non-invasive medium of saliva rather than blood to supplement information gathered from the mother. Through the use of microcomputers, this interview data will be merged with the laboratory analyses of saliva specimens to determine both the reported vaccination status and the measured immunization status of the survey participants. The WHO advocates similar studies for describing the prevalence of human immunodeficiency virus (HIV) infection and for evaluating poten-

tial intervention strategies (Harris et al. 1991; Wawer et al. 1994); rather than blood, saliva will probably become the medium of choice for both functions in field surveys of HIV infection (Frerichs et al. 1994).

Computer-assisted telephone interviews, which have been used extensively in the United States (Berrios et al. 1993; Valdiserri et al. 1993), are related to rapid surveys. The cost and convenience of interviewing by telephone and entering the data directly into the computer contributes to the popularity of this approach (Derr et al. 1992). Rather than interviewing subjects face to face, other surveyors have chosen to use microcomputers to query subjects directly on sensitive items, with favourable results. For example, Locke et al. (1994) have used a computer-based interview to detect factors related to the risk of HIV among potential blood donors. They found that a computer interview was much more successful in identifying either behaviour associated with a risk of acquiring HIV or symptoms compatible with AIDS than the standard American Red Cross procedures for assessment of donor suitability (written questionnaires and face-to-face interviews).

Evaluating vaccine effectiveness

Primary prevention of many infectious diseases is brought about by vaccination. Yet, while the efficacy of vaccines is often known based on clinical or vaccine trials, the effectiveness in a field setting may vary for a wide variety of reasons. Orenstein et al. (1985, 1988) have summarized factors that influence vaccine effectiveness and have presented several useful formulae for epidemiologists who need to estimate the effectiveness of an immunization programme. In this section, we shall describe the immunization formulae and demonstrate how a spreadsheet program can be used to estimate what is happening in a population, given the uncertainty of existing surveillance or survey data. We shall first describe the formulae and then show a spreadsheet program that derives useful measures for epidemiologists and programme managers.

Explanation of formulae

Vaccine effectiveness (VE) is the extent to which a vaccine prevents disease among vaccinated persons in the community. The formula for VE is a version of the more general formula for the prevented fraction among those exposed to a preventive factor:

$$PF_c = \frac{I_u - I_c}{I_u} \qquad (1)$$

where PF_c is the prevented fraction among the exposed, I_u is the incidence of disease among the unexposed, and I_c is the incidence of disease among the exposed. By substituting v (vaccinated) for e and uv (unvaccinated) for u, PF_c becomes PF_v, the prevented fraction among the vaccinated or the proportion of vaccinated persons who did not develop the disease. A more common term for PF_v is vaccine effectiveness (VE), equivalent to one minus the risk ratio, which compares the incidence of disease among those who are vaccinated and those who are not vaccinated:

$$PF_v = VE = 1 - \frac{I_v}{I_{uv}} = 1 - \qquad (2)$$

The prevented fraction attributed to vaccination can also be derived for the total population:

$$PF_{p,v} = \frac{I_{uv} - I_p}{I_{uv}} \qquad (3)$$

Here we see that the prevented fraction in the population attributed to vaccination ($PF_{p,v}$) is equal to the incidence of the disease among the unvaccinated (I_{uv}) minus the incidence in the total population (I_p) divided by the incidence in the unvaccinated. A more common term for $PF_{p,v}$ is community effectiveness (CE), i.e. the effectiveness of an immunization program in the total community. CE is dependent on both effectiveness and coverage:

$$PF_{p,v} = CE = VE \times PPV \qquad (4)$$

where VE is vaccine effectiveness and PPV is the vaccinated proportion of the population (i.e. coverage). The related concept of preventable fraction in the population among the unvaccinated ($PF_{p,uv}$) is used less often. This term measures the proportion of the disease incidence in a population that is preventable if all had been vaccinated,

$$PF_{p,uv} = \frac{I_p - I_v}{I_p} \qquad (5)$$

where $PF_{p,uv}$, I_p, and I_v are as defined previously. The preventable fraction in the population is related to both vaccine effectiveness and coverage:

$$PF_{p,uv} = \frac{(1 - PPV) \times \left(\dfrac{VE}{1 - VE}\right)}{(1 - PPV) \times \left(\dfrac{VE}{1 - VE}\right) + 1}$$

There are other methods of measuring vaccine effectiveness without having detailed information on the incidence of disease among both the vaccinated and unvaccinated. As described by Orenstein et al. (1985; 1988), the proportion of disease cases that are vaccinated is mathematically related to both vaccine effectiveness and coverage:

$$PCV = \frac{PPV - (PPV \times VE)}{1 - (PPV \times VE)} \qquad (7)$$

where PCV is the proportion of cases that had been vaccinated, and PPV and VE are as previously defined. Orenstein et al. presented the relationship between PCV, PPV, and VE in a nomograph to be used by field epidemiologists when information is known for only two of the three variables. While their graph is useful, we feel that the relationship between these parameters might be easier to understand if derived in a spreadsheet program, with results presented in the form of a bar graph.

Before presenting the spreadsheet program, we first need to rearrange the terms in eqn (7) to calculate VE and PPV. Those who manage vaccination programmes will probably not be interested in deriving the proportion of cases that are vaccinated (i.e. PCV). Instead, epidemiologists will probably use surveillance data on vaccinated cases and survey data on vaccine coverage to calculate vaccine effectiveness:

$$VE = \frac{PPV - PCV}{PPV(1 - PCV)} \qquad (8)$$

Epidemiologists might also want to estimate vaccine coverage in the population, using existing surveillance data on vaccinated cases and a priori knowledge about the effectiveness of the vaccine as presented below:

$$PPV = \frac{PCV}{VE(PCV - 1) + 1} \qquad (9)$$

The computer spreadsheet program

Using a simple spreadsheet program, epidemiologists can calculate the missing information if they know the values of at least two of the following three variables: PCV, PPV, or VE. Once the values for all three variables are known, the program also derives the proportion of potential cases in the population that have been prevented by vaccination ($PF_{p,v}$ or CE) and the proportion of actual cases in the population that would have been preventable if all had been vaccinated ($PF_{p,uv}$).

Assume that an epidemiologist is responsible for a population of 100 000 children with incidence and vaccination characteristics for measles as shown in Table 19.2. During the time period of interest, 12.5 per cent of the children developed measles. Earlier, 65 per cent had been vaccinated. The incidence of measles was 1.5 per cent among those who had been vaccinated and 32.9 per cent among those who had not been vaccinated. Since vaccination prevents measles, the risk ratio comparing vaccinated children with unvaccinated children is less than 1.0 (actual value is 0.047). The vaccine was 95.3 per cent effective in preventing measles among those children who were vaccinated. Among all children, the vaccine

Table 19.2 Incidence of measles by vaccination status in an example population of children

	Measles	No measles	Total		
Vaccinated	1000	64 000	65 000	I_v	= 0.0154
Unvaccinated	11 500	23 500	35 000	I_{uv}	= 0.3286
	12 500	87 500	100 000	I_p	= 0.1250

Risk ratio $RR = I_v/I_{uv}$	= 0.0468
Vaccine effectiveness VE	= 0.9532
Prevented fraction in population $PF_{p, v}$	= 0.6196
Preventable fraction in population $PF_{p, uv}$	= 0.8769

prevented 62.0 per cent of the measles cases that theoretically would have occurred if there had been no vaccinations. Finally, nearly 88 per cent of the cases that did occur could have been prevented if all the children had been vaccinated.

The epidemiologist would probably not have known these values; however, information from a measles surveillance system for assessing vaccination status among cases (PCV) and a two-stage cluster survey for vaccination coverage in the community (PPV) might have been available. With these two items, the epidemiologist can derive vaccine effectiveness by using the spreadsheet program shown in Table 19.3. Even if the values of VE and PCV are known, the epidemiologist might have wanted to determine PPC. When

Table 19.3 Spreadsheet entry screen for vaccine effectiveness calculations

	A	B	C	D
1	Field observations	Enter observed value	Calculated value	
2				
3				
4				
5	Proportion of CASES who report			
6	having been vaccinated	0.08	PCV =	0.080
7				
8	Proportion of POPULATION who report			
9	having been vaccinated	0.65	PPV =	0.650
10				
11	VACCINE EFFECTIVENESS		VE =	0.953
12				
13				
14	Proportion of potential CASES in population			
15	that have been PREVENTED by vaccination		$PF_{p, v}$ =	0.620
16				
17	Proportion of actual CASES in population			
18	that are PREVENTABLE by vaccination		$PF_{p, uv}$ =	0.877

Table 19.4 Formulae in vaccine effectiveness spreadsheet

	B	C	D
1	Enter observed value		Calculated value
2			
3			
4			
5			
6	0.08	PCV =	@IF(B6>0,B6,(B9-(B9*B11))/(1-B9*B11)))
7			
8			
9	0.65	PPV =	@IF(B9>0,B9,B6/((B11*(B6-1))+1))
10			
11		VE =	@IF(B11>0,B11,(B6–B9)/(B9*(B6-1)))
12			
13			
14			
15		$PF_{p,v}$ =	+D11*D9
16			
17			
18		$PF_{p,uv}$ =	((1-D9)*(D11/(1-D11)))/((1-D9)*(D11/(1-D11))+1)

any two of the three variables are entered, the program calculates the remaining variable as well as the effectiveness of vaccination in the community ($PF_{p,v}$) and the proportion of existing cases that could have been prevented if prior vaccination coverage had been 100 per cent ($PF_{p,uv}$). The equations for these calculations are shown in Table 19.4. Finally, the spreadsheet program creates a graph that shows the findings of the five variables, making it easier to share the results with programme staff (Fig. 19.3).

While useful for insight and education, the spreadsheet program can also be used by programme staff to monitor the effectiveness of vaccination efforts over time. If local officials carry out periodic vaccination surveys and regularly monitor the reported vaccination status of disease cases, they can use a spreadsheet program to estimate changes in vaccine effectiveness in Fig. 19.4. In this example, the vaccination coverage has remained constant over time, as has the percentage of cases that are vaccinated, at least for the first six quarters. Thereafter, PCV increases, suggesting that the vaccine is no longer as effective as previously estimated. Reviewing this graph should stimulate the staff to investigate the reasons for these changes.

Use of available data

Storage media for microcomputers, such as high-density diskettes (with the ability to use compressed format data) and CDs, make compiled data sets available for use by epidemiologists for further research on the respective studies or simply as an information resource when needed. Fortunately, with the advent of the microcomputer, compatible data formats for many types of hardware and software are more readily available. Many large databases have

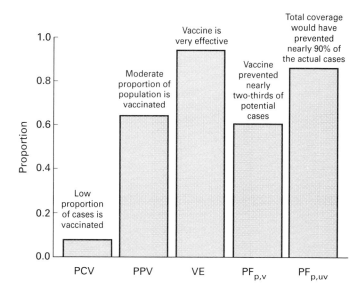

Fig. 19.3 Measures of vaccine effectiveness.

information available for public health researchers. Examples include the following.

- Collection of perinatal studies (particularly randomized clinical trials) which allows epidemiologists to engage in meta-analysis or in reanalysis of data (Chalmers *et al.* 1986).

- Census data available on CD so that epidemiologists have access to detailed data tables and can print them out or import them into spreadsheet programs or word-processing programs.

- Contracted reports, which may be given to the contractor on diskette, such as a needs assessment funded by several hospitals and affiliated institutions covering a multi-county region. The report for such a study could contain a variety of data, collected from many sources, in table and graph format.

Agencies involved receive prepared text and tables or graphs on microcomputer diskettes. The data, which they paid to have collected and organized, become available to them in a convenient format for preparing their own reports mandated by federal guidelines. Therefore epidemiological and public health data are no longer exclusively available to highly trained professionals. Epidemiologists are recognizing the need to learn how to prepare materials for their colleagues in other health professions in order to facilitate understanding and the proper use of these data.

Surveillance

Epidemiologists traditionally carry out surveillance and monitoring activities. The microcomputer can help to increase the speed of the data-reporting function which, in turn, should decrease the time between assessment and taking action to prevent emerging problems. An example of this is the microcomputer-based program Epi Net (Exposure Prevention Information Network) used by hospitals to evaluate prevention activities and to compare injury rates from sharp objects.

This program, which was developed by Dr Janine Jagger (Jagger and Pearson 1991; Anonymous 1992; Editor 1993), provides a set of

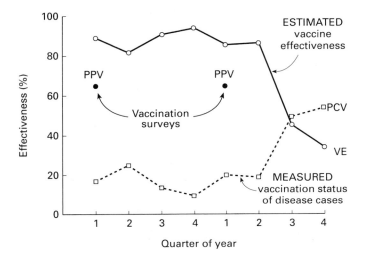

Fig. 19.4 Using survey and surveillance data for estimating vaccine effectiveness.

shared data via computer, which allows interested parties to document events of exposure when they happen, identify the source, and, through surveillance, identify useful prevention practices. One version was developed especially for use in operating rooms; the program is also suitable for use in labour and delivery rooms. This software assists health care institutions in standardizing information collection and reporting about percutaneous injuries and blood and body fluid contacts (Editor 1993). Its primary goal is to reduce the incidence of needlesticks, the principle mode of exposure in most hospitals to HIV and hepatitis B and C virus infections (Jagger and Pearson 1991). Epi Net provides users with incident report forms and preprogrammed software for data entry and report writing. When combined with a statistical–surveillance software package, the program can generate analyses of the data for reports.

Each institution using the microcomputer-based program can function as a 'closed system', i.e., the program and the basic information are kept within the institution. Information derived from one institution can be compared with data from another by creating a combined database or by simply comparing reports generated by the software. In some countries, information from the program is transmitted directly to a national database (Anonymous 1993; Editor 1993), while others use the program for sharing surveillance data on communicable diseases (Grant and Eke 1993). Thanks to microcomputer technology, institutions can operate independently of one another or participate in a network.

Using a common surveillance system allows hospitals to share experiences, eliminating the need to carry out separate product trials at each participating institution. Individually conducted trials often have too few cases during a one-year period to draw meaningful conclusions. Working in a collaborative way, combining cases and experiences from several institutions, permits hospitals to draw conclusions about safe practices and devices more quickly than would be the case for any one institution working alone.

The rules and protocols originally written to prevent needlesticks were not based on data about the effectiveness of changes in practice or devices. After the introduction and use of the Epi Net program, several common practices were shown to be totally ineffective in preventing needlesticks (Editor 1993). It became apparent that health workers needed blood-collection devices that actually lessened the probability of being stuck with a needle.

Within the first six months of use, the Epi Net software program facilitated the collection of enough data to show the effectiveness of a particular device in preventing needlesticks. The device had been in use for about five years, but there had been no consistently collected data to show its effectiveness and many institutions were not using it. Epi Net changed all this. It is simple to use, and careful attention was given to including the minimum number of data items needed for proper evaluation.

In conclusion, the microcomputer is a useful tool, but the programming and preparation of simplified and effective software is a time-consuming task. Effective tools such as Epi Net serve epidemiologists very well and certainly make surveillance more efficient (Grant and Eke 1993).

Telecommunications

The growth of the telecommunications industry and technology will lead public health professionals into an interconnectedness that was not previously possible. The speed and ever-decreasing costs of this technology mean that now we can work globally rather than regionally. Individuals interested in similar issues from various geographic sites can form groups via microcomputer networks, exchange ideas, and work together on related projects.

Epidemiologists can more easily communicate with their colleagues through the worldwide availability of electronic mail. For epidemiologists operating alone in a city or even a country, the ability to consult via e-mail or computer networks will be very helpful. While many offices already have local area networks (LANs) which allow users to share program and data files and send e-mail to each other, the ability to expand LANs around the world via Internet, a collaboration of networks that allows users to communicate across organizational and geographic boundaries, is a more recent development (Nicoll 1994a, b, c). Many international agencies already maintain contact with their grantees and collaborators via computer networks such as Internet. An epidemiologist in Maine, on the east coast of the United States, could use Internet to search MELVYL, the extensive library database which includes the 7.5 million titles and 11.7 million holdings of the University of California and California State University systems, more than 3000 miles away (Nicoll 1994a).

Epidemiologists are collaborating internationally on article writing via computer networks, whose speed of contact makes this form of collaboration possible. Investigators can discuss issues and reach consensus via an almost instantaneous written format, which is available to them regardless of time of day. Many investigators feel that the written e-mail style format is preferable to the telephone style of collaborative work.

Distance learning

Distance learning occurs when the teacher and the learner are separated geographically. The most frequently used media for distance learning are television, video tapes, and computer networks. Currently, distance-learning techniques are being used to teach epidemiology and update professionals as part of continuing education; it will be a format used more frequently in the future in schools of public health. Some areas without schools of public health or similar concentrations of epidemiologists have already established remote-learning sites where classes are held, some in international settings.

Proper use of distance-learning mechanisms calls for carefully prepared teaching materials (Cyrs and Smith 1991). The microcomputer is a useful aid, since materials preparation often involves the use of publication software and clip-art, all available on microcomputers.

Many teachers prepare simulation exercises for students using existing microcomputer software. Increasingly, epidemiologists are trained using outbreak investigation simulations, some of which are now available on microcomputers. An exciting aspect of this is that educators can prepare their own exercises using locally relevant examples, and students can carry out the exercise on microcomputers or paper, depending on available resources.

View of the future

The computer revolution is continuing at such a rapid pace that many epidemiologists look back with nostalgia at favourite computers from the past, with the past being five years earlier. An individual investigator, equipped with broad-ranging expertise and a microcomputer, can now conduct epidemiological studies that previously would have been too expensive or complex to complete. However, this empowerment is not easy to acquire. The epidemiologist must be willing to learn new approaches to gathering, processing, and analysing study data. The microcomputer has rapidly become an essential component for working epidemiologists that will help them to conduct efficient investigations or to assist planners or policy-makers in most countries of the world.

The applications mentioned in this chapter are intended mainly to stimulate the imagination rather than provide a detail protocol for the respective studies. With some exceptions, we have focused on the future, relying on the continuing evolution of both computer hardware and software to maintain a contemporary focus. With an open mind and proper training, there is no reason why the approaches that we have outlined should not become the reality for epidemiologists throughout the world.

We have hesitated to mention specific computers or software in this chapter because of these rapid changes—specific items are likely to be obsolete by the time this chapter is read. Instead, we have focused on general categories of hardware and software that should be available in the future as well. In addition, we have described seven applications of epidemiological importance using current technology in ways that were not possible even a few years ago. Now it is time to look into the future.

Hardware

The next generation of desktop microcomputers will have 64 MB of RAM (i.e. space for 64 000 000 characters); a 4000 MB (4 GB) hard-disk drive, which serves as a holding area for 20 GB of erasable optical storage, a 20 MB 3.5 inch floppy disk drive, and a monitor with 1400×2200 pixel screen resolution and the ability to create thousands of on-screen colours. an internal modem will be built in and will be able to transmit data routinely at 36 000 bits per second. A microphone will attach to the CPU for dictating and converting oral words to written words. Both a page scanner and electronic pencil will be common for entry of written documents, photographs, and hand-written notes.

Portable or laptop computers will also be more powerful, although not as powerful as desktop machines. Colour screens will be the norm on all portable computers, except the PDA, and will weigh 3–5 pounds (1.4–2.3 kg), depending on advances in battery technology. Less expensive subnotebook computers, which rely on solar power to charge the internal batteries and are equipped with black-and-white screens, will become widely available in developing countries.

Printers will be capable of producing a wide variety of colours using mainly laser technology, although some high-resolution dot-matrix printers will still be popular for personal use and printing multiple-copy forms. Portable printers will use ink-jet technology to create high-resolution black-and-white text and graphs as well as colour graphs. As with portable microcomputers, the size and weight of portable printers will depend on advances in battery design.

Software

Most of the applications described earlier in this chapter are available today, but epidemiologists will probably not use them as single programs. Typically, applications will be fitted together in combinations, depending on the needs of each epidemiologist. Word-processing software can integrate complex statistical formulae, graphs, photographs, and handwritten notes into documents and print an image on paper in the same format as it appears on the computer monitor. Software will facilitate professional communication by becoming better at translating material written in English, Spanish, French, German, or other languages. While analyses will be completed faster than before, the basic statistical and analytical methods will still be the same, although the programs will be easier to use once the statistical or analytical methods are understood. Current information on specific diseases will become increasingly available in the United States and, possibly, other countries with the aid of modems and telecommunications software or direct network linkage to the computers at the United States Center for Communicable Diseases or the National Library of Medicine.

Probably the most dramatic changes are occurring in graphics software. In addition to the conventional bar and line charts, epidemiologists are able to visualize complex relationships in three-dimensional forms with a wide variety of shapes and colours. Mapping programs are common and will continue to be used by public health agencies to view disease patterns organized by basic geographic units.

As technology changes and prices decline, microcomputers will become almost as common as calculators are today among epidemiologists throughout the world. Those keeping abreast of changes and using this technology will find that communication and performing epidemiological investigations are easier, faster, and more accurate than ever before. Herein lies the promise of microcomputers for both epidemiologists and society.

References

Anonymous (1992). EPINet: a computerized blood and body fluid exposure reporting system from Dr. Janine Jagger. *Healthcare Hazardous Materials Management*, 5, 5–8.

Anonymous (1993). Canada adopts nationwide needlestick surveillance system-EPINet. *Infection Control and Hospital Epidemiology*, 14, 605.

Ariawan, I. and Frerichs, R.R. (1994). Csurvey: a cluster sampling utility for IBM-compatible microcomputers. Unpublished, University of California, Los Angeles, CA.

Bennett, S., Woods, T., Liyanage, W.M., and Smith, D.L. (1991). A simplified general method for cluster-sample surveys of health in developing countries. *World Health Statistics Quarterly*, 44, 98–106.

Berrios, D.C., Hearst, N., Coates, T.J., Stall, R., Hudes, E.S., Turner, H., et al. (1993). HIV antibody testing among those at risk for infection. The National AIDS Behavioral Surveys. *Journal of the American Medical Association*, 270, 1576–80.

Brown, D.W., Ramsay, M.E., Richards, A.F., and Miller, E. (1994). Salivary diagnosis of measles: a study of notifed cases in the United Kingdom, 1991–3. *British Medical Journal*, 308, 1015–17.

Chalmers, I., Hetherington, J., Newdick, M., Mutch, L., Grant, A., Enkin, M., et al. (1986). The Oxford Database of Perinatal Trials: developing a register of published reports of controlled trials. *Controlled Clinical Trials*, 7, 306–24.

Cyrs, T.E. and Smith, F.A. (1991). Interactive study guides with word pictures for teleclass teaching. *Tech Trends*, 36, 37–9.

Dean, A.G., Dean, J.A., Burton, A.H., and Dicker, R.C. (1991). Epi Info: a general-purpose microcomputer program for public health information systems. *American Journal of Preventive Medicine*, 7, 178–82.

Derr, J.A., Mitchell, D.C., Brannon, D., Smiciklas-Wright, H., Dixon, L.B., and Shannon, B.M. (1992). Time and cost analysis of a computer-assisted telephone interview system to collect dietary recalls. *American Journal of Epidemiology*, 136, 1386–92.

Editor (1993). National data-sharing network shows efficacy of safer needle device. *Hospital Employee Health*, 12, 106–8.

Epidemiology Program Office (1994). *Epi Map*. United States Centers for Disease Control and Prevention, Atlanta, GA.

Frerichs, R.R. (1989). Simple analytic procedures for rapid microcomputer-assisted cluster surveys in developing countries. *Public Health Reports*, 104, 24–35.

Frerichs, R.R. and Selwyn, B.J. (1991). Microcomputer applications in epidemiology. In *Oxford textbook of public health* (2nd edn), (ed. W.W. Holland, R. Detels, and E.G. Knox), Vol. 2, pp. 271–84. Oxford University Press.

Frerichs, R.R. and Tar, K.T. (1989). Computer-assisted rapid surveys in developing countries. *Public Health Reports*, 104, 14–23.

Frerichs, R.R., Silarug, N., Eskes, N., Pagcharoenpol, P., Rodklai, A., Thangsupachai, S., and Wongba, C. (1994). Saliva-based HIV antibody testing in Thailand. *AIDS*, 8, 885–94.

Grant, A.D. and Eke, B. (1993). Application of information technology to the laboratory reporting of communicable disease in England and Wales. *Communicable Disease Report Review*, 3, R75–8.

Harris, D.R., Lemeshow, S., Lwanga, S.K., et al. (1991). Evaluation of a standardized survey design proposed for use in epidemiological research on AIDS. *International Journal of Epidemiology*, 20, 1048–56.

Jagger, J. and Pearson, R.D. (1991). Universal precautions: still missing the point on needlesticks. *Infection Control and Hospital Epidemiology*, 12, 211–13.

Lemeshow, S. and Robinson, D. (1985). Surveys to measure programme coverage and impact: a review of the methodology used by the Expanded Programme on Immunization. *World Health Statistics Quarterly*, 38, 65–75.

Locke, S.E., Kowaloff, H.B., Hoff, R.G., et al. (1994). Computer interview for screening blood donors for risk of HIV transmission. *MD Computing*, 11, 26–32.

McNichols, C.W. and Rushinek, S.F. (1988). *Database management: a microcomputer approach*. Prentice-Hall, Englewood Cliffs, NJ.

Nicoll, L.H. (1994a). An introduction to the Internet. Part I: History, structure, and access. *Journal of Nursing Administration*, 24(3), 9–11.

Nicoll, L.H. (1994b). An introduction to the Internet. Part II: Addresses and resources. *Journal of Nursing Administration*, 24(5), 11–13.

Nicoll, L.H. (1994c). An introduction to the Internet. Part III: The Internet and other online services. *Journal of Nursing Administration*, 24(7–8), 15–17.

Orenstein, W.A., Bernier, R.H., Dondero, T.J., et al. (1985). Field evaluation of vaccine efficacy. *Bulletin of the World Health Organization*, 63, 1055–68.

Orenstein, W.A., Bernier, R.H., and Hinman, A.R. (1988). Assessing vaccine efficacy in the field: further observations. *Epidemiologic Reviews*, 10 212–41.

Perry, K.R., Brown, D.W., Parry, J.V., et al. (1993). Detection of measles, mumps, and rubella antibodies in saliva using antibody capture radio-immunoassay. *Journal of Medical Virology*, 40, 235–40.

Rothman, K.J. (1986). *Modern epidemiology*. Little Brown, Boston, MA.

Selwyn, B.J. (1985). Graphic packages and graphs in epidemiology. *Epidemiology Monitor*, 6, 3.

Selwyn, B.J., Frerichs, R.R., Smith, G.S., and Olson, J. (1989). Rapid epidemiologic assessment: the evolution of a new discipline—introduction. *International Journal of Epidemiology*, 18 (Suppl. 2), S1.

Smith, G.S. (1980). Development of rapid epidemiologic assessment methods to evaluate health status and delivery of health services. *International Journal of Epidemiology*, 18 (Suppl. 2), S2–15.

US CDC (United States Centers for Disease Control) (1992). Rapid health needs assessment following Hurricane Andrew—Florida and Louisiana, 1992. *Morbidity and Mortality Weekly Report*, 41, 685–8.

Valdiserri, R.O. Holtgrave, D.R., and Brackbill, R. (1993). American adults' knowledge of HIV testing availability. *American Journal of Public Health*, 83, 525–8.

Wawer, M.J., Sewankambo, N.K., Berkley, S., et al. (1994). Incidence of HIV-1 infection in a rural region of Uganda. *British Medical Journal*, 308, 171–3.

20 Public health surveillance

Ruth L. Berkelman, Donna F. Stroup, and James W. Buehler

Public health surveillance is the epidemiological foundation for modern public health. Surveillance data resulting from the continuous monitoring of the occurrence of a disease or condition, such as acquired immunodeficiency syndrome (AIDS) or tuberculosis, underlie what public health actions are taken and whether these actions are effective. The term 'surveillance' is derived from the French word meaning 'to watch over' and, as applied to public health, means the close monitoring of the occurrence of selected health conditions in the population. Although surveillance methods were originally developed as part of efforts to control infectious diseases, basic concepts of surveillance have been applied to all areas of public health. Public health surveillance has been expanded to include not only information on diseases, injuries, and other conditions but also information such as the prevalence of risk factors, both personal and environmental.

Definition

In 1963 Alexander Langmuir defined disease surveillance as 'the continued watchfulness over the distribution and trends of incidence through the systematic collection, consolidation, and evaluation of morbidity and mortality reports and other relevant data' together with timely and regular dissemination to those who 'need to know'. In 1968 the 21st World Health Assembly described surveillance as the systematic collection and use of epidemiological information for the planning, implementation, and assessment of disease control; in short, surveillance implied 'information for action' (WHO 1968). The role and concept of public health surveillance continue to evolve as the scope of surveillance broadens and as increasingly sophisticated methods are applied (Thacker *et al.* 1989; Thacker and Stroup 1994).

Surveillance should begin when there exists or is likely to occur a public health problem for which programmes for prevention and control of a health event have been or may need to be initiated. A critical component of the definition of surveillance is that surveillance systems include the ongoing collection, analysis, and use of health data. Thus, health information systems (for example, registration of births and deaths, routine abstraction of hospital records, general health surveys in a population) that are general and not linked to specific prevention and control programmes do not, by themselves, constitute surveillance. However, data collected from ongoing health information systems may be useful for surveillance when systematically analysed on a timely basis.

History

Recording of deaths is the oldest form of data collection for monitoring public health. John Graunt is generally recognized as the first person to describe use of numerical methods for this purpose in his treatise *Natural and political observations on the bills of mortality* (1662). In 1776 Johann Peter Frank advocated a more extensive monitoring of health in Germany that would support public health efforts related to schoolchildren's health, prevention of injuries, maternal and child health, and public water and sewage disposal.

William Farr is recognized as the founder of the modern concept of surveillance. As Superintendent of the Statistical Department of the General Registrar's Office in Great Britain from 1839 to 1879, he collected, analysed, and interpreted vital statistics and disseminated the information in weekly, quarterly, and annual reports. He did not stop with publication of official reports, but regularly contributed papers to medical journals and even used the public press to achieve effective action (Langmuir 1976). Thus, he took the responsibility of seeing that action was taken on the basis of his analyses.

In the nineteenth century, Farr's efforts at health monitoring were extended by Edwin Chadwick, who investigated the relationship between environmental conditions and disease. Chadwick was followed by Louis René Villerme, who analysed the relationship between poverty and mortality in Paris. Lemuel Shattuck also published data in the United States that related deaths, infant and maternal mortality, and infectious diseases to living conditions. He further recommended standardized nomenclature for cause of disease and death, and the collection of health data that included sex, age, locality, and other demographic factors. The first international list of causes of death was developed in 1893 (Eylenbosch and Noah 1988).

Increasingly, elements of surveillance were applied to aid in detecting epidemics and in preventing and controlling infectious diseases. In 1899 the United Kingdom began compulsory notification of selected infectious diseases. National morbidity data collection on plague, smallpox, and yellow fever was initiated in 1878 in the United States, and by 1925 all states were reporting weekly to the United States Public Health Service on the occurrence of selected diseases. In a public health context, the term surveillance was increasingly applied to programmes of reporting selected infectious diseases in a population, with less emphasis on its application to quarantine of individuals (Langmuir 1963).

Table 20.1 Acute and chronic disease surveillance

	Common characteristics	Acute disease surveillance	Chronic disease surveillance
Purpose	Monitor trends Describe problem and estimate health burden	Emphasis on weekly or monthly variations to detect outbreaks	Emphasis on year-to-year trends
	Direct/evaluate programmes for prevention and control		
Data	Regular	Reliance on notification by health care providers/laboratories	Greater use of existing databases (e.g. vital statistics, hospital discharges)
Data analysis	Descriptive statistics for time, place, person	Emphasis often on case counts	Emphasis usually on rates
Data dissemination	Regular; frequency reflects data collection	More frequent	Less frequent
	Audience targeted		

Similar reporting activities were occurring in Europe at about the same time. In 1907 the Office International d'Hygiene Publique, predominantly composed of European member states, was created (WHO 1958). The office was to disseminate information in a monthly bulletin on the occurrence of selected diseases, most notably cholera, plague, and yellow fever. In the succeeding decades, other diseases were recommended for surveillance in step with the International Sanitary Regulations. However, many of the morbidity and mortality reporting systems were not systematic and were still largely developed for long-term archival functions.

Since the early 1950s, the critical importance of surveillance to public health efforts has been demonstrated frequently. In 1955 acute poliomyelitis among recipients of the poliomyelitis vaccine in the United States threatened national vaccination programmes that had just begun. In collaboration with state health departments, the United States Centers for Disease Control (US CDC) developed an intensive national surveillance system, and at one point a daily report was being issued regarding poliomyelitis cases. The surveillance data assisted epidemiologists in demonstrating that the problem was limited to a single manufacturer of the vaccine and allowed the vaccination programme to continue with a resulting dramatic decline in cases of acute poliomyelitis in the United States in successive years (Langmuir 1963). During the worldwide malaria control programme, surveillance was used to determine areas of continued transmission and to focus spraying efforts, as well as to document those areas without malaria (Raska 1966). With the subsequent decline in malaria control efforts, surveillance data have shown the re-emergence of malaria in many areas of the world.

Surveillance was also the foundation for the successful global campaign to eradicate smallpox. When the campaign began in 1967, efforts were focused on achieving a high vaccination level in countries with endemic smallpox; however, it was soon evident that a programme based on surveillance to target vaccinations in limited areas would be more efficient. Smallpox reporting sources, usually medical facilities, were contacted on a routine basis, and thus a reporting network was firmly established in most countries. In

addition, other reporting sources were often established, including markets, schools, police, agricultural extension workers, and others. In 1973, as the goal of eradication neared, a systematic house-to-house search for cases was established in India and subsequently used widely in Pakistan and Bangladesh (Henderson 1976). Well-designed surveillance systems for data collection, tabulation, and routine feedback were vital to the success of the programme.

In 1981, shortly after the disease later named AIDS was recognized, national surveillance was begun in the United States and other countries. Even before the aetiological agent, human immunodeficiency virus (HIV), was identified, surveillance data contributed to identifying modes of transmission, population groups at risk for infection, and, equally important, population groups not at risk for infection. These data have been instrumental in directing public health resources to programmes, preventing further spread of HIV, and averting widespread public hysteria (Jaffe et al. 1983).

The potential usefulness of surveillance as a public health tool to address problems beyond infectious disease was emphasized in 1968 when the 21st World Health Assembly recommended the application of surveillance principles to a wider scope of problems including cancer, atherosclerosis, and social problems such as drug addiction (WHO 1968). Many of the principles of surveillance traditionally applied to acute infectious diseases have also been applied to chronic diseases and conditions, although some differences in surveillance techniques have been observed (Thacker et al. 1995) (Table 20.1). Even though chronic diseases may have long latency periods, trends in their incidence may change relatively quickly, and surveillance can play a key role in detecting these changes when effective interventions are applied (Berkelman and Buehler 1990).

In addition to the increased scope of health problems under surveillance, the methods of surveillance have expanded from general disease notification systems to include survey techniques, sentinel health provider systems, and other approaches to data collection (Thacker and Berkelman 1988; Thacker and Stroup

Table 20.2 Purposes of public health surveillance

To characterize disease patterns by time, place, and person

To detect epidemics

To suggest hypotheses

To identify cases for epidemiological research

To evaluate prevention and control programmes

To project future health care needs

1994). The assimilation of microcomputers into the workplace has also made possible more efficient data collection as well as more rapid and sophisticated analyses. In the United States all state health departments are linked to the US CDC by computer for the routine collection and dissemination of selected data on notifiable health conditions (US CDC 1991). In France the utility of computers in office-based surveillance of various conditions of public health has been demonstrated (Valleron *et al.* 1986). In developing countries, computers are increasingly being used with epidemiological programs for analysis and mapping (Frerichs 1991; Dean *et al.* 1993).

Purposes of surveillance

A surveillance system should be designed to meet the needs of a prevention and control programme (Table 20.2). These needs usually include a description of the temporal and geographic trends in the occurrence of a health event in a particular population. Most importantly, surveillance systems should identify changes in disease occurrence. The data should be useful for substantiating patterns of both endemic and epidemic disease.

The role of surveillance in guiding public health programmes is illustrated by the first major national activity initiated by the US CDC—the Malaria Eradication Programme. Surveys in the mid-1930s had established malaria to be an endemic problem deeply rooted in the southeastern part of the United States. An extensive chlorophenothane (DDT) spraying programme was launched after the Second World War, and surveillance was instituted in 1947. It was established quite rapidly that endemic malaria had essentially disappeared, probably even before the DDT programme was under way (Langmuir 1963). In this case, surveillance was used as the basis for dismantling a public health programme and redirecting public health resources to problems of higher priority.

However, the need for surveillance itself may continue for a disease even when prevention and control programmes are cut back, particularly for infectious diseases such as tuberculosis, dengue fever, or malaria whose incidence may change quickly. Generally, the more quickly re-emergence of a disease is detected, the more quickly and efficiently it can be controlled (US CDC 1992*a*; PAHO 1994).

Surveillance data are also useful for evaluating the effectiveness of prevention and control programmes (US CDC 1992*b*) and of regulations or laws modified or initiated to address public health concerns (for example safety of food and water, alcohol-related motor vehicle injuries). Monitoring of changes in the incidence of the disease or condition is necessary, and monitoring of associated risk factors (food and water sanitation, self-reports of drinking and driving) may also be useful. The rapid decline in morbidity from many infectious diseases in certain populations has been related directly to vaccination campaigns that were conducted as a result of surveillance data on disease incidence. Direct correlation of a single intervention to a specific disease outcome may be difficult when the aetiology of the disease is multifactorial, but the impact of an intervention on disease outcome, including its incidence and severity, remains the ultimate test of policy.

Assessment of the burden of disease, including its incidence (i.e. the number of people newly affected each year) and its current and projected prevalence (i.e. the number of people affected by the disease at any point in time), is essential to planning public health programmes. For example, surveillance for AIDS has been critical to the forecasting of the future burden of that disease in the United States (Gail and Brookmeyer 1988; Institute of Medicine 1988). With the ageing of the population, projections of disease prevalence in the elderly are needed to determine future health care needs.

Surveillance may be initiated to identify risk factors associated with disease and to suggest hypotheses for further investigation; cases identified through surveillance are sometimes used in case–control studies, as in the early studies of toxic shock syndrome and the AIDS epidemic (Shands *et al.* 1980; Jaffe *et al.* 1983). Effective preventive actions were formulated based on such research even before the aetiological agents, a toxigenic strain of *Staphylococcus aureus* and HIV, were discovered.

Establishing a surveillance system

Establishing a surveillance system requires a statement of objectives, definition of the disease or condition under surveillance, and implementation of procedures for collecting, interpreting, and disseminating information. Surveillance systems can be considered as information loops, or cycles, that involve health care providers, public health agencies, and the public. A weakness in any part of the loop or information chain weakens the entire surveillance process. For example, if public health measures mandate that infectious conditions such as cryptosporidiosis must be reported, the surveillance system will be successful only if laboratories have the capacity to diagnose the infection (Berkelman 1994). Likewise, if the diagnosis on a hospital discharge record is coded incorrectly, surveillance data based on hospital discharge records will reflect the inaccuracies.

The information cycle begins when cases occur and is completed when information about these cases is made available and is used for prevention and control. This process may involve multiple cycles, ranging from the local response to individual cases to the development of national policies based on information aggregated from many cases. Essential to the completion of the surveillance cycle is the return of information to those who 'need to know' (Langmuir 1963), and thus attention must be directed not only to procedures for collecting data but also to procedures for ensuring that useful information is returned to constituents (Fig. 20.1).

The likelihood that clearly effective interventions can be found, can prevent the occurrence of disease, or can alleviate the course of existing disease is an important consideration in determining whether a surveillance system will be useful. However, even in the absence of a currently effective intervention, surveillance data can point to the need for legislation (for example the use of surveillance

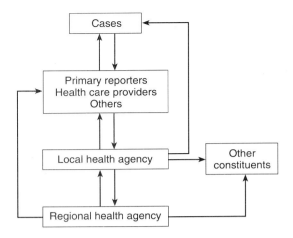

Fig. 20.1 Cycle of information flow in surveillance systems.

data on firearm injuries to influence legislation regarding gun control) (Loftin *et al.* 1991) or to the need for more resource allocation if a problem poses an increasing health threat (for example development of a pneumococcal vaccine for children less than two years old becomes more urgent as the incidence of multi-drug-resistant pneumococci increases). A surveillance programme is less likely to succeed if no clearly effective control or prevention measures are defined.

Health priorities for surveillance must be continually evaluated as new infections emerge (for example *Escherichia coli* O157:H7), the population is exposed to new hazards (for example new consumer products, environmental contamination), and other health conditions change. Surveillance for both the disease or condition, as well as for associated risk factors and prevention services, should be considered.

System objectives

Defining the objectives of a surveillance system depends on what information is needed, who needs it, and how it will be used. Implementing a system will require a balance of competing interests, and a clear statement of objectives will provide a framework for subsequent decisions. For example, the desire to collect detailed information about cases may compete with needs to assess the number of cases rapidly. Thus, if the primary objective is to obtain rapid case counts, then less information would be collected about each case to avoid delays in reporting. The objectives of a surveillance system will be shaped by its target population, its constituents, the nature of prevention and control programmes, and the health problem under surveillance.

Target population

A surveillance system seeks to identify health events within a specified population. This population may be defined on the basis of where persons live, work, attend school, or use health care services, for example. Alternatively, the population may be defined on the basis of where health events occur. For example, a surveillance system that monitors newborn health as a measure of prenatal care services would focus on deliveries to women who live within a community and not on women who live elsewhere but deliver in the community's hospitals. In contrast, surveillance of traffic injuries

aimed at identifying roadway hazards could include all injuries that occur in a community, regardless of whether affected persons are community residents.

Constituents

Surveillance systems are likely to have many constituents, including clinicians, health agencies, academics, politicians, media reporters, and others with diverse perspectives and uses for surveillance data. Because these diverse needs cannot always be satisfied, the primary or most important constituents should be identified.

Public health programmes

The objectives of surveillance systems will be shaped by the objectives and capabilities of the public health programmes they serve. For example, a programme to eliminate an infectious disease requires intensive surveillance that emphasizes identification of all persons with the disease in the final stages of the programme. This strategy was used in the smallpox eradication programme and has also been employed in the poliomyelitis eradication programmes in the Americas (Foege *et al.* 1975; Biellik *et al.* 1992). In contrast, an educational programme to influence behaviour may depend on a surveillance system that describes the practices of a sample of persons in a community (Remington *et al.* 1988).

Health problems

It is necessary to decide exactly what disease or health problem will be under surveillance. Surveillance may frequently be conducted for any of several points along a spectrum ranging from exposure to an adverse outcome. One should consider which manifestation(s) or stage(s) of a disease should be under surveillance. For example, manifestations of ischaemic heart disease include abnormal diagnostic tests in the absence of symptoms, angina pectoris, acute myocardial infarction, and (sudden) death. If the goal of surveillance is to assess the burden of the disease on health care systems, a broad definition that encompasses various manifestations may be appropriate. If the purpose is to monitor trends in the disease, a more limited and severe manifestation, such as myocardial infarction, may be the appropriate target for surveillance. If resources are limited, surveillance based on analyses of death certificates may be most feasible; however, interpretation of trends may be complicated by independent trends in the occurrence of the disease, advances in treatment, or changes in coding of vital records. Alternatively, attention may be focused on risk factors for cardiovascular disease, such as hypertension, smoking, cholesterol levels, or physical activity. For surveillance of infections carried by animals or arthropods (such as rabies and encephalitis), surveillance of infection in the reservoir host may be as important as surveillance in the human population.

Case definition

The case definition is fundamental to any surveillance system, since it is the formal answer to the question of what manifestations of a disease or condition are under surveillance (US CDC 1990*b*). It is both a criterion for determining who is counted and a guide to local health departments for case investigations and follow-up. It ensures that the same measure is used across geographic areas. The case definition must be sufficiently inclusive (sensitive) to identify persons who require public health attention but sufficiently exclusive (specific) to avoid unnecessary diversion of that attention. In addition, the case definition must be usable by all persons on whom the system depends for case reporting. There is no ideal case definition for any particular disease or condition.

The following are two possible case definitions that could be used in conducting surveillance for hepatitis A.

Definition 1

Illness characterized by jaundice, elevated liver enzymes, and serological detection of immunoglobulin M (IgM) antibodies against hepatitis A.

This definition presumes that affected persons will have access to health care services, including diagnostic testing. The definition does not include persons with asymptomatic hepatitis A infection. An alternative may be to limit the definition to persons with a positive test for IgM antibodies against the hepatitis A virus. However, this approach would exclude persons who have an epidemiological and clinical picture consistent with hepatitis A but who lack serological testing. To accommodate these possibilities, the case definition may be subdivided to allow for symptomatic versus asymptomatic cases or for gradations based on certainty of diagnosis (confirmed case, presumptive case, possible case).

Definition 2

Yellow eyes.

This definition is simple and may be appropriate in a setting where hepatitis A transmission has been documented and where there is limited access to diagnostic services, where field staff have little formal training, and where there is an emergent need to assess a population rapidly (for example a refugee camp). With this definition, hepatitis case counts may include some persons with jaundice due to other conditions, but the lack of specificity may not substantially affect the usefulness of the overall information.

Neither of these two definitions or possible variations is inherently better than the other, and each may be appropriate in a given setting. The first definition is more specific but may lack utility in geographic areas where laboratory testing is unavailable. The second definition would not be appropriate for a population vaccinated against hepatitis A.

Thus the definition must be geared to the circumstances that govern each surveillance system. The definition must also remain current as conditions change. During the course of the poliomyelitis eradication campaign, different definitions have been used, with a less specific definition needed when cases of poliomyelitis are common. Following successful vaccination campaigns and a large reduction in disease incidence, case definitions for poliomyelitis require more specificity, which in turn requires laboratory confirmation of cases of acute flaccid paralysis (Andrus et al. 1992).

A similar range of possible case definitions also exists for surveillance systems that focus on adverse health exposures rather than disease outcomes. For example, in a surveillance system that addresses occupational hazards, exposure to a harmful substance may be monitored by self-report of workers, by company log-books of manufacturing procedures, or by routine measurement of substances in the work environment, on workers' clothing, or in specimens collected from workers. Each of these possible case definitions would require different levels of co-operation from the company or workers, and each may be subject to unique limitations that could bias surveillance.

The flow of information

Surveillance systems depend on the sequential flow of information through the full surveillance cycle. Each facet of this process should be carefully planned, as described below.

Reporters

Persons responsible for reporting cases may be all health care providers in a defined area, selected providers, or persons at specific institutions (for example clinics, hospitals, schools, factories). In addition to communicating case reports, reporters may be responsible for collecting specimens needed by public health agencies for laboratory confirmation or application of molecular epidemiological techniques (for example determining whether a case of poliomyelitis has been caused by a vaccine strain or a wild-type poliomyelitis virus).

Forms

The desire to collect detailed information must be tempered by the need to limit data to items that can be reliably and consistently collected over the long term. Forms that are too detailed and too complicated will not be welcomed by those on whom the surveillance system must depend.

Timing

Surveillance systems provide data on a regular basis, ranging from daily to annually. Whatever periodicity is used should be specified and adhered to by participants in all phases of the surveillance loop, even when the number of reported cases is zero. To contain an outbreak of meningococcal meningitis, the health department must receive reports of cases quickly (i.e., within 24 hours) so that necessary control measures may be taken immediately. In contrast, a breast cancer registry evaluating the effectiveness of targeted screening services for breast cancer may collect and analyse data on a quarterly basis or even less frequently. The timing most appropriate to achieve the objective of the surveillance should be selected.

Aggregation of data

Surveillance data may be in the form of individual patient records or aggregate counts and tabulations. For example, there may be a need at the local level to maintain records on individual persons to direct follow-up services. However, there may be no need to maintain records on the individual at a regional level, and aggregate counts or tabulations may be sufficient. However, aggregate data do not permit the same flexibility of analysis as individual data.

Data transmission

The mode of data transmission will depend on both the need for timeliness and communications resources. Increasingly, computers, and particularly microcomputers, are being used in surveillance systems, permitting transmission of data in electronic formats such as telecommunication or mailing data storage devices (Valleron et al. 1986; US CDC 1991). The rapidity of data transmission afforded by computers may not be necessary, however, and postage of forms may be sufficient. If very limited volumes of data, such as simple case counts, are being sent, communication by telephone or fax may be sufficient.

Computerization is only a tool to facilitate transmission of data and does not replace the need for regular contact between health care providers, public health professionals, and others who participate in the information loop. Reporting of disease outbreaks and insights into disease occurrence are often best and most promptly communicated through personal contacts.

Data management and dissemination

The following issues in data management and dissemination should be considered in planning for storage, analysis, and dissemination of surveillance information.

Updating records

Surveillance data often need to be updated. Information that was initially unattainable may become available, follow-up investigations yield supplemental information, persons initially classified as meeting or not meeting a case definition may be reclassified, errors in reporting may be identified and corrected, and duplicate case reports may be recognized and culled. One approach to handling these and other changes is to maintain both provisional and final records, including separate publications for provisional and final data. Thus provisional reports may satisfy immediate information needs, while final and more delayed reports can accommodate corrections and updates to a reasonable limit and can serve an archival function.

Selecting measures for time and place

A case report may include such dates as those of the onset of disease, the diagnosis, the report to local health authorities, and the report to regional or national health authorities. Tabulations of surveillance data may be based on the date of any of these events. However, if there are, for example, long delays between dates of diagnosis and report, analyses of trends based on date of diagnosis will be unreliable for the most recent periods. Similarly, surveillance data may be tabulated on the basis of the site of occurrence of the health event, the site of diagnosis, or the residence of persons reported. The selection of these measures for time and place may also differ for provisional and final surveillance reports.

Detail in published reports

The value of surveillance activities can best be measured by the extent to which the information obtained is used in public health practice: the usefulness of data is dependent, in part, on the ease of interpretation of the presentation. Thus the goal of published reports should be simple and easily interpreted analyses. Surveillance data may be published in either tables or graphs and maps (Dean et al. 1993). The advantages of tables are that more detail can be provided and that numbers are available for readers to use in further calculations and analyses. The disadvantage is that more time and effort are required to extract summary points from a table than from a good figure. The advantage of figures is that one or more key points can be visualized by a reader almost instantly; the disadvantage is a loss of detail. Thus the intended audience must be considered in selecting tables, figures, or a combination of both for published surveillance reports.

Confidentiality

Preventing inappropriate disclosure of surveillance data is essential both to the privacy of persons with reported cases of disease and to the trust of participants in the surveillance system. The protection of confidentiality begins with limiting data collection and transmission to a minimum and includes ensuring the physical security of surveillance records, the discretion of surveillance staff, and legal safeguards (Federal Committee on Statistics 1994). In addition, summaries of surveillance data should not present data in a manner that would permit identification of individuals. For example, data should not be reported in cross-tabulations when the population represented is small and the report may lead to identification of individuals.

Initiating and maintaining participation

Public health agencies depend on the ongoing co-operation of others to identify and report cases in most surveillance systems. Regardless of whether reporting is required by law, is voluntary, or is financially rewarded, it takes time and effort. Any approach requires personal contact and dissemination of reports that document the usefulness of surveillance data, which are likely to be a key to initiating and maintaining participation in the system.

For certain diseases, reporting is often required by law. While legal mandates may not guarantee reporting, they establish the authority under which health agencies conduct surveillance. In addition, reporting laws and regulations may identify not only those who are required to report cases but also those who may report cases without fear of liability for violation of privacy. Statutes may also protect health agencies from forced disclosure of the identity of persons with particular diseases.

Organizational structure

If the surveillance loop of data collection, analysis, interpretation, and feedback is to function as a continuous process, an organizational structure is required. Such a structure depends on the resources available (including the number of skilled and unskilled personnel), the technology available for communication and data management (for example computers), and financial constraints, as well as the number and type of diseases under surveillance. In its simplest form, the organizational structure requires health care providers to report a single disease or health event on a regular basis to a co-ordinating public health authority. A more complex form would include a network of reporting units dealing concurrently with problems related to many diseases. In any case, the structure must allow data to be gathered from various sources and evaluated by epidemiologists in time for appropriate action to be taken. These data must be routinely disseminated to a targeted audience; therefore reproduction or telecommunication equipment is usually needed.

The structure should provide support for training of key personnel in surveillance through seminars or other meetings that give field and central staff the opportunity to review procedures and to resolve operational problems. Appropriate technical support, such as provision of diagnostic reagents, laboratory space, and computer equipment, must also be ensured. The need for regular evaluation of the surveillance systems should also be recognized.

Delegating tasks to international, national, regional, and local health authorities should depend on information needs and resources at each level. Particular attention should be directed to the local level because primary responsibility for information collection and public health responsibilities are local. Central agencies are responsible for guiding, as well as co-ordinating, data collection procedures to ensure that surveillance data are collected using sound methodology so that they can be reliably compared from one area to another and aggregated into regional or national summaries. Also, because many monitoring efforts for non-infectious conditions (for example traffic injuries, water pollution) are dealt with by governmental agencies other than public health agencies (for example police authorities, environmental protection agencies), there needs to be effective co-ordination between health authorities and other appropriate authorities; for this purpose, procedures may need to be established to ensure the necessary communication.

Data collection

Public health surveillance data are collected in many ways, depending on the nature of the health event under surveillance, potential methods for identifying the disease, the population involved, the resources available, and the goals of the programme. Some surveillance systems may rely on a single source of data with alternate data sources being used periodically to evaluate or to enhance the completeness of routine surveillance data.

Notification systems

Notifiable disease reporting is the surveillance approach traditionally used by public health programmes. A system of notification is based on laws or regulations by health authorities that require reporting of selected diseases, usually infectious, to the health department to support and direct prevention and control programmes. Notification reporting may be instituted at many levels (local, national, and international). Ultimately, under a system of notification, the reporting will be most useful and most accurate for diseases if surveillance is supported and emphasized at a local level. Persons or institutions with responsibility for reporting to the public health authority often include physicians, other health care providers, coroners and medical examiners, laboratories, and hospitals. Historically, physicians have been most important to systems of notification, but reliance on laboratory reporting has been increasing.

In any country, the extent of notification activities depends on the availability of facilities and resources—trained staff, laboratory and other equipment, epidemiological services, and liaison with health care providers—as well as the health priority of the disease and method of diagnosis (Berkelman et al. 1994). Reports are often initiated by the health care provider or other reporting source; for some diseases for which more complete reporting is sought, public health professionals may contact major reporting sources and/or review laboratory or other relevant records to ensure that cases are ascertained. These systems of reporting have been described as passive and active, respectively, but the distinctions are not always clear. Data for many surveillance programmes represent a mixture of both reports elicited by public health professionals contacting health care providers or reviewing records and reports submitted by health care providers to public health officials without direct solicitation.

Reporting is generally incomplete for most notifiable diseases (Hinman 1977; Vogt et al. 1983). If persons are asymptomatic or have only mild symptoms, they will not usually seek health care. Patients and physicians may conceal diseases that carry a social stigma such as sexually transmitted diseases. Health care providers may also fail to report because they may be unaware of regulations or because they may treat the symptoms without a complete laboratory investigation. Completeness of reporting may also be significantly influenced by factors such as medical community interest and publicity; the most important is probably intensity of surveillance efforts, which is closely linked to availability of resources (Davis and Vergeront 1982; Buehler et al. 1992).

Many incomplete data may serve their purpose, however. Epidemics, as well as general temporal and geographic trends, can be determined as long as the proportion of cases detected remains consistent over time and across geographic areas.

A comparison in Israel between cases of viral hepatitis reported by practitioners in private practice and cases reported in a population covered by an insurance plan demonstrated that, although completeness of reporting by the physicians was only 37 per cent, the distribution of reported cases by season and age was similar to that recorded in the insured population (Brachott and Mosley 1972). However, under-reporting may affect representativeness; a study of under-reporting of acute viral hepatitis in the United States demonstrated that homosexual men with hepatitis B and blood transfusion recipients with non-A non-B hepatitis were less likely than members of other risk groups to be reported (Alter et al. 1987). Thus, surveillance data acquired through reports initiated by health care providers may not accurately reflect the risk for specific populations.

Unless infectious diseases are eradicated (for example smallpox), the potential for re-emergence requires continued vigilance and capacity to respond, even though the control programme may not be a high public health priority (for example plague). As new infectious agents are recognized, the need to expand the surveillance system to control these agents effectively has been recognized in many countries. Furthermore, as international travel and commerce facilitate the rapid spread of pathogens from one part of the globe to another, the need for improved international disease surveillance has become apparent (Institute of Medicine 1992; US CDC 1992d, 1994a).

Although infectious conditions have dominated the list of notifiable diseases in most countries, other diseases and conditions may also have to be reported. Adverse drug reactions, occupational injuries, poisonings, and specified malignancies, among others, may be required to be reported, particularly in developed countries (Faich et al. 1987; De Bock 1988; Freund et al. 1989).

In settings where the infrastructure does not exist to support accurate case reporting systems yet there is a need to assess the impact of a disease on morbidity, an alternative and potentially simple and rapid approach is to survey hospitals periodically for the number of admissions attributed to a particular condition (DeCock et al. 1989). Another crude but inexpensive surveillance system for diseases with high morbidity rates and for which notification may not be appropriate (for example gastrointestinal illnesses or influenza) may be based on absenteeism from schools or industry, depending on the ages of the affected populations.

Health care provider networks

Networks of health care providers have been organized in recent years primarily to gather information on selected health events. Most have been organized by practising physicians on a voluntary basis; in many European countries, these networks have formed firm relationships with both public health authorities and academic centres, and often form the basis for morbidity surveillance (Valleron *et al.* 1986). In 1979 the Ministry of Public Health in China and the Chinese Academy of Preventive Medicine initiated a sentinel network of surveillance sites to address the need for more timely and representative data (Cheng 1992; Yang 1992). The strengths of such a system include the commitment of the participants, the possibility of collecting longitudinal data, the flexibility of the system to address a changing set of conditions, and the ability to gain information on all patient–provider encounters, regardless of severity of illness. The most severe limitation of this type of system is that the population served by these physicians may not be representative of the general population. In addition, the illness must be fairly common to provide representative incidence data from a small sample of physician contacts.

Example: A voluntary network of general practitioners in Belgium was initiated in 1978 (Stroobant *et al.* 1988). Practitioners were selected who were representative of Belgian general practitioners according to age and sex and who were geographically distributed to ensure coverage of the country. Participants report weekly, and the results are sent to the participants on a quarterly basis. The list of health problems has included selected vaccine-preventable diseases, respiratory conditions, and suicide attempts, with some health problems such as mumps and measles reported continuously and others on a less frequent basis. An excellent level of participation has been documented, with the degree of form completion and continuity of reporting as criteria for assessment. The network has been evaluated in terms of its possible biases, such as non-participation of practitioners and difficulties in estimating the population at risk for the health problems under study; methods have been developed to reduce these biases (Lobet *et al.* 1987).

Example: The British Paediatric Surveillance Unit (BPSU 1993) was initiated in 1986 through the collaboration of several agencies: the British Paediatric Society, the Public Health Laboratory Service Communicable Disease Surveillance Centre, and the Department of Epidemiology at the University of London. The BPSU has also added collaborators from specialty groups such as orthopaedics, rheumatology, and dermatology. The BPSU has enabled paediatricians to participate in the surveillance of infections and infection-related conditions and in studies of uncommon disorders. It also provides a mechanism by which new diseases can be detected quickly and monitored. The reporting system involves the mailing of a monthly card that contains the disorders currently being surveyed. Examples of conditions under surveillance have included HIV infection and AIDS, insulin-dependent diabetes mellitus, acute flaccid paralysis, and Kawasaki disease in children. In 1992 over 1000 paediatricians participated in the BPSU.

Laboratory surveillance

Surveillance of routinely collected laboratory reports has been particularly useful for certain infectious conditions. For instance, in the United States, reporting from many public health laboratories is automated (Bean *et al.* 1992). In England nearly all microbiology laboratories report positive identifications of specified infections each week to the Communicable Disease Surveillance Centre. The advantages of the laboratory reporting system are its specificity, its flexibility in adding new diseases, its rapidity, and the amount of

detail about the infectious agent that can be provided. Reports indicate trends or the appearance of rare infections originating from a common source that could not be identified by a single laboratory. One disadvantage is that the number of persons from whom specimens are tested is usually not reported. In addition, the persons tested may not be representative of the population at risk. For some infections, such as toxic shock syndrome, there is no suitable laboratory test, and for many common illnesses a specimen may not be taken (for example influenza).

Nosocomial infection surveillance is often based on review of laboratory records by an infection control nurse or other designated staff (Brachman 1982). In 1970 the National Nosocomial Infection Study was initiated to monitor the frequency and trends of nosocomial infection in United States hospitals. Over 160 hospitals participate in what is now a voluntary national surveillance system, with microbiology studies reported on 90 per cent of infected patients (Gaynes *et al.* 1991). A network of laboratories of different medical centres around the world has been established to conduct surveillance of antibiotic resistance for various pathogens (O'Brien *et al.* 1986).

Disease registries

Registries are comprehensive listings of individuals with particular conditions. They often include detailed information about diagnostic classification, treatment, and outcome. Registries were initially established primarily for epidemiological research on individual diseases or conditions to develop aetiological hypotheses and to identify cases for further research (Weddell 1973). Registries have also been used to ensure the provision of appropriate care and to evaluate changing patterns of medical care; unlike other disease information systems, they cut across the different levels of severity of illness and may provide information over time about individual persons. Recently, the value of registries for monitoring disease incidence and its distribution, as well as for evaluating the effectiveness of targeted screening programmes, has been more widely recognized.

In focusing on selected diseases or conditions, registries often develop a constituency that promotes participation and reporting. Most registries rely on numerous sources of data for case detection including, but not limited to, hospitals, laboratories, and death records; few registries rely primarily on physician notification. Public health professionals probably have the most experience with cancer registries and registries for congenital malformations.

Cancer registries generally have relied on multiple sources of data, including notification by health care providers, hospital discharge abstracts, treatment records (especially from oncology or radiotherapy units), death certificates, and pathology reports. Elaborate population-based registries for all cancers, such as registries developed by the United States National Cancer Institute in discrete geographic areas, have been particularly useful for national trend estimates and epidemiological research (Horm *et al.* 1984). Less sophisticated registries have been developed by state and local governments or by physician initiatives (Parkin 1988; US CDC 1994*b*; Pommerenke *et al.* 1994).

Surveillance for birth defects was first initiated in many parts of the world in response to the thalidomide tragedy; registries were established to provide reliable baseline rates for specific birth defects and to detect increases in the prevalence of birth defects as a means of rapidly identifying human teratogens (Kallen et al. 1984; Holtzman and Khoury 1986). The US CDC has conducted birth defects surveillance in metropolitan Atlanta since 1967 using multiple sources of ascertainment of all serious birth defects observed in stillborn and liveborn infants or recognized by signs and symptoms apparent in the first year of life (Edmonds et al. 1981; US CDC 1993). The US CDC also conducts national birth defects surveillance using newborn discharge diagnoses from about 1200 hospitals (Edmonds et al. 1981; US CDC 1993). Because the coverage and the quality of the nationwide system are not optimal, use of a birth defects registry system in metropolitan Atlanta has been a valuable additional resource for monitoring rates of change of specific defects (Yen et al. 1992) and for conducting numerous genetic and epidemiological investigations of risk factors for birth defects (Mulinare et al. 1988; Erickson 1992). Moreover, the registry has become a model to over 20 states currently conducting or considering birth defects surveillance activities (Lynberg and Edmonds 1992).

Internationally, about 25 countries are now conducting birth defects surveillance activities and are members of the International Clearinghouse for Birth Defects Monitoring Systems (1991), which regularly conducts collaborative surveillance activities and epidemiologic studies. In developing countries, birth defects surveillance has been conducted using a few large maternity hospitals relying on voluntary reporting from collaborating health care professionals (Castilla et al. 1991).

Health information systems

Surveillance systems may, and should, use existing health data collection systems when possible. However, lack of accuracy and specificity remain a major concern, and most surveillance systems require a separate data collection system to meet the needs of specific prevention and control programs (Calle and Khoury 1991).

Data from medical claims records, death certificates, and other existing databases may not contain enough information to define public health priorities for reducing disease incidence. For example, an increase in deaths from cirrhosis, not otherwise specified, may be the result of an infectious agent, alcohol use, or other toxin. The occurrence of bladder cancer may or may not be related to a particular environmental exposure. These data are often most useful as an adjunct to surveillance systems designed more specifically for prevention and control programmes.

Vital records

Mortality statistics serve as the most accessible source of data for comparisons of many health problems. In most developed countries, registration of deaths is compulsory and largely complete. Records include basic demographic information, the cause or causes of death, and other descriptive information about the circumstances of death. In other countries, registration may be conducted only in major cities, or not at all. In all countries, the accuracy and specificity of many diagnoses is limited, and changes in the use of diagnostic categories and codes over time, together with variation in the quality of information, are limiting factors. For example, a study by the United States National Cancer Institute revealed that seven countries in Europe and North America coded the underlying cause of death the same for only 53 per cent of a

sample of 1246 death certificates sent to these countries (Percy and Dolman 1978). Despite these limitations, vital statistics, particularly mortality statistics, are used to support many surveillance activities.

Example: Death certificates have been used in maternal mortality surveillance as a source of data to demonstrate progress toward reduction in maternal mortality in association with increased use of prenatal care and other factors. Analyses of death certificates in the United States have highlighted racial differences in mortality rates over time and differences in maternal mortality rates for women more than 35 years old. Because maternal mortality rates are often based on number of live births, this surveillance system also depends on birth certificate information (Kaunitz et al. 1984).

There is frequently a lengthy interval between death and collection and analysis of death certificates, which may make such vital statistics less useful for surveillance purposes when more current data are needed. However, summary vital data can be rapidly collected. For example, weekly telephonic reporting of deaths from 121 American cities to US CDC has been integral to the surveillance of influenza epidemics in that country (Choi and Thacker 1981).

Medical examiner and coroner reports

For a more detailed description of circumstances surrounding deaths (including autopsy reports, toxicology studies, and police reports), medical examiner and coroner records may be useful. In the United States, these reports are most representative of deaths caused by intentional and unintentional injuries and other unnatural causes. These records have been particularly useful in surveillance of heat-wave-related mortality, sudden unexplained death syndrome in Southeast Asian refugees, and alcohol-related injuries (Jones et al. 1982; Berkelman et al. 1985; Parrish et al. 1987).

Medical care records

Hospital records and other medical care records may be useful sources of information on diagnoses, surgical procedures, and patient demographic characteristics. However, with increases in length and complexity of the medical record, retrieval of information is often difficult and time consuming. Although computerization of parts of these records has allowed their use for routine surveillance, a major limitation has existed when no identifiers are recorded since repeat admissions and discharges by individual patients usually cannot be identified.

Hospital discharge records have been useful for surveillance of many medical care technologies, such as trends in the use of hysterectomies in the United States (particularly by geographical region), in the rate of coronary artery bypass graft procedures by sex, and in the assessment of outcome with carotid endarterectomies (Sattin et al. 1983; Thacker and Berkelman 1986; Caper 1987). More recently, hospital discharge record systems have been used as an alternative data source to evaluate surveillance data sets.

Relying exclusively on measurements of mortality from death certificates and morbidity from medical records can produce an underestimate of the impact of many diseases or conditions. A more complete estimate of the impact of disease has been attempted by including a measure of the loss of healthy life resulting from disability (World Bank 1993) for such conditions as malaria and arthritis, which may not result in contact with medical care providers.

Insurance records and workers' compensation

Insurance records and workers' compensation claims have been useful for surveillance of injuries in specific geographic locales. Because regulations governing completion and submission of forms differ both among and within countries, data derived from these systems cannot easily be compared. In addition, the use of medical claims data for surveillance may be limited by the accuracy of diagnostic recording as well as the problem of comparing different health systems (Pollack and Ringen 1992).

The severity of reported injury varies, and is influenced by legislation related to compensation, medical care, rehabilitation of those injured at work, and the degree of fear of job loss resulting from absence from work.

Example: In an evaluation of claims for workers' compensation as an adjunct to an occupational lead surveillance system, the usefulness of claims was demonstrated: the likelihood that a company had a case of lead poisoning strongly correlated with the number of claims against the company (Seligman *et al.* 1986).

Surveys of health behaviour and physician utilization

Household surveys of the general population, such as the National Health Interview Survey conducted in the United States (National Center for Health Statistics 1985) or the General Household Survey in England and Wales (Fraser *et al.* 1978), have provided information at the national level on personal health practices such as alcohol use and smoking, on disabilities, and on physician encounters. In the People's Republic of China, in addition to mandated information on acute infectious conditions, sentinel sites, known as disease surveillance points, are chosen through a statistical sample of provincial areas. These sites collect data on health events and medical encounters for the entire population within their jurisdiction (Cheng 1992; Yang 1992).

Although national estimates may be gained more efficiently from such surveys, local programmes may benefit from involvement in data collection and the flexibility to adapt data collection to their particular needs. Interview surveys conducted by telephone and in person in the United States can obtain personal health-related information with only minor differences in the reported prevalence of various health conditions. Telephone interviews have the advantages of lower cost and ease of supervising interviewers (Siegel *et al.* 1991).

Hazard and exposure surveillance

In addition to surveillance of health outcomes, two other types of surveillance are also used: hazard surveillance and exposure surveillance. Hazard surveillance has been defined as the 'assessment of the occurrence of, distribution of, and the secular trends in levels of hazards (toxic chemical agents, physical agents, biomechanical stressors, as well as biological agents) responsible for disease and injury' (Wegman 1992). Exposure surveillance is the monitoring of a population for the presence of an agent or the clinically non-apparent effects of an environmental hazard (e.g., lead) or infectious agent (e.g., HIV) in individuals within a population (Weniger *et al.* 1991). These types of surveillance may be complementary.

Indeed, the optimal strategy for preventing or reducing the impact of a specific public health problem sometimes dictates the use of all three types of surveillance. For example, although hazard surveillance is the first measure available to detecting potential health threats, exposure and outcome surveillance may provide valuable information for the evaluation of the effectiveness of hazard and exposure-reduction regulations.

Remote sensing and geographic information system technologies are now being used as an adjunct to disease surveillance (Barinaga 1993; Washino and Wood 1994). A major goal of this approach is the identification of environmental parameters that affect the patterns of disease risk and transmission.

Example: In 1993 the southern Kerio Valley of Kenya experienced the first cases of yellow fever ever recorded in that country. The virus had recently infected the monkey population in the valley, and forest-dwelling mosquitoes were passing the virus from monkeys to persons entering the forest. The human population in the area was vaccinated, but the question remained as to whether the inhabitants of the nearby cities also required vaccination. Satellite photographs are being used to determine whether continuous forest corridors to any of the cities exist through which the virus can travel from one monkey population to another.

Analysis of surveillance data

The uses of public health data often derive from a simple analysis of surveillance data according to the basic epidemiological parameters of time, place, and person. Analysis of data over time can reveal trends in disease or injury upon which public health actions or the need for such actions may be evaluated.

The approach to the prevention and control of disease and injury is often determined by circumstances unique to 'place': the geographic distribution of the disease or of its causative exposures or risk-associated behaviour.

The characteristics of the people or groups who develop specific diseases or sustain specific injuries are important in understanding the disease or injury, identifying those at high risk, and targeting intervention efforts. For example, disparities in health (incidence or severity of disease) among members of different population groups highlight the need to identify cultural, economic, or social factors associated with these health problems (Hahn and Stroup 1994).

When combined with appropriate population information, morbidity or mortality rates can be calculated to compare risks of disease. Often rates are examined in broad age groups that are selected to reflect the different sets of conditions affecting mortality rates in each group (Doll 1974). Proper analysis of surveillance data can assist in determining aetiology, modes of transmission, risk factors associated with disease, and opportunities for prevention or control, can detect epidemics, can monitor long-term trends, can follow seasonal patterns, and can make projections of future disease occurrence.

Once descriptive techniques are used to determine basic characteristics, more sophisticated methods can be used, for example to make forecasts using regression and time series analyses for the surveillance of influenza (Serfling 1963; Choi and Thacker 1981; Lui and Kendal 1987) or to combine information from several surveillance series (Newhouse *et al.* 1986; Stroup *et al.* 1988). In addition, modern methods (for example Bayesian techniques) that incorporate information in addition to the data themselves, such as changes in a surveillance case definition or surveillance information from contiguous data (Stroup and Thacker 1993), can be useful when applied to public health surveillance data.

Epidemic detection and cluster analysis

Many epidemics are detected by astute health care providers who note or suspect an increase in disease occurrence often before disease reports are received, assembled, and reviewed by health departments. The ongoing surveillance process between health practitioners and health departments increases the likelihood that providers will contact the health department when they suspect an outbreak or any unusual occurrence of disease.

Surveillance is most likely to detect epidemics in situations where cases, despite their aetiological link, are occurring over a wide geographic area (Cliff et al. 1992), over a relatively gradual period (Nobre and Stroup 1994), or among a well-defined sub-group with links among cases often unrecognized by individual practitioners.

Example: Laboratory-based surveillance of Salmonella serotypes has identified outbreaks in which unusual serotypes and/or anti-microbial patterns identify an outbreak of diarrhoeal disease that might otherwise have gone undetected, such as the outbreak of drug-resistant *Salmonella newport* in a large geographic area of the United States, which originated from animals fed antimicrobial agents (Holmberg et al. 1984).

Example: Age-adjusted oesophageal cancer mortality rates in white men and women in the United States have remained fairly steady during the period between 1950 and 1980 but nearly doubled for African-Americans during the same period. Oesophageal cancer has gradually become one of the most common malignancies in African-American men under the age of 55, while still a relatively rare cancer in white men of a similar age (Blot and Fraumeni 1987).

A frequent concern of the analysis of surveillance data is whether an apparent cluster of health events in time is significant and unlikely to have occurred by chance alone. Statistical methods can be applied to this problem (US CDC 1990a). Most of these methods involve a comparison of observed incidence with a historical baseline and may involve clustering in time (Wallenstein 1980; Gallus et al. 1986; Stroup et al. 1993), clustering in space (Cliff and Ord 1981), or clustering in both time and space (Klauber 1974).

Statistical limitations of surveillance data

Surveillance data have traditionally had specific characteristics that have made application of standard statistical techniques difficult. First, reporting bias may produce data that are not representative of the population. For example, severe or otherwise noteworthy cases are more likely to be reported than minor illnesses. Rubella in a woman of child-bearing age is more likely to be reported than rubella in a man, and a patient in some clinics may be more likely to be reported than patients seen in other settings, particularly if the disease is socially stigmatizing. Health care provider networks may have a biased sample of physicians (Lobet et al. 1987).

Second, under-reporting may be considerable, particularly in a voluntary system of notification. When another independent source of data is available (for example hospital discharge, vital statistics), the total number of cases actually occurring can be estimated (Chandra-Sekar and Deming 1949; Cormack 1963) to determine, for example, the sensitivity of two systems for detecting vaccine-preventable diseases (Orenstein et al. 1986). In addition, specific information for each case may be incompletely reported (Buehler et al. 1989).

Provisional data increase the timeliness and hence may increase the usefulness of public health surveillance data to epidemiologists; however, provisional data may differ markedly from final data that have been confirmed. To enhance the usefulness of provisional data for recent periods, epidemiologists may compare these data retro-spectively with confirmed data to estimate what final data for recent periods will eventually reveal (Thacker et al. 1989). A model can incorporate this consistent under-reporting to permit more accurate estimation of the final data from provisional data. In addition, when provisional data are used to examine temporal trends, current provisional data should be compared with historical provisional data rather than with final data to avoid bias.

Role of surveillance data in evaluation of community interventions

The ease with which trends in disease occurrence can be linked to interventions depends on both the disease and the intervention. The success of an immunization campaign can usually be easily inferred from surveillance data; however, such inferences become difficult when several factors contribute to a change in disease occurrence. Analyses are also difficult because of constraints such as migration and variable acceptance of interventions in the community. Programme evaluation may be improved by monitoring risk factors as well as various stages of morbidity. In addition, combining data from several communities with similar public health programmes will strengthen the assessment of programme effectiveness.

Mathematical models can be used to elucidate the complexities of evaluating community interventions. Such models have been used most extensively for infectious diseases. However, models for predicting the decline of mortality rates given changes in risk factors have also been developed for mortality due to cirrhosis using population changes in levels of consumption of alcohol (Skog 1984), for cardiovascular disease using changes in cigarette consumption in a population (Kullback and Cornfield 1976), and for blood lead levels given changes in legislation banning lead from petrol (Annest et al. 1983).

Linkage of surveillance data to other information sources

Given the complexity of establishing new data and information systems, there is increasing interest in the combination of existing databases for surveillance purposes. Techniques involved in data linkage are complex and are based on matching records by comparison of key data fields (Newcombe 1988). In some countries, a unique number may be assigned to an individual at birth to serve as a reference number for any contact with health care services (Paterson 1988). In other countries, a number may be assigned only for use at a single health care facility or hospital. When record systems are linked, the probability that the record linkage is correct must be determined, with the degree of certainty of a correct linkage depending on the comparisons of the individual identifiers such as name or initials, date or year of birth, sex, and race/ethnicity. Names may be converted to a code (e.g., Soundex) to allow for errors in spelling. If all identifiers match exactly, the degree of assurance that the linkage is correct is high. The existence of few similarities argues against a correct linkage. Any linked set will normally contain a small number of pairs that should not have been linked and, conversely, will have missed a few pairs that should have been linked.

Linkage of data sets has facilitated calculation of rates, such as birth-weight-specific death rates that can be calculated following linkage of birth and death certificates (McCarthy *et al.* 1980).

Dissemination of data

Communication of surveillance data is an essential step in the surveillance chain. The purpose of the communication and the audience targeted must be defined. Appropriate feedback must be given to those providing the data to demonstrate their usefulness and to stimulate further reporting. Persons providing the data should be credited for their contributions and acknowledged for their provision of accurate and complete data. Public health professionals, policy-makers, or others who may be responsible for taking action or setting direction of public health programmes in response to surveillance data must receive the information that they need from the surveillance system on a timely basis and in an appropriate format for their use.

The data must be provided on a regular basis, with the frequency of surveillance reports dependent on the nature of the surveillance system, the characteristics of the disease process (for example surveillance reports on measles are required more frequently than reports on cancer), and the public health impact of the disease. For diseases and other health events requiring major policy decisions (for example removal of lead from petrol), it may be useful to provide frequent updates to remind policy-makers of the potential for prevention. In general, reports need not be issued at more frequent intervals than the data are collected from reporting sites. Provisional data should be accepted for dissemination, since rapid turn-round of data is usually more important than absolute accuracy and completeness; rarely have provisional data driven major public health decisions in directions different from those that would have been based on final data.

The format for dissemination varies with the target audience, but in any case the design of the communications should be as creative as possible without losing essential information. A creative design will help to make the information stand apart from other documents and receive greater attention. Most policy-makers and clinicians would prefer to see the data interpreted using graphics accompanied by an abbreviated summary text; the important role that graphs can play in visually decoding large quantities of data has been clearly demonstrated, with graphic displays giving the reader an understanding of large and complex data sets not conveyed easily in other ways (Tukey 1977; Tufte 1983; Cleveland 1985). Microcomputer graphics, in particular, have made the results of data analysis far more useful to private and public policy-makers in their planning and management of health care resources (Caper 1987). However, many epidemiologists and other scientists, including mathematicians projecting the future course of diseases, find

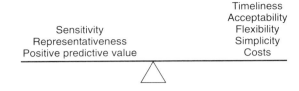

Fig. 20.2 Balance of attributes in surveillance systems.

the more detailed raw data in tabular format or on electronic media most useful. Comparison with previous years or previous periods (for example experience of the last 12 months compared with experience of the previous 12 months) is often helpful.

Maps are useful in providing rapid insight into the geographic occurrence of diseases, and there is currently a strong interest in computer mapping and graphic displays. Mapping both absolute counts of disease occurrence and rates of disease for more common conditions may be useful, particularly when geographic areas are quite variable in their population density.

Evaluation of surveillance systems

Surveillance systems should be periodically evaluated to ensure that important public health problems are under surveillance and that useful information for disease prevention and control is collected. An evaluation of a surveillance system should include a review of its objectives, a detailed description of its operation, an assessment of its performance, and recommendations (US CDC 1988).

The performance of surveillance systems can be judged using a series of attributes, including sensitivity, timeliness, representativeness, positive predictive value, acceptability, flexibility, simplicity, and costs. The importance of individual attributes will vary among systems, and efforts to improve on a system's performance on one attribute may compete with efforts to improve its performance on another. Thus the evaluation of surveillance systems should not focus solely on the extent to which each attribute is achieved but rather on the attainment of the appropriate balance of attributes (Fig. 20.2). The ultimate impact of improvements in surveillance should be assessed in terms of improvements in health (Thacker *et al.* 1986).

Sensitivity

The sensitivity of a surveillance system can be judged by its completeness of case reporting. If all persons with the condition under surveillance in the target population are detected by a surveillance system, then its sensitivity is 100 per cent. Sensitivity of surveillance systems can be measured by comparing routinely collected case reports with data obtained by special case-finding methods. For example, the sensitivity of AIDS surveillance has been assessed through detailed review of death certificates and various hospital records, such as laboratory data, patient logbooks, and computerized discharge diagnoses (Chamberland *et al.* 1985; Rosenblum *et al.* 1992).

Timeliness

Timeliness refers to the entire surveillance cycle, ranging from how quickly cases are reported to the distribution of surveillance reports.

Representativeness

Representativeness is a measure of how well reported cases in a population reflect all cases that actually occurred in the population. This comparison often requires independent surveillance, which ascertains as many cases as possible in the population for a given time period (Klaucke 1994). Surveillance reporting is rarely complete, and cases that are reported may differ from unreported cases in terms of demographic characteristics, site or use of health care services, or risk exposures (Alter *et al.* 1987). Representativeness of surveillance data is also affected by the quality of descriptive data that accompany case reports. Incomplete or incorrect data on surveillance forms limit representativeness.

Positive predictive value

Persons with reported cases of disease may not actually have the disease in question. This may reflect incorrect diagnoses (false positives), a lack of specificity in the case definition, or errors in the interpretation of the case definition. If all persons reported as cases indeed had the disease in question, then the positive predictive value would be 100 per cent. Positive predictive value depends both on the specificity of diagnostic tests and the case definition and on the prevalence of the condition under surveillance. Evaluation of the positive predictive value is difficult and requires a careful review of cases detected through routine methods. For example, hospital-based stroke surveillance based on readily available admission diagnoses was found to include a substantial proportion of persons without cerebrovascular disease when more stringent diagnostic criteria were applied (Barker *et al.* 1984).

The concept of positive predictive value can be extended to the detection of epidemics in a surveillance system. If change in disease occurrence is used as an indicator to trigger investigations, then a high frequency of 'false alarms' would indicate a low predictive value for epidemic detection.

Acceptability

Surveillance systems depend on the co-operation of many people over a long period. If procedures are easy to follow and useful information is returned to participants, then acceptability is likely to remain high. Other factors, such as protection of confidentiality of individual cases, are also important.

Flexibility

The circumstances under which surveillance systems operate are subject to change, ranging from logistic constraints to information needs; surveillance systems should have sufficient flexibility to accommodate these changes. For example, surveillance for AIDS has been ongoing during a period of rapid evolution in the understanding of the disease, during the introduction of a diagnostic test for HIV infection, and during changing diagnostic and treatment practices as a once rare disease has become more common. Surveillance for AIDS has been flexible as revisions to the case definition were needed (US CDC 1992*c*).

Simplicity

Simplicity is desirable throughout the entire cycle in surveillance systems and is closely tied to other attributes such as acceptability, flexibility, and costs.

Costs

Surveillance systems incur costs in time, equipment, and supplies, which may be difficult to judge relative to their public health value. Evaluation of the costs and benefits of aggressive versus less aggressive case-finding methods in surveillance of selected notifiable diseases has yielded different conclusions that vary according to specific local circumstances (Hinds *et al.* 1985; Vogt *et al.* 1986). Generally, standard cost–benefit analysis is inappropriate for disease surveillance systems; indeed, it is the surveillance data themselves that are used for determining cost–benefit analyses of various public health strategies adopted to control or prevent disease. However, a description of the time requirements and costs of a surveillance system is useful for its evaluation (Hinds *et al.* 1985; Vogt *et al.* 1986; Stroobant *et al.* 1988).

The evaluation of a surveillance system should conclude with an assessment of its structure and usefulness, considering its mix of attributes in relation to its objectives. Recommendations should state whether the system should be continued and what specific changes, if any, should be made.

Conclusion

Public health surveillance has historically galvanized prevention and control programmes ranging from smallpox eradication and immunization campaigns for childhood diseases to HIV infection and AIDS. Surveillance is also taking on increased visibility and importance in evaluating and directing prevention and control efforts for non-infectious diseases and conditions. Surveillance systems represent information loops, with data flowing from local to central agencies and back. Surveillance provides a stimulus to keep prevention and control activities moving rapidly and in the right direction, guiding the response to individual cases as well as public policy.

Effective public health interventions depend upon a continuing and reliable source of information. The data must be timely and representative of the population; they must be analysed and interpreted with feedback to the reporters and dissemination to those formulating and implementing public health policy. Resources necessary for the maintenance of the surveillance systems and for their regular evaluation should be allocated, balancing needs for data to direct prevention activities with needs for resources to implement those activities.

References

Alter, M.J., Mares, A., Hadler, S.C., and Maynard, J.E. (1987). The effect of underreporting on the apparent incidence and epidemiology of acute viral hepatitis. *American Journal of Epidemiology*, **125(1)**, 133–9.

Andrus, J.K., de Quadros, C., Olive, J.M., and Hull, H.F. (1992). Screening of cases of acute flaccid paralysis for poliomyelitis eradication: ways to improve specificity. *Bulletin of the World Health Organization*, **70**, 591–6.

Annest, J.L., Pirkle, J.L., Makuc, D., *et al.* (1983). Chronological trend in blood lead levels between 1976 and 1980. *New England Journal of Medicine*, **308**, 1373–7.

Barinaga, M. (1993). Satellite data rocket disease control efforts into orbit. *Science*, **261**, 31–2.

Barker, W.H., Feldt, K.S., and Feibel, J. (1984). Assessment of hospital admission surveillance of stroke in a metropolitan community. *Journal of Chronic Diseases*, **37**, 609–15.

Bean, N.H., Martin, S.M., and Bradford, H. Jr. (1992). PHLIS: an electronic system for reporting public health data from remote sites. *American Journal of Public Health*, **82(9)**, 1273–6.

Berkelman, R.L. (1994). Emerging infectious diseases in the United States, 1993. *Journal of Infectious Diseases*, **170**, 272–7.

Berkelman, R.L. and Buehler, J.W. (1990). Public health surveillance of non-infectious chronic diseases: the potential to detect rapid change in disease burden. *International Journal of Epidemiology*, **19**, 628–35.

Berkelman, R.L., Herndon, J.L., Callaway, J.L., *et al.* (1985). A surveillance system for alcohol- and drug-related fatal injuries. *American Journal of Preventive Medicine*, **1**, 21–8.

Berkelman, R.L., Bryan, R.T., Osterholm, M.T., LeDuc, J.W., and Hughes, J.M. (1994). Infectious disease surveillance: a crumbling foundation. *Science*, **264**, 368–70.

Biellik, R.J., Bueno, H., Olive, J.–M., *et al.* (1992). Poliomyelitis case confirmation: characteristics for use by national eradication programmes. *Bulletin of the World Health Organization*, **70(1)**, 79–84.

Blot, W.J. and Fraumeni, J.F. Jr. (1987). Trends in oesophageal cancer mortality among US blacks and whites. *American Journal of Public Health*, **77(3)**, 296–8.

(BPSU) (British Paediatric Surveillance Unit) (1993). *Seventh Annual Report 1992*. BPSU, London.

Brachman, P.S. (1982). Surveillance. In *Bacterial infections of humans* (ed. A. S. Evans and H. H. Feldman), pp. 49–61. Plenum Medical, New York.

Brachott, D. and Mosley, J.W. (1972). Viral hepatitis in Israel: the effect of canvassing physicians on notifications and the apparent epidemiological pattern. *Bulletin of the World Health Organization*, **46**, 457–64.

Buehler, J.W., Stroup, D.F., Klaucke, D.N., *et al.* (1989). The reporting of race and ethnicity in the National Notifiable Diseases Surveillance System. *Public Health Reports*, **104**, 457–65.

Buehler, J.W., Berkelman, R.L., and Stehr-Green, J.K. (1992). The completeness of AIDS surveillance. *Journal of Acquired Immune Deficiency Syndromes*, **5**, 257–64.

Calle, E.E. and Khoury, M.J. (1991). Completeness of the discharge diagnoses as a measure of birth defects recorded in the hospital birth record. *American Journal of Epidemiology*, **134**, 69–77.

Caper, P. (1987). The epidemiologic surveillance of medical care. *American Journal of Public Health*, **77(6)**, 669–70.

Castilla, E.E., Lopez, J.S, Dutra, G.P., and Paz, J.E. (1991). Birth defects monitoring in undeveloped countries: an example from Uruguay. *International Journal of Risk Safety in Medicine*, **5**, 271–88.

Chamberland, M.E., Allen, J.R., Monroe, J.M., *et al.* (1985). Acquired immunodeficiency syndrome in New York City: evaluation of an active surveillance system. *Journal of the American Medical Association*, **254**, 383–7.

Chandra-Sekar, C. and Deming, W.E. (1949). On a method for estimating birth and death rates and the extent of registration. *Journal of the American Statistical Association*, **44**, 101–15.

Cheng, C.M. (1992). Disease surveillance in China. In *Proceedings of the 1992 International Symposium on Public Health Surveillance* (ed. S. F. Wetterhall). *Morbidity and Mortality Weekly Report*, **41** (Suppl.), 111–22.

Choi, K. and Thacker, S.B. (1981). An evaluation of influenza mortality surveillance, 1962–1979. I. Time series forecasts of expected pneumonia and influenza deaths. *American Journal of Epidemiology*, **113**, 215–26.

Cleveland, W.S. (1985). *The elements of graphing data*. Bell Telephone Laboratories, Murray Hill, NJ.

Cliff, A.D. and Ord, J.K. (1981). *Spatial processes, models, and application*. Pion, London.

Cliff, A.D., Haggett, P., and Stroup, D.F. (1992). The geographical structure of measles epidemics in the northeastern United States. *American Journal of Epidemiology*, **136(5)**, 592–602.

Committee on National Statistics, Commission on Behavioral and Social Sciences and Education, National Research Council, and Social Science Research Council (1993). *Private lives and public policies: confidentiality and accessibility of government statistics*. National Academy Press, Washington, DC.

Cormack, R.M. (1963). The statistics of capture–recapture. *Ocean Marine Biology Annual Review*, **6**, 455–506.

Davis, J.P. and Vergeront, J.M. (1982). The effect of publicity on the reporting of toxic-shock syndrome in Wisconsin. *Journal of Infectious Diseases*, **145**, 449–57.

Dean, A.G., Dean, J.A., Burton, J.H., *et al.* (1993). A word processing, database and statistics program for epidemiology on microcomputers (computer program). *Epi Info*, Version 6. Centers for Disease Control and Prevention (US CDC), Atlanta, G. A.

De Bock, A. (1988). Surveillance for accidents at work. In *Surveillance in health and disease* (ed. W. J. Eylenbosch and N. D. Noah), pp. 191–201. Oxford University Press, New York.

DeCock, K.M., Odehouri, K., Moreau, J., *et al.* (1989). Rapid emergence of AIDS in Abidjan, Ivory Coast. *Lancet*, **334**, 408–11.

Doll, R. (1974). Surveillance and monitoring. *International Journal of Epidemiology*, **3**, 305–14.

Edmonds, L.D., Layde, P.M., James, L.M., *et al.* (1981). Congenital malformations surveillance: two American systems. *International Journal of Epidemiology*, **10**, 247–52.

Erickson, J.D. (1992). Teratology data from the Atlanta birth defects case-control study. *Teratology*, **43**, 41–51.

Eylenbosch, W.J. and Noah, N.D. (ed.) (1988). *Surveillance in health and disease*. Oxford University Press.

Faich, G.A., Knapp, D., Dreis, M., and Turner, W. (1987). National adverse drug reaction surveillance: 1985. *Journal of the American Medical Association*, **257**, 2068–70.

Federal Committee on Statistics (1994). *Private lives and public policies*. US Department of Health and Human Services, Washington, DC.

Foege, W.H., Millar, J.D., and Henderson, D.A. (1975). Smallpox eradication in West and Central Africa. *Bulletin of the World Health Organization*, **52**, 209–22.

Fraser, P., Beral, V., and Chilvers, C. (1978). Monitoring disease in England and Wales: methods applicable to routine data-collecting systems. *Journal of Epidemiology and Community Health*, **32**, 294–302.

Frerichs, R.R. (1991). Epidemiologic surveillance in developing countries. *Annual Reviews in Public Health*, **12**, 80–257.

Freund, E., Seligman, P.J., Chorba, T.L., *et al.* (1989). Mandatory reporting of occupational diseases by clinicians. *Journal of the American Medical Association*, **262(21)**, 3041–4.

Gail, M.H. and Brookmeyer, R. (1988). Methods for projecting course of acquired immunodeficiency syndrome epidemic. *Journal of the National Cancer Institute*, **80(12)**, 900–11.

Gallus, G., Mandelli, C., Marchi, M., and Radaelli, G. (1986). On surveillance methods for congenital malformations. *Statistics in Medicine*, **5(6)**, 565–71.

Gaynes, R.P., Culver, D.H., Emori, T.G., *et al.* (1991). The national nosocomial infections surveillance system: plans for the 1990s and beyond. *American Journal of Medicine*, **91(3B)**, 116S–20S.

Hahn, R.A. and Stroup, D.F. (1994). Race and ethnicity in public health surveillance: criteria for the scientific use of social categories. *Public Health Reports*, **109(1)**, 7–15.

Henderson, D.A. (1976). Surveillance of smallpox. *International Journal of Epidemiology*, **5**, 19–28.

Hinds, M.W., Skaggs, J.W., and Bergeisen, G.H. (1985). Benefit cost analysis of active surveillance of primary care physicians for hepatitis A. *American Journal of Public Health*, **75(2)**, 176–7.

Hinman, A.R. (1977). Analysis, interpretation, use and dissemination of surveillance information. *Pan American Health Organization Bulletin*, **11**, 338–43.

Holmberg, S.D., Osterholm, M.T., Senger, K.A., and Cohen, M.L. (1984). Drug-resistant *Salmonella* from animals fed antimicrobials. *New England Journal of Medicine*, **311**, 617–22.

Holtzman, N.A. and Khoury, M.J. (1986). Monitoring for congenital malformations. *Annual Review of Public Health*, **7**, 237–66.

Horm, J.W., Asire, A.J., Young, J.L. Jr., *et al.* (1984). *SEER program: cancer incidence and mortality in the United States, 1973–1981*. NIH Publication No. 85–1837. US Department of Health and Human Services, Bethesda, MD.

Institute of Medicine (1988). *Approaches to modeling disease spread and impact.*

Report of a workshop on mathematical modeling of the spread of human immunodeficiency virus and the demographic impact of acquired immune deficiency syndrome, 15–17 October 1987. National Academy Press, Washington, DC.

Institute of Medicine (1992). *Emerging infections: microbial threats to health in the United States*. National Academy Press, Washington, DC.

International Clearinghouse for Birth Defects Monitoring Systems (1991). *Congenital malformations worldwide*. Elsevier, Amsterdam.

Jaffe, H.W., Choi, K., Thomas, P.A., *et al*. (1983). National case control study of Kaposi's sarcoma and *Pneumocystis carinii* pneumonia in homosexual men: epidemiologic results. *Annals of Internal Medicine*, **99**, 293–8.

Jones, T.S., Liang, A.P., Kilbourne, E.M., *et al*. (1982). Morbidity and mortality associated with the July 1980 heat wave in St. Louis and Kansas City, Missouri. *Journal of the American Medical Association*, **247**, 3327–31.

Kallen, B., Hay, S., and Klinberg, M. (1984). Birth defects monitoring systems: accomplishments and goals. In *Issues and reviews in teratology* (ed. H. Kalter), Vol. 2, pp. 1–22. Plenum, New York.

Kaunitz, A.M., Rochat, R.W., Hughes, J.M., *et al*. (1984). Maternal mortality surveillance, 1974–1978. *Centers for Disease Control Surveillance Summaries*, **33** (1SS), 5SS–8SS.

Klauber, M.R. (1975). Space–time clustering tests for more than two samples. *Biometrics*, **31**(3), 719–26.

Klaucke, D.N. (1994). Evaluating public health surveillance. In *Principles and practice of public health surveillance* (ed. S. M. Teutsch and R. E. Churchill), pp. 158–74. Oxford University Press.

Kullback, S. and Cornfield, J. (1976). An information theoretic contingency table analysis of the Dorn study of smoking and mortality. *Computers and Biomedical Research*, **9**, 409–37.

Langmuir, A.D. (1963). The surveillance of communicable diseases of national importance. *New England Journal of Medicine*, **268**, 182–92.

Langmuir, A.D. (1976). William Farr: founder of modern concepts of surveillance. *International Journal of Epidemiology*, **5**, 13–18.

Lobet, M.P., Stroobant, A., Mertens, R., *et al*. (1987). Tool for validation of the network of sentinel general practitioners in the Belgian health care system. *International Journal of Epidemiology*, **16**(4), 612–18.

Loftin, C., McDowall, D., Wiersema, B., *et al*. (1991). Effects of restrictive licensing of handguns on homicide and suicide in the District of Columbia. *New England Journal of Medicine*, **325**, 1615–20.

Lui, K.-J. and Kendal, A.P. (1987). Impact of influenza epidemics on mortality in the United States from October 1972 to May 1985. *American Journal of Public Health*, **77**(6), 712–16.

Lynberg, M.C. and Edmonds, L.D. (1992). Surveillance of birth defects. In *Public Health Surveillance* (ed. W. Halperin, E. L. Baker, and R. R. Monson), pp. 157–77. Van Nostrand Reinhold, New York.

McCarthy, B.J., Terry, J., Rochat, R.W., *et al*. (1980). The under-registration of neonatal deaths: Georgia, 1974–1977. *American Journal of Public Health*, **70**, 977–82.

Mulinare, J., Cordero, J.F., Erickson, J.D., and Berry, R.J. (1988). Periconceptional use of multivitamins and the occurrence of neural tube defects. *Journal of the American Medical Association*, **260**, 3141–5.

National Center for Health Statistics (1985). *The National Health Interview Survey design, 1973–84, and procedures, 1975–83. Vital and Health Statistics*, Series 1, No. 18, Department of Health and Human Services Publication no. PHS 85–1320. US Government Printing Office, Washington, DC.

Newcombe, H.B. (1988). *Handbook of record linkage*. Oxford University Press.

Newhouse, V.F., Choi, K., D'Angelo, L.J., *et al*. (1986). Analysis of social and environmental factors affecting the occurrence of Rocky Mountain spotted fever in Georgia, 1961–75. *Public Health Reports*, **101**(4), 419–28.

Nobre, F.F. and Stroup, D.F. (1994). A monitoring system to detect pattern changes in public health surveillance data. *International Journal of Epidemiology*, **23**(2), 408–18.

O'Brien, T.F. and the International Survey of Antibiotic Resistance Group (1986). Resistance to antibiotics at medical centres in different parts of the world. *British Society for Antimicrobial Chemotherapy*, **18** (Suppl. C), 243–53.

Orenstein, W.A., Bart, S.W., Bart, K.J., *et al*. (1986). Epidemiology of rubella and its complications. In *Vaccinating against brain syndromes: the campaign against measles and rubella* (ed. E. M. Grunberg, C. Louis, and S. E. Goldson), pp. 49–69. Oxford University Press, New York.

PAHO (Pan American Health Organization) (1994). Dengue fever in Costa Rica and Panama. *Epidemiological Bulletin*, **15**(2), 9–10.

Parkin, D. (1988). Surveillance of cancer. In *Surveillance in health and disease* (ed. W. J. Eylenbosch and N. D. Noah), pp. 143–65. Oxford University Press.

Parrish, R.G., Tucker, M., Ing, R., and Encarnacion, C. (1987). Sudden unexplained death syndrome in southeast Asian refugees: a review of CDC surveillance. *Centers for Disease Control Surveillance Summaries*, **36** (1SS), 43SS–53SS.

Paterson, J.G. (1988). Surveillance systems from hospital data. In *Surveillance in health and disease* (ed. W. J. Eylenbosch and N. D. Noah), pp. 49–61. Oxford University Press.

Percy, C. and Dolman, A. (1978). Comparison of the coding of death certificates related to cancer in seven countries. *Public Health Reports*, **93**, 335–50.

Pollack, E.S. and Ringen, K. (1992). Risk of hospitalization for specific non-work-related conditions among laborers and their families. *American Journal of Industrial Medicine*, **23**(3), 417–25.

Pommerenke, F.A., Miller, R.W., Srivastava, S., and Ackermann, S.P. (1994). Targeting cancer control: the state cancer control map and data program. *American Journal of Public Health*, **84**(9), 1479–82.

Raska, K. (1966). National and international surveillance of communicable diseases. *World Health Organization Chronicle*, **20**, 315–21.

Remington, P.L.S., Smith, M.Y., Williamson, D.F., *et al*. (1988). Design, characteristics and usefulness of state-based behavioral risk factor surveillance: 1981–1987. *Public Health Reports*, **103**(4), 366–75.

Rosenblum, L., Buehler, J.W., Morgan, M.W., *et al*. (1992). Completeness of AIDS case reporting, 1988: a multisite collaborative surveillance project. *American Journal of Public Health*, **82**(11), 1495–9.

Sattin, R.W., Rubin, G.L., and Hughes, J.M. (1983). Hysterectomy among women of reproductive age, United States, update for 1979–1980. *Centers for Disease Control Surveillance Summaries*, **32**, 1SS–7SS.

Seligman, P.J., Halperin, W.E., Mullan, R.J., and Frazier, T.M. (1986). Occupational lead poisoning in Ohio: surveillance using worker's compensation data. *American Journal of Public Health*, **76**, 1299–1302.

Serfling, R.E. (1963). Methods for current statistical analysis of excess pneumonia-influenza deaths. *Public Health Reports*, **78**, 494–506.

Shands, K.N., Schmid, G.P., Dan, B.B., *et al*. (1980). Toxic-shock syndrome in menstruating women: association with tampon use and *Staphylococcus aureus* and clinical features in 52 cases. *New England Journal of Medicine*, **303**, 1436–42.

Siegel, P.Z., Brackbill, R.M., Frazier, E.L., *et al*. (1991). Behavioral risk factor surveillance, 1986–1990. *CDC Surveillance Summaries, Morbidity and Mortality Weekly Report*, **40** (SS-4), 1–23.

Skog, O. (1984). The risk function for liver cirrhosis from lifetime alcohol consumption. *Journal of Studies on Alcohol*, **45**, 199–208.

Stroobant, A.W., Van Casteren, V., and Thiers, G. (1988). Surveillance systems from primary-care data: surveillance through a network of sentinel general practitioners. In *Surveillance in health and disease* (ed. W. J. Eylenbosch and N. D. Noah), pp. 62–74. Oxford University Press.

Stroup, D.F. and Thacker, S.B. (1993). A Bayesian approach to the detection of aberrations in public health surveillance data. *American Journal of Epidemiology*, **4**(5), 435–43.

Stroup, D.F., Thacker, S.B., and Herndon, J.L. (1988). Application of multiple time series analysis to the estimation of pneumonia and influenza mortality by age: 1962–1983. *Statistics in Medicine*, **7**(10), 1045–59.

Stroup, D.F., Wharton, M., Kafadar, K., and Dean, A.G. (1993). An evaluation of a method for detecting aberrations in public health surveillance data. *American Journal of Epidemiology*, **137**(3), 373–80.

Thacker, S.B. and Berkelman, R.L. (1986). Surveillance of medical technologies. *Journal of Public Health Policy*, **7**, 363–77.

Thacker, S.B. and Berkelman, R.L. (1988). Public health surveillance in the United States. *Epidemiologic Reviews*, **10**, 164–90.

Thacker, S.B. and Stroup, D.F. (1994). Future directions of comprehensive public health surveillance and health information systems in the United States. *American Journal of Epidemiology*, **140**(5), 383–97.

Thacker, S.B., Redmon, S., Rothenberg, R.B., *et al.* (1986). A controlled trial of disease surveillance strategies. *American Journal of Preventive Medicine*, **2**, 345–50.

Thacker, S.B., Berkelman, R.L., and Stroup, D.F. (1989). The science of public health surveillance. *Journal of Public Policy*, **10**, 187–203.

Thacker, S.B., Stroup, D.F., Rothenberg, R.B., and Brownson, R.C. (1995). Public health surveillance for chronic conditions: a scientific basis for decisions. *Statistics in Medicine*, **14**, 629–41.

Tufte, E.R. (1983). *The visual display of quantitative information*. Graphics Press, Cheshire, CT.

Tukey, J.W. (1977). *Exploratory data analysis*. Addison-Wesley, Reading, MA.

US CDC (US Centers for Disease Control) (1988). Guidelines for evaluating surveillance systems. *Morbidity and Mortality Weekly Report*, **37** (S–5).

US CDC (US Centers for Disease Control) (1990a). Guidelines for investigating clusters of health events. *Morbidity and Mortality Weekly Report*, **39** (RR–11).

US CDC (US Centers for Disease Control) (1990b). Case definitions for public health surveillance. *Morbidity and Mortality Weekly Report*, **39** (RR–13).

US CDC (US Centers for Disease Control) (1991). National electronic telecommunications system for surveillance—United States, 1990–1991. *Morbidity and Mortality Weekly Report*, **40**, 502–3.

US CDC (US Centers for Disease Control) (1992a). Meeting the challenge of multidrug-resistant tuberculosis: summary of a conference. *Morbidity and Mortality Weekly Report*, **41** (RR–11), 49–57.

US CDC (US Centers for Disease Control) (1992b). A framework for assessing the effectiveness of disease and injury prevention. *Morbidity and Mortality Weekly Report*, **41** (RR–3).

US CDC (US Centers for Disease Control) (1992c). 1993 revised classification system for HIV infection and expanded surveillance case definition for AIDS among adolescents and adults. *Morbidity and Mortality Weekly Report*, **41** (RR–17).

US CDC (US Centers for Disease Control) (1992d). Public health surveillance and international health. *Morbidity and Mortality Weekly Report*, **41** (SS–4).

US CDC (US Centers for Disease Control) (1993). Congenital malformations surveillance. *Teratology*, **48**, 545–730.

US CDC (US Centers for Disease Control) (1994a). *Addressing emerging infectious disease threats: a prevention strategy for the United States*. US Department of Health and Human Services, Public Health Service, Atlanta, GA.

US CDC (US Centers for Disease Control) (1994b). State cancer registries: status of authorizing legislation and enabling regulations—United States. *Morbidity and Mortality Weekly Report*, **43**, 71–5.

Valleron, A.J., Bouvet, E., Garnerin, P., *et al.* (1986). Computer network for the surveillance of communicable diseases: the French experiment. *American Journal of Public Health*, **76**(11), 1289–92.

Vogt, R.L., LaRue, D., Klaucke, D.N., and Jillson, D.A. (1983). Comparison of active and passive surveillance systems of primary care providers for hepatitis, measles, rubella and salmonellosis in Vermont. *American Journal of Public Health*, **73**, 795–7.

Vogt, R.L., Clark, S.W., and Kappel, S. (1986). Evaluation of the state surveillance system using hospital discharge diagnoses, 1982–1983. *American Journal of Epidemiology*, **123**(1), 197–8.

Wallenstein, S. (1980). A test for detection of clustering over time. *American Journal of Epidemiology*, **111**, 367–72.

Washino, R.K. and Wood, B.L. (1994). Application of remote sensing to arthropod vector surveillance and control. *American Journal of Tropical Health and Hygiene*, **50** (6 Suppl), 134–44.

Weddell, J.M. (1973). Registers and registries: a review. *International Journal of Epidemiology*, **2**, 221–8.

Wegman, D.H. (1992). Hazard surveillance. In *Public health surveillance* (ed. W. Halperin and E. L. Baker Jr.), pp. 62–75. Van Nostrand Reinhold, New York.

Weniger, B.G., Limpakarnjanarat, K., Ungchusak, K., *et al.* (1991). The epidemiology of HIV infections and AIDS in Thailand. *AIDS*, **5** (suppl. 2), 271–85.

WHO (World Health Organization) (1958). *The first ten years of the World Health Organization*. WHO, Geneva.

WHO (World Health Organization) (1968). Report of the technical discussions at the twenty-first World Health Assembly on 'national and global surveillance of communicable diseases', 18 May 1968, A21. WHO, Geneva.

World Bank (1993). *World Development Report 1993: investing in health*. Oxford University Press, New York.

Yang, G. (1992). Selection of DSP points in second stage and their representation. *Chinese Journal of Epidemiology*, **13**(4), 197–201.

Yen, I.H., Khoury, M.J., Erickson, J.D., *et al.* (1992). The changing epidemiology of neural tube defects in the United States. *American Journal of Diseases in Children*, **146**, 857–61.

III Social science techniques

21 Social policy and the welfare system

Nicholas Mays

Introduction

The operation of social policies by governments and other major social institutions (for example, insurers, pension funds, and business corporations) has a considerable bearing on the health of the population in Western countries. This influence and how it is studied by social scientists are the twin topics of the chapter which follows. Much of the material on which the chapter is based relates to United Kingdom policy and research. In part, this is because the study of social policy as a distinct academic discipline is more clearly delineated in the United Kingdom and the British Commonwealth than in other parts of the world and partly because a short chapter could not do justice to the wide variation in the details of policy in different countries. Despite this limitation, the ground covered is of general importance for public health research and practice.

The chapter is in four main sections. The first attempts to show how students of social policy define what are 'social policies' and distinguish them from other sorts of public policy. The second section looks at the nature of the academic discipline which has developed to study social policy and its implementation. Analysts of social policy have contributed much to the study of health policy and how health care systems work. The third section gives representative examples of the specific contribution of social policy analysis to the study and practice of public health.

The fourth section of the chapter brings the discussion of social policy in Western countries up to date by considering the challenge posed to traditional, post-Second World War thinking and practice in the welfare system from feminists and from the neo-conservative and neo-liberal New Right. Far from ending state involvement in setting social policies, the New Right critique of the 1980s is shown to have led to experiments in a number of countries with new forms of welfare provision. The principles and methods of an idealized free market in goods and services are increasingly being introduced into publicly funded health and social services. The chapter concludes by arguing that it is important for the public's health and well-being to continue to monitor and analyse the consequences of these ideological and organizational shifts in the field of social policy. Social policy analysis and public health practice should remain closely allied enterprises.

What are social policies?

Analysts of social policy have articulated a range of definitions of what it is they profess to study from administrative definitions of social policy, through more sociological definitions which extend beyond the formally recognized institutions of the welfare state, to perspectives based on Marxist political economy. The first part of this chapter will attempt to set out these different definitions of what social policies are. At the risk of imposing consensus where none exists, most but by no means all students of social policy today would probably accept a very general definition that social as opposed to economic policy consists in collective intervention to improve, maintain, or promote the welfare of individuals or society as a whole. However, beyond this high level of generality, definitions diverge and have altered over time.

Formal institutional definition

T.H. Marshall's classic view from the 1940s and 1950s stressed that social policy was distinguished from economic policy which was directed at the commonwealth, by its focus on securing individual welfare by means of government action to provide services or income through the formal mechanisms of the welfare state, such as the National Health Service (NHS) in the United Kingdom and the social security system (Marshall 1975). The role of these institutions was to relieve citizens of their anxiety in the face of the future threats to their well being posed by life course events such as illness, disability, unemployment, and retirement, by ensuring national minimum standards of living. Marshall's (1975) approach to defining social policy appears somewhat dated at the very end of the twentieth century with its emphasis on government action to provide services or income. The contemporary welfare state in most Western countries embodies a plurality of arrangements for the financing, provision, and regulation of key services such as education, housing, and health involving combinations of public, private, and voluntary sector action. Social policy is no longer confined to the direct provision by the state of publicly funded services.

Integrative and moral definition

In another classic definition of social policies, Titmuss (1968) drew attention rather to the social values reflected in social policies. He stressed the integrative and stabilizing functions of social policies defining them as the 'different types of moral transactions, embodying notions of gift-exchange, of reciprocal obligations, which have developed in modern societies in institutional forms to bring about and maintain social and community relations' (Titmuss 1968, pp. 20–1). One way in which social policies could achieve social harmony was by providing a degree of compensation for the personal costs associated with economic and technological development (for example, unemployment). This implies that social policies frequently include an element of redistribution both horizontally (for example, between those who are well to those who are sick) and vertically (between the better-off and poor) in society in accordance with some notion of 'need'.

Needs-based definition

Indeed, an alternative to Titmuss' (1968) definition of social policy focuses on its characteristic in the meeting of human needs (Rein 1976; Mishra 1977, 1981; Donnison 1979). Thus, Mishra (1977, 1981, p. xi) defined social policies as ' . . . those *social* arrangements, patterns and mechanisms that are typically concerned with the distribution of resources in accordance with some criterion of *need*'. Mishra's (1981) definition includes within the sphere of social policy actions other than those of the government (for example, by industry, commerce, and the voluntary sector) and reflects many of the criticisms which were levelled at earlier formulations by those who took a broader, more sociological view of the nature and scope of social policy. However, it continues to limit social policy to the distribution of resources rather than the way in which they are produced.

Social structural definition

Townsend (1976) criticized the 'traditional' view of authorities such as Marshall (1975) for its parochialism in defining social policy in terms of the specific institutions of the social services in the United Kingdom, for its assumption that collective policies can only emanate from the government, for its assumption that collective policies are inevitably beneficial in terms of welfare, for implying that social policies can operate according to different principles from the market principles dominant in capitalist societies without contradiction or conflict, for assuming that social policy is exclusively concerned with the distribution of the surplus and has no part to play in modifying the nature of relations on the production side of the economy, and for overlooking important sources of social inequality and disadvantage which lie outside the sphere of control of welfare agencies (Townsend 1976, pp. 2–9).

Townsend (1976) built on Titmuss' (1963, pp. 34–55) 'social division of welfare' thesis (see below) to highlight the existence of 'social policies' pursued by institutions outside the framework of the state which produced results which frequently threatened the pursuit of welfare state objectives such as social justice or equality of opportunity, furthering instead the goals of the dominant economic system. In his 'structuralist' analysis, Townsend (1976) was also sensitive to questions of the distribution of power in society and the ability of those with power to prevent issues reaching the realms of practical policies (Bachrach and Baratz 1970). Thus, for Townsend (1974, pp. 31–3), social policy is concerned with the production and distribution of a wide range of social resources, including cash income, savings, property, employment benefits, services in kind such as health, and education, environment, status, and power. It includes ' . . . the underlying as well as the professed rationale by which social institutions and groups are developed or created to ensure social preservation or development' (Townsend 1976, p. 6). This more radical approach focuses on the hidden intentions as well as the explicit goals of policy, all the social institutions which determine the production and distribution of resources and opportunities, and the differential status, power, and rewards which exist along gender, class, and ethnic lines in society.

Walker (1981) summarized his version of this position, with its strong emphasis on the distributional role of social policy, as follows: ' . . . "Social policy" might be defined therefore as the rationale underlying the development and use of social institutions and groups which affect the distribution of resources, status and power between individuals and groups in society' (p. 239).

Marxist definition

The approach exemplified by Townsend (1976) and Walker (1981) recognizes that social problems such as poverty are related to the class structure of society rather than technical malfunctions in the bureaucratic system (Townsend 1979). Yet, it has been criticized by Marxists for not making explicit the strong links between the state and the capitalist economy and the scale of the material obstacles to large-scale redistributive policies required to overcome social problems such as poverty (Gough 1978).

The Marxist perspective on the nature of social policy differs from the preceding definitions in regarding social policy as intimately bound up with the functions of the modern capitalist state in

1. accumulation, maintaining conditions favourable to the accumulation of capital;

2. reproduction, ensuring a healthy, skilled work-force which is at the same time disciplined;

3. legitimization, maintaining political stability, social harmony, and social control (O'Connor 1973).

From a very different theoretical stance, economists such as Barr (1987) have also pointed out that the welfare state can contribute to the achievement of goals of productive efficiency, as well as simply distributing resources and opportunities between social groups. For example, state involvement in education may ensure that the work-force is sufficiently well educated to be able to adapt to changing occupational demands in a way which employers themselves could not achieve.

However, as Gough (1978, 1979), a leading British Marxist theorist of welfare pointed out, welfare programmes are rarely straightforwardly functional in the maintenance of capitalism. First, the functions of accumulation, reproduction, and legitimation may come into conflict with one another, for example when the level of taxation and public expenditure required for investment in reproduction (for example, through spending on health services and education) is perceived by owners of capital to threaten the current profitability of their enterprises. Second, certain aspects of the welfare state may be attributable not so much to the self-interested actions of the ruling class and its agents, as the result of working-class struggles to improve social conditions under capitalism (Navarro 1978). Navarro (1989) explained the emergence of social insurance in Western European countries such as Germany from the 1880s onwards in terms of the political pressure exerted on governments by organized labour.

What is social policy and administration?

. . . The term 'Social Administration' is a misleading one; we are not experts in office management and social book-keeping, nor are we technicians in man manipulation (Titmuss, 1968, p. 20).

The previous section of this chapter has shown how definitions of what constitutes 'social policies' have changed over time and provoked controversy. Similarly, defining the nature and scope of the academic discipline of 'social administration' or 'social policy', as it now tends to be referred to, has never been straightforward. Definitions have changed as the discipline itself has developed. It remains to be seen whether its practitioners will ever agree on a single definition. At its simplest, the discipline comprises the academic study of human welfare and the social institutions which shape the welfare of members of societies rich and poor. These include formal structures of welfare assembled under the title of the 'welfare state'.

Evolution of the discipline

As a separate and distinctive university discipline, social policy and administration originated primarily in universities in the United Kingdom and later in the British Commonwealth (Canada, New Zealand, Australia, etc.). By contrast, in the United States, for example, the study of social policy and its effects tends to take place in university departments of urban studies, planning, political science, policy analysis, government, sociology, social work, applied economics, and a range of research institutes, rather than in departments explicitly focused on the study of social policy. In some cases, the older term of 'political economy' may be more appropriately used. For example, the eminent North American economist J.K. Galbraith represents this tradition in his work which persistently links an analysis of the economy to the wider political and social system in which it is embedded (Galbraith 1972).

The early growth of the separate discipline of social policy and administration was closely tied to the development of a collective, state infrastructure of policies and institutions devoted to tackling the social problems thrown up by early twentieth-century Western capitalism. Courses in social science were established in the United Kingdom early in the twentieth century to train students who wished to work in the newly established social services. For example, a School of Social Studies was established in Liverpool as early as 1904, followed by courses at Birmingham in 1908 and the London School of Economics in 1913.

In this period, the study of social administration in Britain was decisively shaped by members of the Fabian Society, particularly Beatrice and Sidney Webb. Fabianism was characterized by an emphasis on using the techniques of empirical social investigation to develop practical proposals aimed at alleviating social problems such as poverty. Fabians believed in gradually moving towards socialism by means of a programme of social reform implemented through state intervention in the economy and in the distribution of income, wealth, and services.

The subject expanded rapidly after the Second World War linked to the emergence of welfare states in Western Europe committed to using their political power to supersede, supplement, or modify the workings of the free market in order to improve the quality of life and living standards of their peoples. The discipline flourished in the relative consensus which existed until the mid-1970s as to the purposes and instruments of state welfare. The role of social administration in this period was to train the staff who would operate the new institutions of welfare while, at the same time, improving the working of the welfare state through empirical analysis.

In the 1940s and 1950s the discipline in the United Kingdom was dominated by the work of Richard Titmuss (1907–1973). Titmuss has subsequently been criticized for taking an atheoretical approach and for his unself-conscious adherence to the values of Fabian collectivism (Reisman 1977; Walker 1988). Yet for all the limitations of his approach, as judged with the benefit of hindsight, Titmuss ensured that the study of social administration extended beyond the formal social services and their administration to encompass the full range of mechanisms by which social needs are met and benefits distributed in society. In much of his empirical work he showed that the supposed redistributive intent of the welfare state in Britain was imperfectly realized. Perhaps his most influential piece, 'The social division of welfare', first published in 1956, showed how an analysis of the impact of social policies was incomplete unless it included the fiscal (tax reliefs) and occupational (fringe benefits) systems of middle-class welfare as well as the more conventionally identified statutory social services (Titmuss 1963, pp. 34–55). While Titmuss and his younger colleagues used this material to argue for reform of the welfare state, the results were also employed later by opponents of extensive state provision to argue for radical change and the development of more individualistic approaches to welfare (see the discussion of the New Right below).

Normative and explanatory concerns: identifying models of welfare

Titmuss (1974) and his followers also emphasized the normative aspects of social policy analysis, based on a recognition that social policy decisions involve choices between different objectives based on conflicting value systems. The means chosen to achieve policy goals are at least as important as their immediate consequences since they carry highly visible messages as to the sort of society we wish to create. In *The gift relationship*, Titmuss (1970) contended that the system of voluntary blood donation in the NHS fostered altruism, whereas the commercial system in the United States had the opposite effect, commodifying a moral transaction as well as producing an inefficient and unsafe system.

Contemporary writers in the Fabian tradition are more critical of the bureaucratic, centralizing tendencies of state provision than Titmuss' generation (Deakin 1987). While a moral commitment to social improvement has remained a feature of much academic social policy analysis ever since (distinguishing it, perhaps, from other less applied social sciences such as sociology), later analysts have increasingly recognized the need to elucidate a wider range of perspectives than Fabianism, for example by acknowledging developments in both Marxist and neo-liberal (New Right) theory and critiques of the welfare state. A leading contemporary theorist in the field of social policy has argued that the discipline of social policy is distinguished by an attempt to develop both normative theory (social philosophy) and explanatory theory (social science) concerning welfare (Mishra 1986). Under normative theory, Mishra (1986) included the study of values such as liberty, equality, justice, security, and social integration which are either implicitly or explicitly the objectives of specific social policies. Under explanatory theory, Mishra (1986) included the analysis of how social

Table 21.1 Models of welfare

Reference	Models of welfare identified			
Wilensky and Lebeaux (1958)	Residual			Institutional
Pinker (1971)	Residual			Institutional
Titmuss (1974)	Residual	Industrial Achievement–Performance		Institutional–Redistributive
Parker (1975)	*Laissez-faire*	Liberal		Socialist
George and Wilding (1976, 1985)	Anticollectivist	Reluctant Socialism	Fabian Socialist	Marxist
Mishra (1977, 1981)	Residual	Institutional		Structural (Normative in 1977)
Pinker (1979)	Market	Mercantilist–Collectivist		Socialist
Room (1979)	Liberal	Social democratic		Marxist
Taylor-Gooby and Dale (1981)	Individualist	Reformist		Structural

policy develops and with what consequences, intended or unintended. For example, the distributional impact of the welfare state would constitute an important theme for explanatory studies.

As the study of social policy has developed beyond the purely vocational training of welfare practitioners such as social workers and probation officers, so interest in knowledge building based on theory and empirical testing of theory has quickened (Pinker 1971; George and Wilding 1976, 1985; Mishra 1977, 1981; Pinker 1979; Room 1979; Taylor-Gooby and Dale 1981). A wide range of 'models of welfare' or welfare paradigms has been identified which include elements of normative and explanatory theory (see Table 21.1). Each represents an ideological prescription for the development of social policies based on a particular set of value preferences and views about the nature of humanity and society (Mishra 1986). In addition, each embodies a set of factual propositions which ought in principle to be testable empirically. Each can be seen to occupy a different position on a continuum of social policy from the absence of any collective responsibility for individual needs to a socialist idea of 'to each according to his/her needs'. Mishra (1986) contended that these models can be logically reduced to three basic or ideal–typical models: a 'market' model, a 'mixed' model, and a 'need' model of social welfare. Since all forms of welfare could be said to meet need in different ways, the 'need' model might be better titled a 'planned' or 'command' model (see Table 21.2). For Mishra (1986, p. 35), therefore 'It is the central task of social policy analysis to tease out the normative and factual propositions or assumptions (directly relevant to welfare) associated with each model and to subject them to close scrutiny.'

Hence, following Titmuss (1968, pp. 20–3), the discipline is concerned with the objectives of social policy (normative), its development (positive), and its consequences (normative and positive). The model-based approach offers the basis for a social science discipline which goes beyond the study of individual services or particular social problems, to study normative and positive aspects of social policy in widely differing settings taking account systematically of the effect of different economic, ideological, political, and government structures on the precise form of social policies in different countries (Walker 1981).

Walker (1988) elaborated Mishra's very general guide to the tasks facing social policy analysts in terms more comprehensible to those working at the mid- and micro-levels on the details of particular policies or services. At these levels, social policy analysis is formulated as, 'the pluralistic evaluation of policy... and understanding of the outcomes of policy set against a knowledge of the aspirations and intentions of the various actors involved in the policy process' (Walker 1988). A notable example of such a study in the health field is Smith and Cantley's (1985) explicitly pluralist evaluation of the success of a new NHS psychogeriatric day centre which incorporates the differing perspectives of the range of groups involved in the service such as patients, their relatives and carers, medical staff, nurses, paramedics, the health authority, and

Table 21.2 Three ideal–typical models of welfare

	Market	Mixed	Planned/command
Methods of securing welfare	Minimal collective responsibility for welfare	Pragmatic mix of market and need criteria	Total collective responsibility for welfare
Pre-eminent values	Liberty	Mixed values	Equality
Factual propositions (empirically testable)	Free enterprise/the market best promotes economic growth and welfare of the population	A 'mixed economy' optimizes welfare by stimulating economic activity and at the same time mitigating the adverse effects of unfettered markets	State planning best secures the welfare of the population

From Mishra (1986).

the local authority. The study demonstrated that a comprehensive assessment of the costs and benefits of the innovatory service had to cope with the often conflicting objectives held by different groups. For example, medical and nursing staff tended to view success in terms of 'patient flow' through the centre to avoid the service 'silting up', whereas for the relatives of confused patients, the opposite was the case. They had little or no interest in seeing patients discharged to their full-time care at home! Pluralistic evaluation is inevitably controversial since it highlights conflicts of interest and perception between those involved in any programme. It lacks the level of scientific respectability accorded to quasi-experimental designs such as cost-effectiveness analysis. None the less, its fidelity to the reality of local agency conflict which can undermine policy innovations has led to its adoption in a number of other studies (Means and Smith 1988).

Use of theoretical insights from other social sciences

Smith and Cantley's (1985) study demonstrated the growing theoretical sophistication of the discipline as it becomes less preoccupied with descriptive accounts of statutory welfare agencies and more explicitly analytic. A major thrust is to measure, explain, and evaluate patterns of service distribution and outcome by building on theory derived from the other social sciences, for example, Merton's (1968) concept of manifest (recognized and intended) and latent (unrecognized and unintended) functions of action, or rival elitist (Mills 1956), pluralist (Dahl 1961), and corporatist (Cawson 1982) theories of policy making.

As an instance, Merton's (1968) concepts have been fruitful in yielding insights into the operation of welfare organizations. The observation that one of the latent functions of such organizations is to provide satisfying work for the staff and that this may conflict with their manifest functions of meeting the needs of patients, clients, and users draws on a Mertonian analysis. A specific application in the health field occurs in Calnan's (1982; quoted in Forder et al. 1984, pp. 128–9) study of accident and emergency departments in the British National Health Service (NHS) in which the professionally desired development of the service into a specialized area of medicine with a clear career structure and area of expertise was found to be in conflict with the public expectation of the service as a convenient alternative to visiting a primary care physician.

Corporatism generally refers to an arrangement in which the state plays a positive role in directing the economy and in providing or subsidizing services in close cooperation with a limited number of key interest groups. Klein's (1977) interpretation of the development of the NHS in the 1970s provides an example of a broadly corporatist analysis. He argued that decision making was the outcome of relatively stable bargaining arrangements between the state and the medical profession, the most powerful 'quasi-feudal occupational barony' in the health sector (Klein 1977, p. 179, 1983, 1989a). It remains to be seen whether a corporatist account of this relationship will still hold good at the end of the 1990s after the introduction of competitive market principles into the NHS following the 1989 Government White Paper *Working for patients* (Secretaries of State for Health, Wales, Northern Ireland and Scotland 1989).

In the 1970s and 1980s there was a rapid development in theoretically informed studies of the social policy process at different levels from formal, explicit central government decision making through to the day-to-day, discretionary decisions of professional staff working in field agencies (for example, Donnison and Chapman 1965; Hall et al. 1975; Allen 1979; Banting 1979; Hunter 1980; Ham 1981). In a pioneering series of case studies, Donnison and Chapman (1965) showed how official policy changes were frequently no more than codifications and explicit recognition of changes in practice worked out previously by local service providers. A decade later, Hall et al. (1975) set the analysis of social policy change on a mature footing by exposing the limitations of simplistic accounts of policy development in terms of either 'social conscience' or 'rationality'. In six United Kingdom case studies they showed that policy developments were profoundly shaped by the manner in which the claims of an issue were assessed in terms of its 'legitimacy', 'feasibility', and 'support', the characteristics of the issue itself (for example, the scope of an issue and its links with other issues), the political context, and the resultant conflicts which surrounded the issue. For example, in their account of the struggle which preceded the 1956 Clean Air Act in the United Kingdom, they attempted to show why it was that, despite seemingly good prospects for early and effective legislation, the attitude of the government was characterized by 'reluctance, apprehension and tardiness' (Hall et al. 1975, p. 371). The pressures for change appeared to have been generated entirely outside the traditional government bureaucracies since there were other pressing political priorities preoccupying the official government machine at the time and no well-established interest in the issue among civil servants. The medical profession as a whole showed little sense of outrage and there was no well-developed medical interest group concerned primarily with the consequences of atmospheric pollution. Precise, hard evidence of the health effects of polluted air was also not yet available, although it was widely agreed that polluted air was harmful to health. For these and other reasons, including the Conservative Government's reluctance to embark on domestic controls having been elected to remove wartime restrictions on private life, the campaign for clean air took 4 years to reach the statute book.

Theoretically informed studies of the health services

In the fields of health policy and management, there have been a series of important studies by social policy analysts of the United Kingdom NHS which have applied and tested a range of conceptual schemes derived from sociology and political science in order to shed light on the persistent problems of implementation deficit in the service. For example, Allen (1979) attempted to explain the origins and implementation of the 1962 Hospital Plan which was directed at building district general hospitals in under-provided areas of the country in terms of the three different rational, incremental, and bureaucratic political models of public policy making derived from the work of American political scientists such as Lindblom (1959) and Allison (1971).

Hunter (1980) studied the difficulties faced by authority members and officials in Scottish Health Boards in making more than incremental resource shifts between services for different care groups despite clear national guidance to revise past patterns of spending. The decision process was problematic because it was 'complicated', involving large numbers of people at different levels, all representing different interests, it was 'fragmented' by the demarcations between administrative bodies, and it was 'disjointed' in that decision makers tended not to follow plans, but to allocate development funds in small amounts to different clinical interest groups as part of an intuitive approach based on crisis management and appeasement. Faced with the dilemma of either allocating development funds to change the direction of policy in line with national 'priorities' for neglected services or responding to the clamour for more resources for existing, well-established services, the demands from existing services normally prevailed.

Ham (1981) explained the politics of 'conflict without change' and the pre-eminence of matters of acute, curative medicine over the needs of the so-called 'priority care groups' in the actions of the Leeds Regional Hospital Board through the 1960s and early 1970s in terms of American sociologist Alford's (1975) theory of the power relations between the three key structural interests identifiable in all modern health care systems: the professional monopolists (who were traditionally 'dominant'), the corporate rationalizers (planners and managers who were normally to be found 'challenging' the professionals), and the public (who were currently a 'repressed' interest). Ham (1981) showed how the hospital professionals effectively defined the limits of practical politics and used their resources of technical knowledge and social prestige to neutralize policies articulated further up the NHS hierarchy which threatened to disturb the historic centrality of acute medicine.

Delineating the subject matter of social policy studies

The study of policy making and implementation, of course, comprises only one part of the terrain of contemporary social policy and administration. Just as definitions of the intellectual and theoretical core of the discipline remain controversial (see below for yet further feminist and neo-liberal critiques), so, too, are accounts of the subject matter of the discipline closely debated. The primary focus for many students of social policy remains the study of the formal and visible institutions of the welfare state as the embodiment, however imperfect (Brown and Madge 1982; Ringen 1987), of social justice and notions of shared citizenship. Indeed, Brown (1983) warned of the danger of an excessive broadening of the subject matter of the discipline lest it become unmanageable and lose its distinctive identity.

In the United States, social policy studies tend to be organized and defined in terms of the heterogeneous and ever-changing group of topics which American society regards as 'social problems' (for example, unemployment, drug addiction, urban decay, the underclass, etc). The 'social problems approach has been criticized for producing an incoherent, unstable, and parochial basis for the discipline.

An alternative approach is to define and organize the subject matter of the discipline of social policy around a series of key concepts such as need, stigma, universality, selectivity, citizenship, social justice, etc. (Forder 1974). Like the 'social problems' approach, the 'key concepts' approach tends to produce an arbitrary set of concepts and to isolate the study of social policy from its wider societal context.

In an address to the first meeting of the United Kingdom Social Administration Association (now the Social Policy Association),

Richard Titmuss, one of the main founders of British academic social policy analysis, put forward eight areas of study for students of social administration.

1. Analysis and description of policy formation and its consequences, intended and unintended.

2. Study of the structure, function, organization, planning, and administrative processes of institutions and agencies, historical and comparative.

3. Study of social needs and of problems of access to, utilization of and patterns of outcome of services, transactions, and transfers.

4. Analysis of the nature, attributes, and distribution of social costs and disadvantage.

5. Analysis of distributive and allocative patterns in command-over-resources-through-time and the particular impact of the social services.

6. Study of the roles and functions of elected representatives, professional workers, administrators, and interest groups in the operation of social welfare institutions.

7. Study of the social rights of the citizen as contributor, participant, and user of the social services.

8. Study of the role of government (local and central) as an allocator of values and of rights to social property, as expressed through social and administrative law and other rule-making channels (Titmuss 1968, pp. 22–3).

Although Titmuss' (1968) definition of the subject matter of social administration was broad by comparison with many of his contemporaries, he was at pains, none the less, to distinguish social policy clearly from economic policy as a distinctive area of government activity. Later attempts to delineate the field of study have broadened its scope towards 'political economy' to include, for example, general socioeconomic changes and macro-economic policy in so far as these impinge on social welfare. Reflecting this view, Donnison's (1979) list of topics for social policy studies compiled 12 years later is still broader and reads as follows.

1. The social services (including the private and voluntary sectors).

2. The impact of changes in industrial structure and employment on workers.

3. The distribution of income, wealth, public expenditure, and incidence of taxation.

4. Changing patterns in the family.

5. Administrative, legal, economic, and political issues relating to points 1 to 4 above.

6. The interaction between social change and institutions set up to cope with social change (Donnison 1979).

Walker (1981) argued even more forcefully that by placing the explicit welfare activities of the government too close to the centre of their attention, social policy specialists were in danger of missing the important welfare consequences of non-governmental agencies and social institutions such as multinational corporations, financial enterprises, and their interrelationships with the macro-economic policies of government. Predictably, Walker's (1981) widening of the scope of the subject to include broad questions of economic, political, and social theory and the change of name from 'social administration' to the less dreary, more theoretical and more political 'social policy' have not gone unchallenged. Glennerster (1988) argued that scholars have been distracted by theorizing and failed the ordinary consumers of welfare by not devoting sufficient time to analyse in-depth how welfare bureaucracies actually work at the local level in order to help them work better in the future.

The persistent preoccupation with defining the nature and scope of the discipline, is in part a reflection of its eclecticism. 'Social administrators' tend to come from many different backgrounds in the social sciences. Much of their research takes place on the bounds of welfare economics, law, sociology, politics, and public administration. Social policy and administration, as currently thought of, draws on philosophy to clarify definitions of terms, to identify value positions, and to elucidate the objectives of policy, on statistics and methods of social investigation to establish the incidence of and trends in social phenomena, on sociology to understand the nature of social structure, organizational behaviour, and social change, on psychology to assess the impact of policies on individuals, on economics for insights into macro-economic policy, resource constraints, and methods of evaluation such as cost-effectiveness and cost-benefit analysis together with assessing the theory and practice of different mechanisms for resource allocation, including markets, quasi-markets (see below), and conventional command bureaucracies, on history and political science to explain the origins and development of social policies and for public choice theories of government behaviour, and, finally, on government and public administration to describe contemporary political and governmental process.

The contribution of the discipline of social policy and administration to the practice of public health

Almost any factor which can be identified as creating human suffering, distress, or reduced well-being is also highly likely to affect health adversely. Thus, the public health implications of many social policies are so much a part of those policies that they are often taken for granted. For example, it may be assumed that improvements in housing standards, higher levels of social support, a reduction in poverty, and the minimization of unemployment will all improve the health of the groups affected. However, few if any welfare programmes derive their justification exclusively from their direct impact on health. Warm, dry housing, for example, is an unequivocal social benefit irrespective of the strength of the evidence linking poor housing conditions such as dampness to particular aspects of ill health (Platt et al. 1989). Recent research showing that the links between housing inequalities and health inequalities have remained despite the postwar expansion of public housing in the United Kingdom serves only to reinforce the existing case for high quality modern housing (Byrne et al. 1986; Blackman et al. 1989).

None the less, social policy researchers have an important contribution to make in showing how changes in parts of the system of welfare outside the health sector (for example, housing, income maintenance, pensions, etc.) affect the physical, social, and economic circumstances of individuals and ultimately their health. For example, there is a long tradition of research linking social administration and epidemiology, dating back to the 1930s, which looks at the living standards and health of unemployed people (Morris and Titmuss 1944; Moser et al. 1984). In the same vein, in the 1980s, work in the United Kingdom on social security showed how a seemingly minor change in the rules surrounding the payment of board and lodging allowances to elderly people on income support who were in residential care had accelerated the growth of private nursing homes, directly contrary to the Government's avowed policy of community care, as well as leading to a huge unplanned increase in public expenditure. Concerns were raised that elderly patients were leaving their own homes to go in to inappropriate residential settings where they risked becoming unnecessarily dependent and that existing regulatory mechanisms were inadequate to monitor the quality of care in the private sector (Day and Klein 1987). This interest in tracing the unintended consequences of a policy change in one area on the effectiveness of policy in another is typical of an important strand in social policy research.

Contemporary social policy research with a bearing on health and health services covers a wide range of themes relevant to the practice of public health. It is impossible to summarize it all here (see Volume 3, Chapter 25). Instead, a number of contrasting studies will be described to give an indication of the contribution of the discipline, to add to the studies already referred to earlier in the chapter. The studies cover three characteristic concerns of the discipline relevant to the study and practice of public health: the problems of policy implementation in complex organizations, the patterning of and explanation for social inequalities in health, and the success of welfare services in meeting the needs arising from these inequalities.

Policy implementation in health care organizations

The 'administrative anthropology' of organizations delivering welfare services has long represented a significant part of the research effort in social administration. The replacement of multidisciplinary consensus management in the NHS with commercial-style general management in 1984 following the recommendations of the Griffiths report on the management of the service (NHS Management Enquiry 1983), was widely regarded at the time as a more fundamental change than the succession of structural reorganizations which had preceded it (Day and Klein 1983). A qualitative study was undertaken in the later 1980s to assess whether the implementation of the Griffiths 'revolution' had succeeded in changing the substance as well as the form of management in an organization dominated by professional rather than bureaucratic values (Pollitt et al. 1988). The Griffiths reforms included a commitment to involve clinicians more closely in the management process as budget holders. Pollitt et al. (1988) found that inadequate attention had been given to convincing clinicians, who were usually suspicious of budgeting and others, who were only occasionally in favour of such schemes (for example, nurses), of the merits of the proposed changes. Instead, the scheme had been regarded largely as a technical exercise in developing appropriate information systems to the exclusion of behavioural issues and questions of organizational politics (Hunter 1990).

Further major changes occurred in the NHS in the early 1990s following the government White Paper *Working for patients* (Secretaries of State for Health, Wales, Northern Ireland and Scotland 1989) which resulted in the introduction of a quasi-market system (see below) which split the service into purchasers of care (health authorities and large general practices) and providers (for example, semi-autonomous hospitals) with the aim of improving the efficiency and responsiveness of the service to patients. Members of the earlier research team attempted to trace the impact of these wider developments on the relative power of managers and clinicians. By the mid-1990s, they were able to conclude that clinicians were subject to greater control by general managers than they had been in the 1980s, but that further growth of managerial control was likely to be increasingly constrained for a variety of reasons (Harrison and Pollitt 1994). For example, managers were still far from being able to render clinical activity predictable, capable of standardization, and, therefore, visible to external scrutiny.

Social inequalities in health

Both public health and the applied social science of social administration in the United Kingdom share a tradition of research, some of it collaborative, describing and seeking to explain the variations in health, for example between different geographical areas in relation to their relative prosperity (M'Gonigle and Kirby 1936; Titmuss 1938). Work on geographical inequalities since the Second World War quickened in the period immediately before and after the implementation of the Resource Allocation Working Party (**RAWP**) formula for distributing financial resources fairly in relation to population need in the NHS in England (Department of Health and Social Security 1976) and the introduction of other similar formulas in Scotland, Wales, and Northern Ireland. The **RAWP** formula represented the fruitful coming together of epidemiology and Fabian social administration to produce an explicit and rational system for reallocating finance.

Another related research tradition involving applied social scientists, social epidemiologists, and public health doctors has been the study of the relations between health and socioeconomic conditions, particularly the explanation of occupational social class gradients in ill health with a view to informing a wide range of policy (Stevenson 1923; Brotherston 1976; Black Report 1980; Whitehead 1992). A study undertaken in the Northern Region of England between 1984 and 1986 built on both traditions to investigate the health differences between the 678 electoral wards of the region and ascertain the extent to which differences in health were matched by differences in material and social conditions. The differences in health and in deprivation between wards were found to be very wide. Poor health and material deprivation were found to be strongly associated with one another. Analysis of poor health at the ward level (as measured by rates of mortality, people permanently sick and unable to work, and low birth weight) in relation to the ward characteristics of material deprivation explained more of the idiosyncrasies in area variations in health than could be explained by an analysis based simply on occupational social class variations between wards (Townsend *et al.* 1988). The authors

concluded by noting that the inequalities in health and affluence which were observed by M'Gonigle and Kirby (1936) in the 1930s within the urban areas of the region persisted 50 years later.

With the growing recognition that occupational social class is inadequate as a means of stratifying the population socioeconomically, particularly in the case of women (Whitehead 1992), increasing attention has been given to studies using other socioeconomic indicators such as housing tenure and ownership or not of a car. In these studies, differences in chronic ill health and death rates have been shown to exist not just between the most and least disadvantaged groups, but in a stepwise gradient throughout the entire distribution of socio-economic circumstances. For example, the standardized mortality ratio (**SMR**) for 1976–1991 for women aged 15–59 years in England and Wales who had access to a car and were owner–occupiers was 78 compared with an SMR of 106 for those who were owner-occupiers, but did not have access to a car. Women with access to a car but living in the publicly rented sector had an SMR of 99 as against those without access to a car who had an SMR of 138 (Goldblatt 1990). In the same analysis of mortality, even the number of cars available to the household appeared to be associated with noticeable differences in life expectancy.

The results of this sort of study not only reinforced the conclusion of the earlier Black Report (1980) in the United Kingdom that material circumstances played a predominant role in explaining inequalities in health, but also provided up-to-date evidence of how far the United Kingdom had still to go before the World Health Organization (**WHO**) goal of equity in health status could be secured.

It is characteristic of the applied nature of the discipline of social policy and administration that the large volume of social and epidemiological research on health inequalities in the United Kingdom and elsewhere has been deployed in an attempt to influence the shape of social policies (Whitehead and Dahlgren 1994). It is increasingly possible to identify those socioeconomic, behavioural, and environmental factors which have a bearing on different aspects of health and which are potentially remediable. A range of policy developments has been proposed to improve the health of the least healthy concerned with improving housing, relieving family poverty, reducing income inequality, controlling smoking, mitigating the ill effects of unemployment, and reorienting the health services towards meeting the needs of vulnerable groups (Benzeval *et al.* 1995). However, the challenge facing public health practitioners and social policy analysts in implementing the results of research is daunting, since the principal determinants of levels of population health and differences in health between socioeconomic groups lie in broader societal changes outside the sphere of the health services (Smith and Jacobson 1988).

The success of the health and social services in meeting needs

As well as a strong interest in health inequalities, one of the major themes of recent studies in social policy relevant to public health has been the distribution of public expenditure on the health and social services between different population groups and whether spending relates to population needs. The belief that public spending on welfare services such as housing, education, health, and social security could promote a fairer society by overcoming the inequalities resulting from the market process was an important spur to the development of the welfare state (Crosland 1956, p. 519). A major programme of work on the effects of the welfare state in the United Kingdom between 1973 and 1993 concluded that welfare arrangements, while by no means perfect, had succeeded in redistributing income and services in kind between rich and poor households over the period (Hills 1993). Benefits in kind (for example, publicly funded health services) were less concentrated on the poor than cash benefits but, none the less, households at the bottom of the income distribution still received more in absolute terms than those at the top. For example, there was evidence that poorer people reported higher levels of chronic and acute illness, but also consulted their NHS general practitioners more frequently than better-off people (Le Grand et al. 1990). This is contrary to earlier work which had suggested that, for example, access to and use of the NHS together with public education, housing, and transport services were not correlated with relative need and that the welfare state had, therefore, largely failed in its redistributive aims (Le Grand 1982). This alteration of perspective on the welfare state demonstrates the importance of sustained social policy research which monitors the consequences at a population level of complex, interactive policy changes in a range of welfare institutions over time.

Critical perspectives on contemporary social policy

The breakdown of consensus

The early conviction within the discipline of social policy and administration that the publicly provided, professionalized, social services of the post-Second World War welfare state would successfully achieve society's objectives and be intrinsically beneficent in their impact has been tempered since by the accumulation of empirical work on the practical operation of welfare services and societal limits on what they can achieve. Within the study of social policy and administration, newer critical perspectives on the welfare system have been developed, often based on the experiences of users themselves who may have found services unnecessarily bureaucratic, remote, unresponsive to individual needs, sexist, or racist. The emergence of these perspectives has coincided with significant changes in the economic context of welfare, the tenor of the political debate surrounding welfare and the type of innovations being made in welfare systems. Since the world economic crises of the mid-1970s, governments in the Western world have been continuously preoccupied with restraining the level of resources available for state welfare. The political truce between Left and Right over the economic and social merits of the welfare state has largely broken down and the role of values in making social policy has become more explicit. A change of emphasis has occurred in the prevailing policy debate and to a lesser degree in the actual provision of welfare towards 'welfare pluralism' or 'the mixed economy of welfare' (Johnson 1987). Although such terms are imprecise, they tend to refer to a system in which services are provided by the voluntary, informal, and commercial sectors, as well as through state agencies with the state becoming less dominant. This is accompanied in some versions of welfare pluralism by measures to decentralize resource allocation decisions and encourage wider participation by clients and employees in planning services (Hadley and Hatch 1981).

The New Right critique

Although the antibureaucratic and antiprofessional themes in welfare pluralism appeal to Left and Right, the most potent welfare pluralists have come in the form of Conservative Governments imbued with ideas derived from what is now known the the 'New Right'. The New Right combines the economic liberalism of Hayek and Friedman with the social authoritarianism of neoconservatives such as Roger Scruton and is associated in the United Kingdom particularly with the work of the Institute of Economic Affairs and the journal the *Salisbury Review* (Green 1987). The principal New Right critique of the welfare state highlights the lack of individual choice and control suffered by patients and clients which is exacerbated by the lack of alternatives to state provision. It is argued that the monopoly position of conventional welfare bureaucracies makes them wasteful and inefficient. They are operated by paternalistic professionals and administrators whose self-interest dictates that need is constantly redefined so that the welfare state can expand without limit. This leads to excessive taxation which stifles economic growth and overall prosperity suffers (see George and Wilding (1985, Chapter 2) for a more detailed summary of these views).

Three broad categories of remedy to the ills of the postwar welfare state are proposed from the New Right: incentives to the private sector to develop a range of user-friendly rivals to state provision, privatization or contracting out of state welfare services to the private and voluntary sectors, and the introduction into state welfare of the principles of the private market-place through competitive strategies such as voucher schemes or competition between provider organizations (Enthoven 1985). These challenges to orthodox welfare thinking from *laissez-faire* liberals have elicited a response, particularly from economists interested in social policy. Economists have strongly influenced recent thinking and debate in the discipline of social policy and administration by promoting the view that a distinction can be drawn between the possible ends of social policy (such as efficiency, social justice, and community) and the range of means available to realize these ends (for example, conventional welfare bureaucracies, private markets, and quasi-markets) (Barr 1987; Le Grand et al. 1992; Le Grand and Bartlett 1993). The separation of ends and means is thus an attempt to reconcile the New Right critique with a defence of the welfare state as a means of giving all members of society access to a comprehensive range of social services and income support. Over the next few years, it should become clearer whether longstanding goals of social policy, particularly of equity, can be pursued through seemingly inimical methods such as quasi-markets without being compromised (see below).

The feminist critique

A further challenge to the philosophy of state intervention and the academic discipline which grew up around it, has come from feminist critics of the welfare state (Wilson 1977; Ungerson 1985; Pascall 1986). Feminists from a variety of positions have drawn attention to the way in which the major institutions of the welfare state in Western societies have either failed to give women the help they needed or reinforced material and ideological aspects of their subordination and dependency as users of welfare and as workers in the welfare services (Williams 1989, p. 10). In this analysis, the state is both capitalist, in that it manages the reproduction of the work--

force and patriarchal, in that it sustains family forms, a domestic division of labour, patterns of paid work, and a benefits system which contribute to women's oppression. Rose (1986) summed up the development of the welfare state in Western Europe as ' . . . an accommodation between capital and a male-dominated labour movement . . . ' (quoted in Williams 1989, p. 63).

Feminist analysts of welfare have been particularly active in the health field in areas where the existence of biological differences has been used in the past to justify divisions of labour and of power between men and women. In the area of reproductive technology, for example, the feminist critique has focused not on the new technologies themselves, but on creating the political and cultural conditions in which the technologies can be used to realize women's own definitions of reproduction rather than those of predominantly male doctors (Stanworth 1987).

Another area where the feminist critique of what is biologically given and what is conditioned by material circumstances and ideology has challenged existing welfare provision, lies in the analysis of the gendered nature of caring and the separation between paid work in the formal, visible economy and unpaid work in the informal, invisible economy of caring and how the state plays a part in the structuring of work in both sectors. These forms of analysis have led to a wide range of proposals for social policy change which challenge the existing sexual division of labour and the sharp distinction between paid (male) and unpaid (female) work, such as schemes to promote the rights of women to receive benefits in their own right, the introduction of payments for married women caring for dependent relatives, and policies for better nursery and day care for children. Analyses of policy cast in a broadly feminist mould have had a major impact in questioning fashionable policies for 'community care' of elderly, frail, and disabled people which rest in part on a greater use of informal sources of care. The recognition by feminists that much community care relies on the unpaid work of women which can seriously undermine their own health and well being is a crucial insight for the development of humane policies for the care of dependent groups (Finch and Groves 1983).

Conclusions

Research in the field of social policy and administration over the last 40 years has provided much of the raw material for the contemporary reaction in Western Europe against the provision of health and social services by large, monolithic, bureaucratic organizations in which professional power prevails over individual wishes. There are signs that the role of the state in welfare will persist despite the critics, but that it is changing from near-monopoly provider of many social services to that of regulator and auditor of services provided in the public, voluntary, and commercial sectors with a variety of public and private sources of funding (Klein 1987). Yet, the majority position within the discipline of social policy and administration hitherto has tended to be identified with conventional state provision despite its limitations and failures. As a result, the New Right political philosophers and economists appear to have succeeded for the moment, not so much in dismantling Western welfare states, but in promoting an alternative vision. Market-style, competitive solutions are promoted as the only feasible means to realize people's desires for choice, autonomy, and flexibility in their dealings with welfare services, while at the same

time making the professionals accountable for the quality, appropriateness, and cost of their services (Taylor-Gooby; 1987 Harris 1988). However, it is interesting to note that in most Western countries, the New Right critique has not greatly dented popular support for publicly subsidized services in mainstream fields such as health and education and for a comprehensive system of income maintenance. None the less, questions such as who funds and in what proportion, who provides, and who regulates welfare services and how, which were taken for granted in the last 50 years are now up for debate as it is increasingly recognized that these roles need not be undertaken by a unitary public agency, nor, indeed, exclusively by the state at all. Developments in information technology, for example, offer public authorities the potential to enforce notions of accountability on providers of services without direct, face-to-face control (Klein 1989b).

Thus, one of the principal tasks for social policy analysis in the late 1990s and beyond will be to respond to this changing scene by evaluating the consequences for the complex range of objectives underlying each welfare system of applying the principles of market competition and new forms of organization such as purchaser–provider contracting, to areas such as health and social care. While issues of efficiency, flexibility, and responsiveness of services, together with client choice, are currently pre-eminent in the minds of policy makers, the impact of social policy change on other enduring principles such as equity, social justice, minimum standards, individual rights, and democratic participation cannot and should not be ignored. Social policy research must assess the extent to which fashionable changes in the form of welfare produce the empirical results predicted by their proponents, but must also evaluate their side-effects and wider normative implications. In the health field, the major reforms of the United Kingdom NHS which began with the 1989 White Paper *Working for patients* (Secretaries of State for Health, Wales, Northern Ireland and Scotland, 1989) are a notable example of the emerging trend towards quasi-market reforms of cherished welfare institutions which were initiated with little rational analysis of options. The changes aimed to inject the characteristics commonly associated with private commerce such as dynamism, a willingness to innovate, and a responsiveness to consumer views, into public health care through the development of an untried 'quasi-market', sometimes referred to as a 'provider market' (King's Fund Institute 1989), in which public and private health care operators compete for the business of providing health services for the populations of health authorities and general practice budget holders which act as publicly financed purchasing agencies on behalf of patients. Similar proposals have been developed elsewhere, for example in New Zealand (Maxwell 1988), The Netherlands, and Sweden (Saltman and von Otter 1987). The idea of giving groups of GPs budgets for secondary care was, in part, inspired by the development of health maintenance organizations (**HMOs**) in the United States, which attracted policy makers because of their theoretical incentive to provide high quality care while also controlling their costs. Unlike the conventional third-party payer system of health insurance in which neither doctor nor patient has any incentive to control costs at the time of use of services, the HMO combines the role of insurer and health care provider. Typically, patients enrol through the payment of an annual fee set in advance and the HMO contracts to provide all necessary care for the coming year.

These important and complex changes in different countries throw up numerous questions for social policy research; for example, is it possible to apply business methods and incentives to the NHS without damaging the essential principles underlying the service (in so far as these continue to command popular support)? If so, what combinations of state, voluntary, and commercial funding, provision, and regulation are most likely to achieve this?

Empirical and theoretical research on these questions is beginning to become available (Le Grand and Bartlett 1993; Glennerster *et al.* 1994; Robinson and Le Grand 1994). Overall, the United Kingdom research suggests that innovations such as giving GPs budgets to purchase a range of non-emergency services for their patients as part of the NHS have the potential for improving efficiency and the responsiveness of services to individual need, but that they may have a detrimental effect on providing an equitable service. For example, care will have to be taken to ensure that sicker, more expensive users of health care are not discriminated against by budget-holding GPs. Similarly, the rising administrative costs of operating a quasi-market in the NHS based on contracting between purchasers and providers will have to be monitored closely.

Similarly challenging research agendas exist in many other fields of social policy relevant to the public health at a time of rapid socioeconomic and policy change in Western countries. It would be naive, however, to be too optimistic that the results of research on the consequences of market and quasi-market solutions will be responded to enthusiastically by Western governments. There is little evidence of a commitment at present to the use of the results of rational, applied social research by governments in countries such as the United Kingdom and the United States where policy is more explicitly ideologically driven than it has been for several decades (Booth 1988). None the less, it is important that the discipline maintains its distinctive contribution to intellectual life by continuing to document and explain the impact on life chances and welfare of the interaction between socio-economic change and the social policy response.

References

Alford, R.R. (1975). *Health care politics*. University of Chicago Press, Chicago.

Allen, D. (1979). *Hospital planning*. Pitman Medical, London.

Allison, G.T. (1971). *Essence of decision*. Little Brown, Boston.

Bachrach, P. and Baratz, M.S. (1970). *Power and poverty*. Oxford University Press, New York.

Banting, K.G. (1979). *Poverty, politics and policy*. Macmillan, London.

Barr, N. (1987). *The economics of the welfare state*. Weidenfeld and Nicholson, London.

Benzeval, M., Judge, K., and Whitehead, M. (ed.) (1995). *Tackling inequalities in health*, King's Fund Institute, London.

Black Report (1980). *Inequalities in health: report of a research working group*. Department of Health and Social Security, London.

Blackman, T., Evason, E., Melaugh, M., and Wood, R. (1989). Housing and health: a case study of two areas in West Belfast. *Journal of Social Policy*, **18**, 1–26.

Booth, T. (1988). *Developing policy research*. Gower, Aldershot.

Brotherston, J. (1976). Inequality: is it inevitable? In *Equalities and inequalities in health* (ed. C.O. Carter and J. Peel), pp. 73–104. Academic Press, London.

Brown, M. (1983). The development of social administration. In *Social policy and social welfare: a reader* (ed. M. Loney, D. Boswell, and J. Clarke), pp. 88–103. Open University Press, Milton Keynes.

Brown, M. and Madge, N. (1982). *Despite the welfare state*. Heinemann, London.

Byrne, D., Harrison, S., Keithley, J., and McCarthy, P. (1986). *Housing and health: the relationship between housing conditions and the health of council tenants*. Gower, London.

Calnan, M. (1982). The hospital accident and emergency department: what is its role? *Journal of Social Policy*, **11**, 483–503.

Cawson, A. (1982). *Corporatism and welfare*. Heinemann, London.

Crosland, C.A.R. (1956). *The future of socialism*. Cape, London.

Dahl, R.A. (1961). *Who governs? Democracy and power in the American city*. Yale University Press, New Haven, CT.

Day, P. and Klein, R. (1983). The mobilisation of consent versus the management of conflict: decoding the Griffiths report. *British Medical Journal*, **287**, 1813–16.

Day, P. and Klein, R. (1987). Quality of institutional care and the elderly: policy issues and options. *British Medical Journal*, **294**, 384–7.

Deakin, N. (1987). *The politics of welfare*. Methuen, London.

Department of Health and Social Security (1976). *Sharing resources for health in England: the report of the Resource Allocation Working Party*. HMSO, London.

Donnison, D. (1979). Social policy since Titmuss. *Journal of Social Policy*, **8**, 145–56.

Donnison, D.V. and Chapman, V. (1965). *Social policy and administration*. Allen & Unwin, London.

Enthoven, A.C. (1985). *Reflections on the management of the National Health Service*. Nuffield Provincial Hospitals Trust, London.

Finch, J. and Groves, D. (ed.) (1983). *A labour of love: women, work and caring*. Routledge & Kegan Paul, London.

Forder, A. (1974). *Concepts in social adminstration*. Routledge & Kegan Paul, London.

Forder, A., Caslin, T., Ponton, G., and Walklate, S. (1984). *Theories of welfare*. Routledge & Kegan Paul, London.

Galbraith, J.K. (1972). *The new industrial state* (2nd edn.) André Deutsch, London.

George, V. and Wilding, P. (1976). *Ideology and social welfare*. Routledge & Kegan Paul, London.

George, V. and Wilding, P. (1985). *Ideology and social welfare* (2nd revised edn). Routledge & Kegan Paul, London.

Glennerster, H. (1988). Requiem for the Social Administration Association. *Journal of Social Policy*, **17**, 83–4.

Glennerster, H., Matsaganis, M., Owens, P., and Hancock, S. (1994). *Implementing GP fundholding*. Open University Press, Buckingham.

Goldblatt, P. (1990). Mortality and alternative social classifications. In *Longitudinal study: mortality and social organization* (ed. P. Goldblatt), pp 163–92. HMSO, London.

Gough, I. (1978). Theories of the welfare state: a critique. *International Journal of Health Services*, **8**, 27–40.

Gough, I. (1979). *The political economy of the welfare state*. Macmillan, London.

Green, D.G. (1987). *The New Right: the counter-revolution in political, economic and social thought*. Harvester Wheatsheaf, Brighton.

Hadley, R. and Hatch, S. (1981). *Social welfare and the failure of the state*. Allen & Unwin, London.

Hall, P., Land, H., Parker, R., and Webb, A. (1975). *Change, choice and conflict in social policy*. Heinemann, London.

Ham, C. (1981). *Policy-making in the National Health Service: a case study of the Leeds Regional Hospital Board*. Macmillan, London.

Harris, R. (1988). *Beyond the welfare state*. Institute for Economic Affairs, London.

Harrison, S. and Pollitt, C. (1994). *Controlling health professionals: the future of work and organization in the NHS*. Open University Press, Buckingham.

Hills, J. (with the LSE Welfare State Programme) (1993). *The future of welfare: a guide to the debate*. Joseph Rowntree Foundation, York.

Hunter, D. (1980). *Coping with uncertainty: policy and politics in the National Health Service*. Research Studies Press, Wiley, Chichester.

Hunter, D. (1990). Organizing and managing health care: a challenge for medical sociology. In *Readings in medical sociology* (ed. S. Cunningham-Burley and N.P. McKeganey), pp. 213–36. Tavistock/Routledge, London.

Johnson, N. (1987). *The welfare state in transition: the theory and practice of welfare pluralism.* Harvester Wheatsheaf, Brighton.

King's Fund Institute (1989). *Managed competition: A new approach to health care in Britain.* King's Fund Institute, London.

Klein, R. (1977). The corporate state, the health service and the professions. *New Universities Quarterly*, **31**, 161–80.

Klein, R. (1983). *The politics of the National Health Service.* Longman, London.

Klein, R. (1987). Towards a new pluralism. *Health Policy*, **8**, 5–12.

Klein, R. (1989a). *The politics of the National Health Service* (2nd revised edn.), Longman, London.

Klein, R. (1989b). *Social policy agendas of the 1980s: an overview.* Paper delivered to a plenary session of the 23rd Annual Conference of the Social Policy Association, University of Bath, 10–12 July 1989.

Le Grand, J. (1982). *The strategy of equality: redistribution and the social services.* Allen & Unwin, London.

Le Grand, J. and Bartlett, W. (ed.) (1993). *Quasi-markets and social policy.* Macmillan, London.

Le Grand, J., Winter, D., and Woolley, F. (1990). The NHS: safe in whose hands? In *The state of welfare: the welfare state in Britain since 1974* (ed. J. Hills), pp. 88–134. Clarendon Press, Oxford.

Le Grand, J., Propper, C., and Robinson, R. (1992). *The economics of social problems* (3rd edn). Macmillan, London.

Lindblom, C.E. (1959). The science of 'muddling through'. *Public Administration Review*, **19**, 79–99.

Marshall, T.H. (1975). *Social policy in the twentieth century* (4th revised edn). Hutchinson, London.

Maxwell, R.J. (1988). New Zealand proposals to unshackle hospitals: suggestions to make regional health authorities purchasers of services. *British Medical Journal*, **297**, 1214–5.

Means, R. and Smith, R. (1988). Implementing a pluralistic approach to evaluation in health education. *Policy and Politics*, **16**, 17–28.

Merton, R.K. (1968). *Social theory and social structure.* Free Press, New York.

M'Gonigle, G.E.N. and Kirby, J. (1936). *Poverty and public health.* Gollancz, London.

Mills, C.W. (1956). *The power elite.* Oxford University Press, New York.

Mishra, R. (1977). *Society and social policy.* Macmillan, London.

Mishra, R. (1981). *Society and social policy* (2nd revised edn). Macmillan, London.

Mishra, R. (1986). Social policy and the discipline of social administration. *Social Policy and Administration*, **20**, 28–38.

Morris, J.N. and Titmuss, R.M. (1944). Health and social change: the recent history of rheumatic heart disease. *Medical Officer*, **2**, 69–71, 77–9, 85–7.

Moser, K.A., Fox, A.J. and Jones, D.R. (1984). Unemployment and mortality in the OPCS longitudinal study. *Lancet*, ii, 1324–8.

Navarro, V. (1978). *Class struggle, the state and medicine: an historical and contemporary analysis of the medical sector in Great Britain.* Martin Robertson, Oxford.

Navarro, V. (1989). Why some countries have national health insurance, others have national health services and the U.S. has neither. *Social Science and Medicine*, **28**, 887–8.

NHS Management Enquiry (1983). *Report (Chairman: Sir Roy Griffiths).* Department of Health and Social Security, London.

O'Connor, J. (1973). *The fiscal crisis of the state.* St James's Press, New York.

Parker, J. (1975). *Social policy and citizenship.* Macmillan, London.

Pascall, G. (1986). *Social policy: a feminist analysis.* Tavistock, London.

Pinker, R. (1971). *Social theory and social policy.* Heinemann, London.

Pinker, R. (1979). *The idea of welfare.* Heinemann, London.

Platt, S., Martin, C.J., Hunt, S.M., and Lewis, C.W. (1989). Damp housing, mould growth and symptomatic health state. *British Medical Journal*, **298**, 1673–8.

Pollitt, C., Harrison, S., Hunter, D., and Marnoch, G. (1988). The reluctant managers: clinicians and budgets in the NHS. *Financial Accountability and Management*, **43**, 213–33.

Rein, M. (1976). *Social science and public policy.* Penguin, Harmondsworth.

Reisman, D.A. (1977). *Richard Titmuss: welfare and society.* Heinemann, London.

Ringen, S. (1987). *The possibility of politics: a study in the political economy of the welfare state.* Clarendon Press, Oxford.

Robinson, R. and Le Grand, J. (ed.) (1994). *Evaluating the NHS reforms.* King's Fund Institute, London.

Room, G. (1979). *The sociology of welfare.* Basil Blackwell, Oxford.

Rose, H. (1986). Women and the restructuring of the welfare state. In *Comparing welfare states and their futures* (ed. E. Owen). Gower, Aldershot.

Saltman, R.B. and von Otter, C. (1987). Re-vitalizing public health care systems: a proposal for public competition in Sweden. *Health Policy*, **7**, 21–40.

Secretaries of State for Health, Wales, Northern Ireland and Scotland (1989). *Working for patients.* HMSO, London.

Smith, A. and Jacobson, B. (ed.) (1988). *The nation's health: a strategy for the 1990s.* King Edward's Hospital Fund for London, London.

Smith, G. and Cantley, C. (1985). *Assessing health care: a study in organizational evaluation.* Open University Press, Milton Keynes.

Stanworth, M. (ed.) (1987). *Reproductive technologies: gender, motherhood and medicine.* Polity Press, Cambridge.

Stevenson, T.H.C. (1923). The social distribution of mortality from different causes in England and Wales 1910–1912. *Biometrika*, **15**, 382–400.

Taylor-Gooby, P. (1987). Welfare attitudes: cleavage, consensus and citizenship. *Quarterly Journal of Social Affairs* **3**, 199–211.

Taylor-Gooby, P. and Dale, J. (1981). *Social theory and social welfare.* Edward Arnold, London.

Titmuss, R.M. (1938). *Poverty and population: a factual study of contemporary social welfare.* Macmillan, London.

Titmuss, R. (1963). The social division of welfare: some reflections on the search for equity. In *Essays on the welfare state*, pp. 34–55. Allen & Unwin, London.

Titmuss, R. (1968). The subject of social administration. In *Commitment to welfare*, pp. 13–24. Allen & Unwin, London.

Titmuss, R. (1970). *The gift relationship.* Allen & Unwin, London.

Titmuss, R. (1974). *Social policy.* Allen & Unwin, London.

Townsend, P. (1974). Poverty as relative deprivation: resources and style of living. In *Poverty, inequality and class structure* (ed. D. Wedderburn), pp. 15–41. Cambridge University Press, London.

Townsend, P. (1976). *Sociology and social policy.* Penguin, Harmondsworth.

Townsend, P. (1979). *Poverty in the United Kingdom.* Penguin, Harmondsworth.

Townsend, P., Phillimore, P., and Beattie, A. (1988). *Health and deprivation: inequality and the North.* Croom Helm, London.

Ungerson, C. (ed.) (1985). *Women and social policy: a reader.* Macmillan, London.

Walker, A. (1981). Social policy, social administration and the social construction of welfare. *Sociology*, **15**, 225–250.

Walker, R. (1988). Syllogism based on licensed premises. *The Times Higher Education Supplement*, **18 March**, 15.

Whitehead, M. (1992). *The health divide.* Penguin, Harmondsworth.

Whitehead, M. and Dahlgren, G. (1994). Why not now? Action on inequalities in health. *European Journal of Public Health*, **4**, 1–2.

Wilensky, H.L. and Lebeaux, C.N. (1958). *Industrial society and social welfare.* Free Press, New York.

Williams, F. (1989). *Social policy: a critical introduction. Issues of race, gender and class.* Polity Press, Cambridge.

Wilson, E. (1977). *Women and the welfare state.* Tavistock, London.

22 Sociological investigations

Myfanwy Morgan

Introduction

Most issues in the field of public health have an important social dimension. These range from traditional epidemiological concerns regarding the social causes of disease and its distribution among social classes, ethnic groups and other social categories, to a consideration of health and illness in a broader context, including patients' subjective assessments of health and quality of life and the social meanings and responses to chronic and stigmatizing illness. Issues relating directly to the organization and provision of health services and the design of effective preventive programmes also pose questions of a social nature, including the social characteristics and priorities of communities, the social influences on health and illness behaviours, and the requirements for the successful implementation and adoption of organizational change. Sociological research has also contributed more broadly to analyses of the social forces that shape prevailing medical institutions and approaches to health.

Health and medicine as a specialized field of sociological enquiry has partly developed alongside epidemiology and shared its concerns. Thus both epidemiologists and medical sociologists frequently trace the origins of their common interests in the role of economic, social, political and cultural factors in health and disease patterns to the nineteenth century struggles of physicians like Virchov in Germany, Chadwick in the United Kingdom, Shattuck in the United States, and Coronel in The Netherlands. Moreover the empirical enquiries undertaken by these physicians and other nineteenth century social reformers laid the foundations for the development of both sociology and epidemiology by establishing the social survey as a method of investigation. Collaboration of social scientists and epidemiologists in carrying out research on questions of the social distribution and causes of non-infectious conditions such as lung cancer, bronchitis and coronary heart disease, and questions relating to the organization and provision of health services probably dates from the 1940s in both Britain and the United States. The particular contribution of social scientists was in terms of their skills in social survey techniques and in their knowledge of social variables, such as social class, housing conditions, poverty etc. This co-operation between epidemiologists, sociologists, statisticians, economists, and others in undertaking research on issues relating to disease, illness and health care has continued. It is encouraged by the increased recognition of the social, psychological, and economic dimensions of health and health care, and the greater involvement of governments in the planning and provision of health services and the funding of research.

The other major influence on the growth and development of sociological enquiries in the field of health and medicine has stemmed from the growth of sociology itself as an academic discipline. This has provided large numbers of people trained in the theories and methods of sociological investigation and has been associated with the development of specialist sub-fields in medicine, the family, deviance, education, race relations, and other aspects of society.

The strength and development of medical sociology as a specialism has varied between countries. This reflects differences in the strength of sociology as an academic discipline, the collaboration which exists between epidemiologists and social scientists in studying public health issues, and the level of funding of research concerned with the health of participants and the organization and provision of health care. The period of rapid growth in medical sociology as a sub-field started in the 1950s in the United States and about a decade later in the United Kingdom, and continued until the late 1970s. In both countries, medical sociology (or the sociology of health and illness as it may be more appropriately described) forms the largest sociological sub-field in terms of the numbers of people involved. Although developing rather more slowly in many other countries, it now forms an important specialism for social scientists, while the main international journal *Social Science and Medicine* was founded in 1966.

There is considerable overlap between the concerns of epidemiology and sociology, since both have a common interest in the factors contributing to the distribution, prevalence and incidence of illness and disease, and its prevention and cure, and each employs concepts from the other discipline. Both epidemiologists and social scientists are therefore frequently engaged in similar areas of research and each group draws on concepts and methods developed in other disciplines. Moreover sociologists frequently participate in multidisciplinary teams and bring a particular expertise and knowledge of the nature and measurement of social variables. However while acknowledging this overlap and the large body of research undertaken on a collaborative basis, this chapter focuses on what is distinctive about sociological investigations in terms of their perspectives, methods of investigation, and focus of research.

Sociological perspectives

The basic framework for epidemiological investigations is provided by the biomedical model of disease, with biological inferences being derived from observations of disease occurrence and related phenomena in human population groups. In contrast, the broad

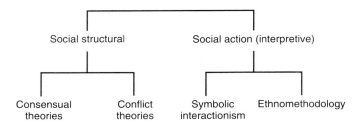

Fig. 22.1 Sociological perspectives.

conceptual framework for sociologists is provided by their perspective concerning the nature and workings of society. However, an important feature of sociology is that it is characterized by a range of theories about the nature and workings of society rather than a single unified approach. These theories play an important role in drawing attention to different aspects of society and helping to explain or give meaning to observations. As O'Brien (1993) explains: 'Different theories bring different aspects of the world into view: theories are like the lenses of the kaleidoscope; when you slot different ones into place things you could not see before suddenly become visible; patterns that were indistinct become sharper' (p. 11).

Sociological theories can be broadly divided into those that adopt a structural perspective which emphasize the broad structures and functioning of society, and those which adopt an interpretative perspective and are primarily concerned with how individuals perceive their social world (Fig. 22.1). These theories are briefly outlined below to demonstrate how different 'ways of seeing' the social world leads to different types of questions and explanations, and different methods of research. This diversity of perspectives and approaches forms an important aspect of sociological investigations in public health as in other fields of enquiry.

Structural theories

Modern structural theories in sociology had their origins in the late nineteenth century, which was a time of unprecedented social upheaval in Europe associated with agricultural production giving way to industrialization, a movement of people into urban areas, and a decline in traditional institutions of power such as the church and nobility. Aware of this rapid transformation of society, Emile Durkheim, Karl Marx and others were concerned to identify the dynamics of social change and the basis of social order and stability. Each presented their own theories regarding the nature and workings of society, which have been further developed and elaborated over this century. These theories may be broadly divided into consensual theories, which emphasize the way that societies are characterized by common interests, values and goals, and conflict theories which emphasize the differences in interests and struggles for advantage between groups in society.

A consensual view of society guided sociological analyses during the 1950s and early 1960s. This was mainly associated with functionalist theory which derives from early anthropological writings and the works of Emile Durkheim and Talcott Parsons within sociology. Parsons presented the most complete analysis of society from a functionalist perspective in 'The Social System' (1951). He viewed the functioning of society in terms very much

akin to the functioning of a physical organism and regarded social relationships as being structured and organized in terms of various social institutions, such as the family, the economy, the health system, and the educational system, which are each concerned with meeting the basic needs of society. These social institutions although concerned with particular spheres of social life are regarded as interrelated to form a system in which the different parts influence each other and contribute towards the efficient functioning of the whole. This was viewed as being very much like the way the heart, lungs and other organs each perform a specific function and contribute to the well-being of the body. For example the existence of social stratification was explained in functionalist terms as serving the general interest of society. This is because it is necessary to motivate the most able people to enter those positions requiring considerable skill and long periods of training and motivate them to perform well. As a result such positions attract greater status and economic rewards, which thus functions to promote the well-being of society as a whole (Davis and Moore 1945). The special position of doctors and other professions is similarly explained in functionalist terms as reflecting their requirements for specialist knowledge, and their special position in using this expert knowledge in the community's interest and adopting an altruistic and service orientation. In repayment for this special role they are accorded higher status than other groups and a high level of financial reward (Parsons 1951). These examples illustrate a central tenet underpinning functionalism in terms of the assumption of a consensus of values and goals, which forms the basis of social solidarity and co-operation. Value consensus in turn is maintained by the process of socialization whereby values are internalized and transmitted from one generation to the next, and are translated into specific directives in terms of roles and norms which define socially expected behaviours. For example, the nuclear family is made up of the interconnected roles of husband, father, wife, mother, son and daughter, while health care involves various professional and patient roles. Those who deviate from society's values and prescribed roles are subject to mechanisms of social control, which serves to ensure a high level of conformity and the smooth functioning of social institutions.

This functionalist perspective had an important influence on the early development of medical sociology and was compatible with the prevailing reformist approaches to health services care. The writings of Talcott Parsons (1951) were central to the development of a functionalist approach to health and medicine, and arose from his general question of how society minimizes the disruptive effects of illness. Parsons regarded illness as deviance not merely in biological terms but also in social terms, as sick people are not able to perform their normal social roles. The existence of such deviance on a large scale would therefore threaten the smooth functioning of society. Parsons identified society's mechanisms for handling sickness, so that it does not place too great a strain on the social system, as being to institute a special status and social role for sick people (the 'sick role') and a complementary role for doctors. Like all social roles these carry both rights and obligations. The obligations on the sick person are that they are expected to be motivated to want to get better as quickly as possible, rather than malingering in the sick role. To this end they are expected to seek technically competent help and co-operate with medical experts. The privileges of the sick role are that the sick person is given exemption from the performance of normal duties and responsibilities, relative to the nature and severity of the illness (for example the person may be allowed or even required to take time off work) and they are also regarded as being in need of care. Complementing the sick role is the role of the doctor, which also involves both rights and obligations. These include the expectation that doctors will apply a high degree of knowledge and skill to the problems of illness, act for the welfare of the patient rather than in their own self-interest, be objective and emotionally detached, and be guided by the rules of professional conduct. In return for these obligations, doctors are granted the right to examine patients physically and enquire into intimate details of their physical and personal life. They also enjoy considerable autonomy in relation to the patient and occupy a position of authority.

Parsons's theoretical analysis of society's response to illness is generally regarded as marking the beginning of health and medicine as a sociological specialism. This is because it extended the view of illness from a purely biological state to the social sphere, and identified a specific set of rights and obligations that surround the sick person. These ideas have since been widely employed and developed in the analysis of illness. For example, the often ambivalent responses of the public and medical staff to conditions such as alcoholism, overdoses and AIDS can be explained in terms of their unwillingness to view such conditions purely as sickness requiring treatment and therefore to grant people with these conditions the privileges of the sick role. Instead there is a tendency to ascribe notions of responsibility and thus of punishment to people with such conditions and possibly to their close relatives (Pollack 1992). Similarly, Parsons's portrayal of the relationship between doctors and patients as a social relationship and not merely a technical relationship has been important in focusing attention on the ways in which this social relationship can be improved, so as to promote the diagnostic and therapeutic process and increase patients' satisfaction with the consultation (Tuckett et al. 1985). This has included the development and extension of Parsons's model to identify different types of relationship between doctor and patient, depending on the relative power and control exercised by both doctors and patients (Stewart and Roter 1989).

Whereas functionalist theory was influential during the early development of medical sociology, by the beginning of 1970s it had become largely replaced by conflict theory. This was partly because of its promise to provide answers which functionalism failed to provide and partly because it was more in keeping with the tenor and mood of the times. Rather than depicting society as based on shared values and altruism, these theories drew attention to the conflict that exists in terms of the struggle for advantage between groups in society. However, they differ in their views of the distribution of power and the nature of conflicting groups.

Conflict theory was initially informed by historical materialism (Marxist theory) which offers a radical alternative to functionalism as a general theory of society. Historical materialism emphasizes the basic divisions in society along class lines, and the conflict which characterizes their relationship, since each can only gain at the expense of the other. Social classes are regarded as reflecting the basic divisions associated with a system of economic production which involves the participation of two major groups, namely a capitalist class who own the means of production (land, factories, etc) and dominate and exploit a working class who are simply a source of labour in the production process. Moreover the interests of the dominant group in the economic sphere and its ideology is regarded as shaping the political, legal, medical, educational and other institutions in society. These functions thus serve to reinforce and support interests of the ruling class and justify its power and privilege.

In the health field, materialist perspectives have been particularly influential in relation to analyses of the social causes and distribution of disease, and have considered the ways in which the organization of work in capitalist economies exposes workers to risks of ill health. For example, Doyal (1981) examines the various physical health risks arising from the 'safe' levels set for exposure to chemicals, gases, dusts and other toxic substances, and ascribes such conditions to the interests of the owners and controllers of industry who operate on the basis of 'acceptable' risks for a given return on investment. The fairly limited and fragmentary nature of health and safety legislation, with little priority assigned by the government to its enforcement is similarly attributed to the way in which the economic interests of the capitalists and ruling class have priority over considerations of the health risks for the workforce. Other writers have focused on the feelings of alienation and stress associated with the routinization of work and lack of control. For Navarro (1982) this produces a need among workers to acquire satisfaction through consumption, thus encouraging cigarette smoking and other behaviours harmful to health. Demands for these products are also regarded as being and promoted by the needs of the economic system, which requires to be sustained by a high level of demand for its products. Other writers emphasize the adverse health effects of psychological stresses and low self-esteem arising from an organization of work which denies workers autonomy and control (Schwalbe and Staples 1986). A general implication of such analyses is thus to focus on the structural determinants of ill health, and to make links between a specific form of economic organization and both the social distribution of ill health and the dominance of individual interventionist approaches to promoting the health of populations (Crawford 1977).

Analyses of issues in the health field are now commonly influenced by a conflict model. However, this is generally derived from elite or power group theories. These view power as distributed among several groups who may differ in their interests, agendas and goals, rather than reflecting broad class interests and divisions. The interests of the medical profession, owners and controllers of industry, and government departments may thus converge on some issues but diverge on others, reflecting their differing structural position and interests. An example is Calnan's (1984) analysis of the voluntary and fairly limited government controls on the tobacco industry in the United Kingdom with the emphasis on self-regulation. Rather than explaining this in terms of class interests, Calnan draws attention to the conflicts of interests which exists among those with power. For example, the tobacco industry and the Department of Trade and Treasury have opposed stricter controls on the tobacco industry, as a result of economic considerations in terms of the effects on profits and government revenue. In contrast, the Department of Health, the medical profession, and various pressure groups have been important in pressing for and achieving the restrictions on advertising and the health warnings that do exist, reflecting their concerns with the health risks of smoking. Similar differences in approach characterize explanations of the nature of the broader health care system. Historical materialist analyses emphasize the way in which the organization of health care systems and their reform in capitalist societies reflect class interests (Navarro 1989), whereas power group theories identify the differing interests and influence of the medical profession, corporate interests, health planners and other groups (Alford 1985; Starr 1982).

Whereas functionalist and conflict theories have been described in broad outline, in practice each of these theories or theoretical frameworks encompasses a number of differing interpretations. However, what is of importance is an appreciation of the ways in which different theoretical perspectives serve to focus on different questions and aspects of social reality, and may also suggest different explanatory links. They thus serve to inform theories of the middle range which deal with delimited aspects of social phenomena and the development and explanation of concepts. For example, Parsons's functionalist analysis contributed notions of illness as social deviance, the sick role, and medicine and social control. These notions have subsequently been developed and elaborated through empirical research assessing their applicability in relation to different settings and conditions (Morgan *et al.* 1985). These social phenomena have also been viewed from a conflict perspective, which in turn has highlighted different aspects. For example, whereas Parsons depicted the doctors' function in officially legitimizing illness and controlling access to the sick role in purely positive terms, conflict theories emphasize the conflicts inherent in doctors' roles and have also drawn attention to the possible negative aspects of the doctors' gatekeeper function in officially legitimizing illness and determining access to the sick role (Morgan 1991). More generally, recognition of the social meanings and significance of medical diagnosis or 'labels' has been associated with analyses of both the positive and negative effects of an expansion of the medical sphere to encompass conditions such as alcoholism, drug addiction, infertility and hyperactivity among children (Zola 1975; Conrad 1976). Such analyses have served a sensitizing function and increased awareness of the possible social and psychological costs and benefits of defining these conditions as medical problems requiring treatment. This now forms an important consideration in relation to evaluations of blood pressure detection and treatment programmes, treatment for high cholesterol levels and the greater involvement of doctors in providing lifestyles advice and other preventive strategies which involve an expanded role for medicine (Macdonald *et al.* 1984; Stoate 1989; Stott and Pill 1990).

As this section shows, different theories of society give rise to differing explanations of the characteristics of social phenomena, such as social class inequalities, the characteristics of professions, and the characteristics of health care systems. They are also associated with differing recommendations for health policies and social change, based on their underlying assumptions and models of society (see chapter on Social Administration). However structural theories all share a common focus on the structure of society and its institutions and the objective nature of social phenomena. They also regard society as shaping the beliefs, values and patterns of behaviour characteristic of social groups. The social expectations guiding the behaviour of for example doctors and patients, parents and children, and men and women, are thus seen as largely a social product learned through a process of socialization. Various pres-

sures are also placed on people to conform to the practices and values of society. This contrasts with social action theories which take the individual as the centrepoint of analysis and view social life as essentially subjective or interpretive. Individuals' actions are thus seen as guided by their own social meanings and interpretations of the social world rather than responding more passively to the demands of the social system.

Social action theories

A social action perspective is based on the premise that human action is meaningful to those involved. An understanding of social behaviour therefore requires an interpretation of the meanings which people give to the social world. Max Weber (1864 to 1920), a German sociologist, is regarded as founding the social action or interpretive school of sociology, in that he emphasized the importance not merely of focusing on objective structures but also of understanding individuals' perceptions and meanings to know why they acted in a particular way. This emphasis on the need to understand meanings as a form of explanation was later developed through sociological theories known as interactionism and ethnomethodology which have been influential since the early 1960s (Fig. 22.1). These theories differ in the extent to which they acknowledge and incorporate notions of an objective structure which shapes individuals perceptions and experiences, although sharing a 'common' interpretive perspective in their emphasis on subjective meanings as a central focus of sociological enquiry (Layder 1994).

One example of 'the way of seeing' associated with an interpretive perspective is provided by its approach to official statistics. Rather than accepting the objective nature and facts conveyed by such 'hard' data, an interpretive approach focuses on the social construction of these social facts. For example, data demonstrating variations in morbidity or mortality rates from specific causes between social groups or geographical areas raises questions of how far the observed variations may be a product of various decision-making processes. Whereas epidemiologists acknowledge such potential sources of bias and artefacts, writers adopting an interpretive approach have taken this as a focus of investigation and examined the social processes involved in the production of official statistics. For example, they have examined how coroners reach the decision to categorize a death as 'suicide' or 'accidental', and how diagnostic decision rules are interpreted and applied by coders in local areas (Pryor 1985). This approach also focuses on the ways in which doctors' application of diagnostic labels and treatment decisions are influenced by the social meanings of medical conditions, and the social images and categorization of patients. For example, the negative meanings of 'stigma' surrounding alcoholism, overdoses and AIDS, often results in an associated condition being recorded on the death certificate, thus saving the family from feelings of shame (King 1989). Treatment decisions undertaken in situations where the need to balance supply and demand leads to rationing, may also be influenced implicitly if not explicitly by social as well as medical criteria, and involve social judgements and evaluations based on age, employment position, family responsibilities and other criteria (Challah *et al.* 1984). Images of particular conditions, such as the common perception of heart disease as a disease of affluence and its association with executive stress among men, may also have a self-fulfilling prophecy by increasing doctors' readiness to diagnose and treat patients in these presenting categories. As these examples illustrate, human actions can be viewed as responding to meanings, while such meanings can be viewed as a social product or construction which may vary over time and between societies and social groups, rather than forming an inherent attribute and unvarying characteristic of a condition or behaviour.

An interpretive approach has not only served to focus on social meanings and their influence on behaviours, but also challenges the notion of a single dominant value system and emphasizes the plurality of beliefs and values. This has been associated with an acknowledgement of patients' or lay views as important realities in their own right, rather than comprising an inferior form of medical knowledge. For example, patients non-use or irregular use of prescribed medication was traditionally viewed from a biomedical perspective as deviance from a medical norm. Major reasons for such non-compliance apart from problems of drug side-effects, were hypothesized to be patients forgetting to take the tablets, and problems created by patients' lack of understanding of medication instructions from the doctor or of the significance of the medical condition. However, these traditional factors failed to account for more than a small proportion of patients' non-compliance, with the result that educational interventions although increasing knowledge often failed to change behaviours and achieve greater conformity with medical advice or treatment (Morris and Schulz 1992). A more complete understanding of individual's 'non-compliance' has been provided by research adopting a more patient-oriented perspective, which views patients' non-adherence as largely 'reflective' non-adherence based on their own beliefs and evaluations and the everyday life situation in which the illness occurs and the treatment is used (Conrad 1985; Donovan and Blake 1992). The aim is thus to understand patients' own logic and the reasons for their behaviours. This approach has identified a variety of factors that influence patients' decision making which extend beyond the traditional medical model. These include what are often strongly felt concerns about the possible long-term harmful side-effects of drugs, and fears of becoming dependent on drugs both physically and psychologically. Many patients also wish to deny the condition and thus not be reminded of it by regular medication use, or do not wish to draw attention to a potentially stigmatized condition. Medication use may also be incompatible with other valued activities such as eating and drinking with friends. Patients and doctors thus often differ in their priorities and goals of treatment, with patients being more willing to accept or live with some symptoms or the possibility of future health risks, and may regard this as preferable to long-term drug use and acceptance of a patient role. This approach thus broadens the focus of traditional compliance research and suggests that an understanding of such patient held beliefs and meanings forms an important basis for increasing the acceptability and effectiveness of medical care, and acknowledges that patients' beliefs, values and priorities form a social reality that requires to be accepted and responded to.

The content of lay or patients' perspectives has traditionally formed a major focus of investigation. However, attention is now also increasingly being given to understanding the perspectives of doctors and other health workers. This reflects an acknowledgement that although formally engaged in a common medical task, different occupational groups and specialties may vary in their interests, and hold differing criteria of success or priorities associated with their particular location within the health care system. This has important implications for the organization and success of multidisciplinary health teams, as well as for the adoption of new policy initiatives which may be resisted by those whose interests are threatened. Thus an important task is to make explicit and where possible respond to the needs and concerns of different occupational or provider groups. For example, the apparent reluctance among nurses to enter day surgical nursing was identified as a barrier to the more widespread adoption of this form of surgical organization in the United Kingdom. This reluctance on the part of nurses could not be explained by surgeons who viewed day surgery as providing a favourable environment for nurses, especially given the convenience of the hours. However, a study of nurses' perspectives showed that a major problem was the low status in which day surgery was held by nurses in general. This was based on a common misconception of day surgery as mainly minor surgery concerned with 'lumps and bumps', whereas day surgery in the United Kingdom is a rapidly growing area and is concerned with groin hernia repair, varicose veins stripping, laparoscopy, arthroscopy and other formerly inpatient procedures. Other problems arose because day surgery was not well integrated into the career structure for nurses, which restricted opportunities for advancement, and of importance for younger nurses was the lack of overtime which reduced financial rewards. By examining day surgical nursing from the perspective of nurses themselves it thus became clear why this specialty as currently organized was of limited attractiveness for many nurses (Morgan and Reynolds 1991).

An interactionist perspective does not overlook the existence of social roles and formal organizational structures, but instead portrays these as relatively fluid. There is thus seen to be room for bargaining and negotiation, since roles can rarely be so tightly defined that they are not open to interpretation and interpersonal processes based on social meanings. For example, negotiation over responsibilities often occurs between different categories of hospital staff involved in patient care (Strauss 1963). Opportunities for negotiation are often greater in medical than surgical specialties, as treatment and management decisions in medical specialties are less clear-cut and different professional groups seeks to co-ordinate activities as part of a team. Despite the relative powerlessness of patients, they may nevertheless also negotiate with medical staff. Thus studies of the doctor–patient relationship have examined the ways in which both patients and doctors may persuade, bargain and negotiate and achieve their own goals. They illustrate how both verbal and non-verbal strategies in terms of gestures and the conveying of interest or lack of interest, may be employed, especially by doctors, to control the consultation. Indeed it has been calculated that in a normal two-person conversation the verbal component carries less than 35 per cent of the social meaning of the situation and more than 65 per cent is carried by the non-verbal component (Pietroni 1976). For example, a doctor's continued rifling through notes, fidgeting with pens, and failure to look directly at the patient may be viewed as a sign of disinterest by patients and influence the information they communicate in the consultation.

These examples illustrate the ways in which an interpretive perspective provides a framework for research which focuses on

social meanings and processes. It thus complements more traditional sociomedical enquiries and structural approaches by raising
different questions regarding health, illness and the provision of
health care, and in this way has contributed new 'ways of seeing' as
well as new concepts and explanations.

Methods of research

Sociological investigations employ both quantitative and qualitative
methods. At one level these may be regarded as merely differences
in research techniques. However, they can also be viewed as
deriving from different philosophical positions regarding the
nature of the social world and its appropriate methods of study.
This section briefly outlines the assumptions and methods of both
quantitative and qualitative research. Particular attention is paid to
the methodology of qualitative research, as this approach involves
radical departures from the assumptions and methods of the
scientific model generally employed by epidemiologists and the
clinical sciences.

Quantitative research

Quantitative methods derive from a positivist philosophy, of which
a key element is the view that social phenomena are objective and
external to the individual and thus take the form of social 'facts'.
These social facts are therefore studied in much the same way as
phenomena in the natural world through the application of the
scientific method, with the aim of producing valid and generalized
findings and thus a science of society. The assumptions of
quantitative research therefore accord with structural theories in
sociology and the biomedical model, with their common emphasis
on the objective nature of social phenomena and aim to establish
how much, how many and what is the association or cause–
effect?

A fundamental difference between the social and natural worlds
is that human beings react to situations, and may for example
change their behaviour if they are aware they are being observed or
give what they perceive to be socially acceptable answers in
interview surveys. However, this is generally regarded from a
quantitative stance as a problem to be overcome or at least reduced
through appropriate research methods. Emphasis is therefore
placed on ways of reducing bias and ensuring the repeatability of
findings and the validity of instruments. Second, although human
beings have feelings and imbue situations with meanings, these are
not regarded as an important focus of the study. Instead the
emphasis is on the ways in which predetermined variables (such as
age, access, and knowledge) influence behaviour.

The basic framework guiding quantitative sociological investigations is provided by the scientific method (Table 22.1). This
requires that hypotheses are specified at the outset, or at least
precise research questions formulated. The relevant variables are
then 'operationalized'; that is, defined in ways that are measurable.
For example, the hypothesis that unemployed men with high levels
of social support will experience fewer health problems than
unemployed men lacking high levels of social support, requires that
the concepts of unemployment, high level of social support, and
health problems are each defined in ways that are measurable. Data
are collected from the entire population of interest, or from a
representative sample based on statistical principles of sampling, to
test the hypothesis or examine the research question. The relation-

Table 22.1 Quantitative and qualitative research

	Quantitative	Qualitative
View of social world	Social reality exists as objective, measurable phenomena, external to the individual (Positivism)	Social reality is subjectively interpreted and experienced (Interpretive)
Logic of enquiry	Deductive based on testing formal hypotheses to establish casual relationships	Inductive reasoning with understanding of social processes derived from data
Research design	Quantitative, with sample selection, data collection and analysis based on scientific procedures and ensuring repeatable and generalizable results	Qualitative, based on detailed study of beliefs and behaviours of groups of interest to elicit their interpretations and responses
Validity	Corresponds to an objective reality	Corresponds to a subjective reality

ship between variables is then analysed statistically, with the aim of
establishing cause–effect associations between variables and the
achievement of generalizable results.

The data employed in quantitative research may be derived from
a number of sources (Table 22.2). In some cases this consists of
available or 'secondary' data in the form of routinely collected
statistics or other written records. However, many research questions can only be answered through the collection of first-hand or
primary data. This generally involves the use of a structured
questionnaire, which is self-completed by the respondent or
administered by an interviewer. An important feature of the
structured questionnaire is that it is designed to be administered in
exactly the same way to all respondents. Interviewers are therefore
given no discretion as to how to ask the questions or in what order,
and are required to conduct each interview in exactly the same
manner. The questions are also often precoded and allow only a
limited range of responses. In this way, subjectivity and the effects
of interviewer variability are reduced, and the results obtained

Table 22.2 Sources of data in sociological investigations

Secondary data	Primary data
Routine statistics (e.g. mortality data, hospital statistics)	Structured questionnaire Semi-structured interview
Government surveys and other *ad hoc* enquiries	Unstructured (or focused) interview
Written records (including historical and literary sources)	Group interview (focus group)
	Diary method
	Observation

through the use of this standard approach are regarded as repeatable. Interviews are usually conducted face-to-face, preferably with the respondent alone. However, telephone interviews are increasingly being employed, especially as an initial screening interview, given that this is relatively quick and inexpensive compared with a household survey and allows respondents to be interviewed at times most convenient to them. However, the feasibility of telephone interviewing and the possible bias introduced depends on the proportion of households with phones in the community (McCann *et al.* 1984).

Observation is occasionally employed as a method of data collection in quantitative research. However, an important limitation is regarded as the small number of people or situations that it is generally feasible to observe, which raises questions of the generalizability of the results. Observation when employed in quantitative research is usually tightly defined with the aim of achieving a uniform, standardized method of data collection. The observer is therefore required to record only certain types of predefined behaviours or comments. An example is Clark and Bowling's (1989) study designed to test the hypothesis that small nursing homes would provide long-stay elderly patients with more personal attention and freedom of choice compared with hospital wards, and that the nursing home environment would therefore provide a better quality of life. The study employed observation as one of several forms of data collection. Observation required that the observers logged activities, interactions, and moods in 15-minute blocks. A total of 232 observational sessions were conducted over a 3-month period, in four settings. The types of activities and interactions recorded included meal times, serving of tea/coffee, presence of visitors, playing of radio/television/music, interaction with professionals, etc. The recording was undertaken by two observers and in order to achieve a high level of inter-observer reliability they piloted the observational schedule until they achieved consistent ratings.

A variant of direct observation which is sometimes employed to minimize the intrusive effect of an observer, is video or audio tape recording. When employed in quantitative research, the material is translated into numerical data for analysis. This is achieved by classifying data into categories, based on the content of responses or by using rating scales. For example in a study of the effects of differences in the length of medical consultations on the amount and type of communication which occurred, 623 consultations were recorded. This material was then analysed by classifying both doctors and patients statements into categories. These included, statement by doctor explaining treatment, statement interrupting patient, question asked by patient, etc. This produced a count of the frequency with which different types of statements occurred and thus provided data in quantitative form (Roland *et al.* 1986).

The diary method in which people record feelings or activities, usually daily, in a 'diary' or record book, is occasionally employed in quantitative research for collecting data on symptoms and illness behaviours (Richardson 1994). An example of the use of health diaries as one of several forms of data collection is a study of self-care in 107 households in Denmark (Bentzen *et al.* 1989). The diaries were structured for daily entries and required the recording of symptoms for each household member. For each illness respondents also recorded their self-care activities, activity restrictions and professional care sought. Altogether information was completed for 998 households (94 per cent) with 2661 members over 52 weeks. This allowed quantitative statements to be made, concerning, for example, how many people experienced particular types of symptoms, such as headaches, backpain, and feverishness, and how many consulted the doctor about their symptoms. The use of health diaries is regarded as particularly well suited to the study of self-care, in that less salient events and activities than those requiring professional care are picked up far better in prospective health diaries than in retrospective questionnaire-based surveys.

Quantitative research thus relies on different sources and methods of data collection, with the choice depending on the precise questions being investigated. However, what is important is that the method of data collection and analysis takes place within a framework which is guided by scientific principles of research, with the aim of producing results that are repeatable and generalizable and which conform to an objective reality. The acceptance by epidemiology and to a large extent by sociology of the scientific model of research has formed an important bond promoting their collaboration in the study of public health issues. Probably the main difference between their approaches is the greater reliance by epidemiologists on an experimental design in the form of randomized controlled trials (RCTs). Sociologists rarely regard an experimental design as either feasible or ethical in relation to their particular research questions. They therefore more often undertake descriptive studies, which are designed to examine one or more research questions rather than to test a single tightly defined hypothesis.

Qualitative research

Qualitative research has a long tradition in sociology and characterized many of the early sociological studies undertaken in the United States in the 1940s, as well as forming the general method of anthropological research. However, the application of qualitative methods to the field of public health mainly dates from the early 1970s. This was associated with a more general development of a social action approach or interpretive perspective within sociology, with its emphasis on social reality as subjectively perceived and experienced. Thus whereas quantitative research focuses on objective facts and is concerned with establishing statistical relationships, a social action or interpretive position emphasizes insight and understanding and is concerned with the beliefs, motivations and actions of people, organizations and institutions. These differences in subject matter in turn require a different logic and methods of research.

Central to an interpretive approach is the use of inductive reasoning or a 'ground-up' approach. This means that rather than specifying hypotheses and defining concepts as the first stage of the research and then collecting data to test the hypothesis, the data themselves suggest concepts and explanations and draw attention to social processes thus leading to the generation or refinement of theories (Table 22.1). Glaser and Strauss (1967) termed this 'grounded theory' as it arises out of the categories that the participants themselves use to order their experience, rather than being based on categories that are defined at the outset by the researcher and may therefore fit poorly with the participants' perspectives.

This aim of seeing the world through the eyes of their subjects also requires that forms of data collection are relatively open and unstructured, so as not to confine responses to inappropriate categories. Various methods of data collection are employed including both primary and secondary sources (Table 22.2). Interviews provide the main source of data in qualitative research, as they do in quantitative research. The difference is that rather than involving structured questionnaires with precoded answers, a much freer format is adopted with interviews taking more the form of a conversation and they are usually tape recorded. Various terms are employed to describe the types of interviews undertaken in qualitative research and are identified here as semistructured and unstructured (or focused) interviews. In semistructured interviews respondents are asked a series of open-ended questions by interviewers trained in qualitative research. Rather than following a standard format, the order in which questions are asked or topics addressed can be varied to assist the flow of the interview. Interviewers are also free to probe as necessary to amplify and clarify responses and to follow up interesting ideas and explanations. Unstructured (or focused) interviews involve an even freer format, with respondents often being asked about a particular topic, such as their recent experience of hospital care or their views about the causes of ill health. However, the discussion is guided by the interviewer so as to focus on topics of research interest, and is therefore not completely unstructured. Focused interviews are employed when the subject matter is particularly complex or covers areas that have not previously been described. An example is Cornwell's case studies (1987) of the ideas and theories about health, illness, and health services held by people in East London. Although some standard questions were put to everyone, the interviews largely involved following up and exploring the individual's ideas. A notable feature of this study is that more than one interview was undertaken, with the second and third interviews allowing some of the themes identified in the initial interview to be explored in greater detail and therefore related to an individual's previously expressed ideas and explanations. In all 24 people were interviewed and a total of 70 hours of interviewing recorded, with notes of a further 60 hours spent in people's homes.

Another technique increasingly adopted in academic research is the use of focus groups. These are group discussions organized to explore a specific set of issues, such as people's views and experiences of health services, mental illness, AIDS, or nutrition (Morgan 1993). Most researchers rely on four or five groups with about 8 to 10 participants in each, and with the researcher acting as facilitator of the group discussion. Individual groups are generally selected to be relatively homogeneous in their social characteristics so as to promote open discussion. These normally last for one to two hours and are usually tape recorded with additional notes also being made. Focus group discussions can be particularly useful as a quick way of establishing the range of perspectives on an issue of importance among different groups. They may also encourage open conversation about embarrassing subjects and facilitate the expression of ideas and experiences that might be left underdeveloped in an interview. However, focus groups are generally viewed as stronger on breadth than depth, and tend to be influenced by general group dynamics. They are therefore often employed in the initial exploration of a topic and then followed by personal interviews (Kitzinger 1994).

Other forms of data collection occasionally employed in qualitative research are observation and the diary method. In both cases the data to be collected are less precisely defined at the outset than in quantitative research. For example, Clark and Bowling (1989) in their evaluation of the quality of life in hospitals and nursing homes, supplemented their structured observations with a less structured approach. The latter required the researchers in their role as non-participant observers to write an account of events, interactions, and moods as well as their overall impressions and remarks. Participant observation in which the researcher participates as part of the group being studied is less common, given the practical problems and ethical issues that may arise. However a notable example of this approach is Goffman's classic study of the cultural and social organization of a psychiatric hospital, based on his observations while employed as assistant to the athletic director of a large American mental hospital. This led him to develop the concept of a 'total institution' and to analyse both its causes and effects for patients and staff (Goffman 1961).

The numbers of people and settings studied using qualitative methods is generally quite small, with the emphasis being on their in-depth study and analysis. In terms of the selection of respondents, one approach is to ensure that what are perceived as relevant variables (age, sex, social class etc) are represented to ensure that the range of responses will be identified (Fitzpatrick and Boulton 1994). Another approach is to control for such variables at the outset of the study. The research may therefore focus on a particular age group, ethnic group, medical diagnosis, and so on, with the aim of studying people who are 'typical' of a defined population and thus generalizing findings to this group. The numbers of people who should be interviewed in qualitative research is often difficult to determine in advance. This is because it depends on the range of responses, which is not predetermined through the structuring of response categories. Interviews therefore often continue until the 'theoretic saturation' point is reached and further interviews do not identify new themes or explanations (Murphy and Mattison 1992).

Data in qualitative research usually consist of text (that is written words), often in the form of interview transcripts. Analysing text requires that it is first coded and classified in terms of the investigators initial concepts and categories and those arising from the material. These categories may then be regrouped to produce meaningful typologies that fit the data and associations identified (Bryman and Burgess 1993). Traditionally such analysis was undertaken manually and involved the researcher in a scissors and paste exercise in which data relating to particular themes was identified and assembled from individual transcripts, as well as being viewed within the wider context of the interview. This process is now assisted by computer programs, such as Ethnograph, which are designed for the analysis of qualitative data (Fielding and Lee 1991; Tesch 1990).

Analysing qualitative data is time consuming, as it involves a process in which text is used to both develop and test ideas. As Fitzpatrick and Boulton (1994) observe: 'A variety of intimidating terms have been developed to describe the logic of qualitative analysis including "analytic induction" and "grounded theory". In different ways such accounts emphasize one common feature – namely, that qualitative analysis is iterative. The investigator goes back and forth between his developing concepts and ideas and the raw data of texts, or ideally, fresh observations of the field.' (p. 111).

The analysis of qualitative data thus requires that the researcher is immersed in the text and is engaged in posing questions of the data and analysing responses across the study group, paying particular attention to cases that do not seem to fit. As a result of this process, new questions and more refined categories are developed until analysis and explanation have been systematically and thoroughly accomplished (Malterud 1993).

An example of the nature of the conceptual generalizations arising from qualitative research is provided by the study of Scambler and Hopkins (1990) of 108 people with epilepsy. The respondents comprised people aged 16 years and over, who were identified from general practice records as having experienced at least one epileptic seizure in the last two years and/or were on anticonvulsant drugs and had more than one non-febrile seizure in the past. Through semistructured interviews, the researchers elicited detailed accounts of people's beliefs, worries and experiences of this condition. Content analysis of this interview data led Scambler and Hopkins to develop the notions of 'felt' and 'enacted' stigma to describe the social meanings of epilepsy and its implications for their lives. Felt stigma referred to the shame associated with 'being epileptic', and most significantly to the fear of being discriminated against solely on the grounds of an imputed cultural unacceptability or inferiority, while enacted stigma refers to actual discrimination of this kind. Felt stigma was shown to lead to non-disclosure and concealment which in turn placed considerable costs on individuals. However, the success of these strategies reduced their likelihood of encountering enacted stigma or the actual experience of discrimination and exclusion. As a result, felt stigma was more disruptive of people's lives and well-being and formed for many people the major burden of their epilepsy. This research thus identified generalizable social meanings and process relating to the experience of epilepsy and made an important contribution at this conceptual level. However, questions of the prevalence of felt and enacted stigma and their distribution among different age groups or by other social or medical variables, would require a larger quantitative study in which notions of felt and enacted stigma were precisely operationalized and measured using a structured questionnaire. This has formed an important further stage leading on from the initial identification of these concepts and meanings (Jacoby 1992).

Whereas some qualitative enquiries contribute new conceptual categories and classifications, a more general contribution of qualitative research is in terms of the explanations and understandings that are derived. These often differ from the findings of quantitative methods, as the freer format of interviews is more likely to elicit people's 'private account', or the way in which a person would respond if thinking only what he and the people he knows directly would think and do. In contrast, structured questionnaires elicit what Cornwell (1984) refers to as individuals' knowledge or 'public account', in terms of the aspects of their ideas, experience and values that people believe are acceptable. As Cornwell acknowledges, both types of accounts are selective and partial, while the extent to which they differ depends on the degree of perceived acceptability of an individual's private account. For example, when asked about their use of prescribed medications in a quantitative study, patients frequently report what they regard as medically expected behaviours which generally has the effect of overestimating 'compliance'. However, in open interviews patients often describe their personal beliefs and medication practices, even though aware that this departs from professional expectations (Morgan and Watkins 1988). A second difference is that whereas quantitative data are subjected to reductionist techniques and analysed as individual variables, qualitative research is based on content analysis which involves examining beliefs and actions in their broader context and may thus contribute differing understanding and explanations.

Differences between qualitative and quantitative research in the nature of the data and forms of analysis is also associated with differences in the presentation of research findings. Quantitative data is analysed statistically and presented in tabular form, whereas research papers based on qualitative methods often include case material in terms of verbatim statements to convey the main themes and ideas discussed. Quantification when employed is limited to identifying the numbers of people who share similar experiences, views or behaviours. In contrast with quantitative research, the findings of qualitative research are generally discussed as they are presented. This format thus departs from the rigid distinction between results and discussion that is characteristic of the scientific model, and underlines the differing philosophies and approaches of these two research methodologies.

Assessment of qualitative research

Epidemiology and the clinical sciences have traditionally been critical of qualitative research. This is because its assumptions and methods diverge from the traditions of scientific research that underpin their own disciplines and which have yielded significant contributions to knowledge. In contrast, qualitative research is seen as less rigorous or objective, and less generalizable, and therefore as less meritorious. As a result, opportunities for funding and publication in public health and medical journals have traditionally been limited.

One of the main criticisms of qualitative research relates to the small numbers of respondents or situations that are studied (usually 12 to 100 respondents), which is regarded as limiting the generalizability of the results. However, this criticism largely reflects a misunderstanding of the aims of qualitative research. Qualitative research does not aim to achieve statistical generalization in terms of X per cent with Y characteristic. Rather the aim is conceptual generalization in terms of identifying general social categories, processes and explanations. These differing aims thus have different methodological requirements in terms of sample size and methods of data collection, analysis and validation. However, although qualitative research is based on relatively small numbers of people, it is important that their selection and characteristics are clearly described, so that the applicability of the findings is clear.

A second common criticism of qualitative research concerns the possibilities of bias. The requirement for researchers to be actively involved in directing interviews and probing ideas and explanations is regarded as affording particular scope for individuals' personal beliefs and values to influence the information elicited, while the close involvement of the researcher with those being studied is also recognized to place considerable demands on the researcher (Oakley 1981; Cannon 1989). However, although the subjective influence of the investigator on the conduct of research is greater in qualitative research, this subjectivity is not excluded in quantitative research given that the researcher's beliefs and values influences the

selection of variables for study and the construction of questionnaires thus determines the research framework. The researcher
also makes choices regarding the analyses undertaken, and is
frequently engaged in a process of interpreting responses to very
specific questions which involves supplying meaning in idiosyncratic or culturally patterned ways (Cicourel 1964). Research of
whatever form is thus a social act. However, a major difference and
often greater problem for qualitative research is that the choices
and decisions made by the investigators are generally less apparent
or subject to formal rules. It is therefore important that researchers
give clear details of the research process, including the characteristics and selection of study groups, and the ways in which they
conducted the analysis, as well as taking account of cases that do
not fit categories or explanations developed. In addition, researchers employing qualitative methods should adopt a vigorous
approach to checking their findings and assessing validity. In
qualitative research this refers to assessing the validity of second-
order constructs, or meanings and explanations derived from the
data, rather than assessing the validity of the data on which they
were based.

One approach to checking the validity of explanations developed
in qualitative research is through 'triangulation', which literally
involves looking at things from more than one direction (Denzin
1978). This requires that data are collected from multiple sources
to corroborate an overall interpretation and is therefore fairly
similar to the process of establishing construct validity in quantitative research. For example, an investigation by Dent (1990) of the
ways in which the clinical division of labour between doctors and
nurses in the renal units of two hospitals shaped the ways in which
the computer system was utilized, was based on tape recorded
semistructured interviews, observations of meetings, clinics and
nursing activities, and the review of the documents and minutes of
meetings. He also employed what is termed respondent validation.
This requires that the study subjects or other respondents are given
an opportunity to comment on the constructs and explanations
derived by the researcher, so as to check that they accord with
people's experiences and perceptions and are therefore credible in
these terms.

As Guba and Lincoln (1981) note, credibility rather than
internal validity in the quantitative sense is the criterion by which
the true value of qualitative research requires to be evaluated. As
they state: 'A qualitative study is credible when it presents such
faithful descriptions or interpretations of a human experience that
the people having that experience would immediately recognize it
from those descriptions or interpretations as their own'. This form
of respondent validation was undertaken by the author in relation
to a study of white and Afro-Caribbean hypertensive patients
(Morgan and Watkins 1988). Large numbers of Afro-Caribbean
patients acknowledged that they regularly 'left off' the prescribed
antihypertensive drugs for a few days each week, or for a week or
two at a time. This did not appear to reflect a lack of knowledge of
medical expectations, or a lack of awareness and concern about
their high blood pressure and increased risks of cardiovascular
disease. Instead their medication practices could be understood in
terms of their traditional cultural beliefs and practices, which
appear to both have heightened their concerns about possible long-
term harmful effects of drug treatment, and also provided an
alternative resource in terms of their continued use of herbal

remedies. This explanation for non-adherence with antihypertensive medication among Afro-Caribbean patients was checked with
other Afro-Caribbean people to ensure that the researchers' analysis and interpretation 'made sense' to them. The study findings
were also presented to local general practitioners who found that as
a result they felt able to overcome a cultural barrier and 'open up'
the consultations with their Afro-Caribbean hypertensive patients,
thus achieving what they regarded as a more successful encounter
(Morgan 1995). This provided further evidence of the validity of
the research findings and corresponds to what has been referred to
as pragmatic validity, which means that a hypothesis or theory is
valid when it is applicable in further studies or in everyday practice
(Kvale 1987). However, occasionally participants may have various
reasons for not agreeing with analyses of their behaviours, which in
itself may comprise further data (Silverman 1993).

In common with research generally, the most important means
of ensuring the validity of qualitative studies is through the rigour
of the methods employed. It is also important that researchers
provide the reader with a clear description of the methods,
including how the subjects were selected, the interviewing or other
techniques employed, how the analysis was carried out, and
whether any themes (especially counter themes) have been excluded
from the analysis (Sandelowski 1986).

A further problem for qualitative research is the tendency to
designate as 'qualitative' any research that does not satisfy the
requirements of quantitative research, for example in terms of
sample size. The term is also often applied fairly loosely to include
the exploratory interviews undertaken to develop a structured
questionnaire, or the inclusion of a few open questions in an
otherwise structured questionnaire. These uses of open questions
do not comprise qualitative research but rather provide exploratory
or illustrative material for use within a quantitative framework.

Whereas quantitative and qualitative research are often depicted
in terms of a conflict of methods, what is important is to
acknowledge their differing contributions, and to employ in a
rigorous way whichever research methodology is appropriate in
relation to the particular questions being asked. Quantitative and
qualitative research may also occasionally be incorporated within a
single project to address different questions. This is illustrated by
a study of disability in the community (Patrick and Peach 1989), in
which the main emphasis was to assess the prevalence of disability,
the demands on services and the effects of disability on income
levels and working practices – all quantitative methods. However,
this material was complemented by a study based on semistructured interviews with 24 people who were moderately to
severely disabled by rheumatoid arthritis. These interviews examined peoples perceptions of the impact of rheumatoid arthritis on
their life and life prospects, and their ways of coping with the
condition and the disability and disadvantage it caused, and thus
complemented the quantitative data by giving greater insight into
the meanings of arthritis for this group of people.

A second way in which quantitative and qualitative approaches
may directly complement each other is when the concepts and
explanations developed in qualitative studies are subsequently
operationalized and measured using structured questionnaires and
standard rating scales, to assess the prevalence of these characteristics and categories. For example, research identifying the meanings of stigma has enabled the development of stigma rating scales

and their application in large-scale surveys (Macdonald 1988; Jacoby 1992). Studies of the subjective experience and impact of ill health similarly identified the social and psychological outcomes of disease, and were the basis for the conceptualization and measurement of disability and of subjective health status (Bowling 1991; Jenkinson 1994). More generally, qualitative research may often reorient research in new directions by providing new explanations and understandings which may then be examined using quantitative as well as qualitative methods.

Few studies have attempted to integrate systematically quantitative and qualitative methods and data within a single study, with the notable exception of the Brown and Harris (1978) study of the causes of depression among middle-class and working-class women. This research investigated the influence of various vulnerability and protective factors on risks of developing depression, including the women's experience of life events and the quality of their social support, and thus focused on one of the central issues of social epidemiological research. The approach adopted by Brown and Harris was informed by the requirements of quantification. For example, the women were drawn from households selected at random from local authority records, depression was identified using a shortened version of the Present State Examination, and the effects of various risk and vulnerability factors were examined using statistical methods. Their approach to the measurement of life events and social support was unique in combining the quantification of these concepts with an assessment of their subjective meanings for individuals.

Traditionally life events have been quantified in epidemiological studies using the Holmes–Rahe Social Readjustment Rating Scale (Holmes and Rahe 1967) or one of its many modifications. This consists of a standard checklist of life events in which each event is assigned a score to indicate its severity, defined as the amount of readjustment required, with these scores being derived on the basis of previous scaling studies. The use of uniform scores, while recognizing that events differ in their severity, nevertheless assumes that everyone experiencing a particular type of life event (such as widowhood, divorce, changing job, moving house, etc) undergoes a similar amount of readjustment. In the same way, social support is usually assessed by asking respondents a series of questions about the number and types of social contacts they experience. Respondents are then assigned a support score based on the researcher's fairly arbitrary method for combining this data, with no assessment being made by respondents of the adequacy of their level of support (Cohen and Syme 1985). In contrast to this traditional approach, Brown and Harris (1978) wished to elicit the women's own views about their life events and support, recognizing that the stressfulness of life events and the quality of support depend on individuals' subjective assessments. They therefore first elicited the respondents' own feelings and experiences of their life events and social support in in-depth interviews. This material was then analysed by employing carefully defined criteria by which to assess the women's personal experience of life events. This included the perceived short-term threat of a life event, its long-term threat, the feelings of anxiety it produced, etc. The quality of their social ties was similarly elicited through interviews and rated numerically on predefined scales. This use of standard rating scales meant that a uniform method of assessment was applied to the women's own descriptions of their experiences and was preferable to requiring

the respondents themselves to make judgements of the severity of the life events they experienced, or the strength of their social support. This is because the criteria employed in making such judgements is likely to vary between respondents and may also be influenced in retrospective assessments by whether or not the life event resulted in subsequent illness. These considerations emphasize the problems of measurement in social science research, and the particular difficulties that may arise in establishing causality using quantitative methods, given that human beings actively interpret situations and respond on the basis of subjective meanings.

Whereas the insights derived from qualitative social science research have influenced thinking in the field of public health over many years it is only fairly recently that qualitative methods have begun to gain official recognition and acceptance. This change is marked by papers in key medical and public health journals devoted to a consideration of qualitative research methods and their potential contribution to health service issues and medical care. For example, Black (1994) in an editorial in the *Journal of Epidemiology and Community Health* entitled 'Why we need qualitative research', identified several ways in which this form of research may enhance our understanding of health service issues. Fitzpatrick and Boulton (1994) present a similar message in the *Journal of Quality in Health Care*, as do Pope and Mays (1993) in the *British Medical Journal*. The contribution of qualitative research has also formed the subject of recent editorials in epidemiological and family practice journals (Murphy and Mattison 1992; Britten and Fisher 1993; Holman 1993). As Holman (1993) notes, what is important is that the methods employed should fit the question asked, not vice versa. However, he believes that the almost sole recognition given to quantitative methods has delayed the development of essential medical knowledge, and concludes that: ' . . . good medical research requires recognizing the complementary and interpenetration of quantitative and qualitative methods of inquiry. When qualitative methods are clearly established in our research repertoire, the advance of medical knowledge will be greatly accelerated.' An example he cites is the contributions of qualitative research to an understanding of the meaning of chronic illness for patients, which has implications for both the design of treatment programmes and the programmes' success.

Areas of sociological investigation

Sociological investigations in the field of public health cover a broad area, given that most aspects of health, disease and illness, and the organization, provision and evaluation of health services have important social aspects and dimensions. A broad classification of research themes by Spruit and Kromhout (1987) based on the 1985 volume of *Social Science and Medicine* provides an indication of the range of sociological research (Table 22.3). However, the specific content of these themes and their relative importance tends to vary between countries and changes over time, reflecting what are currently perceived as problems, priorities and areas of concern. New areas of research in recent years include sociological investigations of beliefs about HIV/AIDS and studies of sexual behaviours as a basis for understanding patterns of transmission of this condition and for developing appropriate health education materials and service provision in response to the new threat of this disease. Likewise, developments in DNA probes and genetic

Table 22.3 Research themes in social science and medicine

Health care structure, behaviour, policy etc.

Social categories, structural factors and disease

Patient behaviour, doctor–patient relationship, health care utilization

Behaviour, sociomedical factors/characteristics, health and sociomedical consequences

Psychosocial and other consequences of disease and disability

Social construction of health, illness and patienthood

Health and illness behaviour and beliefs

Based on analysis of 1985 volume by Spruit and Kromhout (1987)

screening have opened up new areas of research concerned with the social and psychological outcomes of different screening strategies and styles of counselling. Similarly, the changes occurring in many countries in the financing and organization of health services had led to research concerned with implementing and evaluating these new forms of provision, as well as greater concerns with issues of the quality and acceptability of health service provision. Although sociological investigations in the field of public health are often responsive to changes in patterns of disease, new clinical technologies, and developments in health policies, priorities and provision of services, they are also influenced by more general developments in sociology itself including new theories, methods of research, and concepts developed by sociologists specializing in other subfields.

It is difficult to determine precise disciplinary boundaries or their contributions to public health, as epidemiology, sociology, psychology, anthropology and other disciplines frequently draw on and share common concepts, explanations and measures, while research is often based on multidisciplinary teams. However, while recognizing the complex overlapping between different disciplines and bodies of knowledge, this section will identify some of the ways in which sociology has contributed to particular areas and issues within the public health field.

Social patterning and causes of disease

Both epidemiology and sociology have a common interest in the social causes of disease. For epidemiology a principal aim is to uncover risk factors for specific diseases by studying the distribution of disease in populations. Themes in epidemiology thus often centre around particular diseases or disease groups, like respiratory diseases, cardiovascular diseases and cancer. Factors like age and sex, ethnicity, socio-economic group, and personal behaviours such as smoking, diet and alcohol intake, are all regarded as potential risk factors for disease, as are genetic and environmental factors. The emphasis is thus to identify the association and causal pathways between these individual risk factors and specific diseases and to achieve biological inferences. However, the finding that for example coronary heart disease is related to socio-economic status raises questions of what particular aspects of socio-economic position may be responsible for this association, thus drawing on sociological knowledge of the concept and meanings of socio-economic position. In this way sociology contributes directly to epidemiological questions.

The questions posed for sociologists in relation to the social causes of disease relate more broadly to the general social pattening of mortality and morbidity rates (Macintyre 1986, 1994). For example, there is a general pattern across most countries of increasing mortality rates with declining socio-economic position, with this holding for most individual causes of death and fitting a linear rather than a threshold model. This raises questions of when such differences begin in the life cycle, and how they are caused in terms of the particular aspects and characteristics of socio-economic status that increase health risks and produce higher morbidity and mortality rates (Davey et al. 1992). Other social categories including gender, marital state and ethnicity are similarly associated with a social patterning of disease. For example, across countries and over time there is a general pattern of lower age standardized mortality rates among married compared with non-married people for almost all causes of death, with the highest rates usually occurring among divorced people (Morgan 1980). Moreover in all contemporary industrial countries men have higher death rates and a shorter expectation of life than women, whereas women appear to have higher morbidity rates, leading to a situation in which 'women get sick and men die'. A small component of this pattern is probably attributable to physiological sex differences which protects women from some genetic disorders and other conditions with high risks of death, although rendering them more vulnerable to disorders of the reproductive system and conditions associated with considerable morbidity but low mortality rates. However, a more important factor is regarded as being the differences in the social expectations, lifestyles and behaviours of men and women, and thus in gender differences (Verbrugge 1985; Wingard et al. 1989).

These associations between social position and rates of morbidity and mortality thus raise questions of the ways in which these social categories influence their occupants' general susceptibility or risks of disease and death. One type of explanation focuses on the conditions of life of different social groups and their association with differences in mortality risks. For example, explanations of inequalities in health among socio-economic groups raises questions of the effects of differences in their material conditions of life for both mental and physical health, including differences in housing conditions, working conditions, environmental conditions, and the effects of poverty both in current and previous generations (Whitehead 1987). Similarly, the ways in which the social roles of men and women, particularly the nature of their work roles, influences health and illness behaviours has formed a major area of research (Arber *et al.* 1985). Second, there are questions of the nature and effects of differences in life-styles among social groups, including differences in diet, patterns of exercise and smoking, and the uptake of medical care and preventive health services. Third, there is a possibility that less fit people may be selected into (or out of) particular marital or socio-economic groups, thus contributing to the maintenance of the observed differentials. There is some evidence to support this notion (compatible with a functionalist theory of stratification) of more healthy women being recruited to or remaining in a higher socio-economic position at marriage, and less healthy people experiencing downward drift or a lack of upward mobility (Illsley 1980). Fourth, notions of the social construction of official statistics have focused on possible artefactual explanations. For example a factor that may contribute to the relatively high recorded mortality rates among unskilled workers in the United Kingdom is the difference surrounding the recording of occupational position at census (the denominator) and death registration (the numerator), which may serve to increase the recorded numbers of deaths and mortality rates in the lowest socio-economic group (Macintyre and West 1991). Similarly, the higher recorded morbidity rates among women may partly reflect the differing social images of men and women, and result in doctors more readily labelling women as 'sick' and prescribe drugs, thus increasing their officially sanctioned and recorded morbidity (Verbrugge and Steiner 1985).

Research examining the relationship between social categories and rates of morbidity and mortality at a macro-level and investigations of the causes and effects of particular subgroups, such as the unemployed and homeless, has served to complement and expand epidemiological enquiries by 'unpacking' these social variables and identifying those aspects of their conditions of life or behaviours associated with increased health risks. Knowledge of the extent and causes of variations in smoking, diet and other health behaviours among social groups has also been of importance in informing the design of health promotion strategies (Thorogood 1992), while investigations of the structural sources of inequalities in health provides a framework for the formulation of effective policies for their alleviation or control, and thus contributes to the broader role of public health in promoting the health of populations (Blane 1985; Ashton and Seymour 1988).

Measures of health status and quality of life

Health status measures consist of multidimensional measures which cover physical, social and psychological aspects of ill health. They are regarded as subjective measures in that they consist of a schedule of questions which record individuals' perception of their own health, rather than relying on clinical measures. These measures may be designed to assess the impact and experience of particular medical conditions (disease specific measures) or be more broadly based to be applicable to a wide range of diseases (generic measures). A large number of health status measures of each type are now available and differ in their length, the content of questions, the method of weighting or assessing severity, and whether the results are presented as category scores or an overall global score can be derived (for reviews see McDowell and Newell 1987; Bowling 1991). The three most widely used generic health status measures are the 38 item Nottingham Health Profile (NHP) which covers 6 domains of health (Hunt and McEwen 1980), the 136 item Sickness Impact Profile which covers 12 areas of health (Bergner *et al.* 1981), and the 36 item Short Form (SF36) developed from the Rand Corporation Medical Outcomes Study (Ware 1993).

There is no precise definition of the content and coverage of health status measures, or what are often referred to as measures of health related quality of life. Instead these terms tend to be applied to patient assessed measures of health which cover more than one dimension of physical function, social function, emotional or mental state, burden or symptoms and some of well-being. However, a general trend over time has been the expansion in the scope and coverage of patient assessed measures. Whereas early measures mainly focused on limitations in self-care they now generally include a large number of activities and feeling states (Ziebland *et al.* 1993). Second, whereas such health measures were initially 'subjective' purely in terms of recording patients' self-assessments rather being completed by an observer or clinician, these items are now generally derived from data collected in informal interviews examining the impact of ill health for lay people in social, psychological and behavioural terms. Similarly, the severity weights attached to items in areas such as the NHP and SIP are derived from empirical rating studies and thus to some extent reflect lay assessments. Recently a third approach has been developed which allows greater personal subjectivity. This replaces a uniform schedule of questions and severity weights with a Patient Generated Index (PGI). The PGI is developed for individual patients in three stages. First, patients list the five most important areas or activities of their life affected by their condition. Second, they are asked to rate how badly they are affected in their chosen areas on a scale from zero to 100. Third, they are given 60 points to choose to spread across one or more areas to reflect the relative importance they attach to improvements in these areas. These different ratings can then be used to calculate an individual's quality of life index and are summed across patients (Ruta and Garratt 1994).

Sociologists involvement in the field of health status measurement came partly at a technical level through their participation in multidisciplinary teams concerned with developing, testing and applying these measures in evaluative studies. However, sociological investigations also provided a conceptual framework which encouraged the development of subjective health status measures by demonstrating the differences between medical definitions of disease as assessed by various clinical indicators and peoples' experience of ill health. For example, individuals' subjective assessment and experience of ill health was shown to be more closely related to illness behaviour than were clinical measures of disease severity, with the effects of ill health on their everyday activities being a major trigger influencing professional help-seeking (Zola 1973). It has also frequently been demonstrated that individuals' experience and assessments of their health do not necessarily correlate with clinical measures. For example, spirometric measures of lung function tend to be only weakly related to the experience of breathlessness, physical disability and the psychosocial aspects of life among patients with chronic respiratory disease (Williams 1993). Such diversities between patients' evaluations and clinical measurements were often regarded as evidence of patients' lack of knowledge and ability to assess their health state. However, an interpretive approach within sociology, with its acknowledgement of multiple realities and focus on individual meanings provided the basis for patient centred measures through studies of the content of patients conceptions of health and their subjective experience of ill health.

A pioneering study examining lay conceptions of health was conducted by Herzlich (1973) in the 1960s based on semistructured interviews with 80 adults in France. This identified four conceptions of health held by lay people. Health as the 'absence of disease' formed just one, with others consisting of health as 'functional fitness' (with assessments of ill health thus depending on the extent to which a condition is disruptive of their ability to perform their everyday activities) the notion of a 'reserve' of overall health (determined in large part by the individual's constitution), and health as a positive state of 'well-being'. Lay evaluations of health, thus reflect concepts and criteria which often differ from a medical model, with health assessed in terms of a reserve of health or well-being often being perceived as compatible with the presence of chronic disease. Similarly, studies of patients' experience of chronic illness and disability identify the ways in which the impacts of medical conditions extend beyond the biomedical sphere, in terms of their effects on physical functioning, social interactions and relationships, emotional well-being and other aspects of quality of life (Albrecht 1976; Locker 1983).

Studies of patients' concepts and experiences of health and illness thus identified important differences between lay and medical perspectives, and encouraged the adoption of a broader social model of health and patient-based evaluations. The rapid expansion in research in this area also reflects the increased prevalence of chronic conditions, causing considerable disability, and the greater emphasis on the evaluation of health outcomes so as to provide more effective provision and a greater efficiency of resource use.

Social processes and organizational efficiency

A central concern of health services research is to increase the efficiency and effectiveness of service provision. This requires that efficient and effective methods of service organization and delivery are identified and that they are then widely adopted and implemented. The traditional means of establishing the effectiveness and efficiency of new procedures or forms of organization is through conducting randomized controlled trials (RCTs). Sociological investigations have been important in expanding the range of outcomes assessed in such trials to include patient satisfaction, and to supplement conventional clinical outcome measures by subjective health status measures (Hopkins and Costain 1994). Both these aspects have now achieved the status of a general expectation and requirement of evaluative studies. New directions and contributions of sociological investigations are stemming from the demonstration of the value of qualitative methods and pluralistic models in contributing to an understanding of social processes, which assists with both the identification of organizational problems and the implementation of change.

One example of the way in which an understanding of social processes may contribute to organizational efficiency is provided by research on waiting lists. In the United Kingdom waiting lists for surgery are common and both their length and waiting times are of great public and professional concern. Most research on waiting lists has been quantitative and has been concerned with examining the characteristics of waiting lists and identifying ways of reducing

their size and time. However, most interventions to reduce the waiting list backlog have had little long-term impact (Morgan 1992). This may largely reflect the organization of lists, which have traditionally been viewed by both patients and professionals as akin to a bus queue in which someone joins the end and works their way up to the front. A qualitative study involving interviews with patients, doctors and administrative staff and observation of hospital records departments led to the identification of several limitations of rational queue theory as applied to waiting lists, and showed that the actions of hospital personnel and patients mitigate against an orderly queue (Pope 1991). A different conceptual model was therefore put forward. This viewed waiting lists as more akin to a 'store', with those who work within it acting as storekeepers. Doctors select from the store so as to provide a mix of cases on their operating lists and to make efficient and effective use of their skills. Given that waiting lists functioned as a sign of demand and therefore prestige, doctors also did not have powerful incentives to reduce their lists. Waiting lists clerks have a different set of priorities, with their main goal being the smooth running of the office. They were therefore less likely to select patients who are not on the phone, or have been on the list for a long time, often years, and are therefore difficult to contact, or patients who refused one offer of admission. As a result, such 'difficult' patients comprised the waiting list backlog, which has not been substantially affected by computerization or other new management techniques. Of importance in reducing waiting lists was thus the need to influence the way in which lists were managed, which formed a product of the varying interests of the different occupational groups involved.

A second example of the role of qualitative research in uncovering underlying social processes is Bloor's research on adenotonsillectomy (Bloor 1976). This study examined the causes of the different profile of surgical work performed by different surgeons, as represented in the well documented variations in rates of common operative procedures between hospitals and geographic areas (Wennberg et al. 1987). Bloor's observational study of ear, nose and throat out-patient clinics showed there to be systematic variations between consultants in their assessment routines, which were rooted in differences in their informal decision-making rules. This underlying cause of the observed variation in surgical rates had been largely omitted from and neglected by previous research This is because the main emphasis of traditional quantitative studies was to explain the variations in rates of operative procedures in terms of hypothesized differences in 'need', arising from the morbidity of populations and differences in the availability of surgical beds.

The demonstration of differences both within and between professional groups in their interests, priorities, philosophies of care and training, has implications for the successful implementation and adoption of change both at an individual and organizational level. For example, barriers to the successful introduction and implementation of clinical guidelines and audit, include the differences in priorities and practice styles that may exist among doctors, especially between hospital specialists and primary care physicians. New forms of service organization, such as an increased emphasis on community based services, or a greater involvement of nurses in clinical work, may also be resisted by doctors if these changes are perceived as reducing their status, job satisfaction, patient contact or other aspects of their work (Black and Thomson 1993). The importance of acknowledging and responding to such beliefs and concerns as part of the process of implementing change is increasingly recognized. However, this contrasts with the traditional rational model of change, which assumed that the provision of information and education or clinical guidelines identifying optimum care, and the demonstration of efficient forms of organization will necessarily be accepted and change behaviours in the desired direction. Similarly, Smith and Cantley (1985) advocate that the differing interests, interpretations of success, and strategies employed by key groups within an organization should be identified and incorporated into organizational evaluations. They demonstrate this approach in their evaluation of a psychogeriatric day hospital. This evaluation involved interviews with different groups of staff and a sample of patients' relatives, data extracted from hospital records, and observations of meetings and of the general activities and life of the day hospital. Smith and Cantley believe that such 'pluralistic' evaluations will lead to a better understanding of why failures or successes occur, and how performance might be improved. They also note that all too often the results of evaluative exercises are dismissed because the criteria employed in their assessments do not accord with the criteria of success held by many groups within the organization.

Conclusions

The areas of sociological research in public health are wide-ranging, given that health, disease and illness, the organization and provision of medical care and the development and implementation of preventive programmes, all have important social aspects and dimensions. The contributions of sociology arise from its techniques of enquiry and its body of knowledge concerning the nature and influence of social factors and social processes such as social class, disability, and illness behaviour both at a micro-level and in terms of broader social structures. Some research is concerned with the measurement and application of these social variables, while other research aims to develop new understanding of social phenomena drawing on particular theories of society and may be informed by a structural or social action perspective.

It is difficult to determine precise disciplinary boundaries and their contribution to public health, as each discipline draws on concepts and methods developed in other disciplines. The concepts, insights and explanations derived from a particular disciplinary perceptive thus often become incorporated over time into the general body of knowledge in the field. For example, socio-psychological knowledge of stressful life events and coping, sociological concepts of social support, social mobility and stigma, and epidemiological knowledge of the distribution and risk factors for specific diseases, all now form part of a general body of knowledge in the field. As Spruit and Kromhout (1987) observe: 'medical sociological research has established that attitudinal, behavioural and structural factors do influence disease, so epidemiology has to include this in its philosophy. Also, the distribution of disease is part of empirical health and illness reality, so medical sociology has to include epidemiology in studying this reality' (p. 586). Second, an important contribution of sociology has been to perform an enlightenment function by drawing attention to new ways of viewing aspects of health, illness and medical care, which again may become part of the accepted wisdom in the field. For example, the

distinction between disease and patients' experience of illness is now commonplace, and subjective health status measures are employed routinely in assessing the outcome of medical care. Similarly, the problem of institutionalization associated with long-term care in rigidly organized institutions is widely acknowledged, as are the social costs to families of community care. Effective health education is also accepted to require not merely the provision of health advice, but also to address people's personal beliefs and take account of the situation and context of their lives. However, the influence of research on thinking and policy decisions is often the result of a cumulative effect rather than the product of a single study. The impact of research also often depends on the compatibility of its findings with the current economic and political framework, and with prevailing interests, priorities and concerns, and thus reflects the broader social context of the research.

Future trends in sociological research in the field of public health may include a greater emphasis on studies informed by an interpretive approach and employing qualitative methods, reflecting a greater acceptance of the value of such studies and their contribution to an understanding of social behaviours and processes. Sociological research may also increasingly be conducted within a pluralist framework, which acknowledges the importance of taking account of the interests and expectations of different groups in society in understanding behaviour and implementing changes in the health care field. More generally, the growth of new medical technologies, and changes in health care systems and in patterns of disease will continue to raise new issues for research with important social dimensions.

References

Albrecht, G.L. (ed.) (1976). *The sociology of disability and rehabilitation*. University of Pittsburgh Press, Pittsburgh.

Alford, R. (1985). *Health care policies*. University of Chicago Press, Chicago.

Arber, S., Gilbert, N., and Dale, A. (1985). Paid employment and women's health: a benefit or a source of role strain? *Sociology of Health and Illness* 7(3), 375.

Ashton, J. and Seymour, H. (1988). *The new public health*. Open University Press, Milton Keynes.

Bentzen, N., Christiansen, C., and Pedersen, K.M. (1989). Self care within a model of demand for medical care. *Social Science and Medicine*, 29, 185–93.

Bergner, M., Bobbitt, R.A., Rollard, W.E., Martin, D.P., and Gibson, B.S. (1981). The Sickness Impact Profile: development and final revision of a health status measure. *Medical Care*, 18, 787.

Black, N. (1994). Why we need qualitative research (editorial). *Journal of Epidemiology and Community Health* 48, 425–6.

Black, N.A., Thompson, E. (1993). Attitudes to medical audit: British doctors speak. *Social Science and Medicine* 36, 849.

Blane, D. (1985). An assessment of the Black Report's explanations of health inequalities. *Sociology of Health and Illness* 7, 423.

Bloor, M. (1976). Bishop Berkeley and the adenotonsillectomy enigma: an explanation of variation in the social construction of medical disposals. *Sociology* 10, 43.

Bowling, A. (1991). *Measuring health: a review of quality of life measurement scales*. Open University Press, Buckinghamshire.

Britten, N. and Fisher, B. (1993). Qualitative research and general practice. *British Journal of General Practice* (Editorial), 43, 270–71.

Brown, G.W. and Harris, T. (1978). *The social origins of depression: a study of psychiatric disorder in women*. Tavistock Publications, London.

Bryman, A. and Burgess, R. (eds.) (1993). *Analysing qualitative data*. Routledge, London.

Calnan, M. (1984). The politics of health: the case of smoking control. *Journal of Social Policy* **13**, 279.

Cannon, S. (1989). Social research in stressful settings: difficulties for the sociologist in studying the treatment of breast cancer. *Sociology of Health and Illness* **11**, 62.

Challah, S., Wing, A.J., Bauer, R., Morris, R.W., Schroeder, S.A. (1984). Negative selection of patients for dialysis and transplantation in the United Kingdom. *British Medical Journal* **284**, 1119.

Cicourel, A.V. (1964). *Method and measurement in sociology.* Free Press, New York.

Clark, P. and Bowling, A. (1989). Observational study of quality of life in NHS nursing homes and a long stay ward for the elderly. *Ageing and Society* **9**, 123.

Cohen, S. and Syme, L. (ed.) (1985). *Social support and health.* Academic Press, New York.

Conrad, P. (1976). The discovery of hyperkinesis. *Social Problems* **23**, 12.

Conrad, P. (1985). The meaning of medications: another look at compliance. *Social Science and Medicine* **20**, 29–37.

Cornwell, J. (1984). Hard earned lives: accounts of health and illness from East London. Tavistock Publication, London.

Crawford, R. (1977). You are dangerous to your health: the ideology and politics of victim blaming. *International Journal of Health Services* **7**, 663.

Davey Smith, G. and Egger, M. (1992). Socio economic differences in mortality in Britain and the United States. *American Journal of Public Health* **82**, 1079.

Davis, K. and Moore, W. E. (1945). Some principles of stratification. *American Sociological Review* **2**, 242.

Dent, M. (1990). Organization and change in renal work: a study of the impact of a computer system within two hospitals. *Sociology of Health and Illness* **12**, 413.

Denzin, N.K. (1978). *The research act in sociology.* Aldine, Chicago.

Donovan, J. and Blake, R. (1992). Patient non-compliance: deviance or reasoned decision-making? *Social Science and Medicine* **34**, 507.

Doyal, L. (1981). *The political economy of health.* Pluto Press, London.

Fielding, N. and Lee, R. (eds.) (1991.) *Using computers in qualitative research.* Sage, London.

Fitzpatrick, R. and Boulton, M. (1994). Qualitative methods for assessing health. *Quality in Health Care* **3**, 107.

Glaser, B.G. and Strauss, A.L. (1967). *The discovery of grounded theory: strategies for qualitative research.* Aldine, New York.

Goffman, E. (1961) *Asylums: essays on the social situation of mental patients and other inmates.* Doubleday, New York.

Guba, E.G. and Lincoln, Y.S. (1981). *Effective evaluation.* Jossey-Bass, San Francisco, CA.

Herzlich, C. (1973). *Health and illness.* Academic Press, London.

Holman, H.R. (1993). Qualitative enquiry in medical research. *Journal of Clinical Epidemiology* **46**, 29.

Holmes, T.H. and Rahe, R.H. (1967). The social readjustment rating scale. *Journal of Psychosomatic Research* **11**, 213.

Hopkins, A. and Costain, D. (1994). *Measuring the outcomes of medical care.* Royal College of Physicians and Kings Fund Centre, London.

Hunt, S. and McEwen, J. (1980). The development of a subjective health indicator. *Sociology of Health and Illness* **2**, 231.

Illsley, R. (1980). *Professional or public health?* Nuffield Provincial Hospitals Trust, London.

Jacoby, A. (1992). Felt versus enacted stigma: a concept revisited. Evidence from a study of people with epilepsy in remission. *Social Science and Medicine* **38**, 269.

Jenkinson, C. (ed.) (1994). *Measuring health and medical outcomes.* UCL Press, London.

King, M.B. (1989). AIDS on the death certificate: the final stigma. *British Medical Journal*, **298**, 734.

Kitzinger, J. (1994). The methodology of focus groups: the importance of interaction between research participants. *Sociology of Health and Illness* **16**, 103.

Kvale, S. (1987). Validity in the qualitative research interview. *Journal of Human Science* **1**, 37–72.

Layder, D. (1994). *Understanding social theory.* Sage, London.

Locker, D. (1983). *Disability and disadvantage.* Tavistock Publications, London.

Macdonald, L. (1988). The experience of stigma: living with rectal cancer. In *Living with chronic illness,* (ed. R. Anderson and M. Bury), Chapter 8, Allen and Unwin, London.

Macdonald, L.A., Sackett, D.L., Haynes, R.B., and Taylor, D.W. (1984). Labelling in hypertension: a review of the behavioural and psychological consequences. *Journal of Chronic Disease* **37**, 933.

Macintyre, S. (1986). The patterning of health by social position in contemporary Britain: directions for sociological research. *Social Science and Medicine* **23**, 393.

Macintyre, S. (1994). Understanding the social patterning of health. *Journal of Public Health Medicine* **16**, 53.

Macintyre, S. and West, P. (1991). Lack of class variation in health in adolescence: an artefact of an occupational measure of social class? *Social Science and Medicine* **32**, 395.

Malterud, K. (1993). Shared understanding of the qualitative research process: guidelines for the medical researcher. *Family Practice* **10**, 201.

McCann, K., Clark, D., Taylor, R., and Morrice, K. (1984). Telephone screening as a research technique. *Sociology* **18**, 393.

McDowell, I. and Newell, C. (1987). *Measuring health: a guide to rating scales and questionnaires.* Oxford University Press, New York.

Morgan, D. (ed.) (1993). *Successful focus groups.* Sage, London.

Morgan, M. (1980). Marital status, health, illness and service use. *Social Science and Medicine* **14A**, 633.

Morgan, M. (1991). The doctor–patient relationship. In *Sociology as applied to medicine* (3rd edn) (ed. G. Scambler), Ballière Tindall, London.

Morgan, M. (1992). Waiting lists. *In The best of health? The status and future of health care in the UK.* (ed. E. Beck, S. Lonsdale, S. Newman, and D. Patterson), Chapter 11. Chapman and Hall, London.

Morgan, M. (1995). The significance of ethnicity for health promotion: the use of anti-hypertensive drugs in inner London. *International Journal of Epidemiology,* **24** Suppl., 579–84.

Morgan, M. and Reynolds, A. (1991). Day surgery units: Are they attractive to nurses? *Journal of Advances in Health and Nursing Care* **1**, 59–74.

Morgan, M. and Watkins, C. (1988). Managing hypertension: beliefs and responses to medication among cultural groups. *Sociology of Health and Illness* **10**, 556.

Morgan, M., Calnan, M., and Manning, N. (1985). *Sociological approaches to health and medicine.* Routledge and Kegan Paul, London.

Morris, L.S. and Schulz, R.M. (1992). Patient compliance – an overview. *Journal of Clinical Pharmacy and Therapeutics* **17**, 283.

Murphy, E. and Mattison, B. (1992). Qualitative research and family practice: A marriage made in heaven? *Family Practice* **9**, 85.

Navarro, V. (1982). The labor process and health: A historical materialist interpretation. *International Journal of Health Services* **12**, 5.

Navarro, V. (1989). Why some countries have national health insurance, others have national health services, and the U.S. has neither. *Social Science and Medicine* **28**, 887.

Oakley, A. (1981). Interviewing women: a contradiction in terms. In *Doing feminist research,* (ed. H. Roberts). Routledge and Kegan Paul, London.

O'Brien, M. (1993). Social research and sociology. In *Researching social life,* (ed. N. Gilbert). Sage, London.

Parsons, T. (1951). *The social system.* Free Press, New York.

Patrick, D.L. and Peach, H. (ed.) (1989). *Disablement in the community.* Oxford University Press, Oxford.

Pietroni, P. (1976). Language and communication in general practice. In *Communication in the general practice surgery,* (ed. B. Tanner). Hodder and Stoughton, London.

Pollack, M., Poucheler, G. and Pierret, J. (1992). *AIDS: A problem for sociological research.* Sage, London.

Pope, C. (1991). Trouble in store: Some thoughts in the management of waiting lists. *Sociology of Health and Illness* **13**, 193–212.

Pope, C. and Mays, N. (1993). Opening the black box: an encounter in the corridors of health services research. *British Medical Journal* **306**, 315–18.

Pryor, L. (1985). Making sense of mortality. *Sociology of Health and Illness* **7**, 167.

Richardson, A. (1994). The health diary: an examination of its use as a data collection method. *Journal of Advanced Nursing* **19**, 782.

Roland, M., Bartholomew, J., Courtenay, M.F.J., Morris, R.W., and Morrell, D.C. (1986). The 'five minute' consultation: effect of time constraints on verbal communication. *British Medical Journal* **292**, 874.

Ruta, D.A. and Garratt, A.M. (1994). Health status to quality of life measurement. In *Measuring health outcomes*, (ed. C. Jenkinson). UCL Press, London.

Sandelowski, N. (1986). The problem of vigour in qualitative research. *Advances in Nursing Science* **8**, 27.

Scambler, G. and Hopkins, A. (1990). Generating a model of epileptic stigma: the role of qualitative analysis. *Social Science and Medicine* **30**, 1189–94.

Schwalbe, M.L. and Staples, C.L. (1986). Class position, work experience, and health. *International Journal of Health Services* **16**, 583.

Silverman, D. (1993). *Interpreting qualitative data*. Routledge, London.

Smith, G. and Cantley, C. (1985). *Assessing health care: a study in organizational evaluation*, Open University Press, Milton Keynes.

Spruit, I.P., and Kromhaut K., (1987). Medical sociology and epidemiology: convergences, divergences and legitimate boundaries. *Social Science and Medicine* **25**, 579.

Starr, P. (1982). *The social transformation of American medicine*. Basic Books, New York.

Stewart, M. and Roter, D. (1989). *Communicating with medical patients*. Sage, New York.

Stoate, H. (1989). Can health screening damage your health? *Journal of Royal College of General Practitioners* **39**, 193.

Stott, N. and Pill, R. (1990). 'Advice yes, dictate no'. Patient's own views on health promotion in the consultation. *Family Practice* **7**, 125.

Strauss, A. (1963). The hospital and its negotiated order. In *The hospital in modern society*, (ed. E. Freidson), Chapter 6. Free Press, New York.

Thorogood, N. (1992). What is the relevance of sociology for health promotion? In *Health promotion: disciplines and diversity*, (ed. R. Burston and G. Macdonald). Routledge, London.

Tesch, R. (1990). *Qualitative research: analysis types and software tools*. The Falmer Press, New York.

Tuckett, D., Boulton, M., Olson, C., and Williams, A. (1985). *Meetings between experts: an approach to sharing ideas on medical consultations*. Tavistock, London.

Verbrugge, L.M. (1985). Gender and health: an update on hypothesis and evidence. *Journal of Health and Social Behaviour* **26**, 156.

Verbrugge, L.M. and Steiner, R.P. (1985). Prescribing drugs to men and women. *Health Psychology* **4**, 79.

Ware, J.E. (1993). Measuring patients' views: the optimum outcome measure. SF36: a valid, reliable assessment of health from the patient's point of view. *British Medical Journal* **306**, 1429.

Wennberg, J., Freeman, J.L., and Culp, W.J. (1987). Are hospital services rationed in New Haven or over-utilised in Boston? *Lancet* **i**, 1185.

Whitehead, M. (1987). *The health divide*. Health Education Council, London.

Williams, S. (1993). *Chronic respiratory illness*. Routledge, London.

Wingard, D.L., Cohn, B.A., Kaplan, G.A., Cirillo, P.M., and Cohen, R.D. (1989). Sex differentials in morbidity and mortality risks examined by age and cause in the same cohort. *American Journal of Epidemiology* **130**, 601.

Ziebland, S., Fitzpatrick, R. and Jenkinson, C. (1993). Tacit models of disability underlying health status instruments. *Social Science and Medicine* **37**, 69.

Zola, I. (1973). Pathways to the doctor: from person to patient. *Social Science and Medicine* **7**, 677.

Zola, I. (1975). In the name of health and illness. *Social Science and Medicine*, **9**, 83–8.

23 Health education, behaviour change, and the public health

Keith Tones

Most health and medical professionals will have formed some opinion about the nature and pretensions of health education and health promotion. However, it would not be surprising if there was some confusion about the precise meaning of these two interrelated activities since they can have a multitude of meanings and philosophies. It is hoped that this chapter will help to clarify these conceptual uncertainties.

Again, even those who have only the sketchiest acquaintance with health education and health promotion are likely to raise the issue of effectiveness and ask whether health promotion 'works' and, if so, which tactics work best. Since all medical interventions should be subjected to such scrutiny, it is quite legitimate to expect health promotion to provide answers to these questions. Of course, this is not meant to be a text on evaluation and therefore only limited discussion is possible. None the less, some consideration will be given to the important matters of effectiveness and efficiency. However, the analysis of the various psychological, social, and environmental influences on human behaviour in health and illness, which is the main purpose of this chapter, should offer valuable insights into just what it means to develop an effective intervention. It is hoped that this will generate more thoughtful and realistic expectations of what health promotion might be expected to achieve.

Accordingly, in this chapter we aim to illuminate the contribution that human behaviour makes to health and illness. More particularly, we shall consider how health might be promoted and disease prevented by the judicious application of educational strategies. Prior to doing this, some brief consideration will be given to the part played by health education in the new health promotion 'movement' and how it might contribute to the public health.

Having examined the social, psychological, and environmental factors that typically influence people's health and illness behaviour, we shall describe strategies and tactics that might be adopted to influence health choices. This will involve a macrolevel analysis of how communities come to adopt new ideas and practices. It will also include a more detailed and individual focus on the principles of effective communication and will provide guidelines for the educational process.

Finally, key features of the systematic design of community-wide health promotion programmes will be discussed. This will incorporate a review of the potential as well as limitations of key settings and strategies such as mass media, school, and workplace.

Reference will also be made to the importance of the skilful use of appropriate educational methods and techniques—and, in accordance with our commitment to give some thought to the question of efficiency, some final remarks will be devoted to the thorny issue of evaluation.

Health promotion and the people's health

Health education: the ascendancy of prevention

Before considering further the role of health education in influencing people's health choices, it may be helpful to provide a reminder of certain historic circumstances that have contributed to its recent development. Over a period of some 150 years, what might be described as a rise, fall, and resurrection of public health occurred in 'developed' countries. During this time three phenomena with special significance for health education and health promotion were recorded: first, there was a substantial improvement in the health of the population (as measured by increased life expectancy and a reduction in premature death); second, there was a general rise in living standards; third, the status, power (and cost) of curative medicine was significantly enhanced. Health education has figured at various stages in this 'public health career'—if not as a star performer, then at least in a supportive role.

Some form of education (or, more accurately, propaganda!) was present in the great days of the first public health movement in the nineteenth century. Typically, this took the form of pamphleteering and what would now be called 'advocacy' for the implementation of various social and sanitary reforms. However, health education emerged as a professional activity sometime later and paralleled an increasing disillusionment with what many considered to be the failure of curative medicine to fulfil its early promise. It is neither desirable nor possible to do justice here to the well-rehearsed arguments about the limitations of modern medicine. However, these might be summarized as follows.

- Medicine was not succeeding in curing the 'new generation' of chronic degenerative diseases.

- Its attempts to do so were involving escalating cost (together with a degree of iatrogenesis and, arguably, a loss of its traditional caring function).

- What might not be cured should be prevented.

- Human behaviour was intimately implicated in the aetiology and management of preventable disease.

- People should be persuaded to adopt life-styles and behaviours in the interest of disease prevention and (particularly latterly) in order to save money for increasingly hard-pressed health services.

Thus health education became closely involved with preventive medicine. Its twofold task was to prevent disease at the primary, secondary, and tertiary levels and to promote the proper use of medical services. In order to achieve these aims, it was expected to cajole or coerce people into adopting life-styles that would prevent, according to contemporary epidemiological wisdom, the onset of any given disease. The populace should also be persuaded to use appropriate screening services to detect precursor deviations from normality and asymptomatic disease. Finally, they should learn how to deal with signs and symptoms in an approved fashion, for example by taking treatable conditions to a medical practitioner at an early stage while accommodating to 'trivial' or self-limiting conditions and/or subscribing to sensible self-medication.

In addition to its secondary prevention function, health education also had a role in tertiary prevention. This would include such measures as fostering compliance with medication regimes in order to prevent relapse and helping people readjust to normal life after having experienced some disabling condition.

The values and practices associated with the form of health education described above constitute what is typically described, for obvious reasons, as a **preventive medical model**. It is important to note at this juncture that this preventive model has been subjected to sharp criticism for a number of reasons. In short, while the importance of preventing disease has not been challenged, the traditional preventive approach to health education outlined above is considered to be of very limited effectiveness. Moreover, its ideological foundation—the values and assumptions about people and society on which it is based—is considered to be inappropriate to a modern democratic society. This critique is particularly important in the context of the present chapter since it reflects the philosophy to which the World Health Organization (WHO) subscribed in its *Health for All* movement (of which health promotion could legitimately be called its 'militant wing'). Accordingly, we shall now briefly consider the main features of health promotion and its relation to health education.

The meaning of health promotion

A full discussion of the nature of health promotion and its relationship with health education cannot be entertained here. A more complete analysis is provided by Tones and Tilford (1994). First of all, we should note that the concept of health promotion is essentially contested; it has a variety of meanings and thus is used to describe a number of different activities, many of which may be based on different philosophies. For instance, the 'health promotion clinics' recently created in British general medical practice could best be described in terms of the preventive medical model described above. In contrast, the model of health promotion used in this chapter incorporates the key features of the concept as developed by the WHO (1984) and embodied in the Ottawa Charter (WHO 1986).

Health promotion and the health field concept

One of the influences on the concept of health promotion was a notion popularized by the Lalonde (1974) report on the health of Canadians, which described the **health field**. This simple map of 'health territory' asserts that there are four main 'inputs' to individual health:

- genetic predisposition

- the health services

- individual behaviour and life-style

- environmental circumstances.

Health promotion is typically involved with three of these inputs: it is concerned to promote health by seeking to influence life-style, health services, and, above all, environment. Apart from some passing consideration of genetic counselling, the 'inherited' aspects of health receive little attention. It is the environment that is considered to have the major influence on individual health.

Health promotion is concerned not only with the physical environment but also with the cultural and socio-economic circumstances that substantially determine health status. Accordingly, a major emphasis of the Ottawa Charter (WHO 1986) is placed on the importance of 'building healthy public policy'. In short, just as the nineteenth-century public health movement owed its success to legislative, economic, and engineering measures, these same measures should be deployed to address late-twentieth-century health problems. To be sure, problems such as pollution and environmental degradation may have a different character in the twentieth century, but they are still problems. Moreover, the age-old problems of poverty and inequity are still with us. Accordingly, if we are serious about health promotion, then what is rather glibly called the 'political will' must be harnessed to the task of tackling unhealthy environments and implementing healthy policy. Following the precepts of health promotion, health services must be revitalized. This involves two related measures. First, it should be recognized that a whole range of public services and institutions have an effect on health which is often substantial. Housing, transport, and economic policies, for example, can all promote or militate against health. Secondly, medical services should be 'reoriented' to meet the real needs of consumers.

The 'empowerment' of communities and individuals figures prominently in the WHO's lexicon of health promotion principles: people should become actively involved in fostering the health of their communities; they should be helped to acquire an increasing sense of control over their lives. Accordingly, as part of the related process of demedicalization, there should be a shift in the balance of power between doctor and client. Co-operation and empowered patient choice should replace the traditional emphasis on 'compliance'. Human dignity, quality of life, and quality of care should be central concerns for health services. In short, five principles encapsulate the WHO's ideology of health promotion.

- Health is a positive state; it is an essential commodity, which people need in order to achieve a socially and economically productive life.

- Substantial progress in health promotion depends on rectifying inequalities in health within and between nations.

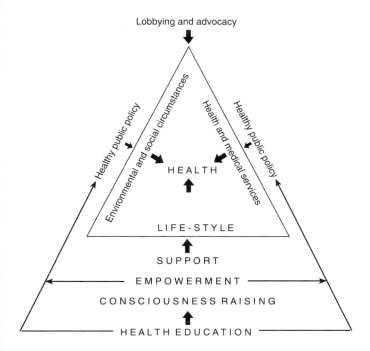

Fig. 23.1 The contribution of education to health promotion.

- Health promotion depends on the existence of an active empowered community.

- Medical services should be reoriented; the focus should be on empowerment, co-operation, and quality of life.

- Health is not just an individual responsibility. To seek to cajole individuals into taking responsibility for their own health, while ignoring the social and environmental circumstances which conspire to make them ill, is a fundamentally defective strategy—and unethical. 'Healthy public policy' is at the heart of health promotion.

The contributions of health education

So far we have considered the key features of health promotion and indicated how it seeks to revive the halcyon days of the nineteenth-century public health movement. We have also noted some of the limitations of the narrow individualistic focus of the preventive model of health education. Bearing in mind this criticism, we shall now consider the features of an expanded approach to health education, which will be consistent with the principles of health promotion outlined above. The requirements of such an approach are summarized in Fig. 23.1.

In short, one of the major functions of a 'revitalized' health education is that of influencing individual health choices. However, its purpose and techniques differ quite fundamentally from the more traditional preventive approach discussed earlier. The emphasis is less on persuasion and more on support. The goal is not one of manipulation and compliance but, rather, empowerment and facilitation of choice. Admittedly, the meanings of some of these terms are a little vague but they will be made more explicit when the psychological and social determinants of health-related behaviours are examined later in this chapter. For now, we may observe from Fig. 23.1 that health education is still concerned with

promoting appropriate use of health services. However, consistent with the principles of health promotion, one of its important functions will be to expand the horizons of service users and providers. It will seek to broaden the definition of health services and raise awareness of the important role that various organizations and services have to play in enhancing public health. At the same time, it will maintain its traditional function of helping to provide those communication and educational skills that professionals and lay people alike need to provide effective health education for their colleagues, clients, and the public at large. As a result of the educational enterprise and the judicious use of advocacy, it is hoped that services of all kinds will be accessible and responsive to the genuine needs of the population that they serve.

Although a redefinition of the meaning of health services may be quite novel, a more radical health education function appears in Fig. 23.1. This is directly congruent with the Ottawa Charter's exhortation to 'build healthy public policy'. No doubt, it is self-evident that the creation of new health policy is frequently a task of mammoth proportions, particularly in the face of counterpressures from the various vested interests which are, from time to time, described as the 'anti-health lobby'. Moreover, there are a number of well-recognized political ploys and procedures for influencing policy; these include lobbying by more or less powerful individuals and organizations, either on their own behalf or on behalf of those who are relatively powerless. Indeed, 'advocacy', 'mediation', and lobbying in general form a central part of the recommendations that the Ottawa Charter makes for building healthy public policy and remedying disadvantage. However, our assertion here is that only the concerted force of public pressure (and perhaps the ballot box) might be sufficient to bring about the kinds of substantial policy change needed (for example to influence levels of unemployment or the health problems associated with poverty). For this reason, one of the essential functions of health education is not merely to bring health issues to the attention of the public but rather to generate the kind of indignant concern that is encapsulated in Freire's term **critical consciousness raising** (Freire 1974).

Enhanced consciousness about social issues may be necessary for community action, but it is not sufficient. It must be supplemented by that mix of beliefs, attitudes, and competences that contribute to an 'active empowered community'. Accordingly, one of health education's major supportive functions is to enhance self-confidence and provide the variety of skills needed by individuals and their communities to influence the policy-making process and to make a positive contribution to the public health.

The dynamics of empowerment will receive further consideration as we focus on the more 'technical' features of health education later in this chapter. However, before we do that, it is worthwhile to revisit briefly the effectiveness issue in pursuit of our concern to shed some light on the vexing question of whether and how well health education 'works'.

The values of health promotion and the question of effectiveness

Of course, the assessment of effectiveness is the purpose of evaluation. At its simplest, evaluation seeks to ascertain the extent to which **valued** outcomes have been achieved. Therefore, before addressing the effectiveness issue, we should be clear about the nature of these valued outcomes; we need to ask just what success would look like if it were achieved.

In fact, we have noted two basic sets of values: first the values underpinning the preventive medical model, and second the more ambitious complex of health promotion values in its 'WHO approved' form. The first set of values can be stated quite unequivocally as the prevention of disease. The second set of values is, as we have seen, more holistic, more ambitious, and generally more imprecise! In short, successful health promotion would ultimately increase the prospects of individuals leading socially and economically productive lives. A comprehensive discussion of what exactly constitutes a socially and economically productive life cannot be addressed here, of course, but it is not unreasonable to claim that people need to be healthy in order to achieve it! As we have observed, health status is considered by WHO and the health promotion movement as having positive aspects associated with **quality of life**. Again, this is a concept open to multiple interpretations and definitions. Suffice it to say that once it has been defined, it is usually possible to measure it, and thus to gauge the success of interventions designed to achieve the outcome in question.

However, since these broader conceptualizations of health are beyond the scope of this chapter, we shall merely make two assertions:

- premature mortality and morbidity and the experience of disease militate against health, however it is defined;

- taking account of quality of life (for instance avoiding wherever possible assaults on patients' dignity) must be viewed as an integral part of effective health-promoting medical interventions.

Therefore it follows logically that, whatever else it concerns, health promotion must be concerned with the prevention and management of disease—the traditional goals of a preventive medical model. Indeed, few health promoters would take issue with the following widely accepted conceptualization of **health gain**:

- adding years to life—reducing avoidable deaths

- adding health to life—reducing disease and disability

- adding life to years—enhancing quality of life.

Following the requirement for efficiency that is typically built into the notion of health gain, the means used to achieve these outcomes should be feasible and practicable.

However, we should note that health promotion will differ from traditional models in the methods it advocates for achieving these health gain goals and, possibly, its view of human nature. For instance, it would be churlish to deny that therapeutic interventions contributed to the promotion of health. None the less, in so far as medical practitioners viewed the disease as solely due to patients' stupidity, ignorance, or perverseness, and treated them in paternalistic fashion while demanding compliance with 'doctors' orders', then they would not be acting in accordance with the principles of health promotion. Moreover, as we shall suggest later, the medical practitioners in question would be less likely to achieve their medical or preventive goals by acting in such a manner.

Even if we were to adopt a narrower set of goals centring on the primary, secondary, and tertiary prevention of disease (whilst perhaps acknowledging the legitimacy of broader, 'positive', and holistic health outcomes), we should still need to recognize the importance of certain key sub goals espoused by health promotion. For instance, if we accept that failure to achieve preventive outcomes is substantially due to socio-economic factors and lack of empowerment, then we would expect to assess the effectiveness of health promotion by the extent to which healthy public policies have been implemented in order to:

- remove unjustified inequalities in the distribution of disease and its socio-economic determinants

- create 'reoriented' (i.e. demystified, accessible, and responsive) services.

At first glance, these subgoals might appear as grandiose and unattainable as the phantasmagoric visions of positive health or well-being. However, if our assertion that these are the stepping stones leading to preventive outcomes is true, then the aims and pretensions must be operationalized and translated into precise objectives; these objectives, then, would guide health promotion practice and provide a series of indicators that may be used as criteria for judging the success or failure of interventions.

Therefore we shall make a start on this 'translation' process by offering a technical analysis of health education which will describe key features of human behaviour in health and illness, and thus provide guidelines for improving communication between client and health professional and for enhancing the design and implementation of health education programmes.

Health education: a technology

So far, we have described the contribution that health education might make to the broader strategy of health promotion. It will be obvious that it has a central part to play. Indeed, we might distil the concept of health promotion into the following 'quintessential' formula:

health promotion = health education × healthy public policy.

As we have noted, the discussion of health education thus far has been fundamentally ideological. In other words, we have considered what the purpose of health education should or should not be. The simple preventive model has been challenged and the principles of health promotion, in general, have been espoused. However, we may and should consider health education as a technical activity—as a set of procedures designed to achieve whatever goals have been generated by ideological preference. All these often conflicting goals will have one thing in common: their concern is to influence human decision-making and behaviour. Indeed, a technical definition of health education is not difficult to provide and, for the purposes of this chapter, the following is proposed.

Health education is any intentional activity that is designed to achieve health or illness-related learning, i.e. some relatively permanent change in an individual's capability or disposition. Thus, effective health education may produce changes in knowledge and understanding or ways of thinking; it may influence or clarify values; it may bring about some shift in belief

or attitude; it may facilitate the acquisition of skills; and it may even effect changes in behaviour or life-style.

Before we can specify the requirements for efficient communication and effective education, we need to understand how constructs such as those in the above definition can be applied in a social context and how they interact to influence behaviour. For example, we need to know how knowledge relates to practice, how beliefs influence attitudes, and which skills are necessary for empowered decision-making. Therefore, we shall now give some consideration to the factors influencing health choices and the broader question of human behaviour in health and illness.

Human behaviour in health and illness

Health and illness: a career-line perspective

As we have noted, the purpose of health education is to promote learning and influence the kind of choices that individuals make when they are healthy or ill. Certainly, from the perspective of the medical practitioner, the choices that are habitually made leave a lot to be desired—frequently being characterized as neither logical nor rational! While this is not necessarily true, the frustrations of health workers can be understood by considering briefly what conventional research wisdom tells us about the major influences on individuals' progress from health to illness and, it is hoped, their return to their former health status. This process will be embodied in an idealized **sickness career**.

In formulating this sickness career, we should first acknowledge the relevance of three concepts from medical sociology: the notions of **health behaviour, illness behaviour,** and the **sick role.** Health behaviour refers to any activities that individuals might undertake while believing that they are healthy in order to minimize the likelihood of future disease (for instance by adopting a healthy life-style or taking steps to detect asymptomatic disease). In other words, appropriate health behaviour should result in primary prevention.

Illness behaviour, however, refers to those activities undertaken by individuals in response to symptom experience. It typically includes mental debate about the significance and seriousness of those symptoms, lay consultation, decisions about action, including self-medication, and possibly contact with health professionals. Therefore the adoption of appropriate illness behaviour should result in the attainment of secondary prevention goals.

The notion of sick role was developed to describe the behaviours of those people—typically in Western societies—whose contact with health professionals resulted in the legitimation of their illness status. Conferment of the sick role involves both rights and duties. Patients have the right to claim exemption from normal activities (such as work), and they can also expect help from other people, especially medical practitioners. However, patients are expected to make every effort to recover and are duty bound to comply with medical advice.

Depending on the nature and stage of the disease, conformity to the sick role may result in either secondary or tertiary preventive gains. For instance, compliance with prescribed medication should reverse the disease process and/or prevent more serious consequences; compliance with recommendations for rehabilitation should result in patients relinquishing the sick role and viewing

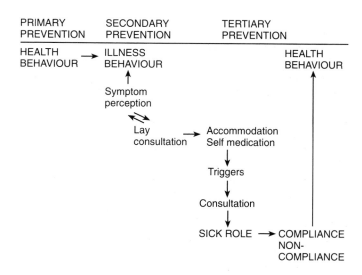

Fig. 23.2 The sickness career.

themselves as healthy even though they have some residual disability or functional impairment.

Kasl and Cobb (1966) provide a seminal review of the various concepts that are integral to the sickness career (summarized in Fig. 23.2).

When we consider the progress of a hypothetical individual along the sickness career, it is important to observe that there is quite commonly a major discrepancy between the subjective world of this 'actor' and the relatively objective reality represented by medical diagnosis and the logical and rational analyses and recommendations typically made by health educators. Not infrequently, there is also a substantial gap between people's knowledge of what healthy living entails and their actual health practices—just as there may be a hiatus between the information presented by health practitioners and their clients' compliance with this medically approved advice. Some indication of the extent to which individuals adopt appropriate health behaviour is provided by a recent survey of the health and life-style of a national sample of British men and women (Blaxter 1990). About 15 per cent of the sample practised healthy behaviour in four key areas: smoking, alcohol consumption, diet, and exercise (although it was reported that 'only about 5 per cent had totally "unhealthy" lives' in those respects.) From the same study, we should also note that interpretations of the meaning of health and the values attached to these varied widely: notions such as quality of life and well-being exist in the world of lay interpretations of health, and it would be unwise to ignore these when making judgements about 'prudent' life-styles! In short 'objective' prescriptions of **health** behaviour are always paralleled by 'subjective' interpretations of **healthy** behaviour.

Thus it seems quite likely that the health behaviour of our hypothetical individual will not gladden the heart of health professionals. What might we expect of his or her illness behaviour as we move further along the sickness career? At the risk of lapsing into caricature, we shall rapidly summarize a number of research results in this area. First, we should record the fact that a substantial majority of people are experiencing symptoms at any given point in time. If illness were the same thing as disease experience, then most people would appear to be ill most of the time! We can do no better than repeat the results of a survey by Wadsworth *et al.* (1971) of 1000 randomly selected people in two London boroughs; this research discovered only 49 individuals who had not experienced at least one painful or distressing symptom during the previous 14 days. However, when asked to rate their health in general, a very different situation was revealed. Thirty-five per cent of this apparently diseased and distressed population considered that they were in 'perfect health'! A further 34 per cent rated their health as 'good', while only 21 per cent and 10 per cent believed they were in 'fair' or 'poor' health respectively.

Of course, the process of symptom perception is not a kind of routine physiological activity. In fact, it is similar to the process involved in interpreting an educational message. Attention is paid to the stimulus in question and an active attempt is made to decipher its meaning. An hypothesis is entertained about symptom significance and a decision is made on the basis of sensory evidence. As with, say, the interpretation of a message on a poster, symptom perception can be accurate or inaccurate. It can be biased by expectation, prejudice, and wishful thinking. Moreover, as we know from instances of mass psychogenic illness and so-called 'medical students' disease', symptoms can be illusory; bodily symptoms may be either invented or grossly misinterpreted.

Symptom perception has a well-recognized social and even ethnic dimension. Zola's classic research into illness behaviour demonstrated consistent differences among the responses of Americans of Italian, Irish, and Anglo-Saxon descent to symptoms presented at ear, nose, and throat or eye hospital outpatient clinics (Zola 1973). For example, 'Italians had significantly more complaints of greater variety, and in more places than did the Irish . . . Italians [claimed] that the symptoms interfered with their general mode of living and the Irish just as vehemently [denied] any such interference'. Moreover, Italians much more often considered that pain constituted a major part of their problem.

Zola described the process of translating symptom into action rather elegantly.

> Virtually every day of our lives we are subject to a vast array of bodily discomforts. Only an infinitesimal amount of these get to a physician. Neither the mere presence nor the obviousness of symptoms, neither the medical seriousness nor objective discomfort seems to differentiate those episodes which do and do not get professional treatment (Zola 1973, p. 679).

In the survey by Wadsworth *et al.* (1973) referred to earlier, 188 symptomatic individuals took no action while 562 of the 1000 sample took 'non–medical' action. Accordingly, we can reiterate Zola's observation that only a relative minority of individuals consult a health professional. Furthermore, the majority of those consulting present with minor conditions and those with serious or potentially life-threatening conditions are equally well represented outside treatment.

Of those who are symptomatic but do not seek a professional consultation, a majority either accommodate to the symptoms or employ self-medication. In any event, the process of lay referral is widespread. Indeed, Freidson (1970) posited the existence of a 'lay referral system', which involves a network 'of potential consultants from the intimate confines of the nuclear family through successively more select, distant and authoritative laymen until the "professional" is reached'. Freidson also asserted that the likelihood of individuals utilizing any given health service depended on two interacting variables:

- the density of the social network;
- the extent to which the values and beliefs of the members of that network were congruent with those of the professional practitioner.

For instance, if a particular community was characterized by an 'extended lay referral system' of close-knit kith and kin (and if that community considered that medical treatment was the appropriate way to treat any given symptom), there was a strong likelihood that the individual experiencing those symptoms would yield to interpersonal and social pressure and report rapidly to the local doctor.

Zola is also responsible for pointing out that accommodation to symptoms—perhaps after a long delay incorporating lay consultation—can break down and result in a possibly reluctant consultation. He noted what he called 'non-physiological patterns of triggers to the decision to seek medical aid':

- the occurrence of an interpersonal crisis
- perceived interference (by the symptoms) with social or personal relations
- sanctioning (approval or pressure from some significant other person)
- perceived interference with vocational or physical activity.

Zola also noted a fifth, and somewhat different, trigger which he called 'temporalizing of symptomatology'. He illustrated this phenomenon by describing a fairly typical way in which patients from an 'Anglo-Saxon' background would set external time criteria for action—such as, 'If it isn't better in 3 days, or 1 week, or 7 hours, or 6 months, then I'll take care of it'. The relevance of temporalizing, and indeed the other triggers, for the problem of delay in presenting potentially treatable and serious conditions is doubtless self-evident.

Finally, let us consider the latter part of the sickness career and examine what frequently happens once patients embark on their consultations. First, it is not uncommon for people not to present all their symptoms, including those of greatest concern. This may be due in part to a tendency to accumulate symptoms, like money in a savings bank, until there is a sufficient balance to justify a visit to the doctor. Alternatively, it might merely be an excuse to seek counselling for a personal or social problem unrelated to any of the symptoms presented.

Unfortunately, despite a fairly common tendency, at least in the United Kingdom, for patients to be satisfied with their doctor in general, something of the order of 40 to 50 per cent will be dissatisfied with their most recent consultation and, more significantly, an equal percentage will not comply with the advice that they receive. If it is assumed that the advice is sound, this statistic should be a cause for concern, implying, as it does, that approximately half the professional resources utilized in the consultation are wasted.

The purpose of this review of the sickness career has been to highlight the complexities and uncertainties associated with human behaviour in health and illness. Unless health practitioners have insight into these complexities and what often appear to be merely irrational decisions, they cannot hope to deliver efficient health education; their health promotion strategies will be fundamentally flawed. In the remainder of this chapter we shall examine the psychological, social, and environmental factors that govern health-related decisions. We shall then seek to identify how, through effective communication and education, healthy choices can be facilitated. Before commencing this process, we summarize the implications for public health of the facts embodied in the sickness career.

- We need to influence health behaviour in such a way that individuals are empowered to adopt life-styles and make choices that contribute to the primary prevention of disease while at the same time maximizing their quality of life and their own subjective health goals.

- We need to help individuals to make correct interpretations of symptoms and facilitate decisions about their management. In so doing, we should ensure that health professionals are consulted when they can offer genuine cure or palliation of disease and attempt to reduce delay to a minimum.

- In the context of tertiary prevention, we need to promote those measures that maximize potential and quality of life.

For reasons that will be examined later, all three measures listed above require an emphasis on co-operation rather than compliance. They also require a combined approach in which education directed at individuals is supported by favourable environmental circumstances.

Understanding health choices
The health action model

Common sense tells us that we need to have some understanding of the factors that influence human behaviour in health and illness before we can develop efficient health promotion programmes. Many people (either consciously or intuitively) subscribe to a simple but outmoded notion embodied in the so-called 'K–A–P formula'. This formula asserts that the mere provision of knowledge (K) is insufficient to persuade individuals to adopt sound health practices (P). An intermediate stage must be supplied, which involves the development of attitudes (A) favourable to the adoption of the approved healthy practices. While it is undeniable that failure to make healthy choices typically cannot be attributed to lack of knowledge, the notion of attitude is itself oversimplistic and limited. Reality is much more complex, and a more sophisticated conceptualization than the K–A–P formula must be found.

In fact, there is a plethora of more complex theories and models that seek to explain human decision-making, both in general and in relation to health and illness. In this chapter, the **health action model** will be used as an explanatory framework, since it was originally developed to provide theoretical guidelines for health education programmes (Tones 1979). It was subsequently updated so that it could take account of the emerging concept of health promotion (Tones 1987; Tones and Tilford 1994, pp. 87–103).

The main features of the health action model are summarized in Fig. 23.3, which shows how an individual's intention to undertake any given health action is influenced by three main systems: a set of

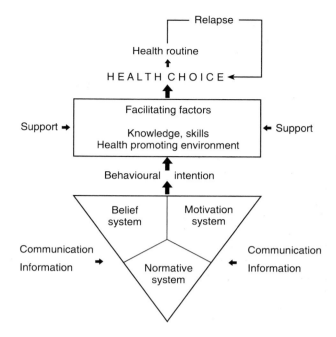

Fig. 23.3 The health action model.

beliefs, a cluster of motivational factors, and various normative pressures. It also makes the important point that before intention can be translated into practice, a variety of facilitating factors must be in place. These may comprise additional knowledge or key skills. More importantly, perhaps, the environment itself must be favourable if the healthy choice is to be the easy choice. As we have observed earlier, one of the prime goals of health promotion is the construction of healthy public policy in order to create supportive environments which reduce the impediments to healthy decision-making. We shall now elaborate on the importance of these different systems in turn.

The importance of health beliefs

Influencing health beliefs is a main concern of health education. A belief is a subjective probability judgement that describes the extent to which an individual considers that a particular circumstance or relationship is true. For example, in the context of current public health concerns, one of the main tasks of education would be to convince people that the following examples of medically received wisdom are indeed true.

- Human immunodeficiency virus (HIV) is transmitted by exchange of body fluids.

- Acquired immune deficiency syndrome (AIDS) is a fatal disease.

- Intravenous drug users are susceptible to infection.

- Smoking is related to a number of serious diseases.

- Immunization will protect against a variety of specific childhood diseases.

- Having a mammogram will involve only minor discomfort and provide peace of mind.

The importance of beliefs is not merely limited to an individualistic preventive model. In pursuit of healthy public policy, it would be hoped that the population might be persuaded to accept the following.

- Poverty and unemployment are inextricably associated with preventable death and disease.

- A ban on tobacco advertising will contribute to improvements in public health.

- If a government is reluctant to take action against unhealthy commercial interests, writing a protest letter to a Member of Parliament might well contribute to a change in policy.

The importance of several of the beliefs listed above can be illustrated by reference to a well-known model of some historic importance, which was originally developed to explain why people did or, more significantly, did not use medical services. The model in question is the **health belief model** (for a recent discussion, see (Becker 1984)), which posits that individuals will not take appropriate health actions unless:

- they believe that they are susceptible to a given disease;

- they consider the disease to be serious;

- they accept that the recommended preventive measures will actually be effective;

- undertaking the recommended action will not incur excessive costs or disadvantages.

If these conditions prevail, the probability of action will be enhanced; however, some trigger (for example, similar to those ascribed to Zola earlier in this chapter) may also be needed.

A comprehensive review of the important but complex subject of health beliefs is not possible here. However, three further kinds of belief should receive some brief consideration if we are to gain a more complete insight into the requirements of behaviour change strategies. They are beliefs about the causes of disease, beliefs derived from perceptions of risk, and beliefs about 'affect'.

It would seem self-evident that one of the tasks of education is to ensure that disease causation or the nature of the risk factors associated with diseases should be properly understood. It is perhaps less obvious how these causal beliefs (sometimes termed 'causal attributions' or 'theories of illness') might indirectly influence health decisions. Let us consider the role of beliefs in promoting early diagnosis of skin cancer.

Before seeking medical help, individuals must be aware of the potential implications of the symptom that they are experiencing; they must believe that this might be cancer. The chances of seeking help will also be increased if they believe that they are susceptible to skin cancer—perhaps as a result of having accepted that their particular skin type is at increased risk of damage from exposure to the sun.

However, action may well be inhibited by the long-recognized phenomenon of 'cancerophobia', i.e. an unrealistic level of fear about the disease, which, in turn, derives from a number of subordinate beliefs. One of these is the belief that treatment is (i) generally ineffective because cancer is essentially incurable and (ii) painful and distressing.

It is frequently difficult to provide an educational 'treatment' for pessimism about cancer—largely due to a failure to recognize root causes, including inappropriate causal attributions (i.e. believing 'myths' about the nature and origin of cancers). We need to probe further before structuring an educational programme. If we do so, we should then recognize that people may have a variety of 'theories' about the cause of cancer. For example, a 'retribution' theory describes a conviction that cancer is a kind of punishment visited on the individual for past sins and moral transgressions. In contrast, the 'seed and trigger theory' infers that everybody has cancer within them in a dormant form, like a seed, merely waiting for some event (almost any event such as a knock, stress at work, family upset) to trigger it.

Less dramatic perhaps but equally important is the fact that many people consider cancer to be a single undifferentiated disease. Thus if people know that, in some cases, treatment usually seems to fail—and believe that all cancers are the same—then pessimism is a logical outcome. Therefore the educational task (preferably carried out in the school setting) is one of providing appropriate biological understanding.

Returning briefly to the health belief model, the concept of susceptibility needs a rather more critical analysis than it usually receives. It certainly seems to make sense that those at risk of disease or other negative consequences must believe that they are susceptible to those consequences before they will be inclined to take preventive action. However, we not only need to understand why people may not accept the level of risk to which they are exposed (for example because of a tendency to overestimate the likelihood of the unlikely and underestimate the real frequency of quite common threats), but we must also acknowledge that many people actively seek risk. In short, these 'risk takers' would not be keen to undertake the behaviour in question unless they believed that they were susceptible to possible negative consequences! Various explanations have been advanced for the motivational effect of risk taking: these range from hypothesised 'addiction' to endorphins to a desire to demonstrate control (arguably, a healthy trait!). Lyng (1990) described the exercise of control in this way as **edgework**. A prerequisite for the satisfaction experienced in exerting control in hazardous circumstances (such as sky-diving) was the belief that there was 'a clearly observable threat to one's physical or mental well-being or one's sense of an ordered existence . . . in which the individual's failure to meet the challenge at hand will result in death or, at the very least, debilitating injury'.

The third example of the need to take account of a key belief in order to develop appropriate educational methods has to do with **affect**. Affect refers to various, generally motivational, states or feelings. In certain circumstances, beliefs about affect might materially influence an individual's intention to adopt a particular health-related behaviour. For instance, a national survey of British smoking attitudes and behaviour demonstrated that one of the more significant determinants of individuals' intention to give up smoking was whether or not they believed that they would be able to cope with the negative affect of withdrawal or relinquish the positive affect associated with emotional and 'physiological' gratification derived from their habit (Marsh and Matheson 1983).

In a similar vein, Davis (1992) has suggested that the main reason militating against the rehabilitation of 'addicts' is not so much their physiological addiction and fear of withdrawal but the belief that they are addicted.

Values, attitudes, and feelings

In addition to a **belief system**, Fig. 23.3 incorporates a **motivation system**—a complex of different affective elements. These affective elements ultimately determine an individual's intention of adopting a particular course of action.

Individual's values form an important part of the motivation system. Values are affectively charged sets of beliefs referring to significant aspects of experience. They are culturally determined; they are acquired through the processes of socialization and underpin all significant health choices. For instance, religious and moral values influence gender and sexual behaviour in particular social groups; thus they are likely to determine whether or not condoms are used as contraceptives or prophylaxis against AIDS. Socially created values may influence food choice, the acceptability of exercise, or the choice of breast feeding.

Attitudes, however, are more specific entities; they describe the importance attached to particular actions and issues. Each value will generate a variety of attitudes, and the acquisition of new beliefs may create new attitudes which are 'energized' by an individual's value system. For example, a belief that breast feeding would militate against a full sharing of the parental role might contribute to a negative attitude to it (other things being equal) in a household in which gender equality was highly prized.

In addition to values and attitudes, the motivation system recognizes the fact that certain basic and powerful influences may override socially acquired values and attitudes. The term 'drive' is used to refer to such largely inherited and 'instinctive' species-specific motivational factors as hunger, sex, and pain. It is also used here to describe acquired motivators having drive-like qualities, such as those arguably ascribed to the addictive state. The importance of drives in determining behaviour is self-evident. For example, a teenager might believe in her susceptibility to an unwanted pregnancy, accept the benefits of using condoms, and have acquired the skills needed to use them. However, even if she also has a well-developed moral sense, her values and attitudes may succumb to the imperative of sexual passion.

Frequently, there may be no obvious drive influencing intention to act; none the less, the presence of certain emotional states may signify the existence of motivational factors derived from drives. Thus guilt and anxiety, in this context, may be viewed as a fractionated or 'diluted' version of pain or fear. Everyday experience confirms the importance of such emotional states in determining action. Indeed, as we shall see, the problem of maintaining post-decisional healthy behaviours, and of managing relapse, is one of the more difficult tasks facing health professionals.

Before considering the third major set of influences on behavioural intention—the normative system—it is important to emphasize the interaction of these various systems. As we have seen, sets of beliefs that are congruent with people's value systems create positive attitudes and intentions. Conversely, values and attitudes frequently influence beliefs. 'Autistic thinking' (believing what it is

comfortable to believe) is a common phenomenon, and we often resolutely refuse to accept apparently rational arguments about, say, the hazards of smoking because to do so would create too much uncomfortable dissonance. Indeed 'wish fulfilment' and defensive avoidance typically may lead to selective attention and biased perception, causing people to misinterpret verbal advice and to ignore or even 'fail to see' threatening posters.

The normative system

The normative system should need little explanation. It is almost a truism to say that, despite our own beliefs and personal preferences, our intentions may be influenced for good or ill by other people. The normative system subdivides these social influences into general social norms and the more direct impact of significant others (i.e. individuals or groups of individuals having special significance, such as spouse, family, or peer group). The common-sense assertion is made that general social norms conveyed via mass media will have less impact than observations of normal practices in our own community, which, in turn, will exert less pressure than direct interpersonal interaction with those close to us.

What is less obvious is the separate but interrelated function of belief and motivation. First, our intention to act is affected by our beliefs about social norms and our anticipation of how significant others are likely to react to our intended actions. Second, these beliefs will only influence our intentions if we value the reaction of other people and/or are motivated to comply with their wishes (real or imagined) or feel that it is important to conform to social norms. For example, a person's intention to adhere to recommended alcohol limits will depend not only on the belief that a friend would approve but also on a desire to please that friend.

Again, whether or not an individual decides to wear protective headgear while cycling could be influenced not merely by a belief that very few people appear to wear crash helmets but also by the extent to which that individual is prepared to tolerate the possible ridicule that might result from deviating from normal practice.

The **lay referral system**, which features in the normative system in Fig. 23.3, has already been discussed in the context of a sickness career. Therefore we need only note here that this concept provides a useful explanation of the ways in which normative pressures in a given type of community might influence utilization or non-utilization of particular health services.

Empowering health choices: providing support

Reference to empowerment has already been made on several occasions. Not only is it an ideological *sine qua non* for health promotion, it is an essential element within that cluster of psychosocial and environmental variables that determine whether or not we adopt behaviour leading to primary, secondary, or tertiary outcomes. We have also argued that concepts such as empowerment must be operationalized if we are to develop precise and measurable objectives in health promotion. We shall now attempt to do just that: we shall identify and review the ways in which environmental circumstances and related factors may enable or inhibit empowered choices.

Personality, self-empowerment, and health choices

Personality (i.e. that relatively enduring cluster of personal traits and attributes that can provide a holistic profile of any given individual) is not considered to be a particularly useful concept in helping to explain human behaviour in health and illness, at least not in terms of potential application to the design of health education programmes. Although such personality traits as hypochondriasis or emotional stability may have an important bearing on individual health, there is little evidence that these factors materially influence the adoption of healthy life-styles. However, there is one cluster of characteristics that is considered to be highly relevant to health promotion, both ideologically and technically. It involves two complementary attributes: self-esteem and locus of control.

In order to explain the relationship between locus of control and self-esteem, we should recall the dichotomy between the belief and motivation systems in the health action model. In addition to specific beliefs about, for example, the costs and benefits of adopting a course of action, each individual has a complex set of beliefs about self. The sum total of these beliefs forms what is often defined as 'self-concept'. As with any other belief or belief system, self-concept describes the extent to which any given person accepts that he or she truly possesses a number of attributes—positive or negative. Hence self-concept may be realistic or unrealistic. Self-concept also includes beliefs about the body or physical appearance (i.e. body image).

Self-esteem is a complementary feature of the self-concept and is one of the most important and powerful values in the motivation system. It refers to the extent to which the individual values the attributes that make up the self-concept. Just as we formulate attitudes to any aspect of our world in accordance with our value system, we develop attitudes to ourselves. The sum of these attitudes defines our self-esteem.

The central relevance of self-esteem for healthy decision-making can be summarized readily. At one level of reasoning, a quite common-sense assertion can be made: presumably if people possess a good measure of self-worth, they are more likely to respond to the exhortation of preventive medicine to 'look after themselves'. Again, the acquisition of self-esteem (based on a realistic self-concept and taking account of the rights of others!) can be confidently identified as one of the less illusory and contentious goals of 'positive' mental health promotion.

More specifically, the possession of self-esteem has been associated with a tendency to have the courage of one's convictions (and hence an increased capacity to resist social pressure to do unhealthy things). It has also been suggested that persons with higher self-esteem are more able to handle threat in a productive manner. For instance, in response to fear-arousing educational messages, those having high self-esteem are more likely to be able to cope with threat rather than resort to defensive avoidance behaviour.

Furthermore, it also seems likely that people enjoying high self-esteem will experience greater dissonance when acting in a manner inconsistent with their beliefs and values. For instance, an individual having high self-esteem, and who also values health, would feel considerably more uncomfortable knowing that he or she were overweight than someone having a lower level of self-worth.

Dissonance is one of those emotional states incorporated into the motivation system. It may not be quite as uncomfortable as guilt, embarrassment, or anxiety; none the less we prefer to avoid it if at all possible.

Empowerment and the notion of control

Self-esteem has many sources, such as the way that our parents have treated us in the past and the way that our peers react to us at present. Self-esteem also seems to be closely related to the extent to which we feel in control of our lives. As we noted earlier, beliefs about control are central to health promotion's ideological goal of active and empowered people and communities. However, there are different types and degrees of beliefs about control. We shall briefly consider some of the most important of these.

Reference was made earlier to attributional beliefs, i.e. how we explain the nature and causes of disease and illness. One particular application of attribution theory centres on how people explain the various vicissitudes that they experience during their lives. Of special importance is the extent to which they explain what happens to them in terms of their own agency rather than the agency of other people or mere fate.

The notion of perceived locus of control is perhaps the most widely known of the psychological constructs associated with beliefs about control. Rotter (1966) defined the essence of this concept in a seminal paper, which argued that people could be differentiated according to the extent to which they believed that their lives were controlled by chance or powerful others rather than by their own efforts. Although, no doubt, people are distributed normally on this trait, those who by and large consider that they are influenced by external forces are considered to have an external locus of control. However, those who have confidence that whatever happens to them, pleasant or unpleasant, is substantially within their domain of influence are said to have a predominantly internal locus of control. A more complete review is not appropriate here. Suffice it to say that the development of a health locus of control scale has resulted in research demonstrating that there is, indeed, an association between internality and the likelihood of making healthy choices (Wallston and Wallston 1978; Tones 1992).

Conversely, it seems fairly clear from the work of Seligman (1975) and others that the state of 'learned helplessness', which derives from a belief that events are not influenced in any way by individual action, is both intrinsically unhealthy and militates against decision-making of any kind.

At a more specific level, two further situations in which beliefs about control can have a positive influence will be mentioned here. First, the feeling of control resulting from receiving information, involvement in decision-making, and the acquisition of competences to influence events (aversive or otherwise) can enhance not only the likelihood of making healthy decisions but also the achievement of therapeutic outcomes (Egbert et al. 1964; Langer and Rodin 1976). The second situation relates to a particularly relevant and practically applicable aspect of control described as **self-efficacy**.

The construct of self-efficacy is associated with Bandura (1977, 1986). People who have self-efficacy expectations believe that they are capable of performing a particular activity. Whereas locus of control is a generalized trait, self-efficacy is specific. For example, while someone might believe that she is generally not in control of her life, she might be persuaded that she could actually come for her mammogram and leave her children in the crèche (thoughtfully provided by the health centre). However, another person might feel generally in charge of his life but, because of a belief that he could not cope with the loss of affect associated with giving up smoking, would be convinced that he would not be able to make that particular healthy choice. Therefore, according to one simple formulation, people must not only believe that a health decision is beneficial and worthwhile, but they must also believe that they are capable of implementing it. Therefore influencing self-efficacy beliefs must be accorded a high priority educationally.

Facilitating decision-making: the provision of support

One of the more illuminating components of **social learning theory**, with which Bandura (1977, 1986) was closely associated, was the concept of **reciprocal determinism**, which states that there is a reciprocal relationship between human action and environmental circumstances. On the one hand, most people can exert some degree of influence on their environment; on the other hand, we do not operate in a vacuum and must take account of those environmental constraints and limitations which can act as barriers to free choice.

As we noted in the health action model, health promotion is not only concerned with influencing beliefs, motivation, and intention to act, but it has a responsibility to do all it can to ensure that intention is translated into practice. Accordingly, Fig. 23.3 reveals the necessity to facilitate choice by taking account of a number of factors that can either increase the likelihood of sustained healthy behaviour or, alternatively, act as barriers to its attainment. The first and, arguably, the most significant of these factors is the environment.

The environment can be viewed at a macrolevel in terms of the broad range of circumstances addressed in our earlier discussion of health promotion—in other words, the major physical and socio-economic aspects of the social system that require the application of healthy public policy at various levels 'to make the healthy choice the easy choice'. The importance of this cannot be overestimated, but needs no further consideration here.

However, following the principle of reciprocal determinism, we need to emphasize the significance of what could be termed the micro-environment. By this we mean the immediate social and physical circumstances that can influence health choices. For example, the intimate environment of the home can serve to trigger smoking and must be actively managed in order to facilitate smoking cessation. Conversely, the availability of social support can help individuals to succeed in their determination to change their behaviour. A substantial literature on the health benefits of social support has accumulated in recent years (Gottlieb and McLeroy 1992), although a detailed review is not possible here. However, at this point we might comment on the importance of, say, a general practitioner arranging supportive social environments for patients. For instance, the spouse and family might be involved in discussions about how best to support a family member's behaviour change programme, or a ' buddy system' might be introduced into a self-help group (for example, participants in a smoking clinic might be asked to maintain contact with each other between

meetings in order to support their mutual resolve to give up smoking).

Providing skills and preventing relapse

One of the points emphasized in the health action model is the importance of providing the knowledge and skills that people need to ensure that any given health action will materialize and be sustained. Knowledge is clearly important. For example, unless the patient knows how, when, and how much medication to take, it will be difficult for them to comply with their medication regime. Less obviously, perhaps, is the need for skills acquisition. Necessary skills may include psychomotor competences, such as dexterity in the use of a condom or the efficient practice of first-aid techniques. These will also include social interaction skills. An intention to communicate assertively with a partner about safer sex practices will collapse unless verbal and non-verbal skills have been practised enough that a high level of proficiency has been achieved.

Sustaining behaviours that involves loss of gratification or some degree of initial discomfort is one of the most difficult tasks that health education seeks to facilitate. In addition to managing the micro-environment, as indicated above, training in the use of 'self-regulatory' skills will usually be required. For instance, the difficulties intrinsic to the control of 'addictive behaviours' have been well documented. Accordingly, a variety of techniques associated with behaviour modification approaches have been evolved to help people monitor their behaviours and environmental circumstances, avoid temptation, and discover substitute gratifications and rewards for successful maintenance of the healthy activities that they have chosen to adopt.

A 'revolving door' model has been developed by DiClemente and Prochaska (1982), which provides a useful insight into the ways in which heavy smokers, for example, might move round a kind of cyclical trajectory before they eventually succeed in giving up smoking (see also Prochaska 1992). According to the model, they may move through five stages of change. The first three are called **precontemplation**, **contemplation**, and **action**. Some clients will move on to **maintenance**, while many others will find themselves in the **relapse** stage. The assumption is made that many will return to the contemplation stage and move on to maintenance.

A system of 'motivational interviewing' or counselling has been based on the analysis developed by Prochaska and DiClemente. However, it seems probable that the acquisition of self-regulatory skills would minimize the likelihood of relapse, and further reference to this kind of skill will be made later in the chapter. Self-regulation is a significant notion within the general body of theory known as **behaviour modification**; a discussion of the theory and practice of behaviour modification is not possible here, although a wide variety of texts are available for further consultation (Kanfer and Karoly 1972; Watson and Tharp 1989).

So far, then, we have provided, in the form of the health action model, a kind of map on which we might plot the multitude of psychological, social, and environmental determinants of any particular health- or illness-related behaviour. Therefore it is opportune at this point to revisit the evaluation question and to ask to what extent our discussion of these psychosocial and environmental factors might have increased the sophistication of our thinking on matters of measurement. In brief, we ought to remark that these very factors can provide a number of intermediate indicators of effectiveness and efficiency. For instance, both preventive and empowerment goals will require evidence of successful learning; in other words, the acquisition of relevant beliefs, the clarification of values, shifts in attitude, and the adoption of skilled behaviours. Bearing in mind the importance of the environment, we should also look for evidence that policies have been successfully initiated and implemented. For instance, the following intermediate indicators would provide partial and proximal measures of longer-term success: the number of no smoking areas provided in a workplace, the ready availability of condom machines, or the provision of a responsive user-friendly service in an outpatient clinic.

Behaviour change: influencing health choices

The communication process: lessons from failure

We have stated that successful learning is at the heart of the successful health promotion enterprise and the educational encounter. However, learning is not possible without efficient communication. Accordingly, we shall now give some detailed consideration to this important matter.

There is no universally agreed definition of communication, although effective communication is almost unanimously believed to be a universally good thing. However, we might remark that the term is often used in two different senses in the context of health promotion. On occasions it is used to describe the whole process of influencing behaviour change. Communication failure, according to this conceptualization, would describe failure to change life-style or comply with recommended advice. Alternatively, use of the term communication may be restricted to the provision of information. This narrower definition is employed here, and the process is described in Fig. 23.4.

Communication consists of the transmission of messages from a given source to an audience. The audience may comprise one or more individuals. In the classic research situations described below, the communicators are health professionals (usually doctors), while the audience consists of patients or clients. Effective communication occurs when the audience's interpretation of the message matches that of the communicator.

Given the difficulties people frequently experience in interpreting communications, the notion of 'coding' is highly appropriate. This code may be symbolic, pictorial, or participatory. Normally, a symbolic message would be in either spoken or written form. Alternatively, or additionally, some pictorial presentation may be used, for example in the form of a visual aid. Less commonly (often in educational settings), the audience may be invited to participate actively for the sake of more effective communication. For example, role play might be used to convey emotional impact.

When people respond successfully to a communication, the message must first reach their senses; they must be able to see and hear it. Secondly, the message must attract and sustain their attention. Thirdly, it must be correctly interpreted—a process involving perception.

The feedback loop shown in Fig. 23.4 is an essential feature of the communication process. Communication cannot be successful

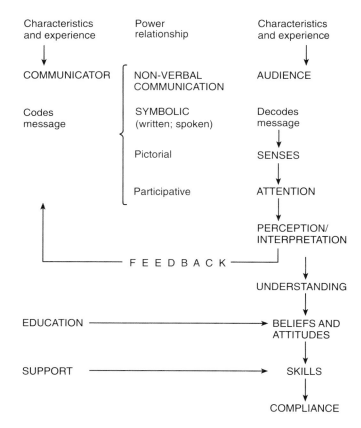

Fig. 23.4 Communication and the education process.

unless communicators check the effectiveness of the process during and/or immediately after the interaction by asking questions or noting non-verbal reactions.

We can also see from Fig. 23.4 that the communication process is materially affected by the expectations, emotional state, and other characteristics of both source and audience. For instance, patients' anxiety may well result in their selectively attending to a particular message or misperceiving it. The ways in which certain attributes of doctors might affect the consultation will be considered later.

Figure 23.4 includes an important feature of the communication process—non-verbal communication. In many instances, aspects of non-verbal communication (such as facial expression, tone of voice, or posture) may be more important than the spoken word, particularly in conveying attitudes and feelings. Moreover, it is often through non-verbal communication that communicator and audience exchange impressions about their characteristics. For completeness, we should perhaps state the obvious point that the roles of audience and communicator will reciprocate in accordance with the ebb and flow of conversation. The doctor will ask a question and the patient, in responding to it, then becomes the communicator. The doctor then has the task of decoding the resulting message.

Factors associated with failure in communication and education

There has been a good deal of research into communication failure. A substantial proportion of such research has focused on the doctor–patient encounter. The reasons for this partiality are not absolutely clear; it is probably not because doctors are worse communicators than other professionals but rather that the outcome of failure may be more dramatic! We should also give credit to the large numbers of doctors who have exposed themselves to scrutiny in this way. In all events, the results of such research are revealing and serve to highlight the requirements of effective educational interventions. In research on failure, the distinction between communication and education is often unclear and, typically, includes examples of both unsuccessful communication and unsuccessful education (defined as a failure to promote health- or illness-related learning).

An extensive literature review is not appropriate here, but Ley (1990) provides a useful analysis. None the less, we give a brief description of some key research findings below.

As we observed in our earlier comments on the sickness career, there appears to be a good deal of dissatisfaction with medical communications and a high level of non-compliance. Ley (1990) reviewed 33 different investigations into the level of patient dissatisfaction with communication: this ranged from 5 per cent to 82 per cent with a mean rate of some 37 per cent. Ley also summarized four reviews of compliance in the late 1970s and noted their mean non-compliance rates for four areas: medication, clinic attendance, diet, and 'miscellaneous'. The average non-compliance across all these studies was of the order of 46 per cent.

As Pascoe (1983) cogently demonstrates, the notion of patient dissatisfaction is rather vague; it has been used here merely to describe the extent to which patients like or dislike the communication that they have received from medical practitioners. However, it is clear that the relationship between non-compliance and dissatisfaction is tenuous. Indeed, Ley found a correlation of only +0.26 between these two variables. We must look elsewhere if we are to explain people's failure to follow advice.

One factor that, logically, would militate against compliance is misperception of the message communicated by the health professional. Tuckett, et al. (1985), who investigated doctor–patient interactions in 1000 consultations in primary care, provide valuable insights not only into patient misperception and misinterpretation of communications but also into two other important areas directly relevant to education. In summary, they demonstrated not only a high level of misinterpretation of messages but also a not insubstantial 'lack of commitment' by patients to courses of action that they had understood. They also checked the extent to which patients had forgotten what their doctor had told them. In all, there were some 34 per cent of consultations in which the patient either 'did not remember or make sense "correctly" or was not "committed" to key points'.

The extent to which patients actually forget the information that they have been given is a matter of some debate. In his comprehensive literature review Ley (1990) reported that the mean percentage of information recalled after medical consultations was approximately 60 per cent in hospital patients and 65 per cent in general practice patients. In other words, patients appear to forget about 40 per cent of what they have been told. However, Tuckett et al. found only 10 per cent of consultations after which the patient was unable to correctly recall key points. Moreover, they ascribed some of this memory deficit to the fact that patients were not committed to the advice offered! Therefore, according to Tuckett et al., factors other than memory failure must account for failure to comply with medical advice.

Explaining non-compliance

In providing a cogent explanation for non-compliance, we need to bear in mind that three sets of key actors are involved. First there is the doctor or health professional, second there is the patient, client, or learner, and finally there is what might be best described as lay opinion, which will include not only the lay referral system mentioned earlier but also a kind of background noise of information coming from mass media and other educational agencies, formal or informal. Therefore it is certainly wrong to consider non-compliance merely as patient failure. Indeed, one further example from Ley is an intriguing analysis of what he calls 'noncompliance by health care professionals with rules for good patient care'! He examined 19 research studies into the activities of psychologists, pharmacists, nurses, dentists, emergency medical technicians, and medical practitioners. The mean proportion of professionals not complying with recommended practice was about 60 per cent —rather higher than the patients' failure rate!

Hopefully, it is now clear that compliance will not happen if communication fails, i.e. if the message does not reach the senses, if patients do not pay attention, and if they misinterpret the message. At the next stage, that of influencing client learning and behaviour, we need to give a little further consideration to the comments of Tuckett et al. (1985) on the lack of commitment to doctors' advice which many patients demonstrated in their research. What does this lack of commitment mean?

In short, lack of commitment is best understood in terms of attitude theory; the patient has a negative attitude to the course of action recommended by the doctor. This negative attitude may be understood, in turn, by reference to key beliefs. One of these beliefs will be similar to the notion of self-efficacy mentioned earlier. For instance, although patients might accept that a recommended course of action, such as a period of bed rest, will be beneficial, if they know that bed rest is incompatible with environmental circumstances and domestic duties, then, inevitably, there will be a lack of commitment and non-compliance. To reiterate a point made earlier, educational programmes must include environmental analysis and support.

We shall draw on the health action model again to explain a second reason for a possible lack of commitment to action—and this is a point which Tuckett et al. themselves emphasized. First we recall that the majority of patients consulting a doctor or nurse will have already made their own diagnosis of their presenting problem and probably will have identified beforehand the kind of prescription needed (doubtless some form of medication). Failure to confirm the patients' expectations is likely to be a cause for dissatisfaction and, possibly, non-compliance. More significant, though, is the reason why patients make their diagnosis in the first place. The explanation frequently derives from patients' causal attributions and what Tuckett et al. preferred to call 'theories of disease'. An example will serve to clarify this observation.

Consider the case of a patient who presented with a rash on his leg. The doctor diagnosed a self-limiting allergic condition of no great significance and prescribed an emollient cream. Later, at interview, it became clear that the patient was not committed to the recommended advice, although he had understood it thoroughly and had complete recall of key points. The reason for the non-compliance followed a self-diagnosis, which had its roots in a dimly formed association of the complaint with phlebitis. This, in turn, had a kind of metaphorical association with the bite of a flea and the resultant association with a blood disorder. The latter was described in terms of the blood being too 'rich' (owing to too rich a diet). The patient believed that his rash was symptomatic of this underlying disorder. Accordingly, he was reluctant to comply with the doctor's recommended treatment, and this led him to formulate his own treatment plan. His own (very logical) preferred remedy would have been a medicine to 'cleanse the blood'; medication was his treatment of choice. Alternatively, he would have accepted a recommended change in diet, even if he had been unwilling to cope with the loss of gratification! The patient duly made some marginal dietary changes, such as cutting down sugar intake. In due course the rash disappeared, as it was indeed self-limiting as the doctor had predicted, thus confirming the patient's diagnosis and his theory of illness!

The educational implication of incidents such as this is made abundantly clear by Tuckett *et al.*: if they want to reduce non-compliance, practitioners must first explore patients' theories of illness—a process involving negotiation and co-operation rather than prescription and compliance.

Before leaving the realm of patients' beliefs, the reader should note that a number of beliefs identified in the health action model are applicable to the context of compliance with medical advice. These will not be repeated here, but we shall remark, by way of example, that the health belief model would be highly relevant. The probabilities of compliance will be substantially increased to the extent that patients accept their own (or their children's) susceptibility to a medical condition, rate it as serious, and believe that the prescribed measures will be effective without, at the same time, entailing too many costs (in terms of such barriers to action as inconvenience, discomfort, loss of money, and the like).

Before leaving the question of non-compliance, it is worth recalling that aspect of the health action model that was concerned with facilitating the translation of intention into practice. Assuming that a patient is committed to the advice provided and believes that the recommended action is manageable in his or her social and environmental circumstances, then it is essential to ensure, as far as humanly possible, that those circumstances are, in fact, conducive to compliance. For this reason, the educational encounter should include, where necessary, the provision of any skills needed by the patient together with the requisite environmental and social support.

We are now in a position to translate the various constructs and processes described in Fig. 23.4 into a more detailed set of guidelines for an educational consultation. Before doing this, however, it is important for us to give some thought to a key issue that bears on both the question of empowerment, which, we have argued, is central to the practice of health promotion, and the whole matter of patient compliance.

Communicator credibility and the power relationship

We have already indicated that patient commitment may depend on whether patients prefer to believe their doctors or would rather rely on their own theories of illness and the lay referral system from which they derive. In short, we have witnessed a kind of credibility clash between professional and lay referents.

Clearly, communicator credibility is a phenomenon of some importance in the educational process, and it has long been recognized that there are at least two different varieties of source credibility. One of these has been variously described as 'legitimate' or 'expert' authority; thus credibility is bestowed on a person who is perceived to have a high level of relevant (and often technical) expertise, particularly if supported by some formal status conferred by state institutions. Obviously, doctors (and, to a lesser extent, teachers) would be included in this category.

Alternatively, the lay referral system has been granted formal status as a kind of 'referent authority.' Rogers and Shoemaker (1971) coined the word **homophily** to explain the way in which referent authority operates. In summary, the principle of homophily states that members of a social group are most likely to be influenced by 'opinion leaders' who embody the norms of that particular community and are perceived to share those characteristics of community members that are deemed to be important. Like influences like.

According to this principle, all professionals whose social group and background are different, by definition, from their clients' social milieu will find it difficult to influence anyone from a different social class or ethnic group. While clients might accept the doctor's superior knowledge about illness (provided that it does not conflict with lay wisdom and everyday experience), they will be reluctant to believe that doctors can really appreciate the problems that their patients face as unemployed single parents living in a slum. Therefore advice will be treated with a degree of scepticism!

However, and very significantly, the principle of homophily has a rider that states that it is possible for people from different circumstances to have credibility provided that they also have **empathy**. Since empathy is a recognized social interaction skill, it can be taught. The implications for training health professionals should be apparent. None the less, the acquisition of homophily by the medical profession is beset with certain difficulties deriving from the very power and status that give doctors their 'legitimate authority'. Therefore we shall consider briefly some features of what might be called a power bind for doctors who wish to acquire the empathy and social interaction skills associated with effective communication and education.

Any health educator working face to face with clients, either singly or in a group setting, needs a repertoire of social interaction skills. Central to the socially skilled response is the capacity to interpret key aspects of the client's mental state correctly by appropriate use of questioning and sensitivity to non-verbal communication. Therefore the successful communicator and educator should be capable of responding flexibly to the perceived needs of the client—in short, to provide 'different strokes for different folks'. Key components of the skilled response and the mental set underlying those skills is what has often been called the 'holy trinity' of counselling: respect, empathy, and genuineness. Empathy, as we have suggested, is a social skill which can be learned; respect and genuineness are less easily acquired. Indeed, it has been argued that respect and genuine interest in a client cannot be faked; any attempt to do so usually will be detected by the client, probably as a result of 'non-verbal leakage.' In short, the implications for effective education are that health professionals must have a genuine interest in their clients and possess a variety of communication and social interaction skills.

In the context of the doctor–patient interaction, there is strong evidence that patient satisfaction is associated with a liking for the doctor's interpersonal skills, even if this is only described in terms of 'perceived friendliness'. It also seems likely that many doctors lack the flexibility of response associated with a socially skilled performance. Indeed, it is all too easy for professionals to stereotype clients in the educational or caring setting (for example in response to perceptions of ethnic status or social class).

In an important British study, Byrne and Long (1976) made a distinction between doctor-centred and patient-centred modes of social interaction in the consultation. The former approach focused primarily on gathering information by questioning, probing, and analysing. However, the patient-centred approach demonstrated key features of the skilful educational encounter and was characterized by various 'micro-skills': active listening, providing the patient with a breathing space in which to think and speak, asking 'open' clarifying questions rather than closed questions requiring merely the answer 'yes' or 'no', and empathic reflection of patients' concerns and feelings. Byrne and Long also described a significant tendency of doctors to use only one interaction style with a variety of different patients—the antithesis of providing 'different strokes for different folks'.

As we noted earlier, Tuckett et al. (1985) urged practitioners to explore patients' theories of illness if they wished to maximize co-operation with their advice. The patient-centred techniques presented above are exactly those needed to investigate client theories, perceptions, beliefs, and attitudes. Although the most frequently cited reason given by doctors for not undertaking health education is lack of time, it is very likely that investment in a patient-centred educational approach will pay dividends in reducing the problem of non-compliance.

Tuckett et al. also noted that patients had an irritating tendency to expect that their doctors would divine, somehow magically, their uncertainties, anxieties, and concerns. If and when the doctors failed to do so, patient satisfaction plummeted. The researchers asked these patients why they did not question their doctors or, if they were not committed to the advice offered, whey they did not explain their doubts or even challenge the doctor's point of view. Their answers revealed a decidedly low level of empowerment.

- Sixty per cent of the respondents identified questions that they would have liked to have asked the doctor, but did not do so; they gave a total of 104 reasons for staying silent.

- Thirty-three per cent of respondents had doubts that, again, they did not express; they gave 44 reasons for keeping quiet. Most of these reasons reflected the nature of the power relationship between doctor and patient. They included the following specific statements:

  - felt hurried

  - frightened of a bad reaction from the doctor

  - frightened that the doctor will think less well of the patient

  - felt that it was not up to the patient to ask/mention.

Tuckett and co-workers examined the level of patients' participation in the consultation in some detail and recorded this level of involvement with reference to what they identified as five key **consultation tasks**. For example, two of these tasks were associated with patients' theories of illness and the extent to which they expressed doubts about doctors' advice. Forty-four per cent of patients showed 'no sign' of expressing doubts; 73 per cent made no attempt at all to explain their ideas about their symptoms and the underlying illnesses.

Bearing in mind the oft-repeated importance of empowerment in health education (and the ways in which various environmental or social 'structural' factors may militate against active community participation), perhaps we should give some further consideration to the notion of the sick role and its associated requirement for patient compliance with 'doctor's orders'.

Compliance and the sick role

In a classic analysis, Parsons (1951) specified a 'proper role' for doctor and patient in Western society. Sociologically, his stance was 'functionalist': in other words, he argued that the peculiar relationship between doctor and patient existed because it was functional —it met an important social need. As mentioned earlier, patients are accorded certain privileges when their 'sickness status' has been legitimized by the medical profession. They are excused from normal duties but are expected to make every effort to recover and resume the role of healthy person by complying assiduously with medical advice.

However, it should be mentioned that this Parsonian perspective has been challenged as oversimplistic and idealistic. Freidson (1970) argued that the interaction between practitioner and patient is characterized by conflict rather than compliance. On the basis of our review of the research in this area, both points of view seem to obtain in real life. On the one hand, patients frequently disagree with their doctors and do not comply with advice; on the other hand, they tend to be reluctant to engage in a process of negotiation and bargaining for fear of being labelled 'bad patients'.

The justification for the Parsonian view of the unequal distribution of power between patient and doctor (and, more generally, between medicine and society in general) is quite simple. The doctor assumes power in the best interest of the patient since there is a 'competence gap' between health professional and client; this gap is the result of the complex and esoteric body of knowledge that the physician acquires through a long process of training and socialization. In the words of DiMatteo and DiNicola (1982), the 'disparity in power and control carves an emotional chasm between physician and patient—a chasm that is bridged only by the physician's altruism and orientation to serving people'.

Clearly there is an alternative view, which applies generally to the process of professionalization. Following George Bernard Shaw's observation that the 'professions are a conspiracy against the laity', doctors seek to maintain this imbalance in power and resort to mystification in a purely self-seeking way. Whatever the truth may be, from a health promotion perspective there are major disadvantages inherent in patients' adoption of a sick role. First, primary prevention requires people to look after themselves and adopt a prudent life-style. They must make day-to-day decisions and cannot merely comply with a simple medical prescription. Second, in so far as there is no simple one-off cure for a majority of contemporary diseases and a good deal of doubt and uncertainty surrounds the very notion of risk factors, co-operation rather than compliance is an absolute necessity. Furthermore, the notion of 'affective neutrality' embodied in the traditional prescription for the relationship between doctors (and professions allied to medicine) and their patients actively militates against the requirements for effective education and counselling. It is not possible to maintain emotional distance and, at the same time, display respect, empathy, and genuineness. For example, Zola's (1986) description of the 'language of endearment, familiarity and/or belittlement', which characterizes a 'top-down' approach to communication, is completely at odds with the need to encourage clients and patients to be assertive and take responsibility for their health.

A disparity of power is not only bad for patients, but is not good for doctors. Apart from the little matter of the high non-compliance rate, doctors who wish to be empathic and encourage patients to be assertive may find it extremely difficult to cast off their heavy burden of legitimate authority because patients may not let them do so. The solution from a health promotion perspective is not difficult to formulate, although not at all easy to implement in practice. On the one hand, all health practitioners can be trained in counselling skills, provided that they are convinced of the benefits of relinquishing some of the less productive aspects of their professional socialization. On the other hand, the general public should be sufficiently well educated about health and illness that they will not only be able to make reasoned decisions about their health and illness behaviour but will also have a more realistic appreciation of what medicine can achieve.

Of course, this general education about health and the health services is entirely congruent with WHO's desire to reverse the process of medicalization and achieve a reorientation of health services. As we have seen, it is an integral part of the ideology of health promotion. We should also note that, at a stage in the history of the welfare state when increasing concern is being shown about escalating cost (and an associated need for some sort of rationing), an educated public will not only be more consumer-oriented but should also be more willing and able to make democratic decisions through the ballot box about the kind of health service that it wants.

In the shorter term, more specific measures typically would be recommended to enhance understanding of and co-operation with medical advice. For instance, patients should be encouraged to have a friend accompany them to the surgery as a kind of advocate and memory jogger. They should be advised to write down their symptoms together with the questions they would like to ask. Above all they should be provided with a valuable commodity with multiple health-related applications—they should be given assertiveness training.

The reference made above to the general public's need for health education will serve as an introduction to the next section in this chapter, which will provide a wider perspective on influencing health and illness decisions. In brief, we shall consider some aspects of mounting community-wide programmes in a number of different settings and contexts. We shall then devote some time to a consideration of specific educational techniques, many of which will be relevant to the needs of effective communication and education in the encounters between health professionals and patients. However, before tackling this issue, let us see whether we have accumulated any further insights into the issue of assessing effectiveness and efficiency.

We noted previously the need to use intermediate indicators of success by measuring patients' or clients' beliefs, attitudes, and skills. We have now added an extra dimension in the form of so-called **process evaluation**. For example, if doctors' social interaction skills influence patients' beliefs and attitudes and increase the likelihood of their co-operating with recommended advice, then it is reasonable to use an assessment of the extent to which health professionals exhibit an appropriate level of such skills not only as an intermediate indicator of patient adherence to a prescribed regime, but also as a staging post on the route to longer-term reductions in mortality and morbidity. Accordingly, an evaluation of this process can provide a valuable quality audit of practitioner performance.

Influencing behaviour: strategies, settings, and contexts

Before discussing specific communication techniques and the educational methods needed to influence behaviours in the specific milieu of primary care, we shall provide an overview at the macrolevel of key settings and contexts for the 'delivery' of health education. Prior to doing this, a few important generalizations can usefully be made about how social systems or communities tend to change.

Change at the macrolevel: the adoption of innovations

One of the most useful reviews of community-level change is provided by the **communication of innovations theory** (Rogers and Shoemaker 1971). It generalizes from seven major research traditions and seeks to illuminate the process whereby 'an idea, practice, or object perceived as new by an individual' comes to be adopted (or rejected) by a community or, more precisely, a social system. Typically, the social system is defined graphically but it may be 'relational,' for instance a 'community' of doctors within a particular region. A number of generalizations can be made about the communication of innovations, and these are concerned with five phenomena:

- the rate of adoption

- the nature of the social system

- the characteristics of potential adopters

- the characteristics of 'change agents'

- the characteristics of the innovation.

First, it is salutary to note that the rate of adoption of new practices is characteristically slow. Additionally and irrespective of the time taken, the process is described by an 'S-shaped' curve which demonstrates the fact that the rate of change is initially slow, then gathers momentum, and finally tails off. This fact, in turn, has been ascribed to different adopter attributes. So-called **innovators** (amounting to perhaps 2.5 per cent of the population) seize on the innovation eagerly; they are followed by a category of **early adopters** (arguably 13.5 per cent of the population), who are then followed by an **early** and a **late majority**, who account for 68 per cent of the whole group. Finally, a collection of some 16 per cent diehard **laggards** bring up the rear! Of course, these findings reflect only a situation in which the innovation is sufficiently attractive to create social change.

The above observations are quite valuable in that they should curtail unrealistic expectations of rapid change in response to public communication exercises. They also have implications for the continuous monitoring of the effect of such communications. Perhaps there are more significant implications to be drawn from the remaining three phenomena under consideration.

It is probably self-evident that the rate of adoption of an innovation will be influenced by the characteristics of the social system itself. In short, it is argued that a 'traditional' community will always take longer to adopt an innovation than a more modern 'cosmopolitan' population. Of greater significance, though, is the importance of taking account of the community's **felt needs**. For instance, if a given social group recognizes that it has a particular need and discovers a remedy for that need, change will be relatively rapid and will not involve any interference from external change agents. If those change agents manage to supply the solution to a problem that the members of a community have identified, again the innovation will be relatively speedy. However, an attempt to impose an externally generated solution on a community that does not believe that it has a problem is doomed to failure. However, if a sensitive community development programme is employed, the community worker/health educator may, as mentioned at the beginning of this chapter, gradually raise the level of critical consciousness of a community such that it becomes aware of a need that it has not yet managed to articulate. Subsequently, the effective educator or community worker will act as facilitator, provide support, and work as an advocate to meet the newly awakened need.

It is unnecessary to discuss the characteristics of the change agent further, other than providing a reminder of the paramount importance of credibility and the principle of homophily. Just like doctors, teachers, or nurses, community workers must possess the social skills associated with communicating respect, empathy, and genuineness. They must enlist the support of community opinion leaders and others who already enjoy credibility in the eyes of the people.

Last but not least, we turn to the real and perceived attributes of the innovation itself. Ideally, it should have a number of characteristics.

- It should be seen to be simple rather than complex.

- People should believe that it can be readily tried and the beneficial effects should be observable sooner rather than later.

- Importantly, the innovation should be compatible with existing culture and norms, and should have a fairly clear advantage compared with current practice.

- It should not appear to incur any substantial costs, financial or otherwise.

It is a salutary exercise to check any given health promotion measure (such as condom use or the adoption of vigorous cardio-protective exercise) against this list of criteria for successful innovation.

Mass media: limitations and potential

We shall now consider some of the broader strategies and settings in which health promotion seeks to foster the adoption of health- and illness-related innovations. The strategic use of mass media will be the first subject for discussion.

One of the most confident assertions emerging from communication of innovations theory is that interpersonal channels of communication are more effective than mass media publicity when it comes to persuading communities to change their practices. Use of the mass media is more than frequent in health promotion; it is often viewed as a panacea. Therefore it is important here to provide a rather rapid summary of the capabilities of this extremely important strategy for public education.

The main characteristics of mass media are quite simply defined. First, they have the potential for reaching a mass audience (and therefore, in principle, might influence very large numbers of individuals 'at a stroke'). Second, they mediate the educational message using such channels as television or the printed word. Because of the mediated nature of the message, there is no possibility for receiving immediate feedback from the audience, and we argued earlier that immediate feedback is a prerequisite for effective communication. In other words, mass media cannot provide 'different strokes for different folks', nor is it possible for producers and presenters to react creatively to the many different audience responses to the message.

Lazarsfeld and Merton (1948) identified three major conditions in which mass media were most likely to have a substantial effect on a given population. They were described as **monopolization**, **canalization**, and **supplementation**. In other words, mass media would not be influential unless the following conditions were satisfied.

- The recipient of the media messages lived in relative social isolation or was not exposed to counter-messages.

- They canalized or built on already existing motivation.

- They were used to supplement and support other initiatives such as interpersonal education and/or policy developments.

Therefore, we can say that, in the absence of these circumstances, mass media are unlikely to be effective in changing attitudes and behaviours, particularly where these involve some loss of gratification or are perceived to result in discomfort or major inconvenience. They cannot teach complex skills nor provide understanding of complex issues. However, they can raise awareness and reinforce other initiatives very successfully.

Clearly, there are many different types of media and therefore the generalizations listed below should be treated with caution. For a more comprehensive account of the complex theoretical and practical dimensions of mass media, those interested should consult MacShane (1979), Salmon (1989), Backer et al. (1992), and Tones and Tilford (1994, pp. 87–103).

Generalizations about mass media use in health promotion

- Different mass media can achieve different effects.

- There is a major difference between the persuasive use of mass media and 'documentaries' or 'educational broadcasting'.

- Various incidental effects of media (for example the portrayal of alcohol use in soap operas) may have a negative influence on health. Healthy public policy is needed to regulate any demonstrably harmful effects.

- In general, persuasive advertising will have a minimal effect on beliefs, attitudes, and behaviour, particularly when the behaviour in question involves a loss of gratification, inconvenience, or discomfort.

- Mass media have a limited potential for teaching complex concepts or providing psychomotor or social interaction skills.

- Mass media can have a valuable 'climate setting' role and can be extremely effective in 'agenda setting' or critical consciousness raising.

In fact, on the basis of a substantial amount of research into social marketing in general and the use of mass media for health promotion in particular, we are in a position to make a number of specific observations and recommendations. Given the 'panacea tendency' mentioned above, a list of these recommendations is probably justified! This is as follows.

- More effective campaigns use multiple media.

- More effective campaigns use mass media as part of community-wide programmes to support other activities—in school, primary care, etc.

- More effective campaigns are co-ordinated with direct service delivery (for example information 'hotlines' and support services).

- More effective campaigns involve key power figures and groups in mass media organizations and government.

- Role models should be carefully selected; it is essential to be sure that the target group identifies with the models selected and that the models continue to retain their appeal and credibility.

- Consultative collaboration should be used as part of a broad health promotion strategy in order to influence media policy and thus mitigate negative effects of the portrayal of health matters in the media.

- Campaigns should emphasize positive behaviour change rather than negative consequences and current rewards rather than the avoidance of distant negative consequences.

- Any anxiety-provoking media messages should be accompanied by mechanisms for reducing that anxiety.

- More effective campaigns utilize educational messages in entertainment contexts.

- Campaign timing is very important.

- Repetition of a single (simple) message is more likely to create an impact.

- Campaigns should use key marketing principles—such as audience segmentation, setting modest and realistic goals, formative evaluation, and message pretesting.

- Audience segmentation is likely to be more productive if it is based on 'psychographics' (for example exploration of beliefs or values using qualitative research techniques) rather than demographics (broader focus on such variables as social class using quantitative techniques) as part of the pretesting strategy.

- A good deal of thought and effort should be devoted to media advocacy using creative epidemiology.

- Wherever possible, health promotion should obtain value for money by generating newsworthy stories which create unpaid advertising.

It should be clear from the above discussion of the use of mass media that perhaps their major function is to support general community-wide initiatives that centre on interpersonal education techniques supported by healthy public policy. Accordingly, we shall provide a fairly cursory review of the various key settings and contexts in which these interpersonal methods typically operate.

Key settings and contexts for health promotion

Health promotion can be employed in a number of settings and contexts, for example schools, local authority institutions, youth clubs, workplaces, pharmacies, and of course by the various provisions of the health and medical services. Two principles will guide the discussion that follows. The first of these emphasizes the importance of a 'healthy alliance' between the various delivery systems and the second makes the common-sense assertion that each particular context and setting has its own strengths and specific potential for promoting health and, conversely, its own limitations.

The concept of intersectoral collaboration figures prominently in WHO's formulation of health promotion practice, and at the time of writing the notion of a **healthy alliance** is enjoying a degree of popularity in the United Kingdom health service. There is nothing particularly startling about the rationale for the healthy alliance, which rests on the assumption that there will be a synergistic effect if each and every possible avenue through which health promotion might be provided is maximally exploited, i.e. substantial benefits should accrue for the public health.

Two kinds of collaborative endeavour are worth noting. The first of these is often described in relation to a notional 'health career'. For example, it is helpful to construct a 'smoking career' as a basis for devising a coherent programme of smoking education. The smoking career identifies the progress made by individuals who, at some point, are recruited to smoking as 'experimental smokers', become 'regular smokers', and, subsequently, either give up their habit (thus swelling the ranks of 'ex-smokers') or continue along their career as regular and probably dissonant smokers concerned at their increased risk of tobacco-related disease or premature death.

A number of important influences on the smoking career have been identified. These include the extent to which parents 'model' smoking by their example or encourage it by their *laissez-faire* attitude or positive approval. They also include peer group example and the various psychological and social needs that lead to young people exposing themselves to the pressures of one peer group rather than another. They include the normative pressures of the workplace and the general background 'noise' provided by mass media.

Macrolevel factors such as socio-economic status exert a continuing and, typically, mediating effect. Of course, it is a truism to observe that people in unskilled manual occupations have a higher level of smoking than those from the upper echelons of management and the professions. Even more substantial rates of smoking are apparent in the unemployed or those who experience some other form of social deprivation.

A more detailed analysis of the smoking career is beyond the scope of this chapter, but sufficient has probably been said to demonstrate the significance of the career-line analysis for the systematic planning of health promotion programmes. In short, if the tendency to adopt and sustain smoking results from the combined and cumulative effects of socialization and a variety of environmental circumstances, then health promotion not only needs to take account of these various pressures but must also develop a competing programme. Such a programme should have, in addition, a cumulative effect by ensuring that a variety of agencies, formal and informal, operate in a compatible and synergistic fashion. In this manner, the school programme builds appropriately on antenatal and child-care initiatives undertaken in primary care and sets the scene for later mass media campaigns and efforts in the workplace and wider community.

The second kind of synergistic programme mentioned earlier is cross-sectional rather than longitudinal. It has to do with establishing healthy alliances and intersectoral collaboration. We have mentioned this before, but it is well worth reiterating the point that collaboration between those involved in providing health education (i.e. seeking to influence people's behaviours) must be supplemented by supportive healthy public policy if the maximum synergistic effect is to be achieved. We shall bear this principle in mind as we now consider a number of important health promotion settings and give some thought to the particular contribution that they might make to the general collaborative effort.

Inevitably, the following review will be somewhat cursory; more complete treatments of health promotion settings and strategies have been given by Bracht (1990), Glanz *et al.* (1990), Whitehead and Tones (1991), and Tones and Tilford (1994, pp. 87–103).

The workplace

In the United States the workplace has been viewed as an important location for health promotion for many years, and there are signs that its popularity has increased in recent years in Europe as well. In commenting on the workplace, reference will be made to the two recurrent themes in this present review:

- the advantages and limitations of any given setting for establishing health promotion programmes;

- the importance of incorporating complementary health policy.

We should begin by making the fairly obvious point that all settings contribute to health whether or not they have a health promotion policy. The influence may be good or bad. For instance, if the workplace has poor safety procedures, creates stress in the work-force through poor staff relationships or the threat of redundancy, and offers only unhealthy food in smoke-clouded canteens, it could hardly be considered as health promoting!

Certainly, the workplace has been an attractive proposition for health educators since it offers a great opportunity for gaining access to a large proportion of the adult population (some 26 million people in the United Kingdom) in a well-defined and, it is hoped, supportive setting.

However, certain problematic aspects must be taken into account. The organizational goals of the workplace are fundamentally different from the goals of health promoters. Indeed, the sole purpose of the commercial sector is to maximize profit. Fortunately, managers seem to be increasingly convinced that health promotion in their workplace will actually increase profit. Their rationale is as follows: a health promotion programme as part of workers' welfare provision enhances the public image of the company; it enhances staff morale and reduces turnover and its associated retraining costs; sickness absence rates should decline and productivity should improve. Moreover, in the United States at least, insurance costs should be reduced dramatically. In fact, there is a good deal of evidence that these managerial perceptions are justified.

Clearly, in the United Kingdom the public sector employs a substantial proportion of the workforce, and the profit motive is perhaps less significant. The National Health Service provides a particularly apposite example of such a workforce, and it is a matter of some interest that one of the more important requirements of WHO's 'health promoting hospital' initiative is that health service institutions and organizations develop an 'exemplary' occupational health service incorporating health education, empowerment, and supportive health-promoting policy.

Clearly, for any health promotion programme to be completely effective, it must be fully incorporated into the normal day-to-day working of a given organization. Even if the resources were available, outside health professionals should not be expected to provide a direct service. However, although an occupational health service might be an obvious candidate for the health promotion task, provision can be patchy, particularly in small industries and organizations. This fact leads us to the second of the two themes mentioned earlier: the policy imperative.

Policy is important at two levels. The possible lack of a proper occupational health service has implications for macro-level policy in terms of financial support, legislation, and nurse training. At the local level, the importance of policy has been emphasized thoroughly. For many years it has been acknowledged that blaming accidents on workers' carelessness or failure to take proper precautions is a classic example of victim blaming, and there has been a corresponding improvement in safety legislation and environmental protection schemes. More recently, a good deal of progress has been made in the adoption and implementation of health policy in areas related to other aspects of life-style: smoking policies are now commonplace, alcohol policies are increasingly being implemented, and a start is being made in providing healthy eating and, less frequently, exercise facilities.

The health-promoting school

The school is conventionally regarded as an obvious place for teaching about health, and the emergence of any particular health concern is likely to lead to the somewhat aggrieved question: 'What are the schools doing about it?'

Again, the question of designing and implementing health education curricula in schools has a long pedigree. It has a substantial theoretical and practical base and an extensive associated literature. A wide variety of teaching materials, curriculum planning guides, and training initiatives have been launched. Some further insights into this sophisticated world are provided by Ryder and Campbell (1988) and Nutbeam *et al.* (1991). A few, perhaps obvious, points are worth making.

The major advantage for ensuring a sound health promotion presence in the school curriculum is the fact that young people spend a long time in this setting (some 15 000 hours in the United Kingdom). Moreover, schoolchildren are at a relatively early stage in their health career. Logically, this should be a prime opportunity for influencing attitudes and behaviours at a formative stage.

Much more important, however, is the possibility for schools to provide horizontal rather than vertical health education programmes. One of the major implications of the kind of analysis that we conducted earlier in discussing the health action model is a need to take a sophisticated look at the factors contributing to health and illness behaviours. In short, quite basic attributes and competences such as self-esteem, locus of control, or the possession of various 'life-skills' will influence all kinds of health decisions. Accordingly, rather than focusing on current epidemiological priorities, and professionally defined health problems (as exemplified by the five key areas highlighted by the Department of Health's review of England's health (Department of Health 1992)), we should focus on root causes and solutions. This point has been more extensively argued elsewhere (Tones 1993*a*), but we would assert that a broad horizontal programme of school-based personal, social, and health education will lay a proper foundation for empowered decision-making. This will be both more productive and more economical than concentrating solely on vertical programmes such as accident prevention or cancer education.

In the context of our continuing emphasis on supportive public policy, one of the recent features of school health education has been the formal acknowledgement of a need to ensure that health teaching is not inconsistent with the general life of the school. The existence of a 'hidden curriculum' has always been acknowledged by general theory and practice in education. It has been part of the conventional wisdom of the school sector that the school's 'ethos' can have substantial effects for good or ill. The relatively recent accentuation of this phenomenon in the health context characterizes contemporary definitions of the health-promoting school. Following this principle, it is important that schools should deliberately formulate policies that will complement teaching; nutrition education should not take place in a setting where only unhealthy snacks and school meals are on offer. Exhortations about self-worth will have relatively little impact in an ambience where only the academically outstanding appear to be valued.

The health-promoting hospital

Reference has already been made to the health-promoting hospital initiative, which represents the most significant recent setting in which attempts are being made to ensure that healthy public policy supports other health endeavours. Clearly treatment features prominently in this context, although education is assuming an increasingly higher profile. The origin of the health promoting hospital was the Healthy Cities movement, and its 'ratification' was the Budapest Declaration (1991). The main features of hospitals subscribing to the principles of the Budapest Declaration are summarized below.

- The Health Promoting Hospital has an integrated policy for promoting positive health for patients, staff, and visitors covering all aspects of the hospital environment and the transactions occurring within it.

- The Health Promoting Hospital should be seen as part of the local community it serves and should maintain active links and alliances with community groups and agencies.

- The Health Promoting Hospital should have a model occupational health service which provides an example of good practice for other workplaces.

- The Health Promoting Hospital is characterized not only by effective communication and good patient education; it strives to empower the patients in its care.

The pedigree and rationale of the four principles listed above are doubtless self-explanatory. However, the notion of positive health emphasized by the Budapest Declaration and the empowerment question do merit a little further elaboration. The concept of positive health is by no means clearly articulated but is closely associated with the condition of empowerment. Macleod Clark's (1993) distinction between 'sick' nursing and 'health' nursing is clearly germane to this debate. The evolutionary, or perhaps revolutionary, move from sick nursing behaviours (which are 'dominating, generalized, prescriptive, reassuring, directive') to health nursing would be entirely consistent with the goals of a health-promoting hospital. Macleod Clark's description of health nursing is also congruent with our earlier recommendation for effective doctor–patient consultations. Unlike sick nursing, it involves the processes of 'collaboration, negotiation, facilitation, the provision of support, and the individualisation of communication'.

Indeed, this accentuation of empowerment in the hospital setting is intriguing if we bear in mind that, traditionally, the hospital has provided a classic example of a 'total institution'. According to Taylor (1979), a hospital is one of the few places where an individual forfeits control over virtually every task that he or she customarily performs.

Interestingly, the Management Executive of the British National Health Service apparently has taken the notion of the health promoting hospital very seriously in their publication of guidelines (National Health Service Management Executive 1994) and provision of general support. This level of commitment was illustrated by a nursing officer from the Department of Health who cited the results of departmental research into health education and health promotion in nursing in acute areas. She quoted the following extract:

> The data revealed that the ward climate needs to be such that nurses feel valued, supported, autonomous and empowered members of the ward team. This appeared to facilitate health education and health promotion via increasing morale and enabling nurses to support and empower their patients rather than maintain traditional role distinctions and the unequal balance of power inherent in these. (Weeks 1993)

Community development

The final example of a setting or context is that of community development. Again, this is a complex and often contested concept. It is difficult, in a brief review, to avoid stereotyping and over-simplification. At one level, we can view community development as a setting that differs from other settings merely in its informality of approach. However, the most significant feature of the approach is its ideology.

Community development should not be confused with so-called 'community-wide' programmes, which involve the deployment of the widest possible range of agencies in a common cause (such as the prevention of coronary heart disease). Community development does not equate with those 'outreach' programmes that deliver services to those members of the community who do not use existing facilities, and it is not synonymous with educational programmes that use community workers to 'get through to' the 'hard to reach'. Community development does involve working with those so-called 'resistant' groups in settings characterized typically by urban squalor, disadvantage, and deprivation.

Community development is of particular relevance to health promotion since its concern is, above all, with empowerment and its ideology is best described in terms of a 'radical model', as defined at the beginning of this chapter. In short, the ideological imperative is with remedying disadvantage and achieving a fairer distribution of resources in society. It typically operates by employing community change agents to work with people in relatively small geographic areas. Their task is to help the community identify its 'felt needs'. A successful intervention would raise people's consciousness and concern over their social circumstances; their beliefs and perceptions should change and they should feel more confident in their ability to agitate for social and environmental change, and they should acquire skills to help them achieve the changes that had been identified as important. In short, they would be empowered.

Although they do not match this pure and idealized form of community development, many community health projects embody the 'bottom-up' empowering stance of the ideal type. Since they often start with well-recognized public health issues, they may bypass the stage of identifying felt needs, although they would consider it essential to consult the community extensively about its perception of need within the somewhat narrower domain of health and prevention. Therefore community health projects do not attempt to 'colonize' a community with health workers whose purpose is to infiltrate and manipulate networks in order to achieve predetermined goals and meet specific targets imposed in an authoritarian way, as will be clear from the following list of the characteristics of community health projects (derived from Rosenthal 1983):

- firmly based outside health professions;
- concerned with addressing inequalities in health and health care provision;
- concerned to promote collective awareness of social causes of ill health;
- assert that the monopoly of information about health and ill health by professionals must be challenged both individually and collectively;
- activities centre on work with small groups of local people;
- projects have a catalyst function in stimulating local health, social, and educational services.

Bearing in mind that the main purpose of this chapter is to illuminate the various factors and approaches that may influence behaviours, at this juncture we ought to reaffirm that the use of empowering techniques, whether in community or hospital, does not merely serve ideological ends. If successful, the empowering effects of community health projects are more likely to lead to the adoption of medically approved preventive behaviours than are competing disease-focused vertical programmes delivered in a traditional way.

The requirements of systematic programme design

Microlevel analysis would reveal that a variety of specific communication techniques and educational methods are usually used in all the settings explored above. Before considering the appropriate selection of these methods, the relationship between settings and methods in the context of a systematic approach to designing health education programmes is shown in Fig. 23.5.

Any given programme involves an assessment of need, either explicitly or implicitly. Figure 23.5 contrasts 'normative' (i.e. professionally prescribed) needs with a community's 'felt needs'—and notes that both might be overruled by the superior force of political imperatives! At all events, a process of prioritizing competing demands must take place. The process of assessing need and the associated resource implications would be followed typically by identification of aims and an analysis of the relative contribution to be made by health policy measures and health education within a variety of different settings. Where a programme involves a synergistic amalgam of both policy and education, programme design and evaluation will be considerably facilitated by the statement of precise and detailed objectives. Therefore, since the purpose of health education is to facilitate learning, the educational task would be expressed as 'learning objectives'. Both sets of objectives would be stated with respect to the target group(s) or individuals who, it is hoped, will benefit from the programme. This procedure should be preceded by a process of pretesting (or assessment of 'learning readiness') to determine relevant characteristics of the target group, including such features as existing practices, levels of knowledge, and attitudes. Ideally, a picture or profile of the community itself would be developed to illuminate programme planning. The construction of both kinds of profile

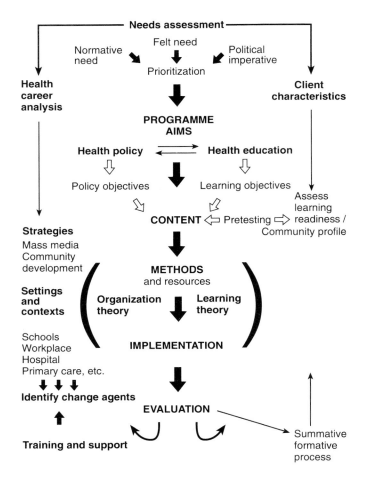

Fig. 23.5 Relationship between settings and methods.

should form part of the general database on which decisions might be made about health promotion strategies and the methods needed to translate educational and policy objectives into practice.

A **health career analysis** provides a useful developmental perspective for planners in identifying the mix of strategies and settings that should maximize the chance of an effective outcome. For instance, the construction of a smoking career would identify important influences on recruitment to smoking—such as family, socio-economic group, community values and social network, school ethos, peer group, and mass media. Accordingly, a programme designed to prevent the adoption of smoking would employ strategies and initiate programmes in settings that would ensure the provision of education, supported by facilitative policies, at the most productive points on the health career.

Ideally, of course, there would be 'intersectoral collaboration' to maximize their cumulative impact between the various agencies and institutions contributing at various stages on the health career. At the same time 'healthy alliances' might be formed at any given point in time between health workers in the various settings mentioned above. Increasingly, this kind of alliance is described as a 'community coalition' (*Health Education Research* 1993), although the term 'community' is used somewhat loosely. At all events, it is argued quite logically that the formation of a coalition that includes the great and the good together with key local decision-makers, health

professionals, representatives of important organizations, and lay members is likely to provide a powerful impetus for change.

Figure 23.5 also shows how change agents within the various settings and contexts might be identified. These are the potential health educators or advocates for change. The extent to which they have the necessary motivation, knowledge, skills, and competences will vary quite substantially from context to context. Accordingly, they might well need training prior to programme implementation. As we shall see later in the chapter, evaluation of the success of that training may provide one of a series of 'indirect' indicators of programme efficiency.

Since health promotion programmes may range from regional campaigns to a single clinical consultation to a series of group sessions within a health promotion clinic in primary care or even to an entire school curriculum, their content will vary dramatically in both comprehensiveness and style. None the less, decisions should be made after consideration of the requirements of given settings or modes of delivery but before the specification of methods and the selection of adjuvant learning resources or visual aids, such as videos or leaflets.

The development of policies rather than education programmes would follow a similar general pattern. Policy objectives would be translated into content, and various tactics and techniques would be employed to achieve implementation. In many instances this developmental process will occur in tandem with supportive education. The achievement of both policy and educational goals will be facilitated by consulting relevant theory. For instance, organizational theory might provide valuable insights for initiating change in factory or business setting, whereas learning theory should be used to guide choice of programme content and teaching method. Reference was made earlier to the health action model, and this might offer useful guidelines for the decision-making process.

Not surprisingly, the final stage in the process of systematic programme design is one of evaluation. Three kinds of evaluation are shown in Fig. 23.5: summative, formative, and process. Further reference will be made to these in the final section of this chapter. We may merely note here that summative evaluation will assess programme effectiveness by noting the extent to which learning objectives have been achieved. Formative evaluation monitors progress and, where necessary, supplies guidelines for 'remedial work'. Ideally, process evaluation would make available detailed documentation of the processes and procedures that happened during the programme in order to provide 'illumination' and insight into possible reasons for its successes or failures.

The microlevel: selecting methods for facilitating learning and changing behaviours

So far, we have considered the general nature and philosophy of health promotion and health education. We have considered the relationship between these two complementary procedures and the ways in which people and communities make decisions, and perhaps even change their behaviours. We have also analysed in some depth the processes of communication and education and described the requirements of successful learning. Subsequently, the various contexts and settings in which health promotion and health education typically operate have been explored, and we have identified the key requirements for designing systematic health promotion programmes.

This part of the chapter is concerned with educational methodology which, as we have noted, is an integral component within a systems approach to health education. Methods are relatively specific and operate at the microlevel rather than the macrolevel of strategic planning. Very similar methods may be used in a variety of the several contexts or settings considered above. For example, they may form part of community development or be used as a supplement to mass media. In their turn, particular audiovisual aids or learning resources may be used as adjuncts to methods. For instance, group discussion may be facilitated by a short trigger video. Of course, a video used on its own (for example at a display in a health fair) falls into the category of mass media.

There is only one logical justification for using one or more educational methods, and that is to supply the conditions necessary for efficient learning. The line of reasoning should be as follows: (i) identify the kind(s) of learning involved in a particular programme, (ii) specify the conditions that must be supplied in order to promote the kind of learning identified (i.e. a 'relatively permanent change in capability or disposition'), and (iii) select the educational method or methods most suitable for supplying the conditions in question. For instance, if the health education goal is only to produce understanding of the risk factors associated with coronary heart disease, then good question-and-answer technique together with clear well-programmed explanation supported by an appropriate visual aid and a written *aide-memoire* will probably suffice. Indeed, this basic teaching form is usually present in most 'cocktails' of rather more exotic techniques.

However, less traditional methods will usually be needed to achieve the specific goals of health promotion. For example, 'experiential' learning would be considered a better tactic for influencing beliefs and attitudes and for equipping learners with skills. Experiential learning was referred to earlier in this chapter in discussing alternative modes of 'coding' messages in the communication process (for a more thorough discussion, see Tones (1993*b*)). Health education is more than the mere provision of information; it involves the skilful selection and practice of particular techniques illustrated below in specific examples.

Experiential learning and skills training

Despite the etymology of the word 'doctor', it is relatively uncommon to use the term 'teaching' in a health context. None the less, since teaching involves the efficient promotion of learning, this is exactly what is happening in any successful educational encounter. Moreover, teaching should not be equated with a didactic presentation of information by an expert source. Teaching involves deliberately engineering opportunities for learning (including such activities as explaining or counselling), but which may well consist of providing experiences for the learner. As an example, we shall consider a notional drugs course.

A group of adolescents are required to work in pairs. They are given a pack of different cards that separately depict different types of information about drugs. The pack includes a card with only the words 'legal' or 'illegal' printed on it. Another card describes the effects of an unnamed drug. A further card describes the effects of an unnamed drug on the user. Yet another card includes a

description of a 'typical' hypothetical user. Each pair of young people then proceeds to match a set of, say, 12 commonly used drugs with the various attributes on the cards mentioned above.

Clearly, a teacher could have told them the facts (which would have been decidedly boring) or given them a list to read later (which may or may not have happened!). However, the experiential expedient ensures participation and attention. Of course, they are not expected to remember the information but are given a copy of the correct matching once they have completed their problem-solving task. Furthermore, because coffee, alcohol, and cigarette smoking are included in the list of drugs, they begin to learn, incidentally, something about the socially constructed definition of substances.

The next procedure might be to take nine drugs cards and arrange them in some kind of priority order with respect to their seriousness and social acceptability. The cards now become a learning resource for triggering debate and discussion to help the learners clarify their opinions and values about drug misuse as part of the process of facilitating decision-making.

Role play is a commonly used method in health education that admirably illustrates the principles of experiential learning. It is part of the broader methodological category of simulation and gaming. Its particular strengths derive from the opportunities that it provides for problem solving and attitude change. For example, trainee town planners (an important group of health promoters) might be provided with a detailed but fictitious case study of a mental health dispute. This could represent the not uncommon 'not-in-my-backyard' syndrome in which local residents are angered by the potential siting of a half-way house for the mentally ill in their neighbourhood. The participants in the role play are then required to act out various parts: the mental health worker, the local councillor, the angry local resident, the local general practitioner, and so on. Hopefully, the exercise should not only provide good insights into this kind of problem but may also generate a more positive attitude to the half-way house and even influence beliefs, concerns, and general attitudes relating to mental illness itself.

Turning to the question of skills training, it will be quite apparent to anyone who has had the task of teaching another person a psychomotor skill that the skill cannot be readily acquired by merely providing information. For example, consider the learning requirements of teaching young people first-aid procedures as part of a harm-minimization strategy in drug education. They will not only have to see these procedures properly modelled by a competent practitioner, but will also need to practice the procedures and receive rapid feedback so that they can correct their errors and internalize correct responses.

The requirements of learning social interaction skills are less obvious. For instance, as part of a series of health promotion 'clinics' designed to reduce coronary heart disease risk, it is clear that the commitment of group members to following 'sensible drinking' guidelines requires the support of appropriate social interaction skills, as was noted earlier in Fig. 23.3. In short, they need to acquire competences in refusing an alcoholic drink in the difficult context of a 'round-buying' culture. They might readily learn four rules of verbal assertiveness (be clear in your own mind what you want to say; state your position; state your reason; acknowledge the other person's position or feelings). However, in order to apply these rules in a real-life scenario, they will need to learn not only what to say but how to say it. They will need social skills, and these would be provided by following the kind of techniques that would be used to teach cardiopulmonary resuscitation skills; in short, demonstration and modelling followed by repetition, feedback, correction of errors, and reinforcement of good practice. Accordingly, they will have to practice four rules of non-verbal assertive behaviour: using an appropriate tone of voice, correct eye contact, facial expression consistent with verbal message, and proper body language. Practice followed by consolidation through role play should establish the newly learned competence.

Learning in groups

Our discussion of educational methodology in this chapter will be concluded with a brief review of the two most common situations in the health care context: the face-to-face consultation and the group teaching session. As indicated earlier, any specific method might be 'nested' within another method. For instance, group work on mental health promotion would typically include a practice of skills element in which individuals learn techniques of relaxation. Our discussion here will focus on some of the key features of group work *per se* and will use the example of an antenatal class to exemplify these.

Any review of group work provided here will inevitably be somewhat superficial. Even the definition of 'group' creates problems. For the purpose of this discussion, however, we shall consider the group as a kind of minicommunity involving a relatively small aggregate of people sharing a particular complex of interpersonal interactions and dynamics.

The most obvious comparative advantage of group teaching is its potential for quite intensive interpersonal interaction. At the simplest level, it is possible to involve every group member in the learning task, gain immediate feedback about the current state of participants' learning, and provide the 'different strokes' to which reference has been made more than once in this chapter. While intensity of interaction over a given period of time will be greater in the one-to-one circumstance, there are two extra dimensions in the group. The first of these is the expertise and experience of other (lay) members; the second is the often very powerful effect of group norms.

Let us assume that the subject of the antenatal class is infant feeding. Since three major factors appear to influence intention to breast or bottle feed, it would seem logical to centre discussion on those factors. In short, breast feeding is typically influenced by beliefs about the benefits of the practice for the baby's health and beliefs about its costs with respect to inconvenience and, more importantly, embarrassment. Accordingly, although some explanation by a group leader (for example a midwife) will be necessary at some stage, the main thrust of the class should be to allow the mothers to explore the beliefs and values that they share about feeding babies, particularly in relation to the three factors mentioned above. In this context, beliefs and attitudes may change as the views and experiences of other group members are discussed. Of course, complementary learning experiences may be built into the class. A nursing mother might serve as a credible communicator and could model breast feeding. Moreover, as breast feeding is clearly a psychomotor skill, an opportunity must be provided, at a

later support stage, to practice that skill—probably in the confines of a ward in a health-promoting hospital!

It will be evident that the activities of the antenatal class are entirely consistent with an empowerment approach; the goal is to help women make a choice of breast or bottle feeding. On the one hand, group dynamics might be exploited deliberately by zealous health educators determined to instil the desirability of breast feeding. The best example of this is the work of Lewin (1958) and later Bond (1958), who employed the group discussion–decision technique. Lewin demonstrated that this method was superior to a lecture in persuading housewives to change their family's diet (not surprising, perhaps) and also (more surprising) better than face-to-face advice from a dietitian. The effect, it has been argued, is due to two factors: first the effect of an individual group member's commitment (possibly in public) to a course of action, and second the impact of group pressure. Clearly, the method can misfire dramatically if the group norm swings against the outcome that the group leader is seeking to manipulate!

As a final observation in our discussion of the value of group methods, we shall reiterate the necessity for the group leader/facilitator to have a knowledge of both group dynamics and those social interaction skills needed to manage the learning experiences of the participants.

One-to-one encounters: the consultation

Here an attempt will be made to integrate earlier observations about the complementary and, to some extent, consecutive processes of communication and education. To this end, Fig. 23.6 summarizes the key features of these processes.

Although these processes are applicable to a greater or lesser extent to all educational methods, the dyadic encounter between doctor/health worker and client epitomizes them.

The principles of effective communication are quite readily stated. In order to ensure that clients correctly interpret the communication, the communicator must check clients' existing knowledge, beliefs, and attitudes (in an empathic manner) and 'encode' the message in an appropriate format. Particular care must be taken with non-verbal communication. The communicator must try to ensure that, where necessary, messages are remembered and, above all, check that they have been correctly interpreted and understood.

The requirement for the teacher/health educator to ensure client recall or remembering features twice in Fig. 23.6. First it appears in the context mentioned above (i.e. to minimize forgetting important information), and second it appears at the later stage of motivating and facilitating client choice. By definition, learning involves change; as change is stored in memory, it merits some brief consideration.

Remembering and forgetting

In an earlier reference to the importance of forgetting in the context of communication failure, we noted the existence of two different viewpoints. On the one hand, Tuckett *et al.* (1985) considered that inability to recall information made an insignificant contribution to patients' lack of commitment to recommended actions. However, Ley (1990) apparently demonstrated that patients forgot about 40 per cent of the information provided. How can these seemingly conflicting observations be reconciled?

EDUCATIONAL TASK **CLIENT TASK**

Communication

Check felt needs/need for
information
Establish rapport using
counselling skills: active
listening etc.
Take account of non-verbal
communication
Check for understanding
Check intelligibility of written
information
Take steps to maximize
recall/provide aide memoire if
necessary

Receive message: pay attention
Perceive and interpret message
correctly

**Motivation:
facilitating decision making**

Explore existing beliefs,
attitudes, skills; seek to modify
beliefs and attitudes where
appropriate
Provide information; provide
skills: decision making;
psychomotor; social and lifeskills
Check learning and recall
Analyse environmental
circumstances
Negotiate and agree 'contract'

Form appropriate beliefs (e.g.
about causes and nature of
disease and health issues;
about susceptibility, seriousness,
costs, and benefits of
recommended actions)

Develop self-efficacy beliefs
Acquire skills
Agree contract

**POSITIVE ATTITUDE/
INTENTION TO ACT**

Provide support

Provide opportunity for acquiring
supportive knowledge, social
and self-regulatory skills
Help mobilize social and
environmental support
Act as advocate for social and
environmental change
Check client's progress

Acquire new information and skills

**ADOPT AND SUSTAIN
HEALTH ACTION**

IMPROVED HEALTH

Fig. 23.6 Health promotion and the consultation.

The fact is that human information processing systems have a limited capacity. Therefore people can recall only a limited amount of data at any one time. Indeed, Miller (1951) argued convincingly that the actual amount of information that could be handled was 'seven plus or minus two' bits. Thus, it is not surprising that a substantial proportion of certain kinds of information will be forgotten. It is equally clear that the amount remembered may be enhanced by the use of various mnemonics, and Ley (1990) advised doctors to employ a variety of such devices in order to optimize patient recall. These memory-enhancing techniques included, for example, simple repetition of items of information, emphasizing particularly important items, and using 'explicit categorization'. The last-mentioned technique involves the practitioner providing a kind of advance warning of advice to come in the form of particular categories. For instance, a doctor might say: 'First of all, I am going to tell you the results of the tests that you had last week; I will then tell you what is wrong with you; we will next discuss the implications of this, and so forth'. There is reliable evidence that the adoption of these rather mechanical measures are indeed

effective in increasing the amount that patients can recall after the consultation.

Before leaving the subject of remembering and forgetting, it is worth drawing attention to another tradition of psychological research which does not focus on the quantitative aspects of forgetting but rather seeks to describe and explain qualitative changes. In short, forgetting does not merely consist of data loss; it involves a process of active reconstruction. Just as the process of perception is no mere photographic phenomenon but consists of an energetic striving to make sense of the world, the process of remembering incorporates 'effort after meaning' and interpretation. People reconstruct their imperfect memories until they make sense. In doing so, they often fail to remember what actually happened but recall what they expected to happen and/or would have liked to happen. Doctors have often been surprised and sometimes alarmed at patients' spurious recollections of earlier consultations and their firm conviction about the reality of diagnoses that were never made and advice that was never given!

Whether we consider the quantitative or the qualitative aspects of memory, there is one consistent finding of paramount significance: people will have more complete and accurate recall if the information provided can be assimilated into existing understanding. Thus two observations may be made: first, a population that has received general health education should have superior recall; second, the highly recommended counselling practice of exploring clients' theories and beliefs will not only diminish attitudinal barriers but should result in better understanding and, as a consequence, a diminished chance of forgetting important information.

Doubtless, it will be self-evident that even if recommendations for healthy actions have been provided in an insightful and meaningful fashion, people will still have difficulty in recalling detailed lists of data, no matter how useful. One solution to this problem is to employ some of the mnemonics mentioned above. A simpler alternative would be to provide an appropriate *aide-memoire* in the form of a leaflet (hopefully, checked for 'reading ease').

Persuasion or supporting decision-making?

Returning now to our consideration of the educational process shown in Fig. 23.6, we can see that a key element in the checklist centres on the motivation of the learner and the facilitation of decision-making. We are illustrating, in an operational form, two principles of health promotion: first, that health promotion is concerned to empower rather than to coerce; second, that healthy choices are more likely to result from making this healthy choice the easy choice than from the deployment of techniques to change attitudes.

Motivation is obviously an essential precursor to action but should be achieved as follows:

- ensuring access to necessary information;

- checking clients' beliefs, attitudes, and skills, i.e. their learning readiness;

- remedying information deficit, influencing beliefs, and providing skills;

- Conducting a thorough analysis of environmental and situational factors that might militate against client choice;

• Establishing a contract with the client.

Earlier in this chapter we discussed the central role of beliefs and other psychosocial factors in motivating people to adopt healthy behaviours. None the less, at this juncture, the interactions among environmental analysis, skills acquisition, and self-efficacy beliefs deserve further emphasis. As we have shown, individuals must believe that they are actually capable of undertaking recommended actions before they will invest time and effort in complying with these recommendations. Since persuasion and exhortation alone are unlikely to convince the doubtful, some or all of the following procedures will be needed. First, the practitioner and the client, in counselling mode, must examine critically the social and environmental circumstances in which the client will have to undertake the proposed behaviour. Assuming that the client has already been motivated as a result of previous exploration of values and beliefs, necessary skills must be provided. These might include psychomotor competences, such as the skills needed to exercise safely and beneficially after myocardial infarction. They might include cooking and even shopping skills to support a healthier diet. As noted above, social interaction skills will frequently be essential—perhaps to help a parent cope with a troublesome adolescent!

If behaviours have been modelled by a credible communicator (as described in the earlier observations on group teaching) and skills have been acquired, clients may come to believe that they might actually achieve the goal that they desire. However, people must be reasonably convinced that environmental conditions are not so negative that, even with skills, they are bound to fail. The result of this interaction should be a contract accepted by both the health educator and the learner. The contract may be in written form, in which case it may serve not only to enhance commitment but might also provide a useful *aide-memoire*.

Situational support and the problem of relapse

As shown in Fig. 23.6, the final phase of the one-to-one educational consultation involves the provision of support. It is assumed that if things have gone according to plan, the contract will have resulted in the client's adopting the healthy behaviours specified therein. As their contribution to contracting, health professionals will do whatever is feasible to engineer actual changes in the environment as well as giving clients the skills that they need to manage situational barriers to action. Clearly, there are limits to what even the most dynamic health worker can achieve, although, as we suggested before, a commitment to health promotion implies the adoption of an advocacy role which involves pressing for policies to reduce unhealthy social circumstances. At the very least, health workers can usually marshal social support even if they are unable to have much effect on major environmental problems.

As we observed in our discussion of the health action model, one of the more useful analyses of behaviours liable to relapse has been provided by Prochaska and DiClemente (1986). People are not expected to make a once-and-for-all decision to adopt and sustain the healthy course of action; relapse is considered to be a likely result. However, the individual is also expected to make a renewed commitment to addiction-free living at some time in the future.

A particular technique of 'motivational interviewing' is associated with the 'revolving door model' proposed by Prochaska and DiClemente. In short, standard counselling skills are employed in accordance with the counsellor's perception of the client's particular stage on the spiral of precontemplation to relapse. The techniques are well described by Rollnick *et al.* (1992).

In order to minimize the problem of relapse, insights from behaviour modification may be used to equip the client with self-regulatory skills prior to undertaking the desired behaviour change. A discussion of the theory and practice of behaviour modification is not possible here. However, a wide variety of texts are available for further consultation (Kanfer and Karoly 1972; Watson and Tharp 1989). These skills are designed to help people gain control over the various powerful drives and emotions that are inconsistent with their values and attitudes. In summary, self-regulation normally consists of monitoring the reciprocal relationship between environment and behaviours. People are helped to monitor and record their actions (for instance, noting the circumstances that trigger their smoking and the degree of pleasure or relief that they gain from any particular cigarette). They are taught to monitor any gaps between the goals that they have set themselves and their actions. They learn how to control their environment in order to avoid temptation and to break well-established unhealthy routines. They are helped to identify substitute gratifications (often an exceedingly difficult task!), for instance acquiring relaxation skills as an alternative to smoking as a stress management device. Finally, clients are encouraged to consolidate healthy behaviour by rewarding themselves for achieving their targets.

Education and communication skills

The purpose of this section has been to explore the complexities of human behaviour in health and illness and to examine the contribution that health education might make to broader health promotion programmes. Hopefully, we have demonstrated the difficulties involved in influencing behaviour as well as provided a framework for effective action in various settings and contexts. A wide range of methods is available for those who seek to undertake the complementary tasks of communication and education. Consideration of the detailed techniques that are required in the various interpersonal encounters between health and education workers and their different client groups should lead to the conclusion that a high level of skill is needed to influence and support health choices. While demystification is both possible and desirable, we cannot expect effectiveness and efficiency without competence.

Success in health promotion: assessing effectiveness
A rationale for evaluation

In this chapter we have made several passing references to the assessment of success in health promotion and health education and noted that the reader must consult specialists texts for a thorough treatment of evaluation (Green and Lewis 1986; Sarvela and McDermott 1993; Tones and Tilford 1994). Again, in order to acquire greater and more detailed insight into the levels of success that have been recorded for different kinds of health education intervention, readers might usefully consult the extensive 14 volume review provided by the International Union of Health for Health Promotion and Education (1994). However, given the increasing demands for 'proof' of the effectiveness of health promotion at a time when resources for traditional medical interventions are failing to meet demand, it would be remiss not to give some consideration to this issue.

We should insist that merely to ask whether or not health promotion works is a naïve or even crass question. We do not usually ask, for instance, whether politics works! Yet, to ask whether health promotion works is a question of a similar level of generality. People may well ask whether health services are successful, but most serious researchers would consider that question as ingenuous. They would expect to know at least which services were to be investigated and require further specification of client groups, situations, and attendant circumstances.

Therefore, bearing in mind that the term 'evaluation' refers to the process of measuring the extent to which certain valued outcomes have been achieved, we must be clear about what success means for those concerned with health promotion. At one level, this is not difficult to specify. For example, as we noted earlier, we might look for evidence that programmes had achieved greater equity or (to give the issue a British flavour) we might look for progress toward slaying William Beveridge's 'five giants of disease, idleness, ignorance, squalor, and want'. Of course, such broad goals are not only remarkable difficult to achieve but are also too general to be used as indicators of success.

Before giving further consideration to the selection of more appropriate indicators of health promotion success, it is worth recalling the main reasons for evaluating any given programme.

Efficacy, effectiveness, and efficiency

Typically, three broad criteria are used in defining programme success: these are **efficacy**, **effectiveness**, and **efficiency**. The term efficacy is used here in accordance with Brook and Lohr's distinction: 'Efficacy refers to the probability of benefit to individuals in a defined population . . . **under ideal conditions of use**' (Brook and Lohr 1985, p. 711, present author's emphasis). Effectiveness simply refers to the extent to which a programme has achieved its goals. The distinction is important to note and, although Brooke and Lohr were considering general health service research, it is particularly apposite to health promotion since it is rare to find programmes operating under ideal circumstances. For instance, we might argue that a particular alcohol education intervention would need supportive fiscal policy to reduce consumer demand for alcohol. We might also specify the need for a long-term programme involving parental modelling and effective teaching in primary school as a prerequisite for work with adolescents. Again, (ideally) we would want to ensure that adolescents had received a properly structured course of assertiveness training before we explored their values and attitudes about alcohol, and we would want to provide them with the understanding and competences needed to refuse all offers of alcohol at a party as part of their particular role as 'designated driver'. Needless to say, such ideal conditions rarely obtain, and so even if we are convinced that such a programme would achieve its stated goal, we would normally have to make do with a much more limited situation in which we had only four school sessions to devote to alcohol.

The matter of efficiency takes us into the domain of relative effectiveness. In other words, efficiency describes the extent to which a given programme has achieved its goals by comparison with some alternative or competing intervention. For instance, if a

course of drugs could reduce population cholesterol levels more quickly and completely than dietary change, it would be a more efficient strategy. Again, it could well be the case that consistent and repeated price increases on cigarettes might be superior to education as a strategy for reducing tobacco consumption. Yet again, if health education delivered by the primary health care team could substantially lower the prevalence of smoking in young women, it would be a more efficient procedure than building smoking education programmes into schools. As a final example, if we could show that using a 'group discussion–decision' method with a practice nurse leader resulted in a higher adoption and maintenance of breast feeding than authoritative advice from a doctor in general practice, then the group work should be judged to be the method of choice.

On cost effectiveness

One of the most important criteria for appraising the efficiency of programme interventions is by calculating the relative financial costs of competing interventions (cost-effectiveness analysis). Cost-benefit analysis, in contrast, not only states the costs in monetary terms but also seeks to place a price tab on the benefits accruing from the programme. A calculation of the cost per given benefit is then possible (typically expressed as a cost-benefit ratio). Now, on the one hand, there is quite firm evidence that health promotion can achieve results that demonstrate not only cost effectiveness but also commendable cost-benefit ratios. On the other hand, cost effectiveness can be a double-edged weapon. We shall provide some brief elaboration of these assertions, but we might note that cost is by no means always used as a criterion for action. For instance, Mooney (1977) demonstrated the truth of this observation quite convincingly when he showed that cost per life saved for a variety of preventive measures ranged from £50 for stillbirth screening to £20 million for alterations to high-rise flats following the collapse of the Ronan Point tower block!

Returning to evidence of financially sound interventions, as long ago as 1974, Green showed how a specific health education programme resulted in a saving of US $7.81 per dollar invested in a hypertension screening and education programme; he also demonstrated that using group discussion techniques to educate asthmatic patients about the best means of controlling their condition resulted in a cost-benefit ratio of 1:5.

More recently, a British study of the effectiveness of family planning services (Laing 1982) identified conservative benefit-to-cost ratios of 1.3:1 for preventing 'typical unplanned pregnancies', a ratio of 4.5:1 for preventing pregnancies among mothers of three or more children, and a ratio of 5.3:1 for unplanned premarital conceptions. As the author put it, 'for every £100 spent on family planning services, the public sector can expect a benefit of £130, £450, and £530, respectively'.

In relation to smoking education programmes, Townsend (1986) argued that if a hypothetical mass media programme were to result in 1000 people giving up smoking permanently, 10000 giving up temporarily, 2000 cutting down, and 15000 seriously considering giving up, then 2991 life years would be saved at a cost of £84 per life. Admittedly, this is a hypothetical example, but Phillips and Prowle (1993) offered a more tangible analysis of benefits by calculating the costs and benefits of the Heartbeat Wales programme. They were unable to ascribe precise cause and effect.

However, on a 'pessimistic worst case' assumption that the programme had only a 10 per cent impact rate on the actual decline in smoking in Wales over a four-year period (1985–1989), they estimated that the 'net cost per working life year saved . . . worked out at approximately £64'.

Finally, recent studies in the United Kingdom have demonstrated the efficiency of advice about methods of stopping smoking provided by doctors in general practice in accordance with quite stringent economic criteria. For a budget of £1 million, a relatively straightforward and simple intervention has been calculated to result in some 59 888 quality-adjusted life-years (QALYs) compared with, for example, a much lower figure for breast screening (302 QALYs). Again, it is generally considered that hip replacement is a highly efficient and appropriate surgical procedure, yet it costs £750 per QALY compared with £167 for physician-provided smoking-related advice (Godfrey *et al.* 1989).

Despite this cheering evidence of effectiveness, we commented that economic indicators of success should be treated with caution. Even allowing for 'discounting'—the process whereby future costs are considered less important than current costs—it seems likely that in the last analysis really effective health promotion, which defers death and generates a large elderly population, will increase the substantial medical costs involved in treating very old people as well as increasing the pensions and benefits bill. Perhaps the most useful approach to this dilemma is to follow the recommendations made by Cohen (1981). Prevention (and health promotion) should be treated as a **merit good**, i.e. something which satisfies a **merit want**. According to Musgrave (1959) (cited by Cohen), merit wants are 'so meritorious that their satisfaction is provided for through the public budget over and above what is provided for through the market and paid for by private buyers'. Clearly, such a view has particular significance at this time in the development of thinking about health services and the marketplace.

At all events, health promotion can demonstrate its capacity to satisfy quite stringent measures of efficiency. However, we need to examine more critically which indicators of its effectiveness and efficiency are most appropriate for those seeking to evaluate success.

Epidemiological indicators

We have argued that health promotion has different goals, including that of empowerment. However, we have also acknowledged that the orientation of this chapter is towards the prevention of disease. Even so, a major principle underlying the evaluation of health promotion initiatives is that traditional epidemiological indicators are inappropriate, and even behavioural outcomes may not be the most useful way of appraising general efficacy.

The above assertion might seem a little surprising. After all, if health promotion has a useful contribution to make to achieving preventive outcomes, is it not reasonable to assess success in terms of reductions in mortality and morbidity? There are two main reasons for not doing so. First, some degree of uncertainty is often associated with the postulated links between particular behaviours and specific disease outcomes. At any rate, on a population basis it would be unreasonable to claim that health promotion has been ineffective if it has influenced life-style but the changes in behaviour had not led to a reduction in disease. For instance, given the uncertainty associated with postulated links between saturated

fat consumption and breast cancer, it would be unwise to measure the success of dietary interventions in terms of a decline in breast cancer mortality. Indeed, given the fact that risk factors for many diseases may fail to explain a substantial amount of the variance in mortality and morbidity, a one-to-one relationship between behaviour change and 'medical' outcome would not be expected to occur.

At first glance, it might be argued that failure to establish clear epidemiological links casts doubts on the wisdom of undertaking behaviour change programmes. This is manifestly untrue; in the example provided above, dietary changes of unproven benefit for preventing breast cancer might well be effective in preventing other disorders. Moreover, even if behaviour change were insufficient on its own to achieve a given preventive outcome, it may well be a necessary component in a broader programme of interventions.

The importance of intermediate indicators

Even life-style changes or other behavioural indicators may not be appropriate indicators of the success of health promotion. While in some instances it would be reasonable to expect to see a change in behaviour after a particular educational intervention (for example a school-based smoking programme might, if properly conducted, delay the onset of smoking in school pupils), in other cases behavioural outcomes would not be feasible. One such instance is provided by programmes where a particular educational input could not be expected to influence a given outcome for many years. For instance, a successful cancer education programme, which effectively teaches children about the nature of cancers in such a way as to contribute to a reduction in cancerophobia, could not be expected to have an impact on a woman's utilization of mammography screening until the young women in question had reached middle age!

An even more important reason for using intermediate indicators derives from the fact that decisions about health or illness have multiple determinants. Hopefully, by now readers might agree that health education is not at all like a drug. Even a relatively straightforward face-to-face consultation between nurse and patient is much more complex and sophisticated than administering pills and potions. As we have seen, health decisions are not the result of a simple linear progression from provision of knowledge through attitude change to the adoption of healthy practices. Accordingly one single input, simple or complex, is unlikely to achieve a desired output. Consider the case of one of the more simple educational interventions—a mass media commercial seeking to influence dietary practices. At the very least, the following chain of events would take place before a successful outcome might be achieved: first, the target audience would need to be adequately exposed to the message and become aware of its existence; they would need to interpret it correctly and understand it; they would need to believe it and assess its personal relevance; typically, they would consider the possible costs and benefits involved in undertaking the changes in diet recommended by the programme and then assess the likelihood of their having the expertise and stamina needed to make those changes. If these several steps have been negotiated successfully and the audience has not been antagonized or made anxious by the message, a positive attitude to adopting a health diet might result. Of course, before that attitude can be translated into practice, the client group will doubtless need a variety of skills and additional knowledge, and of course they must be able to find the healthy products and be able to afford them.

Let us simplify the above process into the following sequence: awareness–knowledge–beliefs–attitudes–support–action. If we were to assign hypothetical probabilities of each stage being satisfactorily negotiated (expressed as a percentage of the population achieving the requisite goal), then the likelihood of success in terms of behaviour change might be depicted as follows:

awareness – knowledge – beliefs/attitudes – support = action
30 per cent 85 per cent 31 per cent   40 per cent = 3 per cent

This 'formula' is based on 30 per cent of the audience having become aware of the message, 85 per cent of that particular group understanding it, 31 per cent of the 85 per cent believing it and being committed to the recommended action, but only 40 per cent having appropriately supportive environmental and social circumstances. The result (quite creditable if judged by the standards of commercial advertising) is a 3 per cent change in behaviour. Perhaps we should note that the figures presented above are not completely hypothetical. The percentages for awareness, knowledge, and beliefs/attitudes are based on the average figures expected for well-pretested cancer education materials (Romano 1984). The assumption that 40 per cent of those exposed to the media programme will receive the necessary social, environmental, and educational support that they need is hypothetical—and probably somewhat optimistic!

In order to improve effectiveness, the mass media input would need to be complemented by a variety of different educational interventions. These would be designed to achieve different learning outcomes and be delivered over a period of time in a variety of contexts and settings. Ideally, the educational programme would be supplemented by appropriate healthy public policy. Accordingly, it makes sense to assess each of these inputs separately; for example, understanding of the nutritional information on which dietary decisions are based might best be provided in schools, and assessed there. Empowerment-related beliefs and attitudes could also be supplied by food labelling in the supermarket, in the personal and social education programme within the school, and/or in the works canteen.

Indirect indicators

On some occasions, even intermediate indicators may not be necessary for valid appraisal of effectiveness of inputs. For instance, we may need to assess the efficiency of a communication skills course provided for practice nurses (see training 'input' in Fig. 23.5). If the course is sound, the trainees will become more skilled in educating their clients. Ultimately, their new skill, will, in turn, be reflected in more effective work with patients. In the longer term they, and the course that they have completed, may contribute to clients' behaviour change—and may even have some small impact on the prevalence of disease!

Clearly, important decisions have to be made regarding the selection of particular intermediate and indirect indicators. These decisions can be based only on good-quality theories derived from research. In the light of earlier remarks about the relevance of epidemiological indicators, it will probably come as no surprise

when we assert that the evaluation designs that traditionally have been associated with medical research are frequently not relevant to the needs of health promoters seeking to enhance the quality of their programmes.

Research design: key issues

As we have seen, health promotion programmes should not be seen as 'one-shot' activities; they require complex, cumulative, and sophisticated subprogrammes. For this and other reasons, traditional epidemiological research designs are frequently not appropriate for evaluating health promotion work. Furthermore, a quantitative approach to the analysis and description of research results will often be less useful than qualitative measures.

First, we must acknowledge that the randomized controlled trial has been and still is the 'gold standard' for rigorously assessing the effectiveness of interventions. We might also note recent observations by the Executive Director of the Welsh Health Planning Forum about the limited extent to which a whole range of currently accepted health care initiatives can be said to be of proven value—using the randomized controlled trial gold standard. According to his so-called 'health gain rhomboid' (Warner 1994), only some 20 per cent of these initiatives are of proven effectiveness, some 20 per cent have been shown to lead to a proven reduction in health gain, while equal proportions either 'appear unpromising' or have 'uncertain effects.' He cites Brook and Lohr (1985, p. 711) to support his claim that only 20 per cent have been evaluated by randomized controlled trial.

The equivalent of the randomized controlled trial in behavioural sciences and education is the **true experimental design**, which employs techniques of randomization and uses one or more control groups. Such designs probably have to be somewhat more sophisticated than the randomized controlled trial because of the more complex nature of the inputs, as mentioned above. For instance, an educational programme would not just involve recording whether or not an input had been provided but typically would assess the extent to which a number of objectives had been achieved. Evaluation tools of this kind are readily available, but in recent years there has been increasing doubt about the value of using experimental designs. Indeed, prevailing evaluation practices in education were challenged by Hamilton et al. (1978) in an important publication revealingly entitled Beyond the numbers game. For present purposes, only three issues associated with the randomized controlled trial or true experimental design will be noted.

- For the kind of community-wide intervention that is likely to maximize the impact of a health promotion programme, it is virtually impossible to identify a valid control or comparison area. In part, this is for ethical reasons (as with certain medical randomized controlled trials); if it is reasonably clear that communities will benefit from the intervention, it is unethical to withhold it. More importantly, perhaps, it is virtually impossible to avoid 'contamination' of the comparison area since the programme in the experimental area is likely to trigger similar enterprises in the proposed control community—a fact clearly demonstrated by the Heartbeat Wales coronary heart disease prevention programme (Nutbeam et al. 1993).

- It is a fundamental error to equate a 'medical' with an educational initiative. The presence of human volition introduces a substantial degree of uncertainty into the proceedings and requires a complex and sophisticated programme completely unlike the administration of medication or a surgical procedure.

- It is important not only to know that a given intervention has achieved success (or failure), but it is imperative to discover why the initiative might have been effective or ineffective. In short, even when an experimental design is feasible, process evaluation (see earlier comments on evaluation in relation to Fig. 23.5) will also be needed. For example, if a group teaching session conducted by a practice nurse was more successful in increasing patients' commitment to take exercise than one-to-one sessions in which the doctor was the key educator, it would be valuable to know just why this might have been the case. The '5W + H formula' could beneficially be applied: Who did What to Whom, When and Where —and How? This could only be assessed in practice by observing and recording what went on in these sessions.

The qualitative dimension

Qualitative research techniques tend to be associated with process evaluation and are often considered to be alien to the allegedly more rigorous methods associated with randomized controlled trial. Only a cursory series of observations can be made here about qualitative methodology, but, given its importance in health promotion and the degree of controversy associated with its use, it may be helpful to provide the following summary.

- Qualitative methods are particularly useful at the pretesting stage of programmes for assessing learning readiness and needs, providing rich insights into underlying reasons for people's health-related actions, formulating hypotheses, and testing theory.

- **Formative evaluation** monitors the progress of groups and individuals by providing a series of assessments, which are then used to modify educational inputs in order to maximize the chance of success. Although quantitative techniques might be used to do this, qualitative methods are better able to provide readily applicable information about not only the nature and extent of change in the clients but also about attendant circumstances, such as the characteristics and effect of a group leader or health educator.

- **Summative evaluation** records the effect of the whole intervention, typically by administering some form of post-test and comparing the results of this with a pretest. Randomized controlled trial or experimental design would be employed where possible to allow health promoters to claim credit for any apparent changes in the target group. In such an instance, qualitative methods would usually be appropriate for recording 'process'.

- Qualitative methods do not have to sacrifice the rigour associated with quantitative approaches; indeed, validity and reliability can be achieved through the use of appropriate techniques. Of particular importance is the technique of 'triangulation' which, for example, pools information from a variety of different sources in order to assemble multifaceted 'evidence' on which to base decision-making.

So, can health promotion be effective?

Before drawing this chapter to a close, we should bear in mind that there are three major reasons for conducting programme evaluations:

- to assess programme effectiveness and efficiency;

- to use the results of evaluation research on specific programmes to improve the programme, to build better theory, to add to the general body of health promotion knowledge, and thus to improve the general quality of decision-making about programme design;

- to respond to various 'political imperatives'!

The political imperatives to which reference is made above are well known. Frequently the initiation of research and the reporting of results are driven largely by the need to gain future funding and/ or ensure the survival of a programme! Alternatively, research might be commissioned with the often covert purpose of accumulating evidence in order to close down a programme of work. In both instances, contradictory results may be 'massaged' or even suppressed. Furthermore, many programmes have been launched over the years despite evidence that they were unlikely to be effective; clearly, in this latter instance there are implicit, even concealed, effectiveness outcomes having little to do with the programme itself. If the performance indicators of these sorts of programmes were ever to be made public, their political nature might be revealed; for example a logically appropriate measure of success might be an acceptable percentage increase in government popularity in the opinion polls!

Of course, our concern here is with health promotion rather than political outcomes. Hopefully, although this chapter has not assembled a comprehensive and detailed review of effectiveness studies, it should be clear from the incidental examples provided that there is quite consistent evidence that health promotion can frequently be effective when the right conditions have been met (i.e. it can be efficacious). However, we should note that this does not happen too often, and we might legitimately speculate about the degree of success that might be achieved if programmes were to incorporate all that we know about good practice! For example, we should expect much more impressive results where a synergistic input of both education and healthy public policy were to be provided since, as we have seen, both together will achieve more than either type of intervention operating singly.

At this juncture, we ought to enter a caveat: we must recall that if people are genuinely empowered, their choice may not reflect the prevailing concerns of medicine! We should also repeat our assertion that the risk is worth taking since, by and large, empowered people will be more rather than less inclined to adopt medically approved actions—and if the principles of empowerment have been properly operationalized, more rather than less success will be experienced.

Let us complete this chapter by reporting three different perspectives on success, each of which provide valid evidence of health promotion's potential effectiveness. The first relates to traditional preventive goals but refers to a situation in which policy measures and education are inextricably linked. Warner (1989) makes the following observation (in a United States context): 'In the absence of the antismoking campaign, adult per capita cigarette consumption in 1987 would have been an estimated 78–89 per cent higher than the level actually experienced'. As a result, he noted, 'an estimated 789 200 Americans avoided or postponed smoking-related deaths and gained an average of 21 additional years of life expectancy each'.

In the second example, a school- and community-based health education programme in South Carolina demonstrated specific relationships between input and output. It showed rather conclusively that, compared with three comparison counties, statistically significant reductions occurred in adolescent pregnancy rates (Vincent *et al.* 1987). According to the researchers, the target county showed a 'remarkably sustained decline . . . not observed in comparison counties', whose unwanted pregnancy rates increased during the same period.

The final example is drawn from a study by Durrant (1993). It reports the result of using drama in the (perhaps unlikely) setting of a doctor in general practice. It used qualitative methodology to describe what appears to be clear gains in empowerment by patient participants. It also provides a few hints and suggestions about possible longer-term health gains. We cite one of the participating physician's own reports on the impact of the programme:

> We have seen people grow in confidence, make important decisions, get on better with their families, have more patience with their children, make friends, and grow as people.

A community worker associated with the venture provides a little 'triangulated' corroboration of the benefits:

> As they gain confidence in the sessions, they take this out onto the street, and this is seen in their daily lives. They feel they can apply for jobs they thought they never could have applied for, moved to better houses, taken on the council about the poll tax or the water meters, or allowances. We have people here now who wouldn't think twice about making a banner and campaigning outside the Town Hall to save local amenities.

References

Backer, T.E., Rogers, E.M., and Sopory, P. (1992). *Designing health communication campaigns: what works?* Sage, Newbury Park, CA.

Bandura, A. (1977). Self-efficacy: toward a unifying theory of behavioural change. *Psychological Review*, **64**(2), 191–215.

Bandura, A. (1986). *Social foundations of thought and action: a social cognitive theory*. Prentice-Hall, Englewood Cliffs, NJ.

Becker, M.H. (1984) (ed.) *The health belief model and personal health behavior*. Charles B. Slack, Thorofare, NJ.

Blaxter, M. (1990). *Health and lifestyles*. Tavistock, London.

Bond, B.W. (1958). A study in health education methods. *International Journal of Health Education*, **1**, 41–6.

Bracht, N. (ed.) (1990). *Health promotion at the community level*. Sage, Newbury Park, CA.

Brook, R. and Lohr, K. (1985). Efficiency, effectiveness, variations and quality. *Medical Care*, **23**, 710–22.

Budapest Declaration on Health Promoting Hospitals. WHO Business Meeting, Budapest, Hungary, 31 May–1 June 1991.

Byrne, P.S. and Long, B.E.L. (1976). *Doctors talking to patients*. HMSO, London.

Cohen, D. (1981). *Prevention as a merit good*. Health Economics Research Unit, University of Aberdeen.

Davis, J.B. (1992). *The myth of addiction*. Harwood, Switzerland.

Department of Health (1992). *Health of the nation*. HMSO, London.

DiClemente, C.C. and Prochaska, J.O. (1982). Self change and therapy change of smoking behaviour: a comparison of processes of change in cessation and maintenance. *Addictive Behaviours*, **7**, 133–42.

DiMatteo, M.R. and DiNicola, D.D. (1982). *Achieving patient compliance: the psychology of the medical practitioner's role*. Pergamon Press, New York.

Durrant, K. (1993). *The creative arts and the promotion of health in community settings*. M.Sc. Dissertation, Leeds Metropolitan University.

Egbert, J., Battit, G.E., Welch, C.E., and Bartlett, M.K. (1964). Reduction of post operative pain by encouragement and instruction of patients. *New England Journal of Medicine*, **270**, 825–7.

Freidson, E. (1961). *Patients' views of medical practice*. Russell Sage, New York.

Freire, P. (1974). *Education and the practice of freedom*. Writers and Readers Publishing Cooperative, London (originally published in Portuguese, 1967).

Glanz, K., Lewis, F.M., and Rimer, B.K. (ed.) (1990). *Health behavior and health education: theory, research and practice*. Jossey-Bass, San Francisco, CA.

Godfrey, C., Hardman, G., and Maynard, A. (1989). *Priorities for health promotion: an economic approach*. Discussion Paper 59, Centre for Health Economics, University of York.

Gottlieb, N. and McLeroy, K.R. (1992). Social health. In *Health promotion in the workplace* (2nd edn.) (ed. M.P. O'Donnell). Delmar, New York.

Green, L.W. (1974). Toward cost-benefit evaluation of health education: some concepts, methods and examples. *Health Education Monographs*, **2**, 34–64.

Green, L.W. and Lewis, F.M. (1986). *Measurement and evaluation in health education and health promotion*. Mayfield, Palo Alto, CA.

Hamilton, D., *et al.* (ed.) (1977). *Beyond the numbers game: a reader in educational evaluation*. Macmillan, London.

Health Education Research: Theory and Practice (1993). Special issue on Community Coalitions, 8(3).

International Union for Health Promotion and Education (1994). *Improvement of the effectiveness of health education and health promotion; a series of publications and a database*. IUHPE Regional Office for Europe, JC Utrecht.

Kanfer, F.H. and Karoly, P. (1972). Self-control: a behavioristic excursion into the lion's den. *Behavior Therapy*, **3**, 398–416.

Kasl, S.V. and Cobb, S. (1966). Health behavior, illness behavior and sick role behavior. *Archives of Environmental Health*, **12**, 246–66.

Laing, W.A. (1982). *Family planning: the benefits and the costs*. Publication 607, Policy Studies Institute, London.

Lalonde, M. (1974). *A new perspective on the health of Canadians*. Government of Canada, Ottawa.

Langer, E.J. and Rodin, J. (1976). The effects of enhanced personal responsibility for the aged. *Journal of Personality and Social Psychology*, **34**(2), 191–8.

Lazarsfeld, P.F. and Merton, R.K. (1975). Mass communication, popular taste and organized social action. In R. McCarthy (ed.), *Alcohol education for classroom and community*. McGraw-Hill, New York. (Reprinted from *The communication of ideas*, Institute for Religious and Social Studies, New York (1948).

Lewin, K. (1958) Group decision and social change. In *Readings in social psychology* (eds. Maccoby, F.E. *et al.*). Holt Rinehart and Winston, New York.

Ley, P. (1990). *Communicating with patients*. Chapman and Hall, London.

Lyng, S. (1990). Edgework: a social psychological analysis of voluntary risk taking. *American Journal of Sociology*, **95**(4), 851–86.

Macleod Clark, J. (1993). From sick nursing to health nursing: evolution or revolution? In *Research in health promotion and nursing* (ed. J. Wilson-Barnett and J. Macleod Clark). Macmillan, London.

MacShane, D. (1979). *Using the media*. Pluto Press, London.

Marsh, A. and Matheson, J. (1983). *Smoking attitudes and behaviour*. HMSO, London.

Miller, G. (1951). The magical number seven, plus or minus two: some limits on our capacity for processing information. *Psychological Review*, **63**, 81–7.

Mooney, G.H. (1977). *The valuation of human life*. Macmillan, London.

National Health Service Management Executive (1994). *Health promoting hospitals: a guidance document*. HMSO, London.

Nutbeam, D., Haglund, B., Farley, P., and Tilgren, P. (1991). *Youth health promotion: from theory to practice in school and community*. Forbes, London.

Nutbeam, D., Smith, C., Murphy, S. and Catford, J. (1993). Maintaining evaluation designs in long term community based health promotion programmes: Heartbeat Wales case study. *Journal of Epidemiology and Community Health*, **47**, 127–33.

Parsons, T. (1951). Illness and the role of the physician: a sociological perspective. *American Journal of Orthopsychiatry*, **21**, 452–60.

Pascoe, G.C. (1983). Patient satisfaction in primary health care: a literature review and analysis. *Evaluation and Programme Planning*, **6**, 185–210.

Phillips, C.J. and Prowle, M.J. (1993). Economics of a reduction in smoking: case study from Heartbeat Wales. *Journal of Epidemiology and Community Health*, **47**, 215–23.

Prochaska, J.O. (1992). What causes people to change from unhealthy to health enhancing behaviour? In *Preventing Cancers* (ed. T. Heller, L. Bailey, and S. Pattison). Open University Press, Milton Keynes.

Prochaska, J.O. and Di Clemente, C. (1986). Toward a comprehensive model of change. In *Treating addictive behaviors: processes of change* (ed. W.R. Miller and N. Heather). Plenum, New York.

Rogers, E.M. and Shoemaker, F.F. (1971). *Communication of innovations*. Free Press, New York.

Rollnick, S., Heather, N., and Bell, A. (1992). Negotiating behaviour change in medical settings: the development of brief motivational interviewing. *Journal of Mental Health*, **1**, 25–37.

Romano, R. (1984). *Pretesting in health communications*. National Cancer Institute, Bethesda, MD.

Rosenthal, H. (1983). Neighbourhood health projects: some new approaches to health and community work in parts of the United Kingdom. *Community Development Journal*, **13**(2), 122–31.

Rotter, J.B. (1966). Generalised expectancies for internal versus external control of reinforcement. *Psychological Monographs*, **80**(1), 1–28.

Ryder, J. and Campbell, L. (1988). *Balancing acts in personal, social and health education*. Routledge, London.

Salmon, C.T. (ed.) (1989). *Information campaigns: balancing social values and social change*. Sage, Newbury Park, CA.

Sarvela, P.D. and McDermott, R.J. (1993). *Health education evaluation and measurement: a practitioner's perspective*. Brown and Benchmark, Madison, WI.

Seligman, M.E.P. (1975). *Helplessness - on depression, development and death*. W.H. Freeman, New York.

Taylor, S.E. (1979). Hospital patient behavior: reactance, helplessness, or control? *Journal of Social Issues*, **35**(1), 156–84.

Tones, B.K. (1979). Past achievement, future success. In *Health education: perspectives and choices* (ed. I. Sutherland). Allen and Unwin, London.

Tones, B.K. (1987). Devising strategies for preventing drug misuse: the role of the health action model. *Health Education Research*, **2**(4), 305–18.

Tones, B.K. (1992). Health promotion, empowerment and the concept of control. In *Health education: politics and practice*. Deakin University Press, Victoria, Australia.

Tones, B.K. (1993a). The importance of horizontal programmes in Health Education. *Health Education Research*, **8**(4), 455–9.

Tones, B.K. (1993b). Changing theory and practice: trends in methods, strategies and settings in health education. *Health Education Journal*, **52**(3), 126–39.

Tones, B.K. and Tilford, S. (1994). *Health education: effectiveness, efficiency and equity*. Chapman and Hall, London.

Townsend, J. (1986). Cost effectiveness. In *Smoking control: strategies and evaluation in community and mass media programmes* (ed. J. Crofton and M. Wood). Health Education Council, London.

Tuckett, D., Boulton, M., Olson, C., and Williams, A. (1985). *Meetings between experts*. Tavistock, London.

Wadsworth, M., Butterfield, W.J.H., and Blaney, R. (1971). *Health and sickness: the choice of treatment*. Tavistock, London.

Wallston, K.A. and Wallston, B.S. (ed.) (1978). Health locus of control. *Health Education Monographs*, **6**(2), 107–17.

Warner, K.E. (1989). Effects of the antismoking campaign: an update. *American Journal of Public Health*, **79**(2), 144–51.

Warner, M.W. (1994). Present needs and future context: forces for change in health care in the United Kingdom. In *Health care systems in Canada and the United Kingdom* (ed. K. Lee). Keele University Press.

Watson, D.L. and Tharp, R.G. (1989). *Self-directed behavior: self-modification for personal adjustment*. Brooks/Cole, Pacific Grove, CA.

Weeks, V. (1993). The Department of Health view. In *Promoting health: Is there a role for hospital staff?* Health of the Nation Unit, Oxford Regional Health Authority.

Whitehead, M. and Tones, B.K. (1991). *Avoiding the pitfalls*. Health Education Authority, London.

WHO (World Health Organization) (1984). *Health promotion: a discussion document on the concepts and principles*. WHO Regional Office for Europe, Copenhagen.

WHO (World Health Organization) (1986). *Ottawa Charter for Health Promotion: an international conference on health promotion*. WHO Regional Office for Europe, Copenhagen.

Zola, I.K. (1973). Pathways to the doctor—from person to patient. *Social Science and Medicine*, **7**, 67–689.

Zola, I.K. (1986). Illness behaviour—a political analysis. In *Illness behavior: a multidisciplinary model* (ed. S. McHugh and T.M. Vallis). Plenum Press, New York.

24 Beyond quantitative measures: the relevance of anthropology for public health

H.K. Heggenhougen and Duncan Pedersen

Introduction

Until recently, people both inside and outside public health institutions could not quite understand what anthropologists and anthropological perspectives—including the use of qualitative methods—had to do with public health, nor why some anthropologists were even employed in public health institutions. A remark sometimes heard in the corridors of governmental or academic institutions was: '. . . anthropology is jolly interesting, so long as it doesn't get in the way of "the real stuff"'!' For many of those working in international public health 'the real stuff' was represented by biomedicine and rigorous epidemiology grounded in biostatistics, and these, and only these, would reveal the patterns of disease and the groups at risk. The qualitative research carried out by anthropologists and other social scientists was considered 'soft' and the results interesting—even fascinating 'stories'—but it was not 'the real stuff'. Yet, social epidemiology notwithstanding, it turned out that the 'real stuff' was not very good at explaining the reasons why particular disease patterns existed, why certain people became ill while others did not, or why people behaved as they did. It was not so successful in making public health problems understandable in terms of the total (sociocultural, political, and economic) context of people's lives. There have been significant public health success stories without attending to these matters—the smallpox eradication campaign (which was carried out in an almost military fashion) is a well-known example. However, the partial or total failure of scores of other public health interventions can be linked to the lack of an understanding of, and attention to, 'meaning' and to the wider sociocultural context of people's lives.

Even though the book, *Health, culture and community*, edited by the anthropologist Benjamin Paul (1955) while at the Harvard School of Public Health, and Polgar's seminal article 'Health and human behaviour: areas of interest common to the social and medical sciences', published in 1962 (see also Polgar 1963), marked a watershed for the establishment of medical anthropology and for the increased involvement of anthropologists in public health, it was not really before the middle to late 1980s that the relevance of anthropology and the use of qualitative approaches to understanding and helping to solve public health problems were readily recognized. Despite the growth of social epidemiology from the 1950s and 1960s onwards, and the Alma-Ata Declaration on primary health care in 1978 (WHO/UNICEF 1978), the 'new'

public health, which avoids reductionism and deals with the complexities of health issues, and understands these through both quantitative and qualitative research, has emerged only very recently.

Despite its long history, 'public health' still evokes different representations in the collective imagination, often laden with ambiguities (which have strongly influenced the professional identity of its practitioners). The globalization of the economy, the implementation of structural adjustment programmes, and the subsequent transformation and collapse of the state and public services have finally brought the notion of 'crisis' to the public health arena. It is relatively recently that international experts have agreed to discuss the 'crisis of public health' (PAHO 1992) within the context of the dismantling of the welfare state. However, we would like to discuss collective health from a different perspective: that of a new stage in the relentless process of change which expands the horizons of the 'conventional' public health field. If we take a brief look at the recent history of the dominant ideologies in public health, the first half of this century was dominated by the notions of hygiene and sanitation. After the Second World War advances in the prevention and treatment of infectious diseases and in epidemiology characterized what we may call the biomedical model of public health. By the 1970s this had evolved into an ecological model of health, with an emphasis on ecology and the natural environment which, combined with the relatively recent incorporation of the social sciences, led to the transition towards the now prevailing socio-epidemiological model (Frenk 1992). On the threshold of the twenty-first century, we face the need to develop a new paradigm for the understanding of the health and disease process of individuals, communities, and societies which, for the purposes of this chapter, we have labelled 'new' public health. In order to achieve this, we must review and renovate the mandate, substance, and methods which will force us to redraw the traditional boundaries of public health, including its relationships with medicine and the social sciences (Pedersen 1994).

Despite advances made by research in reducing disease and death and in developing cost-effective interventions, many problems remain unsolved. At the same time, as part of the health transition, 'new' patterns of morbidity and mortality have emerged, changing the face of the international health agenda. The increased importance of mental and behaviour-related conditions (Desjarlais *et al.* 1995), the threatening AIDS pandemic, and the resurgence of 'old time' diseases, such as cholera, malaria, dengue, and tuberculosis, within specific regions and populations, coupled with the appearance of various forms of resistance to antibacterial agents and the deleterious impact of institutionalized health care on certain disease conditions, all represent major new challenges for the international health sector. As we approach the turn of the century, renewed efforts are being made to regain control over a (sombre?) world health scenario, where the construction of a 'new' public health should now lead the way. Anthropological perspectives and innovative action initiatives in international health must play an increasingly vital role in accomplishing these goals.

Of course, the increased recognition of the influence of lifestyles and human behaviour in the health status of individuals and populations, and particularly the primary health care movement in the late 1970s and 1980s which received some prominence amongst scientists at the time (Engel 1977), influenced the character of public health discourse and reconnected it to its historical past and the wider perspectives drawn by the public health theorists of the last century, among whom Virchow, Snow, Farr, Engels, and Durkheim are well known. Yet it was the unexpected advent of AIDS which made a significant impact, possibly being the most important single factor contributing to the growing acceptance of anthropological perspectives and methods for public health.

Since the early 1990s the character of public health has also been strongly influenced by a third major phenomenon, namely the belated prominence of a linkage between health and human rights. This interconnection is not new; for example, Vincente Navarro (1974a,b) has long pointed to the relationship between human rights abuses—of structural (and direct) violence—and health. The World Health Organization's (WHO's) definition of health in terms of physical, psychological, and social well-being, and not just the absence of disease, has also clearly marked this interconnection, as has the work of such groups as Physicians for Human Rights. Yet, it is only in the 1990s when, not coincidentally, Amnesty International and Rigoberta Menchu were awarded Nobel Peace Prizes, and with the launching of the journal *Health and Human Rights* in 1994 and the establishment of a Center for Health and Human Rights at the Harvard School of Public Health in the same year, that this relationship—of 'the impact of health policies, programs and practices on human rights' on the one hand and that 'human rights violations have health impacts' on the other, leading to the conclusion 'that promotion and protection of human rights and promotion and protection of health are fundamentally linked'—has entered the centre stage of public health discourse (Mann *et al.* 1994, p. 13). It is now quite widely accepted that the epidemiology resulting from the direct and 'hidden' human rights abuses points to a worldwide epidemic of pandemic proportions. Any understanding of epidemiological patterns—any efforts to improve the health of people showing low health indicators—must consider, and attempt to affect, human rights and inequitable sociopolitical and economic conditions. The recent focus of national and international public health debates on 'violence and health' and 'health and human rights' is a promising development (Heggenhougen 1995, pp. 281–2).

Suddenly, what Benjamin Paul had said 40 years ago, and what Virchow, Snow, and others a century before that, was rediscovered: not only was human behaviour important for public health, but behaviour itself was strongly influenced by cultural parameters, as well as by social, economic and political dimensions. The AIDS epidemic represents a prime example of this assertion. Sexual practices were recognized as being influenced by cultural norms. Due to the sensitivity of subjects related to HIV transmission, research on sexual practices and intravenous drug users had to be carried out differently than had been usual for more conventional quantitative survey studies, with greater emphasis on building rapport, concern for confidentiality, and understanding behaviour from the point of view of the actors involved. As discussed below in more detail, the so-called KAP (knowledge, attitudes, and practices) survey questionnaires were increasingly found to be of limited use. They simply did not reflect reality.

This book is about public health and thus there is no need to define it in great detail. For the purposes of this chapter, it is sufficient to state that public health is concerned with the determinants of health and disease, with the spatial and social distribution of diseases, with the identification of areas and population groups at risk, and with the development of appropriate interventions to improve the health status of populations, with (all things being equal, which they usually are not) particular attention given to areas and groups with the worst health indicators which, presumably, are in most need.

Anthropology is particularly concerned with the study of human beings within a culture. Culture can be simply defined as 'a set of beliefs and behaviour shared by a group of people' or that 'culture provides people with a way of perceiving the world at large and with ways of coming to terms with the problems they face: this includes attitudes about the body and ways in which a person should be treated when ill'. Anthropology is certainly concerned with culture, but anthropologists are not mere 'culturists' (reductionists in their emphasis on culture). Rather, their main concern remains with the overall context in which individuals and groups are situated—with the ways that people (have to) live their daily lives within local worlds, that is within webs of local factors which are themselves influenced by larger, sometimes national and even international, forces. What is the context within which people exist and act? What is the context within which people, consciously or as a matter of course, practice or do not practice preventive and health promotional activities? What is the context within which epidemiological patterns are embedded? These are prevalent questions asked by anthropologists. This focus on the interlocking web of factors, and the qualitative research methods that may be used to arrive at a better and a more valid understanding of this web, may be the major contribution of anthropology to the required collaborative approach for the 'new' public health. Incidentally, this contribution does not necessarily depend on taking 'years of time', for which anthropologists have been shunned.

Anthropology, in its concern with 'stepping into a different reality', with gaining an insider's perspective, with establishing rapport, and with understanding 'the other' (and thus also understanding 'ourselves' better), is particularly suitable for assisting in the identification of health needs within a holistic appreciation of the meaning of illness and the context of people's lives.

Before ending this section, it is worth noting the differences between anthropology and sociology. This difference is frequently blurred as there are sociologists who act very much like anthropologists, both in terms of the focus of their attention and the research methods used, and there are anthropologists who at times also take what might be called a sociological approach. However, to stereotype the two we may say that anthropologists are concerned with understanding (the culture of) microenvironments and using qualitative methods to gain an (emic) insider's perspective, whereas sociologists are concerned with understanding the organizations and social structures of macroenvironments and using primarily quantitative methods to gain an (etic) outsider's rigorously examined perspective (Foster 1974).

A short history of anthropology and public health

Historically, most anthropologists concerned with public health (and medical anthropologists in general) see their own work, as well as that of social epidemiologists (Janes *et al.* 1986; Trostle, 1986*a,b*), as being rooted in the concerns of the European social theorists of the last century. The German pathologist Virchow (as well as the sociologist Durkheim and the sociopolitical critic Engels) has received particular historical prominence (Eisenberg 1984). For example, the following statement made by Virchow in 1849 was used as the introductory quotation to Landy's (1977) *Culture, disease and healing*, one of the earliest collections of articles on anthropology and health following Paul's (1955) volume:

> In reality, if medicine is the science of the healthy as well as the ill human being (which is what it ought to be), what other science is better suited to propose laws as the basis of the social structure, in order to make effective those which are inherent in man himself? Once medicine is established as anthropology, and once the interests of the privileged no longer determine the course of public events, the physiologist and the practitioner will be counted among the elder statesmen who support the social structure. Medicine is a social science in its very bone and marrow. (P. Virchow, *Die Einheitsbestrebungen*, 1849)

The encompassing concerns of the social theorists were overtaken by the bacteriological era at the end of the nineteenth century and only re-emerged with some force in the late 1960s and 1970s, although efforts had obviously been made prior to that. George Foster (1982), who, with Benjamin Paul (both now in their mid 80s), is the elder statesman of anthropology and international public health, has reviewed some of the early involvement of, primarily American, anthropologists in public health in this century. In the United Kingdom, many of the early efforts concerned nutrition and dietary habits and its consequences for health. In 1934, Raymond Firth, a major figure in British anthropology, published 'The sociological study of native diet' (see also Firth 1957). This was followed by similar publications by Richards (1939) and Malinowski (1961). In the United States two of the best known American anthropologists, Ruth Benedict (see, for example, *Patterns of culture*, published in 1935) and Margaret Mead, were involved in the Committee of Food Habits established by the National Research Council in 1940.

In terms of institutional connections by American anthropologists, one of the earliest was Esther Brown who in 1930 was hired by the Russell Sage Foundation and specifically asked to explore with schools of public health, medical schools, and nursing schools whether they wanted anthropologists on their faculties. The receptivity at that time was not overwhelming! In 1943,

Richard Adams, George Foster, and Ozzie Simmons joined the Smithsonian Institute in Washington, DC, and began work related to public health in Latin America. However, it was not until 1951 that Benjamin Paul was hired by the Harvard School of Public Health (where he did not receive tenure), followed by L. Saunders (1954), a sociologist, who joined the University of Colorado School of Medicine in 1954.

In 1950, Cora DuBois was the first anthropologist hired by the WHO. This was a short-lived experience, since she left disappointed after a year. Except for having an anthropologist working in contraceptive practices within the Special Programme on Human Reproduction in the late 1970s, it is only quite recently that a more positive attitude has developed within international organizations such as the WHO, with anthropologists now working in its Global Programme on AIDS and the Tropical Disease Research Programme (WHO/TDR). Social scientists and anthropologists have also been (and still are) involved as short-term consultants with WHO's Expanded Programme on Immunization, the control of malaria, diarrhoeal diseases, and acute respiratory infection, maternal and child health care, and the (now redesigned) Essential Drugs Programme. Other United Nations agencies, such as UNICEF, have also invited the collaboration of anthropologists in the development of child survival programmes (Scrimshaw and Hurtado 1987). Within the last 20 years or so, bilateral agencies, especially the Scandinavian aid agencies, as well as USAID and a growing body of non-governmental organizations, have hired anthropologists to work in various social sectors, including education and public health.

A history of anthropologists in public health must also mention their involvement with the health programmes for Amerindian peoples. Associated with this is the early work of Leighton and Leighton (see *The Navaho door*, published in 1944), Adair and Deuschle (see 'Some problems of the physicians on the Navajo reservations', 1958; also 1988), and C. Richards ('Cooperation between anthropologists and medical personnel', 1960).

There is now a considerable body of literature dealing with anthropology and public health to substantiate the relevance of this interrelation. In addition to those already mentioned, many of the pioneers published their work during the first half of this century. These pioneers were often physicians, anthropologists, or social scientists working in remote traditional societies where they became interested in health beliefs and traditional medicine practices yet in relative isolation from the newly emerging public health and anthropology of the time. Although this is not the place to trace back the origins of what is now the broad field of social sciences and medicine, anthropology, and public health, we cannot overlook these susbtantive contributions to the field.

In Latin America, for example, there are the early works of Valdizán, on mental illness among indigenous populations (Valdizán 1915) and his comprehensive study of popular medicine practices in Peru (Valdizán and Maldonado 1922) (*La Medicina Popular Peruana*). Seguin (1959, 1979), Chiappe (1968), and Dobkin de Rios (1968) in Peru, Othón de Mendizábal (1946), Aguirre Beltrán (1955), García Manzanedo (1983) and, recently, Campos Navarro (1992) in Mexico, and Reichel-Dolmatoff (1953, 1959), Fals Borda (1964) and more recently, Taussig (1979, 1980) in Colombia, are all prime examples of the many contributors to this field of enquiry. Today, there are several Latin American review articles, bibliographies, and periodicals, which reflect the increase in the number of anthropological studies of health and illness over the last three decades. See, for instance, de Souza Queiroz and Canesqui's (1986) review article for Brazil, the series of *Estudios de Antropología Médica* (Mexico), *La medicina moderna y la antropología médica en la población fronteriza mexicano-estadounidense* (Velimirovic, 1979), and two (among many others) annotated bibliographies, *Antropología Médica y Medicina Tradicional en Colombia* (Herrera and Lobo-Guerrero 1982) and the *Selected bibliography in medical anthropology for health professionals in the Americas* (OPS/OMS1978).

In North America, the works of Rivers (1924), Clements (1932, 1959), and Ackerknecht (1971) represent some of the earliest of the twentieth century literature. Subsequent books and reviews, such as those of Caudill (1953), Scotch (1963), Fabrega (1972, 1974), Lieban (1977), Foster and Anderson (1978), McElroy and Townsend (1979), Young (1982), and Helman (1984), should also be included.

More recent publications include Coreil and Mull (1990), Nichter (1989), Chrisman and Maretzki (1982), Janes *et al.* (1986), and van der Geest and Whyte (1991). The volumes published in the 'Comparative Studies of Health Systems and Medical Care' series of the University of California Press since 1976 (for example, Leslie 1976; Justice 1986), in the 'Culture, Illness and Healing—Studies in Comparative Cross Cultural Research', series of the Reidel Press since 1981 (for example, Eisenberg and Kleinman 1981), and the recently established (1992) 'Theory and Practice in Medical Anthropology and International Health' series published by Gordon and Breach should also be mentioned. Well-established journals such as *Social Science and Medicine*, *Medical Anthropology Quarterly*, *Medical Anthropology*, *Culture, Medicine and Psychiatry*, and *Curare* have long published papers in this field. A recently published book by Desjarlais *et al.* (1995), concerned with promoting an international mental health agenda, should also be mentioned as the main authors are primarily anthropologists.

To conclude this short history of anthropology and public health it may be fitting to point to just two of a number of examples showing that some progress has been made in terms of the role of anthropology in public health since the short tenure of Benjamin Paul at the Harvard School of Public Health: first, at the 1994 conference of the American Society of Tropical Medicine and Hygiene, Dr Barnett Cline, in his presidential address, spent at least a quarter of his time discussing the need for collaboration with anthropologists; second, in January 1995 the anthropologist Susan Scrimshaw became the Dean of the School of Public Health at the University of Illinois, Chicago. There may now be less need to demonstrate the relevance of anthropology for public health than simply to get on with the collaborative work of improving peoples' health.

Why are people sick? The web of causation

Why are people sick? The answer quite rightly points to the exposure to agents of various kinds. Viruses, bacteria, parasites, and other infectious agents, as well as diverse sources of stress including malnutrition, make us sick. However, while this may be so, the answer to this question should not stop here. We cannot ignore the wider ecological contexts of people's lives which are crucial in influencing the risk of being affected by these vectors. Such ecological contexts include not only the physical and biological environments but also the sociocultural (including political and economic) environment.

With the advent of primary health care we have been encouraged to take a more encompassing view of health and to focus on the web of interrelated factors which contribute to ill health. Acknowledging a 'web of causality' and a 'web of healing' quite clearly recognizes that social and cultural environments are important components of such webs, and thus that anthropology is essential for identifying health needs and for formulating and implementing appropriate treatment and public health interventions. When we ask why people become sick in the light of this perspective, different types of noxa or 'insults' (Audy and Dunn 1974), beyond the commonly recognized agents, are revealed. These include afflictions such as hunger, cold, and lack of shelter. Poverty and violence (direct and structural) are clearly major health problems in the world today. The inability of the majority of the world's population to share equitably in available resources (including heath services) creates 'sores that fester'. Thus increasing the scope of the discussion to issues of community participation, self-reliance, and even empowerment in health begins to make sense.

While other diseases resulting from poverty and poor environmental conditions, such as diarrhoea or tuberculosis, have often been 'medicalized' (transforming largely social and political problems into strictly biomedical concerns) and subject to massive technological interventions, mental disorders and the newly emerging, behaviour-related problems challenge conventional medical solutions and demand a different approach. As shown in carefully conducted studies, the course and outcome of severe mental disorders depend not solely on hospital facilities, medication, skills, and the availability of professional care, but also on the reactions, care, and support provided by family members and the immediate social network of community resources. Likewise, many behaviour-related disorders (that is, street and domestic violence, child sexual abuse, including sexually transmitted diseases such as AIDS, and so on) have no simple, effective, and readily available biotechnological solution, but require changes in individual and group behaviour as well as interventions directed to both 'microsocial processes' and the broader social context, where anthropologists are a critical resource in growing demand.

From this viewpoint, epidemiological patterns can be seen as reflections of the manner in which people (have to) live their lives, which in turn is influenced by cultural and sociostructural norms as well as by powerful local and global political and economic factors (for example, Dunn 1979). Thus public health perceptions and interventions for improving health must also understand 'risk' and the presence of aetiological factors in terms of the wider sociocultural contexts in which they are embedded.

Of course, this holistic view of health is not a novel idea. It has been essential in much of traditional medicine practices, as well as in the Greek origins of 'Western' medicine. However, it is only recently that a growing number of studies have made it unarguably clear that our ' . . . social environment is a component in the etiology of nearly all diseases and [that] the outcome of treatment depends equally upon how favorable that social environment is' (Berkman and Syme 1979). In summary, given a social context and as part of the history of a given population, each society would construct specifically its own experience of disease and illness, as well as a more or less appropriate set of responses for its control and resolution. There is a continuity between the context, the social determinants of health and disease, the illness experience, and the initiatives and actions taken for improving the health status. Thus, to identify the health needs of different communities, it is important to gain an understanding of the social and cultural contexts of people's lives and local worlds in order to identify needs from within and in terms of such contexts and worlds.

Improvements in public health inevitably require change. Changes in behaviour and in cultural practices are frequently suggested and often relevant. However, improving health in hierarchical structured countries where social inequity is the rule also calls for more fundamental (socio-economic and political) changes. It requires an attack on the persistence of a system of functional apartheid (Heggenhougen 1995), elimination of overt state-sponsored repression, violence, and torture, and a move towards a much more equitable system of distribution of resources and employment compensation. How this can be done without putting people at further and greater risk must be included in such a consideration. It may also be inappropriate for foreigners to direct such interventions, although on the basis of a fundamental and universal human rights credo (that is, the UN Charter on Human Rights) outsiders do have a responsibility to voice their concern and to assist those who are beginning to improve the overall conditions of their lives and to improve their health. Primary health care strategies and the current concern with health and human rights are two sides of the same coin, namely that basic equity, social justice, human rights, and human dignity are essential to achieving health. It is with these issues, including of course the provision of easily accessible (available, affordable, and acceptable) health services, that action must be taken.

Within the field of international health, the Alma-Ata Declaration on primary health care in 1978 served as a watershed for a wider perspective in thinking about why and how people become sick and for a reformulation of efforts to improve health. However sceptical we may be of the official primary health care policies now professed by most countries in the world, and although we may lament the rather limited nature of the selective rather than comprehensive primary health care interventions which exist at present, the interconnection of human rights, socio-economic factors, and health has been legitimized and stimulated—again, brought onto centre stage—by this declaration. However, precisely because the concepts of equity and social justice are central to the primary health care philosophy, it becomes difficult to implement comprehensive primary health care programmes since these must ultimately question and try to correct inequitable social relationships. We are left with the question of whether primary health care will be allowed to succeed (Heggenhougen 1984).

No matter how expert we are in our own disciplines, or how important specific technical interventions may be, we must insist on looking at, and attempting to improve, people's health through a matrix of sociocultural (including political, economic, and historical) factors, not the least of which involve the examination and the consequences of functional apartheid and human rights abuses.

Medical anthropologists working within public health and in collaboration with epidemiologists have generally concentrated on the significance of cultural factors in explaining epidemiological patterns and in promoting successful public health interventions. In the most negative sense anthropologists have been used to finding the culturally relevant buttons to push in order to market preconceived 'effective and necessary' public health interventions successfully. In a more positive light, anthropologists have been 'cultural brokers', that is interpreters and intermediaries ensuring that public health interventions are mutually agreed upon and culturally appropriate.

Other contributions have concerned the health impact of stress amongst immigrant and refugee populations, and the relationship between degrees of acculturation and health. Such work has obviously been of great significance and continues to be of importance. Culture does influence disease patterns and the illness experience. However, despite the prominence of these relationships, human rights and socio-economic (class) issues must also be included. This is a fundamental notion in the 'new' public health.

Anthropologists certainly do not have a monopoly of working in this arena, nor are they always in the forefront relative to these concerns. However, the point of discussing these fundamental notions in a chapter on anthropology and public health is not so much to assert the prominent expertise of anthropologists in dealing with these issues nor to claim that they necessarily command the ethical 'high ground', but rather to note that because of the prevalent anthropological concern not only with culture but with context, anthropologists, although focusing on 'local worlds' and the 'micro-environment', nevertheless constantly attempt to understand the 'big picture'. The very nature of the anthropological enterprise is to understand and assign meaning to (and to make whole) the web of interrelated factors. It is this very notion that is essential to public health: anthropologists can help to remind us of the importance of interrelationships and to warn against the tendency to overestimate the influence of any single, 'isolated' causative factor.

Context, nuance, diversity, and ambiguity

Anthropologists avoid talking in absolutes. They are interested in detail, as well as in diversity and the nature of the differences, and thus they may work well with epidemiologists who look for universal factors and overall patterns.

Anthropologists are generally sceptical of reified 'facts' or universal laws, often preferring to respond to these with, 'Well, it all depends. . .'. ('There is no law which is universally applicable, including this one' is a statement which is uttered only partially in jest.) Their traditional training makes this position rather difficult for physicians and other public health personnel to comprehend. Physicians tend to be both uncomfortable and intolerant of ambiguity and relativism. However, not only anthropologists indicate the need to be sensitive to nuance and ambiguity if we are to understand the lives of people in specific situations. The social epidemiologist John Cassel (1964) postulated that 'Factors which may be causal under certain circumstances may under other circumstances be neutral or perhaps even beneficial'. The concepts of nuance and ambiguity are important in the presentation of the daily lives of people in real communities, including their 'beliefs, attitudes and behaviour'. While recognizing the importance of the broad strokes in guiding planning and implementation, attention to detail and specificity are important precisely for the success of such implementation.

The insistence of anthropologists on context, nuance, and ambiguity is not adopted to be difficult or to put 'spanners in the wheels of "progress" ', but rather to warn against deceptive and simplistic solutions, even as we begin to understand major 'belief systems' and cultural norms. It is precisely because we want plans and interventions to be the most appropriate in terms of social development, and to have a sustainable effect in improving people's health, that these concerns are emphasized.

In our age of specialization we have tended to see solutions in a vacuum—medicine and public health have been particularly accused of this—and thus things such as new filtering systems, for example, become adequate, or even satisfactory, answers to our pollution problems, and more and more sophisticated curative health technologies become solutions to health problems. If such a segmented view continues to prevail, then even concern for the 'ecological crisis' becomes a 'cop-out' and an avoidance of more basic realities—a dread of facing more unpleasant problems. An overemphasis on a 'magic bullet' approach denies the relevance of the more basic social, psychological, economic, and political factors influencing health and welfare. Of course, technological solutions to problems are necessary but, by themselves, they are hardly sufficient.

More than 20 years ago, the American statesman Adlai Stevenson (1965) called most eloquently for the re-establishment of harmony between all the elements in the web of interdependence within which we exist:

> We travel together, passengers on a little spaceship, dependent on its vulnerable supplies of air and soil; all committed for our safety to its security and peace, preserved from annihilation only by the care, the work and I will say, the love we give our fragile craft.

In retrospect, this statement may seem both 'rosy' and incredibly naïve, yet it pinpoints a crucial problem for the public's health. People's actions do not often verify their sense of interconnectedness with people in different parts of the world, nor with those, albeit close at hand, in circumstances different from their own. Individualistic and competitive striving contradicts our inherent interdependence. The concept of 'commerciogenic pathology' is no longer a strange and exotic joke but is increasingly voiced. All too often we forge ahead with our sights set on short-term gains with little thought for long-term consequences. There is a saying, voiced by the WHO a few years ago: 'Think globally, act locally!'. However, although we act locally and internationally, our thinking is seldom global, seldom holistic, and seldom integrated. There is a need to re-establish balance.

Those who ask what this has to do with people dying of measles, malaria, diarrhoea, and other diseases 'for which there are technical solutions' are only partially correct in their insistence 'to get on with it', depoliticizing health while providing technical solutions, and to transfer technical knowledge, be it for immunization or for 'raising the standard of living' through economic growth. They then neglect the immediate and larger contexts in which these ailments exist and persist, contexts where technical interventions alone are not enough to correct and lead to the sustained improvement of the health status.

Anthropologists constantly introduce examples of how culture and health are interrelated, and maintain that cultural characteristics are often reflected in specific epidemiological patterns (Dunn and Janes 1986). However, most anthropologists do not want to be 'boxed in' by culture alone (Kaufert 1990). People are not tin soldiers uniformly marching to the tune of any one cultural norm. It is also important to move beyond culture as such, in the limited sense of that word, to a concern for the total context, including social status and economic and power relationships, in which people live their everyday lives in their local worlds, including, of course, a concern for the wider forces which impinge upon that world. This should be self-evident not only to the so-called 'critical medical (or "therapeutic") anthropologists' (Heggenhougen 1979; Singer 1986) but to most public health professionals as well as anthropologists. However, although this may be (theoretically) self-evident, and despite the Alma-Ata Declaration having imbued the current international public health 'language' with such an ecological perspective, the focus of prevalent public health activities makes it clear that this perspective cannot be taken for granted and that we need to continue to impress upon our biomedical and public health colleagues its relevance for practice.

This overall context, and particularly its sociocultural dimensions, can usually best be studied in a different way from studying the life-cycle of the schistosome, for example (Lock and Scheper-Hughes 1990). It may require not only more qualitative than quantitative methods, but a combination of the two, and some of the other approaches discussed in the later sections of this chapter. Putting this knowledge into practice and beginning to foster required changes in the sociocultural environment, in the wider context of people's lives, is much more difficult and potentially more dangerous than implementing more technical biomedical interventions, yet it is essential if we are to affect the root causes of disease and to take the public's health seriously.

A discussion of anthropology and public health must at least also touch on the myth of a value-free science. If we recognize the importance of context for the health of people, and if we take issues such as social justice and health, and human rights and health, seriously, we can not be dispassionate and neutral.

James Thurber's quip that 'A critic is a person who looks in the microscope and discovers his own eye!' may hold true not only for some anthropologists but also for many in the 'hard sciences' as well. This is important to keep in mind not only in terms of the specific research itself, but relative to the very choice of studying what we study, of funding one set of research questions rather than another. Such choices are value laden. We cannot escape that, but we must ask whose values are operating in a cross-cultural public health setting—ours, theirs, or both? However, recognition of this does not imply that we compromise the rigour of our scientific research. (For a discussion of objectivity in anthropological research see Maquet (1964)).

Anthropological methods

- Emphasizing quality and validity

- Looking for questions as well as answers

- Gaining an insider's perspective

- Being open to expect the unexpected

There is no one research method which serves all situations or best helps solve every problem. Different problems require different approaches. Additionally, since ill health is caused by a combination of factors, different methodological approaches may best be able to reveal different aspects of any one problem. Thus an interdisciplinary approach, using a combination of methods, can usually be employed as the most beneficial procedure. A multi-method approach, both qualitative and quantitative, is also important in ensuring validity as well as replicability and generalizability.

Given that what researchers do is, in essence, very straightforward—to look, to ask, to read, and occasionally to think—we should not forget that observation, interviews, questionnaires, and other tools, under the title of research methods, are not necessarily quantitative or qualitative *per se*. Any attempt to quantify involves a qualitative judgement and, vice versa, qualitative statements imply a certain hierarchy, number, and magnitude which give form to meaning (Davies *et al.* 1985; Pedersen 1990).

Whereas surveys in industrialized nations were carried out to determine the population's opinion with regard to a given aspect of social and political life, their use in the countries of Africa, Asia, and Latin America responded to other needs, more related to the process of domination, control, and exploitation of resources. It is quite clear that the first colonial nations, and later the countries of the North, needed specific baseline information about the native populations—demographic data and information about what people say or do, have or have not—for the purpose of planning and executing administrative functions. In this way they were able to establish the terms for economic and cultural exchange, or religious and ideological imposition or domination. The implicit purpose of the surveyors was to collect information from those who had no decision-making powers in order to make decisions for them. Political authorities, administrators, the military, religious orders, and later, of course, social scientists and public health professionals all collaborated for this purpose.

Despite the popularity of survey research, it was soon realized that what is needed to survey and measure one population, ethnic group, or social class, is not necessarily valid in another population, ethnic group, or socio-economic group. The questions that the surveyors asked over and over again were whether the same survey instruments could be used in different population groups and contexts. Later, when the need to adapt or develop new survey instruments became evident, surveyors asked themselves whether data collected in this way were reliable and comparable, and moreover, whether they were representative of the general population.

Unlike the surveys used in the industrialized nations, there was a need in less developed countries to adapt survey forms to a different social context. Population sampling and the application of questionnaires from standardized surveys are two techniques which were developed to facilitate the generalization of results, to reduce errors and biases, to shorten time frames and lower costs, and to establish a basis for comparison between the population under survey and the referral group (Pedersen 1990).

We would like this historical perspective to reveal not only how methods and techniques evolved as societal aims changed, but more importantly, we want to stress the transformation which came about with the process of appropriating knowledge. In other words, research evolved from asystematic and isolated observations into a systematic series of observations and comparisons, with increasingly technical interpretations of reality. This process led to the transfer of the power to create knowledge from the people to those who held the required skills and controlled the application of methods and techniques (Hall 1979).

The problems and limitations of survey research

The dissatisfaction experienced with conventional approaches to survey research led to the search for new approaches, strategies, and alternative research methods. We shall now review some of the general limitations recognized by different researchers, and point out others that are more specific to health research (see Pedersen 1990).

One general limitation attributed to survey research is the oversimplification of social reality. The arbitrary design of questionnaires and multiple-choice questions with preconceived categories represents a biased and overly simplistic view of reality. Individual responses to questions, and their addition and subtraction, lead to the arithmetic manipulation of figures, creating frequencies, averages, and rates, which represent 'average replies', ratios, or proportions, which bear no real significance on their own and rather mystify reality (for example 37.5 per cent of respondents reported a health problem within the last 2 weeks, or 68.2 per cent of the population have a latrine). Cross-sectional surveys lead to the reading of a static or 'photographic' image of what is, in reality, an interactive and dynamic process.

On the other hand, the inconsistency of data can be attributed not only to the oversimplification of reality caused by the methods and instruments used, but also to the dynamic and genuine variability or fleeting occurrence of the phenomenon under observation (for example, blood pressure, simple morbidity episodes, and so on).

Finally, when dealing with interviews or structured questionnaires, inconsistencies can be attributed to the lack of truth or consistency in the replies. Questions can be well intentioned (for example, collecting basic information or designing effective intervention, or evaluating a health programme), but end up being inadequate or even irrelevant with respect to the culture and values of the informants. Despite the appearance of new methods, research techniques are clearly blemished by prejudices, or influenced by the ideology and value system of the researchers. Although sampling strategies and changes in questionnaire construction have improved the application and representativity of surveys, they have proved once again to be insufficient in overcoming these prejudices.

A large proportion of health research corresponds to cross-sectional and KAP surveys on samples of rural or urban populations undergoing acculturation and rapid change. These studies often involve the collection of information about births, deaths, and reproduction, sexual practices, food intake, child-rearing and child-care practices, contraceptive use and abortion, use of drugs, alcohol, and tobacco, defecation and the disposal of solid waste, and other more or less sensitive or 'stigmatized' behaviours. Survey research often demands clear-cut answers to questions related to illness perception, beliefs, and health-seeking behaviours, patterns of resort and therapeutic usages, and reasons for using or not using available health technologies and services. This kind of survey study, which explores the intimate and discreet behaviour of everyday life, leads to questionable results, and about half of collected data is considered to be erroneous or misleading (Zola 1983, 1991; Bernard *et al.* 1984) and therefore of poor reliability.

The use of closed-ended questionnaires and precoded forms not only presents problems of validity and reliability, but often their formulation elicits an incorrect, evasive, or deliberately wrong answer. There are a few references to the occurrence and importance of elusive or lying informants in field research (Evans-Pritchard 1940; Salomone 1984; Bleek 1987), and most agree that respondents do not lie without good reason. Often, deliberate distortion or simply 'lying' is resorted to as a mechanism of escape from an embarrassing situation created by the nature of the subject that the question raises (Pedersen 1990).

Many authors have reported that information given by mothers on past illness episodes of their children, health care and child-rearing practices, or utilization of health services show such large discrepancies with reality that they invalidate about a third of all responses. The conclusions speak for themselves: the reliability of responses given by a segment of the population decreases with the lengthening of the recall period (telescopic memory effect), and whether because of omission, imprecision, or deliberate distortion, half of the what is reported bears little resemblance to behaviour actually adopted (Bernard *et al.* 1984; Husband and Foster 1987).

In summary, experience of using health surveys on populations in low-income countries has demonstrated limitations in their application and problems with regard to reliability and validity. The point in question is whether this is due to the conceptual perspective, the types of questions and methods used, the researchers themselves, the culture of the respondents, or a combination of all these factors. We can add two epistemological approaches to this debate, one based on the social science paradigms and the other on natural science paradigms, expressing either in numbers or in words what people say and do.

However, closed and quantitative oriented methods seem to predominate through the use of the ever pervasive closed-ended KAP survey studies. Of course, such studies will provide answers; most members of rural communities are polite and will respond when approached by outsiders, particularly those representing institutions of some power. However, although beautiful graphs, statistics, and χ^2 calculations can be obtained from such answers, the validity of information obtained by such means through a brief interchange must sometimes be strongly questioned (Campbell *et al.* 1979). It is not that quantitative methods do not have merit, but only that they are not creditable for every purpose. When first trying to understand a community, and the obvious as well as the more hidden health needs, more sensitive and qualitative methods are required, particularly as the problem may involve areas not readily revealed.

The importance of asking the right questions is central to effective international public health research. It must simply be said that epidemiologists and other public health professionals only receive answers to the questions that they ask! This seems obvious, and not particularly problematic. Questions are based on professional knowledge and are not plucked out of thin air. However,

the questions asked may not always be the most useful, particularly if they are formulated in the comfort (and isolation) of the researcher's study. For example, asking about sexual abstinence without realizing that for some people this term does not exclude a great many sexual practices may not be very important and may in fact result in quite misleading data (Huygens *et al.* 1996).

If we are serious about truly understanding people's health situations and needs within the wider context of their lives, we must be willing to assume not only that we lack answers, but also that we may not have all the appropriate questions. When trying to understand the sociocultural context within which people live their everyday lives and within which health problems occur, and by which these problems are shaped and even generated, it is important to start with an open mind, making as few assumptions as possible. Anthropological research is relevant because of its willingness to expect the unexpected. Anthropologists are not only (nor primarily) interested in receiving answers to their preconceived questions (although that is important of course), but by beginning research in an open-ended exploratory fashion, they are able to discover the most meaningful questions which will truly lead to a comprehensive understanding of the particular problem of concern—whether it is how best to reduce the incidence of diarrhoea, or bilharzia, or AIDS. Such initial comprehension can best be obtained from in-depth qualitative probing and the use of a range of other qualitative methods.

Some of these methods include participant observation, in-depth and key-informant interviewing, the use of open-ended questionnaires and conversational guidelines, and focus group discussion, to mention some of the most common. Descriptions of these anthropological methods and of the relevance of the anthropological perspective in general are given by Campbell *et al.* (1979), Casley and Lury (1981), Ellen (1984), Feuerstein (1986), Folch-Lyon and Frost (1982), Foster (1984), Miles and Huberman (1984), Peacock (1986), Pelto and Pelto (1978), Scrimshaw and Hurtado (1987), Soon Young Yoon (1986) Spradley (1979, 1980), and Stromquist (1984).

Questions are as important as answers! The important questions arise from 'being there', from understanding the context of people's lives from 'the inside', and from valuing their priorities and norms (Foster 1987; Schambra 1990). Anthropological researchers try to be receptive to the importance of seemingly unrelated factors which, upon greater reflection, may turn out to be very significant.

Of course, anthropologists are concerned with more than finding the right questions to ask. Whether answers to even the most appropriate of questions will reflect the reality of people's lives and accurately guide effective interventions will depend not only on the questions we ask, but on how we ask them. Have we established rapport with the people with whom we wish to work? Have we even gone so far as to consider participatory research leading to mutual planning and collaborative implementation (Fernandez and Tandon 1981; Feuerstein 1986)? How we ask the questions that we have come to believe are important depends on the characteristics of the population with whom we work, the general topic, and the detailed questions that we feel it is important to ask.

Qualitative methods are probing. They are useful in generating hypotheses, and in discovering the most important questions to include in random sample questionnaires. Qualitative approaches are concerned with why things are the way that they are and with what meaning they have for the people concerned. Thus, as well as being used in preparatory research for the purpose of best being able to formulate more broad-based questionnaires, qualitative methods can also be used after surveys to reveal the reasons for, and the meaning of, particular results from larger quantitative approaches. A dialectical process of interaction between a range of different quantitative and qualitative methods may be the most productive (Brewer and Hunter 1989). This interactive process will in itself lead to the pertinent questions and answers.

Since anthropological research is primarily explanatory, it is a dynamic process which adds new questions and can shift the focus of inquiry as further knowledge, particularly new associations, are discovered and obtained. In this way it is critically different from rigorous epidemiological and other survey research, and because its purpose and methods are different the efficacy of these methods, which are not less rigorous, cannot be judged by the same criteria. It must be noted here that because qualitative research is open-ended, exploratory, and even opportunistic, it is not casual or 'just common sense'. Detailed note-taking, categorization, and analysis are constant activities, and this in itself points to another distinction, namely that analysis is an ongoing process leading to the exploration and re-examination of new clues.

The strength of a qualitative approach rests on validity, which depends greatly on how questions are asked, by whom, where, and after what effort at establishing rapport. Qualitative methods do not pretend to test generalizability (other methods can do that), but they are particularly effective in understanding a problem 'from the inside'. Combination of the results of qualitative methods with those of quantitative methods allows a more accurate perception (both in terms of depth and breadth) of public health problems to be achieved and viable intervention to be developed.

The importance of trying to obtain an insider's perspective—to bridge the gap between 'us' and 'them'—guards against formulating research instruments entirely according to 'our' paradigms and predetermined hypothesis. The qualitative nature of the research and the way that it is carried out—the concern for rapport between researcher and the persons being researched—facilitate the entrance into another reality and an ability to understand the meanings of actions and phenomena within disparate sociocultural environments, which is a prerequisite for appropriate interventions. Of course, this is not necessarily foreign to epidemiologists. Again, to quote Cassel (1957), 'Health workers should have an intimate, detailed knowledge of people's beliefs, attitudes, knowledge, and behaviour before attempting to introduce any innovation into an area'.

Finally, it has been claimed by those who are anxious for rapid results that anthropological researches take too long. Certainly, carrying out a fully fledged ethnography of a community and a cultural group will take time, but a researcher living in a community for only a week, particularly someone who is familiar with the culture and knows the language (that is, a more 'focused' ethnography) can produce significantly more valid and comprehensive data for other (public health) purposes than those obtained by a score of field-workers arriving by car and carrying out a large set of interviews in half a day.

In closing this section, it may be worthwhile indicating some areas of convergence and discrepancy with the application of the rapid rural assessment method to health research (see Pedersen 1990). In order to do this, we should bear in mind the premises which uphold rapid assessment strategies and ask ourselves what benefits will be obtained from proposing an abbreviated time frame and a 'new' set of field research tools in health–disease.

First, rapid rural assessment should be recognized as an effective strategy for finding wider acceptance for qualitative and phenomenological research in the scientific community and amongst health professionals. Although the 'triangulation' strategy has been applied successfully to health research, resistance is still met when it comes to adopting innovations in the use of qualitative methods. The incorporation of qualitative methods in research is a *sine qua non* for expanding the conventional epidemiological and biomedical model of public health, for reorienting health plans and programmes, and for designing more effective interventions.

It has been said more than once that rapid rural assessment is rather more than organized common sense. Chambers was right to warn rapid rural assessment enthusiasts of the dangers of superficiality and error in this method. Above all, rapid assessment techniques are not supposed to save time, but ' . . . should release time for more contact with and learning from the poorer rural people' (Chambers 1985).

In reviewing the premises on which 'rapid' methods of research and assessment are based, it becomes evident that prolonged field-work leads to the unnecessary accumulation of ethnographic material which is not always relevant to the subject under study. As a result, it is proposed that field visits be shortened and efficiency increased so that only information considered necessary is collected. In order to do this, a list or 'prescription' of subjects considered to be universally relevant is drawn up, suggestions are made for adaptation to local realities, and recommendations are made for the combined use of quantitative and qualitative methods in the collection of data. The underlying assumption is that the adherence of the researcher to this 'prescription' or list of subjects, and the use of combined methods, will render data collection both efficient and scientifically rigorous.

However, it is difficult to distinguish between necessary and superfluous information *a priori*. Moreover, this assumes that other prejudices and sources of error in the research process (choice of theoretical framework, relationship between interviewer and interviewee, analysis and interpretation of data) either do not exist or are neutralized by the effects of the method and by the type of information gathered.

The rapid rural assessment methodology represents a first approximation. Information collected transversely and over a short period of time may be efficient from the researcher's viewpoint, but it runs the risk of being incomplete and of presenting a static image of reality. Research in general ' . . . should be a dialectic process, a dialogue over a long period of time' (Hall 1979), and the 'dialogue' cannot be restricted to certain stages, like the collection of data. The process of collecting and interpreting is iterative, which is why it should be done on a continuum, with each process helping the other. This does not mean that field-work and analysis should be extended indefinitely, but the time allotted should be sufficient to allow for the analysis of information *in situ* and if necessary to return to gather additional data.

Another unsolved problem with regard to rapid rural assessment is the interpretation of information and the use of data collected. Various alternative routes can be followed in the interpretation of data. Results can be laid out in such a way that they describe a programme or interpret a health problem or assess the impact of an intervention, but data have to be analysed not only in order to understand, evaluate, and explain reality, but also to transform it.

A central premise of the 'rapid' methods is that the objective reality exists 'out there' and, although independent of human perception, can be laid bare by the rigorous, and accelerated, application of methods. This is an incomplete premise, and today we should take it upon ourselves to review this partial (and reductionist) conception of scientific research. A broader approach departs from the assumption that each phase or stage in the research process is in dynamic interaction with the other phases and components, and simultaneously with the whole. Again, we have to insist on the adoption of an 'expanded' view of scientific rigour and the research–assessment process as a whole (Ratcliffe and Gonzalez del Valle 1988).

Scientific rigour in research cannot (and should not) be restricted to the discussion of data-collecting methods, nor to the efficiency or rapidity with which it is carried out. Therefore scientific rigour would not be tied down to the selection of techniques and the proportions to which the quantitative and qualitative methods be applied, but rather to the quality of decisions which researchers make throughout the research process. The definition of the problem, the conceptual framework, the generation of hypotheses, field-work, and the analysis and interpretation of results all form an integrated whole, to which data-collecting methods and instruments are added.

Secondly, the generation of new methods, and the substitution of some research techniques by others does not solve the problem of the monopoly of knowledge. We would like to suggest that all research and assessment (either 'rapid' or conventional) should involve the people and the community who have been excluded from the process up to now. This leads us to ask once again: What do we really need in order to conduct health research? A greater number of researchers qualified in the application of more 'scientific research techniques' does not appear to be a sufficient answer.

Rapid assessment methods should not replace the knowledge and experience of local researchers and informants. The participative research approach is an 'alliance' which brings together professional researchers and representatives from the local community in the research process, representing a valid alternative for increasing efficiency, reducing time frames, and democratizing the process of production and utilization of knowledge.

In the quest for the 'good' society

In a recent lecture delivered in Cardiff, Wales, Professor John K. Galbraith in reviewing major world social and economic changes, said in referring to the advanced countries and the quest for a 'good' society:

'The great political dichotomy, the capitalist and the working masses, has retreated into the shadows. In place of the capitalist is the modern great corporate bureaucracy. Not capitalists but managers . . . Politically dominant now are the managerial bureaucracy, the public bureaucracy, and the lawyers,

physicians, educators, members of the many other professions . . . We have a now a new class structure that embraces, on the one hand, the comfortably situated just mentioned who have replaced the once-dominant capitalist and, on the other, a large number of less affluent or often impoverished who do the work and render the services that make life pleasant, even tolerable, for what I have elsewhere called the culture of contentment. The modern equivalent of the one-time industrial proletariat is an underclass in the service of the comfortably situated . . . In the good society there cannot, must not, be a deprived and excluded underclass.' (Galbraith 1994).

We fully agree with Galbraith in pointing to the ethics of international health and development that if we are to build a new, compassionate society with greater solidarity—a 'good' society as he call it—then the more affluent countries must bear strongly in mind those who live on the other side of our wellbeing. He went on to say ' . . . And out of the resources and experience that so favour us we must extend help. Conscience cannot allow us to do less—to be less than concerned, less than generous. And it is thus, over time, that we will help to assume for others and for ourselves a more peaceful world' (Galbraith 1994).

As part of that vision of a good society which must extend help to others, a more balanced and wider perspective in public health, international health, and development is beginning to emerge, with the following features.

1. A move towards the construction of a 'new' public health, including the development of a biosocial model as a new paradigm of health and illness, based on the growing recognition of the political, economic, and social aspects of health advancement and of the interplay of the social with the biological dimension of health and disease.

2. The need to expand the international health research agenda to incorporate qualitative methods: to monitor progress, to evaluate performance, to guide experimentation and innovation, and to cast light on the broader social, cultural, and political issues, as well as the microsocial processes influencing the health status and the illness experience of large segments of the world population (Pedersen, 1994).

3. The increasing recognition of human rights as a central issue in the public health discourse.

4. The adoption of a 'militant' participatory strategy, in both research and action in collective health, through establishing an alliance between public health workers and the local communities with whom they are working.

Alliances for public health

In many respects, people the world over are similar; they are often preoccupied with meeting the same basic needs and aspirations, and we all face the possibilities of disease (although the type and rate of risk varies greatly). Despite certain similarities, it is also clear that people are quite different (at times almost 'deceptively' so). This is particularly true in the sphere of public health. We acknowledge such differences as obvious, and may even be annoyed that this is emphasized yet again. However, it is equally clear that we do not always act on this knowledge, in our everyday interactions and in our public health work, as we are often convinced of (the superiority of) our own norms and by the clarity of the proper application of our particular professional training and scientific knowledge.

Primarily owing to differences in their cultural and socio-economic situations people react differently to the same symptoms and exhibit different health-seeking behaviours. In some settings it is the sick person who is the main decision-maker and his or her ailment is the only or the singular concern. Elsewhere the sick individual has only a minor role in deciding what should be done—a 'therapy management group' (Janzen 1978) may be the deciding entity and the sick individual may not even be the central concern since an entire social group may be considered as 'the patient'. A whole range of popular, folk, and professional (including professional traditional) health care resources may be used at the same time or sequentially in different settings (Kleinman and Sung 1979).

People also have different social representations (explanatory models) for their ailments as well as for appropriate sick roles and behaviours concerning management and prevention. These are derived from the norms of their cultural and socio-economic environments, and often include spiritual, psychological, and social as well as physical factors. These differences between cultural groups, and between different segments within any one culture, must be recognized, as must be the differences usually existing between public health workers and the groups of people whose health they attempt to improve.

The concept of 'therapeutic alliance' (Kleinman et al. 1978; Helman 1984) is usually mentioned relative to a one-to-one patient–doctor interaction—the effectiveness and appropriateness of the therapeutic process is believed to depend quite significantly on the strength of the alliance (the therapeutic alliance) established between the healer and the patient. This is an alliance which must bridge the gap of cultural and socio-economic differences, including differences in explanatory models. Similarly, we can also talk about the need for public health workers to establish therapeutic, or public health, alliances with the communities in which they work or which they try to affect. Again, this obviously includes bridging cultural and socio-economic differences—a process which depends on an understanding of 'the other', that is an understanding of the characteristic norms of the group of people concerned, of the particular problems (including health) that they face, and of the particular context of their lives. Anthropologists, whose profession it is to cross borders and to understand those different from themselves, may be particularly useful in providing insight for the establishment of such alliances.

An understanding of the conditions of daily life of specific communities is also important for the formulation of effective health education programmes. There are many strategies for health education and social marketing (Kotler 1982; UNICEF/EAPRO 1986) including adapting 'Madison Avenue' methods for the promotion of public health activities.* We should keep in mind that health education is different from propaganda and should include understanding (or provision of new knowledge) as well as motivation for specific action. Different behavioural models guide the formulation of health education material. The health belief model (Rosenstock 1974; Rosenstock et al. 1988) and the diffusion of innovation model are just two of these which are quite widely known.† However, these methods have been found to be inadequate because factors other than beliefs about disease and appropriate treatment may influence people's behaviour and actions.

Mention should also be made of what has been called an 'experience near' form of health education, aspects of which also appear in other approaches, including social marketing. In this approach messages are promoted using idioms and symbols which are familiar to the target population together with examples and stories that are immediately recognizable by this population (Were 1985).

Anthropologists, who can serve as cultural interpreters and who can provide insiders' information and perspectives, can obviously facilitate the effectiveness of health education and social marketing strategies of various types. However, this should be done consequent to, and as a result of, the establishment of a public health alliance with the communities with whom we are working. Otherwise we may be guilty not only of paternalism but also of manipulation. Approaches which do not necessarily result from such an alliance—from working 'with the people' (Gish 1979)—may work to some degree and for a period of time, but in the long run their impact will be limited.

Paulo Freire's method of 'conscientization' is an approach which appears to integrate therapeutic alliance, social and community empowerment, and health education through a process of self-discovery. With the help of a facilitator, groups of individuals are involved in the process of (1) reflecting on aspects of their reality, (2) looking behind immediate problems to their root cause, (3) examining the implications and consequences of these issues, and (4) developing a plan of action to deal with problems collectively. Accordingly, the facilitators (or 'teacher–learners') follow a series of steps: (a) tuning in to the 'vocabulary universe' of the people (through use of an anthropological approach of participant observation and living with the people for an extended period), (b) initially working with small groups searching for 'generative themes' (key words suggestive of the hopes and concerns of the people), and (c) synthesizing the ideas of the people and codifying them in visual images, and returning these symbols and images back to the people

---

* It has been argued that if we understand what influences different populations to perceive different health care options in particular ways and what motivates them to make certain health care choices, this could (and perhaps should) be used to perfect social marketing techniques to bring about changes both in perception and in disease prevention and health-seeking behaviour. The UNICEF social marketing literature (UNICEF/EAPRO 1986) indicates that sociocultural, political, and economic factors are uncontrollable variables and that social marketing techniques should focus instead on the controllable variables of place, price, and promotion of the product (the four Ps) and thus be able to make an impact no matter what the character of the uncontrollable

factors. Such assumptions are not without foundation and can be adopted in countries of quite varied sociopolitical character, but, as indicated by the Alma-Ata Declaration and other documents, is it not precisely the sociocultural, political, and economic factors which are the direct determinants of health. Even though social marketing techniques may make significant contributions, this should not prevent us from examining and attempting to affect the larger (so-called uncontrollable) context in which ill health occurs.

† Briefly, the premise of the health belief model is that those most receptive to attempts to change their behaviour have the following beliefs: (1) their susceptibility to a particular disease is high; (2) if acquired, the disease could have very serious consequences; (3) the action indicated by a health education message is the most effective way of preventing the disease; (4) there are no serious barriers inhibiting such action.

The diffusion of innovation model indicates that the acceptance of an innovation is a three-step process of (1) initial awareness, (2) deciding to adopt the innovation, and (3) acting on that decision. Thus health education should (1) make people aware of specific public health innovations or measures, (2) persuade them of the need to adopt these measures, and (3) make the innovation or measures easily available (that is, immunization services).

for decoding through 'cultural circles', that is groups of people who look at the causes, consequences, and possible solutions to their problems and the 'generative themes' that they have identified (Freire 1973, 1985; Minkler and Cox 1980; Freire and Faundez 1989).

As we attempt to educate and to bring about change, even to transform communities, which is ultimately what public health is all about, both anthropologists and public health professionals may be informed by reflecting on two aspects of the history of anthropology when considering the public health roles that the former are sometimes asked to play.

As already mentioned, one aspect of the history of the role of anthropologists is that of having been 'brokers' or 'servants' to colonial administrators. Anthropological insights were used to understand better, and thus to control better, the lives of the 'natives', and thus to administer colonial enterprises more effectively. This heritage remains despite the interventions of some anthropologists to abate the cultural imperialism of colonial powers.

Today, this time in the service of public health, there is again a tendency to use anthropologists as cultural brokers. They are asked to find the correct buttons to push to make the 'natives' jump, this time, presumably, for their own good—for their own health and well-being. Such, albeit well-meaning, use of anthropological knowledge is no less manipulation of people than that used 50 or more years ago and often disregards the perspectives (and values) of the 'native' people themselves. It defeats the practice of the 'art of the possible' (Ramalingaswami 1986) in that it does not equitably join two disciplines, but rather employs one for the implementation of the 'scientifically correct' interventions of the other. Recognizing the importance of the alliance (with different disciplines and with the 'target population') should guard against this distortion.

History provides direction as well as caution. Another historical root shows the anthropological enterprise arising from a sense of alienation and dissatisfaction with one's own society. It was, and still is, a search for alternatives, rather than a way to engage in a 'missionary' conversion to 'our models'. It allows us to examine our own values and cultural characteristics in juxtaposition to those of others, and to recognize that there is a difference. It provides a two-dimensional gaze for self-criticism with which to look at ourselves and others, and to engage with them (Diamond 1974), without presuming that our values are always to be used as the norms, particularly as we interact with those different from ourselves, whether in a foreign country or 'across the street' (from a school of public health). This two-way perspective is essential in establishing 'public health alliances', which are fundamental to the development of the 'new' public health, and even more importantly for improving people's health.

Bibliography

In preparing this chapter the first author relied on a number of his previous publications.

Heggenhougen, H.K. (1984). Will primary health care be allowed to succeed? *Social Science and Medicine*, 19(3), 217–24.

Heggenhougen, H.K. (1985). The future of medical anthropology. In *Technical manual on medical anthropology* (ed. C. E. Hill), pp. 130–6. American Anthropological Association, Washington, DC.

Heggenhougen, H.K. (1986). Ten best books in medical anthropology. *Health Policy and Planning*, 1(2), 176–7.

Heggenhougen, H.K. (1990). Whither medical anthropology? A cautionary note. *British Medical Anthropology Society Newsletter*, **Spring**, 1–3.

Heggenhougen, H.K. (1991). Role of anthropological methods to identify health needs. In *Primary health care*, (ed. C. A. K. Yesudian), pp. 68–76. Tata Institute of Social Sciences, Bombay.

Heggenhougen, H.K. (1992). The interlocking web of development, environment and health—the relevance of anthropological methods for public health research. In *Health and environment in developing countries* (ed. A. Manu), pp. 127–47. University of Oslo Press, Oslo.

Heggenhougen, H.K. (1993). PHC and anthropology: challenges and opportunities. *Medical Culture and Psychology*, 17, 281–9.

Heggenhougen, H.K. (1993). Joining community struggles for health: anthropological notes on learning from 'the other'. In *A new dawn in Guatemala——toward a worldwide health vision* (ed. R. Luecke), pp. 135–50. Waveland Press, Prospect Heights, IL.

Heggenhougen, H.K. and Clements, C.J. (1987) *Acceptability of childhood immunization*. London School of Hygiene and Tropical Medicine, and WHO, Geneva.

Heggenhougen, H.K. and Clements, C.J. (1990). An anthropological perspective on the acceptability of immunization services. *Scandinavian Journal of Infectious Diseases (Supplement)*, 76, 20–31.

Heggenhougen, H.K. and Draper, A. (1990). *Medical anthropology and primary health care*. London School of Hygiene and Tropical Medicine.

Heggenhougen, H.K. and Shore, L. (1986). Cultural components of behavioural epidemiology. *Social Science and Medicine*, 22(11), 1235–45.

References

Ackerknecht, E. (1971). *Medicine and ethnology: selected essays*. Johns Hopkins Press, Baltimore, MD.

Adair, J. and Deuschle, K. (1958). Some problems of physicians on the Navajo Reservation. *Human Organization*, 16(4), 19–23.

Adair, J. and Deuschle, K. (1988). *The people's health: medicine and anthropology in a Navajo community*. University of New Mexico Press, Albuquerque, NM.

Aguirre Beltrán, G. (1955). *Programas de salud en la situación intercultural*. Instituto Indigenista Interamericano, Mexico City.

Audy, J.R. and Dunn, F.L. (1974). Community health. In *Human Ecology* (ed. F. Sargent), pp. 345–63. Elsevier, Amsterdam.

Benedict, R. (1935). *Patterns of culture*. Routledge and Kegan Paul, London.

Berkman, L. and Syme, S. (1979). Social networks, host resistance, and mortality: a nine year follow up study of Alameda County residents. *American Journal of Epidemiology*, 109(2), 186–204.

Bernard, H.R., Killworth, P.D., Kronenfeld, D., and Sailer, L. (1984). The problem of informant accuracy: the validity of retrospective data. *Annual Review of Anthropology*, 13, 495–517.

Bleek, W. (1987). Lying informants: a fieldwork experience from Ghana. *Population Development Review*, 13(2), 314–22.

Brewer, J. and Hunter, A. (1989). *Multimethod research: a synthesis of styles*. Sage, New York.

Campbell, J.G., Shrestha, R., and Stone, L. (1979). *The use and misuse of social science research in Nepal*. Center for Nepal and Asian Studies, HMG Press, Kathmandu.

Campos Navarro, R. (ed.) (1992). *La Antropología Médica en México*. Instituto Mora, Universidad Autonoma Metropolitana, San Juan, Mixcoac, Mexico.

Casley, P.J. and Lury, D.A. (1981). *Data collection in developing countries*. Oxford University Press, Oxford.

Cassel, J. (1957). Social and cultural implications of food and food habits. *American Journal of Public Health*, 47, 732–40.

Cassel, J. (1964). Social science theory as a source of hypotheses in epidemiological research. *American Journal of Public Health*, 54, 1482–8.

Caudill, W. (1953) Applied anthropology in medicine. In *Anthropology today: an encyclopedic inventory* (ed. A. L. Kroeber), pp. 771–806. University of Chicago Press, Chicago.

Chambers, R. (1985). Shortcut methods of gathering social information for rural development projects. In *Putting people first: sociological analysis in rural development* (ed. M. M. Cernea), pp. 399–416. Oxford University Press, New York, for the World Bank.

Chiappe, M. (1968) El Curanderismo en la Costa Norte del Peru. In *Anales del V Congreso Latinoamericano de Psiquiatría.* (ed. C.A. Seguin). pp. 76–93. Ediciones Ermar, Lima, Peru.

Chrisman, N.J. and Maretzki, T.W. (ed.) (1982). *Clinically applied anthropology.* Reidel, Dordrecht.

Clements, F.E. (1932). *Primitive concepts of disease. University of California Press publications in archaeology and anthropology,* Vol. 32, pp. 185–252. University of California Press, Berkely, CA.

Coreil, J. and Mull, J.D. (ed.) (1990). *Anthropology and primary health care.* Westview Press, Boulder, CO.

Davies, B., Corbishley, P., Evans, J., and Kenrick, C. (1985). Integrating methodologies: if the intellectual relations don't get you, then the social will. In *Strategies in educational research: qualitative methods* (ed. R. G. Burgess), pp. 289–321. Falmer Press, London.

de Souza Queiroz, M. and Canesqui, A.M. (1986). Contribucoes da Antropologia a Medicina: uma revisao de estudos no Brazil. *Revista de Sande Publica,* **20**(2), 141–51.

Desjarlais, R., Eisenberg, L., Good, B., *et al.* (1995). *World mental health —problems and priorities in low-income countries.* Oxford University Press, New York.

Deuschle, K. and Adair, J. (1958). An interdisciplinary approach to public health on the Navajo Indian Reservation: medical and anthropological aspects. *Annals of the New York Academy of Sciences,* **84**, 887–904.

Diamond, S. (1974). *In search of the primitive—a critique of civilization.* Transaction Books, New Brunswick, NJ.

Dobkin de Rios, M. (1968). Folk curing with a psychodelic cactus in Northern Peru. *International Journal of Social Psychiatry,* **15**(1), 23–32.

Dunn, F. (1979). Behavioural aspects of the control of parasitic diseases. *Bulletin of the WHO,* **57**, 499–512.

Dunn, F.L. and Janes, C.R. (1986). Introduction: medical anthropology and epidemiology. In *Anthropology and epidemiology* (ed. C. R. Janes, R. Stall, and S. M. Gifford), pp. 3–34. Reidel, Dordrecht.

Eisenberg, L. (1984). Rudolph Virchow, where are you now that we need you? *American Journal of Medicine,* **77**, 524–32.

Eisenberg, L. and Kleinman, A. (1981). *The relevance of social science for medicine.* Reidel, Dordrecht.

Ellen, R.F. (1984). *Ethnographic research: a guide to general conduct.* Academic Press, London.

Engel, G. (1977) The need for a new biomedical model: a challenge for biomedicine. *Science,* **196**, 129–36.

Evans-Pritchard, E. (1940). *The Nuer.* Clarendon Press, Oxford.

Fabrega, H. (1972). Medical anthropology. In *Biennial review of anthropology* (ed. B. J. Siegel). Stanford University Press, Standford, CA.

Fabrega, H. (1974). *Disease and social behaviour.* MIT Press, Cambridge, MA.

Fals Borda, O. (1964). Las Ciencias Sociales en la Enseñanza y en la Investigación Médica. In *Medicina y Desorrollo Social* (ed. T Mundo). pp. 23–57. ASCOFAME, Bogotá.

Fernandez, W. and Tandon, R. (ed.) (1981). *Participatory research and evaluation: experiments in research as a process of liberation.* Indian Social Institute, New Delhi.

Feuerstein, M.-T. (1986). *Partners in evaluation: evaluating development and community programs with participants.* MacMillan, London.

Firth, R. (1934) The sociological study of native diet. *Africa,* **7**, 401–14.

Firth, R. (1957). Health planning and community organization. *Health Education Journal,* **15**, 118–25.

Folch-Lyon, E. and Frost, J.F. (1982). Conducting focus group sessions. *Studies in Family Planning,* **12**(12), 443–9.

Foster, G.M. (1974). Medical anthropology: some contrasts with medical sociology. *Medical Anthropology Newsletter,* **6**(1), 1–6.

Foster, G.M. (1982). Applied anthropology and international health, retrospect and prospect. *Human Organization,* **41**(3), 189–97.

Foster, G.M. (1984) Anthropological research perspectives on health problems in developing countries. *Social Science and Medicine,* **18**(10), 847–54.

Foster, G.M. (1987). World Health Organization behavioral science research: problems and prospects. *Social Science and Medicine,* **24**(9), 709–17.

Foster, G.M. and Anderson, B. (1978). *Medical anthropology.* Wiley, New York.

Freire, P. (1973). *Education for critical consciousness.* Continuum, New York.

Freire, P. (1985). *The politics of education: culture, power and liberation.* Bergin and Garvey, South Hadley, MA.

Freire, P. and Faundez, A. (1989). *Learning to question: a pedagogy of liberation.* World Council of Churches, Geneva.

Frenk, J. (1992). The new public health. In: PAHO/WHO, The crisis of public health: reflections for the debate. (Scientific Publication No. 540), pp. 75–94. Pan American Health Organization, Washington.

Galbraith, J.K. (1994). The good society considered: the economic dimension. *Journal of Law and Society,* 3–4.

García Manzanedo, H. (1983). *Manual de investigación aplicada en servicios sociales y de salud.* La Prensa Médica Mexicana, Mexico City.

Gish, O. (1979). The political economy of primary health care and 'health by the people': an historical exploration. *Social Science and Medicine,* **13C**, 203–11.

Hall B. (1979) Breaking the monopoly of knowledge: research methods, participation and development. In *Creating knowledge: a monopoly?* (ed. B. Hall, A. Gilletto, and R. Tandon) pp. 132–49. International Council for Adult Education, Toronto.

Heggenhougen, H.K. (1979) 'Therapeutic anthropology'—reaction to Shiloh's proposal. *American Anthropologist,* **81**(3), 647–51.

Heggenhougen, H.K. (1984) Will primary health care be allowed to succeed? *Social Science and Medicine,* **19**(3), 217–24.

Heggenhougen, H.K. (1995). The epidemiology of functional apartheid and human rights abuses. *Social Science and Medicine,* **40**(3), 281–4.

Helman, C. (1984). *Culture, health and illness.* Wright, Bristol.

Herrera, X. and Lobo-Guerrero, M. (1982). *Antropología Médica y Medicina Tradicional en Colombia: Temario-Guía y Bibliografía Anotada.* Centro Cultural Jorge Eliecer Gaitan (mimeo).

Husband, R. and Foster, W. (1987) Understanding qualitative research: a strategic approach to qualitative methodology. *Journal of Human Education and Development,* **26**(2), 51–63.

Huygens, P., Kajura, E., Seeley, J., and Barton, (1996). Rethinking methods for the study of sexual behaviour. *Social Science and Medicine,* **42**(2), 221–31.

Janes, C.R., Stall, R., and Gifford, S.M. (1986). *Anthropology and epidemiology: interdisciplinary approaches to the study of health and disease,* Reidel, Dordrecht.

Janzen, J. (1978). *The quest for therapy in Lower Zaire.* University of California Press, Berkeley, CA.

Justice. J. (1986). *Policies, plans and people.* University of California Press, Berkeley, CA.

Kaufert, P.A. (1990). The 'box-ification' of culture: the role of the social scientist. *Sante, Culture, Health,* **7**(2–3), 139–48.

Kleinman, A. and Sung, L.H. (1979). Why do indigenous practitioners successfully heal? *Social Science and Medicine,* **13B**, 7–26.

Kleinman, A., Eisenberg, L., and Good, B. (1978). Culture, illness and care: clinical lessons from anthropologic and cross-cultural research. *Annals of Internal Medicine,* **99**, 25–58.

Kotler, P. (1982). *Marketing for non-profit organizations,* Prentice-Hall, Englewood Cliffs, NJ.

Landy, D. (ed.) (1977). *Culture, disease and healing,* Macmillan, New York.

Leighton, A. and Leighton, D. (1944). *The Navaho door. An introduction to Navaho life.* Harvard University Press, Cambridge, MA.

Leslie, C. (1976). *Asian medical systems: a comparative study.* University of California Press, Berkeley, CA.

Lieban, R. (1977) The field of medical anthropology. In *Culture, disease and healing,* (ed. D, Landy), pp. 13–31. Macmillan, New York.

Lock, M. and Scheper-Hughes, N. (1990). A critical-interpretive approach in medical anthropology. Rituals and routines of discipline and dissent. In *Medical anthropology. Contemporary theory and method* (ed. T. M. Johnson and C. F. Sargent). Praeger, New York.

McElroy, A. and Townsend, P.K. (1979). *Medical anthropology in ecological perspective.* Duxbury Press, North Scituate, MA.

Malinowski, B. (1945). Problems of native diet in the economic setting. In *The Dynamic of culture change. An inquiry into race relations in Africa.* (ed. B. Malinowski). Yale University Press, New Haven CT.

Malinowski, B. (1961). *Argonauts of the Western Pacific.* Dutton, New York.

Mann, J.M., Gostin, L., Gruskin, S., Brennan, T., Lazzarini, Z., and Fineberg, H.V. (1994). Health and human rights. *Health and Human Rights*, 1(1), 6–23.

Maquet, J.J. (1964). Objectivity in anthropology. *Current Anthropology*, 5(1), 47–55.

Miles, M.B. and Huberman, M. (1984). *Qualitative data analysis: a sourcebook of new methods.* Sage, Newbury Park, CA.

Minkler, M. and Cox, K. (1980). Creating critical consciousness in health: applications of Freire's philosophy and methods to the health care setting. *International Journal of Health Services*, 10(2), 311–22.

Nations, M. (1986). Epidemiological research on infectious disease: quantitative rigor or rigor mortis? Insights from ethnomedicine. In *Anthropology and epidemiology interdisciplinary approaches to the study of health and disease* (ed. C. R. Janes, R. Stall, and E. M. Gifford), pp. 97–123. Reidel, Dordrecht.

Navarro, V. (1974a). The underdevelopment of health or the health of underdevelopment: an analysis of the distribution of human health resources in Latin America. In *Imperialism, health and medicine* (ed. V. Navarro), pp. 15–36. Baywood, Farmingdale, NY.

Navarro, V. (1974b). The economic and political determinants of human (including health) rights. In *Imperialism, health and medicine* (ed. V. Navarro), pp. 53–76. Baywood, Farmingdale, NY.

Nichter, M. (1989). *Anthropology and international health.* Kluwer, Dordrecht.

OPS/OMS (1978). *Bibliografía seleccionada en antropología médica para las protesionales de salud en las Américas,* OSP, Oficina de Campo de la Frontera Mexicano-Estadounidense, El Paso, TX.

PAHO (Pan American Health Organisation) (1992). *La crisis de la salud pública: reflexiones para el debate.* Scientific Publication 540, OPS, Washington, DC.

Paul, B. (1955), *Health, culture and community.* Sage, New York.

Peacock, J.L. (1986). *The anthropological lens.* Cambridge University Press, Cambridge.

Pedersen, D. (1990). Qualitative and quantitative: two styles of viewing the world or two categories of reality. In *International Conference on Rapid Assessment Methodologies for Planning and Evaluation of Health Related Programs.* (ed. N. Scrimshaw), pp. 72–90, United Nations University, UNICEF and PAHO/WHO, Tokyo.

Pedersen, D. (1994). *The development of teaching and research in public health,* Technical Report Series, Universidad de Buenos Aires–OPS/OMS. OPS, Buenos Aires.

Pelto, P.J. and Pelto, G.H. (1978). *Anthropological research: the structure of enquiry.* Cambridge University Press, Cambridge.

Polgar, S. (1962). Health and human behaviour: areas of interest common to the social and medical sciences. *Current Anthropology*, 3(2), 159–206.

Polgar, S. (1963). Health action in cross-cultural perspective. In *Handbook of medical sociology* (ed. H. Freeman, S. Levine, and L. Reeder). Prentice Hall, Englewood Cliffs, NJ.

Ramalingaswami, V. (1986). The art of the possible. *Social Science and Medicine*, 22, 1097–103.

Ratcliffe, J. and Gonzalez Del Valle, A. (1988). Rigor in health related research. Towards an expanded conceptualization. *International Journal of Health Services*, 18(3), 361–92.

Reichel-Dormatoff, G. (1953). Prácticas obstétricas como factor de control social en una cultura de transición. *Anales de la Sociedad de Biología de Bogotá (BICAN)*, 6(1), 30–7.

Reichel-Dormatoff, G. (1959). Nivel de salud y medicina popular en una aldea mestiza colombiana. *Revista Colombiana de Antropología (BICAN)*, 7, 201–49.

Richards, A. (1939). *Land, labour and diet in Northern Rhodesia.* Oxford University Press, Oxford.

Richards, C. (1960). Cooperation between anthropologist and medical personnel. *Human Organization*, 19, 64–7.

Rivers, W.H.R. (1924). *Medicine, magic and religion.* Harcourt Brace, New York.

Rosenstock, I.M. (1974). The health belief model and preventive health behaviour. *Health Education Monographs*, 2, 354–85.

Rosenstock, I.M., Strecher, V.J., and Becker, M.H. (1988). Social learning theory and the health belief model. *Health Education Quarterly*, 15(2), 175–83.

Salomone, F. (1984). The methodological significance of the lying informant. *Anthropology Quarterly*, 50(3), 117–24.

Saunders, L. (1954). *Cultural difference and medical care: the case of the Spanish-speaking people of the Southwest.* Sage, New York.

Schambra, P.E. (1990). Seeking new dimensions in international health research. *Journal of the American Medical Association*, 263(24), 3325–7.

Scotch, N. (1963). Medical anthropology. In *Biennial review of anthropology* (ed. B.J. Siegel). pp. 1183–1213. Stanford University Press, Stanford, CA.

Scrimshaw, S.C.M. and Hurtado, E. (1987). *Rapid assessment procedures for nutrition and primary health care: anthropological approaches to improving program effectiveness,* UCLA Latin American Center Publications, University of California, Los Angeles, CA.

Seguin, C.A. (1959). Presente y perspectivas de la Psiquiatría en el Peru. *Revista Psiquiátrica Peruana*, 1(2).

Seguin, C.A. (1979). *Psiquiatría Folklórica.* Centro de Proyección Cristiana, Lima.

Singer, M. (1986). Developing a critical perspective in medical anthropology. *Medical Anthropology Quarterly*, 17(5), 128–9.

Spradley, J.P. (1979). *The ethnographic interview.* Holt, New York.

Spradley, J.P. (1980). *Participant observation.* Holt, New York.

Stromquist, N. (1984). Action research: a new sociological approach in developing countries. *IDRC Report*, 13(3), 5–19.

Taussig, M. (1979). Folk healing and the structure of conquest in southwest of Colombia. *Journal of Latin American Lore*, 6(2).

Taussig, M. (1980). *The deveil and commodity fetichism in South America.* University of North Carolina Press, Chapel Hill.

Trostle, J. (1986a). Early work in anthropology and epidemiology. In *Anthropology and epidemiology: interdisciplinary approaches to the study of health and disease* (ed. C. R. Janes, R. Stall, and S. M. Gifford), pp. 35–96. Reidel, Dordrecht.

Trostle, J. (1986b). Anthropology and epidemiology in the twentieth century. In *Anthropology and epidemiology: interdisciplinary approaches to the study of health and disease* (ed. C. R. Janes, R. Stall, and S. M. Gifford), Chapter 3. Reidel, Dordrecht.

UNICEF/EAPRO (1986). *Social marketing. Handbooks in communication and training for CSDR.* 7. East Asia and Pakistan Regional Office, Bangkok.

Valdizán, H. (1915). La alienación mental entre los primitivos Peruano. Tesis de Doctorado, Universidad Mayor de San Marcos, Lima. (Reprinted in Valdizán, H. (1990). *Paleopsiquiatría del Antiguo Perú.* Universidad Peruana Cayehano Heredia, Lima.).

Valdizán, H. and Maldonado, A. (1922). *La Medicina Popular Peruana,* 3 vols. Impenta Torres Aguirre, Lima.

van der Geest, S. and Whyte, S.R. (1991). *The context of medicines in developing countries—studies in pharmaceutical anthropology.* Het Spinhuis, Amsterdam.

Velimirovic, B. (ed.) (1979). *La medicina moderna y la antropología médica en la población fronteriza mexicano-estadounidense.* OPS, Washington, DC.

Were, M. (1985). Communicating on immunization to mothers and community groups. *Assignment Children*, 69/72, 429–42.

WHO/UNICEF (1978). The Alma-Ata Conference on Primary Health Care. *WHO Chronicle*, 32(11), 431–8.

Young, A. (1982). The anthropologies of illness and sickness. *Annual Review of Anthropology*, 11, 257–85.

Young Yoon, S. (1988). *Concepts of health behaviour research,* SEARO Regional Health Paper 13, WHO, New Delhi.

Zola, I. (1983). *Socio-medical inquiries: recollections, reflections, and reconsiderations.* Temple University Press, Philadelphia, PA.

Zola, I. (1991). Bringing our bodies and ourselves back in: reflections on a past, present and future 'medical sociology'. *Journal of Health and Social Behavior*, 32(1), 1–16.

25 Demography and public health

C.M. Suchindran and Helen P. Koo

Introduction

The field of public health is very broad, being dedicated to applying scientific and technical knowledge to prevent disease and promote the health of the population (or subpopulations or communities) (Institute of Medicine 1988). The field encompasses many disciplines or activities, such as the investigation of the causes of disease, surveillance of the health of the population (including the collection and analysis of vital statistics), immunization against communicable disease, protection against hazards in the workplace, environmental sanitation, educational campaigns to encourage healthful behaviours, development of health policy and organization of health care delivery and financing. The field of demography is much narrower, being the study of the size and distribution of human populations, and of processes that bring about change in these population parameters – in particular, the processes of fertility (births), mortality (deaths), and migration.

The two fields of public health and demography intersect at many points, however, because they are concerned with some of the same processes (notably births and deaths) and for both, the population is the primary unit of concern.

Two out of the three population processes studied by demographers – mortality and fertility – are fundamental processes that involve every human being. These processes form integral parts of the health of populations and are thus of central concern to the public health field. The interest of the two fields in these processes is fueled by different motivations, however. Demographers investigate mortality and fertility (along with their determinants and components) as an end unto itself, with the object of understanding these as processes of population change. The implications of these processes, including public health implications, are also of concern to demographers, but they are secondary ones. In contrast, public health professionals' primary interest in mortality, fertility and their components lies in these phenomena's bearing upon the health of the people. The object of public health professionals' interest in these processes is to measure them to assess the health of the population, and to study them as a basis for developing policies and designing public health programmes and services to improve the public health.

Both fields are centrally concerned with some of the same phenomena at the level of populations and, therefore, some of their activities overlap. One of the fundamental functions of the public health field is to monitor and assess the health of populations. For this, public health professionals collect and analyse a variety of data – vital statistics, administrative records, survey and census data.

Demographers also collect and use these types of data, and perform similar analyses; these will be described later in this chapter.

The two fields are also linked because population change can profoundly affect the need for public health services, and conversely public health measures can change population size or processes. For example, in the United States and other developed countries, the low fertility rates of recent decades, combined with increased longevity, have dramatically raised the proportion of older people in the population. As a result, a significantly increased share of public health resources has been directed at the prevention of the chronic and degenerative diseases suffered by older people. As another example, the migration of foreign workers into selected states of the United States, and, within the country, the increased concentration of minority populations in inner cities, have meant that additional public health facilities and services need to be located where these at-risk populations can be served. Conversely, public health programmes have affected population structure and processes. For example, in the past handful of decades, public health programmes have contributed to a great reduction in deaths of infants and children, thereby helping to alter the age composition of the population.

The purpose of this chapter is to present an overview of the basic measures and foci of demography, and the concerns of demography especially in economically developed countries. It is our hope that this overview will provide public health practitioners and researchers with a better understanding of how demographers measure and study population structure and change. We hope that this, in turn, will stimulate an appreciation by public health professionals of what the tools and measures of demography can do to further their understanding of the complexities of the public's health status and its determinants, and of special at-risk populations for whom public health programmes need to be targeted.

Synopsis of demography

Before discussing various aspects of demography, we first present a summary of its subject areas and of the methods of analysis used. A subsequent section reviews the data collected and analysed by demographers. Then we consider various parts of demography, in turn. The discussion necessarily includes only some of the measures, tools, data, concepts, and topics of demography – chosen because they represent fundamental aspects of the field, or because they have particular relevance to public health. Thus this chapter does not attempt to present a comprehensive or balanced view of demography. It complements the broad account of the field given in Volume I (Chapter 5). Similarly, the references cited in the present chapter should not be seen as a comprehensive or balanced selection. We have preferred to cite review articles, or if none was available to us, we have selected only a few examples of a much vaster body of literature. These references are intended as an entree for interested readers into the fuller literature.

As stated earlier, demography centres on the study of population size and structure, and changes in these. Three processes bring about population change: fertility, mortality, and migration. For that reason, a basic objective of demography is to study trends over time and variation across regions or subgroups in these population processes. Furthermore, demographers investigate the factors that cause changes in time or differences among subgroups or individuals in these processes. Fertility and mortality are biological processes. As such, their occurrence depends in part on a number of biological precursors or factors that are linked to these precursors; demographers call these 'proximate determinants' (for example, proximate determinants of fertility include the physiological ability to conceive, breastfeeding, and use of contraception). In addition, demographers study the dependence of mortality, fertility and their proximate determinants on a variety of social, cultural, economic, psychological, environmental and behavioural or life-style factors – including, in some cases, access to or use of health services. The public health field also considers a similar, broad range of factors that impinge on health or the avoidance of premature morbidity and mortality. Thus, the two fields intersect in some of their research, and both can profit from building on each others' results.

Besides studying the determinants of population change, demographers also investigate the consequences of change in population processes. For example, they have examined the implications of the aging of the population for the labour force and the economy, the consequences of childbearing in the adolescent and older ages for women's and children's health and well-being, and the implications of population movements for the epidemiology of diseases.

Formal demography is the study of population size and structure, and change in these. Formal demography relies primarily on analysing descriptive measures such as rates, ratios and life table measures, and also on analytical growth models such as stable population models. These growth models examine the interrelationships among fertility, mortality, and migration. In addition, formal demography uses computer simulation models to study population growth.

In the study of determinants and consequences of population processes, social demographers use conventional regression techniques (such as multiple linear regression, logistic and probit regression) and categorical data analysis techniques (such as log-linear models). Recently, several statistical techniques have been adapted by demographers (United Nations Population Fund 1993). These include hazards modelling, a method for analysing duration data (such as intervals between births or length of life) that are subject to censoring. Hazards modelling can be thought of as a technique of multivariate analysis of life-table probabilities (Namboodiri and Suchindran 1987). Another relatively recent advance is the use of models that include unobservable heterogeneity or frailty. These models take into account factors that put people at variable risk of having the event of interest (such as death, birth) but that have not been measured, such as genetic predispositions or susceptibility as a result of cumulative exposures to environmental influences (Heckman and Singer 1982; Vaupel *et al.* 1979).

Longitudinal data have become more commonly available and thus require special statistical techniques. Techniques for analysis of longitudinal data that examine correlated outcomes include mixed linear models and longitudinal logistic models such as Generalized Estimating Equations (GEE) models (Zeger *et al.* 1988; Tsui *et al.* 1993).

Demographers also use multilevel models that include both individual-level variables (such as a person's sex, education) and contextual or community-level variables (such as distance from the community to nearest hospital, density of medical personnel in the community). These models capture the influence of both individuals' characteristics or experiences and those of the physical or cultural community in which they live (Entwistle and Mason 1985). In addition, demographers use grade-of-membership (GOM) models to classify individuals within heterogeneous populations into special risk-groups on the basis of multiple characteristics. This method differs from cluster analysis in that GOM models do not assign each person into one specific group. Instead, individuals are given 'degree of similarity' or 'grades of membership' scores, which indicate the degree to which an individual resembles each of a set of ideal profiles or 'pure groups'. GOM models are useful where populations include many subgroups that differ in their vulnerability to a disease, and where classifying people into specific groups is impossible (Berkman *et al.* 1989). Finally, demographers have begun to use geographic information systems (GIS) to perform spacial analyses of population processes (see section below on 'Population Distribution').

Data used by demographers

Demographers collect and analyse several types of data, which are outlined below. A further discussion, including consideration of data collection problems, is given in Volume I (Chapter 5).

National population censuses (typically conducted every 10 years) provide a complete count of the population by location and also obtain selected characteristics of the individuals, families, and households in the country at a specified time. Census data are used for estimating many basic demographic measures such as the size of population at risk of mortality, fertility, migration, marriage, divorce, etc. (that are the denominators for many basic rates and ratios). Census data are also used for sampling frames for selecting samples for health, demographic and other surveys. Furthermore, census data form the basis for making population projections.

Vital registration systems record all births, deaths (including fetal deaths), marriages and (in some countries) divorces occurring in each vital registration area. These systems also obtain basic characteristics of the people experiencing these events. For example, birth certificates in the United States obtain demographic information about the mother, prenatal care, obstetric conditions, lifestyle behaviours of the mother (such as smoking and alcohol use), the birthweight and health conditions of the newborn. Death certificates in many countries obtain demographic data about the decedent and about medical causes of death. Marriage certificates collect sociodemographic data about both partners. Divorce certificates may obtain demographic and socio-economic information about both partners, children from the union, etc.

Vital registration data provide the basic information for measuring these vital events. They are also often used for analysing interrelationships between demographic and socio-economic factors and the occurrence of the events.

Data from the vital registration system have been made even more useful in recent years by linking them with data from other sources. For example, death certificate data have been linked to birth certificate data. Also, data from medical or health insurance records have been linked to death and birth registration data. Vital registration data have also been merged with administrative records such as tax and social security (pension) records.

Continuous registration systems record on a continuous basis information about vital events and in- and out-migration. Data from these systems are used for obtaining current knowledge about the size and distribution of the population, complementing and checking the census, and in some cases, replacing the census. These data are also used for historical demography. Continuous registration systems are found mostly in Scandinavia.

A wide variety of retrospective, cross-sectional sample surveys have been conducted to collect more detailed information about fertility, mortality, and migration and components such as family planning, and about their determinants. These surveys are conducted at one time and obtain retrospectively the histories of respondents and their families about topics of concern (childbearing, contraceptive use, deaths, moves, etc.). In some cases, surveys use a calendar method to record retrospectively information on various types of events that could have occurred concurrently (for example births, contraceptive use, breastfeeding, infant deaths) so that the timing of the events may be explicitly related and used to help the respondents to recall them (Goldman *et al.* 1991). Retrospective survey data provide in-depth information about these processes and about their correlates.

For example, household surveys have been conducted worldwide in the past three decades to collect information on women's histories of childbearing and contraceptive use. These surveys, notably the World Fertility Survey (WFS), and its successor, the Demographic and Health Survey (DHS), have provided the major data for analysing international trends and variations in fertility, as well as their determinants. In the United States, national fertility surveys have taken place periodically since 1955. The federal government conducted the most recent series, known as the National Survey of Family Growth (NSFG), in 1973, 1976, 1982, 1988, and 1994.

The Current Population Survey of the United States is a series of surveys that has been conducted almost every month for the past 50 years. The surveys generally cover the same topics at annual intervals, including marital status, family and household composition, residence, mobility, school enrolment and educational attainment. Special supplements periodically include childbearing and marital histories. The results of these surveys, published in the *Current Population Reports*, provide current descriptions of the population on an ongoing basis.

Other smaller scale or specialized surveys have been conducted for various purposes, including the study of migration and mortality.

Although these cross-sectional surveys have provided a wealth of information about the population and about population processes, they face the limitation of any data collected at one time. In particular, they do not obtain adequate information about changes

in factors influencing the processes captured in the retrospective histories, and the histories may not be accurately recalled.

To overcome the weaknesses of retrospective surveys, prospective, longitudinal sample surveys have also been conducted to collect demographic information. These surveys obtain information about the same people at two or more times. Longitudinal survey data are useful for studying changes in demographic behaviour and the effects of past experience on later behaviour. Prospective surveys enjoy certain advantages over the retrospective surveys: the reporting of the events of interest does not depend on memory over a long period; they allow the study of change, permit the calculation of incidence rates, and allow the observation of many outcomes. Prospective surveys also have some disadvantages. For example, they are costly; attrition and loss of subjects occur; and criteria and methods for data collection can change over time.

Several longitudinal surveys conducted in the United States for other purposes have contained sufficient information about family formation and childbearing that they have been extensively used for investigating the determinants and consequences of fertility. They include the National Longitudinal Survey of Young Women (NLSYW) and the National Longitudinal Survey of Youth (NLSY). Both surveys' primary purpose was to study entry into the labour force. The young men and women in these surveys have been interviewed annually or biennially since 1968 (NLSYW) or 1979 (NLSY). The Panel Study of Income Dynamics (PSID) has followed members of two samples of United States households with annual interviews since 1968.

To investigate factors related to poor pregnancy outcome, the National Maternal and Infant Health Survey (NMHIS) used vital registration information to obtain a national sample of women who had live births, late fetal deaths, or infant deaths in 1988. Questionnaire data supplied by the mothers were linked to the vital registration information; data were also obtained from prenatal care providers and hospitals of delivery. To study the development and care of the children born in the sample, the Longitudinal Follow-up in 1991 surveyed the mothers who had delivered live births, their paediatric care providers and hospitals named by the mothers as the ones that had provided care to the children (Sanderson *et al.* 1991).

Another way of obtaining longitudinal data is to match cross-sectional survey data with vital registration data. For example, the National Longitudinal Mortality Study (NLMS) included people surveyed in the Current Population Surveys in the United States from 1973 to 1985 (and also a sample of people from the 1980 United States Census). The survey data of these participants were matched with data from death certificates from 1979 to 1986 for any who died during that period (Rogot *et al.* 1992). Researchers use these data for detailed analysis of factors associated with mortality and causes of death.

A reverse example is the series of National Mortality Followback Surveys (NMFS) of 1961, 1964 to 1965, 1966 to 1968, 1986, and 1993 (Seeman *et al.* 1993). For a sample of death certificates, relatives or other informants are surveyed to obtain information about the decedents' characteristics and behaviours while alive, and a variety of other information (including health care and medical facilities), the nature of which varied by year. The data from these surveys provide valuable information about mortality determinants and trends that death certificate data alone could not.

Longitudinal survey data can also be linked with other types of data. For example, the data from the 1983, 1984, and 1989 National Long-Term Care Surveys (NLTCS) were linked to data from respondents' claims submitted to Medicare (the United States health insurance system for the elderly). Investigators use these data for studying changes in the elderly's health and use of services.

Demographers recognize that survey and vital registration data have had limited success in explaining variation in many population phenomena and in elucidating the mechanisms through which factors captured in such data work their influence on population processes (for example the basis for persistent differences among racial and ethnic groups in levels of adolescent pregnancy, low birthweight and infant mortality). Thus demographers have recently turned to more qualitative methods of data collection. These include focus groups, in which a small purposive sample of people is gathered for discussions of defined topics, and ethnographic approaches. Such methods allow for gathering information that is more diverse, that may be more culturally appropriate, and that may be motivated by the subjects' suggestions or behaviours (rather than information that is specified beforehand, as in the quantitative methods of data collection). Such data can be used to elaborate on results obtained from more quantitative methods, especially the mechanisms behind relationships, or to suggest preliminary hypotheses to guide the collection of quantitative data suitable for testing these hypotheses.

Examples include the use of home-based observational methods to investigate the effect of mothers' age on the quality of parenting (Chase-Lansdale *et al.* 1994), ethnographic studies of patterns of care in families with pregnant adolescents (Burton 1993), and small-scale anthropological investigations to explore fertility behaviour and fertility control (Caldwell *et al.* 1994).

The various types of data described above have been used to varying degrees to study population processes. We turn below to discussing these processes and selected topics in demography.

Demographic processes

The size of a population is determined by the three basic processes: mortality, fertility, and migration. (See Volume I, Chapter 5 for another discussion of these processes.) That is, the number of people in a geographic unit at a given time is equal to the number of people there at an earlier time, plus the following changes that occur between the two times: the number of births minus the number of deaths, plus in-migrants and minus out-migrants. Growth in population occurs when the number of births and in-migrants exceeds the number of deaths and out-migrants. For example, it was estimated that the black population in the United States numbered 31.4 million at the beginning of 1992, and grew by 536 000 in that year. The increase resulted from 693 000 births, minus 263 000 deaths, plus 107 000 resulting from net migration (United States Bureau of the Census 1994, Table No. 19).

These three processes determine not only the size but also the structure of populations. The most basic dimension of population structure is its age composition. This is determined by past fertility and mortality rates, as well as by migration. Contrary to intuition, fertility and not mortality is the dominant factor in determining age structure. Populations which have recently experienced high birth rates will be young (relatively large proportions of the people are

young), whereas populations which have experienced low fertility will be old (relatively small proportions of the population are young). Demographers often study population structure in terms of the composition of the population by sex, race or ethnicity, marital status, education, and occupation – characteristics selected because they typically do not change. The population composition with respect to these factors is determined by differential rates of the three demographic processes among the subgroups of concern.

In recent decades, the age and sex structure of the United States population has undergone large changes. People age 65 and over comprised 9.8 per cent of the population in 1970. They increased to 11.3 per cent in 1980, and 12.5 per cent in 1990, and are projected to reach nearly 13 per cent of the population by the year 2000. In this age group, there has been a large and increasing deficit of males. The sex ratio (ratio of males to females, multiplied by 100) was 72.1 in 1970; it decreased to 67.6 in 1980 and 67.2 in 1990. It had been 82.8 in 1960 and 89.6 in 1950 (United States Bureau of the Census 1993). The increasing male deficit reflects the growing numbers of women who survive to older ages without a spouse. In 1990, among women age 65 or older, nearly half were widowed at the time of the census, and 42 per cent were living alone. These figures stand in sharp contrast to men in this age group; only 14 per cent of them were widowed and only 16 per cent lived alone. Since married people (especially men) enjoy better health and longevity compared with divorced, widowed, and never-married people, and older people suffer higher rates of chronic diseases and disabling conditions, these changes in the population structure have significant public health implications. In particular, they point out the differential needs of older females in the United States.

The above discussion focused on the effects of population processes on composition. In turn, the composition of the population affects population growth and change. For example, when the age structure is old – when the proportion of the population in the older ages is relatively large – then the number of deaths in the population will be relatively large, because of the higher death rates of the elderly.

The population composition is important to public health because the risk of various illnesses and conditions, as well as the incidence of health risk behaviours (such as smoking, alcohol consumption, reckless driving, unprotected sexual intercourse) vary among different population subgroups. For purposes of planning public health programmes and allocating resources, it is necessary to know the numbers of people in the various risk groups and their geographic distribution. For example, the age–sex composition of the population identifies the size of the young and old populations, and the number of women of childbearing age – each of which is susceptible to different health risks and to whom special programmes or public media campaigns are often targetted. Demographers' studies of the three demographic processes and population composition can provide knowledge of the size of the risk groups, the prevalence and incidence of various conditions, and also an understanding of the anticipated changes in these.

Mortality

As a major component of population change, mortality is an integral part of demography. The level of mortality in a region or of a subpopulation (for example among infants) is also used as a

Table 25.1 Measures of mortality

Term	Definition
Crude death rate	Number of deaths per 1000 people in a population in a given year
Specific death rate	A specific death rate measures the number of deaths among people in a category per 1000 people in that category in a given year
Age-specific death rate	Death rate specific to a given age group
Standardized rates	Overall rates adjusted for the effects of differences in population composition (such as in age, sex)
Infant mortality rate	The number of deaths among infants under one year of age per 1000 live births. (Conventionally births and deaths are measured in the same year). For a cohort based measure, the rate includes the death under one year per 1000 live births
Neonatal mortality rate	Number of deaths of infants under 1 month of age per 1000 live births
Post-neonatal mortality rate	Number of infant deaths between 1 and 11 months of age per 1000 live births
Perinatal mortality ratio	Number of deaths of infants under one week of age plus late fetal deaths per 1000 live births
Life table survival rate	Proportion of a cohort in a life table surviving to a specified age
Life expectancy	The average number of years of life remaining for people who attain a given age. At age zero life expectancy is referred as life expectancy at birth
Life table death rate	Reciprocal of life expectancy at birth. This measure, based on the stationary population model, is an age-standardized measure
Cause-specific death rate	Number of deaths from a given cause occurring during a year per 100 000 people in a population
Cause-specific death ratio	Percentage of all deaths resulting from a particular cause in a given year
Maternal mortality rate	Number of deaths resulting from complications of pregnancy, labour and puerperium per 100 000 live births in a given year

basic public health indicator. This overlap of interest between the two fields of demography and public health should result in major contributions to the understanding and management of human mortality.

Rates and ratios of mortality and pregnancy wastage

Mortality is measured by a variety of death rates, several of which are defined in Table 25.1. There are two basic types of rates: the crude rate, and the death rate specific for a subgroup. The crude death rate (CDR) is the number of deaths per 1000 population. Demographers most commonly estimate death rates specific for various age groups, though they also find rates specific for sex, race, and other groups to be useful. Generally, age-specific death rates (ASDRs) follow a J-shaped pattern: High death rates in infancy and early childhood, declining to a low point by childhood (age 10 in the United States), and climbing with age thereafter.

In the United States, the CDR was estimated to be 8.8 per 1000 population in 1980, and 8.6 in 1990, representing a slight decline. In contrast, the CDR for white females was 7.9 per 1000 females in 1980 and 8.2 per 1000 females in 1989, representing a slight increase (NCHS, 1993a). However, as the CDR is an unreliable measure for detecting or understanding mortality change, this increase does not necessarily mean that female mortality rose. The CDR is the weighted average of the age-specific rates, the weights being the proportions of the population in each age group. In 1989, a larger proportion of the white female population was in the older age classes than in 1980, and these older age groups had higher death rates. This resulted in an increase in the CDR in 1989.

Thus, to detect change, it is necessary to examine changes in ASDRs. For example, the ASDR for white females in 1989 was lower in every age group than in 1980 – the opposite of the direction of change in the CDR. (This phenomenon is known as Simpson's paradox, see Simpson 1951.)

For comparing mortality over time (or across populations), one can also summarize ASDRs into a single measure that adjusts for differences in the age structure – a process called standardization. For example, one could use the age distribution of the population in 1940 as a 'standard population' and apply these age proportions as weights to the 1980 and 1989 ASDRs of white females. Summing these products yields an age-standardized rate.

This standardization yields an adjusted rate of 4.3 for 1980 and 4.0 for 1989. Unlike the crude rates, these standardized rates show the decline in female mortality that occurred during the period.

There are several methods for standardizing crude rates. Among the most commonly used are 'direct standardization' (described above) and 'indirect standardization'. (For details of basic standardization techniques, see Shryock and Siegel 1973.)

Partly because death rates among infants are a particularly sensitive indicator of the health standing of populations, several rates of mortality for infants are commonly studied. As seen in Table 25.1, the infant mortality rate measures death during the first year of life; the neonatal mortality rate, death during the first 28 days; and the postneonatal mortality rate, death during the remainder of the first year. The distinction between the latter two measures is made because neonatal deaths are often caused by congenital or genetic conditions or by complications of childbirth, whereas postneonatal deaths are often attributable to social or environmental factors. The age at infant death is used in these two measures only as an approximate indicator of probable types of causes of death. These two rates are especially useful where data on actual causes of death are not available.

Infant mortality in the United States decreased from 12.6 per 1000 live births in 1980 to 8.9 in 1991. Perpetuating a large gap between the races, the rate of decline was greater for the white population than for the black population. In 1980, the infant mortality rate stood at 21.4 for black and 11.0 for white babies. In 1991, the rate had changed to 17.6 for black and 7.3 for white babies. The neonatal component of the infant mortality rate showed a similar racial discrepancy and differential decline. The neonatal mortality rate for the United States was 8.5 in 1980 and 5.6 in 1991. The corresponding figures for black babies were 14.1 and 11.2, and for white, 7.5 and 4.5 (United States Bureau of the Census 1994, Table No. 120).

Between 1980 and 1991, the percentage of live-born infants weighing less than 2 500 g (babies of low birthweight) increased from 6.8 per cent to 7.1 per cent. For black newborns, however, the percentage remained steady, at the high level of 13.6 per cent. Although the overall infant mortality for black babies is higher than that of white, the death rate among low birthweight babies is lower for black than white (NCHS 1994, Fig. 2).

Despite improvements in the infant mortality rate in the United States, the rate of 8.3 in 1993 was higher than 21 other countries (Wegman 1994).

In addition to measures of infant deaths, pregnancy wastage is also captured in demographic measures. For example, the fetal death ratio is the ratio of the number of spontaneous abortions of fetuses reaching a gestational age of 20 weeks or more per 1000 live births. In 1990, this rate was 7.5 per 1000 live births in the United States. The black population had a higher rate, 11.7.

The rate of pregnancy wastage resulting from induced abortions is usually measured by the abortion ratio, the number of induced abortions per 1000 live births. In the United States this ratio declined from 428 per 1000 live births in 1980 to 379 in 1992 (United States Bureau of the Census 1994, Table No. 113).

An additional measure of pregnancy wastage is the perinatal mortality ratio – the number of deaths of infants under one week of age plus the number of late fetal deaths (usually gestations of 28 weeks or more) per 1000 live births. In the United States, the perinatal mortality ratio was 13.2 in 1980 and 9.6 in 1989. For the black population, however, the corresponding figures were 20.7 and 16.2 (NCHS 1993a).

Life tables

Demographers use life tables to study longevity – the length of time lived before dying – as well as other types of duration data, such as the length of birth intervals, contraceptive use, and durations of marriage or divorce. Life tables have a long history, as discussed in Volume I (Chapter 5). Life tables can be constructed using either duration-specific incidence rates (such as age-specific death rates to construct a life table of mortality) or data on time of occurrence of an event measured from the time the subject is exposed to the risk of experiencing the event (for example the time from women's first birth to their second birth to construct a life table of the length of the second birth interval). (Details of life table construction are found in Namboodiri and Suchindran 1987.)

Several types of life tables are commonly used. An ordinary life table describes attrition from a cohort (such as people born in the same period) resulting from a single factor (such as death). A multiple-decrement life table describes attrition from a cohort because of more than one factor, for example, from various causes of death. A multistate life table allows a cohort to move through different states that could be transient or absorbing (an absorbing state is defined to be one from which an individual cannot move into any other state). In a multistate life table, for example, one can define transient states to be being never-married, married, separated, and divorced, and absorbing states to be death or various causes of death. The distinction between the multiple-decrement and multistate life table is that the multistate life table allows transitions back and forth among the transient states before moving to absorbing states (for example an individual can marry, divorce, return to the married state before dying). In contrast, multiple-decrement life tables allow individuals to move only into absorbing states (for example, in a multiple-decrement life table of disruption of a first marriage, one could define divorce and widowhood as absorbing states). The multiple-decrement life table is a special subset of the multistate life table.

Life table measures of mortality

A life table of mortality is a statistical model for combining age-specific mortality rates. The life table converts ASDRs into measures of longevity, which are easier to interpret. Another advantage of the life table is that it provides measures of mortality independent of the age distribution of the population, and thus avoids the use of standard populations. In addition, the survival rates obtained from a life table can be used to make estimates of a population at a future date.

For an ordinary life table, one uses age-specific death rates to compute the average duration of life remaining at each age, or the expectation of life at birth or at any other specified age. One also commonly computes the survival probabilities (probabilities that a new born baby survives to specific ages). The reciprocal of the life expectancy at birth is the life table death rate. This is an age-standardized mortality rate, and thus can be used for comparing mortality of different populations. (Table 25.1 gives definitions.)

Another measure based on life tables is years of potential life lost, the total number of years a person would have lived based on the life expectancy at the age of death and the number dying at each age in a given calendar year. In 1991, males in the United States lost 18.4 million years (or 16 years per death), and females lost 15.3 million years (or 15 years per death) (United States Bureau of the Census 1994, Table No. 138).

In the United States, the average expectation of life for a baby born in 1991 reached a record high of 75.5 years. Between 1985 and 1991, the difference in life expectancy between the white and black populations widened, from 6.0 to 7.0 years, and the difference between the two sexes narrowed, from 7.4 to 6.9 years. Between 1985 and 1991, life expectancy for white males increased by 1.1 years, to 72.9 years, but for black males, it decreased by 0.4 years, to 64.6 years. For white females, it rose by 0.9 years, to 79.6; for black females, it increased by 0.5 years, to 73.8 years. These figures illustrate the longer longevity of black females than white males, which has occurred since 1970.

The probability of survival from birth to age 40 in 1991 was 0.946 for white and 0.878 for black individuals (United States Bureau of the Census 1994, Tables No. 114, 115). The lower probability for black individuals reflects the higher mortality among this race during infancy, childhood and early adulthood. These differences at the younger ages largely explain the discrepancy in the life expectancy at birth between the two races.

Causes of death

Demographers study death rates as a result of different causes of death, or cause-specific mortality rates, so as to understand the process of mortality. These rates by cause for specific subgroups are often used as indicators of the prevailing risks of death from specific causes in various subgroups of the population. These rates can be used to target major causes of death, and to direct public health efforts at specific groups at high risk of these conditions. Historical variations in causes of death, and in methods of assignment, are discussed in Volume I (Chapter 5).

A cause-specific mortality rate represents the number of deaths resulting from a specific cause per 100 000 population. These rates are often computed for specific subgroups such as those formed by age, sex and race. These rates can be used for comparing for the same population the risk of deaths from specific causes over time, or across populations at one time.

The leading cause of death (the one with the highest cause-specific rate over the entire population) in the United States is heart disease, but the rate of death from this cause is declining. For example, the age-adjusted heart disease mortality decreased among white males from 277.5 per 100 000 in 1980 to 196.1 in 1991. In 1991, heart disease mortality was almost twice as great for white men as for white women. Black men, however, experienced nearly 40 per cent greater mortality from heart disease than did white men.

The rate of death from the second leading cause, cancer, rose during this period. The death rate from strokes, the third leading cause, declined from 1980 to 1991. Between 1987 and 1991, HIV infection climbed from the 15th to the 9th leading cause of death in the United States. The age-adjusted rate more than doubled, from 5.5 per 100 000 to 11.3. Among persons of 25 to 44 years of age, AIDS was the third leading cause of death; but for black males in that age group, it was the leading cause of death (NCHS 1994).

Dying from complications of pregnancy, labour, and the puerperium (period immediately following childbirth) is a cause of death that carries historical and continuing importance. The maternal mortality rate – the number of women dying from these conditions per 100 000 live births – has declined considerably. In the United States, it was estimated to be 9.2 in 1980, and 7.9 in both 1989 and 1990. Black women experienced a higher maternal mortality rate – 21.5 in 1980, 17.5 in 1989, and 18.3 in 1990 (NCHS 1993a).

Another cause-specific mortality measure is the cause-specific death ratio. This is the percentage of all deaths resulting from a specific cause. The cause-specific death ratio can be used as a gauge of the relative importance of a particular cause of death. For example, in the United States in 1991, for people of ages 55 to 64, deaths resulting from diseases of the heart comprised 30.2 per cent

of all deaths, while neoplasms contributed 38.0 per cent (NCHS 1993c, Table No. 5).

The advantage of the cause-specific ratio over the cause-specific rate is that the former does not include the number of people in the population at risk of death, but uses only data about deaths. Therefore, the cause-specific ratio is often used to compare the relative importance of causes of death across countries and subgroups for whom population estimates are not available. The disadvantage of the ratio is that it does not measure the level of occurrence of a particular cause of death. For two groups for whom a specific cause contributes the same or even the largest percentage of deaths, the rate of deaths from that cause may differ widely. Therefore, to select causes of death in specific subgroups to be targetted by public health efforts, it is necessary to examine both the importance of that cause (cause-specific ratio) and its rate or incidence.

An example of the difference between cause-specific ratios and rates is found in comparing the United States population aged 55 to 64 with that aged 65 to 74 in 1991. The share of deaths resulting from neoplasms for the younger group (given above) was 38.0 per cent, and for the older group, 33.3 per cent; thus the share of deaths from this cause is lower for the older group. However, the cause-specific death rates are much higher for the older group. The death rate caused by neoplasms among the 65- to 74-year-olds was 871.6 per 100 000, whereas it was 448.4 per 100 000 for the 55- to 64-year-olds (NCHS 1993c, Table No. 5).

Demographers also construct multiple decrement life tables by causes of death. Such a life table summarizes age- and cause-specific mortality rates. These life tables provide a number of summary measures, including the probability that a person will eventually die from a particular cause. In addition, one can examine the age distribution of deaths for various causes in the multiple decrement life tables to study the age pattern of deaths resulting from specific causes.

Multiple decrement life tables for the United States show that the probability of eventually dying from cardiovascular diseases declined from 0.6065 in 1960 to 0.5514 in 1970, and 0.4831 in 1985. The eventual probabilities of dying from neoplasms increased from 0.1502 in 1960 to 0.1697 in 1970, and 0.2218 in 1985 (Namboodiri and Suchindran 1987; Namboodiri 1991). In the United States, the age pattern of deaths in the multiple decrement life tables for cardiovascular disease and neoplasms usually shows a unimodal curve with the mode occurring at late ages. In contrast, the age pattern of deaths caused by accidents usually displays more than one mode, indicating higher probabilities of deaths from this cause during childhood, early adult years, and old age.

Cause-elimination life tables

To examine changes through time in the risk of death from a specific cause, or to investigate such differences across subgroups, one needs to take into account the interdependence of risks. That is, to face the risk of dying from one cause, one must first avoid dying from another cause. For example, as death from heart disease decreases, the population lives more years to be subject to the risk of other causes, such as cancer. To what extent has the rate of deaths from cancer increased because people of given age groups have experienced increased susceptibility to this cause of death, and to what extent has the rate risen because people who would have formerly died of heart disease are now surviving to encounter the risk of cancer?

To eliminate the effects of competing risks of dying from various causes on the risk of dying from a given cause, so as to measure the 'pure' severity of this cause, demographers construct cause-elimination life tables. For example, one can construct a life table eliminating all deaths from heart disease to compute expectation of life at various ages, in the hypothetical situation in which this cause of death has been completely eradicated. One can also construct life tables that only partially eliminate a given cause (or causes) of death (for example a reduction of heart disease deaths by 25 per cent in certain age groups, 50 per cent in other age groups). Demographers also construct life tables in which all causes are eliminated except one particular cause. This is a useful tool for comparing the mortality of population subgroups, or of the same group through time, because such life tables adjust for the impact of differential risks of dying from other causes that operate in the various subgroups or at different times.

One summary measure from cause-elimination life tables is the expectation of life to be gained from eradicating a particular cause of death. In the United States, it is estimated that eliminating cardiovascular disease, cancer, or motor vehicular accidents in 1970 would result in an addition of expectation of life at birth of 12.36, 2.02, and 0.70 years, respectively (Tsai *et al.* 1978).

Determinants of mortality

Beyond studying rates of death (by cause or all causes together) among population subgroups and trends over time, demographers also investigate factors influencing the likelihood of death. This includes studying the determinants of behaviours that either decrease or increase the risk of mortality.

Research on the effects of factors that affect the likelihood of dying and dying from various causes has investigated demographic and socio-economic variables (such as age, sex, marital status, family size, income, and education), health-related behaviours (such as smoking, alcohol and drug use), and various types of disabilities and diseases (Rogers 1993).

In investigating child mortality in less economically developed countries, research has examined the proximate determinants through which social, cultural, economic, and other factors influence the chances of death. These proximate determinants include maternal factors (such as age, parity and previous spacing of births), environmental conditions, nutritional adequacy, injury, and the treatment of personal illness (Mosley and Chen 1984).

In the United States, recent research has focused on the determinants of infant mortality, and has sought explanations for the racial disparity in infant death rates. This research similarly incorporates a wide range of both biological, social, and behavioural factors (Cramer 1986; Samuels 1986; Rogers 1989; Eberstein *et al.* 1990; Mangold and Powell-Griner 1991; Hummer *et al.* 1992). Part of this research investigates the factors influencing the receipt of prenatal care, which is one health behaviour that influences the health of the fetus and newborn. Much of the research examines determinants of low birthweight, a primary precursor of infant mortality. Public health programmes addressing low birthweight and infant mortality often have as a central objective in encouraging women to obtain prenatal care early in their pregnancy and with regularity.

Fertility

The second major component of population change is fertility, by which demographers mean the frequency of live births in a population. The processes involved in fertility (for example conception, contraception, successful gestation and parturition, and postpartum amenorrhoea) depend to some degree upon the health of the population. Conversely, various aspects of fertility – such as the number of births, the spacing between them, and the age of the mother – influence the health of the population. Thus, demographers' study of fertility yields a variety of information and implications of interest to the public health field.

Measures of fertility

For demographers, the event defining fertility is a live birth (and not conception). They call the physiological capacity of a man, woman, or couple to reproduce fecundity. They define as a woman's fecundability the probability that a non-contracepting, susceptible (not pregnant and not temporarily or permanently sterile) woman will conceive during a menstrual cycle (or during a month). Not all conceptions can be observed and, therefore, most often studies can only estimate the probability that a susceptible woman will have a conception that results in a live birth. This probability is known as the effective fecundability. All these topics of study by demographers are centrally related to women's health, especially reproductive health.

Demographers usually measure the level of fertility in a fixed, cross-sectional time period by period fertility rates, including crude birth rates (CBR) and rates specific for subpopulations. They often compute age-specific fertility rates and rates specific for both age and parity (the number of births a woman has already had), or age- and parity-specific fertility rates. These usually are defined as the number of births occurring to women in the specific age or age-and-parity group per 1000 women in that group. (See Table 25.2 for definitions of various fertility measures.)

In the United States, between 1980 and 1991, the CBR rose slightly, from 15.9 to 16.3 per 1000 population. In 1991, the CBR for the black population was 21.9. As with crude death rates, the CBR should not be used to detect change over time or differences between subgroups. For these purposes, differences in age and sex composition need to be eliminated by standardizing the age-specific birth rates on some population distribution. For example, the CBR in 1989 was 15.0 for the white, and 23.1 for the black population. The age-adjusted fertility rate, however, for the white population was 16.0, and for the black, 22.1. Thus the crude rates overstate the racial difference (NCHS 1993*b*, Tables 1–1 and 1–4).

By examining age-specific birth rates, we see that in recent years in the United States, fertility has risen among both the youngest and oldest women of childbearing age. The age-specific birth rate for female adolescents between 15 and 17 years of age increased from 32.5 per 1000 female teenagers in that age group in 1980 to 38.7 in 1991. The rate for older adolescents also rose, but not as steeply: the age-specific birth rate for women aged 18 to 19 climbed from 85.0 in 1980 to 94.4 in 1991. At the other end of the age spectrum, the birth rate for women aged 35 to 39 jumped from 19.8 in 1980 to 32.0 in 1991. During this period, the birth rate of fourth and higher order births to women aged 15 to 44 also increased, from 6.3 in 1980 to 7.5 in 1991. These increases in the fertility of

Table 25.2 Measures of fertility

Term	Definition
Fertility	Frequency with which live birth occurs in a population
Fecundity	Biological capacity of a man, a woman or a couple to reproduce
Fecundability	Probability that a susceptible woman will conceive in a month (or during a menstrual cycle)
Crude birth rate	Number of births per 1000 population in a given year
General fertility rate	Number of live births per 1000 women age 15 to 49 (or 15 to 44) in a given year
Specific fertility rate	Number of live births per 1000 women in a specified subgroup of population
Age-specific fertility rate	Fertility rate specific to given age groups
Total fertility rate	Average number of children (of either sex) that would be born alive to a group of women during their lifetimes if they passed through their childbearing years conforming to the age-specific fertility rates of a given year
Gross reproduction rate	Average number of daughters that would be born to a group of women during their lifetimes if they passed through their childbearing years conforming to the age-specific fertility rates of a given year
Net reproduction rate	Average number of daughters that would be born to a group of women during their lifetimes if they passed through their childbearing years conforming to the age-specific fertility rates and age-specific mortality rates of a given year
Age-parity specific birth rate	Number of births of a given parity (birth order) to 1000 women of specified age groups in a given year
Parity progression ratio	Proportion of women with a specific parity who will eventually attain the next higher parity in their lifetime
Mean age at birth of specific order	Average age at which live births of a specified order occur to a group of women who have births of that order
Mean birth interval	Average time (usually measured in months or years) elapsed between two consecutive births

the youngest and oldest women and at higher parity present a potential public health problem because of the greater health risks for both mother and child.

To avoid the limitations of the crude birth rates, demographers often compute the total fertility rate (TFR). The TFR is a summary fertility measure obtained by adding the age-specific fertility rates prevailing in a given period for each of the age groups of women in the childbearing ages (usually 15 to 44 or 15 to 49) in the population. The TFR represents the total number of births (completed family size) a woman would have in her lifetime if, at each year of age, she experienced the age-specific birth rates measured in a given year. A TFR of 2.1 is usually regarded as the 'replacement level' fertility for the total population under current mortality conditions; that is, 2.1 is the average number of children women need to have to replace themselves and their partners. The TFR in the United States increased from 1.84 in 1980 to 2.01 in 1989.

The TFR includes births of both sexes. To obtain a more precise measure of replacement fertility, demographers modify the TFR to count only female births. This measure, the gross reproduction rate, measures the number of daughters a woman would have in her lifetime if she experienced the age-specific female birth rates used in the calculation. The net reproduction rate represents a further refinement that takes into account the mortality of mothers. For example, the gross reproduction rate in 1989 was 0.983. The net reproduction rate was 0.964 in that year (NCHS 1993b). Both measures indicated that the fertility of American women was below replacement level.

Birth rates are sometimes calculated specific to married women, but for populations in which a significant number of births occur outside of wedlock, as in the United States, these rates are not as useful.

The birth rates discussed above are based on the age-specific rates prevailing in a given time period, and thus are period measures. Period measures of fertility describe the level of childbearing prevailing during the current period (or past periods of interest) and are useful for determining the level of need for public health services addressed to issues of reproductive and maternal health.

Period measures, however, are of limited usefulness for understanding the dynamics of fertility and the effects of changes in social and health conditions on childbearing patterns. Fertility is made up of two components: the timing of births and the quantity of births. Timing encompasses the age when women begin childbearing, their spacing of births once they have begun, and the age when they finish reproduction. Quantity includes the number of births women have, the proportion of women never having a birth and the proportions having successively higher order births (first, second, etc.). During a given period, women may respond to changing social, economic, or health conditions by altering either their timing or quantity of childbearing, or both. Women are at different stages of their life (or different ages) when a particular condition occurs (during a specific period) and, consequently, their fertility responses or dynamics may vary according to their age. Therefore, period measures (which essentially sum up fertility measures across various age groups) usually are not appropriate for examining the lifetime impact of social change nor for investigating changing fertility patterns.

For these purposes, demographers often employ measures of fertility for cohorts of women, or cohort fertility measures, rather than period measures. A cohort measure of fertility uses the age-specific birth rates actually experienced by a group of women born in a given calendar period (a 'birth cohort'). Such a cohort measure of the level of fertility is the cohort total fertility rate, which is analogous to the period TFR. The parity progression ratio (PPR) also measures the quantity of fertility. For women who have had a birth of a given order (zero, first, second, etc.), the PPR is the probability of ever having a birth of the next order.

For example, in the United States, women born in 1910, who entered the prime child-bearing ages during the Great Depression, had a cohort TFR of 2.2 among white and 2.6 among non-white women (Evans 1986). Even though this cohort bore children during the Great Depression, when fertility was greatly lowered, their TFR was nevertheless above replacement level. This fertility level was achieved despite a large proportion of the cohort remaining childless because those who bore children had a high level of fertility. Thus, 79.4 per cent of white women and 70.5 per cent of non-white women in this cohort had a first birth (that is were not childless). The PPR from the first to second birth was 73.1 per cent for white women and 63.7 per cent for non-white women. Although non-white women had lower PPRs for the first and second births, their PPRs for all subsequent orders of birth were higher than for white women (Suchindran and Koo 1992). It is known that because of poorer health conditions and the prevalence of sexually trans-mitted diseases (STDs) among non-white women, a relatively large proportion of this and other non-white cohorts failed to conceive. The higher fertility of the non-white women was the result of the larger number of children borne by the smaller but more fertile subgroup.

Measures of timing of fertility include mean ages at first, subsequent, and final births, and the length of birth intervals between successive births. The mean ages at first and final births for white women in the 1910 cohort were estimated to be 23.9 and 31.8. The average birth interval, or number of years elapsing between the first and second births, for the 1910 white cohort was 4.6 years, and between the second and third births, 4.5 years. (These means are computed only for women who had the higher order birth.)

Changes in age at first birth have public health implications. A low mean age at first birth (or a large proportion beginning childbearing while very young) means that public health resources need to be dedicated to promoting early and regular prenatal care among the young women. The infants of such young mothers are also at higher risk of low birthweight and other health problems. At the other end of the age spectrum, a relatively old age at final birth means that relatively large proportions of older women face the higher risks of poorer outcomes for both mother and child.

Short birth intervals also produce public health consequences. Infants born soon after a previous birth are in greater danger of morbidity and mortality; mothers of these infants may suffer maternal depletion, leading to higher risks of maternal morbidity and mortality.

Determinants of fertility

In investigating the determinants of fertility and its components of timing and quantity, demographers often focus on the 'proximate determinants'. These include three classes of variables: factors affecting (1) exposure to sexual intercourse; (2) exposure to conception; and (3) gestation and successful parturition. The intercourse variables involve those governing the formation and dissolution of sexual unions that occur during childbearing ages, such as age at entry into sexual unions, proportions ever marrying, and marital dissolution. They also include factors governing exposure to intercourse such as voluntary abstinence, involuntary abstinence (from illness, temporary separations as a result of migration, etc.), and coital frequency. The variables affecting conception include ages at menarche and menopause, fecundity, permanent and temporary sterility (including post-partum amenorrhoea), breastfeeding and use of contraception. Finally, the variables concerned with gestation and successful delivery include both spontaneous and induced abortions, and stillbirths. (See Davis and Blake 1956, and Bongaarts 1978, for discussions of this framework.)

To understand the nature of trends and variations in fertility across time or populations, it is crucial for demographers to measure each of the proximate variables as accurately as possible and to dissect the effects of each of the proximate determinants on fertility. In studying fertility, demographers also investigate the determinants of each of these proximate determinants, including social, economic, cultural, and biological factors.

Thus, demographers devote substantial attention to phenomena that are both biological and behavioural in their research on fertility. They collect information on these variables, model them, and publish the results of this research primarily in demographic journals. Many of these variables are directly public health concerns or have implications for public health; yet public health professionals may be unaware of this body of work.

Examples of proximate determinants that are also public health concerns are fecundability and sterility. A lively debate can be found in the demographic literature about whether the fecundability of women declines with age (after age 30) (Schwartz and Mayaux 1982). The answer to this debate would affect public health education regarding planning pregnancies in older ages. Furthermore, smoking has been found to decrease fecundability (Weinberg and Gladen 1986). Sexually transmitted diseases, infections, and age can produce secondary sterility.

Breastfeeding (lactation) causes hormonal changes that delay the resumption of menses and ovulation, and therefore is a determinant of fecundability. Thus, demographers' interest in breastfeeding has centred on its effect on fertility, especially on the demographic impact of changing breastfeeding patterns across the world (Knodel and Debavalya 1981). Research has also focused on the effects of breastfeeding on infant survival (DaVanzo et al. 1983). Besides the direct implications for public health, what demographers have learned about breastfeeding practices can be useful to public health professionals who are concerned with the nutritional status of infants and mothers (Popkin et al. 1993).

Contraception

The practice of birth control is one of the proximate determinants of fertility and, therefore, a great deal of demographic effort has been directed to measuring contraceptive use (see United Nations 1991) and studying its determinants and consequences, including its demographic impact. The provision of family planning and abortion services improves maternal and infant health by helping women to have children when they want them, and to space them at intervals long enough to avoid depleting the mother's physical and emotional resources. Also, mothers of unwanted pregnancies are often less likely to take good care of themselves and their babies during pregnancy and afterwards (see Klerman and Klerman 1994). Accurate information about contraceptive use and failure that demographers collect and study may help public health professionals in designing and evaluating family planning programmes.

A basic measure describing contraceptive use is the contraceptive failure rate. The rate at which various contraceptives fail to prevent pregnancy, especially among women of different ages and socio-economic classes, is important for individuals to know in choosing a contraceptive, and for public health staff to understand in designing family planning programmes aimed at different subpopulations. In economically advanced countries, where fertility has been low and use of contraceptives high, contraceptive failure is also an important determinant of the level of fertility and of differentials in fertility among subgroups. In less economically prosperous nations, differentials in the desired family size and in the use of contraception are also important determinants.

Contraceptive failure can be defined as the occurrence of an unintended pregnancy while a contraceptive is being used. A narrow definition of method failure restricts failure to the occurrence of an unintended pregnancy while the contraceptive is always used and used correctly. A more practical measure defines use failure to occur under average conditions of actual contraceptive practice. Demographers usually employ life table methods to compute contraceptive use failure rates, defined as the number of unintended pregnancies occurring per person-month of exposure, during each successive month of use. These monthly rates yield a failure rate over a period of time of use (typically 12 months). Life table methods are needed to control for variability in the length of exposure observed for different groups.

One also uses multiple-decrement life tables to calculate rates of contraceptive discontinuation for reasons other than unintended pregnancies, for example discontinuation because of side-effects, medical contraindications, desire to become pregnant, etc. When these discontinuation rates are computed from multiple-decrement life tables (where each cause of discontinuation is treated as a decrement), the rate for one cause depends partly on the rates of discontinuation for other reasons. That is, discontinuation resulting from various reasons are competing risks. For example, the failure rate or rate of discontinuation because of unintended pregnancy tends to be lower when discontinuation for other reasons is high, since a woman who stops use for other reasons is no longer at risk of accidental pregnancy. Thus these rates of failure and discontinuation are not appropriate for comparing populations or subgroups with different rates resulting from various reasons. To adjust for the competing risks, one constructs associated life tables from the multiple-decrement life tables, eliminating competing causes. The rates thus obtained are called 'gross rates' in the demographic literature, but are labelled 'net rates' in the statistical literature.

Failure and discontinuation rates can be computed from retrospective or prospective survey data, or from clinical data. For example, based on the retrospective contraceptive and pregnancy histories obtained in the 1982 National Survey of Family Growth in the United States, the gross use-failure rates (as defined by demographers) for the first 12 months of use of oral contraceptives was 3.7 pregnancies per 100 woman years of exposure; for intrauterine devices, 7.1; for condoms, 10.6; for barrier methods and spermicides, 20.2; and for use of no methods, 43.1 (Grady *et al.* 1986).

Adolescent pregnancy

Although only a minor proportion of all child-bearing occurs at the youngest and oldest ages of the reproductive span (under 20 and over 35), in recent decades a great deal of attention has focused on fertility of women at the two extremes of reproductive age. Concern over the adverse consequences for health and socio-economic outcomes for adolescent mothers and their children has motivated the attention to early child-bearing (Peckam 1993). The possible demographic impact of increased fertility at the older ages, along with consequences for the older mothers and their infants, have fuelled interest in late childbearing.

Among the industrialized countries (excluding the Eastern European countries), the United States has the highest teenage pregnancy rate, much of it attributable to unintended pregnancies (Senderowitz and Paxman 1985; Forrest 1990). For example, in 1987, 35 per cent of pregnancies to teenagers ended in induced abortions, and another 37 per cent were births which were not intended at conception. In 1987, 64 per cent of adolescent births in the United States occurred to unmarried mothers and in 1992, 71 per cent. Among 15- to 19-year-olds, 71 per cent of pregnancies occurred to adolescents who were not using contraception when they became pregnant (Moore *et al.* 1995).

Teenage birth rates declined in the United States during the 1970s but increased again in the 1980s. The birth rate for 15- to 17-year-olds was 38.8 births per 1000 girls in 1970, 32.5 in 1980 and 38.7 in 1991. The birth rate for 18- to 19-year-olds was 114.7 in 1970, 82.1 in 1980, and 94.4 in 1991 (NCHS 1994, Fig. 1). While a substantial proportion of these births resulted from unintended conceptions, presumably nearly all induced abortions did. The legal abortion ratio for girls under 15 was 122.7 per 100 live births in 1980, and 76.1 in 1991. For women aged 15 to 19, the ratio was 66.4 in 1980 and 45.6 in 1991 (United States Bureau of the Census 1994, Table No. 113). In 1991, women under 20 accounted for 12.9 per cent of all live births in the United States (United States Bureau of the Census 1994, Table No. 92) and 25.6 per cent of all legal abortions (United States Bureau of the Census 1994, Table No. 110).

Since the 1970s, as rates of pregnancy and births to young women under the age of 20 rose in the United States, demographers and researchers from other disciplines have highlighted the adverse consequences experienced by both the parents and children when adolescents become parents. Deleterious effects for the mother that have been examined include curtailed educational attainment (Upchurch and McCarthy 1989; Upchurch 1992), economic disadvantage and inferior jobs (Geronimus and Korenman 1993*b*; Hoffman *et al.* 1993*a*, 1993*b*; Grogger and Bronars 1993; Moore *et al.* 1993), lower entry into marriage and higher marital instability (Bennett and Bloom 1993; Astone 1993), and higher subsequent fertility (especially out-of-wedlock births) (Hofferth 1987*a*). Other work has examined the higher rates of complications of pregnancy and delivery, and maternal mortality among adolescent mothers, and their relationship with the quality of prenatal care obtained by adolescents (Senderowitz and Paxman 1985). Researchers have also called attention to another health risk related to sexual activity – sexually transmitted diseases, and, more recently, HIV infection and AIDS (Strobino 1987; DiClemente 1992).

Similarly, investigators have examined the adverse effects for the health of infants born to adolescent mothers (Hofferth 1987*b*; Rosenzweig and Wolpin 1992; Geronimus and Korenman, 1993*a*). Others have studied the impact of adolescent child-bearing on child development (Morrison *et al.* 1992; Horwitz and Klerman 1992). Substantial numbers of adolescent mothers depend on government programmes for their economic support (Aid to Families with Dependent Children and Food Stamps) and health care (Medicaid), and, therefore, the public costs resulting from adolescent childbearing have been investigated (Burt 1986; Caldas 1993). Recently, however, researchers have debated the extent to which the adverse outcomes observed for adolescent mothers are consequences of the youthful childbearing versus the result of family background or other pre-existing conditions that lead to the poorer outcomes (Geronimus and Korenman 1993*b*; Hoffman *et al.* 1993*a*, 1993*b*).

At the same time that researchers investigated the consequences of adolescent pregnancy, a great deal of effort also addressed its determinants. Studies have been done at the aggregate level (for example Singh 1986), as well as at the individual level (Hofferth and Hayes 1987; Miller and Moore 1990). Some studies have combined both contextual factors along with individual ones (for example Qui and Hayward 1993). A large body of literature examines a variety of factors that lead to adolescent pregnancy and its proximate determinants, especially the initiation of sexual intercourse and the use of contraception (see reviews in Hayes 1987; Hofferth and Hayes 1987; Miller and Moore 1990; Santelli and Beilenson 1992). Factors include socio-economic and demographic variables (such as race, ethnicity, religion, educational attainment of teenagers' parents, income); psychological factors (self-esteem, locus of control, value placed on independence, perceptions of risks and benefits of sexual intercourse, contraception, and pregnancy, acceptability of induced abortion, etc.); family influence (such as parent–child communications, adolescents' mothers' early sexual intercourse or childbearing, parental control, parental attitudes); peer influence (attitudes and behaviours of peers); school performance (academic achievement and ability); media exposure (amount of television viewing); risk behaviours (drinking, drug use, smoking, etc.); and physiological influences (levels of male and female hormones, onset of menarche).

The research has only partially worked out the complex mechanisms or pathways through which the various factors exert their effects and, therefore, the relative importance of each factor for various subgroups is not clear. Nevertheless, this body of literature on determinants and consequences of adolescent pregnancy could be useful to public health officials in designing public health programmes both to prevent teenage pregnancies (and STDs) and to improve the care of adolescents before they conceive, during pregnancy, and after giving birth or having induced abortions.

Migration

The third process of population change is migration, or movement of people from one usual (or primary) residence to another that involves crossing an administrative or political boundary (such as a county or state line). Unlike mortality and fertility, migration is not a biologically based process and it is not limited by physiological constraints: people may never move in their lifetime, or may move many times. As a result of this, and because of ambiguities in the definition of 'usual residence' and differences in the definitions of administrative boundaries across countries and over time, migration is the most difficult of the three population processes to measure. (See also Volume I, Chapter 5.)

Migration contributes to the growth of a population if the number of persons migrating into an area exceeds the number migrating out of the area; it contributes to a reduction of a population if the out-migrants exceed the in-migrants. The movement of people can also be a primary factor in population redistribution among geographic subdivisions of a country (internal migration), or among nations (international migration). Furthermore, the characteristics of the people who choose to move into an area, such as retirees, working population with children, etc., affect the composition of the population, and thereby may influence the rate of natural increase of the population (that is, increase from the excess of births over deaths). For example, an area that attracts large numbers of young adults entering their prime reproductive years would consequently experience higher fertility rates.

Where significant migration occurs, the characteristics of the migrants may also have impacts on public health needs and therefore, on public health policy, programme planning, and facilities and staffing. For example, areas receiving large numbers of young children or of the elderly may need to adjust the mix of public health programmes and services to meet the in-migrants' needs. Migration from areas where contagious diseases such as tuberculosis are endemic into areas virtually free of these diseases would require additional efforts in public health surveillance and prevention. Large-scale migration may also produce major changes in the quality of the environment, by increasing pressures upon natural resources or contributing to pollution.

Internal migration (that which occurs within a country) is usually reported as a net migration rate – the balance between in-migration and out-migration during a given period (usually one year or five years, or the period between two censuses, called intercensal migration). This is a cross-sectional or period measure. Migration is also measured on a cohort basis. For example, the migration expectancy measures the average number of migration movements expected over the entire lifetime of members of a cohort. Based on life table estimates using 1982 to 1983 rates, it was estimated that Americans were expected to make 10 to 11 moves during their lifetime (Long 1988).

Changes in the economy, as well as other social forces, substantially affect the rate of migration and its direction, from places of origin to places of destination. Economic booms or favourable restructuring of jobs usually induce migration, as people move to areas or countries where there are more job opportunities or better wages. On the other hand, wars and political or religious persecution have impelled people to migrate from their countries to others as refugees or asylum seekers.

Compared with people who do not move, migrants tend to have particular personal, social, and economic characteristics. For example, the ages at which migration is most likely to take place are linked to the stage of life cycle. Migration rates are the highest during young adult ages, when children leave home to find jobs, marry, and set up their own households. People who have changed marital status are also likely to change residence. People who retire from employment similarly often move (Long 1988; Warnes 1992).

In the United States in 1992, nearly one-third of the 20 to 29 year old population moved in the previous year, but only 5 per cent of those 65 years old or older did so. The propensity to move in the United States also varies by region. Nearly one-quarter of the American population who lived in the West moved in the previous year, in contrast to only 11 per cent of those in the North-East (Hansen 1993).

Demographers study both international and internal migration. Illegal international migration may be substantial, as in the United States, particularly from Mexico in recent years. Estimates of illegal migration are unreliable, however, and limit our knowledge of the extent and distribution of international migration and of the characteristics and status of illegal migrants in the United States. In many countries the international in-migrants – both legal and illegal but especially the illegal ones – tend to be economically disadvantaged, belong to racial or ethnic minorities, may not be fluent in the language of the host country, may not understand its customs, and for all these reasons have limited access to the health care system. Furthermore, compared with the native population, some migrant groups have worse health status, experiencing higher rates of occupational accidents, poor pregnancy outcomes, and infectious diseases (such as tuberculosis, leprosy, sexually transmitted diseases, Hepatitis B, AIDS) (Bollini 1992; Siem 1992). Thus the role of migration in the transmission of infectious diseases may be of concern. With their greater health needs but often facing higher barriers to health care, international migrants often present a special challenge for health education campaigns and public health outreach programmes.

In countries where both fertility and mortality are low, as in economically advanced countries, international in-migration can comprise a large part of the growth of the population. For example, in 1992, international migration accounted for one-third of the population increase in the United States (United States Bureau of the Census 1994, Table No. 4). Therefore, the public health implications of international in-migration can be significant.

Population distribution

Information on the distribution of the population across geographical or political units is useful for planning public health programmes and allocation of resources. To measure population distribution spatially, demographers have traditionally used measures of the size and density of population by geographic subdivisions. They also measure the concentration of a population, its spacing, and the geographic centre of a population (the centre of population gravity for an area). These measures have been subjected both to statistical analysis and cartographic examination (Bailey 1994).

Recently, the field of demography has begun to use geographic information systems (GIS) to study population distribution and its relationships to population processes. GIS can be defined as 'an organized collection of computer hardware, software, geographic data, and personnel designed to efficiently capture, store, update, manipulate, analyze, and display all forms of geographically referenced information' (Environmental Systems Research Institute 1992, pp. 1–2). Information that can be geographically referenced includes any data (frequencies, rates, measures of climate, etc.) to which a geographical unit can be assigned (such as zip codes, communities or counties, or geographic references such as latitude and longitude). Demographers use GIS to study trends and spatial patterns of population processes such as infant mortality and mortality resulting from specific causes. Demographic studies of spatial distribution and its relationships to socio-economic and health factors performed via GIS methods can provide useful insights into the location and distribution of public health needs and resources, and thus can help in planning the location of future public health infrastructure.

Marriage and marital dissolution

Demographers study entry into marriage (or other sexual unions that resemble marriages) and the disruption of these unions because most childbearing occurs within families formed by these unions. The study of nuptiality deals with the frequency of marriages, characteristics of persons joined in these unions, and their dissolution by separation, divorce or death. Nuptiality affects public health not only through its relationship to fertility, but also via its effects on differential mortality and selective migration.

Like mortality and fertility, marriage is measured by crude rates and age–sex-specific rates, standardized rates, as well as rates specific to the order of marriage (first, second, etc.) The timing of marriage (age at marriage) is also an important measure.

The crude marriage rate is the number of marriages in a year per 1000 population. The general marriage rate relates the number of marriages to the age groups who are in the marriageable population, that is, ages 15 and over. The age- and sex-specific marriage rate represents the number of marriages occurring to persons of a given age and sex group per 1000 persons in that group. Each of these rates measures the level of marriage in a population. However, for comparing across populations or over time, the crude and general marriage rates need to be standardized for differences in the age and sex composition.

The order-specific marriage rate expresses the number of marriages of a given order (first, second, etc.) per 1000 persons 15 and over, or, alternatively, per 1000 persons 15 and over who are in the previous order of marriage (never married, first, etc.).

Demographers measure the timing of entry into marriage by the median or mean age at marriage; this could be computed for specific orders of marriage. Age at first marriage is especially important because it usually marks the formation of a family unit that typically produces children.

In 1987 in the United States, the crude marriage rate was 9.9 per 1000 population. For women 15 and older, the marriage rate was 24.2; for men 15 and older, 26.2. The median age at first marriage for women was 23.6 in 1987; for men, 25.3. The median age at remarriage was 33.3 for women who were previously divorced from marriages and married in 1987; it was 36.7 for men (NCHS 1991, Tables 1–1 and 1–8).

The above rates are generally computed for a given period. The acts of marriage, separation or divorce are highly influenced by the socio-economic changes (such as war, depression, recession) and prevailing social climate (such as social disapproval/approval of divorce, cohabitation) and, therefore, these period rates reflect period responses to such changes. They are not, however, reliable guides for understanding the influence of socio-economic and cultural factors on lifetime marital behaviour. For this, cohort measures of nuptiality are required. These need to be distinguished from the period measures.

A number of measures can be computed for a given period or a given cohort. For example, age at marriage could either be computed as a period or cohort measure. Age–sex-specific marriage rates occurring in a given period could be summed to give a period total marriage rate. This represents the experience of a synthetic cohort, that is, a hypothetical group of women or men who experience at each age the age–sex-specific marriage rates prevailing in a given period. Age–sex-specific marriage rates actually experienced by a given birth cohort as it aged over time could also be summed, to yield a cohort total marriage rate. The total marriage rate calculated on the basis of age–sex-specific first marriage rates gives the proportion of the population ever marrying.

Based on a synthetic cohort from marital status life tables, it has been estimated that if women experienced throughout their lifetime the age-specific marriage rates prevailing in the United States in 1988, 86.6 per cent would eventually marry; for men, it was 82.0 per cent (Schoen and Weinick 1993). In contrast, the rates prevailing in 1970 implied that 94.1 per cent of women would marry, and 92.9 per cent of men. Based on the 1988 age-specific marriage rates, the average age at first marriage computed from these life tables was 25.1 for women, and 27.5 for men. From the 1970 rates, the average age for women was 21.8, and for men, 23.4. Thus, the decline in period marriage rates suggest that a much smaller proportion of both men and women will ever marry, and those who married would do so at significantly older ages. These changes could adversely affect the health of the population because of the advantages in health and longevity enjoyed by married people over never-married (and formerly married) people.

Generally, rates of marital separation are not computed in the United States because vital registration there includes only divorce and not separation. Measures of divorce include: crude divorce rates (number of divorces per 1000 population); divorce rates for married persons (number of divorces per 1000 married population) or for married persons of each sex; age–sex-specific divorce rates (number of divorces occurring to persons of a given age- and sex-group in a given year, per 1000 people in that group, or per 1000 married people in that group). The divorce rates for married persons and the age–sex-specific divorce rates can be computed for specific marriage orders.

Divorce rates specific for marital duration represent the number of divorces occurring to marriages of specific durations per 1000 people in each duration group. One measures the timing of divorce, like the timing of marriage, as the median or mean age at divorce (for specific orders of marriage).

The rate of divorce (and annulment) has climbed in recent decades in the United States: 9.2 per 1000 married women aged 15 and older in 1960, 14.9 in 1970, 22.6 in 1980. Since then, it has abated somewhat, to 20.8 in 1987 (NCHS 1991, Table 2–1).

The median age at divorce of husbands divorcing (from all marriage orders) in 1987 was 34.9, and of wives, 32.5 (NCHS 1991, Table 2–5). The median duration of marriage at the time of divorce in 1987 was 7.0 years (United States Bureau of the Census, 1994, Table 143).

Demographers also study marriage, divorce, widowhood, and remarriage using multistate life tables. Unlike the ordinary (multiple decrement) life table, the multistate life table takes into account the age at entry into marriage or divorce in computing measures of average age at divorce and of lifetime probabilities of divorce. In addition, multistate life tables can provide summary measures such as the average number of marriages and divorces occurring by specific ages in the lifetime of a cohort (usually a synthetic cohort) (Namboodiri and Suchindran 1987).

Based on 1988 United States divorce rates, marital status life tables estimated that for males, 42.7 per cent of marriages would end in divorce; and for females, 43.2 per cent. The average age at divorce would be 37.7 for men, and 34.4 for women. If people experienced in their lifetime the rates of remarriage and divorce prevailing in 1988, men who marry would be expected to have 1.58 marriages, while women who marry would have 1.51 marriages. On average, marriages would endure for 24.5 years (for males) or 24.8 years (for females) before ending in divorce. Divorces would last 7.9 years for males, but 13.4 years for females. For men, the percentage of lives spent as a never-married person would be 46.2 per cent; in a currently married state, 44.8 per cent; as a divorced person, 6.2 per cent; and in the widowed status, 2.8 per cent. The corresponding percentages for females are 39.1, 41.2, 9.6, and 10.0 (Schoen and Weinick 1993).

A great deal of demographic research has focused on the determinants of entry into marriage and of the occurrence of marital disruption. Similarly, a large body of research addresses the negative consequences of marital disruption, especially for the woman and children. A related body of work investigates the determinants and consequences of family and household formation – processes closely linked to marriage and marital dissolution.

Public health professionals may find demographic research regarding the effects of marital status on mortality to be of particular interest. Being married appears to protect against death or, alternatively, being unmarried (divorced, widowed, or never married) puts individuals at higher risk of death (Gove 1973; Hu and Goldman 1990; Millman 1993; Smith and Waitzman 1994). Prospective community-based surveys and other evidence have shown that the beneficial effects of marriage on health and mortality are not simply the result of the differential selection of healthier people or people with better health behaviours into marriage (Gove 1973; Goldman 1993). Although selection explains part of the greater mortality of the unmarried, it appears that the social, psychological, and material support enjoyed by those who remain married contributes to the greater longevity of the married.

For example, in the United States in 1980, in all age groups and among both the black and white populations, and among both males and females, people who were married experienced lower rates of death than the unmarried. Males, however, enjoyed greater longevity advantages from marriage than females; and white individuals more than black. Among unmarried white people, the widowed or the divorced had the worst mortality, depending on age; in contrast, among unmarried black people, the never-married men had the worst rates (except at the oldest ages), while the widowed women were more disadvantaged. For the broad age group of 25 to 64 year olds, compared with the currently married, the relative risk of death among white males for the never married was 2.24; for the divorced, 2.89; and for the widowed, 4.18. The corresponding figures for white females were substantially smaller: 1.87, 2.00, and 2.69, respectively. For the same age group of 25- to 64-year-olds, the relative risks among black males were also generally smaller than those found for white males: 2.46, 1.95, and 2.43 for the never married, divorced, and widowed. Black married females derived the smallest longevity advantage; the corresponding relative risks for the three unmarried groups were 1.82, 1.32, and 2.05 (Millman 1993).

Population estimation and projection

The census is the most complete and reliable source of information on the size and distribution of the population of a country and its geopolitical subdivisions. Although demographic processes constantly change, sometimes quite rapidly, a census is taken usually only every 10 years. Thus, during intercensal years, census data are not adequate for assessing public health risks, nor for planning and evaluating programmes. To meet the need for population data between censuses, demographers make population estimates using analytical methods that involve the use of vital statistics data, immigration data, and other data symptomatic of population change. Where such data are not available, demographers often use mathematical models to estimate populations at current and future times.

Three types of estimates are usually made. The first, intercensal estimates, calculate the population intermediate to two successive censuses. Second, post-censal estimates project the population from the last census to the present. These use sources of data on a sample of the current population such as the Current Population Surveys. Finally, population projections project the population into the future. Population projections require making important assumptions about the future course of the components of population growth (fertility, mortality, migration). All three types of population estimates are made for the total population, as well as for subgroups (such as by age, sex, race and ethnicity, and also by other characteristics).

For example, based on the 1980 census count of 226.5 million people in the United States and the 1990 count of 248.7 million, an intercensal estimate for 1987 was 242.3 million (United States Bureau of the Census 1994, Table 26). After the 1990 census, a post-censal estimate for 1992 was 255.1 million (United States Bureau of the Census 1994, Table 26).

Demographers usually make population projections under a range of assumptions about future levels of fertility, mortality, and net migration. For example, the United States Bureau of the Census has made a series of population projections under three sets of assumptions. The 'medium' level of assumptions presupposes a TFR of 2.1, life expectancy of 82.6 in 2050, and a net migration of 880 000 per year. The corresponding figures for the 'low' assumptions are 1.89 TFR, 75.3 years, and 350 000 net in-migrants annually; and for the 'high' series, 2.62 TFR, 87.5 years, and 1.4 million net in-migrants annually. Under the 'middle' series of assumptions, the population of the United States in the year 2000 is projected to be 276.2 million, and in year 2050, 392.0 million. Under the 'low' assumptions, it is 270.3 million in year 2000, and 285.5 million in 2050. Under the 'high' assumptions, the population is expected to reach 282.0 million in 2000, and 522.1 million in 2050 (United States Bureau of the Census 1994, Table No. 3). Obviously, the projected populations vary widely depending on the assumptions made. For planning purposes, people usually use the projections based on the 'medium' series of assumptions.

Other selected topics

In recent years, demographers in the United States have concentrated research attention on other important demographic phenomena with direct implications for public health. We discuss some of these briefly below.

Demography of ageing

In the 1980s, a subdiscipline of demography, focusing on the demography of aging, has emerged (see Suzman et al. 1992; Martin and Preston 1994). This development has been stimulated by the recognition that worldwide, the number of elderly people has increased rapidly. For example, the number of people aged 65 and older in the world was estimated to be 143 million in 1955; it was 328 in 1990; and it is projected to reach 822 million in 2025 (under medium level assumptions) (United Nations 1993). The corresponding numbers for more economically developed regions were 72, 145 and 256; for the less developed regions, 71, 183, and 566. Thus, the growth in the number of elderly between 1990 and 2025 was projected to be 176 per cent for the more developed regions and 309 per cent for the less developed regions. The need to provide for the health care and social and economic support of increasing numbers of elderly has profound implications worldwide for social and health policy and the allocation of resources.

The demography of ageing duplicates in miniature the concerns of the general field of demography, but it also focuses on special features related to the concerns of ageing. Thus, demographers have investigated the interactions of fertility and mortality to produce older age composition and how selective migration has resulted in regional differences in the growth of the elderly population (Horiuchi 1991; Lee 1993; Bean et al. 1993). They have also studied changes among cohorts of the elderly in their educational attainment, marital status and living arrangements, health behaviours and status (Soldo and Agree 1988).

In addition, the demography of ageing has focused on the elderly themselves and their special concerns. Thus, demographers have conducted descriptive studies of the characteristics and status of the elderly, especially in the realms of health, economic status, labour force participation, family and social relationships, and living arrangements (Soldo and Agree 1988). In particular, research efforts have focused on the labour-force behaviour of the aged (Quinn and Burkhauser 1993) and the economic status of older Americans (Holtz-Eaken and Smeeding 1993). Others have examined social class differentials in mortality among the elderly. Evidence suggests that these differentials may not primarily be the result of differential biomedical risk factors, nor to differential access to health care; thus the role of social relations and social--

psychological factors merits further investigation (Preston and Taubman 1993).

Kinship patterns and exchanges among the elderly have received substantial attention. Demographers have examined the effects of past fertility, mortality, and marital disruption on the availability of children to parents when they reach older ages. Furthermore, they have studied the extent of kinship ties actually experienced by the elderly, including residential proximity and coresidence with kin, and their determinants (Wolf 1993). This area of study is important because in the United States, older people, especially the frail elderly, who are not resident in institutions receive much of their assistance with activities of daily living and other care from relatives (Stone et al. 1987; Soldo and Freedman 1993).

Researchers have studied the relationships between the decline of mortality from specific causes and the prevalence of these conditions among the elderly. For example, it has been found that as mortality resulting from heart disease, stroke, and some cancers has declined, the prevalence of these diseases has increased among the aged (Verbrugge 1984; Manton and Myers 1987). However, others think that the result of reductions in risk factors and improvements in medical interventions will mean that people will live longer, but will suffer these diseases for a shorter time-span close to the time of death (Fries 1987). Most recently, evidence has been presented to indicate that the prevalence of disability (physical or mental handicaps resulting in part from previous experience of such diseases) has now declined among the elderly (Crimmins and Ingegneri 1992; Manton and Stallard 1993).

Investigators have also developed models of morbidity and mortality among the aged. Manton and Stallard (1993) have conceptualized a series of models to examine the interactions between public health interventions and individual risk factors for chronic diseases and their impact on the health and functional status of the elderly. These models also investigate interactions among disease, disability, and mortality, and how these relationships change as individuals grow older. Such models that can examine the potential effects of public health programmes and policies, and can prioritize the importance of various risk factors, will be extremely valuable for guiding the development of public health programmes for the increasing numbers of elderly.

Acquired immune deficiency syndrome

Acquired immune deficiency syndrome, or AIDS, is the modern-day public health scourge. It has affected an array of demographic phenomena, including levels and differentials in mortality, sexual behaviour and the use of contraception, fertility and fecundity, and marriage rates.

In 1987, the United States National Center for Health Statistics introduced codes for classifying deaths caused by HIV infection on death certificates. Thus, United States vital statistics data now can be used to study the levels of mortality resulting from HIV infection and differentials by age, sex, race and ethnicity, and region. The crude death rate from HIV infection was 11.7 per 100 000 population in 1991. The death rate from AIDS was 2.3 during the first year of life, declined to 0.3 for ages 5 to 14, rose slightly to 1.7 for ages 15 to 24, 22.1 for ages 25 to 34, and peaked at 31.2 for ages 35 to 44. The rate decreased to 18.4 for ages 45 to 54, 7.4 for ages 55 to 64, and 0.9 for ages 75 to 84 (NCHS 1993d, Table 5).

Demographers have studied the extent to which the appearance of the HIV epidemic has caused changes in contraceptive behaviour (use of condoms and other barrier methods) (Cates and Stone 1992; Ahituv et al. 1993; Tanfer et al. 1993). In addition, demographers and others have investigated variation in sexual behaviour and changes in behaviour undertaken to protect against AIDS (such as decreasing the coital frequency or the number of partners) (Laumann et al, 1994). The contraceptive and sexual behaviours that protect against AIDS also protect against pregnancy, and thus they can decrease fertility. However, the disease processes of AIDS apparently have had little direct effect on the biological ability to conceive (that is fecundity) (Frank and McNicoll 1987).

From their experience with the usefulness of worldwide national fertility sample surveys (for example Knowledge, Attitude and Practice (KAP), World Fertility Survey (WFS) and Demographic and Health Survey (DHS)), demographers suggested the need to conduct comparable surveys to determine knowledge, attitude and beliefs related to sexual behaviour and AIDS. Consequently, the World Health Organization instituted the Global Programme on AIDS (GPA) (Cleland et al. 1992); surveys have been implemented in several countries in Africa. Demographers have also used anthropological–demographic approaches to gather information to help understand the nexus between sexual networking and AIDS in Africa (Caldwell et al. 1994).

The AIDS epidemic has the potential to rend the social and economic fabric of society and, therefore, considerable effort has been devoted to forecasting the future course of the epidemic. Simple extrapolations to the near future have been performed. In addition, more long-term projections have been done that take into account the complex dynamic processes of HIV transmission and progression into AIDS. In these efforts, researchers from various disciplines have applied different methods. Demographers have joined the effort to project the course of the AIDS epidemic and its demographic impact. They have used the demographic technique of cohort components projection model (see for example Bongaarts 1989; Bulatao 1991) or multistate models that consider various states of health, infection, AIDS, and death at various durations (see for example Palloni and Lamas 1991).

Conclusion

The fields of demography and public health diverge in several ways, but in important ways they converge. Even though the two disciplines are concerned with some of the same processes at the population level, they differ in their goals, as discussed in the Introduction to this chapter. Thus, because of its central mission of preventing disease and promoting health, the public health discipline pays much more attention to the processes of illness and disability than does demography. Recently, however, demographers have placed greater emphasis on understanding the 'proximate causes' of mortality, and thus have turned their attention to studies of morbidity and disability, especially as they relate to specific causes of death. This area of demographic research may be expected to grow in the future.

Its central role in population change means that demographers focus more intensively on fertility and all its components than does the field of public health. Even though childbearing and infertility in fact are important components of the population's health status, they constitute only a part of the public health concerns, and thus receive less intensive attention by the field of public health. However, demographers pay less attention than public health professionals to the roles of nutrition and sexually transmitted diseases in the childbearing process.

As one of the three population processes, migration is one of demography's central concerns. As discussed earlier, migration has many important public health effects. These public health connections may not be fully appreciated by the public health discipline.

The discipline of demography has contributed to the public health field in many ways – in the areas of data collection, analytic methods, and substantive studies. Demographic data provide much of the information needed for monitoring health status and identifying populations at risk. Furthermore, demographic measures and methods help in assessing public health needs and status, evaluating impacts of public health programmes, and investigating factors influencing health outcomes. Finally, demographers' studies of the factors affecting mortality, fertility, their proximate determinants, and migration have contributed insights relevant to the field of public health. In particular, demographic knowledge can be of value in identifying socio-demographic groups at high risk of various poor health behaviours and outcomes, targetting and delivering public health services to them, determining the locations where they are concentrated, and projecting these into the future.

As discussed throughout the chapter, the two disciplines have overlapped in several areas. (See also Volume I, Chapter 5.) This convergence will become increasingly important in the future, as the two disciplines appreciate more and more the mutual benefits to be gained from their interaction. One impetus for this interaction comes from the interplay between population processes and the public health. For example, if efforts at reducing infant mortality succeed, then the prominence of genetic and congenital causes of infant mortality will rise and will thus alter the focus of public health efforts and resources. As efforts have reduced deaths resulting from cardiovascular disease, the importance of cancer as a target of public health attention has risen. Generally, as longevity increases, and the health of older people improves (or declines), how will the role of the public health discipline be altered? In the area of fertility, if interventions to decrease adolescent pregnancy succeed, the average length of time elapsing between generations will be prolonged and thus will slow population growth; this will also boost the share of childbearing borne by the oldest mothers. Consequently, the health risks of the oldest mothers and their children, such as the increased risks of genetic diseases, will require additional public health attention. Migration also interacts with the public health, as international in-migration introduces various infectious diseases into the host population and shifts the prominence of various types of chronic and degenerative diseases because migrants are at greater or lesser risk of different diseases.

A second stimulus to the increased interaction between demography and public health derives from the heightened appreciation in both fields of the importance and complexity of the determinants of various biological and health processes. Thus, as both fields have explored the interplay of biological, social, cultural, behavioural, and environmental factors, both have become increasingly inter-disciplinary. This development should lead to greater and more active collaboration between the two disciplines. The fields of demography and public health stand to learn a great deal from each other, to the significant benefit of both – and of the health of the population.

References

Ahituv, A., Hotz, V.J., and Philipson, T. (1993). *Will the AIDS epidemic be self-limiting? Evidence on the responsiveness of the demand for condoms to the prevalence of AIDS*, Discussion Paper No. 93–3. Population Research Center, University of Chicago.

Astone, N.M. (1993). Are adolescent mothers just single mothers? *Journal of Research on Adolescence* 3(4), 353–71.

Bailey, T.C. (1994). A review of statistical spatial analysis in geographical information systems. In *Spatial analysis and GIS*, (ed. S. Fotheringham and P. Rogerson). Taylor & Francis, London.

Berkman, L., Singer, B., and Manton, K.G. (1989). Black/white differences in health status and mortality among the elderly. *Demography* 26, 661–78.

Bean, F.D., Myers, G.C., Angel, J.L., and Galle, O. (1993). Geographic concentration, migration, and population redistribution among the elderly. In *Demography of aging*, (ed. L.G. Martin and S.H. Preston), pp. 319–55. National Academy Press, Washington, DC.

Bennett, N. and Bloom, D. (1993). The influence of nonmarital childbearing on the formation of marital unions. National Bureau of Economic Research, Working Paper Series No. 4564. Cambridge, Massachusetts.

Bollini, P. (1992). Health policies for immigrant populations in the 1990s. A comparative study in seven receiving countries. *International Migration* (Special Issue on Migration and Health in the 1990s) 30, 103–19.

Bongaarts, J. (1978). A framework for analyzing the proximate determinants of fertility. *Population and Development Review* 4, 105–32.

Bongaarts, J. (1989). A model of the spread of HIV infection and the demographic impact of AIDS. *Statistics in Medicine* 8(1), 103–20.

Bulatao, R.A. (1991). The Bulatao approach: projecting the demographic impact of the HIV epidemic using standard parameters. In *The AIDS epidemic and its demographic consequences*, Proceedings of the United Nations/World Health Organization Workshop on Modelling the Demographic Impact of the AIDS Epidemic in Pattern II Countries: Progress to Date and Policies for the Future, 1989, pp. 90–108.

Burt, M.R. (1986). Estimating the public costs of teenage childbearing. *Family Planning Perspectives* 18(5), 221–6.

Burton, L. (1993). Conscripting kin: reflections on family, generation, and culture. In *The politics of pregnancy: adolescent sexuality and public policy*, (ed. A. Lawson and D.L. Rhode), pp. 174–85. Yale University Press, New Haven, Connecticut.

Caldas, S.J. (1993). The private and societal economic costs of teenage childbearing: the state of the research. *Population and Environment* 4(4), 389–99.

Caldwell, J.C., Orubuloye, I.O., and Caldwell, P. (1994). Methodological advances in studying the social context of AIDS in West Africa. In *Sexual networking and AIDS in Sub-Saharan Africa: behavioural research and the social context*, (ed. I.O. Orubuloye, J.C. Caldwell, P. Caldwell, and G. Santow). The Australian National University, Canberra.

Cates, W., Jr. and Stone, K.M. (1992). Family planning, sexually transmitted diseases and contraceptive choice: a literature update, Part I. *Family Planning Perspectives* 24(2), 75–84.

Chase-Lansdale, L.P., Brooks-Gunn, J., and Zamsky, E.S. (1994). Young African-American multigenerational families in poverty: quality of mothering and grandmothering. *Child Development* 65(2), 373–93.

Cleland, J., Carael, M., Deheneffe, J.-C., and Ferry, B. (1992). Sexual behaviour in the face of risk: preliminary results from first AIDS-related surveys. *Health Transition Review*, 2 (Supplementary issue), 185–204.

Cramer, J.C. (1986). Social factors and infant mortality: identifying high risk groups and proximate causes. *Demography* 24, 299–322.

Crimmins, E.M. and Ingegneri, D.G. (1992). Health trends in the American population. In *Demography and retirement: the 21st century*, (ed. A.M. Rappaport and S.J. Schieber). Greenwood Press, Westport, Connecticut.

DaVanzo, J., Butz, W.P., and Habicht, J.P. (1983). How biological and behavioral influences on mortality in Malaysia vary during the first year of life. *Population Studies* 37, 381–402.

Davis, K. and Blake, J. (1956). Social structure and fertility: an analytic framework. *Economic Development and Cultural Change*, 4, 211–35.

DiClemente, R.J. (1992). Epidemiology of AIDS, HIV prevalence, and HIV incidence among adolescents. *Journal of School Health* 62(7), 325–30.

Eberstein, I., Nam, C., and Hummer, R. (1990). Infant mortality by cause of death: main and interaction effects. *Demography* 27, 413–30.

Entwistle, B. and Mason, W.M. (1985). Multilevel effects of socioeconomic development and family planning programs on children ever born. *American Journal of Sociology* 92(3), 616–49.

Environmental Systems Research Institute (1992). *Understanding GIS*. Environmental Systems Research Institute, Inc., Redlands, California.

Evans, M.D.R. (1986). American fertility patterns: white–nonwhite comparisons. *Population and Development Review* 12(2), 267–93.

Forrest, J.D. (1990). Adolescent reproductive behavior: an international comparison of developed countries. *Advances in Adolescent Mental Health*, 4, 13–34.

Frank, O. and McNicoll, G. (1987). Fertility and population policy in Kenya. *Population and Development Review* 13, 209–43.

Fries, J.F. (1987). An introduction to the compression of morbidity. *Gerontologica Perspecta* 1, 5–7.

Geronimus, A.T. and Korenman, S. (1993a). Maternal youth or family background? On the health disadvantages of infants with teenage mothers. *American Journal of Epidemiology* 137(2), 213–25.

Geronimus, A.T. and Korenman, S. (1993b). The socio-economic costs of teenage childbearing: evidence and interpretation. *Demography* 30(2), 281–90.

Goldman, N. (1993). Marriage selection and mortality patterns. *Demography*, 30(2), 189–208.

Goldman, N., Moren, L., Westoff, C.F., and Vaughan, B. (1991). Estimates of contraceptive failure and discontinuation based on two methods of contraceptive data collection in Peru. In *United Nations, measuring the dynamics of contraceptive use*, pp. 171–83. United Nations, New York.

Gove, W.R. (1973). Sex, marital status, and mortality. *American Journal of Sociology* 79, 45–66.

Grady, W.R., Hayward, M.D., and Yagi, J. (1986). Contraceptive failure in the United States: estimates from the 1982 National Survey of Family Growth. *Family Planning Perspectives* 18(5), 200–9.

Grogger, J. and Bronars, S. (1993). The Socioeconomic consequences of teenage childbearing: findings from a natural experiment. *Family Planning Perspective* 25(4), 156–61, 174.

Hansen, K.A. (1993). *Geographical mobility: March 1991 to March 1992*, US Bureau of the Census, Current Population Reports, pp. 20–473. US Government Printing Office, Washington, DC.

Hayes, C.D. (1987). *Risking the future: adolescent sexuality, pregnancy, and childbearing*, Vol. I. National Academy Press, Washington, DC.

Heckman, J.J. and Singer, B. (1982). Population heterogeneity in demographic models. In *Multidimensional mathematical demography*, (ed. K.C. Land and A. Rogers). Academic Press, New York.

Hofferth, S.L. (1987a). Social and economic consequences of teenage childbearing. In *Risking the future: adolescent sexuality, pregnancy, and childbearing*, Vol. II, (ed. S.L. Hofferth and C.D. Hayes), pp. 123–44. National Academy Press, Washington, DC.

Hofferth, S.L. (1987b). The children of teen childbearers. In *Risking the future: adolescent sexuality, pregnancy, and childbearing*, Vol. II, (ed. S.L. Hofferth and C.D. Hayes), pp. 174–206. National Academy Press, Washington, DC.

Hofferth, S.L. and Hayes, C.D. (ed.) (1987). *Risking the future: adolescent sexuality, pregnancy, and childbearing*, Vol. II. National Academy Press, Washington, DC.

Hoffman, S.D., Foster, E.M., and Furstenberg, F.F., Jr. (1993a). Reevaluating the costs of teenage childbearing. *Demography* 30(1), 1–14.

Hoffman, S.D., Foster, E.M., and Furstenberg, F.F., Jr. (1993b). Reevaluating the costs of teenage childbearing: response to Geronimus and Korenman. *Demography* 30(2), 291–6.

Holtz-Eakin, D. and Smeeding, T.M. (1994). Income, wealth, and intergenerational economic relations of the aged. In *Demography of aging*, (ed. L.G. Martin and S.P. Preston), pp. 102–45. National Academy Press, Washington, DC.

Horiuchi, S. (1991). Assessing the effects of mortality reduction on population ageing. *Population Bulletin of the United Nations* 31/32, 38–51.

Horwitz, S. and Klerman, L. (1992). *Antecedents of delinquent behaviors in the adolescent children of school-age mothers*. Paper presented at a conference convened by the National Institute of Child Health and Human Development. Bethesda, Maryland.

Hu, Y. and Goldman, N. (1990). Mortality differentials by marital status: an international comparison. *Demography* 27(2), 233–49.

Hummer, R.A., Eberstein, I.W., and Nam, C.B. (1992). Infant mortality differentials among Hispanic groups in Florida. *Social Forces* 70(4), 1053–75.

Institute of Medicine (1988). *The future of public health*. National Academy Press, Washington, DC.

Klerman, L.V. and Klerman, J.A. (1994). More evidence for the public health value of family planning. *American Journal of Public Health* 84(9), 1377–8.

Knodel, J. and Debavalya, N. (1981). Breastfeeding trends in Thailand and their demographic impact. *Intercom* 9(3), 8–10.

Laumann, E.O., Gagnon, J.H., Michael, R.T., and Michaels, S. (1994). *The social organization of sexuality. Sexual practices in the United States*. The University of Chicago Press.

Lee, R.D. (1993). The formal demography of population aging, transfers, and the economic life cycle. In *Demography of aging*, (ed. L.G. Martin and S.H. Preston), pp. 8–49. National Academy Press, Washington, DC.

Long, L.H. (1988). *Migration and residential mobility in the United States*. Russell Sage Foundation, New York.

Mangold, W.D. and Powell-Griner, E. (1991). Race of parents and infant birthweight in the United States. *Social Biology* 38(1–2), 13–27.

Manton, K.G. and Myers, G.C. (1987). Recent trends in multiple-caused mortality, 1968–1982: age and cohort components. *Population Research and Policy Review* 6, 16176.

Manton, K.G. and Stallard, E. (1993). Medical demography: interaction of disability dynamics and mortality. In *Demography of aging*, (ed. L.G. Martin and S.H. Preston), pp. 217–78. National Academy Press, Washington, DC.

Martin, L.G. and Preston, S.H. (ed.) (1994). *Demography of aging*. National Academy Press, Washington, DC.

Miller, B.C. and Moore, K.A. (1990). Adolescent sexual behavior, pregnancy, and parenting: research through the 1980s. *Journal of Marriage and the Family* 52(4), 1025–44.

Millman, S. (1993). *Sex, marital status, and mortality revised*. Paper presented at the Annual Meeting of the Population Association of America, Cincinnatti, Ohio.

Moore, K.A., Myers, D.E., Morrison, D.R., Nord, C.W., Brown, B., and Edmonston, B. (1993). Age at first childbirth and later poverty. *Journal of Research on Adolescence* 3(4) 393–422.

Moore, K.A., Snyder, N.O., and Glei, D. (1995). Facts at a glance. Child Trends, Washington, DC.

Morrison, D.R., Moore, K.A., and Myers, D.E. (1992). *Maternal age at first birth and children's behavior and cognitive development*. Paper presented at a conference convened by the National Institute of Child Health and Human Development. Bethesda, Maryland.

Mosley, W.H., and Chen, L.C. (1984). An analytical framework for the study of child survival in developing countries. *Population and Development Review* 10 (Supplement), 25–45.

Namboodiri, N.K. (1991). *Demographic analysis: a stochastic approach*. Academic Press, San Diego, California.

Namboodiri, N.K. and Suchindran, C.M. (1987). *Life table techniques and their applications*. Academic Press, San Diego, California.

NCHS (National Center for Health Statistics) (1991). *Vital statistics of the United States, 1987, Vol. III, Marriage and Divorce*, Public Health Service, Washington, DC, DHHS Pub. No. (PHS) 91–1103. US Government Printing Office.

NCHS (1993*a*). *Vital statistics of the United States, 1989, Vol. II, Mortality, part A*, Public Health Service, Washington, DC, DHHS Pub. No. (PHS) 93–1101. US Government Printing Office.

NCHS (1993*b*). *Vital statistics of the United States, 1989, Vol. I, Natality*, Public Health Service, Washington, DC, DHHS Pub. No. (PHS) 93–1100. US Government Printing Office.

NCHS (1993*c*). Births, marriages, divorces, and deaths for March 1993. *Monthly Vital Statistics Report* **42(3)**. Public Health Service, Hyattsville, Maryland.

NCHS (1993*d*). Births, marriages, divorces, and deaths for August, 1993. *Monthly Vital Statistics Report* **42(2S)**. Public Health Service, Hyattsville, Maryland.

NCHS (1994). *Health United States 1993, chartbook*. Public Health Service, Hyattsville, Maryland.

Palloni, A. and Lamas, L. (1991). The Palloni approach: a duration-dependent model of the spread of HIV/AIDS in Africa. In *The AIDS epidemic and its demographic consequences*, proceedings of the United Nations/World Health Organization Workshop on Modelling the Demographic Impact of the AIDS Epidemic in Pattern II Countries: Progress to Date and Policies for the Future, 1989, pp. 109–36.

Peckam, S. (1993). Preventing unintended teenage pregnancies. *Public Health* **107(2)**, 125–33.

Popkin, B.M., Gulkey, D.K., Akin, J.S., Adair, L.S., Flieger, W., and Udry, J.R. (1993). Nutrition, lactation, and birth spacing in Filipino women. *Demography* **30(3)**, 333–52.

Preston, S.H. and Taubman, P. (1993). Socioeconomic differences in adult mortality and health status. In *Demography of aging*, (ed. L.G. Martin and S.H. Preston), pp. 279–318. National Academy Press, Washington, DC.

Qui, Y. and Hayward, M.D. (1993). *Contextual analysis of teenaged first premarital pregnancy in the United States*. Paper presented at the Annual Meeting of the Population Association of America, Cincinnati, Ohio.

Quinn, J.F. and Burkhauser, R.V. (1993). Retirement and labor force behavior of the elderly. In *Demography of aging*, (ed. L.G. Martin and S.H. Preston), pp. 50–101. National Academy Press, Washington, DC.

Rogers, R.G. (1989). Ethnic and birth weight differences in cause-specific infant mortality. *Demography* **26(2)**, 335–43.

Rogers, R.G. (1993). Successful aging: sociodemographic characteristics of long-lived and healthy individuals, Institute of Behavioral Science, Population Program, Working Paper WP–93–4.

Rogot, E., Sortie, P.D., Johnson, N.J., and Schmitt, C. (ed.) (1992). *A mortality study of 1.3 million persons by demographic, social, and economic factors: 1979–1985 follow-up*, US National Longitudinal Mortality Study, Publication No. 923297. National Institutes of Health, Bethesda, MD.

Rosenzweig, M. and Wolpin, K. (1992). *Sisters, siblings, and mothers: the effects of teenage childbearing on birth outcomes*. Paper presented at a conference convened by the National Institute of Child Health and Human Development.

Samuels, B.N. (1986). Infant mortality and low birth weight among minority groups in the United States: a review of the literature. In *Report of the Secretary's Task Force on Black and Minority Health: Infant Mortality and Low Birthweight*, Vol. 6. US Department of Health and Human Services, Washington, DC.

Sanderson, M., Placek, P.J., and Keppel, K.G. (1991). The 1988 national maternal and infant health survey: design, content, and data availability. *Birth* **18(1)**, 26–32.

Santelli, J.S. and Beilenson, P. (1992). Risk factors for adolescent sexual behavior, fertility, and sexually transmitted diseases. *Journal of School Health* **62(7)**, 271–9.

Schoen, R. and Weinick, R.M. (1993). The slowing metabolism of marriage: figures from 1988 US marital status life tables. *Demography* **30(4)**, 737–46.

Schwartz, D. and Mayaux, H.J. (1982). Female fecundity as a function of age. *New England Journal of Medicine* **307**, 404–6.

Seeman, I., Poe, G.S., and Powell-Griner, E. (1993). Development, methods, and response characteristics of the 1986 National Mortality Followback Survey. National Center for Health Statistics. *Vital and Health Statistics* **1(29)**.

Senderowitz, J. and Paxman, J.M. (1985). Adolescent fertility: worldwide concerns. *Population Bulletin* **40(2)**, 1–51.

Shryock, H.S. and Siegel, J.S. (1973). *The methods and materials of demography*, Vol. II. US Bureau of the Census, Washington, DC, US Government Printing Office.

Siem, H. (1992). Introduction. *International Migration* (Special Issue on Migration and Health in the 1990s), **30**, 3–8.

Simpson, E.H. (1951). The interpretation of interaction in contingency tables. *Journal of the Royal Statistical Society, Se. B*, **13**, 238–41.

Singh, S. (1986). Adolescent pregnancy in the United States: an interstate analysis. *Family Planning Perspectives* **18(5)**, 210–20.

Smith, K.R. and Waitzman, N.J. (1994). Double jeopardy: interaction effects of marital and poverty status on the risk of mortality. *Demography* **31(3)**, 487–507.

Soldo, B.J. and Agree, E.M. (1988). America's elderly. *Population Bulletin* **43(3)**, 1–46.

Soldo, B.J. and Freedman, V.A. (1993). Care of the elderly: division of labor among the family, market, and state. In *Demography of aging*, (ed. L.G. Martin and S.H. Preston), pp. 195–216. National Academy Press, Washington, DC.

Stone, R., Cafferata, G.I., and Sangl, J. (1987). Caregivers of the frail elderly: a national profile. *Gerontologist* **27**, 616–26.

Strobino, D.M. (1987). The health and medical consequences of adolescent sexuality and pregnancy: a review of the literature. In *Risking the future: adolescent sexuality, pregnancy, and childbearing*, Vol. II (ed. S.L. Hofferth and C.D. Hayes), pp. 93–122. National Academy Press, Washington, DC.

Suchindran, C.M. and Koo, H.P. (1992). Age at last birth and its components. *Demography* **29(2)**, 227–46.

Suzman, R.M., Willis, D.P., and Manton, K.G. (1992). *The oldest old*. Oxford University Press, New York.

Tanfer, K., Grady, W., Klepinger, D., and Billy, J. (1993). Condom use among US Men, 1991. *Family Planning Perspectives* **25**, 61–6.

Tsai, S.P., Lee, E.S., and Hardy, R.J. (1978). The effects of a reduction in leading causes of death: potential gain in life expectancy. *American Journal of Public Health* **68**, 966–71.

Tsui, A.O., Singh, K.K., Marinshaw, R., and de Silva, S.V. (1993). Surveying marital sexuality in a developing country: effects of design and desire. Paper presented at the Annual Meeting of the Population Association of America, Cincinnati, Ohio.

United Nations (1991). *Measuring the dynamics of contraceptive use*. United Nations, New York.

United Nations (1993). *World population trends and prospects: the 1992 revision*. United Nations, New York.

United Nations Population Fund (1993). *Readings in population research methodology*, Vol. 1–8. United Nations Fund for Population Activities, Chicago.

United States Bureau of the Census (1993). Current population reports, P25–1095, *US population estimates, by age, sex, race and Hispanic origin: 1980 to 1991*. US Government Printing Office, Washington, DC.

United States Bureau of the Census (1994). *Statistical Abstract of the United States: 1994* (114th edn), Washington DC.

Upchurch, D. (1992). Early schooling and childbearing experiences: implications for post-secondary school attendance. *Journal of Research on Adolescence* **3(4)**, 423–43.

Upchurch, D.M. and McCarthy, J. (1989). Adolescent childbearing and high school completion in the 1980s: have things changed? *Family Planning Perspectives* **21(5)**, 199–202.

Vaupel, J.W., Manton, K.G., and Stallard, E. (1979). The impact of heterogeneity in individual frailty on the dynamics of mortality. *Demography* **16**, 439–56.

Verbrugge, L. (1984). Longer life but worsening health? Trends in health and mortality of middle-aged and older persons. *Milbank Memorial Fund Quarterly* **62**, 475–519.

Warnes, A. (1992). Migration and the life course. In *Migration patterns and processes*, (ed. T. Champion and T. Fielding), pp. 175–87. Belhaven Press, London.

Wegman, M.E. (1994). Annual summary of vital statistics – 1993. *Pediatrics* **94(6 Pt 1)**, 792–803.

Weinberg, C.R. and Gladen, B.C. (1986). The beta geometric distribution applied to comparative fecundability studies. *Biometrics* **42**, 547–60.

Wolf, D.A. (1993). The elderly and their kin: patterns of availability and access. In *Demography of aging*, (ed. L.G. Martin and S.H. Preston), pp. 146–94. National Academy Press, Washington DC.

Zeger, S., Liang, K.-Y., and Albert, P. (1988). Models for longitudinal data: a generalized estimating equation approach. *Biometrics* **44**, 1049–60.

26 Economic evaluation

Cam Donaldson and Phil Shackley*

Introduction

Economic evaluation is now an accepted tool for the appraisal of health care programmes (Mooney 1989). Worldwide, there is a growing volume of economic evaluation in the health care field (Drummond 1981; Blades *et al.* 1986; Drummond *et al.* 1986; Blackhouse *et al.* 1992; Elixhauser 1993). Despite this, journal articles often leave little space for detailed presentation of the methods used. Consequently, it may be that little can be learned by non-economists from these articles about how to go about economic evaluation. Also, it is hard for the non-economist to discern general principles from reading the literature as the content of economic evaluations may vary depending on the context of the study and the objectives.

The principles of economic evaluation of health care interventions are clear-cut. Conveniently, these principles can be divided into those addressing two related questions: how to measure the costs of interventions, and how to measure their benefits. In this chapter both of these issues is addressed in detail.

In practice, non-adherence to the principles of economic evaluation is common (Birch and Donaldson 1987; Birch and Gafni 1992). This may be a result of either a lack of understanding of the principles or because full-blown economic evaluation is difficult to put into practice. This chapter is targeted at public health practitioners with an interest in economic evaluation. However, given that some economists can be counted amongst those who have not followed the principles outlined here (as shown in Birch and Donaldson (1987) and Birch and Gafni (1992)), then economists working in public health may also benefit from reading the contents!

In the following section the economic concept of **opportunity cost** is defined. Then, the techniques of economic evaluation that follow from this definition are introduced: they are **cost–benefit analysis, cost–effectiveness analysis**, and **cost–utility analysis**. In the fourth section, a list of costs and benefits, which should be considered for inclusion in any of these types of evaluation, is provided; this is based on the concept of opportunity cost. Principles of measurement and valuation of costs are then outlined. Some of these (in particular **discounting** and **marginal analysis**) also apply to the measurement and valuation of benefits. Despite this, the main issue on the benefit side is how the different techniques of economic evaluation cope with the challenge of

estimating health care benefits. It is this issue on which the section on measuring and valuing the benefits of health care will concentrate. At the end of the chapter, a checklist for measurement and valuation of costs and benefits has been compiled.

The concept of cost in economic evaluation

The concept of **cost** used by economists is important not only as a rationale for the need for economic evaluation but also because it provides a definition of the term 'cost', which is of use in identifying items to be costed in specific evaluations of health care programmes. This concept is more properly called **opportunity cost**. It rests on two prior principles, scarcity and choice, both of which require explanation.

The notion of scarcity used by economists means simply that societies (even those with great wealth) do not have enough resources at their disposal to meet all of their citizens' wants or desires. Modern advanced economies have to meet demands for items as varied as computers, television sets, education, housing, food, and, of course, health care. The list, if not endless, could go on and on until the total implied demands on resources would far outstrip the capacity of the resources to meet them. Resources that were once thought to be 'limitless', such as the environment and airspace for passenger jets, now have to be carefully regulated and rationed. This is also true of specific sectors of the economy, including health care. In the health care sector, even during the best of economic climates, there will not be enough resources to meet all of society's needs. This problem is exacerbated (but not caused) by expensive technological advancement and changing demographic patterns.

This leads to our second concept: as a result of scarcity, choices have to be made about what activities in society should be undertaken and what activities should not be undertaken. Therefore it is inevitable that opportunities to use resources in some activities will be given up or forgone. The benefits (in terms of well-being or satisfaction*) which would have accrued from such forgone opportunities are opportunity costs. Therefore, in economics, the cost of a programme is defined as its opportunity cost. The opportunity cost of the use of resources in a health care programme is equivalent to the benefits forgone in the best alternative use of these resources.

The aim of economic evaluation within the health care field is to

* The Health Economics Research Unit is funded by the Chief Scientist Office of the Scottish Office Department of Health (SODH). The views expressed in this chapter are those of the authors, and not of SODH.

* Often referred to by economists as 'utility', where utility is a measure of preference (or strength of preference) for a commodity.

Table 26.1 Questions of allocative and technical efficiency

Allocative efficiency questions	Technical efficiency questions
	Day surgery versus inpatient stay for tonsillectomy
Surgery for tonsillectomy versus outpatient clinics for asthmatics	Local versus hospital-based clinics for asthmatics

are greater than the opportunity costs of such programmes (i.e. the benefits associated with forgone health care programmes). Thus costs and benefits in health care go hand in hand. Choosing programmes whose benefits exceed their opportunity costs ensures that the amount of well-being (or health) produced by the health care sector will be maximized and its costs minimized.

Techniques of economic evaluation

The economic concept of cost leads to three related techniques of economic evaluation. These are cost–benefit analysis, cost–effectiveness analysis, and cost–utility analysis. Each technique has advantages and difficulties associated with it. However, as Mooney (1989) has said: 'ease cannot be allowed to dictate use; it is a question of what is best for which question'. Therefore, which technique to use should be determined by the question to be addressed in an evaluation.

Principally, economic evaluation is useful in addressing two levels of question: questions of allocative efficiency and questions of technical efficiency. With allocative efficiency, all health care programmes have to compete with each other for implementation. Concern is with whether to allocate scarce resources to a programme or whether to allocate more or less resources to it. Thus, in Table 26.1, surgery for tonsillectomy and outpatient clinics for asthmatics would compete with each other for more (or less) resources.

With technical efficiency, concern is more about how best to deliver a programme or to achieve a given objective. The resources already allocated to the programme are taken as given. Therefore, in the cases outlined in Table 26.1, technical efficiency questions would address how best to deliver surgery for tonsillectomy and how best to provide asthma clinics.

Generally, with allocative efficiency, one group of patients/clients will gain at the expense of another group. With technical efficiency, the same group will be treated, but the question is by which method. The distinction is important, although it often becomes blurred in practice.

Cost–benefit analysis

Cost–benefit analysis is used to determine allocative efficiency. It seeks to answer the following questions:

Is it worth achieving this goal?

How much more or how much less of society's resources should be allocated to achieving this goal or to this type of health care?

Thus cost–benefit analysis can appear to involve looking at one health care programme in isolation (although the alternative of doing nothing, or current practice, is always implied). Looking at one programme alone, cost–benefit analysis addresses the question of whether its benefits are greater or less than its opportunity costs. Looking at several competing projects, comparisons are made on the basis of the costs and benefits of each. If only one project can be funded, that maximizing net benefit should be chosen. If more than one can be funded, the combination that maximizes benefits should be chosen. In both cases, costs and benefits still need to be known.

In principle, the answers to such questions require all costs and benefits to be valued in a commensurate unit (such as money). If everything is measured in one unit, comparisons are straightforward. The valuation of benefits in money terms is the most obvious distinguishing characteristic of cost–benefit analysis. Conceptually, cost–benefit analysis has a very wide range of applicability as, with everything valued in commensurate terms, it could be used to compare health care objectives with each other or with those arising in other sectors of the economy.

In practice, however, the monetary valuation of benefits in cost–benefit analysis is difficult: how can a value be placed on the saving of life or the relief of suffering? Health improvements are traditionally valued in money terms by using one of two approaches: the human capital approach and the willingness to pay approach. The human capital approach values a health improvement on the basis of one's future productive worth to society resulting from being able to return to work (paid or unpaid) after experiencing that health improvement. Productive worth is usually measured by labour costs (i.e. one's future earnings from work). Values can be imputed for activities such as home-making. Consequently, the human capital approach suffers from problems of how to value health improvements for retired people, women who work at home, and unemployed people, and from difficulties in the choice of appropriate earnings data for use in the analysis (Avorn 1984).

The willingness to pay approach values health improvements (or types of health care) on the basis of people's willingness to pay for them. As a result, this approach suffers from two main problems. First, willingness to pay is affected by ability to pay. Rich people have more capacity to pay and hence appear more willing to pay for treatment than poor people; if diseases affect rich and poor in different proportions, and if richer people tend to have different preferences from poor people, then, other things being equal, treatment of diseases of the rich will be 'valued' more highly. This could be erroneous as the higher willingness to pay value will, to an extent, reflect ability to pay as well as strength of preference. It is the latter (strength of preference) that reflects values. Secondly, people are not used to paying for health care in the marketplace and are likely to have problems judging how successful treatment will be (Donaldson 1990). When asked about their willingness to pay in surveys, they have problems in translating health care into health improvements, health improvements into utility, and utility into willingness to pay. Therefore, judging willingness to pay is difficult. However, there are some advantages. Research on willingness to pay is a growing area and therefore it is reviewed in some detail in the section on measurement and valuation of benefits.

Not surprisingly, no ideal cost–benefit analysis has been carried out in the field of health care, despite the name being included in the titles of many articles. In many cost–benefit analyses, the cost of a new intervention is often assessed against 'benefits' measured in terms of cost savings. However, this clearly involves only a comparison of costs. No consideration is given to the difficult issue of valuing health improvements and other benefits in monetary terms (Birch and Donaldson 1987).

Despite such problems, cost–benefit analysis remains a useful tool, particularly in setting out a decision-making problem. By identifying the costs and benefits associated with different health care programmes and valuing what can be valued, one can explicitly observe the trade-offs between tangible and intangible costs and benefits resulting from a decision to implement, or not to implement, a health care programe. A good example of this is the work on costs and benefits of introducing child-proofing of drug containers in the United Kingdom in the early 1970s. In 1971 a decision was taken not to introduce such child-proofing on the basis of its cost (£500 000 per annum at the time). Using conservative estimates, Gould (1971) showed that without child-proofing there would be 16 000 hospital admissions per annum at a cost of £30 per admission, resulting in costs of £480 000 per annum. Thus, the extra cost of child-proofing was £20 000 per annum. If only 20 lives could be saved by child-proofing, the decision not to child-proof would imply that the life of a child was worth less than £1000 per annum.

Such trade-offs would almost certainly have remained implicit in the absence of cost–benefit analysis, thereby not allowing them to be subjected to the same degree of scrutiny. In the absence of such scrutiny, important aspects of efficiency may not be recognized. Cost–benefit analysis, by analysing who receives benefits and bears costs, also opens up important issues of the distribution (or equity) of health and health care which would have remained uncovered. Thus, although economics is often criticized for ignoring equity, it does actually highlight such issues. By quantifying some values and making others explicit, cost–benefit analysis can be a very useful decision-making aid.

It is worth noting at this point that, owing to scarcity of resources, not all desirable health care can be provided. Consequently, decisions about what types of health care to provide cannot be avoided. Thus, although cost–benefit analysis cannot be expected to be perfect in its application, subjecting decisions to the systematic framework that cost–benefit analysis provides is useful. Either way, valuations have to be made. In the absence of cost–benefit analysis, these valuations will be implicit and therefore more prone to error than if they are rendered explicit. Avoiding the analysis does not avoid the need for a decision to be made.

Cost–effectiveness analysis

Because of its relative simplicity, cost–effectiveness analysis is the most common form of economic evaluation in health care. Its use does not require benefits to be valued in money terms. Cost–effectiveness analysis deals with technical efficiency and seeks to answer the following question: Given that it has been decided that a goal is to be achieved, what is the best way of doing so or what is the best way of spending a given budget? Thus, cost–effectiveness analysis always involves comparison of at least two options with the same goal.

Cost–effectiveness analysis can take two main forms. In the first, if the health outcomes of the alternatives to be compared are known to be equivalent, only cost differences need be analysed. The least costly alternative is obviously most efficient as resources are saved which can be put to some other beneficial use without reducing the health outcomes of the client group being studied (Russell et al. 1977). Unfortunately, this type of cost–effectiveness analysis (sometimes referred to as cost–minimization analysis) is often based on the assumption, rather than the knowledge, that the health outcomes of the alternatives to be compared are equal. On closer examination this may not be the case. Therefore, it is preferable for costs always to be considered with benefits. In fact, for all types of economic evaluation, consideration of costs without consideration of benefits, and vice versa, is not valid.

In the second form of cost–effectiveness analysis, alternatives may differ in terms of cost and effect. A ratio is produced for each alternative in which the numerator is cost and the denominator is the health effect under consideration. Health effects are measures of final outcome: they might be life years saved, heart attacks prevented, or improved physical functioning. The cost–effectiveness ratio produced for each alternative is a measure of cost per unit of health effect. The alternative with the lowest cost–effectiveness ratio is best. Within a given budget, more health can be produced by implementing this alternative. For example, Doessel (1978) used a cost per life year saved ratio in comparing alternatives for the treatment of chronic renal failure.

The phrase 'within a given budget' is of crucial importance. Often authors produce a ratio of extra costs per extra unit of health effect of one intervention over another, and call their analysis a cost–effectiveness analysis (e.g. Boyle et al. 1983). However, such studies are not cost–effectiveness analysis studies. Some judgement is required as to whether such extra costs are worth incurring. The resources to meet these extra costs will inevitably come from some other health care programme (i.e. either from another group of patients within the budget or from another budget altogether). This takes us back to broader comparisons, which is the role of cost–*benefit* analysis, not cost–*effectiveness* analysis.

The main limitation of cost–effectiveness analysis (particularly the ratio form) is that the measure of outcome must be one-dimensional. In any study, the outcome measure should be chosen according to the objectives of the interventions evaluated. As a result, however, other important aspects of outcome may be missed by a cost–effectiveness analysis. For example, in evaluating different treatments for chronic renal failure, enhanced (or maintained) quality of life can be as important an outcome as improving life expectancy. Both these aspects of outcome, as the Doessel study demonstrates, cannot be accounted for in a single cost–effectiveness ratio. Also, one should be careful with outcome measures such as cholesterol reduction, blood pressure, and, even more so, cases detected. This is because the relationship between these and final outcome (i.e. health) may be either unclear or not constant across different cases.

Thus cost–effectiveness analysis cannot be used to compare programmes with different goals. Whilst it can be used to compare treatments for chronic renal failure with each other, if we restrict outcome to life years saved, it cannot be used to compare the best chronic renal failure treatment with, say, hip replacements, as the latter mainly affect quality of life.

Cost–utility analysis

Cost–utility analysis lies somewhere between cost–effectiveness analysis and cost–benefit analysis. It can be used to assess not only technical efficiency but also allocative efficiency within the health care sector. The basic outcome in cost–utility analysis is healthy years. The difference between cost–utility analysis and cost–effectiveness analysis is that years of life in states less than 'full health' (e.g. disability) can be converted to healthy years by the use of various techniques. To date, the most common form of conversion is quality-adjusted life-years (QALYs), although another technique, healthy years equivalents (HYEs), is now gaining favour (Williams 1985; Torrance 1986; Mehrez and Gafni 1989; Gafni and Zylak 1990). QALYs are used to combine life-years gained by health care programmes (or existing life-years) with a judgement (usually made by samples of patients or the general population) about the quality of these life-years. Assuming that health-related quality of life can be valued on a scale from zero to unity, where zero is equated with death and unity is equated with full (or normal) health, then 2 years of life in a health state judged to be halfway between these (i.e. valued at 0.5 on the scale) would be equivalent to one year in full health. In this way, life-years are subjected to a quality adjustment, hence the term quality-adjusted life-years. Rather than obtaining a valuation for a health state and multiplying it by the time in that state, HYEs involve describing a scenario of both the state and its duration together. Respondents are asked how many healthy years of life this scenario is equivalent to, hence the term healthy years equivalents. Using HYEs rather than QALYs can have significant effects on priority setting (Gafni and Zylak 1990). Strictly, HYEs are theoretically correct, although there is some debate about this (Culyer and Wagstaff 1993; Gafni et al. 1993). Techniques for eliciting QALYs and HYEs are outlined in the section on measurement and valuation of benefits.

Cost–utility analysis may be seen as an improvement on cost–effectiveness analysis as it attempts to combine more than one outcome measure. Cost–utility analysis can also be seen as an improvement on cost–benefit analysis as it permits comparisons of programmes within the health sector without the need to place monetary values on their benefits. Thus cost–utility analysis addresses allocative efficiency within the health care sector. However, this advantage is limited when non-health benefits and non-health care costs enter into analyses. So far, QALYs and HYEs do not consider non-health aspects of benefit (e.g. utility from process, such as the care environment in long-term care). Likewise, cost–utility analysis can address allocative efficiency within health services if health care costs only are included. Once non-health benefits and non-health care costs are included, a broader framework (cost–benefit analysis) is required for analysis of allocative efficiency.

One of the problems that arises with QALYs is deciding on the best procedure for combining quality of life attributes into a single index; an additional problem is the potential lack of sensitivity of general QALY scales to meaningful change in the health states of people on some health care programmes (Donaldson et al. 1988; Richardson et al. 1990). However, cost–utility analysis is an important technique to use when quality of life is an important outcome. In particular, cost–utility analysis is important where there is the possibility that either one alternative evaluated is better than

others in terms of effects on survival but worse in terms of quality of life, or one alternative is better than others in terms of some aspects of quality of life but worse in terms of other aspects.

Identification of costs and benefits

It is apparent from the previous section that there are several ways of measuring the benefits of health care in economic evaluation. These differences are explored in the section on measurement and valuation of benefits. In this and the following section, our concern is mainly with how to measure costs. However, many of the principles (such as double counting, discounting and marginal analysis) should also be applied to estimation of benefits.

The principles of identifying costs and benefits in cost–benefit analysis, cost–effectiveness analysis, and cost–utility analysis are essentially the same for each type. Identification of relevant costs and benefits involves a listing of all items of resource use and aspects of well-being affected by the project, i.e. in a comparison of the situations with and without the project. This ensures that attention is paid not only to tangible but also to intangible costs and benefits. The process of measurement involves the estimation of amounts of resources used and benefits produced by programmes in naturally occurring units. For instance, staffing resources would be measured in terms of time. The final step involves monetary valuation or estimation of QALYs/HYEs where possible.

Issues of measurement and valuation are discussed in more detail in the section on measurement and valuation of costs. The principles relating to identification are fivefold: to be aware of the question that is being asked, to keep the principle of opportunity cost in mind when identifying costs and benefits, what this implies in terms of categorizing what is a cost and what is a benefit, how far and how wide the analysis should go, and double counting.

What question is being asked?

In any research task, it is important to be aware of the exact nature of the question that is being asked before setting out to collect data in detail. This is no different in an economic evaluation. As Drummond and Mooney (1983) point out, doctors often ask economists the question: Can you please cost this? However, despite this encouraging recognition of the importance of costs, the question is often posed without linking it to the nature of the basic problem to be addressed.

Drummond and Mooney (1983) demonstrate this by reference to a particular example. In one study the answers to a question about the cost of a delivery in a Scottish maternity unit were £540, £510, and £210 (Gray and Steele 1979). To determine which answer is appropriate, we have to look more closely at the basic problem to be addressed. The point is that each of the answers is appropriate, depending on the question being asked. To demonstrate, consider the following questions and answers.

What is the current health service unit cost of a delivery in a Scottish maternity unit? **Answer: £540.**

If we wanted to increase the number of deliveries in Scottish specialist maternity units, assuming that the number of beds are increased, what would be the extra health service unit cost per delivery? **Answer: £510.**

If we wanted to increase the number of deliveries in Scottish specialist maternity units, assuming that the number of beds is fixed, what would be the extra health service cost per delivery? **Answer: £210**.

The first cost is simply an average cost, calculated by dividing the total cost of a unit by the number of deliveries. The other two costs are marginal or incremental costs, which relate to changes in either the size of maternity units or the number of deliveries that can be undertaken within a unit that remains constant in size. Most often, questions relating to economic evaluation are of the latter type, i.e. should we do more or less of this? Obviously, then, it is important to consider marginal costs and benefits. We shall discuss the concept of marginal cost in more detail below. The important point to remember at this stage is that when the question posed is, 'What does X cost?', the first answer is always, 'Why do you want to know?'

Identifying opportunity costs

In keeping with the concept of cost introduced above, items to be identified for inclusion in the cost side of an economic evaluation are any resources that have an opportunity cost as a result of being used in the health care programmes under consideration. This may seem self-evident, but it is not always followed. Instead, analysts sometimes classify any negative effect of a health care programme as costs and positive effects as benefits. Alchian (1972) has noted this tendency:

> to think that because events are valued by comparing the good attributes with the bad, cost must be the bad attributes . . . The value of a given event is obtained by weighing its good and bad consequences against each other . . . but the cost of that event is still not revealed. The highest valued forsaken option must still be ascertained in order to determine the cost . . . What cost really measures is not the bad consequences of an action, but the highest valued forsaken opportunity.

The 'highest valued forsaken' opportunity of an action is of course its opportunity cost. It is the resources used as inputs to health care interventions that have opportunity costs. Such costs are often measured in terms of money, but what we are really concerned with is the benefits of an intervention compared with the benefits we could obtain if that money could be used in another (the next best) activity. Sometimes cost is used to mean burden, but the two are not synonymous in economic evaluation. This means that, beyond resource use, adverse effects of health care on people's well-being should not be counted as costs.

For example, anxiety is often counted as a cost (even though it is rarely valued). A recent example of this has been provided by Buhaug *et al.* (1989). However, anxiety *per se* does not have an opportunity cost—it is not a resource that could be used in some other beneficial activity. This is not to say that anxiety should be ignored; it has a negative effect on well-being and should be counted as such. Assuming all other effects on well-being to be equivalent, if two programmes differ in terms of anxiety and cost, then if one is less costly and incurs less anxiety, it will be more efficient than the other. If one programme is more costly and incurs less anxiety, then a judgement has to be made as to whether the reduction in anxiety is worth the cost incurred. This issue has been the subject of debate in the *Medical Journal of Australia* (Gerard *et*

Table 26.2 Identification of costs for inclusion in economic evaluations

Health care resources

Staffing
Consumables
Overheads
Capital

Other related services

Community services
Ambulance services
Voluntary services

Costs incurred by clients and their families

Inputs to treatment
Out-of-pocket expenses

Time lost from work

Costs borne externally to health and welfare services

al. 1990*a,b*: Stanford 1990). How to measure such effects on well-being is part of the subject matter of the section on the measurement and valuation of benefits.

This example demonstrates that, following Alchian, all negative effects on well-being resulting from a health care programme should be netted out on the benefit side in a cost–benefit analysis, the effectiveness side in a cost–effectiveness analysis, and the utility side in a cost–utility analysis. (Strictly, given that cost–effectiveness analysis may use only one-dimensional measures of outcome, this cannot be done if positive and negative effects are in different dimensions). Likewise, cost savings should be handled as negative costs and netted out on the cost side. In effect, they are savings in resource inputs. This is the only way of ensuring that improvements in well-being, on one side, are compared with their resource (or opportunity) costs on the other. Costs will then reflect resource use, which is correct, as it is resources that have opportunity costs.

Categorizing costs and benefits

General guidance as to what costs should be included in an economic evaluation is given in Table 26.2. All the costs listed relate to resources used. The list is not exhaustive, neither is it appropriate to include the full range of costs listed in Table 26.2 in every evaluation. For instance, community care costs or costs of voluntary workers may often be safely omitted in an evaluation comparing different surgical interventions. Costs included will depend on the objectives and context of the evaluation. Hence, Table 26.2 serves as a checklist. Listing costs in this way represents an attempt to ensure that items that are hard to measure receive as much prominence as easily measurable items.

Health care resource costs are often classified under four main headings: staffing, consumables, overheads, and capital. The most obvious health care resource cost is that of professional staff time, which usually forms the largest part of the running costs of any programme. These costs include doctor, nurse, and other health care professional time spent on the health care programme. Consumable items are those which are used by (or on behalf of) the patient, such as drugs and radiography film, or have to be replaced on a regular basis, such as medical or surgical supplies and equipment.

Less obvious costs are overheads, which are often referred to as non–patient-related costs. Overhead costs are those shared by more than one programme. The most common examples are in hospitals where administration, management, heating, lighting, laundry, linen, and cleaning services are provided centrally. The problem is to determine how much of these costs to allocate to the health care programme being evaluated.

It may be thought that one small programme has no overall effect on such costs, thus presenting an appealing argument for ignoring them. For example, having one less ward is unlikely to change the total financial costs of administration in a large general hospital. However, in the absence of the programme, if people working in centralized departments could have spent their time on some other beneficial activity, there will be an opportunity cost of the programme. This opportunity cost should be valued. Therefore, although the health care programme sometimes does not add to financial costs, it may still have opportunity costs which should be counted. This demonstrates that accounting costs and economic costs are not the same.

Time-scale is also important here. In the short term, admission of some extra patients may have little impact on opportunity costs (i.e. most costs remain fixed). A fixed cost is a cost that does not vary with activity. For example, small numbers of patients admitted to a hospital over a short period of time may have little or no impact on staff costs. In the long run, however, a programme involving a larger number of new patients may have a substantial impact on opportunity costs (i.e. most costs vary with the introduction of the programme). For example, the admission of a large number of patients over time may lead to the employment of extra staff or existing staff working extra hours. What was a fixed cost in one context (i.e. the short term) is now a variable cost in another context (i.e. the longer term). It is variable opportunity costs (i.e. those that change as activity changes) that should be counted in any particular costing context.

Capital items include land and buildings as well as major items of equipment. Health care managers often claim that items of capital and equipment already being used have already been paid for and so should not be included as a cost. This argument is true only when such capital has no alternative beneficial uses (i.e. no opportunity cost). If there is an alternative use, there is an opportunity cost which should be valued in some way. Likewise, even if equipment has no obvious and immediate alternative use, perhaps it could be sold and the proceeds used in another beneficial activity. Again, this opportunity cost should be counted. In addition, time-scale is also important here. The opportunity costs of many capital items may be fixed in the short run but variable in the longer term.

The cost of other related services includes the staffing, supplies, capital, equipment, and overhead costs associated with community, ambulance, and voluntary services. Perhaps the least obvious cost here is that of voluntary services. The argument against their inclusion is based on the reasoning that such services are provided

---

Table 26.3 Identification of benefits for inclusion in economic evaluations

Positive
Health gains (e.g. life-years gained)
Non-health-related effects on well-being (e.g. information, reassurance)
Production gains

Negative
Health deterioration (e.g. side-effects, anxiety)
Non-health-related effects on well-being
Production losses not incurred during treatment

---

free of charge and therefore have a zero cost. However, despite having a zero financial cost, such services will have a positive opportunity cost if their use in one programme prevents their use in another or, indeed, any other activity (e.g. reading, watching television). Once again this is a good example of a case where financial and opportunity costs are likely to diverge.

Clients and families themselves are often used to provide care (for example informal care at home). Once again, such resources are not free and should be counted in an economic evaluation since an opportunity cost is likely to be incurred (Donaldson et al. 1986; Donaldson and Gregson 1989). People caring for elderly relatives may do so at the cost of having paid jobs or participating in some other domestic or leisure activities. It is also important to consider other out-of-pocket expenses, such as transport costs.

All these costs are usually called the direct costs of a health care programme. The identification of the direct costs of a health care programme are often best thought of as a listing of ingredients in a recipe (Drummond et al. 1987). To avoid confusion on the part of the reader, it should be noted at this point that the terms direct and indirect cost are used differently by economists compared with their use by accountants.

Indirect costs of a programme are secondary costs related to paid and unpaid productive activities. Productive activities are those arising from participation in the labour force and from housework. Indirect costs arise because treatment could require confinement to hospital or one's home. This can result in a temporary loss to the community from reduced productive activity. The danger in including such costs is that they may have occurred anyway because of the patient's illness, and so the actual treatment itself does not add to opportunity costs. Thus it is the cost of inputs to treatment that are relevant and not the cost of the patient's illness. The benefit of earlier return to work is a welfare (or well-being) gain to society, which, as we have already established, should be dealt with on the benefit and not the cost side of an analysis.

Costs borne externally to health and welfare services should be recognized. They are rarely included in economic evaluations of health care programmes because they are not easily identifiable and are often very small. An example of such a cost, given by Drummond et al. (1987), is of an occupational health programme that results in higher on-costs of production in a car factory.

Benefits for inclusion in economic evaluations are listed in Table 26.3. This follows directly from the discussion of identifying opportunity costs, including negative as well as positive health effects and negative as well as positive effects in non-health-related well-being. The inclusion of production gains is more controversial, not only because of problems with the human capital approach, but also because it is unclear whether including such gains in addition to other benefits (such as QALYs, HYEs, and willingness to pay) involves double counting, i.e. respondents may have already considered effects on productive activity when giving QALY, HYE, or willingness to pay values.

How far and how wide should we go?

There comes a time when we have to evaluate our own activities, i.e. evaluate the evaluation! Part of this process involves the decision about how extra pieces of information will affect the evaluation. Some costs may not be included in an evaluation, particularly those that are small and difficult to collect. The decision about which costs to include may also depend on the viewpoint of the policymakers. Often health care providers and funders are interested only in costs to the health care system. In other situations, such as evaluation of community care options, it is obviously relevant to examine costs incurred by informal carers or caregivers, such as family and friends. From an economic perspective, the study would ideally take a societal perspective, including as broad a range of costs as possible.

Another common problem here is how far in the future to look. This is a particular problem for preventive programmes. For instance, breast cancer screening may detect breast cancer at an early stage and therefore lengthen life compared with no screening; however, people who survive may develop other conditions in the future. Should the future costs and benefits of treating these (unrelated) conditions be included?

One argument for not including such costs and benefits is that the decision about whether or not to treat a future condition may be separate from the one being taken now and should be based on the costs and benefits of alternative ways of treating the future disease. If the future costs and benefits of treating heart failure make breast cancer screening less efficient than not screening, should we no longer offer screening? With the hope of living longer, people may say 'give me screening but don't treat me if I get heart failure in the future', a perfectly rational and reasonable response, and one that would involve an efficient use of resources.

However, analysts should be careful in evaluating preventive programmes, since life tables are often used to estimate survival owing to the lack of ability to follow up patients over a number of years. These tables permit approximation of survival given certain characteristics (such as age and medical history). Such tables take into account the possibility of such future adverse events as heart failure and the effects (in terms of life-years) of treatment for these adverse events. In principle, the costs of treating future conditions should be included in such cases. In practice, however, there are no cost equivalents to data on life tables. This often makes the estimation of future costs difficult. Despite this, discounting (see the section on the measurement and valuation of costs) of such future costs to present values often reduces their significance to what some analysts have referred to as nothing more than a 'hill of beans' (Bush et al. 1973). Therefore the best approximation may be to use life tables for survival and to ignore future costs of treating other conditions. As a word of caution, the nearer in time such

future costs arise and the more directly related they are to the preventive activity evaluated, the more important it becomes to make some attempt to estimate their magnitude.

Double counting

As well as the problems on the benefit side referred to above, one should be careful to avoid counting the same cost twice. For instance, assume that the aim of a hypothetical economic evaluation is to compare the costs of general practitioners/family doctors versus hospital doctors for minor surgery. For each of these, it may seem appropriate to count the fee paid to doctors and cost the amount of time taken to carry out the procedure separately and then add the two together to obtain a total cost. However, to count costs in such a way would constitute an example of double counting. This is particularly relevant if the fee paid to doctors already accounts for time spent on their activities. To count fees and time costs separately before adding them together would result in an overestimation of the cost of each therapy.

Measurement and valuation of costs
Measurement of costs

After identification comes measurement. In costing, this involves measuring resource use in naturally occurring units. Thus, from Table 26.4, staffing costs will often be measured in units of time, whilst other items of resource use are measured in various other units (e.g. grams of drugs and number of diagnostic tests ordered).

The cost of any item used in a health care programme is made up of the unit cost of the item multiplied by the quantity used. The stage of measurement is important as it involves explicit registration of quantities of items used by programmes being evaluated. Quantities of items used are often more relevant to readers of a report than are expressions of the product of price and quantity, particularly if the reader is from another country or another region of the same country. This is because price and quantity data may vary within and between countries. Costings in which the price and quantity of each item used are expressed separately as well as after they have been multiplied together are more useful. Both prices and quantities can then be adjusted to suit other situations.

Valuation of costs

Many elements of valuing health care costs are straightforward. For instance, we have already said that staffing costs represent the largest component of health care costs. Referring to Table 26.4 again, it is usual to value such costs using wage rates or salaries plus other labour costs. Thus the costs to a programme of a particular grade of nursing staff would be calculated by multiplying hours of nursing time used on the programme by the hourly pay, sick pay, and superannuation. However, although such a procedure may seem straightforward, it is not always advisable simply to accept such monetary figures at face value (see the subsection below on unthinking acceptance of market values). Despite this, market prices are generally accepted as first approximations to the unit cost of most other items within consumable, overhead, and capital categories. Community services, ambulance services, and family/patient expenses should be costed in the same way as health service resources. It should be noted that using patients' and families'

Table 26.4 Measurement and valuation of costs

Resource use	How measured	Basis of valuation
Health services		
Staffing	Time (e.g. hours, months, years)	Wage rates/salaries plus other labour costs
Consumables	Units/amounts consumed	Market prices
Overheads	Units/amounts consumed	Wage rates plus other labour costs/market prices (allocated)
Capital	Units/amounts consumed	Market prices conversion costs/ official valuer's estimate
Other related services		
Community services	Units/amounts consumed	Market prices/ conversion costs/ official valuer's estimate
Ambulance services	Units/amounts consumed	Market prices/ conversion costs/ official valuer's estimate
Voluntary services	Units/amounts consumed	Imputed values for staff costs
Clients and their families		
Inputs to treatment	Hours	Wages rates plus other labour costs imputed values
Expenses	Units/amounts consumed	Market prices/actual expenses
Time lost from work		
	Hours/days/weeks/ years	Wage rates plus other labour costs/imputed values

leisure time also has an opportunity cost. This is difficult to measure. Transport studies have estimated the value of leisure time to be 25 per cent of the local average gross wage rate per hour (Harrison 1974), although a more recent study, specific to health care, has estimated different weights for different types of unpaid activities forgone (Targerson *et al.* 1994).

In finding a monetary value (never mind how good a value) to place on a resource, the greatest problems arise in areas of voluntary care and time lost from housework. No readily available market values exist for such occupations and therefore in most cases a value is imputed from an analogous market. For instance, the wage rate for auxiliary nursing staff has been used to cost inputs by volunteers into respite services for mentally handicapped adults (Gerard 1990). Sometimes it is difficult to find truly analogous markets. For instance, it is difficult to cost housework because of its irregular and long hours, which make it untypical of other occupations. In many cases, average female labour costs may be a more accurate reflection of the opportunity cost of housework.

Despite appearing relatively straightforward, there are a number of principles and pitfalls to take into account in the measurement and valuation of health care costs. These are as follows: counting costs in a base year, discounting, marginal costing, patient-based versus per diem costs, allocation of overhead costs, capital costing, unthinking acceptance of market values, and sensitivity analysis. Each of these is now addressed in turn.

Counting costs in a base year

An obvious but important point about valuation of health care costs is that they should be counted in a base year, i.e. adjusted so as to eliminate the effects of inflation. This should be done because we are interested in real resource use. If the general inflation rate is running at 5 per cent per annum, in one year's time £105 will purchase the same amount of resources as £100 now. Therefore, looking at £105 in a year's time from the perspective of someone now, it is really equivalent to £100. The costs of £100 now and £105 occurring in a year's time are equivalent in real tems (i.e. in terms of the real amounts of resources that they can fund), although their nominal monetary values do not show this to be the case. This is a particular problem when costs of alternative programmes are spread in different proportions across different years, as in the hypothetical example in Table 26.5.

In Table 26.5 surgical and drug therapy are alternative treatments for a hypothetical condition. Each has the same effects but different cost streams with an inflation rate of 5 per cent per annum. With this inflation rate, a cost of £1050 occurring in one year's time is equivalent to £1000 now (i.e. £1050/1.05), and £1102.5 occurring in two years' time is also equivalent to £1000 now (£1102.5/1.05^2).

In this hypothetical example, use of unadjusted costs would result in the conclusion that surgery is more efficient than drug therapy since it is less costly and equally effective. However, the costs of drug therapy appear to be higher only because of inflation. After adjusting costs for the rate of inflation (by adjusting costs to year 0 prices), the two therapies are shown to be equally efficient in terms of resources used.

Costs can also be adjusted to the final year of data collection in an evaluation by inflating costs incurred in previous years. Whether all costs are adjusted to the first or the last year considered will not affect the final result. Also, after undertaking an economic evalua-

Table 26.5 Adjusting costs to base year

Alternatives	Costs arising (£ per person per annum)			
	Year 0	Year 1	Year 2	Total
Surgery	3000			3000
Drug (unadjusted for inflation)	1000	1050	1102.5	3152.5
Drug (adjusted to year 0 prices)	1000	1000	1000	3000

Table 26.6 Hypothetical example of discounting

Alternatives	Costs arising (£ per person per annum)			
	Year 0	Year 1	Year 2	Total
Surgery	3000			3000
Drug (unadjusted for inflation)	1000	1050	1102.5	3152.5
Drug (adjusted to year 0 prices)	1000	1000	1000	3000
Drug (discounted)	1000	952*	907*	2859

* See Appendix.

tion, health care planners may want to reconvert costs to values that are unadjusted for inflation to allow for calculation of the total health care budget for a particular financial year.

Discounting

As stated in the previous subsection, not all costs and benefits of health care programmes occur at the same point in time. The most obvious example is in prevention, where costs are incurred early for the achievement of health benefit later.

The question, then, is should costs (and benefits) occurring at different points in time be given equal weighting? Most economists would say that they should not. This is because individuals in a society display a tendency to prefer to put off costs to the future rather than pay them now. This time preference arises because of the opportunity cost that would arise by allocating funds to paying costs now rather than later and not having those funds available to pursue some other beneficial activity in the meantime. Thus discounting is simply an opportunity cost concept but is applied over time. This myopia partly accounts for the existence of interest rates (i.e. these rates partly reflect the opportunity cost of not being able to use the resources in an alternative way in the meantime).

Other common reasons to explain discounting are diminishing marginal utility of wealth and health. Diminishing marginal utility of wealth refers to the principle that as societies become wealthier over time, the value of an extra £1 in the future is less than the value of an extra £1 now. Likewise, as health improves over time, the value of an extra unit of health improvement in the future is less than that now. At the margin, money and health are worth less over time and therefore future gains and losses in money and health should be discounted.

Summarizing the arguments so far, a cost arising in the future impinges on us less than an equivalent cost arising now. As a result, future costs should be discounted (i.e. given less weighting) in order to reflect this. Similarly, we prefer to have benefits sooner rather than later, and so future benefits should also be discounted.

For example, extending the example given in Table 26.5 to Table 26.6, those costs occurring now (i.e. in year 0) are not discounted. Those occurring in years 1 and 2 are discounted, with year 2 costs

discounted at a higher rate because they are incurred further into the future than year 1 costs. In our example, year 1 and year 2 costs have been discounted back to present values by multiplying the original cost in each year (i.e. £1000) by a discount factor. Usually, discount factors and present values do not have to be calculated as they are often already available in tables, such as that in the Appendix which provides a list of discount factors and present values annually from zero to 50 years at a discount rate of 5 per cent. Some government publications and textbooks contain tables of discount factors at various discount rates (HM Treasury 1982; Drummond *et al.* 1987). The calculation of the discounted costs of our hypothetical drug treatment in years 1 and 2 is explained in the Appendix. From Table 26.6 it can be seen that, after adjusting for inflation and discounting, drug therapy is now less costly (and therefore more efficient) than surgery.

In reality, society's exact discount rate is not known. It is difficult to observe a rate: should it be the rate on long-term government bonds or based on some other interest rates (or average of rates) prevailing in the economy? Drummond *et al.* (1987) recommend a choice of discount rate that is consistent with the following features: it should be consistent with economic theory (between 2 and 10 per cent), include government recommended rates (from 5 to 10 per cent), and be consistent with other published studies and with current practice (from 3 to 10 per cent, but usually 5 per cent).

The recommended rates in England and Scotland are 6 per cent. The Commonwealth Department of Finance in Australia currently recommends a rate of 10 per cent, whilst the Department of Health in Norway recommends a rate of 7 per cent. Given such variation in recommended rates, it is best to test the sensitivity of one's results to variations in the discount rate.

Despite controversy in the United Kingdom, it is conventional (some would say, theoretically correct) to discount benefits (whether or not they are expressed in monetary terms) at the same rate as costs (Cairns 1992; Parsonage and Neuberger 1992).

Marginal or incremental costing

Often decisions relating to health care programmes are not about whether to introduce a programme but, rather, whether to have slightly more or slightly less of a programme. For example, the question may be 'Should we change the screening interval for mammography from three years to one year?' rather than 'Should we have a mammography screening programme at all?'

It follows that it is important to calculate the marginal rather than the average costs of a programme. The marginal cost is the cost incurred or saved from producing one unit more or one unit less of a programme, whereas average cost represents the total cost of the programme divided by total units produced up to the point at which the calculation is made. There is no *a priori* reason to assume that both costs will be equivalent unless total costs rise at a constant rate as the programme is expanded. For instance, although it may cost £25 000 per annum on average to care for an elderly person in hospital, it is unlikely that this amount would be saved if one person less were admitted or that £25 000 would be added to total annual costs if one person more were admitted. This is because certain costs, such as heating, lighting, and some staffing costs, remain fixed and will not vary with small changes in patient load.

Table 26.7 Costs and benefits of strategies to reduce cholesterol

Strategy	(1) Total cost (£)	(2) Total benefit (healthy years)	(3) Added cost (£)	(4) Added benefit (healthy years)	(5) Average cost per healthy year ((1)/(2)) (£)	(6) Marginal cost per healthy year ((3)/(4)) (£)
No action	0	0	0	0		
Population	38 000	3800	38 000	3800	10	10
Combined	40 038 000	4200	40 000 000	400	9530	100 000

Source: Kristiansen *et al.* 1991

To illustrate the principles of opportunity cost and the margin within the context of screening, consider the alternatives for a programme aimed at reducing heart disease in a group of 200 000 men aged 40–49. One alternative is to promote healthy eating in the population in combination with general practitioner screening for high cholesterol levels (serum concentration 6.0–7.9 mmol/l), followed by dietary treatment for those in the relevant range: we shall refer to this as the combined approach. (In the paper cited in Table 26.7, drug treatment was implemented for those with serum cholesterol above 8 mmol/l. This alternative is not considered here.) An alternative is to use population promotion of healthy eating on its own; we shall refer to this as the population approach.

It is assumed that health gain can be measured adequately in terms of healthy years. Table 26.7 shows that the total cost of the combined approach has been estimated at about £40 038 000 with a total benefit of 4200 healthy years, at an average cost of £9530 for each healthy year gained. Whether this represents a reasonable investment is open to question. The question is put beyond doubt, however, when the marginal costs are examined. The second row of data shows that the population approach alone would have yielded 3800 healthy years anyway, at a cost of £38 000 or £10 for each healthy year gained. The additional 400 healthy years are gained by the combined approach at an additional cost of £40 million, a marginal cost of £100 000 for each healthy year gained. The marginal cost for each healthy year gained by the combined programme is over ten times its average cost (thus highlighting the danger of looking at simple averages and hence the importance of marginal analysis!). Reorganization of health care resources to permit the addition of screening and dietary treatment would presumably be judged as not worthwhile. The opportunity cost is too great or, in plainer language, the resources could be better spent on some other health-producing activity.

Another well-known example of the difference between marginal and average costs is that given by Neuhauser and Lewicki (1975), who examined the recommendation by the American Cancer Society that six sequential tests of stool be carried out in order to test for cancer of the colon. The average cost per case of cancer detected after the sixth test was US $2451 (i.e. US $176 337/71.942). However, the incremental gain in cases detected of moving from five to six tests was so small that the marginal cost was US $47 107 214 (i.e. US $13 190/0.0003) per case detected. The study showed that it may not be worth going

beyond two or three tests. It should be noted that the study does not provide an answer to the question of how many tests are worthwhile. It demonstrates what had to be spent to detect an extra case of cancer. In this case policy-makers, not economists, determine what an extra case of colon cancer detected is worth. Although the application of economic principles does not provide an exact answer in such cases, we do end up with a more efficient solution than if the decision were taken in the absence of economic analysis.

Patient-based versus *per diem* costs
Ideally, when comparing two groups of patients consuming alternative types of health care, one would like to follow through each individual's consumption of health care and other resources. Each individual's consumption of resources could then be separately valued and a mean or some other representative cost per patient calculated. What is sought is the difference in resource use with programme patients compared with the alternative situation for these patients.

Valuing opportunity costs is straightforward in some situations (e.g. when nursing is done on a one-to-one basis). Such costing is difficult in other situations because of the problem of joint costing. This problem arises when several patients consume a common resource simultaneously and no rule exists as to how to divide the cost between each individual. For example, a nurse may be providing direct care to one patient on a hospital ward whilst supervising several others. In such circumstances, the cost of the nurse's time cannot be allocated other than arbitrarily. What is required are data on direct contact time with the patient, whether it is a joint activity, and what would have happened in the absence of the patient receiving direct care.

As a last resort, in such cases it is easier to calculate the per diem cost, or cost per bed day, of providing a particular service and multiply this by the length of stay or lengths of use by the patients concerned. For instance, the cost per bed day per annum of a hospital would be calculated by dividing the total cost per annum of running the hospital by the number of bed days per annum used in the hospital.

The problem with using hospital average costs per bed day is that they may not reflect actual resource use by the client group in question if calculated at too general a level. A cost per bed day that is calculated on the basis of that hospital's entire caseload is unlikely to be representative of the cost per bed day for specific conditions. For instance, using a cost per bed day for an entire hospital would

Table 26.8 Simple methods of allocating overhead costs

Department	Method of allocation
Heating, lighting, cleaning	(Square metres taken up by the programme) divided by (square metres taken up by whole hospital) multiplied by (department cost)
Laundry, linen	(Number of requisitions from the programme) divided by (the number of requisitions from the whole hospital) multiplied by (departmental cost)
Administration, management	(Number of cases admitted to the programme) divided by (number of cases admitted to the hospital) multiplied by (departmental cost)

mean that a day spent in intensive care would be credited with the same cost as a day spent in a postnatal ward, or that a day of care for a spinal injuries patient would be costed at the same rate as a day of care for someone recovering from minor surgery.

Therefore it is advisable to isolate costs per bed day for the specialities that are of interest. This is done by isolating total costs per annum at ward level and then dividing by bed days per annum on the ward being costed. The cost of caring for a study patient on that ward would then be calculated by multiplying the number of days that the patient spends on that ward by the cost per bed day for the ward. However, this procedure still requires considerable research effort. For non-hospital or non-institutional settings, such as home nursing or out-patient clinics, similar techniques can be used to calculate a cost per visit. For each study patient, the number of visits would then be multiplied by the cost per visit.

However, it should be remembered that per diem costing, particularly at the hospital rather than the speciality level, is a last resort.

Overhead costs

Overhead costs present us with one of the most difficult valuation problems. These are costs shared by more than one programme but, unlike joint costs, can be divided amongst programmes in an apparently sensible way. As we have said, the most common example arises in a hospital environment where services such as administration, management, heating, lighting, laundry, linen, and cleaning services are provided centrally. The problem for the analyst is to determine how much of the costs of these departments to allocate to the programme being evaluated. Whether one decides to allocate such costs at all will depend on the scale of incremental change considered in the analysis (see the subsection above on marginal or incremental costing).

The solution to this problem is to ensure that overhead costs are allocated to programmes within the hospital on a reasonable basis, i.e. they should represent differences between overhead opportunity costs with and without the existence of the patients concerned. Examples of simple methods of allocation are listed in Table 26.8.

Sometimes these will suffice, although details of more sophisticated overhead allocation mechanisms can be found elsewhere (Drummond *et al.* 1987).

Costing capital

The costs of capital assets, such as land, buildings, and equipment, usually arise at a single point in time. Most frequently this will be at the inception of the programme being evaluated. Despite this, such capital assets are used over time, and at any point in time an asset may be resold for an amount that will be less than its initial cost and that will decrease as time goes by (except for the special case of property in 'boom' periods, which makes no difference to the general approach to dealing with capital costs). Thus, despite an initial one-off outlay, the opportunity costs of capital assets are spread over time. This is accounted for by spreading the opportunity cost of capital assets over the number of years of their life judged relevant in each particular circumstance.

The most common method of doing this is to calculate an equivalent annual cost. Using this method the initial outlay on a capital asset is converted to an annual sum which, when paid over a number of years (usually an estimated or known life of the asset), would add up to the initial value of the capital asset plus the opportunity cost of resources tied up with the asset (because, for example, they could have earned a certain rate of interest if invested). This principle is best understood by relating it to the principle of a mortgage on a house, whereby the cost of the house plus interest charges are reflected in a series of annual (or monthly) equivalent mortgage repayments. As with discount factors and present values, equivalent annual costs do not have to be separately calculated as they are readily available in tables, such as that in the Appendix to this chapter. This table displays the equivalent annual costs of £1 discounted at a rate of 5 per cent for payback periods of zero to 50 years. An example of a conversion of a capital cost to an equivalent annual cost is also provided in the Appendix.

One further problem with costing is in determining a cost for some capital items which can then be converted to an equivalent annual cost. This is not a problem for items that are purchased at the beginning or during the evaluation of a health care programme; these can be costed using the actual purchase prices. Problems arise with items such as land and buildings that already exist at the start of the programme and may have been paid for many years before the programme commenced. Such items should be costed if their use by the health care programme prevents their use in some other beneficial activity. The most common ways of costing such items are to obtain an estimate of the price that the item would attract if made available on the open market, to obtain an estimated cost of replacing the item, or to obtain an estimate of the rental or lease value of the item.

Unthinking acceptance of market values

Economists are often criticized for using market values as a reflection of true opportunity cost. However, such values are often used only as baselines, and adjustments can be made as required. For instance, the readiness of economists to impute values for the unpaid labour of volunteers and home-makers demonstrates that market values are not always accepted at face value (Donaldson *et al* 1986; Donaldson and Gregson 1989). Market values would clearly result in the assignment of zero costs to inputs to care by volunteers and home-makers, despite the fact that these resources have opportunity costs.

One should also be wary of values arising for resources for which markets do exist. For instance, owing to rigidities in modern markets the cost of a doctor is greater than the cost of a nurse. Therefore, other things being equal, a doctor-oriented health care programme will appear to be more costly than a nurse-oriented alternative. However, given the shortage of nurses and the relative glut of doctors in many countries, it may be that investment in the nurse-oriented programme imposes a greater opportunity cost than investment in the doctor-oriented programme. This is because the nurse-oriented programme may attract nurses from other health care specialities, thus reducing or closing down other programmes. Potential benefits to other patients would have to be sacrificed. Therefore, because substantial benefits to other patients are for-gone, a significant opportunity cost is incurred. Alternatively, owing to the glut of doctors, the doctor-oriented programme may involve no opportunity cost to patients in other specialities if it can recruit from the dole queue!

Sometimes it is necessary to attempt to work back to what a market value would have been in the absence of some imposed distortion. For instance, taxes imposed on certain commodities bear no relation to their opportunity cost and often distort the true costs of such commodities. An example of this, cited by Drummond (1980), is in the field of home care versus institutional care for elderly people (see also Wager 1972). In this study, fuel prices were regarded as overstating the opportunity cost of that resource because of the imposition of taxes. Taxes, it was believed, artificially inflated the cost of home nursing relative to institutional care. Therefore the fuel tax was deducted from the estimate of home nursing costs.

These examples demonstrate that, prima facie, market values should be used only as indicators of cost and that analysts should realize that they may not represent true opportunity costs.

Sensitivity analysis

Inevitably, a costing exercise will be subject to some degree of uncertainty. Where one has not been able to estimate costs accurately, some assumptions may have been made about possible values that such costs could take. Sensitivity analysis is useful in such situations as it involves testing the sensitivity of the results (or conclusions) of an evaluation to variations in variables about which one is uncertain.

In situations where the results are not so clear cut, break-even points (where options considered appear to be equally efficient) for the variables subjected to sensitivity analyses should be reported. Readers of a report or article can then judge on which side of the break-even point they lie. A sensitivity analysis can point to where further research is needed for a more accurate estimate of a critical variable.

As an example of sensitivity analysis, Hundley et al. (1995) examined the extra cost of introducing a midwives' unit rather than a consultant-led labour ward in intrapartum care. The baseline extra cost of the midwives' unit was estimated to be £40.71, which would add about 10 per cent to the total costs of delivery. However, there were uncertainties over capital costs and midwife staff costs. For the former it was unclear whether the conversion of rooms for the midwives' unit would have occurred anyway. Deducting this

from the baseline results in an extra cost of £36.89. Similarly, some geographical areas would not require to upgrade midwives as was done in the study location. This would result in an extra cost of £25.01. Combining both these assumptions resulted in an extra cost of £21.19 for the midwives' unit. The midwives' unit would break even only if no extra staff were required as well as no upgrading of existing staff.

The most probable candidates for sensitivity analysis in a costing exercise are production effects, items that have been excluded because of difficulty of collecting data, imputed values, the discount rate, and the lengths of life for capital items. In some cases assumptions about the possible values that a variable can take are arbitrary. On other occasions it may be possible to base a sensitivity analysis on the confidence limits of a statistical estimate of a variable. The effect of such extreme values on results could be tested using upper and lower confidence limits as extreme values. For example, in studying the effects of the use of prophylactic antibiotics on wound infections in Caesarian sections, Mugford et al. (1989) estimated cost effects based on assumptions that the odds of infection would be reduced by either 70 or 50 per cent (the approximate limits of the 95 per cent confidence interval of the odds ratio).

These principles also apply to estimates of benefits. The analyst may be unsure about estimates of life-years gained or quality of life. If so, the sensitivity of results to variation in such estimates should be tested. We now turn to the methods of estimating such benefits.

Measurement and valuation of benefits

Associated with each evaluative technique are particular methods for measuring and valuing benefits. Each of these methods is summarized in Table 26.9 and discussed in this section. The crudest measures of benefit are those used in cost–effectiveness analysis, where benefits are measured in terms of one-dimensional natural units. In cost–utility analysis, benefits are measured not in physical units, but in terms of **healthy years**. Healthy years are represented by a single utility-based health index, which incorporates effects on both quantity and quality of life. The most common measure is the QALY, of which there are two distinct forms —generic QALYs (Williams 1985) and condition-specific QALYs (Torrance 1986). As the names suggest, the former are applicable over a large range of interventions and conditions, while the latter are applied to specific conditions. In recent years an alternative to QALYs, the HYE, has been developed and is becoming increasingly popular (Mehrez and Gafni 1989).*

The most comprehensive (but also the most technically difficult) form of benefit measurement occurs in cost–benefit analysis, where benefits are measured in monetary terms. The two principal methods for doing this are the human capital approach and willingness to pay. The former is rather crude, and in recent years the more sophisticated willingness to pay technique has tended to be favoured. With reference to the subsection on 'cost–benefit analysis' above, even when it is not possible to value all benefits in money terms, cost–benefit analysis can still be useful in setting out

---

* Although used in cost–utility analysis, it should be noted that QALYs and HYEs are narrower concepts of utility than that referred to in the footnote to the first page of this chapter.

Table 26.9 Identification and measurement of benefits in economic evaluation

Evaluative technique	Benefits	Unit of measurement

Cost–effectiveness analysis	Quantity of life
	
	or
	
	Quality of life
		Life-years gained
		
		Natural units:
		  Pain reduction
		  Cases detected
		  Activites of daily living
		  Cholesterol reduction

Cost–utility analysis	Quantity and quality of life	Healthy years:
		  QALYs (generic or
		  condition-specific)
		  HYEs

Cost–benefit analysis	Quantity and quality of life (possibly including some non-health aspects)	Money:
		  Human capital
		  Willingness to pay

a decision-making problem (recall the example of child-proofing of drug containers).

Measures used in cost–effectiveness analysis

As we have said, cost–effectiveness analysis is the simplest form of economic evaluation in health care. In its simplest form, in which costs only are compared, it is necessary to know that the outcomes of alternatives are equivalent or that the less costly alternative is no less beneficial. In such situations it does not matter if outcomes are one-dimensional or multidimensional. For example, in a study comparing different methods of providing long-term care for elderly people, no differences in survival and activities of daily living were found between the alternatives (Bond *et al.* 1989). In view of this, a subsequent study focusing on cost–effectiveness was able to concentrate on cost differences only (Donaldson and Bond 1991).

However, in situations in which cost–effectiveness ratios are used, the outcome (or benefit) in a cost–effectiveness analysis is always measured in terms of one-dimensional natural units. The appropriate measure depends upon the programme being compared. For programmes whose major effect is to extend life, life-years gained would generally be used. In contrast, if the major effect of the programmes is to improve quality of life rather than quantity of life, then some other measure would be more appropriate. For example, in comparing programmes for the prevention of coronary heart disease, unit reductions in serum cholesterol might be an appropriate measure. Similarly, if two antenatal screening programmes are being compared, cases detected might be chosen. The crucial point to note is that only a single measure can be used in the evaluation. Cost–effectiveness ratios cannot measure the effects of a particular intervention on quantity and quality of life, nor can more than one aspect of quality of life be measured in a single ratio. This restriction to a one-dimensional measure of outcome is the main limitation of cost–effectiveness

analysis. Concentration on one aspect of benefit may mean that other important benefits are overlooked. Consider an example in which dialysis is compared with transplantation for the treatment of chronic renal failure. Since a major effect of both interventions is the prolongation of life, they can be compared in terms of cost per life-year gained. However, the two interventions also differ in the extent to which they affect quality of life. In general, quality of life following a successful transplant will be higher than quality of life associated with dialysis (Klarman *et al.* 1968; Doessel 1978). However, by choosing life-years gained as the measure of outcome, these effects on quality of life cannot be incorporated explicitly into the evaluation.

Generic QALYs

The best known and most widely used generic QALY measure is that derived from the Rosser and Watts (1972) classification of states of illness. This classification defines eight levels of disability and four levels of distress (Table 26.10). By combining the disability and distress levels in a 4 × 8 matrix, 32 pairwise combinations of disability and distress (health states) are defined. Of these, only 29 are usable since it is not meaningful to assign levels of distress to the disability state of being unconscious.

Kind *et al* (1982) used a sample of 70 subjects to assign values to each of the 29 states. Six widely dispersed market states were taken as representing the full range of illness. Subjects were initially asked to place these states in rank order of severity. Each subject was then presented with the first two states and asked how many times more ill they thought that a person in the second state was compared with the first. This question was repeated for each successive pair of marker states, and the value for each ratio was multiplied by that for each succeeding ratio. The remaining 23 states were assigned values in a similar way. This method of valuation is known as magnitude estimation (Froberg and Kane 1989). In addition, subjects were asked to assign a score of zero to

Table 26.10 Rosser and Watts classification of states of ill-ness

Disability		Distress	
I	No disability	A	No distress
II	Slight social disability		
III	Severe social disability and/or slight impairment of performance at work. Able to do all housework except very heavy tasks	B	Mild distress
		C	Moderate distress
IV	Choice of work or performance at work very severely limited. House-wives and old people able to do light housework only but able to go shopping	D	Severe distress
V	Unable to undertake any paid employment. Unable to continue any education. Old people confined to home except for escorted outings and short walks and unable to do shopping. Housewives able to perform a few simple tasks		
VI	Confined to chair or to wheelchair or able to move around in the house only with support from an assistant		
VII	Confined to bed		
VIII	Unconscious		

the state to which they thought it reasonable to restore all patients and to locate death amongst the disability/distress states and to place a value on it. The values were transformed and rescaled so that state IA was assigned a value of 1.0 and death was assigned a value of 0.0. The resultant matrix is shown in Table 26.11. States VIIIA and VIID were regarded as being worse than death, and hence were assigned negative values. The value attached to each health state in the matrix can be regarded as a quality adjustment factor (or weight) for that state. If it is possible to chart the progress

Table 26.11 The Rosser index

Disability	Distress			
	A	B	C	D
I	1.000	0.995	0.990	0.967
II	0.990	0.986	0.973	0.932
III	0.980	0.972	0.956	0.912
IV	0.964	0.956	0.942	0.870
V	0.946	0.935	0.900	0.700
VI	0.875	0.845	0.680	0.000
VII	0.677	0.564	0.000	-1.486
VIII	-1.028	n/a	n/a	n/a

of an individual through the matrix over time, the time spent in each state can be multiplied by the appropriate weight and the resultant values summed to produce a QALY score.

This QALY score is the gross number of QALYs generated from the particular intervention being evaluated. However, what is needed is the gain in QALYs from the intervention over and above the QALYs produced from an alternative intervention/existing practice. Therefore it is necessary to estimate profiles for the intervention being evaluated and the alternative intervention/existing practice.

The process of calculating QALYs from the Rosser index is probably best explained with an example (adapted from Gudex and Kind (1988)). Williams (1985) looked at the benefits of coronary artery bypass grafting as an alternative to medical management for the treatment of angina and extensive coronary artery disease. Three cardiologists were asked to judge the health profiles of various patients with angina. The profiles were estimated for surgical management (coronary artery bypass grafting) and medical management, and were expressed in terms of the Rosser index. Table 26.12 shows an example of a profile for an individual suffering from severe angina and left main vessel disease.

For medical management, it was estimated that the individual has a life expectancy of five more years, the first three of which would be spent in a health state equivalent to IVB (quality of life score 0.956) and the last two in a state equivalent to VC (quality of life score 0.900). For reasons explained in the section on the measurement and valuation of costs, a discounted quality of life score was calculated by multiplying each score by an appropriate discount factor (using a 5 per cent discount rate). The total QALYs produced from medical management was found to be 4.049 QALYs. A similar calculation was performed for surgical management (total QALYs produced, 8.165). Therefore the QALY gain from surgical management is $8.165 - 4.049 = 4.116$ QALYs. This total then had to be adjusted. Since 30 per cent of patients have no symptomatic relief after surgery, the maximum QALY gain is $(1.0 - 0.3) \times 4.116 = 2.881$. In addition, adjustment has to be made for the 3 per cent of patients who were expected to die as a result of surgery. These patients lose QALYs that might otherwise have been gained if they had undergone medical management. The QALY loss is $0.03 \times 4.049 = 0.121$. Therefore the net QALY gain per patient from coronary artery bypass grafting over medical management is $2.881 - 0.121 = 2.76$. The cost of coronary artery bypass grafting for severe angina and left main vessel disease over and above medical management was estimated to be £2860. Combining this cost with the QALYs gained allows the calculation of a cost per QALY ratio of £2860/2.76 = £1040, i.e. the cost of producing one QALY from coronary artery bypass grafting is £1040.

Before moving on to discuss condition-specific QALYs, it should be noted that the Rosser index is not the only method of generating generic QALYs. Two other methods are multi-attribute utility models (Torrance et al. 1982) and Euroqol (Euroqol Group 1990; Williams 1993). Multi-attribute utility models have not been widely used, and Euroqol is a relatively recent development. The Euroqol instrument comprises five dimensions of health-related quality of life (mobility, self-care, usual activities, pain/discomfort, and anxiety/depression), each of which has three levels. Health states are described in terms of different levels of the five dimensions. The inclusion of two extra states, unconscious and

Table 26.12 Calculation of QALYs

Years of remaining life	Medical management				Surgical management			
	Quality of life level	Quality of life score	Discount factor	Discounted quality of life score	Quality of life level	Quality of life score	Discount factor	Discounted quality of life score
1	IVB	0.956	0.952	0.910	IIA	0.990	0.952	0.942
2	IVB	0.956	0.907	0.867	IIA	0.990	0.907	0.898
3	IVB	0.956	0.864	0.826	IIA	0.990	0.864	0.855
4	VC	0.900	0.823	0.741	IIA	0.990	0.823	0.815
5	VC	0.900	0.783	0.705	IIA	0.990	0.783	0.775
6	Dead	0.000	0.746	0.000	IIA	0.990	0.746	0.738
7					IIIB	0.972	0.711	0.691
8					IIIB	0.972	0.677	0.658
9					IIIB	0.972	0.645	0.627
10					IIIB	0.972	0.614	0.597
11					IIIB	0.972	0.585	0.596
12					Dead	0.000	0.557	0.000
Total		4.688		4.049		10.80		8.165

dead, means that there are 245 possible health-state descriptions. Health states are valued by means of a visual analogue scale. This is simply a vertical line on a page divided into a hundred equal intervals with the endpoints marked worst imaginable health state and best imaginable health state. Subjects are presented with health-state descriptions and asked to mark on the visual analogue scale how good or bad they think that each is. These values provide the quality adjustment factors (or weights) for use in the calculation of QALYs. Euroqol has been the subject of criticism (Carr-Hill 1992; Gafni and Birch 1993). However, it is still in the developmental stage (more recent work has used another measurement technique—the time trade-off (see below)—alongside the visual analogue scale), and its success or otherwise remains to be seen.

Condition-specific QALYs

The main difference between condition-specific and generic QALYs lies in the way in which health states are described to subjects. With condition-specific QALYs the health-state descriptions focus on the characteristics of the condition being evaluated. This is in contrast with generic QALYs where the health-state descriptions are more general. An important consequence of this distinction is that condition-specific QALYs cannot (should not) be used in league tables (see below).

There are two main methods of generating condition-specific QALYs: standard gamble and time trade-off.

The standard gamble is based directly on the axioms of standard utility theory; it is the classic method of measuring preferences under uncertainty. The technique can be used to measure health-state preferences for chronic and temporary health states. The discussion here focuses on the use of the technique to calculate QALYs for a chronic health state preferred to death. For details of how the standard gamble can be applied to temporary health states and health states not preferred to death see, for example, Froberg and Kane (1989) or Torrance (1986).

An example of the standard gamble framework for a chronic health state preferred to death is shown in Fig. 26.1. To measure

preferences for health state i, subjects are asked to choose between two alternatives. One offers the certain outcome of remaining in the chronic health state for the rest of one's life, whilst the other is a gamble representing a treatment with two possible outcomes. These outcomes are (1) return to full health for the rest of one's life (with an associated probability p of occurring), and (2) immediate death (which has a probability of occurrence of $1-p$). The probability p of a successful outcome is varied by an iterative process until the subject is indifferent (i.e. cannot choose) between the gamble and the certainty. The probability p^* at which the subject is indifferent is used to calculate the utility value of the health state as follows. The outcomes 'return to full health' and 'death' are assigned utility values of unity and zero respectively. At the indifference probability p, the value (measured in terms of expected utility) of the two alternatives is equal, yielding the following simple equation:

$$U(\text{state } i) = p^*U(\text{full health}) + (1-p^*)U(\text{death}).$$

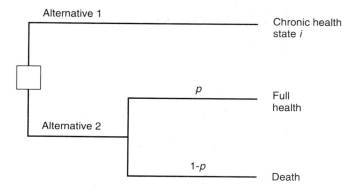

Fig. 26.1 Standard gamble for a chronic health state preferred to death.

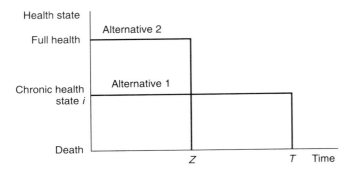

Fig. 26.2 Time trade-off for a chronic health state preferred to death.

Because the utility from full health equals 1.0 and the utility from death equals 0.0, this equation can be reduced to

$$U(\text{state } i) = p^*$$

Therefore, for the case of a chronic health state preferred to death, the utility of the health state is simply p^* (the indifference probability).

The utility of the health state can then be used to calculate the number of QALYs from the treatment. Consider an example of an intervention for treating a chronic condition which, if successful, will result in a return to full health. Suppose that the utility of the chronic health state without the intervention is 0.7 (elicited by presenting an individual with a standard gamble question) and that the individual has a remaining life expectancy of 30 years. If the utility of full health is unity, the gain in QALYs to the individual from successful intervention is given by

$$(1.0 - 0.7) \times 30 = 9 \text{ QALYs.}$$

Time trade-off was developed by Torrance *et al.* (1972) as a substitute for the standard gamble technique. The intention was to develop a technique specifically for use in health care, which gave the same (or similar) values as the standard gamble but which was easier for subjects to understand. Two important differences between time trade-off and the standard gamble should be noted. First time trade-off does not have an axiomatic foundation, and second, subjects are asked to choose between two certain alternatives rather than between a certain outcome and a gamble. Like the standard gamble, time trade-off can be used to elicit health-state preferences for chronic and temporary health states that may or may not be preferred to death. An example of a time trade-off framework for a chronic health state preferred to death is shown in Fig. 26.2. Preferences for health state i are established by eliciting from subjects the number of years in full health (Z years) that is equivalent to spending the rest of their life (T years) in the chronic health state. The value Z^* at which the subject is indifferent between the two alternatives is used to calculate the value of the health state as follows. Full health is assigned a value of unity and death a value of zero. It is assumed that individuals have a value function of the form $V = h_i T$, where h_i is the preference value for health state i ($0 \leqslant h_i \leqslant 1$) and T is remaining years of life.*

---

* A value function assigns a real number to each possible outcome in a choice problem under certainty. Utility functions are appropriate for uncertain choices.

At Z^*, the value functions of the two alternatives are equal, yielding the following equation:

$$V(\text{alternative } 1) = V(\text{alternative } 2)$$

$$h_i T = 1.0 \times Z^*.$$

Therefore the preference value for the chronic health state i is,

$$h_i = Z^* / T.$$

The value of the health state can be used to calculate the number of QALYs from the treatment in the same way as described above for the standard gamble.

Healthy years equivalents

In recent years an alternative to QALYs has been developed—the HYE (Mehrez and Gafni 1989). Like QALYs, HYEs combine quantity and quality of life into a single measure. Unlike QALYs, however, it is claimed that HYEs fully represent individual preferences as they are calculated from the individual's utility function. It is argued that QALYs only partially incorporate patient preferences since utility-based measures are used to calculate health-state weights only. A utility-weighted index (i.e. a QALY) would be a utility function only under very restrictive assumptions (Torrance and Feeny 1989).

The definition of a HYE for a chronic health state is as follows (for a more general definition see Mehrez and Gafni (1989)). Let Q represent the chronic health state of an individual and T the individual's remaining years of life. Let $U(Q,T)$ be the utility function of the individual, which describes the utility of being in health state Q for T years followed immediately by death. Let Q^* represent full health and H^* the healthy years equivalent of (Q,T). The problem is defined as follows:

$$\text{find } H^* \text{ such that } U(Q^*,H^*) = U(Q,T).$$

The solution to the above equation yields a hypothetical combination of H^* years in full health (Q^*), which is equivalent, in terms of utility, to living T years in the chronic health state, Q.

In general, the measurement of HYEs requires the identification and measurement of an individual's utility function over his or her projected lifetime health profile. This is a complex procedure. However, for the case of the chronic health state described above, a simple algorithm has been devised to measure HYEs (Mehrez and Gafni 1991). The algorithm uses the standard gamble technique to measure HYEs directly without the need to assess the utility function first. An example of the algorithm (a two-stage standard gamble procedure) for a chronic health state i is shown in Fig. 26.3. In stage 1 subjects are asked to choose between the certain outcome of remaining in the chronic health state for the rest of their lives and a gamble representing a treatment that will either restore them to full health with probability p or will result in their death with probability $1-p$. The indifference probability p^* is elicited and is carried forward to the standard gamble question in stage 2. Here subjects are asked to choose between a gamble with the outcomes of full health for the rest of their life (probability of occurrence p^*) and death (probability of occurrence $1-p^*$) and the certain outcome of H years in full health. The value of H is varied by means of an iterative process until subjects cannot choose between the gamble and the certain outcome. The value of H at which subjects are

Stage 1

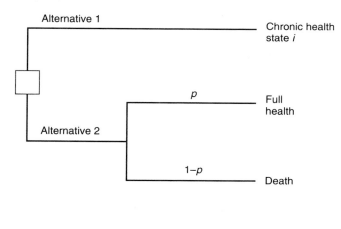

Stage 2

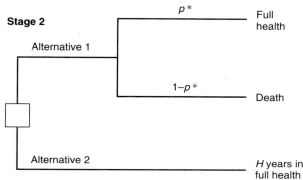

Fig. 26.3 Two-stage standard gamble algorithm for measuring HYEs.

indifferent (H^*) is the healthy years equivalent of the chronic health state i.

It has been argued that this algorithm is merely an unnecessarily complicated way of asking what is essentially a time trade-off question (Buckingham 1993; Johannesson *et al*. 1993). In addition, HYEs have also been criticized at a more general level (Culyer and Wagstaf 1993). Advocates of HYEs have responded to this criticism (in our opinion convincingly), and the interested reader is referred to the debate (Gafni *et al*. 1993; Mehrez and Gafni 1993).

One of the major criticisms of QALYs *vis-à-vis* HYEs is that QALYs are only partially based on individual preferences. To calculate QALYs, the utility weight of a health state is multiplied by the time spent in the health state. The utility weight is based on individual preferences but the duration is not. The conversion of time spent in a particular health state to time in full health is assumed to be linearly related to the time spent in the health state, i.e. one year in a health state with a utility weight of 0.5 is equivalent to six months in full health (utility weight, 1.0). HYEs do not make this assumption. The algorithm for calculating HYEs allows individuals to express their preferences for both the health state and the duration. The linearity assumption of the QALY procedure implies that health states that are very painful but last only a very short time are of negligible effect. However, it is claimed that this assumption is restrictive and in some instances may lead to a potential misrepresentation of patients' preferences. Gafni and Zylak (1990) claim to demonstrate this in a study focusing on a

comparison of ionic and non-ionic contrast media in diagnostic radiology. Short-duration effects in the form of minor reactions are the most comon outcome of using ionic contrast media. The major effect of non-ionic contrast media is to reduce these short-term side-effects. An earlier study by Goel *et al*. (1989) calculated that the cost per QALY gained from introducing non-ionic contrast media was US $64 000. Gafni and Zylak (1990) claim that such a high ratio was a result of there being a very small QALY gain from non-ionic compared with ionic contrast media. They argue that the small gain was attributable to the implicit assumption in the QALY procedure that short-term effects are negligible. The following example was cited to illustrate this claim.

A person has 30 years to live but has to go through a very painful test that takes one hour on average. When asked, the person rates his or her quality of life during the test as being close to death (0.05 when death is defined as zero). Calculating the QALY value of living for 30 years in full health, interrupted by a very painful examination, we find that it is equal to 29.9999 (0.05 × 0.000114 years) + 1.0 (30 years − 0.000114 years). Note that one hour is equal to 0.000114 of a year. It is easy to see that the effect of suffering one hour of pain is negligible.

Based on the assumptions of the earlier study, Gafni and Zylak (1990) calculated a cost per HYE gained from non-ionic contrast media of approximately US $25 000. They argue that the reason that this figure is lower than the cost per QALY figure is that the calculation of HYEs allows individuals to reveal a preference for short-term effects that may not necessarily be negligible.

From a theoretical perspective, HYEs have much to recommend them. However, as yet there have been very few practical applications of the technique. Clearly, more empirical work is necessary before overall judgement can be passed upon whether or not HYEs are to be preferred to QALYs as a measure of health-related quality of life.

Monetary measures

Of the three main techniques of economic evaluation, cost–benefit analysis is, in principle, the most powerful. It is the only form of evaluation that addresses the question of whether or not a particular intervention is worthwhile, i.e. whether the benefits of an intervention exceed its cost. Such a comparison is made possible by the costs and benefits of interventions being measured in commensurate units, with the most common numeraire being money. In theory, all costs and benefits of an intervention should be included in a cost–benefit analysis. However, as we have said, there are difficulties in assigning monetary values to health care benefits. In recent years the most common method of measuring health care benefits in cost–benefit analysis has been willingness to pay. However, the application of willingness to pay to health care is a relatively recent phenomenon, and for many years the dominant measurement technique was the human capital method.

Under the human capital approach individuals are treated like items of capital which are valued because of their potential contribution to future output. Therefore health improvements are valued in terms of future productive worth to society from individuals being able to return to work following the health improvement. Productive worth tends to be proxied by future earnings potential. The human capital approach is seriously flawed. For example, an implication of this approach is that the only reason for providing health care is to enable people to work. The method also discriminates against women, elderly people, and the unemployed. Despite this, the approach has been widely applied in health care and, in particular, to the valuation of human life (Rice and Cooper 1967).

It is generally acknowledged that willingness to pay is a more theoretically correct, and therefore superior, measure of benefit than human capital. The principle of willingness to pay is very simple—the utility that an individual gains from something is valued by the maximum amount that he or she would be willing to pay for that something. The technique of willingness to pay is often criticized for attempting to assign a monetary value to things that are considered by many to be incommensurate with monetary valuation (e.g. the environment, human life, etc.). However, it has to be remembered that such valuations are being made anyway. These valuations arise from the implicit judgements of decision-makers (for example, the US $47 million spent in detecting a case of cancer of the colon, referred to above). What is important is not the unit of value *per se*, but rather the notion of sacrifice embodied in the technique. In economics, something only has value if an individual is prepared to sacrifice something in order to acquire it. In valuing a health care programme, it is difficult to ask respondents what services they would give up to have more of that programme. It is easier to ask individuals to state the maximum amount that they would be willing to pay for more of the programme and for some possible alternative uses of those resources. Thus it is largely for convenience that money is the chosen numeraire.

There have been relatively few published studies using willingness to pay in a health care context (Donaldson 1993). In general, these studies can be divided into those that ask individuals to value health gain (e.g. Thompson 1986; Johannesson 1992) and those in which individuals are asked to value health care (e.g. Easthaugh 1991; Johannesson *et al.* 1991). Willingness to pay for health care can lead to a possible advantage of willingness to pay over other measures of benefit discussed so far in that it provides the opportunity for individuals to value other potential benefits of health care beyond just health gain. The value of a health care intervention can be measured by the maximum amount individuals are prepared to pay for the intervention. Exactly how much individuals are willing to pay will depend upon the perceived benefits to them of the intervention. One of the assumptions of QALYs and HYEs is that the only benefit from health care is improvement in health-related quality of life. However, there is evidence that this is not always the case (Berwick and Weinstein 1985; Mooney and Lange 1993; Donaldson *et al.* 1993). Other possible sources of benefit might include the provision of information (e.g. from screening), dignity (e.g. in long-term care), autonomy (e.g. in community care), and the process of care (e.g. invasive versus non-invasive interventions). Willingness to pay for health care allows individuals to value these (and other) possible sources of benefit whereas QALYs/HYEs do not.

In publicly financed health care systems, such as the United Kingdom National Health Service, individuals do not normally pay for health care at the point of consumption. As such, the elicitation of willingness to pay values usually entails presenting individuals with descriptions of the health care interventions being evaluated and asking them to imagine that they do have to pay. Depending upon the context of the evaluation, there are a number of different ways in which individuals can be asked to imagine they have to pay. These include out-of-pocket payments (Miedzybrodzka *et al.* 1994), one-off extra taxation payments (Olsen and Donaldson 1993), and payments for insurance (Gafni 1991). Willingness to pay values can be elicited either by interviews or by postal questionnaires, although it has recently been recommended that whenever possible interviews should be carried out (Arrow *et al.* 1993). However, this is not always feasible.

As with QALYs, there are a number of different ways of asking willingness to pay questions. These include payment card questions in which subjects are presented with a series of prompts and are asked to select a value which corresponds to their maximum willingness to pay, open-ended questions in which respondents are asked to state their maximum willingness to pay without prompting, and closed-ended questions in which each respondent is presented with a willingness to pay value and asked to indicate whether or not they would be prepared to pay that value. Each method has its advantages and disadvantages, and there is no overall consensus as to which is the best method (Johannesson and Jönsson 1991).

The willingness to pay technique is not without its problems. A frequent criticism is that it is inevitably a function of ability to pay, which, it is argued, could have implications for equity. Ability to pay undoubtedly affects absolute willingness to pay, but there is evidence to suggest that it does not affect relative willingness to pay (Donaldson *et al.* 1994). Another potential problem is that respondents may have difficulty relating to the concept of having to pay for health care. This is a particular problem in publicly financed health care systems (for example, in the United Kingdom).

Despite these problems, the use of willingness to pay in health care evaluation is growing in popularity. One of the main reasons for this is that, unlike the other measures of benefit discussed in this section, willingness to pay allows more to be valued than simply improvements in health-related quality of life.

The use of cost per QALY and willingness to pay data in health care decision-making

So far, we have focused on the measurement and valuation of benefits *per se*. However, it is also important to consider how the different measures of benefit can be used in practice to aid decision-making. In particular, it is useful to discuss the practical applications of cost per QALY and willingness to pay data.

Cost per QALY ratios

Cost per QALY ratios have two principal applications. The first is to compare alternative interventions for the same condition. Here, the intervention with the lowest cost per QALY ratio is the most technically efficient. This is very similar to simple cost-effectiveness analysis, with the main difference being that QALYs are a broader and more sophisticated measure of benefit than life-years gained or some other one-dimensional measure of outcome. In practice the choice between cost–effectiveness analysis and cost–utility analysis will depend upon what is being evaluated and the extra costs of performing the more complicated cost–utility analysis.

The second (and more problematic) use of cost per QALY ratios is to help judge relative priorities across different programmes in health care. Cost per QALY ratios can be calculated for a wide variety of disparate interventions, ranging from general practice advice to give up smoking, chiropody, etc., to renal dialysis and heart transplantation. Because the measure of outcome is the same for all interventions, valid across-programme comparisons can be made. It is possible to construct cost per QALY league tables in which interventions are ranked in terms of increasing cost per QALY ratios, i.e. decreasing relative efficiency. In principle, it should be possible to maximize the number of QALYs from a health care budget by allocating resources to those interventions with the lowest cost per QALY ratios. Indeed, such an exercise has actually been carried out in the state of Oregon in the United States, although not without problems (O'Neill 1990; Dixon and Welch 1991).

QALY league tables have been criticized on a number of grounds, and great care should be taken in their construction and interpretation (Gerard and Mooney 1993; Birch and Gafni 1994). Among the many potential problems of QALY league tables, the following are particularly worthy of note. The most serious problem is that each item in the league table has a different comparator. The cost per QALY gained of programme A may have been produced by comparing programme A with programme B. However, if B is inefficient to begin with, A may also be inefficient. Yet, even if A is inefficient, it may still look good because it was compared with B (another inefficient programme).

League tables also contain programmes of various sizes. Thus a small programme C, which is further down the table, could be combined with a programme D, which is higher up, to produce more QALYs than a larger programme E in the middle. Thus, the opportunity cost of E would be the QALYs forgone from not being able to invest in C and D. Yet the league table would imply that E is to be preferred to C.

Another potential problem is that, to date, QALYs measure only health gain. However, there may be other benefits of health care (such as the provision of information, autonomy, etc.) which are important to patients but which cannot be included in the QALY framework. Implicit in the use of QALY league tables to set health care priorities is the assumption that the only form of benefit relevant to such priority setting is QALYs or health gain. However, it was stated above that this may not always be the case.

An additional problem arising from the assumption that health gain is the only output of health care is that non-health service costs cannot be included in cost per QALY values. Since it is assumed that the only output of health services is QALYs, the opportunity cost of devoting resources to a particular intervention is measured solely in terms of QALYs forgone elsewhere. Other resources such as patient time and travel costs, which have wider opportunity costs than just QALYs forgone, cannot be included. Hence in this respect cost per QALY league tables are limited in addressing questions of allocative efficiency.

Related to the point about comparators, the correct term for QALY league tables is marginal cost per QALY gained league tables; marginal, not average, values are relevant. The margin is defined in terms of changes in costs and benefits of expanding or contracting the existing programme to some higher or lower level of output. This emphasis on the margin means that there are problems in transferring cost per QALY values from one location to another. This is because the basis for comparison will vary between different locations. On the cost side, different locations will tend to have different cost structures and therefore different marginal costs of expansion and contraction. On the benefit side, the capacity of individuals in one location to benefit from a particular intervention will tend to be different from that of individuals in another location, thus leading to different levels of QALYs gained. Because of this potential for variations at the margin between locations, it is likely that a cost per QALY league table used in one location will not be applicable to other locations. Ideally, therefore, if (and it is a big 'if') cost per QALY league tables are to be used for priority setting, they should be locally based. The correct application of a crude locally based league table is preferable to the misapplication of a more sophisticated league table from another location.

It should be apparent that there are problems with QALY league tables. It is likely that the process of constructing a league table may be more important than the table itself, since it provides purchasers with an explicit framework within which to address the problems of priority setting.

Willingness to pay

Like cost–utility analysis, cost–benefit analysis can be used as an aid to priority setting across health care programmes. By comparing the benefits of interventions (measured in terms of willingness to pay) with their costs of provision, it is possible to compare interventions in terms of their net benefits. This method of priority setting is arguably superior to the use of cost per QALY league tables in that the measure of benefit is not restricted to health gain and a wider range of costs can be included (e.g. costs to patients etc.).

A recent example of using willingness to pay to aid priority setting was an evaluation of public sector health care programmes in northern Norway (Olsen and Donaldson 1993). Members of the public were asked their willingness to pay in extra taxation for each of the following: the introduction of a helicopter ambulance service to serve remote communities, an expansion in the number of heart operations performed, and an expansion in the number of hip operations performed. The helicopter ambulance service was considered to be a particularly interesting service on which to perform a willingness to pay study because it possessed certain non-health-enhancing but potentially utility-bearing characteristics: it is a rescue service, which may reduce anxiety among people in rural areas, people may derive utility from knowing that the service is available should it be required, and it contributes to the reduction of regional inequalities of access. Subjects were presented with detailed descriptions of the programmes and were told that only one could be implemented. They were also asked to state the reasons for their willingness to pay responses. The results not only provided information on the relative intensity of people's preferences (willingness to pay for the ambulance service and heart operations was significantly different from that for hip operations), but also indicated that individuals were concerned with more than just health gain from health care. This was shown by subjects' concern for other people's access to care. It appeared that subjects were prepared to express this concern in the values that they ascribed to the ambulance service *vis-à-vis* the other programmes.

The use of willingness to pay is not restricted to issues of allocative efficiency—it can also be used to address cost–

effectiveness questions. A recent example of this is the study by
Meidzybrodzka *et al.* (1994) in which the relative benefits of two
alternative methods of administering an antenatal carrier screening
test for cystic fibrosis were estimated. The study took place in the
context of a randomized trial comparing the two screening methods
(disclosure and non-disclosure). Women in each arm of the trial
were asked their maximum willingness to pay for the method they
received. The results showed no statistically significant difference
between the two methods.

In view of the finding that the overall mean willingness to pay
value for screening was greater than the corresponding cost, it
might be tempting to conclude that carrier screening is worthwhile.
However, such a conclusion should not be drawn. The willingness
to pay values for screening are the absolute values for users of the
service only. The opportunity cost context of the willingness to pay
exercise was restricted to alternative uses of the resources for
screening for cystic fibrosis. Other possible uses of the resources
(i.e. the provision of other health care services) were not considered. Yet the true opportunity cost of the decision to devote
resources to screening for cystic fibrosis is the benefit forgone from
not using those resources in another part of the health care sector.
Therefore the decision to invest in screening is a community
decision. When using willingness to pay values to aid priority
setting (particularly in a publicly financed health care system), the
relative values of members of the community are of importance (see
the northern Norway example above), and not the absolute values
of users. The willingness to pay values of users indicate the
strength of preference of the users for the services being evaluated
and are still useful in that context. For instance, such values could
indicate that the preferences of a minority group are particularly
strong. If this strength of preference is not sufficient to outweigh
that of the majority, such values may still indicate to the decision-
maker that providing both types of care evaluated is the fairest
option. However, it should be remembered that providing such
choice may come at a substantial cost.

Conclusions

The aim of this chapter has been to provide the reader with a step-
by-step guide to the principles of costing and measurement of
benefits in the economic evaluation of health care, and to use simple
examples to illustrate how some of the concepts can be applied. It
is important to follow such principles in order to render such work
relevant to the decision contexts of economic evaluation.

As a result of providing a general overview, not all the principles
outlined in this chapter will be applicable to every evaluation
undertaken. For instance, one would not apply the principle of
discounting to an evaluation of health care alternatives whose costs
and effects occur over a period of only a few months. However, it
is important to use the principles outlined here as a checklist of
which costs and benefits should be valued and how this is to be
done. The checklist basically comprises the questions listed in
Table 26.13. These questions should be addressed in advance of an
evaluation. The answers to each of them will very much determine
the nature of the exercise carried out. However, it is also important
to refer to the checklist whilst an evaluation is ongoing and once it
has been completed.

The task may seem daunting and often is. However, answering
each of these questions will render any evaluation not only easier in

Table 26.13 Checklist for economic evaluation of health care

1   What economic question is being asked?
2   What are the alternatives being evaluated?
3   What changes in service provision are being considered?
4   From whose viewpoint(s) are costs and benefits being esti-
    mated?
5   What resources are used by each of the programmes to be eval-
    uated?
6   Which of these resources incur true opportunity costs?
7   Which groups in society bear the burden of the cost of these
    resources: health services, insurance companies, clients, clients'
    families?
8   What are the benefits and who receives these benefits?
9   Are there any production effects associated with client participa-
    tion in the programme?
10 Are there any costs identified which would have no impact on the
    result of the evaluation or whose collection requires too much
    research effort relative to their potential impact?
11 Can results be expressed in terms of quantities of resources
    used as well as their prices?
12 Do readily available market values exist for items (staffing, con-
    sumable, overhead, capital) costed? If not, from where can
    imputed values be obtained?
13 Are costs and benefits spread over a number of years, thus
    raising the importance of
    • counting costs in a base year?
    • discounting?
14 What is the decision context with respect to marginal costs/
    benefits? Are we talking about the introduction of a totally new
    programme, the expansion of an existing programme, or a com-
    parision of a new with an expanded programme?
15 Can patient-based costing be carried out? If not, how can accu-
    rate per diem costs be obtained?
16 What are the appropriate mechanisms for the allocation of over-
    head costs to the programmes?
17 What is the appropriate length of life to apply to capital assets
    used in the programmes?
18 Do market values accurately reflect opportunity costs?
19 Has sensitivity analysis been carried out? The most likely
    candidates for sensitivity analysis are
    • production effects
    • items excluded because of the effort required to collect data
    • imputed values
    • estimates of future benefits and costs
    • discount rate
    • length of life of capital items
20 What is the appropriate measure of benefit? This will depend on
    • the question being asked
    • whether benefits are multiple or singular (and include more
      than just health gain)
    • whether it is thought that the more beneficial treatment will
      cost more

the long run but also relevant to the decision-making context in
which it is to be applied. Because of the number of questions to be
asked and the detailed nature of many exercises in costing and
benefit estimation, it is recommended that an economist be
involved in any health services evaluation, particularly in the design
stage. If people are to use the techniques of cost–benefit analysis,
cost–effectiveness analysis, and cost–utility analysis, then they
ought to be fully understood. It is hoped that this chapter has shed
some light on such understanding.

Appendix

Discounting

From Table 26.6, the figure £2859 comprises

$$1000 + (1000 \times \frac{1}{1.05}) + (1000 \times \frac{1}{1.05^2})$$

$$= 1000 + (1000 \times 0.95240) + (1000) \times 0.9070).$$

where 0.954 and 0.9070 are discount factors. In general

$$D_n = \frac{1}{(1 + r)^n}$$

where D_n is the discount factor, r is the discount rate, and n is the number of years ahead.

In the example in Table 26.6 the discount rate r is 0.05 (or 5 per cent). Discount factors are obtainable directly from tables such as Table 26.14, which provides a list of discount factors annually from one to 50 years into the future at a discount rate of 5 per cent. The first two values in the column headed Discount factor are 0.9524 and 0.9070. This is because we are interested in discount factors one and two years from year 0 (i.e. now).

Present values

An alternative way of arriving at £2859 would be as follows:

$$£2859 = 1000 \times (1 + 1.8594).$$

The sum of our discount factors (0.9524 + 0.9070) is 1.8594, which is the present value of £1 expended in years 1 and 2.

Thus, if annual costs are all equal, calculation of discounted costs can be speeded up by calculating the present value of the sum of the discount factors and multiplying the present value by the annual amount expended (in this case £1000). In Table 26.14, 1.8594 is the second value in the column headed Present value of £1 per year. This is because we are looking up to two years from year 0.

Equivalent annual costs

Let us assume that our surgical and drug interventions in Tables 26.5 and 26.6 each incurred capital costs of £100 per patient and that the capital assets are costed only for the duration of each programme. From Table 26.14, it can be seen that three annual payments of 37 pence (i.e. 36.72 pence rounded up) discounted at 5 per cent would sum to £1. Therefore three annual payments of £37 discounted at 5 per cent would sum to £100, i.e.

$$\frac{37}{(1.05)} + \frac{37}{(1.05)^2} + \frac{37}{(1.05)^3} = 100.$$

In this example, as capital costs are equivalent in each treatment regimen, their inclusion makes no difference to the final result that drug therapy is more efficient.

Table 26.14 Discount factors, equivalent annual costs, and present values of £1 per year for a discount rate of 5 per cent (base date is year 0).

Year	Discount factor (= present value of £1)	Equivalent annual cost of £1	Present value of £1 per year
1	0.9524	1.0500	0.952
2	0.9070	0.5378	1.859
3	0.8638	0.3672	2.723
4	0.8227	0.3820	3.516
5	0.7835	0.2310	4.329
6	0.7462	0.1970	5.076
7	0.7107	0.1728	5.786
8	0.6768	0.1547	6.463
9	0.6446	0.1407	7.108
10	0.6139	0.1295	7.722
11	0.5847	0.1204	8.306
12	0.5568	0.1128	8.863
13	0.5303	0.1065	9.394
14	0.5051	0.1010	9.899
15	0.4810	0.0963	10.380
16	0.4581	0.0923	10.838
17	0.4363	0.0887	11.274
18	0.4155	0.0855	11.690
19	0.3957	0.0827	12.086
20	0.3769	0.0802	12.462
21	0.3589	0.0780	12.821
22	0.3418	0.0760	12.163
23	0.3256	0.0741	13.489
24	0.3101	0.0725	13.799
25	0.2953	0.0710	14.094
26	0.2812	0.0696	14.375
27	0.2678	0.0683	14.643
28	0.2551	0.0671	14.898
29	0.2429	0.0660	15.141
30	0.2314	0.0651	15.372
31	0.2204	0.0641	15.593
32	0.2099	0.0633	15.803
33	0.1999	0.0625	16.003
34	0.1904	0.0618	16.193
35	0.1813	0.0611	16.374
36	0.1727	0.0604	16.547
37	0.1644	0.0598	16.711
38	0.1566	0.0593	16.868
39	0.1491	0.0588	17.017
40	0.1420	0.0583	17.159
41	0.1353	0.0578	17.294
42	0.1288	0.0574	17.423
43	0.1227	0.0570	17.546
44	0.1169	0.0566	17.663
45	0.1113	0.0563	17.774
46	0.1060	0.0559	17.880
47	0.1009	0.0556	17.981
48	0.0961	0.0553	18.077
49	0.0916	0.0550	18.169
50	0.0872	0.0548	18.256

References

Alchian, A.A. (1972). Cost. In *International encyclopaedia of the social sciences*, Vol. 3 (ed. D. Stills). Macmillan, London.

Avorn, J. (1984). Benefit and cost analysis in geriatric care: turning age discrimination into health policy. *New England Journal of Medicine*, **310**, 1294–300.

Arrow, K., Solow, R., Portney, P.R., *et al.* (1993) Report of the NOAA Panel of Contingent Valuation. *Federal Register*, **58**(10), 4601–14.

Backhouse, M.E., Backhouse, R.J., and Edey, S.A. (1992). Economic evaluation bibliography. *Health Economics* (Suppl.), 1–236.

Berwick, D.M. and Weinstein, M.C. (1985). What do patients value? Willingness to pay for ultrasound in normal pregnancy? *Medical care*, **23**(7), 881–93.

Birch, S. and Donaldson, C. (1987). Applications of cost benefit analysis to health care: departures from welfare economic theory. *Journal of Health Economics*, **6**, 211–25.

Birch, S. and Gafni, A. (1992). Cost effectiveness/utility analyses: do current decision rules lead us to where we want to be? *Journal of Health Economics*, **11**, 279–96.

Birch, S. and Gafni, A. (1994). Cost–effectiveness ratios: in a league of their own. *Health Policy*, **28**, 133–41.

Blades, C.M., Culyer, A.J., Wiseman, J., and Walker, A. (1986). *International bibliography of health economics*, Parts 1 and 2. Harvester Press, Brighton.

Bond, J., Gregson, B.A., and Atkinson, A. (1989). Measurement of outcomes within a multicentred randomized controlled trial in the evaluation of the experimental NHS nursing homes. *Age and Ageing*, **18**, 292–302.

Boyle, M.H., Torrance, G.W., Sinclair, J.C., and Horwood, S.P. (1983). Economic evaluation of neonatal intensive care of very-low-birthweight infants. *New England Journal of Medicine*, **308**, 1330–7.

Buckingham, K. (1993). A note on HYE (healthy years equivalent). *Journal of Health Economics*, **11** 301–9.

Buhaug, H., Skjeldstad, F.E., Backe, B., and Dalen, B. (1989). Cost effectiveness of testing for chlamydial infections in asymptomatic women. *Medical Care*, **27**, 833–41.

Bush, J.W., Chen, M.M., and Patrick, D.L. (1973). Health status index in cost–effectiveness: analysis of a PKU program. In *Health status indexes* (ed. R.L. Berg). Hospital and Educational Research Trust, Chicago, IL.

Cairns, J. (1992). Discounting and health benefits: another perspective. *Health Economics*, **1**, 76–9.

Carr-Hill, R.A. (1992). A second opinion: health related quality of life measurement—Euro style. *Health Policy*, **20**, 321–8.

Culyer, A.J. and Wagstaff, A. (1993). QALYs and HYEs. *Journal of Health Economics*, **11**, 311–23.

Dixon, J. and Welch, H.G. (1991). Priority setting: lessons from Oregon. *Lancet*, **337**, 891–4.

Doessel, D.P. (1978). Economic analysis and end stage renal disease: an Australian study. *Economic Analysis and Policy*, **8**, 21–36.

Donaldson, C. (1990). Willingness to pay for publicly provided goods: a possible measure of benefit? *Journal of Health Economics*, **9**, 103–18.

Donaldson, C. (1993). *Theory and practice of willingness to pay for health care.* Health Economics Research Unit Discussion paper 01/93, University of Aberdeen.

Donaldson, C. and Bond, J. (1991). Cost of continuing-care facilities in the evaluation of experimental National Health Service nursing homes. *Age and Ageing*, **20**, 160–8.

Donaldson, C. and Gregson, B. (1989). Prolonging life at home: what is the cost? *Community Medicine*, **11**, 200–9.

Donaldson, C., Wright, K., and Maynard, A. (1986). Determining value for money in day hospital care for the elderly. *Age and Ageing*, **15**, 1–7.

Donaldson, C. Atkinson, A., Bond, J., and Wright, K. (1988). Should QALYs be programme-specific? *Journal of Health Economics*, **7**, 239–57.

Donaldson, C., Shackley, P., Abdalla, M., and Miedzybrodzka, Z. (1995). Willingness to pay for antenatal carrier screening for cystic fibrosis. *Health Economics* forthcoming.

Donaldson, C., Shackley, P., Abdalla, M., *et al.* (1994). *The use of willingness to pay alongside randomised trials.* Health Economics Research Unit Discussion Paper, 01/94, University of Aberdeen.

Drummond, M.F. (1980). *Principles of economics appraisal in health care.* Oxford University Press.

Drummond, M. (1981). *Studies in economic appraisal in health care.* Oxford University Press.

Drummond, M. and Mooney, G. (1983). *Essentials of health economics.* Northern Health Economics, Aberdeen.

Drummond, M.F., Ludbrook, A., Lowson, K., and Steele, A. (1986) *Studies in economic appraisal in health care*, Vol. 2. Oxford University Press.

Drummond, M.F., Stoddart, G.L., and Torrance, W. (1987). *Methods for the economic evaluation of health care programmes.* Oxford University Press.

Easthaugh, S.R. (1991). Valuation of the benefits of risk-free blood. *International Journal of Technology Assessment in Health Care*, **7**, 51–7.

Elixhauser, A. (1993). Health care cost–benefit and cost–effectiveness analysis (CBA/CEA) from 1979 to 1990: a bibliography. *Medical Care*, **31** (Suppl.), JS1–150.

Euroqol Group (1990). Euroqol—a new facility for the measurement of health-related quality of life. *Health Policy*, **16**, 199–208.

Froberg, D.G. and Kane, R.L. (1989). Methodology for measuring health-state preferences—II scaling methods. *Journal of Clinical Epidemiology*, **42**(5), 459–71.

Gafni, A. (1991). Willingness to pay as a measure of benefits: relevant questions in the context of public decision making about health care programmes. *Medical Care*, **29**, 1246–52.

Gafni, A. and Birch, S. (1993). Searching for a common currency: critical appraisal of the scientific basis underlying European harmonization of the measurement of Health Related Quality of Life (Euroqol). *Health Policy*, **23**, 219–28.

Gafni, A. and Zylak, C.J. (1990) Ionic versus non-ionic contrast media: a burden or a bargain? *Canadian Medical Association Journal*, **143**, 475–8.

Gafni, A., Birch, S., and Mehrez, A. (1993). Economics, health and health economics: HYEs versus QALYs. *Journal of Health Economics*, **11**, 325–39.

Gerard, K. (1990). Economic evaluation of respite care for children with a mental handicap: a preliminary analysis of problems. *Mental Handicap*, **18**, 150–5.

Gerard, K. and Mooney, G. (1993). QALY league tables: handle with care. *Health Economics*, **2**(1), 59–64.

Gerard, K., Salkeld, G., and Hall, J. (1990*a*). Counting the costs of mammography screening: first year results from the Sydney study. *Medical Journal of Australia*, **152**, 466–71.

Gerard, K., Salkeld, G., and Hall, J. (1990*b*). Counting the costs of mammography screening: first year results from the Sydney study (letter). *Medical Journal of Australia*, **153**, 175–6.

Goel, V., Derber, R.B., and Detsky, A.S. (1989). Nonionic contrast media: economic analysis and health policy development. *Canadian Medical Association Journal*, **140**, 389–95.

Gould, D. (1971). A groundling's notebook. *New Scientist*, **51**, 217.

Gray, A.M. and Steele, R. (1979). *The identification of the costs of maternity care: a programme approach to health service expenditure.* Health Economics Research Unit Discussion Paper 03/79, University of Aberdeen.

Gudex, C. and Kind, P. (1988). *The QALY toolkit.* Centre for Health Economics Discussion Paper 38, University of York.

Harrison, A.J. (1974). *The economics of transport appraisal.* Wiley, New York.

HM Treasury (1982). *Investment appraisal in the public sector.* HMSO, London.

Hundley, V., Donaldson, C., Lang, G., *et al.* (1994). Costs of intrapartum care in a Midwife Managed Delivery Unit and a consultant-led Labour Ward. *Midwifery*, **11**, 103–9.

Johannesson, M. (1992). Economic evaluation of lipid lowering—a feasibility test of the contingent valuation approach. *Health Policy*, **20**, 309–20.

Johannesson, M. and Jönsson, B. (1991). Economic evaluation in health care: is there a role for cost–benefit analysis? *Health Policy*, **17**, 1–23.

Johannesson, M., Jönsson, B., and Borquist, L. (1991). Willingness to pay for antihypertensive therapy–results of a Swedish pilot study. *Journal of Health Economics*, **10**, 461–74.

Johannesson, M., Pliskin, J.S., and Weinstein, M.C. (1993). Are healthy years equivalents an improvement over quality adjusted life years? *Medical Decision Making*, **13**, 281–6.

Kind, P. Rosser, R., and Williams, A. (1982). Valuation of quality of life: some psychometric evidence. In *The value of life and safety* (ed. M. W. Jones-Lee). North-Holland, Amsterdam.

Klarman, H.E., Francis, J.O., and Rosenthal, C.D. (1968). Cost–effectiveness analysis applied to the treatment of chronic renal disease. *Medical Care*, **6**, 48–54.

Kristiansen, I.S., Egen, A.E., and Thelle, D.S. (1991). Cost effectiveness of incremental programmes for lowering serum cholesterol concentration: is individual intervention worthwhile? *British Medical Journal*, **302**, 1119–22.

Mehrez, A. and Gafni, A. (1989). Quality adjusted life years, utility theory, and healthy years equivalents. *Medical Decision Making*, **9**, 142–9.

Mehrez, A. and Gafni, A. (1993). The healthy years equivalents: how to measure them using the standard gamble approach. *Medical Decision Making*, **11**, 140–6.

Mehrez, A. and Gafni, A. (1993). Healthy years equivalents versus quality adjusted life years: in pursuit of progress. *Medical Decision Making*, **13**, 287–92.

Miedzybrodzka, Z., Shackley, P., Donaldson, C., and Abdalla, M. (1994). Counting the benefits of screening: a pilot study of willingness to pay for cystic fibrosis carrier screening. *Journal of Medical Screening*, **1**, 82–3.

Mooney, G.H. (1989). Economic evaluation: the Australian road to health service efficiency. In *Health care evaluation, Report of the National Health Care Evaluations Workshop, July 1989*. Public Health Association of Australia, Canberra.

Mooney, G. and Lange, M. (1993). Antenatal screening: what constitutes 'benefit'? *Social Science and Medicine*, **37**(7), 873–8.

Mugford, M., Kingston, J., and Chalmers, I. (1989). Reducing the incidence of infections after Caesarean section: implications of prophylaxis with antibiotics for hospital resources. *British Medical Journal*, **299**, 1003–6.

Neuhauser, D. and Lewicki, A.M. (1975). What do we gain from the sixth stool guaiac? *New England Journal of Medicine*, **293**, 255–8.

Olsen, J.A. and Donaldson, C. (1993). *Willingness to pay for public sector health care programmes in northern Norway*. Health Economics Research Unit Discussion Paper 05/93, University of Aberdeen.

O'Neill, P. (1990). State health plan for the poor stalls. *The Oregonian*, 15 June.

Parsonage, M. and Neuberger, H. (1992). Discounting and health benefits. *Health Economics*, **1**, 71–5.

Rice, D.P. and Cooper, B.S. (1967). The economic value of human life. *American Journal of Public Health*, **57**(11), 1954–66.

Richardson, J., Hall J., and Salkeld, G. (1990) Cost utility analysis: the compatibility of measurement techniques and the measurement of utility through time. In *Economics and health 1990: Proceedings of the 11th Annual Conference of Australian Health Economists* (ed. C. Selby-Smith). Public Sector Management Institute, Monash University, Melbourne.

Rosser, R.M. and Watts, V.C. (1972). The measurement of hospital output. *Journal of Epidemiology*, **1**, 361–8.

Russell, I.T., Devlin, B., Fell, M., *et al.* (1977). Day case surgery for hernias and haemorrhoids: a clinical, social and economic evaluation. *Lancet*, i, 844–7.

Stanford, M. (1990). Counting the costs of mammography screening: first year results from the Sydney study (letter). *Medical Journal of Australia*, **153**, 175.

Thompson, M.S. (1986). Willingness to pay and accept risks to cure chronic disease. *American Journal of Public Health*, **76**, 392–6.

Targerson, D., Donaldson, C., and Reid, D. (1994). Private versus social opportunity cost of time: valuing time in the demand for health care. *Health Economics*, **3**, 149–55.

Torrance, G.W. (1986). Measurement of health state utilities for economic appraisal: a review. *Journal of Health Economics*, **5**, 1–30.

Torrance, G.W. and Feeny, D. (1989). Utilities and quality adjusted life years. *International Journal of Technology Assessment in Health Care*, **5**, 559–75.

Torrance, G.W., Thomas, W.H., and Sackett, D.L. (1972). A utility maximization model for evaluation of health care programmes. *Health Services Research*, **7**, 118–33.

Torrance, G.W., Boyle, M.H., and Horwood, S.P. (1982). Application of multi-attribute utility theory to measure social preferences for health states. *Operations Research*, **30**, 1043–69.

Wager, R. (1972). *Care of the elderly—an exercise in cost benefit analysis commissioned by Essex County Council*. IMTA (now Chartered Institute of Public Finance and Accountancy), London.

Williams, A. (1985). Economics of coronary artery bypass grafting. *British Medical Journal*, **291**, 326–9.

Williams, A. (1993). The Euroqol instrument: a presentation of its key features. Paper presented to the UK Health Economists' Study Group, University of Strathclyde, Glasgow.

27 Operational and system studies

Shan Cretin

Introduction

Operational research was first recognized as a distinct discipline during the Second World War. Scientists, long engaged in the design of weapons, began to apply scientific methods of analysis to the deployment of weapons and to overall military operations, with the goal of providing military commanders with a quantitative basis for decisions (Morse and Kimball 1951). A decision problem (for example, how to search for U-boats in the North Atlantic or what size to make a convoy) was recast into a mathematical model. The key variables in the problem, including the appropriate measure of the effectiveness of the operation, were quantified and the relationships between the variables were described using mathematical expressions. These formulas comprised a mathematical model of the real decision problem and could be manipulated to predict the impact of a given decision on the measure effectiveness. The success of operational research in the Second World War demonstrated that many apparently complex problems could be usefully analysed using simple models to approximate the critical variables and relationships.

After the Second World War operational research was extended to non-military problems. Hospitals and health care systems were quickly identified as fruitful areas for analysis, with the first published reports of health applications appearing in the early 1950s. Bailey (1951, 1952) used the mathematical theory of queues to explore various outpatient appointment systems and to analyse the use of single versus multiple occupancy rooms in hospitals. Other studies applied operational research techniques to models of epidemics (Abbey 1952; Taylor 1958), emergency admissions (Neweill 1954), and inventory control in general hospitals (Flagle 1960) and blood banks (Rockwell et al. 1962; Elston and Pickrel 1963).

Most of these early applications of operational research used mathematical models based on probability or statistical theory. Today, operational research studies use a variety of mathematical tools, some adapted from traditional mathematical fields and some newly developed. The techniques most commonly employed are as follows: probability models, which use queuing theory, Monte Carlo simulations, and statistics, optimization models, which use mathematical programming, dynamic programming, and graph and network theory, differential equation methods and dynamic systems simulation, and decision analyses, which use models based on Bayesian and statistical decision theory, game theory, and utility theory.

The remainder of this chapter will be divided into three parts. The first section will review the most frequently used operational research techniques, with references to sources of more detailed information about each. The second part will review the types of public health problems that have been addressed using operational research methods, with references to some typical studies. The third section will discuss the potential and the problems surrounding applications of operational research methods in public health.

Review of operational research techniques

There are several excellent textbooks surveying the methods of operational research. Duckworth et al. (1977) and Eppen et al. (1987) provided overviews of methods and applications aimed at managers. Hillier and Lieberman (1980) and Wagner (1975) are good references for basic methods. Larson and Odoni (1981) focused on techniques useful in the analysis of urban problems. Warner et al. (1984) stressed methods and applications in health administration. In addition, there are scores of books and hundreds of articles devoted to specific techniques, models, and problems. In the brief review of techniques which follows, reference is made to a few of these more advanced texts.

Probability models

Uncertainty is a feature of life. Many important administrative and policy decisions in health care are complicated by chance elements beyond the control of the decision maker. Recent work by psychologists (Tversky and Kahneman 1974) has demonstrated biases and inconsistencies in our intuition about probabilities. This failure of intuition may explain why operational research models employing probability theory to analyse chance events have resulted in some of the most substantial improvements in operating systems.

Stochastic processes

Stochastic or probabilistic processes evolve over time in a way that is not completely predictable. Some simple probabilistic processes have proved to be useful models of real events. These models have been carefully described and well analysed over the years, so that once the model is known to apply, many results can be inferred. The Bernoulli process (which gives rise to the familiar binomial distribution), the Poisson process, and the Markov process are three models that have been used extensively in health applications.

In the simplest probability models, successive events are assumed to be independent of each other. The classic example is coin flipping, modelled by a Bernoulli process; the outcome (heads or tails) on one toss does not alter the probability of heads or tails on the next toss.

In a Bernoulli process, the outcome is a result of some discrete event. When tossing coins, for example, 'heads' or 'tails' cannot occur at any instant, but only as a result of the action of 'flipping the coin'. For this reason, the Bernoulli process cannot be used to model events which can occur at any moment in time, such as a request for emergency medical service. The Poisson process extends the notion of independent events to continuous time by assuming that the number of events in one time period is independent of the number of events in any other non-overlapping time period. Poisson arrivals (sometimes called 'random arrivals') have been used to model the arrival of women in spontaneous labour at an obstetrics service as well as requests for ambulances or other emergency medical care.

The Poisson and Bernoulli processes are called memoryless. While such memoryless processes may be adequate for many situations, there are times when probabilities of future events will depend on past outcomes. The Markov model is a simple probability model with 'memory'. A Markovian world is assumed to consist of a set of discrete non-overlapping states. For example, a Markovian model of a person's state of health might consist four states: disease free, presymptomatic, symptomatic, and dead. Starting in one of the states, the system undergoes changes of state (or state transitions) according to a set of probability rules. The Markov process is allowed to have a limited memory, that is the probability of transition to a particular state allowed to depend on which state the system is in just before the transition. Some Markovian systems undergo transitions only at discrete times (similar to the Bernoulli process), while others may undergo transitions at any time.

Drake (1967) and Feller (1968) provided introductions to applied theory. Other useful references on stochastic processes are Howard (1960, 1971), Parzen (1960), Bailey (1964), Cox and Miller (1965), and Ross (1970, 1972).

Queuing systems

The application of stochastic models to the analysis of queues for service has been quite fruitful and queuing theory has become a distinct and expanding field of inquiry. A.K. Erlang did much of the early work in this field in conjunction with his studies of the Copenhagen telephone system (Brockmeyer et al. 1948).

The simplest queuing system has one server who handles requests for service sequentially. To simplify the analysis, both arrivals and service are assumed to be 'memoryless'. The arrival of customers is modelled by a Poisson process. Service times for each customer are assumed to be drawn independently from a negative exponential distribution, a distribution with the property that no matter how long service has been in progress, the expected remaining time in service is the same. Given the average arrival rate of customers and the mean service time, we can then calculate the distribution of the length of the queue and the distribution of customer waiting times, as well as characteristics of the server's busy and quiet periods.

More complex queuing systems have been analysed which allow multiple servers, more general arrival and service time distributions, batch arrivals of customers, balking or reneging by customers who wait too long in the queue, tandem queues, or hierarchical queuing networks. Less complete mathematical results are available for these more complex systems, but many approximate results have been obtained. Many complex queuing networks are now analysed using computer simulation methods and this will be discussed in the section on Monte Carlo simulations.

Cox and Smith (1961) provided a concise introduction to queuing theory, while Cooper (1972) and Kleinrock (1975) gave fuller treatment to the subject. Newell (1971) emphasized approximate solution methods.

A special class of queuing models of particular relevance to the analyses of ambulance systems is the spatially distributed queue. In this case, chance is involved not only in the timing of the requests, but also in the location from which the requests originate. The geography of the region is important in describing the location of calls for service and in determining the distribution of response times. Servers are no longer indistinguishable, although they provide the same service, since each potential server may be at a different distance from an incoming call. Models of spatially distributed queues have been developed to analyse the effects of call volume, the number and location of servers, and dispatching strategies on the efficiency and equity of service. Larson and Odoni (1981) gave a description of models and methods. The Rand Fire Project report (Walker et al. 1979) described the use of these and similar models in analysing fire services.

Monte Carlo simulations

The behaviour of systems involving chance elements can often be analysed by simulating the operation of the system. Simulation is also used to analyse complex deterministic systems, as in dynamic systems simulation which is discussed below. Coin flipping could be simulated using digits from a table of random numbers by labelling odd digits as 'heads' and even digits as 'tails'. Alternatively, a computer could be programmed to simulate coin flipping in a similar way using internally generated random numbers.

Simulation is usually an analysis of last resort, which is used when a system is too complex for the simpler mathematical models with closed-form solutions. Complex queuing networks are frequently simulated. In theory a simulation can be carried out 'by hand', but in practice simulations are usually computer operations using one of several simulation languages (SIMSCRIPT, GPSS, or GASP). Simulations in these languages are 'event paced'. First, the logical structure of the system is described and the beginning state of the system is specified. The simulation then focuses on events that change the state of the system (for example, the arrival of a new customer or the completion of service on a current customer). Various statistics describing the operating characteristics of the system are compiled during the simulation and reported when a predetermined span of simulated time has elapsed.

In effect, running a simulation is like collecting experimental data on an operating system. As in any experiment, the interpretation of the result depends on the design of the experiment and the sample size. Interpretation of simulation results may also depend on how the data used in constructing the simulation were obtained. With a little care, a simulation can give a reliable picture of how the model behaves. As with all operational research, the crucial question is also the most difficult to answer: how well does the model represent the real system?

Emshoff and Sisson (1970) and Banks and Catson (1984) provided a general introduction to simulation methods. Manuals for specific simulation languages are also useful guides, for example,

Kiviat *et al.* (1969) on SIMSCRIPT II or Pritsker (1986) on SLAM II.

Competing risk and other life table models

Historically, life tables have been used by demographers and biostatisticians to calculate life expectancies and survival curves. With some modifications the basic life table models can incorporate the notion of competing causes of death (Chiang 1968; Manton *et al.* 1976). The age-specific mortality from and particular cause of death can further be described as a function of various risk factors (such as blood pressure or smoking habits). Several operational research studies have incorporated competing risk/life table methods in larger models designed to estimate the costs and benefits of risk factor intervention programmes (Weinstein and Stason 1976; Berwick *et al.* 1980; Eddy 1980).

Inventory theory

Inventory theory, like queuing theory, is organized around an area of application rather than a method. Inventory models include both deterministic models (which assume that the demand for a good is completely predictable) and probability models (which allow demand and various time lags to be stochastic). The basic components of most inventory models include ordering costs, storage costs for items on hand, shortage costs, outdating costs (for perishable goods, such as whole blood), and the cost of capital. The models are analysed to determine the least-cost inventory policy, including the size and timing of orders.

Inventory models have been developed to analyse one-time ordering decisions, multiple-cycle ordering decisions, and single and multiple product systems. When an inventory problem is too complex to fit any of the existing models, the computer simulation can provide a means of analysis. Buffa and Miller (1979) reviewed inventory theory and practice and Veinott (1966) reviewed theory.

Optimization models

Many of the probability models just discussed are descriptive rather than prescriptive. A queuing model, for example, would be useful in describing the trade-off between customer waiting time and server idle time, but would not indicate the 'optimal' number of servers for a given work-load. The value of the model is in predicting the effects of uncertain events so that a few known alternatives can be evaluated. In some decisions, uncertainty about the outcome of a strategy is not the major difficulty. The outcome for any given alternative is easy to calculate, but the decision maker is cursed with too many choices. In this kind of problem, mathematical modelling can provide an efficient way of finding the optimal alternative from a large (perhaps infinite) number of possibilities. Optimality is defined in terms of a mathematical expression (an 'objective function') which is to be made as large (or as small) as possible.

Mathematical programming

Mathematical programming includes a variety of techniques used to determine the optimal allocation of resources. The form of these models is always the same: maximize or minimize an objective function subject to a series of constraints. The specific techniques (linear programming, quadratic programming, integer programming, or non-linear programming) rest on different assumptions about the mathematical form of the objective function and constraints and therefore involve different solution methods. Linear programming models are usually the simplest to solve and are often used to approximate more complex integer or non-linear problems.

A classic linear programming problem is the 'product mix' decision. Suppose, for example, that a potter has 80 pounds of clay and 10 hours available to prepare pottery for a craft show. They can make vases (each uses a pound of clay and takes 5 minutes) or bowls (each uses a pound and a half of clay and takes 15 minutes). If bowls sell for $20 and vases for $10, how many of each should they make to maximize their revenue.

In this example, the decision variables are the number of vases to be made V and the number of bowls B. The objective is to maximize revenue, which is a linear function of the two decision variables ($20B + 1OV$). There are two constraints, time and material, which can be expressed as linear inequalities:

$$\text{Time: } 11\,V + 4\,B < 10$$

$$\text{Clay: } V + 3\,B < 80$$

If this problem is solved using linear programming techniques, the optimal values for the decision variables will take on fractional values. When it is important to restrict the solution to integral values, the same formulation of the objective function and constraints could be solved using integer programming methods.

In the simple example just given, the decision problem is not very difficult. Once the problem is formulated mathematically, it can be solved by hand using algebraic or graphical techniques. However, many applications of linear programming involve hundreds of decision variables and constraints. The solution of problems of this magnitude only became feasible with the development of the simplex algorithm (Dantzig 1963), which is an extremely efficient solution method when used on high-speed computers. More recently, a new ellipsoid method of solution was introduced (Bland *et al.* 1981).

Although linear programming provides a powerful tool for analysing questions of resource allocation, many practical problems violate the assumptions of the model. A common problem is the need to restrict the solution to integer values. This is demonstrated in the example above and is even more pronounced when the variable represents the number of surgical suites. In other cases, the constraints are not linear. For example, the potter may find that each additional bowl takes a little less time than the preceding bowl, because of a learning effect. While solution methods of non-linear and integer programming problems do exist, except for some rather special cases, these algorithms are far less efficient than linear programming techniques.

Luenberger (1984) provided a valuable introduction to both linear and non-linear programming. Garfinkel and Nemhauser (1972) have produced a good text on integer programming.

Graphs and networks

A graph is a set of nodes or points with lines or branches connecting certain pairs of points. A network is a graph with some type of flow along its branches. A highway system is an example of a network, with roads as branches, intersections as nodes, and traffic flowing along the roads. Network theory provides an excellent means of analysing many problems related to transportation, such as finding the shortest route from one point to another or finding the shortest tour through a network (a path that visits every node). Network theory is also the basis for a technique widely used in coordinating and scheduling interrelated activities. This method has been popularized as programme evaluation and review technique (**PERT**) or critical path method (**CPM**).

PERT systems begin by representing a project as a network. Each node represents an event, for example the beginning of the project, the end of the project, or the completion of some intermediate activity. Each activity or task is represented by a directed branch (a line with an arrow) starting from the node marking completion of all necessary predecessor tasks and ending at a task completion node. If the duration of each subtask is known, network theory can be used to calculate the earliest possible completion time for the whole project, the earliest and latest starting time for each subtask, and the critical path. Activities on the critical path have no slack time, meaning that if the starting time on one of these activities is delayed, the completion of the entire project is delayed.

Although the critical path is found as a result of an optimization technique, the major use of PERT systems is as an aid to scheduling and not as an optimization tool. Sometimes a range of times for each subtask is the basis for 'best-case' and 'worst-case' analyses. Alternatively, the cost of speeding up certain subtasks can be balanced against the effect on project completion time.

Network analyses have also been applied to assignment problems (assigning personnel to tasks) and to facility location problems (finding the best location for fire stations in a region). Assignment problems and certain transportation problems can be solved using adaptations of linear programming algorithms. Ford and Fulkerson (1962) covered network theory in general. CPM and PERT were reviewed by Moder and Phillips (1970). Larson and Odoni (1981) provided a good review of routing problems and facility location problems in the context of urban services.

Dynamic programming

Dynamic programming is a technique for maximizing the overall effectiveness of a series of interrelated decisions. In a dynamic programming problem the decisions take place in stages. The choices available and the results of a decision at each stage depend on the current state of the system. After the decision has been made, the state of the system changes (either deterministically or according to a set of known probabilities). The complexity of the problem is not the result of uncertainty but of the number of possible decision sequences which must be evaluated. If there are only four stages with four possible decisions at each stage, there are 256 distinct sequences.

Finding the optimal solution to a dynamic programming problem is not a simple matter of applying a standard algorithm as was the case for linear programming. Although there is a general approach, it must be tailored to each individual problem. The solution procedure starts by finding the best decisions for each possible state at the last decision stage and works backward. The

best decision set at the nth stage is found by building on the best decisions found for stage $n + 1$.

An extension of dynamic programming to allow an infinite number of recurring decision stages is found in Markovian decision models. Some decisions with continuous outcomes can also be modelled using continuous state dynamic programming. Howard (1960, 1971) discussed both dynamic programming and Markovian decision theory. Denardo (1982) reviewed the theory and applications of dynamic programming.

Differential equations and difference equations

Differential equations and difference equations have been used in modelling electrical, mechanical, and fluid systems for many years. Differential equations are useful in describing systems in which key variables change continuously over time and in which the rate of change of a variable may depend on the level of that variable and on the level and rates of change of other variables. Difference equations are simply approximations to differential equations in which time is only allowed to change in discrete units.

A simple example of a system well modelled by differential equations is a world populated by caterpillars and birds. If some external force suddenly depletes the bird population, the caterpillars will thrive. This, in turn, will allow the small remaining bird population to grow. Such a system may oscillate for some time before reaching a stable equilibrium. The size of the oscillations and the length of time taken for the system to stabilize will depend on the size of the external force and on the exact relationship between the bird and caterpillar populations.

In the late 1950s, Forrester (1961) began using difference equations to model the responses of industrial firms to management policies. Since that time the applications have been extended to many other settings, including health care. The models of such systems are too complex to be solved mathematically and analysis is usually performed using simulation. The computer language DYNAMO was developed especially for this purpose.

Decision analysis

Decision analysis is a general approach to the problem of decision making when there is uncertainty. Embedded in this widely accepted approach to structuring the problem are several thorny and highly controversial topics. How does one estimate the degree of uncertainty in the absence of data? What criteria should be applied in finding the 'best decision'? How does one value outcome, particularly when there are multiple dimensions, for example mortality, money, and impaired function?

Decision analysts structure a problem by first separating decisions, chance events, and outcomes. Decisions and chance events are then displayed using a sequential 'tree'. Branches representing alternatives and chance occurrences radiate from appropriately sequenced 'decision' and 'chance' nodes, respectively. Each end-point of the tree is labelled with the appropriate outcome. Each chance branch is labelled with its probability of occurring. Decision branches are initially unlabelled. At the end of the analysis the 'best' alternative is identified at each decision node.

When the outcome is a single dimension (profit in a business decision or winnings in a gamble), the best decision is often defined as that which maximizes the expected value of the outcome. A common extension of decision analysis uses the decision maker's 'utility' for the outcome, rather than the outcome itself. In this case the best decision is the one which maximizes expected utility.

The concept of utility makes it easier to apply decision analysis to problems with inherently qualitative outcomes and to incorporate multidimensional outcomes. However, the problem of eliciting a decision maker's utilities for complex outcomes is itself quite difficult. The ability of utility theory to model the preferences people express in real decision situations has been challenged in recent years (Tversky and Kahneman 1981).

Another controversial area in the practice of decision analysis is the problem of estimating probabilities in the absence of data. It is common practice to include subjective or intuitive estimates of probabilities when no other means of estimation are possible. However, the method of eliciting these subjective probabilities may bias the estimates (Tversky and Kahneman 1974) and, hence, the analysis. For this reason, many applications of decision analysis include extensive sensitivity analysis to test the stability of the optimal policy. An excellent general introduction to decision analysis is given by Raiffa (1968). McNeil and Pauker (1984) provided a good introduction to public health applications.

Game theory

Game theory involves the analysis of decisions against opponents or competitors. Decisions by one party will interact with decisions by the other party to produce the outcomes. In two-person zero-sum games, the winnings of one party must equal the loss of the opponent. Other games include cooperative games, non-zero-sum games, and games involving more than two players. In game theory (as in decision analysis) the analysis specifies the decision strategy which maximizes one player's gain in the face of the opponents' best strategies. One promising application of game theory is in predicting the behaviour of an industry to changes in regulations or reimbursement methods. Luce and Raiffa (1975) offered an extensive treatment of game theory and decision making.

In the past decade, the rapid development of personal computers has revolutionized the field of operational research. Many of the techniques reviewed above have been incorporated into user-friendly software systems that can be run on desktop or other small computers, allowing decision makers and managers without extensive training in operational research to use and interact directly with models and data. Such 'decision support systems' have sometimes been described as gimmicks (Naylor 1982), but there is no doubt that the computer has been transformed from the exclusive property of the highly trained technician to the office machine. This transformation has aided in the diffusion of operational research applications in health care planning and management (Boldy 1987).

Review of public health applications

Over the last four decades there have been many reviews of health applications of operational research. Some reviewers focused on a particular technique or problem, such as statistics (Bailey 1956), queuing theory (Bailey 1954), mathematical programming (Boldy 1976), decision analysis (Krischer 1980), or facility location (ReVelle et al. 1977). Others have conducted more general surveys leavened with varying degrees of philosophical comment (Flagle

1962; Horvath 1965, 1967; Denison et al. 1969; McLaughlin 1970; Shuman et al. 1975; Fries 1976, 1979, 1981; Boldy 1981; Boldy and O'Kane 1982). Several reviews have looked primarily at applications in hospitals (Nuffield Provincial Hospitals Trust 1955, 1962, 1965; Bailey 1957a; Luck et al. 1971; Stimson and Stimson 1972). Several critical reviews—notably, Stimson and Stimson (1972), Shuman et al. (1975), and Boldy (1981)—have been motivated by the apparent discrepancy between the large number of published studies and the considerably smaller number of successful implementations.

Since there are so many existing reviews I shall not attempt to be comprehensive in this chapter. Rather, for each application area, I shall highlight a few representative studies.

Health facilities management

Many early operational research studies, particularly in the United States, addressed problems that arise in the management of hospitals and clinics. This emphasis can be explained in part by the importance of the hospital and clinic in medical care systems. It is also true that problems in hospitals and clinics (scheduling and inventory control) often have parallels in business and industry. Many hospital applications represented efforts to transfer models and solutions from business to health settings.

Outpatient appointment systems

The design of efficient appointment systems has engaged analysts for three decades. Queuing and simulation studies abound (Bailey 1952; Welch and Bailey 1952; Blanco White and Pike 1964; Welch 1964; Fetter and Thompson 1965; Rockart and Hoffman 1969; Walter 1973; Fries and Marathe 1981) and a considerable amount of data on the performance of operating systems has been collected (Nuffield Provincial Hospitals Trust 1965; United Hospital Fund of New York 1967; Johnson and Rosenfield 1968). Fries and Marathe (1981) used a dynamic programming approach to compare the performance of block appointment systems. Frenkel and Minieka (1982) applied a linear programming model to the problem of outpatient scheduling in a solo ophthalmic practice. Nevertheless, most studies have elaborated (without fundamentally altering) Bailey's original queuing formulation. Given the demand for services and the distribution of service times, the model describes the relationship between patient waiting time and provider idle time under various appointment systems. A wide array of other variables can be added to the basic model: patient and provider punctuality the fraction of patients who arrive without appointments, the fraction of patients who fail to keep appointments, and service times dependent on patient characteristics.

Regardless of the model used or the site of the study, analysts have come to the same general conclusions: patients are quite punctual, but physicians are not and minor changes in clinic procedures will usually eliminate excessive patient delays without significantly increasing the idle time of providers.

Despite the agreement between the analysts, long delays persist in many clinics, including some of those studied. O'Keefe (1985) suggested the importance of determining which policy changes can really be implemented and of educating the participants to accept the proposed changes. Operational research analysts have been quick to assume that the staff and administration of the clinic are interested in reducing patient waiting time and in increasing their own productivity. This may not be the case. Under a system of prepaid health care (the National Health Service (**NHS**) in the United Kingdom or health maintenance organizations in the United States), increasing the number of patient visits will only increase the work-load and not income. Staff may consciously or unconsciously use long patient waiting times to hold down demand for services. Recommended changes, however minor, must be carried out by the staff. If the staff are not interested, the implementation is likely to falter.

When clinic staff recognize a problem in the appointment system, an operational analysis can aid in identifying and evaluating possible solutions (Henderson 1976). In one successful project, staff involvement led to a model which focused on the patient's delay in obtaining an appointment rather than on waiting time in the clinic. The mark of a good operational research analysis is that it solves the problem of interest to the manager, rather than one of interest to the analyst.

Inpatient admission/discharge scheduling

Interest in the efficient scheduling of inpatients arises in over-crowded facilities and also in underutilized facilities. In hospitals with high occupancy rates (90 per cent or more), efficient scheduling can be viewed as an alternative to capital investment in new facilities. Hospitals with low average occupancy face a different problem: wide fluctuations in the size of the patient population are likely to occur, making staffing difficult. In this case, scheduling of patients can result in a more stable operation. Budget cuts and long hospital waiting lists in National Health Service hospitals have stimulated renewed interest in both inpatient scheduling (Worthington 1987) and facility sizing models (Harris 1985; Vassila-copoulos 1985).

Many different models have been used in the analysis of inpatient scheduling: queuing (Worthington 1987), simulation (Smith and Solomon 1966; Webb *et al.* 1977), and Markov probability (Kolesar 1970; Shonick and Jackson 1973; Esogbue and Singh 1976). Some models also employ statistical or time-series forecasting methods in predicting future demand as part of the scheduling problem (Shonick and Jackson 1973; Kao and Poklad-nik 1978).

Despite the variety of models, there is common ground. Most analysts consider at least two classes of admission separately—elective and emergency. A further division into medical versus surgical admissions is frequently used. Future demand in each category is forecast from past experience. Future census is forecast from future emergency demand, future scheduled demand, and length of stay estimates. Measures of the effectiveness of the scheduling system include the resulting inpatient census, rate of turnaway for emergencies, and length of waiting time for elective cases.

The simplest systems generate fixed rules about the maximum number of elective patients who can be scheduled on a given day. The most elaborate systems consider each potential admission separately, using individual patient data to project the length of stay and then scheduling the patient so that the probability of facility overflow never exceeds a preset value (Rubenstein 1976).

The fixed rule systems are most commonly used. The more

complex systems are necessarily limited to hospitals with on-line computerized admission and preadmission systems. Implement-ation studies carried out at two hospitals suggest that systems with heavy day to day data requirements in underutilized hospitals are not as likely to be successful as simpler systems implemented in overcrowded facilities (Griffith *et al.* 1975).

Facility sizing

Most of the scheduling and appointment models discussed assume that the size of the facility is fixed. While efficient scheduling can increase the apparent capacity of a facility, there are times when a hospital or clinic can only meet a growing demand by expanding. Many of the models used in evaluating appointment systems or admissions scheduling systems can be adapted to the problem of establishing an appropriate facility size (Fetter and Thompson 1966; Shonick and Jackson 1973; Esogbue and Singh 1976). These models are limited, however, because they focus on a single facility. A more efficient health system is achieved by fixing the individual facility size as part of a regional plan, as discussed in the section on regional health planning.

Several studies have tried to establish appropriate sizes for various units within a hospital. Using a priority queuing model, Vassilacopoulos (1985) addressed the question of how best to allocate inpatient beds to various hospital departments. Operating suites have been analysed using queuing theory (Whitston 1965), dynamic programming (Esogbue 1969), and simulation (Goldman and Knappenberger 1968).

Maternity services have been analysed using queuing models (Thompson *et al.* 1963) to determine the number of labour, delivery, and postpartum beds required. Markov and semi-Markov probability models have been used to predict the resources needed for coronary patients (Kao 1972). As an example of what might be done using a linear programming model, Dowling (1971) deter-mined the numbers of appendectomies, cholecystectomies, and tonsillectomies that could be performed subject to constraints in the numbers of operating suites, recovery beds, and hospital beds. Responding to National Health Service budget cuts, Harris (1985) used a simulation model to examine the interrelated problems of scheduling operating theatre time and allocating hospital beds.

Most 'size' analyses assume that the pattern of demand for services is fixed. However, reducing the fluctuations in demand through better scheduling may increase the effective capacity of a facility without increasing its size. Simulation studies have been used to evaluate facility size under various scheduling policies, for example surgical suites (Kwak *et al.* 1976) and radiology (O'Kane, 1981). Such comprehensive models are more realistic and therefore more appealing. However, they may be less likely to be used than simpler models. Because complex models take longer to develop and require more extensive data collection, they cannot be used when quick answers are needed.

Staffing

Staffing is a major concern in most health facilities. Nurse staffing, in particular, has been the subject of many operational research analyses, (see, for example Hershey *et al.* 1981). Warner *et al.* (1984) described a three-level classification of staffing decisions: long-range planning of the numbers and types of nursing personnel needed on each unit, deriving work schedules for each individual nurse, and allocation of nurses to units at the start of each shift. In addition, modelling has been applied to a fourth area: predicting the supply of personnel.

A quantitative approach to long-range staffing requires quantification of the nursing tasks needed on a unit. The simplest formulations relate nursing needs to the number of patients. More sophisticated approaches attempt to determine the nursing needs of each patient or class of patients. Simulation or statistical concepts can be used to incorporate the inevitable fluctuation in demand for nursing services (Smallwood *et al.* 1971; Hershey *et al.* 1974).

The scheduling problem consumes considerable time and effort in most hospitals. A common solution is to have each employee rotate through a fixed set of weekly schedules. Various heuristic and mathematical programming techniques have been used to help in formulating sets of schedules that meet staffing needs (Maier-Rothe and Wolfe 1973; James *et al.* 1974). This approach is so simple that it can be implemented on a microcomputer (Rosenbloom and Goertzen 1987). The resulting schedules are fair in that each employee cycles through the same set of schedules; however, it does not exploit differences in personal preferences. Warner (1976) developed and implemented a system to assign schedules based on individual preferences for long weekends, night shifts, and other characteristics. Nurses were asked to assign numerical weights to reflect their preferences and a mathematical programming algorithm was then used to maximize the sum of these weights while meeting minimal coverage requirements.

The need to allocate nurses on a shift by shift basis arises because the number and types of patients assigned to each ward or floor can be expected to fluctuate. In addition, some nurses may be absent from an assigned shift. Many hospitals cope with this problem by having a pool of 'floaters', that is nurses who are not assigned to a particular unit until the start of the shift. Trivedi and Warner (1976) used an integer programming model to assign floaters based on the quantified needs of each unit.

Staffing must also be determined for other areas of the hospital. Queuing and simulation studies have been used in staffing operating rooms (Whitston 1965), messenger services (Gupta *et al.* 1971), and outpatient clinics (Keller and Laughhunn 1973).

The issue of physician staffing has not received much attention. In the United States, most physicians have a voluntary rather than a salaried or contractual relationship with hospitals. Fetter and Thompson (1966) looked at physician staffing in the outpatient clinics of a teaching hospital.

Statistical and probability models have been used to forecast the supply of physicians and other health professionals. The report of the Graduate Medical Education National Advisory Committee (**GMENAC**) modelled both the expected supply of physicians and the anticipated demand (Tarlov 1980*ab*) in order to make national policy recommendations on the need for physicians and other personnel. Kane *et al.* (1980) made similar projections for geriatric manpower.

Patients flow models

Patient flow models do not, in themselves, address operational questions. However, estimates derived from such models may be useful (in conjunction with other models and data) in planning and staffing facilities. Analyses of such operational decisions often hinge on having an explicit model of how patients flow through the facility. Markov and semi-Markov models are frequently proposed as good methods of analysing patient flow. Fetter and Thompson (1965) proposed simulating a Markovian model of patient transition through a facility organized around Progressive Patient Care (a patient classification system based on the nursing needs of the patient). Later, Weiss *et al.* (1982) used a semi-Markov model to predict patient flow through a hospital.

When used to focus on particular patient subgroups, patient flow models blur the distinction between clinical and operational models. Kao (1972), for example, analysed the flow and recovery of coronary patients. Kastner and Shachtman (1982) looked at the flow of patients with hospital-acquired infections.

Ancillary and support services

Ancillary departments of hospitals present special cases of the general problems of sizing, scheduling, staffing, and inventory control. Simulation has been a popular tool for studying the size and operation of radiology departments (Jeans *et al.* 1972), laboratories (Rath *et al.* 1970), outpatient pharmacies (Myers *et al.* 1972), and inpatient drug distribution (Assimakopoulos 1987*a*). A complex hierarchical queuing model was used to study the operation of telemedicine systems (Willemain 1974). A birth-death model was used to describe the problem of medical records storage, allowing an analysis of microfilm policies and development of long-term storage needs (Nimmo 1983).

Inventory theory has proved useful in evaluating drug inventory (Satir and Cengiz 1987) and hospital support services such as oxygen supplies (Kilpatrick and Freund 1967). The costs of ordering, storage, and shortage are considered in determining the best supply policy. Smith *et al.* (1975) used inventory theory to develop a stock control system for hospitals which was widely implemented in the United Kingdom.

The management of a blood bank inventory presents a particularly difficult problem since blood is both a product of unique medical value and one which has a limited shelf-life. Blood banks must manage whole-blood inventories for the eight major blood types and the extraction of blood components (such as platelets, packed cells, and plasma) from whole blood. Prastacos (1984) provided an excellent review of blood inventory management theory and practice, including over 75 published and unpublished studies.

Regional health planning

In the United States regional health planning has fallen in and out of favour several times in the last three decades. Despite these ups and downs, the interest in quantitative models in health planning has grown steadily. Early efforts in modelling health care systems were primarily academic exercises (Navarro 1969). As a result, Shuman *et al.* (1975) found that few operations research models had resulted in useful aids for planners. More recent reports paint a brighter picture. Health planning applications in the United States have addressed resource allocation for mental health using linear programming (Leff *et al.* 1986), primary health care manpower using a semi-Markov Model (Trivedi *et al.* 1987), and a food supplement programme for mothers and children using goal programming (Tingley and Liebman 1984). An equilibrium model was used to model the consumption of 16 different medical services in Quebec Province (Delorme and Rousseau 1987). While these models have been developed using data from operating programmes, they still report hypothetical, rather than actual, use in planning decisions.

A few planning models have been successfully implemented. Pliskin and Tell (1986) developed a model for forecasting the need for dialysis in Massachusetts which was implemented by the Department of Public Health and resulted in a savings of over $5 million between 1978 and 1981. Best *et al.* (1986) described the construction of a broadly formulated planning system for a regional health council in Ontario. Traditional operations research models were incorporated in a strategic planning framework which accommodated multiple objectives, participative decision making, coordination of related decisions, and consideration of the political context. Boldy and Clayden (1979) noted that in the United Kingdom, where regional health planning has long been accepted, the number of operational research projects devoted to 'strategic studies' in health care has increased, while the number of 'hospital-based tactical studies' has declined.

Because the hospital is often the building block in regional planning, there is some interest in determining which populations are apt to be served by which hospital, particularly in multihospital regions. Simple statistical models have been used in defining hospital service areas (Meade 1974; Griffith 1978). In the United States, particularly in regions with an excess number of hospital beds, hospitals have developed 'marketing strategies' to compete for patients (and physicians) based in part on service area statistics.

In both the United Kingdom and the United States, as in other industrialized countries, the emphasis in regional health planning has been on assessing the health needs of a population and then allocating resources to meet those needs most effectively. Operational research models have been used in both the needs assessment and the resources allocation phases of this process. The analysis of ambulance systems has engendered such an extensive literature that we treat it as a separate planning area. There is a growing number of examples of operational research models applicable to the planning needs of developing countries, particularly in the areas of primary care and epidemic control (Blumenfeld 1984).

Population-based needs assessment

Most planning projects start with an estimate of future needs. Because the determination of health needs has proved to be exceptionally difficult, planners have used past utilization (or demand) for health services as a surrogate for needs. Many economists believe that demand, not need, is the most appropriate yardstick for measuring and allocating medical care. Williams (1974), however, found the classical economic concept of demand inadequate and concluded that some of the issues raised by 'methodologists' have merit. Multivariate statistical and econometric methods have been widely used to project future demand for health care from past usage and a few population characteristics such as age, sex, and socio-economic status (Rosenthal 1964; Wirick 1966; Dove and Richie 1972).

Several studies have used probability models, usually Markov models, to predict the need or demand for particular medical services (Navarro 1969; Liebman and Logan 1976). Smallwood *et*

al. (1971) proposed a semi-Markov model of 'disease dynamics' which could be used to project the need for nursing or medical care. The full implementation of this model would require data on the dynamics of scores of disease groupings, however and this limits its practicability.

Another approach to assessing needs has been the use of hybrid models, combining traditional epidemiological methods and data with probability models linking the incidence or prevalence of disease with the need for health services. The HASA Health Care Systems Modelling Team used this approach (Shigan *et al.* 1979). Roberts and Cretin (1980) used life table methods to predict the need for paediatric cardiac surgery, combining epidemiological data on the incidence of congenital heart disease, clinical reports on survival after surgical intervention, and subjective estimates of the fraction of patients operated on at each age. Similar models were presented in a series of reports on the use of health outcomes (usually obtained from vital statistics) as a basis for planning (Harris *et al.* 1977). These techniques have been used in US health systems agencies (for example, Los Angeles County 1978).

Facility location

A wide variety of operational research models have been applied to the facility location problem. Many variants of mathematical programming and network theory have been used to specify sets of hospital locations which would minimize travel time (Calvo and Marks 1973; Elshafei 1977) or maximize consumer preferences (Parker and Srinivasan 1976). Abernathy and Hershey (1972) compared the locations resulting from four different criteria for placement.

Unfortunately, the facility location problem addressed by most existing operational research models is not the problem faced by planners in western Europe and North America. The health planner interested in where to locate facilities faces a complex problem subject to many constraints. Existing facilities are not easily moved and so the question really only applies to new or replacement facilities. Even so, in most urban settings the number of locations actually available for expansion is limited. An additional problem has been the failure to incorporate realistic models of patient and physician behaviour in choosing facilities.

The implementation of new medical systems in developing countries presents fewer constraints in the construction of new facilities than in developed countries, making simple network models more useful. In Ecuador, a location set covering algorithm was used to determine the placement of medical supply centres (Reid *et al.* 1986). The construction of a completely new city in Saudi Arabia presented the opportunity to plan the location and size of primary health care centres using network location theory (Berghmans *et al.* 1984).

Health maintenance organizations have spurred interest in the facility location question, not only for hospitals but also for out patient facilities (Shuman *et al.* 1973). Dokmeci (1977) used a non-linear mathematical programming model to determine the number, size, and location of medical centres, hospitals, and health clinics. This model chose an allocation which minimized the sum of facility and transportation costs. Buchanan (1980) developed a series of algorithms for both the timing and location of expansions for health maintenance organization facilities.

Ambulance system design and operation

Ambulance services present a number of design and operational problems. How many vehicles are needed in a region? Where should the vehicles be stationed? How should they be dispatched? In the last 15 years, all these problems have been addressed with the help of quantitative models, usually simulation, queuing models, or network models (Savas 1969; Fitzsimmons 1973; Larson 1975; Groom 1977; Willemain and Larson 1977). In addition, statistical models have been used to predict demand for emergency medical care (Kamenetzky *et al.* 1982).

Analysts of ambulance systems benefited greatly from the work done in modelling other urban emergency services, mainly fire and police patrol services. Models originally developed for one service were easily adapted to another because the key elements of the systems are the same: vehicles must make their way to emergency calls which may occur at any time and from any location in the region. Although the ultimate goals of the systems are different (to reduce crime, to limit fire damage, and to save lives), the operators of these systems tend to think in terms of the same intermediate objective: minimize response time. The success of operational research models in ambulance systems springs in large part from the fact that emergency medical systems administrators had an agreed-upon easily quantifiable objective which could be incorporated into a mathematical model.

In the case of ambulance systems, the good fit between the mathematical model and the real concerns of the decision makers has borne fruit. In both the United States and the United Kingdom, the recommendations resulting from ambulance system modelling have been successfully implemented (Jarvis *et al.* 1975; Raitt 1981; Eaton *et al.* 1985). The same models have been successfully applied to planning medical transportation requirements for a district in Ghana (Wright *et al.* 1984) and an ambulance system in the Dominican Republic (Eaton *et al.* 1986).

Epidemic control

Epidemiologists and biomathematicians have used mathematical models in investigating the behaviour of epidemics since the nineteenth century (Valinsky 1975). Dietz (1988) reported on a discrete-time model applied to measles epidemics which was developed by P.D. En'ko' and reported in Russian in St Petersburg in 1889. By the late 1950s, both deterministic and probabilistic models of the spread of epidemics had been developed and refined (Abbey 1952; Bailey 1957*b*). The models were so complex that they could not be solved for realistic situations. However, computer simulations of the models were feasible (Taylor 1958; Garg *et al.* 1967; ReVelle *et al.* 1969; Cvietanovic *et al.* 1972; Coffey 1973; Elveback *et al.* 1976).

Simulations of epidemics are closer to dynamic system simulations than to the usual Monte Carlo simulation based on a queuing model and often include an economic component. Differential equations or difference equations are often incorporated to model disease incubation periods and lags in the effectiveness of control programmes (Frerichs and Prawda 1975). Recently, Assimakopoulos (1987*b*) took a novel approach, modelling the spread of hospital-acquired infection as a network in which bacteria from sources of infection are transferred by carriers to susceptible patients. Several hospitals in Athens have used a decision support system incorpo-

rating this model to evaluate proposed measures to reduce the spread of nosocomial infection. The worldwide AIDS epidemic has stimulated many different modelling efforts. The dynamics of the epidemic (May and Anderson 1987; Hyman and Stanley 1988), the incubation period of the virus (Lui *et al.* 1988), the importance of different modes of transmission in different populations (Kaplan 1989), and the effectiveness of proposed interventions (Kaplan and Abramson 1989) have all been explored with the help of mathematical models. The many uncertainties surrounding AIDS, its treatment, and its prevention will only be resolved over a matter of years. In the meantime, models provide a valuable way to evaluate proposals and programmes which, imperfect though they are, may still be able to save thousands of lives if promptly adopted.

Clinical decision making

The study of medical decision making has blossomed in the last decade. Applications of operational research methods, particularly decision analysis, to the diagnosis and treatment of disease are described in several texts (Lusted 1968; Barnoon and Wolfe 1972; Weinstein *et al.* 1980). The use of statistically based algorithms and computeraided diagnosis are widely reported in the medical literature and are well summarized in a recent review (Kassirer *et al.* 1987). In addition, simulation studies, Fourier analysis, and other mathematical techniques are used in the interpretation of data from electrocardiograms (Wolf *et al.* 1977), X-rays (Chan and Doi 1981; Kalender 1981; Kulkarni 1981), and computer-aided tomography (**CAT**) scans (Willis *et al.* 1981).

The early applications of decision analysis to problems of medical management were often too simplistic to be taken seriously by clinicians. While physicians try to decide each case on its individual characteristics, the decision analyst seemed to approach clinical decision making on an aggregate basis, as if there was only one 'best answer' which applied over the whole population. The development of interactive computer programs enabled the physician decision maker to use more complex and therefore more realistic models (Pauker and Kassirer 1981). There is evidence that these decision models are most useful to physicians in training (Walmsley *et al.* 1977; Goldman *et al.* 1981). Clinical decision-making methods have also been extended to the assessment of quality of care (Greenfield *et al.* 1982). With the growing availability of computer systems in hospitals, the place of computer-based decision aids in medical training and medical practice seems secure (Fryback 1986; Crichton and Emerson 1987).

Programme evaluation and policy analysis

The most important public health decisions are those involving the future directions for national health policy. The way in which health care is financed, for example, has consequences for the health and finances of a nation. Decisions regarding national policy on screening or treatment for a specific disease or decisions on which types of biomedical research to fund may also have a major impact on the public's health. These policy decisions are, almost by definition, complex. Decision makers at this level often confront conflicting objectives, competing interest groups, and divergent views of justice, equity, and human behaviour.

What role, if any, can operational research play in the resolution of policy debates? Few analysts (and fewer decision makers) believe that a mathematical model can generate optimal (or even acceptable) solutions to such complex decisions. However, many analysts (and a few decision makers) now believe that mathematical models can be useful in organizing the problem, analysing relevant data, and evaluating the readily quantified consequences of an action.

Most examples of operational research models used in policy analysis involve interdisciplinary projects. Economic and political theories are usually incorporated, as are epidemiological and statistical models. In some of these analyses, operational research plays a relatively minor role, while in others the operational research component is the means for organizing contributions from other fields. In a few examples, the entire analysis revolves around a particular mathematical approach, such as Markov models, dynamic system simulations, or integer programming. Many economic analyses of health care financing and health insurance use simulation (for example, Drabek *et al.* 1974; Feldman and Dowd 1982).

Whether simple or complex, the models are rarely intended to be used as decision-making machines. Rather, they are designed for use in an iterative or interactive mode as an aid to effective decision making. While this caveat applies to every application of operational research, it is especially pertinent when reviewing policy models.

The allocation of research grants in biomedical and health services research was an early area of interest. Utility theory, economic theory, and other scaling techniques were suggested as means of developing funding priorities (Stimson 1969; Keeler 1970; Cutler *et al.* 1973). Shachtman (1980) reported a decision analysis which helped secure funding for a national survey on nosocomial infection. In the United States, the continuing study of the peer review process (Carter 1974) and the use of consensus panels at the National Institute of Health bear the stamp of this earlier work.

Early programme evaluation studies tended to use 'pure' operational research models. Markov models were proposed as a general approach to programme evaluation (Navarro 1969; Ortiz and Parker 1971). Markov models were also proposed to evaluate mental health programmes (Trinkl 1974), tuberculosis control programmes (Bush *et al.* 1972), and geriatric programmes (Meredith 1971; Burton *et al.* 1975) and as a method for generating a measure of benefit for health programmes in general (Chen *et al.* 1975). Dynamic system simulation was used to model narcotics addiction and control (Levin *et al.* 1972), conversion to a health maintenance organization (Hirsch and Miller 1974), and the delivery of dental care (Hirsch and Killingsworth 1975). Mathematical programming models have been used to analyse a voucher system for financing medical care (Whipple 1973). Chen and Bush (1976) used 0–1 integer programming to specify which groups should be screened for phenylketonuria or tuberculosis.

Some of these early simple models have been the foundation for more complex interdisciplinary models. Burton's Markov model of geriatric care has subsequently evolved into a complex methodology for planning geriatric care (Burton and Dellinger 1981). Boldy *et al.* (1981) described the 'balance of care' model used to assist the United Kingdom in allocating resources between various health and social services. Although this is not an optimization model, it grew out of a traditional mathematical programming approach to resource allocation (McDonald *et al.* 1974). Both the geriatric care model and the balance of care model have been used by decision-making agencies.

Nursing homes and long-term care have attracted considerable interest in the United States. Willemain (1980) used modelling to predict the effects of two different reimbursement strategies in nursing homes. Keeler *et al.* (1981) used simple models to explore the mix of long-stay patients in nursing homes.

Case mix in hospitals has been the subject of a series of studies by a group at Yale University (Fetter *et al.* 1980). This work resulted in a set of diagnosis-related groups which form the basis for a hospital reimbursement scheme now being used for Medicare patients in the United States. Klastorin (1982) proposed a very different approach to grouping hospitals for reimbursement or cost-containment purposes. Cluster analysis is used to group hospitals on the basis of price-related variables (prices of inputs, degree of union involvement, and urban versus rural setting).

Several studies have used probability and statistical models to organize a large body of inconclusive scientific data bearing on a policy issue. Cretin (1974, 1977) reviewed the clinical literature on the effectiveness of prehospital cardiac care and hospital coronary care units and then used a hypothetical life table to evaluate the effectiveness of prehospital versus in-hospital care in terms of life-years saved. Weinstein and Stason (1976) used a similar approach in comparing strategies for the screening and treatment of hypertension. They incorporated techniques from decision analysis to arrive at 'quality adjusted life-years' (**QALYs**). Berwick *et al.* (1980) reviewed the literature linking cholesterol and heart disease and analysing alternative policies for screening and treating hypercholesterolaemic children. Eddy (1980) developed a generic Markov model for analysing cancer screening programmes. Using data from the clinical literature to estimate the parameters for specific cancers, he then estimated optimal screening strategies for several major cancers.

Policy models that incorporate extensive reviews of the clinical and epidemiological data can serve two purposes. First, the models can help the policy maker distil the scientific data. This is especially useful when there is an extensive and apparently contradictory body of work. Second, the models can help in identifying the strengths and weaknesses of the scientific evidence, suggesting directions for future studies. Such work has already highlighted one important fact—unanswered questions which are critical to the development of sound public policy in an area are not necessarily the questions of most interest to scientists or clinicians.

This review of health applications of operational research has been of necessity incomplete. The bibliographies mentioned at the beginning of this section are good sources of additional information. In addition, the following journals often include articles using operational research methods: *Health Services Research, Medical Care, Journal of Medical Decision Making*, and *Methods of Information in Medicine*. Operational research journals may also contain reports of health applications, particularly *Interfaces and Management Science. Operations Research, Journal of Operational Research*, and *Operations Research Quarterly* also publish health applications. Unfortunately, the selection of reports for publications is often based on the originality of the modelling approach rather than on the utility of the model to the decision maker. Many good accounts of implementation of operational research receive limited distribution as technical reports.

Problems and prospects

Applications of operational research to public health problems have enjoyed mixed success. Operational research analysts and public health practitioners have worried over the discrepancy between the many published accounts of health applications and the few successful implementations. The problem is a reflection of the gap between academic operational research (theory) and applied operational research (practice) which exists in all areas of application. However, the usual difficulties take a special form in health care systems.

One problem, partly semantic and partly practical, is the notion of 'optimization' inherent in many mathematical methods. Models that optimize are necessarily limited to a single measure of effectiveness. The concepts of 'maximize' and 'minimize' run into difficulty when more than one variable is involved. It is easy to identify the tallest person in a room (the one of maximum height) or the heaviest person (the one of maximum weight). If, however, we define 'bigness' as a two-pat concept involving weight and height, we may not be able to identify the 'biggest' person (unless the tallest is also the heaviest).

The world of public health seems inherently multidimensional. The outcomes of disease inevitably encompass mortality, morbidity, and costs. The goals of health agencies are most often in terms of balancing several outcomes, not in terms of maximizing or minimizing a single variable. We strive for complete physical, psychological, and social well being or for the best possible medical care at the least possible cost. Operational researchers have been quick to point out the logical impossibility of such goals and to recast the goal into a logically acceptable form—minimize the cost of care subject to certain constraints. While such a formulation may, in fact, be adequate for the problem at hand, there is a fundamental difference between the concepts of optimization and balancing which the operational researcher needs to acknowledge.

The analyst also needs to acknowledge that solutions which are optimal in the model are not necessarily optimal in the world. The model is an imperfect representation of the real problem and it is crucial to test the sensitivity of an 'optimal' solution to assumptions and parameters in the model which may well be wrong. For this reason, the best use of operational research models, including optimization models, may be in an interactive mode or, as Boldy (1981) termed it, a 'what if' mode. This may help humble the analyst who claims to have an optimal solution and raise healthy scepticism in the decision maker anxious to believe the claim.

A second difficulty arises because different observers have different opinions about whether health services are inputs to or outputs from the medical care system. Epidemiologists, for example, tend to treat medical services as inputs (or costs) which will eventually produce improved health status as an output (or benefit). Health administrators are more likely to take personnel and facilities as inputs which produce health services as outputs. Operational research studies have tended to follow the latter perspective. Both points of view are valid. However, when differences in perspective are not explicitly recognized, conflict and poor communication may result.

A third problem is the difficulty in quantifying many important parameters. While some analysts think that the main difficulty has been too little quantification, that is reluctance of health practitioners to clear up fuzzy thinking and put a number on some factor, I believe that there has also been too much misleading quantification.

It is relatively easy to quantify concrete things by counting, weighing, or measuring. However, some of the concepts involved in health and the delivery of health services are quite abstract, for example patient satisfaction, quality of care, and health status. The simplicity of the labels belies the richness of the underlying concepts. It is tempting to believe that any concept described by a single word or phrase can automatically be captured by a single number. Unfortunately, this is not the case.

When a concept, such as quality of care, can only be realistically represented by an elaborate measurement scheme, it is appropriate to look for simpler approximate representations. The problem is that approximation of complex concepts has not always been carried out responsibly. This is not solely a problem of operational research and Gould (1981) gave a thorough analysis of the misuse of measures of intelligence.

A good approximation should retain the essential while cutting away the non-essential. This requires that the essential part of a concept be identified with the application in mind. The most critical component of the quality of medical care is different in an emergency department and a nursing home. Approximations are often chosen with little consideration of their appropriateness, but rather because the data are readily available. The problem of using less than adequate approximations is compounded when the analysts fail to distinguish clearly between the underlying concept and the approximate measure. The danger is that the analyst and the decision maker may come to believe that this measure is the concept.

The fourth problem arises in all applications of operational research. Operational research is supposed to be a service to a decision maker. Models are meant to solve the problems perceived by the manager of the system. There is a tendency, particularly among academic operational researchers, to solve problems of interest to the analyst. This problem was exacerbated in health applications of operational research in the United States by the manner in which much of the early work was funded. Individual hospitals, by and large, did not see the possibilities for quantitative analysis. Major funding was through research grants to the analysts. The hope was that these research projects would demonstrate the value of operational research in health and lead operating institutions to fund their own operational research units. This has happened, but very slowly. Many of the projects were never implemented or only implemented with half-hearted support from key decision makers in the organization studied.

Despite the problems, operational research has now become an accepted part of public health, particularly health administration. The maturation and expansion of health operational research has undoubtedly benefited from the expanding role of computers in hospitals. The presence of computers in hospitals encourages the development of more ambitious models which can only be implemented with the help of computers. In addition, the use of the computer to collect and store information in hospitals gives the analyst access to data which were previously unavailable or at least difficult to extract. The ready access to clinical information has contributed to the growth of clinical decision models and computer-aided diagnosis.

Clinicians and administrators have gradually learned the value and the limitations of operational research. Operational researchers have come to respect the uniqueness and complexity of the health field. This atmosphere of mutual respect and realistic expectations bodes well for the effectiveness of future collaborations.

References

Abbey, H. (1952). An examination of the Reed–Frost theory of epidemics. *Human Biology*, **24**, 20.

Abernathy, W. and Hershey, J. (1972). A spatial-allocation model for regional health services planning. *Operations Research*, **20**, 629.

Assimakopoulos, N. (1987a). A medication management system. *Applied Mathematics and Computation*, **21**, 73.

Assimakopoulos, N. (1987b). A network interdiction model for hospital infection control. *Computers in Biology and Medicine*, **17(6)**, 411.

Bailey, N.T.J. (1951). On assessing the efficiency of single-room provision of hospital wards. *Journal of Hygiene*, **49**, 452.

Bailey, N.T.J. (1952). A study of queues and appointment systems in outpatient departments, with special reference to waiting times. *Journal of the Royal Statistical Society Series B*, **14**, 185.

Bailey, N.T.J. (1954). Queueing for medical care. *Applied Statistics*, **3**, 137.

Bailey, N.T.J. (1956). Statistics in hospital planning and design. *Applied Statistics*, **5**, 146.

Bailey, N.T.J. (1957a). Operational research in hospital planning and design. *Operational Research Quarterly*, **8**, 149.

Bailey, N.T.J. (1957b). *The mathematical theory of epidemics*. Griffin, London.

Bailey, N.T.J. (1964). *The elements of stochastic processes with applications to the natural sciences*. Wiley, New York.

Banks, J. and Catson, J.S. (1984). *Discrete-event system simulation*. Prentice-Hall, Englewood Cliffs, NJ.

Barnoon, S. and Wolfe, H. (1972). *Measuring the effectiveness of medical decisions: an operations research approach*. Thomas, Springfield, IL.

Berghmans, L., Schoovaerts, P., and Teghem, J., Jr (1984). Implementation of health facilities in a new city. *Journal of the Operational Research Society*, **35**, 1047.

Berwick, D.K., Cretin, S., and Keeler, E.B. (1980). *Cholesterol, children and heart disease: an analysis of alternatives*. Oxford University Press, New York.

Best, G., Parston, G., and Rosenhead, J. (1986). Robustness in practice—the regional planning of health services. *Journal of the Operational Research Society*, **37(5)**, 464.

Blanco White, M.F. and Pike, M.C. (1964). Appointment systems in outpatient clinics and the effect of patients' unpunctuality. *Medical Care*, **2**, 133.

Bland, R.G., Goldfarb, D., and Todd, M.J. (1981). The ellipsoid method: a survey. *Operations Research*, **29**, 1039.

Blumenfeld, S.N. (1984). The PRICOR project: applications of operations research in PHC planning in developing countries. *Public Health Review*, **12**, 279.

Boldy, D. (1976). A review of application of mathematical programming to tactical and strategic health and social service problems. *Operational Research*, **27**, 439.

Boldy, D.P. (1981). *Operational research applied to health services*. St Martin's Press, New York.

Boldy, D. (1987). The relationship between decision support systems and operational research: health care examples. *European Journal of Operational Research*, **29(2)**, 128.

Boldy, D. and Clayden, D. (1979). Operational research projects in health and welfare services in the United Kingdom and Ireland. *Journal of the Operational Research Society*, **30**, 505.

Boldy, D.P. and O'Kane, P.C. (1982). Health operational research—a selective overview. *European Journal of Research*, **10**, 1.

Boldy, D., Canvin, R., Russell, J., and Royston, G. (1981). Planning the balance of care. In *Operational research applied to health services* (ed. D. Boldy), p. 84. St Martin's Press, New York.

Brockmeyer, E., Halstrom, H.L., and Jensen, A. (1948). *The life and works of A.K. Erlang*. Transaction, Danish Academy of Technical Science, Copenhagen.

Buchanan, J. (1980). Planning inpatient capacity expansion in health maintenance organisations. Unpublished dissertation, Graduate School of Management, University of California, Los Angeles, CA.

Buffa, E.S. and Miller, J.G. (1979). *Production-inventory systems: planning and control* (3rd edn). Irwin, Homewood, IL.

Burton, R.M. and Dellinger, D.C. (1981). Planning the care of the elderly. In *Operational Research applied to health services* (ed. D. Boldy), p. 129. St Martin's Press, New York.

Burton, R.M., Damon, W.W., and Dellinger, D.C. (1975). Patient states and the technology matrix. *Interfaces*, **5**, 43.

Bush, J.W., Fanshel, S., and Chen, M.M. (1972). Analysis of a tuberculin testing program using a health status index. *Socio-Economic Planning Science*, **7**, 49.

Calvo, A. and Marks, D.H. (1973). Location of health care facilities: an analytic approach. *Socio-Economic Planning Science*, **7**, 407.

Carter, G.M. (1974). *Peer review, citations and biomedical research policy: N.I.H. grants to medical school faculty, R–1583–HEW*. Rand Corporation, Santa Monica, CA.

Chan, H.P. and Doi, K. (1981). Monte Carlo simulation studies of backscatter factors in mammography. *Radiology*, **139**, 195.

Chen, M.M. and Bush, J.W. (1976). A mathematical programming approach for selecting an optimal health programme case mix. *Inquiry*, **13**, 215.

Chen, M.M., Bush, J.W., and Patrick, D.L. (1975). Social indicators for health planning and policy analysis. *Political Science*, **6**, 71.

Chiang, C.L. (1968). *Introduction to stochastic processes in biostatistics*. Wiley, New York.

Coffey, R.J. (1973). Model of communicable diseases spread in a rural population. In *Health care delivery planning* (ed. A. Reisman and M. Kiley), p. 287. Gordon and Breach, New York.

Cooper, R.N. (1972). *Introduction to queueing theory*. Macmillan, New York.

Cox, D.R. and Miller, H.D. (1965). *Theory of stochastic processes*. Wiley, New York.

Cox, D.R. and Smith, W.L. (1961). *Queues*. Chapman & Hall, London.

Cretin, S. (1974). *A model of the risk of death from myocardial infarction*. Innovative Resource Planning Project Technical Report No. TR-09-74. MIT Operations Research Center, Cambridge, MA.

Cretin, S. (1977). Cost benefit analysis of treatment and prevention of myocardial infarction. *Health Services Research*, **12**, 174.

Crichton, N.J. and Emerson, P.A. (1987). A probability-based aid for teaching medical students a logical approach to diagnosis. *Statistics in Medicine*, **6**, 805.

Cutler, R.S., Martino, V.A., and Webb, A.M. (1973). Biomedical research relevance assessment. In *Health care delivery planning* (ed. A. Reisman and M. Kiley), p. 89. Gordon and Breach, New York.

Cvietanovic, B., Grab, B., Uemura, K., and Butchenko, B. (1972). Epidemiological model of tetanus and its use in the planning of immunization programmes. *International Journal of Epidemiology*, **1**, 125.

Dantzig, G.B. (1963). *Linear programming and extensions*. Princeton University Press, Princeton, NJ.

Delorme, L. and Rousseau, J.M. (1987). MEMRA: an equilibrium model for resource allocation in a health care system. *European Journal of Operational Research*, **29**, 155.

Denardo, E.V. (1982). *Dynamic programming: models and applications*. Prentice-Hall, Englewood Cliffs, NJ.

Denison, R.A., Wild, R., and Martin, M.J.C. (1969). *A bibliography of operational research in hospitals and the health services*. University of Bradford Management Centre, Bradford.

Dietz, K. (1988). The first epidemic model: a historical note on P.D. En'ko'. *Australian Journal of Statistics*, **30A**, 56.

Dokmeci, V.F. (1977). A quantitative model to plan regional health facility systems. *Management Science*, **24**, 411.

Dove, H.G. and Richie, C.G. (1972). Predicting hospital admission by state. *Inquiry*, **9**, 51.

Dowling, W.L. (1971). The application of linear programming to decision making in hospitals. *Hospital Administration*, **16**, 66.

Drabek, L., Intriligator, M.D., and Kimbell, L.J. (1974). *A forecasting and policy simulation model of the health care sector*. Lexington Books, Lexington, MA.

Drake, A.W. (1967). *Fundamentals of applied probability theory*. McGraw-Hill, New York.

Duckworth, W.E., Gear, A.E., and Lockett, A.G. (1977). *A guide to operational research* (3rd edn). Chapman & Hall, London.

Eaton, D.J., Daskin, M.S., Simmons, D., Bulloch, B., and Jansma, G. (1985). Determining emergency medical service vehicle deployment in Austin, Texas. *Interfaces*, **15(1)**, 96.

Eaton, D.J., Sanchez, H.M., Lantiqua, R.R., and Morgan, J. (1986). Determining ambulance deployment in Santo Domingo, Dominican Republic. *Journal of the Operational Research Society*, **37(2)**, 113.

Eddy, D.M. (1980). *Screening for cancer: theory analysis and design*. Prentice-Hall, Englewood Cliffs, NJ.

Elshafei, A.N. (1977). Hospital layout as a quadratic assignment problem. *Operational Research Quarterly*, **28**, 167.

Elston, R.C. and Pickrel, J.C. (1963). A statistical approach to ordering and usage policies for a hospital blood bank. *Transfusion*, **3**, 41.

Elveback, L.R., Fox, J.P., Ackerman, E., Langworthy, A., Boyd, M., and Gatewood, L. (1976). An influenza simulation model for immunization studies. *American Journal of Epidemiology*, **103**, 152.

Emshoff, J.R. and Sisson, R.L. (1970). *Design and use of computer simulation models*. Macmillan, New York.

Eppen, G.D., Gould, F.J., and Schmidt, C.P. (1987). *Introductory management science* (2nd edn). Prentice-Hall, Englewood Cliffs, NJ.

Esogbue, A. (1969). Dynamic programming and optimal control of variable multichannel stochiastic service systems with applications. *Mathematical Bioscience*, **5**, 133.

Esogbue, A. and Singh, A.J. (1976). A stochiastic model for an optimal priority bed distribution problem in a hospital ward. *Operations Research*, **2A**, 884.

Feldman, R.D. and Dowd, B.E. (1982). Simulation of a health insurance market with adverse selection. *Operations Research*, **30**, 1027.

Feller, W. (1968). *An introduction to probability theory and its applications* (3rd edn), Vol. 1. Wiley, New York.

Fetter, R.B. and Thompson, J.D. (1965). The simulation of hospital systems. *Operations Research*, **13**, 689.

Fetter, R.B. and Thompson, J.D. (1966). Patients' waiting time and doctors' idle time in the outpatient setting. *Health Services Research*, **1**, 66.

Fetter, R., Shin, Y., Freeman, J., Averill, R., and Thompson, J. (1980). Case mix definition by diagnosis related groups. *Medical Care*, **18(2)** (Suppl. 1).

Fitzsimmons, J. (1973). A methodology for emergency ambulance deployment. *Management Science*, **19**, 627.

Flagle, C.D. (1960). The problem of organization for inpatient care. In *Management science: models and techniques*, Vol. 2 (ed. C.W. Churchman and M. Verhulst). Pergamon Press, New York.

Flagle, C.D. (1962). Operations research in the health services. *Operations Research*, **10**, 591.

Flagle, C.D. (1967). A decade of operations research in health. In *New methods of thought and procedure* (ed. F. Zwicky and A.G. Wilson), p. 33. Springer, New York.

Ford, L.R., Jr and Fulkerson, D.R. (1962). *Flows in networks*. Princeton University Press, Princeton, NJ.

Forrester, J. (1961). *Industrial dynamics*. MIT Press, Cambridge, MA.

Frenkel, M. and Minieka, E. (1982). Optimal patient scheduling in a solo practice: an application of linear programming. *Annals of Opthalmology*, **14(9)**, 782.

Frerichs, R. and Prawda, J. (1975). A computer simulation model for the control of rabies in an urban area of Colombia. *Management Science*, **22**, 411.

Fries, B.E. (1976). Bibliography of operations research in health care systems. *Operations Research*, **24**, 801.

Fries, B.E. (1979). Bibliography of operations research in health care systems: an update. *Operations Research*, **27**, 408.

Fries, B.E. (1981). *Applications of operations research to health care delivery systems*. Springer, Berlin.

Fries, B.E. and Marathe, V.P. (1981). Determination of optimal variable sized multiple-block appointment systems. *Operations Research*, **29**, 324.

Fryback, D.G. (1986). A programme for training and feedback about probability estimating for physicians. *Computer Methods and Programs in Biomedicine*, **22**, 27.

Garfinkel, R.S. and Nemhauser, G.L. (1972). *Integer programming*. Wiley, New York.

Garg, M.L., Thompson, D.J., and Gezon, H.M. (1967). Assessing the influence of treatment on the spread of staphylococci in newborn infants by simulation. *American Journal of Epidemiology*, **85**, 220.

Goldman, J. and Knappenberger, H.A. (1968). How to determine the optimum number of operating rooms. *Modern Hospital*, **111**, 114.

Goldman, L., Waternaux, C., Garfield, F. *et al.* (1981). Impact of a cardiology data bank on physicians' prognostic estimates evidence that cardiology fellows change their estimates to become as accurate as the faculty. *Archives of Internal Medicine*, **141**, 1631.

Gould, S.J. (1981). *The mismeasure of man*. Norton, New York.

Greenfield, S.G., Cretin, S., Worthman, L., and Dorey, F. (1982). The use of an ROC curve to express quality of care results. *Medical Decision Making*, **2**, 13.

Griffith, J.R. (1978). *Measuring hospital performance*. Inquiry Book, Blue Cross Association, Chicago, IL.

Griffith, J.R., Munson, F.C., and Hancock, W.M. (1975). *Cost control in hospitals*. Health Administration Press, Ann Arbor, MI.

Groom, K.N. (1977). Planning emergency ambulance services. *Operational Research Quarterly*, **28**, 641.

Gupta, I., Zareda, J., and Kramer, N. (1971). Hospital manpower planning by use of queueing theory. *Health Services Research*, **6**, 76.

Harris, L.J., Keeler, E.B., Kisch, A.E., Michnich, M.E., de Sola, S.F., and Drew, D.E. (1977). *Algorithms for planners: an overview*. R2215/1, Rand Corporation, Santa Monica, CA.

Harris, R.A. (1985). Hospital bed requirements planning. *European Journal of Operations Research*, **25**, 212.

Henderson, K.M. (1976). Some aspects of clinic management. In *Selected papers on operational research in the health services* (ed. B. Barber), p. 161. Operational Research Society, Birmingham.

Hershey, J.C., Abernathy, W.A., and Baloff, N. (1974). Comparison of nurse allocation policies—a Monte Carlo model. *Decision Science* **5**, 58.

Hershey, J., Pierskalla, W., and Wandel, S. (1981). Nurse staffing management. In *Operational research applied to health services* (ed. D. Boldy), p. 189. St Martin's Press, New York.

Hillier, F.S. and Lieberman, G.J. (1980). Operations research (3rd edn). Holden-Day, San Francisco, CA.

Hirsch, G.B. and Killingsworth, W.R. (1975). A new framework for projecting dental manpower requirements. *Inquiry*, **12**, 126.

Hirsch, G.B. and Miller, S. (1974). Evaluating HMO policies with a computer simulation model. *Medical Care*, **12**, 668.

Horvath, W.J. (1965). British experience with operations research in the health services. In *Medical care research* (ed. K.L. White), p. 55. Pergamon Press, New York.

Horvath, W.J. (1967). Operations research in medical and hospital practice. In *Operations research for public systems* (ed. P.M. Morse), p. 127. MIT Press, Cambridge, MA.

Howard, R. (1960). *Dynamic programming and Markov processes*. MIT Press, Cambridge, MA.

Howard, R. (1971). *Dynamic probabilistic systems*, Vols I and II. Wiley, New York.

Hyman, J.M. and Stanley, E.A. (1988). Using mathematical models to understand the AIDS epidemic. *Mathematical Biosciences*, **156**, 189.

James, S., Outten, W., Davis, P.J., and Wands, J. (1974). House staff scheduling: a computer-aided method. *Annals of Internal Medicine*, **80**, 70.

Jarvis, J.P., Stevenson, K.A., and Willemain, T.R. (1975). *A simple procedure for the allocation of ambulances in semi-rural areas.* Technical report TR-13-75. MIT Operations Research Center, Cambridge, MA.

Jeans, W.D., Berger, S.R., and Gill, R. (1972). Computer simulation model of an X-ray department. *British Medical Journal*, i, 674.

Johnson, W.L. and Rosenfeld, L.S. (1968). Factors affecting waiting time in ambulatory care services. *Health Services Research*, 3, 286.

Kalender, W. (1981). Monte Carlo calculations of X-ray scatter data for diagnostic radiology. *Physics in Medicine and Biology*, 26, 835.

Kamenetzky, R.D., Shuman, L.J., and Wolf, H. (1982). Estimating need and demand for prehospital care. *Operations Research*, 30, 1148.

Kane, R., Solomon, D., Beck, J., Keeler, E., and Kane, R. (1980). The future need for geriatric manpower in the United States. *New England Journal of Medicine*, 302, 1327.

Kao, E.P.C. (1972). A semi-Markov model to predict recovery progress of coronary patients. *Health Services Research*, 7, 191.

Kao, E.P.C. and Pokladnik, F.M. (1978). Incorporating exogenous factors in adaptive forecasting of hospital census. *Management Science*, 2A, 1677.

Kaplan, E.H. (1989). What are the risks of risky sex? Modeling the AIDS epidemic. *Operations Research*, 37, 198.

Kaplan, E.H. and Abramson, P.R. (1989). So what if the program ain't perfect? A mathematical model of AIDS education. *Evaluation Review*, 13, 107.

Kassirer, J.P., Moskowitz, A.J., Lau, J., and Pauker, S.G. (1987). Decision analysis: a progress report. *Annals of Internal Medicine*, 106, 275.

Kastner, G.T. and Shachtman, R.H. (1982). A stochastic model to measure patient effects stemming from hospital acquired infections. *Operations Research*, 30, 1105.

Keeler, E. (1970). *Models of disease costs and their use in medical research resource allocation.* Rand Corporation, Santa Monica, CA.

Keeler, E.B., Kane, R.L., and Solomon, D.H. (1981). Short- and long-term residents of nursing homes. *Medical Care*, 19, 363.

Keller, T.F. and Laughhunn, D.J. (1973). An application of queueing theory to a congestion problem in an out-patient clinic. *Decision Science*, 4, 379.

Kilpatrick, K.E . and Freund, L.E. (1967). A simulation of oxygen tank inventory at a community general hospital. *Health Services Research*, 2, 298.

Kiviat, P.J., Villaneauva, R., and Markowitz, H. (1969). *The SIMSCRIPT 11 programming language.* Prentice-Hall, Englewood Cliffs, NJ.

Klastorin, T.D. (1982). An alternative method for hospital partition determination using hierarchical cluster analysis. *Operations Research*, 30, 1134.

Kleinrock, L. (1975). *Queueing systems.* Wiley, New York.

Kolesar, P. (1970). A Markovian model for hospital admission scheduling. *Management Science*, 18, B374.

Krischer, J.P. (1980). An annotated bibliography of decision analytic applications to health care. *Operations Research*, 28, 97.

Kulkarni, R.N. (1981). Monte Carlo calculation of the dose distribution across a plane bone-marrow interface during diagnostic X-ray examinations. *British Journal of Radiology*, 54, 875.

Kwak, N.K., Kuzdrall, P.J., and Schmitz, H.H. (1976). A GPSS simulation of scheduling policies for surgical patients. *Management Science*, 22, 982.

Larson, R.C. (1975). Approximating the performance of urban emergency service systems. *Operations Research*, 22, 845.

Larson, R.C. and Odoni, A.R. (1981). *Urban operations research.* Prentice-Hall, Englewood Cliffs, NJ.

Leff, H.S., Dada, M., and Graves, S.C. (1986). An LP planning model for a mental health community support system. *Management Science*, 32(2), 139.

Levin, G., Hirsch, G., and Roberts, E. (1972). Narcotics and the community: a system simulation. *American Journal of Public Health*, 62, 861.

Liebman, J.S. and Logan, E. (1976). Analysing the start-up effects of new patients on an ambulatory case programme. *Medical Care*, 14, 839.

Los Angeles County (1978) *Health systems plan component, cardiovascular surgery and cardiac catheterization services.* Health Systems Agency, Los Angeles, CA.

Luce, R.D. and Raiffa, H. (1975). *Game and decisions.* Wiley, New York.

Luck, G.M., Luckman, J., Smith, B.W., and Stringer, J. (1971). *Patients, hospitals and operational research.* Tavistock Publications, London.

Luenberger, D.G. (1984). *Linear and nonlinear programming* (2nd edn). Addison-Wesley, Reading, MA.

Lui, K.J., Darow, W.W., and Rutherford, G.W., III (1988). A model-based estimate of the mean incubation period for AIDS in homosexual men. *Science*, 2A0, 1333.

Lusted, L.B. (1968). *Introduction to medical decision making.* Thomas, Springfield, IL.

McDonald, A.G., Cuddeford, G.C., and Beale, E.M.L. (1974). Balance of care: some mathematical models of the National Health Service. *British Medical Bulletin*, 30, 262.

McLaughlin, C.P. (1970). Health operations research and systems analysis literature. In *Systems and medical care* (ed. A. Sheldon, F. Baker, and C.P. McLaughlin), p. 27. MIT Press, Cambridge, MA.

McNeil, B.J. and Pauker, S.G. (1984). Decision analysis for public health; principles and illustrations. *American Review of Public Health*, 5, 135.

Maier-Rothe, C. and Wolfe, H.B. (1973). Cyclical scheduling and allocation of nursing staffing. *Socio-Economic Planning Science*, 7, 471.

Manton, K.G., Tolley, H.D., and Poss, S.S. (1976). Life table techniques for multiple cause mortality. *Demography*, 13, 541.

May, R.M. and Anderson, R.M. (1987). Transmission dynamics of HIV infection. *Nature*, 328, 719.

Meade, J. (1974). A mathematical model for deriving hospital service areas. *International Journal of Health Services*, 4, 353.

Meredith, J. (1971). A Markovian analysis of a geriatric ward. *Management Science*, 19, 604.

Moder, J.J. and Phillips, C.R. (1970). *Project management with CPM and PERT* (2nd edn). Van Nostrand, New York.

Morse, P.M. and Kimball, G.E. (1951). *Methods of operations research* (1st edn, revised). MIT Press, Cambridge, MA.

Myers, J.E., Johnson, R.E., and Egan, D.M. (1972). A computer simulation of outpatient pharmacy operations. *Inquiry*, 9, 40.

Navarro, V. (1969). Planning personal health services: a Markovian model. *Medical Care*, 7, 242.

Naylor, T.H. (1982). Decision support systems or whatever happened to M.l.S.? *Interfaces*, 12, 92.

Neweil, D.J. (1954). Provision of emergency beds in hospitals. *British Journal of Preventive Social Medicine*, 8, 77.

Newell, G.F. (1971). *Applications of queueing theory.* Chapman & Hall, London.

Nimmo, A.W. (1983). A model of medical record storage. *Journal of the Operational Research Society*, 34(5), 391.

Nuffield Provincial Hospitals Trust (1955). *Studies in the functions and design of hospitals.* Oxford University Press, London.

Nuffield Provincial Hospitals Trust (1962). *Towards a clearer view: the organization of diagnostic X-ray departments.* Oxford University Press, London.

Nuffield Provincial Hospitals Trust (1965). *Waiting in out-patient departments.* Oxford University Press, London.

O'Kane, P.C. (1981). Hospital Studies. In *Operational research applied to health services* (ed. D. Boldy), p. 159. St Martin's Press, New York.

O'Keefe, R.M. (1985). Investigating outpatient departments: implementable policies and qualitative approaches. *Journal of the Operational Research Society*, 36(8), 705.

Ortiz, J. and Parker, R. (1971). A birth-life death model for planning and evaluating of health service programmes. *Health Services Research*, 6, 120.

Parker, B.R. and Srinivasan, V. (1976). A consumer preference approach to the planning of rural primary health-care facilities. *Operations Research*, 24, 991.

Parzen, E. (1960). *Modern probability theory and its application.* Wiley, New York.

Pauker, S.G. and Kassirer, J.P. (1981). Clinical decision analysis by personal computer. *Archives of Internal Medicine*, 141, 1831.

Pliskin, J.S. and Tell, E.J. (1986). Health planning in Massachusetts: revisited after four years. *Interfaces*, 16(2), 72.

Prastacos, G.P. (1984). Blood inventory management: an overview of theory and practice. *Management Science*, 30(7), 777.

Pritsker, A.A.B. (1986). *Introduction to simulation and SLAM 11* (3rd edn). Wiley, New York.

Raiffa, H. (1968). *Decision analysis.* Addison-Wesley, Reading, MA.

Raitt, R. (1981). Ambulance service planning. In *Operational research applied to health services* (ed. D. Boldy), p. 239. St Martin's Press, New York.

Rath, G.L., Balbas, J.M.A., Ikeda, T., and Kennedy, G.O. (1970). Simulation of a haematology department. *Health Services Research*, 5, 25.

Reid, R.A., Ruffing, K.L., and Smith, H.J. (1986). Managing medical supply logistics among health workers in Ecuador. *Social Science and Medicine*, 22, 9.

ReVelle, C.S., Feldmann, F., and Lynn, W. (1969). An optimization model of tuberculosis epidemiology. *Management Science*, 16, B190.

ReVelle, C.S., Bigman, D., Schilling, D., Cohon, J., and Church, R. (1977). Facility location: a review of context free and EMS models. *Health Services Research*, 12, 129.

Roberts, N. and Cretin, S. (1980). The changing face of congenital heart disease. *Medical Care*, 18, 930.

Rockart, J.F. and Hoffman, P.B. (1969). Physician and patient behaviour under different scheduling systems in a hospital outpatient department. *Medical Care*, 7, 463.

Rockwell, T.H., Barnum, R.A., and Giffin, W.C. (1962). Inventory analysis applied to hospital whole blood supply and demand. *Journal of Industrial Engineering*, 13, 109.

Rosenbloom, E.S. and Goertzen, N.F. (1987). Cyclic nurse scheduling. *European Journal of Operational Research*, 31, 19.

Rosenthal, G.D. (1964). *The demand for general hospital facilities.* Hospital Monograph Series No. 14. American Hospital Association, Chicago, IL.

Ross, S. (1970). *Applied probability models with optimization applications.* Holden-Day, San Francisco, CA.

Ross, S. (1972). *Introduction to probability models.* Academic Press, New York.

Rubenstein, L.S. (1976). *Computerized hospital inpatient administrations scheduling system—a model.* No. 7S9010, University Microfilms International, Ann Arbor, MI.

Satir, A. and Cengiz, D. (1987). Medical inventory control in a university health centre. *Journal of the Operational Research Society*, 39(5), 387.

Savas, E.S. (1969). Simulation and cost-effectiveness analysis of New York's emergency ambulance service. *Management Science*, 1S, B608.

Shachtman, R.H. (1980). Decision analysis assessment of a national medical study. *Operations Research*, 28, 44.

Shigan, E.N., Hughes, D.J., and Kitsul, P.J. (1979). *Health care systems modeling at IIASA: a status report, SR-79-4.* International Institute for Applied systems Analysis, Laxenburg, Austria.

Shonick, W. and Jackson, J.R. (1973). An improved stochastic model for occupancy-related random variables in general-acute hospitals. *Operations Research*, 21, 952.

Shuman, L.J., Hardwick, P., and Huber, G.A. (1973). Location of ambulatory care centres in a metropolitan area. *Health Services Research*, 8, 121.

Shuman, L.J., Speas, R.D., and Young, J.P. (1975). *Operations research in health care: a critical analysis.* Johns Hopkins University Press, Baltimore, MD.

Smallwood, R.D., Sondik, E.J., and Offensend, F.L. (1971). Towards an integrated methodology for the analysis of healthcare systems. *Operations Research*, 19, 1300.

Smith, A.G., Gregory, K., and Maguire, J.D. (1975). Operational research for the hospital supply service. *Operational Research*, 2, 375.

Smith, W.G. and Solomon, M.B., Jr (1966). A simulation of hospital admission policy. *Communications of the ACM*, 9, 362.

Stimson, D.H. (1969). Utility measurement in public health decision making. *Management Science*, 16, B17.

Stimson, D.H. and Stimson, R.H. (1972). *Operations research in hospitals: diagnosis and prognosis.* Hospital Research and Educational Trust, Chicago, IL.

Tarlov, A.R. (Chairman) (1980a). *Summary report*, Vol. 1. Graduate Medical Education National Advisory Committee, US Government Printing Office, Washington, DC.

Tarlov, A.R. (Chairman) (1980b). *Modeling, research and data technical panel*, Vol. 2. *Graduate Medical Education National Advisory Committee*, US Government Printing Office, Washington, DC.

Taylor, W.F. (1958). Some Monte Carlo methods applied to an epidemic of acute respiratory disease. *Human Biology*, 30, 185.

Thompson, J.D., Fetter, R.B., McIntosh, C.S., and Pelletier, R.J. (1963). Use of computer simulation techniques in predicting requirements for maternity facilities. *Hospitals*, 37, 132.

Tingley, K.M. and Liebman, J.S. (1984). A goal programming example in public health resource allocation. *Management Science*, 30(3), 279.

Trinkl, F.H. (1974). A stochastic analysis of programmes for the mentally retarded. *Operations Research*, 22, 1175.

Trivedi, V.M. and Warner, D.M. (1976). A branch and bound algorithm for optimal allocation of float nurses. *Management Science*, 22, 972.

Trivedi, V., Moscovice, I., Bass, R., and Brooks, J. (1987). A semi Markov model for primary health care manpower supply prediction. *Management Science*, 32(2), 149.

Tversky, A. and Kahneman, D. (1974). Judgement under uncertainty: heuristics and biases. *Science*, 185, 1124.

Tversky, A. and Kahneman, D. (1981). The framing of decisions and the psychology of choice. *Science*, 211, 453.

United Hospital Fund of New York (1967). *System analysis and the design of outpatient department appointment and information systems.* The Fund, Training Research and Special Studies Division, New York.

Valinsky, D. (1975). Simulation. In *Operations research in health care: a critical analysis* (ed. L. Shuman, R. Speas, and J. Young), p. 114. Johns Hopkins University Press, Baltimore, MD.

Vassilacopoulos, G. (1985). A simulation model for bed allocation to hospital inpatient departments. *Simulation*, 45(5), 233.

Veinott, A.F., Jr (1966). The status of mathematical inventory theory. *Management Science*, 12, 745.

Wagner, H.M. (1975). *Principles of operations research* (2nd edn). Prentice-Hall, Englewood Cliffs, NJ.

Walker, W.E., Chaikan, J.M., and Ignall, E.J. (1979). *Fire department deployment analysis.* North-Holland, New York.

Walmsley, G.L., Wilson, D.H., Gunn, A.A., Jenkins, D., Horrocks, J.C., and De Dombal, F.T. (1977). Computer aided diagnosis of lower abdominal pain in women. *British Journal of Surgery*, 64, 538.

Walter, S.D. (1973). A comparison of appointment schedules in a hospital radiology department. *British Journal of Preventive Social Medicine*, 27, 160.

Warner, D.M. (1976). Scheduling nursing personnel according to nursing preference: a mathematical programming approach. *Operations Research*, 24, 842.

Warner, D.M., Holloway, D.C., and Grazier, K.L. (1984). *Decision making and control for health administration* (2nd edn). Health Administration Press, Ann Arbor, MI.

Webb, M., Stevens, G., and Bramson, C. (1977). An approach to the control of bed occupancy in a general hospital. *Operational Research*, 28, 391.

Weinstein, M.C. and Stason, W.B. (1976). *Hypertension: a policy perspective.* Harvard University Press, Cambridge, MA.

Weinstein, M.C., Fineberg, H.V., Elstein, A.S. *et al.* (1980). *Clinical decision analysis.* Saunders, Philadelphia, PA.

Weiss, E.N., Cohen, M.A., and Hershey, J.C. (1982). An iterative estimation and validation procedure for specification of semi Markov models with applications to hospital patient flow. *Operations Research*, 30, 1082.

Welch, J.D. (1964). Appointment systems in hospital outpatient department. *Operational Research*, 15, 224.

Welch, J.D. and Bailey, N.T.J. (1952). Appointment systems in hospital outpatient departments. *Lancet*, i, 1105.

Whipple, D. (1973). A voucher plan for financing health care delivery. *Socio-Economic Planning Science*, **7**, 681.

Whitston, C.W. (1965). An analysis of the problems of scheduling surgery. *Hospital Management*, **99**, 58.

Willemain, T.R. (1974). Approximate analysis of a hierarchical queueing network. *Operations Research*, **22**, 522.

Willemain, T.R. (1980). A comparison of patient-centered and casemix reimbursement for nursing home care. *Health Services*, **15**, 365.

Willemain, T.R. and Larson, R.C. (ed.) (1977). *Emergency medical systems analysis*. Lexington Books, Lexington, MA.

Williams, A. (1974). 'Need' as a demand concept (with special reference to health). In *Economic policies and social goals* (ed. A. Culyer), p. 60. Martin Robertson, London.

Willis, K., du Boulay, G.H., and Teather, D. (1981). Initial findings in the computer-aided diagnosis of cerebral tumours using CT scan results. *British Journal of Radiology*, **54**, 948.

Wirick, G.C. (1966). A multiple equation model of demand for health care. *Health Services*, **1**, 301.

Wolf, H.K., Gregor, R.D., and Chandler, B.M. (1977). Use of computers in clinical electrocardiography: an evaluation. *Canadian Medical Association Journal*, **117**, 877.

Worthington, D.J. (1987). Queueing models for hospital waiting lists. *Journal of the Operational Research Society*, **38**(5), 413.

Wright, D.J., Bandurka, A., Amonoo-Lartson, R., and Lovel, H.J. (1984). Forecasting transportation requirements for district primary health care in Ghana: a simulation study. *European Journal of Operational Research*, **15**, 302.

28 Management science and planning studies: their application to public health

David J. Hunter

To be sure, the fundamental task of management remains the same: to make people capable of joint performance through common goals, common values, the right structure, and the training and development they need to perform and to respond to change. (Drucker 1990, p.214)

If, as the management guru Peter Drucker claims, 'management world-wide has become the new social function' (Drucker 1990, p.218) then this has profound implications for all organizations whether in the business or service sectors. Regardless of whether organizations exist for profit or are non-profit, the responsibilities of the managers running them are essentially the same. They include: defining strategy and goals, developing people, measuring performance, and marketing the organization's services.

Within the health sector, there has been a global revolution in the organization of health services. Management has been held up as the principal instrument through which the supply side objectives of the reforms can be achieved as well as those which seek to shift the emphasis in health policy away from an exclusive concentration on health services and towards the notion of health in its wider sense. In both these spheres public health is seen as having a critical contribution to make to the management task.

The relationship between management, planning, and public health has been a long-standing, and at times difficult, one. In modern health-care systems, public health needs management more than ever but this reliance, not always recognized, often causes offence or a feeling of unease because it is regarded in some quarters as leading to unacceptable compromise in respect of the scientific, knowledge-based bedrock of the specialty of public health medicine. There is no equivalent science of managing since management is contingent upon particular circumstances and contexts and has no universal application. Hardly surprising, therefore, that considerable ambivalence exists in the relationship between public health and management.

The tension set up by the public health medicine ethos of rational scientific inquiry on the one hand and the management ethos of making change happen on the other can be entirely healthy and creative since the excesses of one can be tempered by those of the other. For instance, sometimes management is about achieving change for which there exists no (or incomplete) evidence that it is the right thing to do or will even work. Conversely, public health specialists have been variously accused of not acting on the results of their scientific enquiries, or of taking too long to complete these when the need for action is pressing, and of being managerially weak or incompetent especially when it comes to the need for political skills in winning support for a particular line of action. The consequence has often been a failure to implement policies or to manage change effectively.

But the relevance of management 'science' and planning for public health can only be established if they are seen to contribute to public health's primary purpose of improving the health of populations. Recent developments in management in many health-care systems around the world which have undergone, are undergoing, or can expect to undergo reform create particular difficulties for public health. These have centred on market models directed towards the needs and preferences of individuals as consumers rather than the needs of communities or populations. The needs and wishes of each, though important, may not always coincide which poses a special challenge to public health and managers in securing an acceptable balance between them.

Against this broad context, this chapter is organized into four sections. The first section reviews the notion of management and the management process in general terms. The second considers the evolution of management in the context of health policy and health sector reform in recent years. The third section looks critically at the relationship between public health and management and develops the points made in the two preceding sections. A final section attempts to pull the arguments together and looks ahead to a new synthesis between public health and management in the context of global developments in health-care systems. The implications of management education, training and development for public health, and the need for change in these, are considered and examples given of the kind of training required to equip those in public health with appropriate management skills (see Appendices 28.1 and 28.2).

Management and the management process

What is management?

Management is often thought of as a bag of techniques or tools and as a set of particular skills with which those undertaking management need to be equipped. These skills cover: planning, financing, personnel, marketing, and contracting. While important, they are not a substitute for the 'softer' dimensions of management that stress the importance of essential principles and core values. All too often these cultural aspects are given insufficient attention or are ignored altogether. The 'hard' and 'soft' sides of management must go hand in hand, with prior attention being given to principles and values.

Management thus has four dimensions:

- the culture, principles, and values of management
- the structure of management
- the techniques employed by managers
- the setting, or infrastructure, of management.

Each of these dimensions is considered briefly in turn.

The culture of management

The culture of management is made up of the attitudes and values that help set a pattern of behaviour for actions and opinions. What managers do may be the same in different organizations and countries; how they do it may be quite different. The most important principles and values are as follows:

1. Management is about people—its task is to make people capable of performing jointly, to make their strengths effective and their weaknesses irrelevant.

2. Management is about securing commitment to shared values—its primary task is to think through, set, and exemplify those objectives, values, and goals to which all those working in organizations subscribe.

3. Management is about developing staff—its task is to provide continuous training and development for all members of the workforce.

4. Management is about achieving results—in a hospital, for instance, results are healed or comforted patients.

Traditional notions of management, or administration, particularly in respect of public services, placed the stress on a number of core values such as honesty, fairness, prevention of distortion, inequity, bias, and abuse of office. These values emphasized process controls rather than output controls. In other words, due process was arguably more important than the outputs to be expected from the managerial/administrative arrangements in place. How the job was done was as, or more, important than the results from it.

Conceptions of management since the late 1960s have progressively placed the emphasis on ends rather than means, even if these might be achieved at the expense of guarantees of honesty, neutrality, and fair dealing. It assumes a culture of (public service) honesty as given. In loosening up management, and blurring the division between public and private sectors, the extent to which the new management is likely to induce corrosion in terms of the traditional values listed above remains to be tested. Something of a watershed was reached in Britain in 1994 when the issue of corporate governance rose to the top of the health policy agenda in the midst of enquiries by the House of Commons Public Accounts Committee into allegations of fraud and corruption in the British National Health Service, particularly in the period since the 1991 reforms (National Health Service Executive 1994). The next section returns to this issue of the new management.

Management structure

The structure of management refers to the way organizations are designed. They range from tight bureaucratic structures, with clear command and control relationships and strict rules, to loose networks with a large degree of discretionary decision-making. In between, variants such as project-based and matrix structures may be found. Current notions of management favour increasing individuals' opportunities to make *ad hoc* decisions, that is, empowering them by loosening up the rules and processes to be followed, while at the same time tightening the control of results. Individuals, organizations, and systems are held accountable for the choices and decisions they make in this loose–tight arrangement—one that is loose about means, tight about ends.

Management techniques

Management techniques amount to a bag of tools that managers should master and a range of competencies with which they need to be familiar to be effective. These include in no particular order:

- communication skills (consultation, negotiation, and conflict management)
- management by objectives
- human resource management
- economics, finance and accounting
- (strategic) planning and marketing
- project management
- quality assurance.

To be able to participate in needs assessment and issues concerning clinical effectiveness and health outcomes, which constitute a major component of the management challenge in health care, health-care managers also need knowledge about public health. This issue is taken up in the final section below with a suggested course syllabus in public health management (see Appendix 28.2).

Setting

The setting in which the manager operates is made up of the physical infrastructure such as buildings and technology (especially information technology). These matters are not considered further in this chapter.

Models of management

There are three principal approaches to management (Gunn 1989). They are:

- the business management approach
- the public administration approach
- the public management approach.

The business management approach holds that government has everything to learn from more efficient practices in the private sector and should, literally, become more 'business-like'. The approach is most easily understood in terms of the five Es: economy, efficiency, excellence, enterprise, and effectiveness. The last of these is the most problematic. Measuring effectiveness is much more difficult than measuring economy and efficiency. While business-like approaches may have improved the economy and efficiency of some public organizations, including health services in countries like the United Kingdom, they may not necessarily have enhanced their effectiveness. There may be conflicts between the pursuit of short-term economy and a rather narrow view of efficiency on the one hand and the more fundamental goal of effectiveness in health care on the other.

The public administration approach represents the traditional view that management in the public sector is different from business management and that little, if anything, is to be learned across the sectoral divide. The approach is distinguished by an institutionalist tradition and by a political and ethical context in which public administration exists within a wider framework of accountability relationships and political and moral responsibilities centred on equity, consistency, and equality.

The public management approach is an American concept which is integrative in character, seeking to avoid both the public administration and business management extremes while combining appropriate elements of both. In practice, this means affirming the value basis of public administration while acknowledging that the business approach enables the purpose of public administration to be achieved efficiently and effectively. But there are those who argue that the public management approach has introduced different values and terms (e.g. a focus on cost, price, market, customer) into the dialogue of public administration which may be transforming it (Gray and Jenkins 1995). Indeed, much of public management is hostile to the values of traditional public sector professionals. This is manifested by the imposition of a new management cadre over established professional groups.

Business management is seen, by and large and in most countries, to have limited applicability to public sector services although, as noted, in recent years the move from public administration to public management has been strongly influenced by developments in the business management sector (see below). Traditionally, organizations in the public sector have been administered in a highly centralized, legalistic, institutional manner in which maintaining the status quo was the primary objective. The emphasis in public administration lay on ensuring accountability for decisions and that due process was observed in the conduct of affairs. Public administration was less concerned with management in the sense of having a clear strategic direction and of changing an organization and its practices to achieve it and more concerned with ensuring compliance with the rules and regulations set down. The shift from public administration to public management has its foundations in the notion of government as a 'steerer' rather than a 'rower' (Osborne and Gaebler 1993). Hence the origins of the charge that many public sector organizations were overadministered and undermanaged. But a focus on management and on outputs and results has rapidly begun to hold sway in many health-care systems over the past 15 years or so as the remainder of this section shows.

It cannot be said that a science or profession of management exists (see below) but a number of attributes can be identified which collectively attempt to define public management and its distinctive features. These are that it should

- be close to the citizen and customer
- be able to learn from a changing environment and apply that learning
- be capable of using that learning to determine strategy and policy direction
- work through political processes that steer management action
- devolve responsibility and sharpen accountability
- continually review performance.

Public management possessing these attributes is concerned with survival and with being adaptable. It stresses multiple objectives,

teamwork, high trust relationships, and sharing information. Although it shares some attributes with the business management approach it does not for the most part seek to mimic it in its entirety or sit easily with it. Of the three management approaches, the public management approach is the most challenging and complex. It requires skilled managers who can operate appropriately in situations of extreme political uncertainty, ambiguity, and continuous change. Most health-care systems, and the function of public health within them, possess these features in abundance.

A key issue when considering management in a health-care context is the extent to which health-care organizations, whether publicly funded or not, and their management can be regarded as unique or at least different from other types of organizations, in particular from industrial or business organizations. Shortell and Kaluzny (Shortell and Kaluzny 1983) believe they are and list the key differences as follows:

- defining and measuring output are difficult
- the work involved is felt to be more highly variable and complex than in other organizations
- more of the work is of an emergency and non-deferrable nature
- the work permits little tolerance for ambiguity or error
- the work activities are highly interdependent, requiring a high degree of co-ordination among diverse professional groups
- the work involves an extremely high degree of specialization
- organizational participants are highly professional, and this primary loyalty belongs to the profession rather than to the organization
- there exists little effective organizational or managerial control over the group most responsible for generating work and expenditure: clinicians
- in many health-care organizations, particularly hospitals, there exist dual lines of authority, which create problems of co-ordination and accountability, and confusion of roles.

It is possible to challenge the claim of uniqueness on the grounds that many other organizations, e.g. universities, share many of the characteristics listed above. The uniqueness of health-care organizations can be overstated especially if this implies that little can be done to improve managerial performance in the face of deep-seated and unique impediments. Yet, as Shortell and Kaluzny acknowledge, health-care organizations may at least be unusual, if not unique, in their possession of the above characteristics in combination: 'It is the confluence of professional, technological, and task attributes that makes the management of health-care organizations particularly challenging' (p.14).

The independence of professionals from managerial control is less of a problem in situations where output is readily defined and measured. It is a rather different situation, as in health-care systems, when clear performance criteria do not exist and yet external bodies hold the organization responsible for the activities of the relatively independent group of professionals. Public health doctors stand somewhere in the middle of this complex of centripetal and centrifugal forces and are often placed in the position of trying to secure an effective accommodation between the requirements of the managerial domain on the one hand and those of the professional domain on the other. Indeed, it is this continuous struggle between these two domains which lies at the heart of successive reorganizations of health-care systems around the world, particularly those witnessed in European and Australasian countries over the past 5 years or so. This argument is developed further below in the light of the 'cult of managerialism' which has become a universal feature of virtually all health-care systems and is supported by the World Bank in its review of the health sector in 1993 (World Bank 1993).

The managerial role

The literature on management is rich and diverse. A brief synopsis is offered of key developments in the conception of management and organizations. Classical theorists, such as Taylor (Taylor 1911), viewed organizations in strictly rational, formal, and closed-system terms. They sought to formulate universal principles which would apply in all circumstances. These principles of scientific management consisted of:

- programming the job
- choosing the right person to match the job
- training the person to do the job.

Weber (Weber 1978) took these rational principles further in terms of developing the ideal bureaucratic organization governed by a set of clear rules and requirements. There were five:

- the organization is guided by explicit, specific procedures for governing activities
- activities are distributed among office holders
- offices are arranged in a hierarchical authority structure
- candidates are selected on the basis of their technical competence
- officials carry out their functions in an impersonal fashion.

The aim was to apply the rules in such a way as to ensure uniformity of practice and standards, and impersonality in the fair and equitable application of the rules and standards. Managerial initiative and creativity (sometimes referred to as entrepreneurial flair in current parlance) were seen to be stifled by such rigidities. Moreover, the formal organization was seen as the 'one best way' to structure an organization and it made no allowance for the informal organization which existed alongside the formal organization and was often responsible for what actually happened in practice. Whereas the formal organization was regarded as rational and functional, the informal organization was seen as irrational and dysfunctional.

The closed-system rational model of organization with its principles of management has been powerful in terms of its influence on successive generations of managers and on writers about management. It still lies at the heart of some conceptions of operations research and management. While possessing severe limitations, which natural or organic system theories have challenged, most health-care organizations are organized and managed to some degree along bureaucratic lines. The natural or open-system approach developed as a reaction against the rigidities and other limitations of the rational, closed-system approach.

The rational model of management is based on three stages which are considered to be necessary in the realization of a rationally calculated decision:

- the decision-maker considers all of the alternative courses of action open to him or her
- he or she identifies and evaluates all of the consequences which would flow from the adoption of each alternative
- he or she selects that alternative the public consequences of which would be preferable in terms of his or her most valued ends.

Above all, a rational decision entails clarity and agreement about goals and objectives and a search for the best possible means of attaining them. The development, and application, of management techniques like cost–benefit analysis, programme planning budgeting, management by objectives, operational research, corporate planning, and zero-based budgeting illustrates the successive attempts by reformers to find ways to bring decision-making more in line with the rational model.

Although these and other techniques, invariably peddled by management consultants and economists, are intended to enable a rational choice to be made among a range of alternatives in fact few of the techniques make an impact on actual decisions for the simple reason that the demands of rational analysis are too great despite the sincerest efforts to achieve it.

A rational model, as Allison (Allison 1971) has suggested, presupposes the existence of a consensus within an organization among decision-makers. The greater the degree of rationality in a decision process the greater the emphasis on consensus, on harmony, on a corporate approach to decision-making and on 'technical' criteria for the evaluation of proposals. Allison's rational actor model sees choices in any field of decision-making as being clearly defined and based on rational assessments of public desires—it is merely a matter of fulfilling well-defined goals in an optimal manner. Decisions taken within the framework of the rational actor model reflect a single, coherent and consistent set of calculations about particular problems. The possibility of organizational and political complications fouling the smooth-running machine simply do not enter into the model's orbit, largely because rational models are normative and prescriptive rather than descriptive.

Although of limited value in illuminating how managers operate and decisions are taken, and although inclined to obscure rather than to reveal, an appreciation of rationality can provide further understanding of the management process. The structure of most organizations, including health-care systems, is largely derived from rational theories. Moreover, these theories underlie the public language in which politicians and policy-makers must argue and provide the legitimation of their bargains from whatever motives and interests these result. Similarly, managers may make decisions by doing deals but they would still be obliged to argue in the language of a rational model of the organization's interests. Adherence to a rational paradigm remains strong.

But, in the end, a rational model is flawed because it assumes a unitary view of organizational and managerial relationships and that all those making decisions identify with, and share in, a common superordinate goal. In the case of health services such a goal could be the welfare of patients. Tensions, or clashes of interest, between stakeholders are perceived as irrational and are defined as 'technical' problems, for example, a failure in communication, poor information, incomplete analysis and so on. The unitary perspective denies the existence of sectional interests and is therefore unable to account for the activities and influence of such interests. To do so, a pluralist perspective is required which acknowledges the coexistence of various groups each with its own objectives and interests to pursue.

Not until the late 1950s did the balance begin to shift as a result of a series of studies which sought to focus rather more attention on possible impediments to the efficiency and effectiveness of management and organizational structures. Rational structures of decision-making and managerial control as the primary determinants of organizational life were challenged on the grounds that the empirical evidence from a variety of studies did not support this view of how organizations worked in practice. 'Scientific management' was shown to be severely defective in its explanatory power.

The growth and maturation of the social sciences in the late 1950s marked a new departure in organization and management studies. It was led by Crozier (Crozier 1964), Simon (Simon 1957), March and Simon (March and Simon 1958), and Burns and Stalker (Burns and Stalker 1961). These and other studies all attached importance to the existence of alternative systems of management, one appropriate to relatively stable technological and market conditions (the 'mechanistic' system of management articulated by Burns and Stalker), and the other to situations in which technology and market factors were changing fairly rapidly (the 'organic' system of management). They also demonstrated the importance of concepts like 'bounded rationality' and 'satisficing' in governing the actions of managers since there were cognitive limits on rationality which lead to the adoption of devices to assist the decision-making process. In the 1960s, an important book appeared by Strauss *et al. Psychiatric ideologies and institutions* (Strauss *et al.* 1964). This introduced the concept of 'negotiated order' within organizations whereby the various stakeholders in large psychiatric hospitals had quite different ideas about the appropriate management and care of patients. There had to be some accommodation among these and this was achieved through a process of negotiation. Organizations comprise disparate, decentralized units in which the actors perform with different perspectives and priorities and decisions are made by much pulling and hauling among them and not by a single rational choice.

In later studies of organization and management, the role of politics and power was seen as critically important in the achievement of goals (see Bachrach and Baratz 1962, 1963, 1970; Pfeffer 1981, 1992). For Pfeffer, problems of implementation and management failure are 'problems in developing political will and expertise—the desire to accomplish something, even against opposition, and the knowledge and skills that make it possible to do so' (Pfeffer 1992, pp.7–8). Accomplishing change in organizations requires more than an ability to solve technical or analytical problems. Because change threatens the status quo or a group of stakeholders (possibly more than one), it becomes essential to understand organizational politics if one is to manage change effectively and steer it in the desired direction. Pfeffer warns against ignoring the social realities of power and influence. Unless and until we come to terms with these, then organizational and managerial paralysis, i.e. the failure to mobilize sufficient political support to take action, will become more evident. In place of implementing decisions,

managers will spend endless amounts of time and energy on the decision-making process.

The concern with understanding organizational politics and power centred, as noted above, on the problem of implementation. Pressman and Wildavsky (Pressman and Wildavsky 1973), in a classic study of the issue, raised awareness of the importance of implementation as an area for study, especially in the context of policy-making. Implementation is not a passive process, faithfully enacting a policy. It inevitably reformulates the policy at the same time. Pfeffer (Pfeffer 1992, p.28) argues that implementation is becoming more difficult because

- changing social norms and greater interdependence within organizations have made traditional, formal authority less effective than it once was
- developing a common vision is increasingly difficult in organizations comprised of heterogeneous members.

Pfeffer maintains that managing power is an essential requirement in the achievement of desired goals. A number of steps are involved as follows (Pfeffer 1992, p.29).

1. Decide what your goals are, what you are trying to accomplish.

2. Diagnose patterns of dependence and interdependence; what individuals are influential and important in achieving your goal?

3. What are their points of view likely to be? How will they feel about what you are trying to do?

4. What are their power bases? Which of them is more influential in the decision?

5. What are your bases of power and influence? What bases of influence can you develop to gain more control over the situation?

6. Which of the various strategies and tactics for exercising power seem most appropriate and are likely to be effective, given the situation you confront?

7. Based on the above, choose a course of action to get something done.

These steps, and the whole issue of learning how to manage with power, are especially important in respect of public health when so much of what happens requires an ability to influence (not control) the behaviour of others, to change the course of events, to overcome resistance and non-compliance, and to get people to do things that they would not otherwise do. There are implications for the education and development of those working in public health which are taken up in the final section of this chapter. The converse is also true, namely, that problems of performance and effectiveness are problems of power and politics—power imbalances, powerlessness, and the inability of some groups to get their ideas or suggestions taken seriously. These problems are likely to occur in health-care settings in which performance outcomes are often difficult to assess, especially at the total organizational level, and in which results are likely to be long term.

Studies such as those mentioned above began to show how complex and variegated organizations are. Their management is similarly complex and multifaceted. Organizations were described as ambiguous, contained competing groups, subscribed to vague objectives, and appeared to be pursuing different goals simultaneously. In such settings, policies and decisions were not marked out through formal organizational and managerial structures but were agreed in *ad hoc* fashion through an unending process of discussion, bargaining, and negotiation between the relevant stakeholders. What occurs in practice in organizations can therefore best be described as a 'continuous bargaining-learning process' (Cyert and March 1963).

This convergence of studies of how organizations and managers operated in practice which appeared in the late 1950s and early 1960s was eclipsed through the 1970s and 1980s. Whereas there had been a drawing away from the conception of organization and management embodied in scientific management or Weberian bureaucracy, with important exceptions, like Mintzberg's studies of managerial work, the 1970s and 1980s saw a rekindling of interest in the principles of bureaucracy and scientific management.

As the earlier discussion in this section demonstrated, the management structure of industrial and business organizations was held up as a model for public sector services, like health, to adopt and, in extreme instances, mimic. Simplistic, almost naïve notions about how organizations functioned pervaded the 'new rationalism' which permeated government in the United Kingdom and elsewhere from the 1970s on. Such notions were to some extent a reaction against the studies of organizations which sought to demonstrate how diverse, pluralistic, and multilayered organizations in fact were. But insights of this type were uncomfortable and unsettling for managers and policy-makers intent on the achievement of clear goals and objectives. The undermining of the scientific management school of thought with its comfortable certainties about the nature of organization and management was bound to result in a backlash and a nostalgic harking back to a simpler explanation. This may in large part be responsible for what Burns (Burns 1994, p.xx) has called 'the recrudescence of the hard-line managerialism which has manifested itself in recent years first in America and then in Britain and Europe'. This hard-line managerialism has been to the fore in health-care reform in developed countries in recent years. Developing countries are being attracted to similar solutions (Collins *et al.* 1994). These issues are explored further in the next section.

Summary

If health-care management cannot be said to be unique, although contingency theorists might argue that it is, there is no disputing its distinctiveness or the differences it displays. But there is no general, all-purpose science of management. Nevertheless, certain theories and concepts over the years have influenced in powerful ways the conception and practice of management. In particular, the theory of scientific management, and related notions of rational decision-making, has been a major influence on the design of management systems. Its weakness lies in the evidence that managers in practice do not behave according to the theory. To understand how managers operate it is necessary to turn to the behavioural sciences and to apply concepts like politics, power, and bargaining. These have revolutionized our understanding of management and the context in which managers operate. Yet, rational theories of management continue to inform the public face of

management. They legitimize actions even if they are not the primary determinants of them.

The new rationalism and health

As mentioned above, during the 1970s, a 'cult of managerialism', which remains evident, swept through government in a number of countries. It was directed towards improving the performance of public services which were seen to be overadministered and undermanaged. Allegedly, public services like health had weakly articulated goals and, where they existed, ineffective means of achieving them. The industrial and business sector was looked to as a source of ideas and practical ways forward. There was also a new-found enthusiasm for the mechanistic and rationalistic approaches to management which had been discredited in the 1960s by studies of how organizations and managers in fact operated. Notions of comprehensive rational planning and command and control mechanisms for running organizations were prevalent in the 1970s as politicians wrestled to contain public expenditure and improve the performance of public services. The 1974 reorganization of the British National Health Service was a model example of these concepts and ideas being put into practice on a grand scale (Hunter 1980).

By the 1980s, the political climate had shifted dramatically. Not only were public services being accused of poor management but their very existence was being challenged. The prevailing political ideology was unequivocal in its opposition to monopoly public services and actively sought ways of privatizing them, or parts of them, as a means of containing costs and improving performance through the principle of competition and markets.

These developments have been described by Hood (Hood 1991) as constituting 'the new public management'. As a movement, the new public management has caught the imagination of governments the world over. It constitutes a kind of managerial pandemic, reinforced by the World Bank's endorsement of it as mentioned above. The new public management, argued Hood, 'is one of the most striking international trends in public administration' (Hood 1991, p.3). Its rise is linked with four other administrative trends occurring at the same time:

- attempts to slow down or reverse government growth in public spending
- the shift towards privatization and quasi-privatization and away from core government institutions
- the development of automation, particularly in information technology, in the production and distribution of public services
- the development of a more international agenda, increasingly focused on general issues of public management, policy design, decision styles and intergovernmental co-operation.

New public management, as Hood describes it, is a loose shorthand label for a set of broadly similar doctrines which dominated the management reform agenda in many of the Organization for Economic Cooperation and Development countries from the late 1970s (Pollitt 1990). It sought to replace 'old' public management which with its complex bureaucratic structures and centralizing ethos had failed spectacularly to improve the performance of services. Some observers saw new public management as nothing more than 'a gratuitous and philistine destruction of more than a century's work in developing a distinctive public service ethic and culture' (Hood 1971, p.4).

New public management has seven doctrinal components (adapted from Hood 1991):

- hands-on professional management in the public sector
- standard setting, performance measurement, and target setting, particularly where professionals are involved
- emphasis on output controls linked to resource allocation
- the disaggregation or 'unbundling' of previously monolithic units into provider/producer functions, and the introduction of contracting
- the shift to competition as the key to cutting costs and raising standards
- stress on private-sector management style and a move away from the public service ethic—this includes the introduction of marketing and public relations techniques
- discipline and parsimony in resource use: cost cutting, doing more with less, controlling labour union demands.

New public management derived its theoretical origins from two sources: the new institutional economics, and business-type managerialism. The former helped to generate a set of related reform doctrines built on notions of contestability, user choice, transparency, and incentive structures. Such doctrines were markedly different from traditional notions with their emphasis on orderly hierarchies and the elimination of overlap. The business-type managerialism was merely the latest in a succession of waves of this type which began in the 1970s and were described earlier. It was in the tradition of the scientific management movement, also described above, although it underwent a facelift and image change, and in the process acquired a new jargon. Central to this type of managerialism was a set of common beliefs: professional management (a) was generic and portable; (b) was paramount over technical expertise; (c) required high discretionary power to achieve results; and (d) was central and indispensable to better organizational performance.

There is no single accepted explanation for the considerable appeal of new public management. It would appear to be a response to wider socioeconomic changes with an abhorrence of 'statist' and uniform approaches in public policy and a perception that public services seem to be run more for the convenience of those providing them rather than those paying for and using them. Part of the appeal is that it cuts across party lines and can be seen to be politically neutral.

An emphasis on health sector reform adopting a particular managerial approach based on new public management principles has been encouraged by the World Bank's major review of health (World Bank 1993). The thrust of the Bank's approach has been to promote diversity and competition. A system of 'managed competition' is seen to offer a number of advantages although its limitations and disadvantages are acknowledged in passing. Managed competition or care pursues cost-effective health spending, universal insurance coverage and cost containment through tightly regulated competition among companies that provide a specified package of health care for a fixed annual fee. Evaluations of it show mixed results but Light (Light 1994) regards competing managed care systems as unlikely to tackle the greatest health-care needs of the

twenty-first century and the diseases of chronicity and preventable morbidities.

The World Bank review of the health sector claims that the encouragement of competition in the delivery of health services coupled with effective regulation would increase the effectiveness of health spending. But would it? The transaction costs associated with competitive systems are high and may outweigh any benefits which may be forthcoming. The evidence that competition in health care leads to gains that are not eliminated by other factors does not exist (Maynard 1993).

The World Bank review has proved to be an influential document. Inevitably given the Bank's role as a major donor of aid in developing countries and in those in Central and Eastern Europe. Hardly surprising, therefore, to find countries adopting a similar philosophy of health-care reform derived from market principles. Nor is this redefinition of public management confined to health. It is described in more detail in the next section.

Critics of new public management accuse it of being all hype and no substance. Scratch away the trendy packaging and a fairly orthodox approach to management is all too evident. The language spoken may have changed but beneath it all the old problems and weaknesses remain. The solution to these may lie in carrying new public management to its limits, as has happened in New Zealand, by breaking up public services rather than trying to reform them from within. Other critics claim that new public management has simply led to a rapid growth of managers without evidence of effectiveness in terms either of lowering costs or improving health. Indeed, possibly the only group to benefit from reform has been the new managerialists rather than low level front-line staff or customers.

Wider criticisms of new public management centre on the inappropriate importation of business sector practices into a public service culture. In particular, especially in health care, notions of competition and markets are viewed as anathema and as ultimately leading to the destruction of a public service ethos. The idea that a pure market is possible in health care smacks of the naïvety of those who subscribe to the 'scientific management' school of thought with its simplistic beliefs about rationality and human behaviour. Understanding how markets actually work and the concept of market failure echo the work on 'negotiated order' by Strauss et al. described above. If organizations are political constructs in which various interests jostle for supremacy then markets can be similarly manipulated and subject to the interplay of power between stakeholders. Managers, therefore, need to understand the nature of organizations from such a behavioural perspective if they are going to succeed in moving them closer to agreed goals.

As Handy (Handy 1994, p.17) has written, 'the acceptance of paradox as a feature of our life is the first step towards living with it and managing it'. Whereas Handy, rather like Taylor and his theory of 'scientific management', and Weber with his theory of 'rational bureaucracy', used to think that paradoxes were the visible signs of an imperfect world which demanded to be eradicated, he no longer believes in the possibility of perfection. 'Paradox I now see to be inevitable, endemic and perpetual. The more turbulent the times, the more complex the world, the more the paradoxes' (Handy 1994, p.17). While it may be possible and desirable to minimize the inconsistencies and understand the puzzles in the paradoxes it is not possible to solve them completely. In the final analysis, 'paradoxes are like the weather, something to be lived with, not solved, the worst aspects mitigated, the best enjoyed and used as clues to the way forward. Paradox has to be *accepted*, coped with and made sense of . . . ' (Handy 1994, p.18). It does not have to be resolved—only managed.

What does this mean for managing and planning for health? The buzz-words in the management literature, many of them far from new but dusted down because they resonate with the spirit of the times, are: complexity, paradox, ambiguity, and uncertainty. We are told that successful organizations and managers live with paradox. Organizations have to be planned and yet remain flexible, be differentiated and integrated at the same time, be small in some ways but big in others, be centralized some of the time and decentralized for most of it. Whereas managers used to believe that their task was to choose between such opposites, the task is in fact one of reaching an accommodation between them. It is all a matter of balance and of constantly adjusting and fine-tuning it.

Organic, open systems of management, which Burns and Stalker and others wrote about in the early 1960s, are very much in vogue in the 1990s. Only now, the terms postfordist and postbureaucratic are used to distinguish such forms from their mechanistic counterparts described by Taylor and Weber (Hoggett 1991). In Handy's words (Handy 1994, pp.38–9)

the organizations of the future may not be readily recognizable as such. When intelligence is the primary asset the organization becomes more like a collection of project groups, some fairly permanent, some temporary, some in alliance with other parties.

In such a context there are clear limits to management—it is not a panacea for organizational pathologies and social ills. It is possible we are living through a time called the edge of chaos—a time of turbulence, creativity, and transition out of which a new order may materialize and gel.

Management: science or liberal act?

As a consequence of the foregoing distillation of theories of organization and management over the past 90 years or so it is hardly surprising that establishing an integrated management 'science' in the conventional sense is regarded as highly improbable (Whitley 1988). The low degree of standardization of intellectual objects and concepts in the management sciences is exacerbated by the difficulty in separating them from managerial practices. Management researchers, as Whitley affirms, have not been able to isolate general phenomena and processes which could reasonably be claimed to underlie managerial practices. As the preceding discussion has demonstrated, this is a reflection of 'the necessarily contingent, contextual and relatively unstable nature of managerial tasks and activities' (Whitley 1988, p.54). It is a conclusion shared by Kotter in his study of 15 general managers (Kotter 1982). He states that the data from his sample show a complexity 'which often makes many managerial textbook concepts seem woefully inadequate' (p.9). Even the general managers themselves had difficulty understanding the level of complexity. Management at this senior level looks far more like an art than a science although patterns of behaviour can be discerned.

Management is not independent from the phenomena it seeks to control, influence, or manipulate. It is in fact part of these phenomena. Indeed, these phenomena largely shape and define management and the particular management style adopted. When

these get out of step and lack congruence, as may be happening in health-care services where a particular conception of management borrowed from the industrial sector is overlaid on to a professional organization, then cognitive dissonance is likely to occur as well as attempts to temper that particular management style. To this extent, management is a dynamic activity able to adapt to its environment. Where management cannot adapt it is likely to be recast or overturned through a reorganization, or through a series of individual acts against particular managers.

Drucker (Drucker 1990, p.223) claims that management is a liberal art

'liberal' because it deals with the fundamentals of knowledge, self-knowledge, wisdom, and leadership; 'art' because it is practice and application. Managers draw on all the knowledge and insights of the humanities and the social sciences . . . .

For this reason, management cannot be called a science. For Drucker, because management deals with people and their values it is a humanity.

In short, management is not a distinct activity or function which can be studied in isolation from the context in which it occurs. The notion of a generic management which can be applied to any organizational setting is therefore suspect and ignores the subtle interaction between management and its particular locus. Standardized skills of the type to be found in medicine and law, and other professions, do not exist and are therefore not subject to 'scientification'. Attempts to establish a general 'science of managing' are doomed to failure since managing is not a standardized activity but is highly context-specific. As Kotter (Kotter 1982, p.8) argues,

if 'professional management' means the ability to manage nearly anything well by relying on universal principles and skills and not on detailed knowledge of the specific business involved and close relationships with specific people involved in that business, then *not one* of the effective executives in this study was a 'professional manager'.

Nor did Kotter's managers operate in a well-organized, proactive, and reflective way. Yet their seeming 'irrationality' and disorganization worked.

Planning for health

For the most part, notions of planning and strategy have tended to follow management fads and fashions. So, in the 1960s and 1970s when concepts of management tended to be of the command and control, top-down variety concepts of planning were similarly of a centralized, synoptic rationality type. The subsequent failure of comprehensive rational planning was accounted for by its adherence to a definition of comprehensiveness in a world that lacks any comprehensive political power or institutions. In challenging the somewhat mechanistic and simplistic view of strategy underpinning comprehensive rational planning, Mintzberg's (Mintzberg 1990) notion of strategy as the result of a myriad of decisions and not the logical or inevitable outcome of economic and technical rationality is akin to the bureaucratic politics view of organizational life most ably illuminated by Allison (Allison 1971). Mintzberg (Mintzberg 1988, p.14) defines strategy as what organizations actually achieve and not just what they intend to achieve. 'Defining strategy as a plan in advance of taking action is not sufficient'.

In understanding health planning it is therefore necessary to move away from the corporate planning models prevalent in the 1960s and 1970s in a number of countries, with their emphasis on synoptic rationality, and to look at what managers actually do by way of planning. A distinction, paralleling 'closed' and 'open' systems of management, can be made between planned strategy on the one hand and emergent strategy on the other. McKevitt (McKevitt 1992, p.35) describes the distinction as follows:

Planned strategy emphasizes direction and control of the organization and it is thus more suited to a predictable external environment. *Emergent strategy* . . . puts the emphasis on organizational learning whereby corrective action can be taken to alter strategic direction and to experiment, adapt and review the original decision in the context of changing circumstances.

Given the uncertainty and instability that has overtaken the public sector over the past decade or so, the idea of a clear means–end relationship in policy-making, if indeed it ever did resemble practice, is seen to belong to what might be termed the *Jurassic Park* school of management thinking.

Arguably, it was the failure of the rational, comprehensive model of planning prevalent in many health-care systems that led to widespread disillusionment with health planning of any description and eventually to the various reform moves in the 1980s and into the 1990s with their emphasis on market-type solutions.

Public health was directly involved in these various developments since the notion of planning, whatever interpretation of it was adopted, was seen as essential in getting a grip on the dilemma of rising demand for health care coupled with finite resources. Some form of priority-setting that was transparent and equitable was regarded as essential. Through the 1970s and early 1980s, planners, many of them with a public health qualification, struggled to develop a robust planning framework for health services. Their efforts were always doomed to failure because, rather like the adherents to the theory of 'scientific management', they failed (or forgot) to acknowledge that to secure effective change it is necessary to get ownership for it from those affected by it. It cannot be imposed from above, at least not if it is to be implemented successfully.

For Barnard (Barnard 1991, p.136), the failure of rational central planning in the British National Health Service paved the way for 'the school of thought which in many countries enjoyed ascendancy during the past decade [with its] reaffirmation of the superiority of markets and price mechanisms as the means of satisfying human wants'. Managed competition and devolved management replaced the corporate rationalist approach. The health-care reforms of the 1970s were seen to be overly cumbersome, bureaucratic and belonged to an outmoded rationalist tradition based on Taylorism and his theory of 'scientific management'. Failure, in Barnard's (Barnard 1977) view, was virtually guaranteed since

- there is no single product or range of products in the health service which would allow rationalization in the interests of efficiency
- consumer behaviour is difficult to understand in the health-care context
- conflicting local interests make consultation and collaboration laborious
- the dominant feature of health-care delivery is one which involves concentrating on relieving present problems and not on the provision or attainment of a desirable state of affairs

some time in the future, i.e. 'the urgent' forever drives out 'the important'.

Rathwell (Rathwell 1987) concludes his study of strategic planning in the British National Health Service by cataloguing the reasons for its failure. Chief among these was the separation between management and planning. There was a failure to connect the two. As a consequence, planning was viewed as a highly prescriptive function not keyed into the real world. Management was in practice little more than administration.

With the move in many countries in the late 1980s and early 1990s towards notions of managed markets and a separation of purchaser–provider responsibilities to permit the creation of competition, the planning function passed to the purchaser organization. The separation of roles was seen as desirable because whereas planners in integrated organizations had been regarded as victims of provider capture, under the new arrangements operational responsibilities would pass to providers leaving purchasers free to think and act strategically. The greater clarity of functions was heralded as an important opportunity for public health because its skills would be central to the purchasing task. The emphasis on health gain and the need to demonstrate that medical investments were effective in improving health status gave public health a new lease on life. But the difficulties arising from making the purchaser–provider split work, and the long-term nature of issues associated with effectiveness and outcomes, has rather blunted public health's ability to make a significant impact. However, before pursuing these matters in the context of equipping public health practitioners with appropriate management skills, it is necessary first to reflect upon the nature of management in public health.

Summary

The purpose of this section has been to describe in general terms the evolution of theories of management, planning, and organization and to show how these have impacted upon public management and health-care services. In offering this overview of developments in management, it can be seen that a general science of management is not possible or meaningful because the practice of management cannot be isolated from the context in which it is practised.

The next section adopts a narrower focus and, on the basis of the above discussion on evolving notions of management, examines the specific relationship between management, planning, and public health, and the application of management and planning to public health.

Management and public health

Biomedical systems operate very differently from management systems and are able to subscribe to scientific principles of thought and action, and cause and effect. Perhaps it is their training for this world which makes clinicians, including public health specialists, ill-equipped for a management role, especially of the type studied by Kotter, and described in the previous section. Whereas they may be searching illusively for an understanding of their managerial role rooted in a science of management, in fact what is required is a quite different conception of the management task. Unlike medicine, the nature of managerial skills is not clearly established, nor are they standardized to the same extent. Practitioner controlled knowledge does not exist in management as it does in medicine. As has been shown in the preceding discussion concerning changing theories and conceptions of management, managerial skills deal with much more variable, contingent, and unstable phenomena which include managerial practices themselves. Management's interdependence with the very realities it is seeking to control or influence shapes it.

The tension between bureaucratic and professional models of control was mentioned in the introduction. In the last section attempts to subdue professional autonomy, if not curtail it, through managerial reform were described. The history of health-care reform globally has been one marked by border skirmishes between managers and professions, notably the medical profession. At the core of the management revolution in health care has been the view that doctors must increasingly accept managerial responsibility as well as be managed themselves by non-medical professional managers. In the United Kingdom, the arrival of general management in 1984 heralded a new era of difficult relations between the medical profession and the new breed of general managers. No longer is the medical profession responsible for what happens, and does not happen, in health policy. Bureaucratic politics have eroded the medical profession's authority (Morone 1993).

It seems that Sir Roy Griffiths, architect of general management in the National Health Service, was not altogether happy with this outcome. As he argued in a lecture seven years after the introduction of general management, he never intended his report to be confrontational with the professions (Griffiths 1991). He understood general management 'as shorthand for the introduction of an effective management process. I did not intend that the result should be yet another profession in the NHS to work in parallel with other professions' (p.12).

Even in America, the land of market-led medicine, the medical profession's freedom is strictly curtailed through a variety of management decrees and controls. As Morone puts it, 'control over health policy had passed from providers and legislators to the health bureaucracy' (Morone 1993, p.731). The managed care movement has evolved to monitor in detail the ways in which physicians operate. What was once deemed specialized knowledge is now subject to protocols and guidelines. Professional models of organization are progressively being transformed into managerial ones. This development has led to intense debates among sociologists about the extent to which medicine has become 'deprofessionalized' and 'proletarianized' (Hafferty and McKinlay 1993).

Public health specialists occupy a halfway position between the worlds of management and professionalism. They are therefore partially exempt from the power play between medicine and management because they subscribe to a population-based approach to health care and are more sympathetic to a managerial perspective on matters like planning and priority-setting. For their part, managers are generally more concerned about the collective, that is, about the total population within a locality, and the principle of solidarity.

But if the frontier between medicine and management is shifting perceptibly towards managers as a result of health systems reforms, and related developments in the areas of medical audit and clinical effectiveness, does this not work to the advantage of public health and those who practise it? Or do public health specialists feel threatened by, or oppose, the tighter managerial grip on the grounds that it can operate to compromise their independence and freedom as professionals to speak out and can exert inappropriate pressure to produce quick results?

The speciality of public health medicine is itself ambivalent in its response to these questions. Indeed, there are clear divisions of opinion between those who believe public health must be an active part of the management system with a place at the top table and those who wish public health to remain detached in order to preserve their independence and professional integrity.

Part of the dilemma for public health and its uneasy relationship with management may lie in the model of management which many health-care systems have imported, and only marginally adapted, from the industrial and business sector. As mentioned in the previous section, recent years in virtually all areas of public policy have witnessed a recrudescence of hard-line managerialism. It runs counter to professional conceptions of management which have more in common with postfordist notions. These are now fashionable and may offer a means of resolving the tension between bureaucratic and professional models of managerial control. Rather than polarizing these which recent health-systems reforms have tended to do, unintentionally or not, the issue may in fact be one of finding a new synthesis in which traditional collegiate forms of professional organization are in fact precisely those needed in order to achieve team working, initiative, and collaboration among a range of diverse skills on the basis that complex problems demand complex solutions. As Handy (Handy 1994, p.3) puts it, 'organizations will be flatter, more flexible and more dispersed'. More importantly, he continues (p.174)

the old language of management no longer seems appropriate. It never was appropriate in some quarters. Professional organizations, doctors, architects, lawyers, academics have never used the word manager, except to apply it to the more routine service functions—office-manager, catering-manager. The reason was not just a perverse snobbery but an instinctive recognition that professionals have always worked on the principle of the doughnut.[1] This was necessary because every assignment was slightly different; flexibility and discretion had to be built in.

Arguably, public health has been derailed because it has been forced to conform to an inappropriate 'scientific management' model whereas in fact its own professional instincts might have served it better had it not had to conform to a mechanistic model of management—the 'old' management imported from much, though by no means all, of the business sector. Yet, public health's roots in a scientific medical model of health and disease may have contributed to the dilemma confronting it. Though severely limited in its ability to describe or modify organizational life, scientific management at least resonated with the scientific tradition underpinning public health medicine from which it derived its legitimacy and credibility. Behavioural approaches to management sit uneasily with the scientific tradition. While the 'new' (public) management (see above) with its emphasis on outcomes may come closer to public health's concerns, its simultaneous focus on markets and

---

[1] The doughnut principle (see Handy 1994, pp.65–79). This requires an inside-out doughnut, one with the hole on the outside and the dough in the middle. Organizations have realized that they have their essential core, a core of necessary jobs and necessary people, a core which is surrounded by an open flexible space which they fill with flexible workers and flexible supply contracts. The strategic issue for organizations is to decide what activities and which people to put in which space.

individuals as consumers runs counter to public health's values and responsibilities.

A new managerial paradigm

Public health has flirted with management and in its innocence has been drawn to an inappropriate model which negates the intrinsic strengths of the specialty itself which derive from its roots in the profession of medicine. In this, and other, professions collegiate forms of working operate in place of hierarchy and rigid levels of management. In such a context management is founded on trust whereas the managerialism prevalent in many health services in recent years is founded on distrust. Performance management is centred on providing proof of performance and on individuals and organizations answering for what they fail to do. Concepts like 'chain of command' and 'centralization versus decentralization' are essentially about exercising control.

In contrast to these mechanistic notions, network structures represent a paradigm shift and derive from the flatter, doughnut configured organizations which are emerging in the 1990s. Flexible, organic structures look set to replace rigid, inflexible bureaucratic structures. Given the rapid pace of change, the revolution in knowledge and its transmission via the information superhighway organizational structures which are not extremely adaptable and open to the environment will simply not survive. Structures, and the management systems operating them, will need to be more transitory and *ad hoc* at all levels—operational, strategic, and administrative (Mintzberg 1980).

Network organizations, which function according to the dough-nut principle insofar as they possess a central core surrounded by a constellation of project teams which exist for the duration of particular tasks and then get reformed, will survive. Such structures are flexible and fast moving because they can change quickly as the environment changes. They can also better tap external expertise and knowledge rather than attempt to provide it all inhouse.

Without seeing the disappearance entirely of the traditional bureaucratic type of organization in health services, it is likely that network organizational structures will become more widespread. Developments in health services such as the purchaser–provider separation, management by contract, managed competition, and so on, will most likely encourage the network organization. The idea is not especially new. Writing in the early 1970s about the loss of the stable state and about what might replace it, Schon (Schon 1973) defined the roles of the network manager. Such a person was required in order to allow organizations to be continually rede-signed 'without flying apart at the seams' (Schon 1973, p.172).

In network organizations a new set of roles becomes necessary. They are essential to the design, creation, negotiation, and manage-ment of networks. Schon (Schon 1973, pp.184–6) identifies six roles:

- systems negotiator
- 'underground' manager—maintains and operates informal networks
- manoeuvrer—operates on a project basis
- broker
- network manager—oversees official networks of activities
- facilitator.

These roles are difficult and demand high personal credibility for their successful execution. They are often performed by those who exist on the margins of organizations. As will be suggested in the next section, public health's management function is perhaps best understood by drawing parallels between the expectations of it and the notion of network management described by Schon.

If there is a congruence between the new managerial paradigm described above which is emerging in public services like health-care and professional forms of organization, then public health may, or could, in fact be at the leading edge of developments in management. In reshaping the management roles they assume, public health specialists are in fact part of a broader shift taking place in the nature and definition of management in health care. From attempts in the 1970s and 1980s to strengthen management in order to control professionals, as we move through the 1990s there is evidence of a clear shift towards different managerial forms in which professionals actually have a great deal to offer. This movement seems wholly in keeping with the general management function as Griffiths perceived it in his 1991 Audit Commission lecture (Griffiths 1991).

Summary

The tension between bureaucratic and professional models of control lies at the core of public health's uneasy relationship with management. Arguably, it may not be management *per se* which is the problem but rather the type of management to which public health is expected to contribute. At the same time, notions of management with a behavioural bias can pose problems for a discipline whose origins lie in a scientific, rational model of disease and illness. Yet, of all those practising medicine, only public health specialists appear to be pivotally placed to marry professional, collegiate forms of managing with network management. But before this can happen, public health needs to rid itself of the clutter of outmoded and inappropriate management constructs which have tended to limit its impact over the past 20 years or so.

Perhaps the future lies in a synthesis of public health's tradi-tional professional ethos combined with a grounding in the newer, emerging notions of management. Such a synthesis may be termed public health management. The next and final section considers what is understood by public health management and how it can be brought to life.

Public health and management: towards a synthesis

Improving the health of populations is a challenge confronting all countries in both the developed and developing worlds. Health-care reform has been a catalyst to the long-running debate about how best to improve health because of a renewed emphasis on health as distinct from health-care. The twin specialisms or professions at the centre of these concerns are public health and management.

As health care has become more complex a false antithesis has emerged between public health and health services management. Whereas public health specialists have generally looked outwards towards society and the health needs of the population, health services managers have tended to focus inwards on the organiza-tion, and particularly on the financially demanding secondary and tertiary care sectors. The shift towards a primary care-led health-care delivery system is forcing a rethink. At the same time, many public health practitioners believe that they have become over-identified with health care services.

The notion of public health management is an attempt to bring together public health's planning and management skills but to give them a higher profile and recast them in the light of the discussion in preceding sections on the changing conceptions of management and planning. The concept involves mobilising society's resources, including the specific resources of the health service sector, to improve the health of populations (Alderslade and Hunter 1992, 1994; Hunter 1993; Richardson *et al.* 1994).

The objective of health improvement has a long history among public health practitioners. The discipline of public health medicine has had twin intellectual approaches—knowledge and action—which have gone together. In practice, there has been a tension between knowledge and action, with many practitioners in public health focusing on knowledge rather than action. Public health management seeks to integrate the two approaches so that public health knowledge can be harnessed to action through the deployment of appropriate management and planning skills. These skills are rooted in an open systems approach to management, drawing on related notions of negotiated order and network management described above.

To this end, public health management demands skills other than those generally to be found in public health. Those working in today's public health function are expected to respond to the multisectoral nature of health problems and serve a variety of agencies. Working in a multisectoral arena to develop healthy alliances is akin to the marginal position desired by network managers and discussed by Schon (Schon 1973).

These are heavy demands requiring political and managerial skills in addition to the traditional scientific skills associated with public health. It is a particularly difficult synthesis to achieve not because of the range of skills but because they come from two quite distinct paradigms. The traditional basis of public health medicine belongs to the positivist, biomedical view of scientific enquiry whereas the political and managerial skills base comes from an intuitive, contextual orientation grounded in how organizations work. The tradition is sociological and anthropological rather than biomedical. This may explain why public health specialists may find 'scientific management' theories more immediately appealing than theories of a less 'rational' and more behavioural persuasion where uncertainty, complexity, paradox, and ambiguity figure prominently.

Public health management is, like public health itself, a multi-disciplinary activity. Clear implications flow from this for the direction and type of training in public health medicine and in related areas which have a public health focus.

There is a need for public health physicians, non-medical public health specialists and managers to find an intellectual focus for joint working since each group has a vital contribution to make to the superordinate goal of improved health. Failure to find this can only result in further interprofessional rivalry and a lack of co-ordinated working. Public health management demands knowledge and management skills of the highest order. Public health managers must be able to adopt a strategic approach and be able to describe and understand the health experience of populations and analyse the factors affecting health. To achieve change, skills in leadership and political action are necessary; managers have to operate in a multiprofessional, multiagency environment and be able to achieve multisectoral change. Operating on the margins of their own organizations becomes a prerequisite.

In taking forward this multisectoral approach and health agenda, a number of key processes are involved:

- building alliances and networks with non-health service organizations; relationships will be based on influence rather than on direction and control
- market management: having a strategic framework based on health improvement, the capacity to work within alliances, possessing good market-relevant information
- attention needs to be given to organizational fitness for purpose; it means moving away from functional departments and towards a blending of skills in task forces and in project-managed initiatives—such a team approach will be looser and more fluid than conventional functional departments with their often lengthy hierarchies and multiple layers of management.

Training implications

Moving forward in respect of these processes has implications for management training and development for practitioners of public health management. Certain competencies and qualities are critical although little empirical work has been carried out to identify these in practice-based contexts. A recent Australian study (Lloyd 1994) identified 'key figure' attributes for the effective public health manager as being the following:

charisma, commitment, drive, and an ability to function in a loosely regulated environment while at the same time dealing with bureaucratic processes.

These qualities are regarded as central in attempts to foster fundamental change in the direction of health services towards measurable health gain. There is growing acceptance of the need for political and management skills. The Chief Medical Officer in England, Kenneth Calman (Calman 1993), believes that

the practical implications of public health are an art and require special skills in themselves. Skills need emphasizing and include both management and political skills in the communication of ideas and complex public health issues.

Developing the catalogue of competencies further, Lloyd (Lloyd 1994) reports on the need for competencies relevant to the leadership of complex work groups—communication skills, interpersonal skills, understanding of organizational behaviour, intellect, analytical skills, planning skills, accounting skills, and an understanding of how the system works.

Management education has been a perennial issue for public health. A working party convened some years ago to advise the Faculty of Public Health Medicine in the United Kingdom on the management skills required by public health physicians for their public health role concluded that all such physicians required core management competencies (Nuffield Provincial Hospitals Trust 1990).

But management training for public health needs to be less concerned with theoretical approaches and the prevailing bureaucratic and economic rationalist model of health management and focused instead on social organization, behavioural approaches, and interpersonal skills. This type of management training is weak or non-existent and yet, from the preceding sections of this chapter, it is crucial. A frequent criticism of management training for public health physicians has been its largely mechanistic nature. For the most part, curricula have remained rooted in conventional approaches and management practices applicable to operating in a bureaucratic organization, or in administrative practices, and in a mainly theoretical approach to management. They are based, not surprisingly, on conservative, individualistic principles and reflect the ideology of scientific reductionism emphasizing such activities as organizational delegation, industrial-style negotiation, policy interpretation, and information dissemination. Such processes tend to assume and reinforce the established tradition of élitist management and top-down hierarchical control. As Lloyd (Lloyd 1994, p.192) concludes

it reflects a fundamentally authoritarian, and hence limited, appreciation of what the management role can encompass, as well as having minimal significance in terms of influencing the health of the population.

In contrast, the challenges posed by the new public health demand an approach to management education that emphasizes the dynamic dimension of the learning organization and of managing change (Forster et al. 1994). Management principles derived from conventional health bureaucracies are no longer relevant or appropriate. With organizations being re-engineered, delayered, and right-sized, they are flatter. Managers achieve results through enabling, facilitating, and delegating and not through top-down, hierarchical command and control mechanisms. They need to work in teams and across professional and organizational boundaries. The competencies needed, therefore, centre on building networks and deploying political skills such as networking and manoeuvring to maximize the influence that can be brought to bear on a given problem.

Thompson (1990) makes a similar case when he argues that students of health-care management are not being adequately equipped with a comprehensive range of knowledge and the skills to apply it to real problems. He laments the failure of organization and management research to influence the direction of management (see also Hunter 1988). The impact of most of the findings from management research appear to be on management itself but not on the community being served and how management affects it. Thompson proposes a syllabus for a study of the management of organizations. It is reproduced in Appendix 28.1 as an illustration of what needs to be done. A suggested prospectus for a Masters course in public health management is presented in Appendix 28.2.

Conclusion

The rise of management in health-care systems is a global phenomenon and has been much in evidence over the past 20 years or so. Central to all managerial reforms has been a technocratic faith in improved management and in its capacity to resolve deep-seated, and essentially political, problems. A principal feature of the evolution of management in health-care systems has been the struggle between doctors and managers, whether played out overtly or covertly.

The so-called 'new rationalism' of the 1970s and early 1980s has re-emerged in a new guise in the 1990s albeit with a slightly different focus. This is known as the 'new public management' and it is in large measure a reaction to the perceived failures of what might be called old public management or a traditional public administration approach to public sector management. Part of the search for different management models was fuelled by a loss of faith in comprehensive, or synoptic, rational planning led from central government.

But whatever the perceived failures of old public management, new public management is also flawed. In particular, markets and medicine do not mix well. Markets are of limited utility in health-care systems governed by principles of

- equity or social justice
- access to care at time of need
- comprehensive coverage.

Market failure cannot be dismissed as being of no consequence. The World Bank acknowledges this. However, although new public management may not offer a wholly satisfactory or stable basis for managing health care, its disciplines have, possibly unwittingly, loosened up sclerotic structures and conventions and paved the way for a possible paradigm shift in respect of how we conceive of, and conduct, health policy and management. Public health is critical to these developments but the training for it will require modification in respect of management skills.

In the achievement of health policy goals, particular management skills and competencies are required as well as an orientation that requires that public health and general management progressively overlap and move closer together. They already share a common policy and management agenda, including the following elements

- a focus on health and not just health care
- a focus on outcomes and improvements in health status
- achieving a balance between collective and individual actions.

Given the description in this chapter of health-care systems as political systems where a plurality of interests hold power, there are implications for public health and management. Public health cannot achieve change unless it is prepared to embrace management. Scientific detachment and political innocence alone will achieve little. At the same time, a set of core values and principles is vital if managers are to gain confidence to manage. The paradigm shift, therefore, posits that management and public health are inseparable in the creation and implementation of a change agenda in health care and that this should be reflected in the management education those involved in public health receive.

References

Alderslade, R. and Hunter, D.J. (1992). Forward march. *Health Service Journal*, **19**, 22–3.

Alderslade, R. and Hunter, D.J. (1994). Outward bound. *Health Service Journal*, **27**, 22–4.

Allison, G.T. (1971). *Essence of decision*. Little, Brown, Boston.

Bachrach, P. and Baratz, M.S. (1962). The two faces of power. *American Political Science Review*, **56**, 947–52.

Bachrach, P. and Baratz, M.S. (1963). Decisions and non-decisions: an analytical framework. *American Political Science Review*, **57**, 632–42.

Bachrach, P. and Baratz, M.S. (1970). *Power and poverty*. Oxford University Press, New York.

Barnard, K. (1977). Promises, patients and politics: the conflicts of the NHS. In *Conflicts in the National Health Service*, (ed. K. Barnard and K. Lee), pp.13–25. Croom Helm, London.

Barnard, K. (1991). Trends in health care: beyond market economics? A reflection on 40 years past and 10 years future. In *New directions in managing health care*, (ed. R. Bengoa and D.J. Hunter), pp.135–40. World Health Organization and Nuffield Institute for Health Services Studies, Leeds.

Burns, T. (1994). Preface to the third edition. In *The management of innovation*, (T. Burns and G.M. Stalker), pp.vii–xx. Oxford University Press, Oxford.

Burns, T. and Stalker, G.M. (1961). *The management of innovation*. Tavistock, London.

Calman, K. (1993). The scientific basis of public health. Address to the Annual Conference of the Faculty of Public Health Medicine, Glasgow, 27 June.

Collins, C., Green, A., and Hunter, D.J. (1994). International transfers of NHS reforms: problems and issues. *Lancet*, **344**, 248–50.

Crozier, M. (1964). *The bureaucratic phenomenon*. Chicago University Press, Chicago.

Cyert, R.M. and March, J.G. (1963). *A behavioural theory of the firm*. Prentice-Hall, New Jersey.

Drucker, P. (1990). *The new realities*. Mandarin, London.

Forster, D.P., Acquilla, S., Halpin, J., Hill, P., Watson, H., and Watson, A. (1994). Public health medicine training and the NHS changes. *Public Health*, **108**, 457–62.

Gray, A. and Jenkins, B. (1995). From public administration to public management: reassessing a revolution? *Public Administration*, **73**, 75–99.

Griffiths, R. (1991). *Seven years of progress: general management in the NHS*. Audit Commission Management Lectures No. 3. Audit Commission, London.

Gunn, L. (1989). A public management approach to the NHS. *Health Services Management Research*, **2**, 10–19.

Hafferty, F.W. and McKinlay, J.B. (ed.) (1993). *The changing medical profession: an international perspective*. Oxford University Press, New York.

Handy, C. (1994). *The empty raincoat*. Hutchinson, London.

Hoggett, P. (1991). A new management in the public sector? *Policy and Politics*, **19**, 243–56.

Hood, C. (1991). A public management for all seasons. *Public Administration*, **69**, 3–19.

Hunter, D.J. (1980). *Coping with uncertainty: policy and politics in the National Health Service*. Research Studies Press/Wiley, Chichester.

Hunter, D.J. (1988). The impact of research on restructuring the British NHS. *Journal of Health Administration Education*, **6**, 537–53.

Hunter, D.J. (1993). Public health management: implications for training. *HFA 2000 News*, **23**, 5–7.

Kotter, J.P. (1982). *The general manager*. Free Press, New York.

Light, D.W. (1994). Managed care: false and real solutions. *Lancet*, **344**, 1197–9.

Lloyd, P. (1994). Management competencies in health for all: new public health settings. *Journal of Health Administration Education*, **12**, 187–207.

McKevitt, D. (1992). Strategic management in public services. In *Rediscovering public services management*, (ed. L. Willcocks and J. Harrow), pp.33–49. McGraw-Hill, London.

March, J.G. and Simon, H. (1958). *Organizations*. Wiley, New York.

Maynard, A. (1993). Creating competition in the NHS: is it possible? Will it work? In *Managing the internal market*, (ed. I. Tilley), pp.58–68. Chapman, London.

Mintzberg, H. (1980). Structure in 5s: a synthesis of the research on organization design. *Management Science*, **226**, 332.

Mintzberg, H. (1988). Opening up the definition of strategy. In *The strategy process: concepts, contexts and cases*, (ed. J.B. Quinn *et al.*). Prentice-Hall, New Jersey.

Mintzberg, H. (1990). *Mintzberg on management*. Free Press, London.

Morone, J.A. (1993). The health care bureaucracy: small changes, big consequences. *Journal of Health Politics, Policy and Law*, **18**, 723–39.

National Health Service (NHS) Executive (1994). *Corporate governance in the NHS. Code of conduct. Code of accountability*. Department of Health, London.

Nuffield Provincial Hospitals Trust (1990). Management skills required by public health physicians. *Public Health Physician*, **1**, 6–8.

Osborne, D. and Gaebler, T. (1993). *Reinventing government*. Plume, London.

Pfeffer, J. (1981). *Power in organizations*. Pitman, Massachusetts.

Pfeffer, J. (1992). *Managing with power*. Harvard Business School Press, Boston.

Pollitt, C. (1990). *Managerialism and the public services: the Anglo-American experience*. Basil Blackwell, Oxford.

Pressman, J.L. and Wildavsky, A. (1972). *Implementation*. University of California Press, Berkeley.

Rathwell, T. (1987). *Strategic planning in the health sector*. Croom Helm, London.

Richardson, A., Duggan, M., and Hunter, D.J. (1994). *Adapting to new tasks: the role of public health physicians in purchasing health care*. Nuffield Institute for Health, Leeds.

Schon, D. (1973). *Beyond the stable state*. Penguin, Harmondsworth.

Shortell, S.M. and Kaluzny, A.D. (ed.) (1983). *Health care management: a text in organization theory and behaviour*. Wiley, New York.

Simon, H. (1957). *Administrative behaviour*. Free Press, New York.

Strauss, A., Schutzman, L., Bucher, R., Elrich, D. and Sabatim. M. (1964). *Psychiatric ideologies and institutions*. Free Press, New York.

Taylor, F.W. (1911). *Principles of scientific management*. Harper, New York.

Thompson, D. (1990). Organization studies: time for change. *Health Services Management*, **3**, 270–2.

Weber, M. (1978). *The Protestant ethic and the spirit of capitalism*. Basic Books, New York.

Whitley, R. (1988). The management sciences and managerial skills. *Organization Studies*, **9**, 47–68.

World Bank (1993). *World development report: investing in health*. Oxford University Press, New York.

Appendix 28.1 A syllabus for a study of the management of organizations

The changing management role

The evolution of health-care management from the notion of passive administration to active management and, more latterly, dynamic leadership and even entrepreneurialism; a concern not only with the cost of care but also more active involvement in influencing the quantity, quality, direction, and balance of care

Relevant issues include (a) the balance between powerful providers of care and relatively weak consumer interest, e.g. the place of the internal market in redressing the balance; (b) the pervasive influence of political agendas on health-care management; and (c) the increased awareness of the concepts of excellence and quality in the success of organizations

Concepts of role and an understanding of the approaches to role analysis are key aspects here

The structure of organizations

Organizational structure as a series of roles and relationships, building on insights from the first section; the enduring value of hierarchy, the chain of command and vertical differentiation; the trade-off with horizontal differentiation, the division of labour, and span of control. The problems of organization design

Options for organizational structures—collegiate and matrix forms; advisory relationships; an evaluation of the characteristics of bureaucracy; federal and decentralized forms; the usefulness of job descriptions and organizational charts as descriptions of structure in times of rapid change

Organizational processes

Decision-making and communications; leadership, management and administration

The bases of power, including (a) centralization in tension with local autonomy; (b) the professional as expert; and (c) other forms, e.g. coercive, charismatic, etc.; types of organizational conflict, e.g.

bargaining and bureaucratic, with a consideration of positive and negative aspects

Managing the human resource, especially motivation and group behaviour, team building; task and people orientation

The purpose of organizations

Pluralist and unitary goals; domains and coalitions; levels of purpose, e.g. vision, values, mission statements, business plans, and individual objectives

Assessing performance, especially issues such as means and ends, quality, etc.: (a) organizational aspects, including management control in times of change; monitoring techniques, e.g. performance indicators, medical audit, resource management, etc.; and (b) individual aspects, including objective and characteristic-based review systems, management by objectives, etc.

The changing environment of organizations

The usefulness of the systems and contingency approaches for understanding how an organization interacts with its environment, especially at times of rapid change

The influence of technological, social, political, economic, and demographic changes. The future of organizations

Source: Thompson (1990).

Appendix 28.2 Proposed Masters in public health management: course content

Core module
Foundations of public health management

Topics covered will include: concepts of health, medicine, and public health management; models of behavioural change; management of change; concepts of strategic management; public health, public sector management interface; developing learning skills

Elective modules
Strategic management

Fundamentals of corporate strategy, strategic analysis, strategy implementation within the context of the public sector. Specifically illustrative case material will be based around the British National Health Service. Comparison will be made with examples taken from the commercial sector and commonalities and differences will be explored, explained, and appreciated

Finance, budgets, and markets in health and social care

Topics covered will include: models of purchaser/provider split; markets and competition in health and social care; incentives and perverse incentives; contracting for health and social care; principles of costing and budgets; concepts of casemix; cost centres; care management and resource management; new models of provider internal organization

Economics of health and social care

Topics covered will include: costs, benefits, effectiveness, and utility; inputs, processes, outputs, and outcomes; assessing the costs of planning and implementing strategies; consumer satisfaction and cost utility; costs and benefits of quality circles, cascade training, and educational workshops; costs and benefits of monitoring; assessing and planning

Health and social care policy

Organizational issues surrounding the planning and implementation of strategies in the changing health and social care sectors; managing the service and its relationship with quality, contracting, purchasing, and provider issues

Basic epidemiology and statistics

Topics to be covered will include: types of data, sorting and summarizing data; sampling distributions; hypothesis testing; confidence limits; simple linear regression

Definition of health and disease; quantifying disease and effects; standardization; descriptive, case–control and cohort studies; confounding and bias; paper critique of aetiological studies

Use of epidemiology to form policy in key areas, e.g. ischaemic heart disease; breast screening

Population-based research

Topics to be covered will include: health research, public health and epidemiology; underlying research paradigms; lay and professional public health knowledge; models of health; assessing causation, strengths and weaknesses of population health research approaches; combining methods; participatory research; research and development for public health action

Assessing effectiveness and outcomes

Topics to be covered will include: defining concepts—efficacy, effectiveness, and outcomes; assessing effectiveness; synthesizing studies; undertaking effectiveness research; developing and reviewing outcome measures; assessing outcomes in routine practice; case studies of effectiveness and outcomes research and practice

Optional modules
Medical sociology

This module will be concerned with an examination of sociological theories and empirical studies of the social nature of health and illness. It will do this through a particular focus upon competing perceptions and the way these are resolved in interactions, in a variety of settings, between healers and clients

Ethical issues in health and social care

The module will provide an introduction to ethical issues and ways of thinking about them, examining the moral issues that arise in health and social care. Topics covered in the module will include: justifying action—how actions are justified; distinguishing 'right' from 'good'; current ethical theories; ethics and metaethics. The ethical basis for health and social care—a review of possible ethical bases for the National Health Service in the United Kingdom, other public sector agencies, and the private health-care sector; the implications for the organization and resource allocation. Issues in resource allocation—equity; decisions between populations; decisions between individuals; valuing human life. Issues relating to the person—what constitutes a person?; death and dying; psychiatric care and compulsion

Marketing for health and social care

Areas investigated will include: the development of marketing for non-profit and service organizations; customers, consumers, and patients as decision-making units; the needs, wants, and benefits of the above groups; the meaning for the organization to be 'market oriented'; organizational strategy; development of the marketing mix for services; the marketing environment; business definition and mission statements; marketing planning and its relationship to strategic planning; market research techniques for health and social services; demand management; internal marketing; the introduction of the marketing function into the organization; and marketing communications

Assessing organizational performance

Assessment of performance is a crucial and complex activity, particularly when applied to managerial performance. This is in part due to the breadth of posts that can be generically described as 'managerial', but also because of the problems of identifying specific outcome measures

The module will focus on the principles, techniques, practice, and influential factors that surround the assessment of managerial performance in organizations

Primary and community care

The aim of this module will be to provide a framework for analysing and responding to the post-Griffiths context, and it will address the following issues. Understanding the concept of community care, with particular reference to its organizational, professional, and political constructions. Administrative and funding arrangements at national and local levels, including a critical examination of the marked variation between individual counties in the United Kingdom. Developing comprehensive locally based services and consequences of a mixed economy of provision; critiques of the limitations of community care policies developed in the United Kingdom in the mid-1980s; developing a new framework for the strategic management of community care in the post-Griffiths era; identifying key tasks, skills, and resources

Theories and models of quality assurance

This module will cover definitions of quality and related terms; detailed examination of approaches to quality assurance; and theory and practice of specifying and measuring the quality of care

Health care in an international perspective

The module will examine three major issues: health-care reform, decentralization, and the financing of health services. For each, appropriate theory and case-study material will be explored. Varying models relating to selected countries will be discussed and their relevance to the National Health Service considered

Source: Nuffield Institute for Health, University of Leeds.

IV Environmental health sciences

Toxicology and environmental health

Bernard D. Goldstein and Michael R. Greenberg

Introduction

In recent decades we have witnessed a public outcry against pollution of the environment that parallels the force of the Sanitary Revolution of the mid-nineteenth century. New national and international governmental organizations reflect the political potency of this public concern. The chemical, electronics, and petroleum industries, whose previously steady growth greatly accelerated following the Second World War, are now forced to consider factors other than utility and cost in the development of new products and the marketing of old ones. Substantial societal investments have been made in the developed countries to clean up old environmental pollution problems and to prevent new ones. As with the Sanitary Revolution, part of the rationale has been a developing understanding of the relationship of a foul environment to human ill health, while part is simply a human revulsion to dirty air, tainted water, and a blighted natural environment. Moreover, we have come to recognize that sustainable development of the earth's resources is not possible under the related threats of population growth and environmental degradation.

As we develop more understanding of the Earth, its ecosystems, and the pathways of chemical exposure, problems once thought to be limited to the natural environment have been shown to pose risks to human health, for example contamination of drinking water by hazardous waste dumps.

The most substantial long-range threat to human health posed by environmental chemicals is the alteration of the Earth's atmosphere. Chlorofluorocarbons (CFCs) and other compounds are producing a decrease in the levels of stratospheric ozone which prevents shorter-range ultraviolet light rays from penetrating to the Earth's surface, a protective mantle which has been present through much of evolution. The implications of climatic alterations, such as the greenhouse effect caused primarily by increased fossil fuel use and by agricultural practices, are potentially dire. Together, the secondary effects of the alteration of our global climate could be disastrous to human health and could include major changes in the range and habitat of disease vectors, severe flooding and famine from crop failure (McMichael 1994).

The global climate issue illustrates four points that are pertinent to this chapter.

1. Understanding the effects of chemicals is crucial to environmental health.

2. The system in which chemicals act, whether the human body or planet Earth, is a closed one with only limited response, repair, and regenerative potential.

3. The effects of chemical and physical agents on health are often delayed and indirect, but none the less disastrous.

4. Local, national, and international control efforts have tended to be most effective when dealing with a single pollutant in a single medium directly producing overt effects and least effective when dealing with complex chemical mixtures, with pollutants that cross traditional air, water, soil, and food boundaries, and with effects that are delayed or indirect.

In this chapter we focus on the science of toxicology as it relates to environmental health. We also consider some of the interfaces between environmental health sciences and public policy. Toxicology is the science of poisons (Amdur *et al.* 1991). Knowledge about poisons extends back to the beginning of history as humans became aware of the toxicity of natural food components. The Bible contains injunctions concerning poisons, including how to avoid them. Greek and Roman history gives evidence of the use of poisons as an instrument of statecraft, an approach that was extended in the middle ages with such notable practitioners as the Borgias. Toxicologists tend to view Paracelcus, a seventeenth century alchemist and a bit of a charlatan, as their ancestor, crediting him with the first law of toxicology, that the dose makes the poison (Gallo and Doull 1991). There are two other major maxims that underlie modern toxicology: that chemicals have specific biological effects, and that humans are members of the animal kingdom.

This chapter discusses 'laws' and general concepts of toxicology pertinent to understanding how a chemical or physical agent acts in a biological system. The focus is on the biological response, rather than on the intrinsic property of the agent, although the latter is briefly reviewed (Plaa 1991). The chapter is restricted to human health, although many of the concepts are applicable to ecological health as well.

Laws of toxicology
The dose makes the poison

Central to toxicology is the exploration of how dose is related to response. As a generalization, there are two types of dose–response curves (see Fig. 29.1). One is an S-shaped curve that is characterized by having at lowest doses no observed effect and, as the dose increases, the gradual development of an increasing response. This is followed by a linear phase of increase in response and in relation to dose and, eventually, a dose level at which no further increase in response is observed. Of particular pertinence to environmental toxicology is that this curve presumes that there is a threshold level

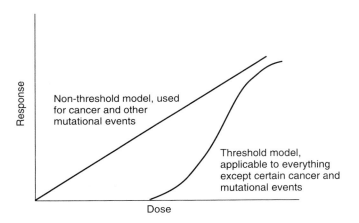

Fig. 29.1 Dose–response curves.

below which no harm whatsoever is to be expected. There is an ample scientific base for the existence of thresholds for specific effects (Aldridge 1986). For example, if undiluted sulphuric acid is splashed on the skin it is capable of producing a severe burn. Yet one drop of pure sulphuric acid in a bathtub of water is sufficiently dilute to be entirely without effect. Thresholds for an adverse effect will differ between individuals based upon a variety of circumstances, some of which are genetically determined and others may represent stages of life or specific circumstances. In the example of sulphuric acid on the skin, there are genetically determined differences in susceptibility related to the protective presence of skin hair, babies being more susceptible than adults, and skin that is already cut being at particular risk. This S-type dose–response curve has generally been found to fit all toxic effects except those that are produced by a direct reaction with genetic material.

The second general type of dose–response curve has no apparent threshold dose. It covers those endpoints caused by persistent changes in the genes. This occurs in cancers, in which a so-called somatic mutation occurring in a single cell results in a clone of cancer cell progeny. Similarly, germ-like mutations can occur in the DNA of cells involved in reproduction. The genetic code can be considered as bits of information strung on a line in such a way that alteration of one single bit of information can have a profound effect on the overall meaning. It is believed that a single change in DNA can alter the genetic code in such a way as to lead to a mutated cell. It therefore follows that any single molecule of a chemical compound or packet of energy of a physical agent, such as ionizing radiation, that can alter DNA is theoretically capable of causing a persistent mutation. If the chemical adduct or other change in DNA is not repaired by cellular enzymes, each molecule or ionizing ray theoretically has the possibility of changing a normal cell to a cancerous cell. The resultant dose–response curve starts at a single molecule, that is it has no threshold below which the risk is zero (Fig. 29.1). There is no absolutely safe dose. In this highly simplified scheme, the shape of the curve is linearly related to dose, such that the risk of two molecules of a DNA-altering chemical causing a mutation is twice that of one molecule and so on until a dose level that results in dead cells. Since dead cells do not reproduce, they cannot be the basis for cancer or for inherited abnormalities Note also that relatively few chemicals are capable of directly altering the DNA of a living cell. Further, the risk of any

one molecule actually causing cancer is infinitesimally small; despite the immense number of carcinogenic molecules in the smoke of one cigarette, only a minority of cigarette smokers ever develop cancer. Yet the assumption that the risk is not zero has a major impact on communicating to the public about cancer risk from chemical and physical carcinogens. Industry has often claimed that a threshold exists for carcinogens and, in some cases, mechanistically based toxicological research has substantiated that claim. The prudent public health approach to known or potential human carcinogens places the burden of proof on an industry making such a claim.

Specificity

That chemical and physical agents have specific effects has been called the second law of toxicology. The concept is no different from recognizing that possession of a gun does not make one a murder suspect if the victim has been stabbed to death. This principle is well understood by the public in terms of medicine: aspirin will help with your headache but is useless for constipation, while laxatives have the opposite specificity. Nevertheless, various surveys suggest that the selectivity of effects of environmental chemicals is not well understood by the public; many believe that a chemical that can cause cancer in a particular organ can cause cancer and other diseases anywhere in the body.

The specificity of effects is due both to chemistry and to biology. Understanding the relationship between chemical structure and biological effect has been a central core of both pharmacology and toxicology. Structure–activity relationships (**SARs**) are often used to design a chemical with a specific effect that might be useful as a therapeutic agent. SARs also are used to predict whether a new chemical being readied for manufacture might be of potential harm. While SARs are a useful tool, the predictive value is too limited to be used without recourse to additional testing of a potentially toxic agent. For example, one methyl group separates toluene from benzene, only the latter causing bone marrow damage and leukaemia, ethanol from methanol, the latter causing acute acidosis and blindness and hexane from either heptane or pentane, with only hexane being responsible for peripheral nerve damage. These differences reflect specificity in the formation of toxic metabolites and in interactions with biological receptors.

Chemical structure is also an important determinant of the specific characteristics of environmental persistence. There is substantial scientific and public concern about agents that accumulate in the human body or in the general environment. Many such compounds have already been banned or severely restricted (for example, dichlorodiphenyltrichloroethane (DDT) and polychlorinated biphenyl (PCBs). There is a consensus that development or use of additional persistent and accumulative agents should be avoided, particularly as standard toxicological approaches cannot predict all untoward effects and it can be decades before reversing the environmental effects of a persistent organic compound is possible. Sometimes, non-persistent compounds may be precursors of persistent agents, such as dioxins and dibenzofurans often produced in the incineration of chlorine-containing wastes. The possibility that such compounds subtly alter oestrogenic hormone function has become a matter of intense interest (Colborn et al. 1993).

Specificity of effects is also conferred by the susceptibility of cellular processes that lead certain cells to be more of a target to environmental agents. For example, the iron-containing protein haemoglobin in red blood cells is responsible for the delivery of oxygen to the tissues in the body. Significant toxicity can occur through several specific mechanisms. Oxidation of the reduced ferrous form to the ferric form of iron in the haemoglobin impairs the ability to carry and release oxygen in the tissues. Various chemical agents oxidize intracellular iron, including nitrites that are common contaminants of well water in agricultural communities. Carbon monoxide, an otherwise relatively inert gas, sufficiently resembles oxygen so that it can bind to the oxygen-combining site of haemoglobin, thereby displacing oxygen. There are many other examples in which a normal body process is disrupted by an exogenous chemical through oxidation, covalent addition, or fitting into a niche designed through evolution to accommodate an internal chemical that it superficially resembles.

Humans are animals

That humans are animals is the third law of toxicology. The conceptual foundation for extrapolating findings in animals to expected effects in humans is a central facet of modern toxicology. The basic principles of cell and organ function are common to all of biology. All cells must obtain energy, build structure, and release waste. The specificity of toxic effects is relatively similar across mammals. In other words, a kidney poison in one species is likely to be a kidney poison in another, although there are exceptions. However, dose–response considerations often vary substantially, reflecting differences in adsorption, distribution, metabolism, excretion, function, and target organ susceptibility between species. Understanding the factors responsible for interspecies differences greatly facilitates extrapolation from animals to humans. Once elucidated, the role of different absorption rates, metabolism, or other factors can be taken into account, often through a mathematical approximation called physiologically based pharmacokinetics (Frantz *et al.* 1994)

Human pathways of exogenous chemicals

A central focus of toxicological science is the assessment of the pathways taken by a chemical from its entrance into the body until its eventual excretion. This process is usually divided into four related processes of absorption, distribution, metabolism, and excretion (Gallo *et al.* 1987).

Absorption

Absorption of a chemical into the body occurs through the mouth, respiratory tract, and skin. Depending upon the specific chemical, the route of exposure can have major implications for absorption into the body and the resultant toxicity. For example, almost 100 per cent of inhaled lead particles are absorbed into the circulation as compared with a much smaller percent of ingested lead. Internal factors can affect absorption, particularly from the gastrointestinal tract. For example, iron and calcium deficiencies, which are common in children in inner city areas where lead is prevalent, both produce an increase in absorption of ingested lead. The milieu of the exposure agent can also have an effect on its bioavailability.

For example, the rate at which benzene in gasoline is absorbed through the skin is increased by the addition of oxygenated components to the gasoline mixture and the extent to which dioxin in soil is absorbed through the gastrointestinal tract differs many hundred-fold depending upon the source of the contaminated soil (Umbreit *et al.* 1986).

Often, a single route of absorption is dominant. Nevertheless, in many instances more than one route is important. For example, exposure due to contamination of well water through a leaky underground storage tank is usually thought of solely in terms of water intake. However, depending upon the height of the water table there may be off gassing into the basement, producing inhalation exposure, and during showering there is likely to be both inhalation and transdermal absorption.

Distribution

Distribution of the chemical, once inside the body, occurs through different pathways. In part this distribution depends upon the route of absorption. Most compounds absorbed in the gastrointestinal tract go directly to the liver and may go no farther, while inhaled agents first go to the lung or other parts of the respiratory tract. Distribution also depends upon the chemical and physical properties of the agents. Small particles tend to be distributed deep within the respiratory tract, while larger particles wind up in the nose or upper respiratory tract. Chemicals that are poorly soluble in water, for example oils, usually distribute within fatty tissues and only certain types of compounds can penetrate from the blood to the brain. Distribution will often depend upon organ-specific factors. For example, the high levels of iodine in the thyroid are due to a specific thyroid pump for the uptake of iodine needed for the synthesis of thyroid hormones.

Metabolism

Metabolism in the narrowest sense of the term refers to alteration of chemicals by the body (Kato *et al.* 1989). The major metabolic function of the body is to alter food into energy or structural materials. Most foods and other exogenous chemicals are metabolized in the liver. All organs have metabolic capability, often related both to organ function and to susceptibility to toxic agents. Understanding the specifics of the enzyme and enzyme families responsible for metabolism within cell types is important to the question of why chemicals have specific effects in specific organs.

Metabolism is often divided into two phases. Phase I reactions usually involve oxidation, reduction, or hydrolysis to convert exogenous chemicals into substances capable of being converted by phase II enzymes into conjugates that can be excreted or into building blocks useful for synthesis of body components. The major family of enzymes involved in phase I reactions are cytochrome P450-containing mono-oxygenases, of which there are multiple forms with varying degrees of specificity.

Metabolism of foreign substances is often protective, converting unwanted absorbed materials into chemical forms that are readily excretable. Thus, a fat-soluble agent can be converted into more water-soluble agents capable of being excreted in the bile or the urine. At times, metabolism is central to toxicity through conversion of relatively inactive compounds into harmful agents (Guengerich and Liebler 1985). A variety of compounds ranging from polycyclic organic hydrocarbon components of soot to the leukae-mogen benzene require metabolic activation to become carcino-genic. In the case of benzene, approximately 50 per cent of the body burden is exhaled unmetabolized and approximately 50 per cent is metabolized into potentially toxic metabolites. Slowing benzene metabolism leads to an increase in the relative amount exhaled rather than metabolized and a decrease in bone marrow toxicity. In contrast, speeding up benzene metabolism increases its toxicity (Snyder *et al.* 1993). For example, alcohol induces an increase in the specific cytochrome P450 responsible for benzene metabolism and has been shown to potentiate benzene toxicity.

Excretion

Excretion from the body can occur through a variety of routes. These include the gastrointestinal tract for unabsorbed ingested components and the urine for water-soluble agents of appropriate molecular weight and charge. The urinary excretion rate can be substantially affected by the state of body hydration. Agents metabolized in the liver are often excreted through the biliary tract. Significant loss of volatile compounds can occur through the respiratory tract, as noted above for benzene. Other routes of excretion include sweat and lactation, the latter unfortunately putting infants at risk when mothers' milk contains toxic agents.

Susceptibility

One of the more difficult problems in toxicology is understanding the basis for differences in human susceptibility to environmental insults (Grandjean 1995). In some individuals, cigarette smoking will cause death at a relatively young age due to lung and other cancers, chronic lung disease, or cardiovascular disease, while other individuals with the same or greater smoking history will survive with relatively minimal damage until much older. A partial explana-tion is that certain environmental toxins act to speed up the effects of impacts that would have occurred later in life due to genetic or other environmental causes. For example, someone who would have died of a heart attack at age 70 years due to an inherited tendency to cholesterol accumulation in the arteries coupled with a high cholesterol intake in the diet, may have a heart attack at age 55 years because of the added insult of cigarette smoking. Understanding of the interaction of genetic and environmental factors in human disease will be greatly abetted by current research on the human genome. While a genetic basis for most diseases will be discernible, it must be emphasized that the inherited factors will usually be necessary but not sufficient to lead to disease. With the exception of certain childhood disorders, environmental factors will usually determine whether and when the genetically determined disease will become manifest.

The known causes of increased human susceptibility to a specific level of a noxious environmental agent fit into four classes: increased uptake into the body, increased delivery of the agent or its metabolite to the target organ, increased susceptibility of the target organ to damage, and increased susceptibility of the individual to a given level of target tissue damage. Increased absorption of an air pollutant may simply represent the difference between sitting on a park bench and jogging in the park. In a snowbound car that has a motor left running, the tragic finding of two dead children in the back seat, while the adults in the front seat are only unconscious, is due primarily to the greater respiratory rate per body size in the

children, leading to a greater uptake of carbon monoxide (Plunkett *et al.* 1992). Genetically determined differences in certain enzymes are well known to affect the rate of metabolism of certain drugs and environmental agents significantly, both detoxification of a noxious compound and activation to a noxious form. For example, acetyla-tion, a common metabolic process, occurs at a relatively fast or slow rate depending upon common variants of the responsible gene and enzyme. Other key metabolic enzymes can have their activity altered by dietary components, alcohol, therapeutic drugs, or previous exposure to the noxious agent. Target organs may also react differently to a given level of an environmental agent or its metabolite. As examples, one in seven black males in the United States has an inherited variant of the enzyme glucose-6-phosphate dehydrogenase that protects against malaria but leaves the red blood cells at particular risk to oxidizing drugs and there are individuals who are at high risk of sunlight-induced skin cancer because they are lacking certain enzymes capable of repairing the DNA damage caused by ultraviolet light. Lastly, individuals may be more susceptible to harm from an environmental toxin not because their target organ response is greater, but because the effect of a loss of function is more deleterious. For example, cigarette smokers have no more and perhaps even less lung responsiveness to inhalation of the air pollutant ozone. This is presumably because the increased mucus in the airway of smokers acts to scrub out the ozone before it reaches the lung cell surface. Yet, because cigarette smokers have so much less overall respiratory capability than do non-smokers, a relatively small ozone-induced additional loss of respiratory capa-bility may have more of an impact on the actual functioning of a smoker than of a non-smoker. Similarly the loss of lung and other organ reserves with ageing will make an elderly individual more susceptible than a younger adult to an identical toxic effect in an organ.

The special problem of mixtures

With the exception of special circumstances, human exposure to potentially toxic chemical and physical agents occurs as part of a mixture. We are well programmed to deal with mixtures—most foodstuffs contain an enormous variety of chemicals. However, the science of toxicology and the regulation of chemicals, has generally focused on individual chemicals rather than the broad mix of agents that are present in contaminated air or water or in such common consumer products as gasoline.

An example of the problem posed by this approach is the recent change in the automotive fuel mixture in the United States to include oxygenates such as methyl tert-butyl ether (**MTBE**). Many people are complaining about non-specific symptoms related to the addition of MTBE to gasoline. These clinical complaints are not well supported by the information in the toxicology database. However, the relevant toxicological database is almost totally restricted to studies of MTBE alone, rather than MTBE in gasoline.

The issue of how to predict the effect of mixtures is not confined solely to a single exposure matrix. As described above, ingestion of alcohol alters the level of metabolic enzymes responsi-ble for the activation or inactivation of a variety of drugs and environmental chemicals. Many other food constituents have such effects, often in different directions to each other. An unexpected finding of the effect of alcohol consumption on the metabolism of a drug was traced to a natural component of grapefruit juice used to dilute the alcohol given to the study participants (Bailey *et al.* 1994).

Most studies of mixtures have found that the effects are additive in that they are predictable by summing up the effects of the individual components of the mixture. This is particularly true when agents have similar effects. At times, the interaction is synergistic. For example, the lung cancer incidence due to cigarette smoking plus occupational asbestos exposure is far greater than should be expected due to the sum of the risks (Selikoff *et al.* 1968). Antagonism also occurs; for example, exposure to toluene plus benzene leads to less benzene toxicity to the bone marrow than if the exposure were to benzene alone (Andrews *et al.* 1977). This is believed to be due to both agents being metabolized by the same metabolic machinery. Benzene is converted into a bone marrow toxin while toluene is converted into a harmless agent. If there is sufficient toluene available to tie up the metabolic machinery, benzene metabolism will be slowed and less toxic metabolite will be formed. Note that no interaction between toluene and benzene occurs when exposure levels are relatively low as there is then sufficient metabolic machinery to handle both of these compounds independently. Potentiation also occurs when one agent, for example alcohol, that has no effect itself increases the effect of another agent.

In view of the almost infinite number of potential combinations of exogenous chemical and physical agents, studying them all is impossible. Two approaches have been developed to deal with this problem. One is to study those combinations to which humans are likely to be exposed, for example gasoline. The other is to focus on understanding the mechanism of toxicity of the individual components so as to predict interactive effects.

The interface between toxicological science and public policy

Toxicology has long been used as a means to estimate the effects of chemicals to protect the public and the general environment. Toxicology has two important roles related to environmental issues: detection of the cause and effect relationships linking environmental chemical and physical agents to adverse effects to humans or the environment and development of techniques capable of preventing these problems. Toxicologists usually approach questions of causation of disease by starting with the chemical or physical agent and studying its effects in laboratory animals or in test-tube systems. One of the more exciting aspects of modern toxicology is the possibility of linking subtle biological markers indicative of exposure with biomarkers showing early effects, thereby providing epidemiologists with powerful early warning tools to evaluate cause and effect relationships between environmental exposure and human diseases (National Research Council 1989).

The use of toxicology to test the safety of chemicals

Assessment of the safety of chemicals has evolved into a relatively standardized approach, particularly when considering new chemicals being developed for the market. The starting assumption is that all chemicals have toxic effects. To protect the public and the

worker it is necessary to know what specific effect occurs at what dose.

A relatively standardized battery of laboratory tests has been developed to assess chemical toxicity. Although varying greatly in effectiveness and cost, they are of value when used with judgement and with understanding of the basic mechanisms of toxicity that govern the ability to predict effects. For certain types of endpoints, such as mutations, there are a variety of apparently effective testing procedures. For other endpoints, such as neurobehavioural effects, we are far less able to predict whether a new agent may have an adverse outcome in humans.

The Ames test for mutagenesis is an example of a short-term test designed specifically to screen for potentially cancer-causing chemicals. By using a bacterial test system that can readily show when a mutation occurs and coupling that to an actively metabolizing fraction of rodent liver, compounds that are capable of producing mutations can usually be detected (Ames *et al.* 1975). Other short-term tests for mutagenesis depend upon mammalian cells *in vitro* or *in vivo*. The classic long-term test lasts almost 2 years, close to the lifetime of a rat or mouse. The dose chosen is one that is maximally tolerated by the laboratory animal in a 90-day trial. The use of a high dose, well beyond that of usual human exposure, has been controversial. Detractors point out that at high doses the toxicological response mechanisms may differ from that at usual doses and that cell toxicity may lead to false-positive findings, particularly of cancer. Supporters point out the effectiveness to date of detecting potential human carcinogens and the statistical impossibility of finding even a 1 in 1000 cancer risk using only at most a few hundred test animals exposed to usual environmental doses (National Research Council 1993). Some of these useful animal tests are under attack by animal rights activists, although for most adverse endpoints there are no validated *in vitro* test procedures capable of protecting the public or, for that matter, capable of protecting pets, such as cats and dogs, that have benefited greatly from the development of chemical products that decrease their suffering and prolong their life.

In some cases, laws and governmental regulations specify the toxicological test information necessary, depending upon the type of product, for example pesticides or food additives. In all cases public concern and the activities of toxic tort plaintiffs' lawyers have produced pressure on chemical industries to screen potential new compounds for adverse effects carefully before they are released to the market.

The role of toxicological information in setting environmental health standards

The setting of environmental health standards depends upon many factors, including legal requirements and political, economic, and social considerations. Certain laws, such as the US Clean Air Act, require the Administrator of the Environmental Protection Agency (**EPA**) to set ambient standards based upon protection of sensitive populations, but with no consideration of the costs to achieve the standard. Other laws, such as the Toxic Substances Control Act, expressly attempt to balance the value to society of new chemical products against the potential risks to human health and the environment from use of these chemicals.

Not surprisingly, there are different levels of toxicological information required by these different laws. As a generalization, chemical agents developed for the market-place can be considered under four headings: agents clearly intended to have a biological impact in humans, primarily therapeutic drugs or vitamins, agents with more limited biological effects in humans, such as cosmetics which alter skin moisture or food additives aimed at the taste bud, agents for which a biological impact is intended, but not in humans, such as pesticides or herbicides, and chemical agents for which no biological effect is desired, such as paints and window cleaners. Before a new drug can be marketed, the Food and Drug Administration (FDA) requires extensive animal studies and then carefully controlled trials in humans. In contrast, premanufacturing notification for a new paint thinner requires little more than identifying the chemical structure and perhaps a few short-term test-tube assays. Usually, the chemical industry is sufficiently concerned about liability issues and the good name of the company so that it will test a new product more extensively before putting it on the market.

Protection factors and weight of evidence

Setting standards for exposure to chemicals has evolved from a rather straightforward arithmetic formulation based upon relatively minimal data in animals to the present day situation where there is often a large body of evidence, including information about humans. As a generalization, the toxicology of the past used a dose–response approach to establish a no observed effect level (**NOEL**) in laboratory animals. The NOEL is in essence the highest tested level below the threshold. Various protection factors, often mislabelled as safety factors (Goldstein 1990), were then applied, usually by dividing the NOEL by factors of 10 each for the greater variability in humans than in inbred laboratory animals, in case of the possibility that humans were more sensitive than the laboratory species under study and even for the possibility that there were unobserved effects in the laboratory animals that were pertinent to humans. The resultant level, usually one-hundredth or one-thousandth of the NOEL, was then used to establish the standard.

Variants of this protective factor approach still exist, often in the more sophisticated form of a reference dose or bench-mark dose. However, particularly in situations where there is a relatively mature database, a more formal approach to the weighing of evidence is often taken. For example, the US Clean Air Act requires that the Administrator of the EPA set an ambient standard for each of six major air pollutants: ozone, sulphur dioxide, particulates, nitrogen dioxide, carbon monoxide, and lead. The standard is required to protect sensitive populations from adverse effects with an adequate margin of safety. The law also set up the Clean Air Scientific Advisory Committee, a seven-member panel that carefully reviews the evidence and makes recommendations to the EPA Administrator, including recommendations concerning the margin of safety. The standards are set without recourse to automatic factors of 10. Rather the available toxicological and epidemiological evidence is carefully weighed as the basis for the recommendation. Because of a rich database, the margin of safety is extremely narrow for most of the criteria air pollutants. These compounds are regulated for non-cancer effects.

The weight of evidence approach is increasingly used to come to judgement about complex issues. Examples include the classification of potential human carcinogens by the International Agency for Research on Cancer (1992) and the recent proposed revision of the EPA's dioxin assessment.

Criteria for evaluating environmental policies

Environmental policies in the United States are neither knee-jerk reactions to mass media coverage of environmental risks, as some claim, nor, as many scientists wish, are they the product of carefully conceived analyses of all the factors that should be considered (Portney 1990; Carlisle and Chechile 1991). Eight criteria for policy formation are described below in the form of questions asked by decision makers or analysts. The first two are always explicitly considered; the last three are often not considered.

1. Health/safety/environmental protection. This is clearly the first criterion. What risks will the proposed policy decrease? Will it increase any risks? To what certainty are these risks known and predictable? In other words, how much uncertainty is there? The greater the uncertainty, the greater the importance of the other seven criteria.

2. Legal/political feasibility. Is the proposed policy consistent with existing legal mandates? Can it be implemented with existing legislative mandates and rules? Does it support national, state, and local political goals? For example, in the United States in the 1990s, will the policy be consistent with a political trend towards less government, less interference with private enterprise, and transfer of authority from the national government to state and local governments, and from government to private enterprise?

3. Reactions from stakeholders. What interest groups are likely to support the proposed policy or oppose the proposed policy? Will elected and agency officials support or oppose it? Can they be persuaded to support it? What will be voter and media reactions?

4. Economic feasibility. Is the policy affordable? Can we prepare an implementation strategy that reaches the ultimate goal in divisible stages? Will the investment of a small amount of money in the initial stages accomplish most of the goals?

5. Benefits/costs. Will the proposed policy yield economic, social, and health benefits that exceed the costs? Are there advantages of using the funds for this purpose rather than another environmental protection policy? Is the proposed approach the least costly or most cost-effective way to obtain the desired benefits?

6. Ethical imperative. Does the proposed policy disproportionately benefit some groups (economic, ethnic, racial, generation, and gender) while placing others at greater risk? How will the consent of the most seriously impacted groups be obtained? Does the policy increase the probability of damaging a unique national or cultural resource?

7. Time pressure. What will happen if the policy is deferred for 1, 5, 10, 20, or more years?

8. Flexibility. Is the policy adaptable to advances in science and engineering and changes in the political climate?

Conclusion

Toxicology occupies an important niche between science and public policy. Its major contribution has been to provide tools and information to policy makers and the public that have prevented what would have been substantially greater environmental degradation, including adverse human health impacts. As society changes due to new technology and to the challenge of sustainable development in the face of increased human population, the role of toxicology in enlightened public policy will become even more important. However, while toxicological information is critical to decision making, it is not the sole determinant of policy, particularly when uncertainty exists.

References

Aldridge, W.N. (1986). The biological basis and measurement of thresholds. *Annual Review of Pharmacology and Toxicology*, **26**, 39–58.

Amdur, M., Doull, J., and Klaasen, C. (ed.) (1991). *Toxicology*, (4th ed.). Pergamon Press, New York, NY.

Ames, B., McCann, J., and Yamasaki, E. (1995). Methods for detecting carcinogens and mutagens with the Salmonella/mammalian microsome mutagenicity test. *Mutation Research*, **31**, 347–64.

Andrews, L.S., Lee, E.W., Witmer, C.M., Kocsis, J.J. and Snyder, R. (1977). Effects of toluene on the metabolism, disposition, and hemopoietic toxicity of ^{3}H benzene. *Biochemistry and Pharmacology*, **26**, 293–300.

Bailey, D.G., Arnold, J.M., and Spence, J.D. (1994). Grapefruit juice and drugs. How significant is the interaction? *Clinical Pharmacokinetics*, **26**, 91–8.

Carlisle, S. and Chechile, R. (ed.) (1991). *Environmental decision making: a multidisciplinary perspective*. Van Nostrand Reinhold, New York, NY.

Colborn, T., vom Saal, F.S., and Soto, A.M. (1993). Developmental effects of endocrine–disrupting chemicals in wildlife and humans. *Environmental Health Perspectives*, **101** (5) 378– 84.

Frantz, S.W., Beatty, P.W., English, J.C., Hundley, S.G., and Wilson, A.G. (1994). The use of pharmacokinetics as an interpretive and predictive tool in chemical toxicology testing and risk assessment: a position paper on the appropriate use of pharmacokinetics in chemical toxicology. *Regulatory Toxicology and Pharmacology*, **19**, 317–37.

Gallo, M. and Doull, J. (1991). History and scope of toxicology. In *Toxicology* (4th ed.), (ed. M.O. Amdur, J. Doull, and C.D. Klaasen), pp. 3–11. Pergamon Press, New York, NY.

Gallo, M., Gochfeld, M., and Goldstein, B.D. (1987). Biomedical aspects of environmental toxicology. In *Toxic chemicals, health, and the environment* (ed. L.B. Lave and A.C. Upton), pp. 170–204. John Hopkins University Press, Baltimore, MD.

Goldstein, B.D. (1990). The problem with the margin of safety: toward the concept of protection. *Risk Analysis*, **10**, 7–10.

Grandjean, P. (1995). Individual susceptibility in occupational and environmental toxicology. *Toxicology Letters*, **77**, 105–8.

Guengerich, F.P. and Liebler, D.C. (1985). Enzymatic activation of chemicals to toxic metabolites. *CRC Critical Reviews in Toxicology*, **14**, 259–307.

International Agency for Research on Cancer (IARC), (1992). *Monographs Evaluating Carcinogenic Risk to Humans*, **237**.

Kato, R., Estabrook, R.W., and Cayen, M.N. (1989). *Xenobiotic metabolism and disposition*. Taylor and Francis, London.

McMichael, A. (1994). Global environmental change and human health: new challenges to scientist and policy-maker. *Journal of Public Health Policy*, **15** (4), 407–19.

National Research Council (1989). *Biological markers in reproductive toxicology*. National Academy Press, Washington, DC.

National Research Council (1993). Use of the maximum tolerated dose in animal bioassays for carcinogenicity. In *Issues in risk assessment*, pp. 15–186. National Academy Press, Washington, DC.

Plaa, G. (1991). Toxic response of the liver. In *Toxicology*. (ed. M.O. Amdur, J. Doull, and C.D. Klaasen) pp. 334–53. Pergamon Press, New York, NY.

Plunkett, L.M., Turnbull, D., and Rodricks, J.V. (1992). Differences between adults and children affecting exposure assessment. In *Similarities and differences between children and adults, implications for risk assessment* (ed. P. Guzelian, C. Henry, and S. Olin). pp. 79–94. ILSI Press, Washington, DC.

Portney, P. (ed.) (1990). *Public policies for environmental protection*. Resources for the Future, Washington, DC.

Schuck, P. (1986). *Agent orange on trial*. Harvard University Press, Cambridge, MA.

Selikoff, I.J., Hammond, E.C., and Churg, J. (1968). Asbestos exposure, smoking, and neoplasia. *Journal of the American Medical Association*, **204** (2), 106–12.

Snyder, R., Witz, G., and Goldstein, B.D. (1993). The toxicology of benzene. *Environmental Health Perspectives*, **100**, 293–306.

Umbreit, T., Hesse, E., and Gallo, M. (1986). Bioavailability of dioxin in soil from a 2,4,5–T manufacturing site. *Science*, **232**, 497–9.

30 Radiological sciences

Arthur C. Upton

Introduction

This chapter reviews the health effects of electromagnetic waves, including ionizing and non-ionizing radiations, accelerated atomic particles, high-intensity ultrasound, and electromagnetic fields. These various forms of energy differ sufficiently from one another in their biological effects so that each is considered separately in the remarks that follow, beginning with a discussion of the effects of ionizing radiation.

Ionizing radiation

Nature, sources, and environmental levels

Ionizing radiation, which consists of those forms of radiation capable of depositing enough localized energy in tissue to dislodge electrons from atoms, comprises: (1) electromagnetic waves of extremely short wavelength (Fig. 30.1) and (2) accelerated atomic particles (for example electrons, protons, neutrons, and alpha particles). Doses of ionizing radiation are measured in terms of energy deposition (Table 30.1).

Natural sources of ionizing radiation include: (1) cosmic rays, (2) radium and other radioactive elements in the Earth's crust,

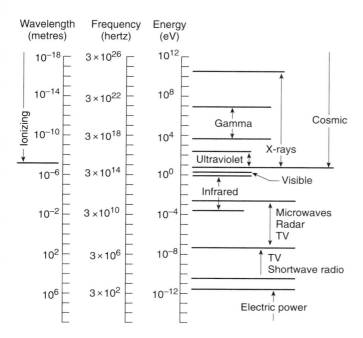

Fig. 30.1 The electromagnetic spectrum (reproduced from Mettler and Upton (1995), with permission).

(3) internally deposited potassium-40, carbon-14, and other radio-nuclides present normally in living cells, and (4) inhaled radon and its daughter elements (Table 30.2). The dose received from cosmic rays can differ appreciably from the value tabulated, depending on one's elevation; that is, it can be twice as high at a mountainous site (such as Denver) as at sea level and up to two orders of magnitude higher at jet aircraft altitudes (NCRP 1987). Likewise, the dose received from radium may be increased by a factor of two or more in regions where the underlying earth is rich in this element (NCRP 1987). It is noteworthy that the largest dose is that which is received by the bronchial epithelium from inhaled radon-222 (Table 30.2), a colourless, odourless α-particle-emitting gas formed by the radioactive decay of radium-226; furthermore, depending on the concentration of radon in indoor air, the dose from radon and its decay elements may vary by an order of magnitude or more (NCRP 1984). In cigarette smokers, moreover, even larger doses [up to 0.2 Sv (20 rem) per year] are received by the bronchial epithelium from the polonium (another α-emitting decay product of radium) that is normally present in tobacco smoke (NCRP 1984).

In addition to the exposure to ionizing radiation that people receive from natural sources, they are exposed to radiation from artificial sources as well, the largest of which is the use of X-rays in medical diagnosis (Table 30.2). Lesser sources of exposure to man-made radiation include radioactive minerals (for example, ^{238}U, ^{232}Th, ^{40}K, ^{226}Ra) in building materials, phosphate fertilizers, and crushed rock; radiation-emitting components of television sets, smoke detectors, and other consumer products; radioactive fallout from atomic weapons (for example, ^{137}Cs, ^{90}Sr, ^{89}Sr, ^{14}C, ^{3}H, ^{95}Zr); and nuclear power (for example, ^{3}H, ^{14}C, ^{85}KR, ^{129}I, ^{137}Cs) (Table 30.2).

In various occupations, workers receive additional doses of ionizing radiation, depending on their job assignments and working conditions. The average annual effective dose received occupation-ally by monitored radiation workers in the United States is less than that received from natural background, and in any given year less than one per cent of such workers receive a dose approaching the maximum permissible yearly limit [50 mSv (5 rem)] (NCRP 1989).

Nature and mechanisms of injury

As ionizing radiation penetrates living cells, it collides randomly with atoms and molecules in its path, giving rise to ions and free radicals which break chemical bonds and cause other molecular alterations that may injure the cells. The spatial distribution of such events along the path of an impinging radiation depends on the

Table 30.1 Quantities and dose units of ionizing radiation

Quantity being measured	Definition	Dose unit*
Absorbed dose	Energy deposited in tissue (1 joule/kg)	Gray (Gy)
Equivalent dose	Absorbed dose weighted for the ion density (potency) of the radiation	Sievert (Sv)
Effective dose	Equivalent dose weighted for the sensitivity of the exposed organ(s)	Sievert (Sv)
Collective effective dose	Effective dose applied to a population	Person–Sv
Committed effective dose	Cumulative effective dose to be received from a given intake of radioactivity	Sievert (Sv)
Radioactivity	One disintegration per second	Becquerel (Bq)

*The units of measure listed are those of the International System, introduced in the 1970s to standardize usage throughout the world (ICRP, 1990). They have largely supplanted the earlier units; namely, the rad (1 rad = 100 ergs per gm = 0.01 Gy), the rem, (1 rem = 0.01 Sv), and the curie (1 Ci = 3.7 ¥ 10^{10} disintegrations per second = 3.7 ¥ 10^{10} Bq).

energy, mass, and charge of the radiation; X-rays and γ-rays are sparsely ionizing in comparison with charged particles, which typically are densely ionizing.

Although any molecule in the cell may be altered by radiation, DNA is the most critical biological target because of the limited redundancy of the genetic information it contains. A dose of

Table 30.2 Average amounts of ionizing radiation received annually from different sources by a member of the United States population[a]

Source	Dose[b]		
	(mSv)	(mrem)	(%)
Natural			
Radon[c]	2.0	200	55
Cosmic	0.27	27	8
Terrestrial	0.28	28	8
Internal	0.39	39	11
Total natural	2.94	294	82
Artificial			
X-ray diagnosis	0.39	39	11
Nuclear medicine	0.14	14	4
Consumer products	0.10	10	3
Occupational	<0.01	<1.0	<0.3
Nuclear fuel cycle	<0.01	<1.0	<0.03
Nuclear fallout	<0.01	<1.0	<0.03
Miscellaneous[d]	<0.01	<1.0	<0.03
Total artificial	0.63	63	18
Total natural and artificial	3.57	357	100

[a] Adapted from National Academy of Sciences, 1990.
[b] Average effective dose to soft tissues, excluding bronchial epithelium.
[c] Average effective dose to bronchial epithelium alone.
[d] Department of Energy facilities, smelters, transportation, etc.

radiation large enough to kill the average dividing cell [2 Sv (200 rem)] causes hundreds of lesions in the cell's DNA molecules (Ward 1988). Most such lesions are reparable, but those produced by a densely ionizing radiation (for example, a proton or an α particle) are generally less reparable than those produced by a sparsely ionizing radiation (such as an X-ray or a γ-ray) (Goodhead 1988). For this reason, the relative biological effectiveness (RBE) of densely ionizing radiations is typically higher than that of sparsely ionizing radiations for most forms of injury (ICRP 1991).

Any damage to DNA that remains unrepaired or that is misrepaired may be expressed in the form of mutations, the frequency of which approximates 10^{-5} to 10^{-6} per locus per Sv (100 rem) (NAS 1990). Because the mutation rate appears to increase as a linear non-threshold function of the dose, it is inferred that traversal of the DNA by a single ionizing particle may, in principle, suffice to cause a mutation (NAS 1990).

Also resulting from radiation damage to the genetic apparatus are changes in chromosome number and structure, the frequency of which increases with the dose in radiation workers and others exposed to ionizing radiation. So well characterized is the dose–response relationship for chromosome aberrations that their frequency in blood lymphocytes can serve as a useful biological dosimeter in radiation accident victims (IAEA 1986).

Radiation damage to genes and chromosomes may be lethal to affected cells, especially dividing cells, which are highly radiosensitive as a class (ICRP 1984). Measured in terms of proliferative capacity, the survival of dividing cells tends to decrease exponentially with increasing dose, 1 to 2 Sv (100 to 200 rem) generally sufficing to reduce the surviving population by about 50 per cent (Fig. 30.2).

Although a dose below 0.5 Sv (50 rem) kills too few cells to cause clinically detectable injury in most organs other than those of the embryo, a larger dose may kill enough of the dividing progenitor cells in a tissue to interfere with the orderly replacement of its senescent cells, thereby causing the tissue to undergo atrophy (Fig. 30.3). The rapidity with which the atrophy ensues will depend in part on the cell population dynamics within the affected tissue; that is, in organs characterized by slow cell turnover, such as the liver and vascular endothelium, the process is typically much

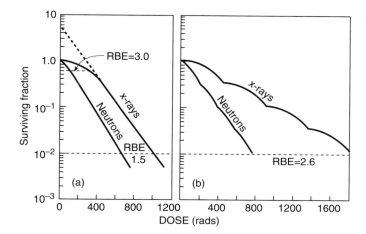

Fig. 30.2 Typical dose-survival curves for mammalian cells exposed to x-rays and fast neutrons (reproduced from Hall (1994), with permission). (a) Single doses, (b) Fractionated doses.

slower than in organs characterized by rapid cell turnover, such as the bone marrow, epidermis, and intestinal mucosa (ICRP 1984). Insofar as the injury is dependent on the extent to which cell renewal in the exposed tissue is impaired, its severity tends to be reduced by the compensatory proliferation of surviving cells when only a small volume of tissue is irradiated or when the dose is accumulated gradually over an extended period of time.

Clinical manifestations of acute injury

After its discovery by Roentgen, in 1895, the X-ray was introduced into medical practice so rapidly that radiation injuries began to be encountered almost immediately. The first such injuries were predominantly acute skin reactions on the hands of those working with the early equipment, but within less than a decade many other types of injury also were observed, including the first cancers attributed to radiation (Upton 1986).

The acute effects of radiation encompass a wide variety of reactions (Mettler and Upton 1995) varying markedly in dose–response relationships, clinical manifestations, timing, and prognosis (Table 30.3). Such reactions generally result from the severe depletion of progenitor cells in affected tissues (Fig. 30.3) and are, consequently, elicited only by doses large enough dose to kill many such cells. Organs in which cells normally turn over rapidly tend to be the most radiosensitive and the first to exhibit injury. Because such reactions are not elicited unless the doses of radiation exceed the substantial thresholds needed to kill many cells, they are viewed as nonstochastic, or deterministic, in nature (ICRP 1984), as opposed to mutagenic and carcinogenic effects of radiation, which are viewed as stochastic phenomena resulting from random molecular alterations in individual cells that increase in frequency as linear non-threshold functions of the dose (NAS 1990; ICRP 1991).

Radiation injury of normal tissue within or adjoining the treatment field occurs to some degree in most radiotherapy patients, although few persons treated with today's methods experience severe or disabling radiation injuries. By the same token, modern safety practices have all but eliminated the injuries resulting from excessive occupational exposure such as were prevalent among early radiation workers. In spite of marked

improvements in radiation protection, however, some 285 nuclear reactor accidents (excluding the Chernobyl accident) were reported in various countries between 1945 and 1987, causing more than 1350 persons to be irradiated, 33 of whom were injured fatally (Lushbaugh *et al.* 1987). In most such accidents, unlike the Chernobyl accident (discussed below), the public was not affected directly.

The Chernobyl accident, by contrast – the most serious reactor accident to date – released enough radioactivity to require the evacuation of tens of thousands of people and farm animals from the surrounding area. This accident, occurring during a reactor test in April, 1986, resulted from the improper withdrawal of control rods and inactivation of important safety systems – in violation of the operating rules – which caused the reactor to overheat, explode, and catch fire (UNSCEAR 1988). The damage to the reactor core and control building allowed large quantities of radiation and radioactive materials to be released during the ensuing 10 days, resulting in radiation sickness and burns in more than 200 emergency personnel and firefighters, 31 of whom were injured fatally. Although the heaviest contamination occurred in the vicinity of the reactor itself and, to a lesser extent, in neighbouring countries of eastern Europe, the population of the northern hemisphere as a whole is estimated to have received a collective dose commitment of 600 000 person-Sv (60 million person-rem), 70 per cent of which is attributed to caesium-137, 20 per cent to caesium-134, 6 per cent to iodine-131, and the remainder to various shorter-lived radionuclides (UNSCEAR 1988). Those living in the vicinity of the reactor were given potassium iodide preparations to inhibit the thyroidal uptake of radioiodine, but infants in a number of areas elsewhere in eastern Europe are estimated to have received an average dose of more than 20 mSv (2 rem) to the thyroid gland, largely through ingestion of radioiodine via cow's milk. The average dose to other organs in such infants, however, was only a fraction of the dose normally received from natural background radiation (UNSCEAR 1988). While the long-term health effects of the released radioactivity cannot be predicted with certainty, non-threshold risk models for carcinogenic effects (discussed below) imply that up to 30 000 additional cancer deaths may occur in the population of the northern hemisphere during the next 70 years as a result of the accident, although, with a few exceptions, the number of additional cancers in any given country is likely to be too small to be detectable epidemiologically (USDOE 1987).

While less catastrophic than reactor accidents, accidents involving medical and industrial γ-ray sources have been far more numerous, some also causing severe injury and loss of life. The improper disposal of a caesium-137 radiotherapy source in Goiania, Brazil, in 1987, for example, resulted in the irradiation of dozens of unsuspecting victims, four of whom were injured fatally as a result (UNSCEAR 1993).

Although a comprehensive discussion of radiation injuries is beyond the scope of this review, prominent reactions of some of the more radiosensitive tissues are described briefly in the following. *Skin.* Owing to the radiosensitivity of cells in the germinal layer of the epidermis, rapid exposure of the skin to a dose of 6 Sv (600 rem) or more produces erythema (reddening) in the exposed area, which typically appears within a day after exposure, lasts a few hours, and is followed 2 to 4 weeks later by one or more waves of deeper and more prolonged erythema, as well as epilation (hair

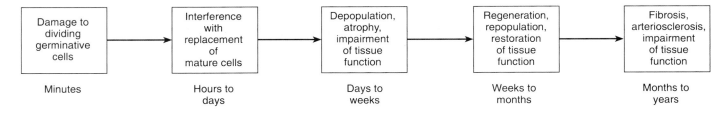

Fig.30.3 Characteristic sequences of events in the pathogenesis of nonstochastic effects of ionizing radiation.

loss). If the dose exceeds 10 to 20 Sv (1000 to 2000 rem), blistering, necrosis, and ulceration may ensue within 2 to 4 weeks, followed by fibrosis of the underlying dermis and vasculature, which may lead to atrophy and a second wave of ulceration months or years later (ICRP 1984).

Bone marrow and lymphoid tissue. Lymphocytes are sufficiently radiosensitive so that a dose of 2 to 3 Sv (200 to 300 rem) delivered rapidly to the whole body results in a marked depression of the lymphocyte count and immune response within hours (UNSCEAR 1988). Haemopoietic cells in the bone marrow are, likewise, killed in sufficient numbers by a comparable dose to cause profound leucopenia and thrombocytopenia to develop within 3 to 5 weeks; after a larger dose, such reductions in white blood cells and platelets may be severe enough to result in fatal infection and/or haemorrhage (Table 30.4).

Intestine. Stem cells in the epithelium lining the small bowel also are highly radiosensitive, an acute dose of 10 Sv (1000 rem) depleting their numbers sufficiently to cause the overlying intestinal villi to become denuded within days (ICRP 1984; UNSCEAR 1988). If a large area of the mucosa is affected, a fulminating, rapidly fatal dysentery-like syndrome results (Table 30.4).

Gonads. Although mature spermatozoa can survive large doses [>100 Sv (10 000 rem)], spermatogonia are so radiosensitive that a dose as low as 0.15 Sv (15 rem) delivered rapidly to both testes will cause oligospermia, and a dose of 2 to 4 Sv (200 to 400 rem) permanent sterility. Oocytes, likewise, are radiosensitive, a dose of 1.5 to 2.0 Sv (150 to 200 rem) delivered rapidly to both ovaries sufficing to cause temporary sterility, and a larger dose permanent sterility, depending on the age of the woman at the time of exposure (ICRP 1984).

Respiratory tract. The lung is not a highly radiosensitive organ, but alveolar cells and pulmonary vasculature can be injured sufficiently by rapid exposure to a dose of 6 to 10 Sv (600 to 1000 rem) to cause acute pneumonitis to develop within the following 1 to 3 months. If a large volume of the lung is affected, the process may terminate in respiratory failure within the ensuing weeks, or in pulmonary fibrosis and cor pulmonale months or years later (ICRP 1984; UNSCEAR 1988).

Lens of the eye. Cells of the anterior epithelium of the lens continue to divide throughout life and are relatively radiosensitive. As a result, acute exposure of the lens to more than 1 Sv (100 rem) may be followed within months by the formation of a microscopic posterior polar opacity, and 2 to 3 Sv (200 to 300 rem) received in a single brief exposure, or 5.5 to 14 Sv (550 to 1400 rem) accumulated over a period of months, may cause a vision-impairing cataract (ICRP 1984).

Other tissues. The tissues mentioned above are generally of higher radiosensitivity than others (Table 30.3). It is noteworthy, however,

that the vulnerability of all tissues is increased when they are in a rapidly growing state (ICRP 1984).

Whole-body radiation injury. If a major part of the body is exposed rapidly to more than 1 Sv, the acute radiation syndrome may result. This syndrome is characterized by: (1) an initial prodromal stage in which there is malaise, anorexia, nausea, and vomiting, (2) an ensuing latent period, (3) a second (main) phase of illness, and (4) finally, either recovery or death (Table 30.4). The main phase of the illness typically takes one of the following four forms, depending on the predominant locus of radiation injury: haematological, gastrointestinal, cerebral, or pulmonary.

Localized radiation injury. In contrast to the clinical manifestations of acute whole-body radiation injury, which are often dramatic and prompt, the reaction to sharply localized irradiation, whether from an external radiation source or from an internally deposited radionuclide, tends to evolve slowly and to produce few symptoms unless the volume of tissue irradiated and/or the dose are relatively large (see Table 30.3). In this connection, it is noteworthy that although some radionuclides (such as tritium, carbon-14, and caesium-137) tend to be distributed systemically and thus to irradiate the whole body to varying degrees, others are characteristically taken up and concentrated in specific organs, producing injuries that are localized accordingly. Radium and strontium-90, for example, are deposited predominantly in bone and injure skeletal tissues primarily, whereas radioactive iodine concentrates in the thyroid gland, which is the chief site of any resulting injury (Stannard 1988).

Carcinogenic effects

The carcinogenicity of ionizing radiation, first manifested early in this century by the occurrence of skin cancer and leukaemia in certain radiation workers, has since been documented extensively by dose-dependent excesses of osteosarcomas and cranial sinus carcinomas in radium dial painters, carcinomas of the respiratory tract in underground rock miners, and cancers of many types in atomic bomb survivors, radiotherapy patients, and experimentally irradiated laboratory animals (Upton 1986).

The growths induced by irradiation characteristically take years or decades to appear and exhibit no known features distinguishing them from those induced by other causes. With few exceptions, moreover, their induction has been detectable only after relatively large doses [>0.5 Sv (50 rem)] and has varied with the type of neoplasm as well as the age and sex of those exposed. In laboratory animals and cultured cells, the carcinogenic effects of radiation have been observed to include initiating effects, promoting effects, and effects on the progression of neoplasia, depending on the experimental conditions in question (NAS 1990). While the molecular mechanisms of these effects remain to be elucidated, the

Table 30.3 Approximate threshold doses of conventionally fractionated therapeutic X-radiation for clinically detrimental non-stochastic effects in various tissues[a]

Organ	Injury at 5 years	Threshold dose (Gv)[b]	Irradiation field (area)
Skin	Ulcer, severe fibrosis	55	100 cm²
Oral mucosa	Ulcer, severe fibrosis	60	50 cm²
Oesophagus	Ulcer, stricture	60	75 cm²
Stomach	Ulcer, perforation	45	100 cm²
Small intestine	Ulcer, stricture	45	100 cm²
Colon	Ulcer, stricture	45	100 cm²
Rectum	Ulcer, stricture	55	100 cm²
Salivary glands	Xerostomia	50	50 cm²
Liver	Liver failure, ascites	35	whole
Kidney	Nephrosclerosis	23	whole
Urinary bladder	Ulcer, contracture	60	whole
Testes	Permanent sterility	5–15	whole
Ovary	Permanent sterility	2–3	whole
Uterus	Necrosis, perforation	>100	whole
Vagina	Ulcer, fistula	90	5 cm²
Breast, child	Hypoplasia	10	5 cm²
Breast, adult	Atrophy, necrosis	>50	whole
Lung	Pneumonitis, fibrosis	40	lobe
Capillaries	Telangiectasis, fibrosis	50–60	—
Heart	Pericarditis, pancarditis	40	whole
Bone, child	Arrested growth	20	10 cm²
Bone, adult	Necrosis, fracture	60	10 cm²
Cartilage, child	Arrested growth	10	whole
Cartilage, adult	Necrosis	60	whole
CNS (brain)	Necrosis	50	whole
Spinal cord	Necrosis, transection	50	5 cm²
Eye	Panophthalmitis, haemorrhage	55	whole
Cornea	Keratitis	50	whole
Lens	Cataract	5	whole
Ear (inner)	Deafness	>60	whole
Thyroid	Hypothyroidism	45	whole
Adrenal	Hypoadrenalism	>60	whole
Pituitary	Hypopituitarism	45	whole
Muscle, child	Hypoplasia	20–30	whole
Muscle, adult	Atrophy	>100	whole
Bone marrow	Hypoplasia	2	whole
Bone marrow	Hypoplasia, fibrosis	20	localized
Lymph nodes	Atrophy	33–45	—
Lymphatics	Sclerosis	50	—
Fetus	Death	2	whole

[a] From Rubin and Casarett, 1972; ICRP, 1984.
[b] Dose causing effect in 1 to 5 per cent of exposed persons.

activation of oncogenes and/or the inactivation or loss of tumour-suppressor genes appear to be implicated in many, if not all, instances (NAS 1990). The carcinogenic effects of radiation also resemble those of chemical carcinogens in being generally modifiable in similar ways by hormones, nutritional variables, and other modifying factors. In combination with chemical carcinogens the effects of radiation may be additive, synergistic, or mutually antagonistic, depending on the specific chemicals and exposure conditions in question (UNSCEAR 1982, 1986).

Because the existing data do not suffice to describe the dose-incidence relationship unambiguously for any type of neoplasm or

to define how long after irradiation the risk of the growth may remain elevated in an exposed population, any risks attributable to low-level irradiation can be estimated only by extrapolation, based on models incorporating assumptions about such parameters (NAS 1990). Of various dose-effect models that have been used to estimate the risks of low-level irradiation, the one that has been judged to provide the best fit to the available data is of the form:

$$R(d) = R_o \left[1 + f(d)g(b) \right]$$

where R_o denotes the age-specific background risk of death from a specific type of cancer, d the radiation dose, f(d) a function of dose

Table 30.4 Major forms and features of the acute radiation syndrome				
Time after irradiation	Cerebral form (>50 Sv)	Gastrointestinal form (10–20 Sv)	Hemopoietic form (2–10 Sv)	Pulmonary form (>6 Sv to lungs)
First day	Nausea Vomiting Diarrhoea Headache Disorientation Ataxia Coma Convulsions Death	Nausea Vomiting Diarrhoea	Nausea Vomiting Diarrhoea	Nausea Vomiting
Second week		Nausea Vomiting Diarrhoea Fever Erythema Prostration Death		
Third to sixth weeks			Weakness Fatigue Anorexia Fever Haemorrhage Epilation Recovery (?) Death (?)	
Second to eighth months				Cough Dyspneoa Fever Chest pain Respiratory Failure (?)

that is linear-quadratic for leukemia and linear for other types of cancer, and g(b) is a risk function dependent on other parameters, such as sex, age at exposure, and time after exposure (NAS 1990). Based on the application of such models to epidemiological data from the Japanese atomic bomb survivors and other irradiated populations, estimates of the lifetime risks of different forms of radiation–induced cancer have been formulated (for example Table 30.5). Such estimates must be used with caution in attempting to predict the risks of cancer attributable to small doses or doses accumulated over weeks, months, or years since experiments with laboratory animals have shown the carcinogenic potency of X-rays and γ rays to be reduced by as much as an order of magnitude when the exposure is greatly prolonged. Also, as has been emphasized elsewhere (NAS 1990), the available data do not exclude the possibility that there may be a threshold in the millisievert dose range, below which the carcinogenicity of radiation is lacking.

It is noteworthy that the above estimates are based on population averages and are not equally applicable to all individuals. Susceptibility to certain types of cancer (notably those of the thyroid and breast) is substantially higher in children than in adults; susceptibility is also increased in some hereditary disorders, such as retinoblastoma and the naevoid basal cell carcinoma syndrome (UNSCEAR 1988; NAS 1990). Such inter-individual

differences notwithstanding, the estimates have been used in compensation cases as a basis for assessing the probability that a cancer arising in a previously irradiated person may have been caused by the exposure in question (NIH 1985).

Studies to ascertain whether the rates of cancer and other diseases do, in fact, vary with natural background radiation levels have been inconclusive so far. A few studies have even suggested an inverse relationship – which some have interpreted as evidence for the existence of beneficial (or hormetic) effects of low-level irradiation – but the relationship has not persisted after controlling for the effects of confounding variables (NAS 1990). While any risks that may result from the low levels of exposure associated with natural background radiation remain to be determined, the available data are consistent with the estimates in Table 30.5, which suggest that no more than 3 per cent of all cancers in the population are attributable to natural background radiation. The possibility that a larger percentage (up to 10 per cent) of lung cancers may result from residential exposure to radon, however, is suggested by the dose-dependent increase in the incidence of such cancers in underground rock miners (NAS 1990; Lubin *et al.* 1994), and although epidemiological studies of the effects of indoor radon have been inconclusive to date – owing in part to uncertainties in dosimetry and difficulties in controlling for the influence of

Table 30.5 Estimated lifetime risks of cancer attributable to 0.1 Sv (10 rem) rapid irradiation[a]

Type or site of cancer	Excess cancer deaths per 100 000	
	(No.)	(%)[b]
Stomach	110	18
Lung	85	3
Colon	85	5
Leukaemia (excluding CLL)	50	10
Urinary bladder	30	5
Oesophagus	30	10
Breast	20	1
Liver	15	8
Gonads	10	2
Thyroid	8	8
Osteosarcoma	5	5
Skin	2	2
Remainder	50	1
Total	500	2

[a] Modified from ICRP, 1991.
[b] Percentage increase in background expectation for a non-irradiated population.

cigarette smoking and other confounding variables – the results of such studies are compatible with the implied exposure–risk relationship (Lubin 1994; NAS 1994) The magnitude of the presumed risks, while yet to be validated epidemiologically, has prompted prudent guidelines for limiting residential radon concentrations in the United States and other countries (for example USEPA 1992).

The occurrence of clusters of leukaemia in children residing in the vicinity of nuclear plants in the United Kingdom has suggested the possibility that such cancers may have resulted from radioactivity released by the plants. However, because the releases are estimated to have increased the total radiation dose to such populations by less than 2 per cent, other explanations are considered more likely (Doll et al. 1994). An infective aetiology for the observed clusters has been suggested by the finding of comparable excesses of childhood leukaemia at sites in the United Kingdom lacking nuclear facilities, but otherwise resembling such sites demographically in having similarly experienced large influxes of population in recent times (Kinlen 1988; Doll et al. 1994). The possibility that the leukaemias in question may have resulted from heritable oncogenic effects caused by occupational irradiation of the fathers of the affected children also has been suggested (Gardner et al. 1990), an hypothesis which is generally discounted for reasons that are discussed below.

In occupationally exposed workers, carcinogenic effects of irradiation are no longer clearly demonstrable – thanks to modern radiation protection practices – except in certain cohorts of underground rock miners who continue to suffer increased mortality from lung cancer (Lubin et al. 1994). In only 1 of 17 recent studies of radiation workers, for example, was a significant excess of leukaemia found, and in none of the studies was a significantly positive dose–response for the disease observed (Upton et al. 1990), suggesting that the average risk of leukaemia in today's radiation workers is no higher than that implied by the estimate in Table 30.5. For multiple myeloma, likewise, no excess has been detected in the majority of cohorts investigated (Upton et al. 1990). Although excesses of other forms of cancer have been reported occasionally in various occupationally exposed cohorts, they too are of equivocal significance because of methodological problems and other sources of uncertainty (Upton et al. 1990).

Among populations exposed to radioactive fallout, carcinogenic effects on the thyroid gland have been well documented in Marshall Islanders who received large doses to the thyroid in childhood [7–14 Gy (700–1400 rad)] and infancy [possibly up to 20 Gy (2000 rad)] from radioactive iodine, tellurium, and external γ-ray emitters in fallout released by a thermonuclear weapons test at Bikini atoll in 1954 (Robbins and Adams 1989). Children living in areas of Belarus and the Ukraine contaminated by radionuclides released from the Chernobyl accident have also been reported to show an increased incidence of thyroid cancer (Prisyazhuik et al. 1991; Kasakov et al. 1992), but these findings are at variance with those of the International Chernobyl Project, which has found no excess of benign or malignant thyroid nodules in children living in the more heavily contaminated areas around Chernobyl (Mettler et al. 1992), and they are also at variance with the published literature, which indicates a minimum latency for radiation-induced thyroid neoplasms of about 5 years (NAS 1990). The basis for this discrepancy, and whether the reported excesses may have resulted from heightened surveillance alone, remains to be determined. In this connection, it is noteworthy that children of south-western Utah and Nevada who were exposed to fallout from nuclear weapons testing at the Nevada test site in the 1950s have shown no significant increase in any type of thyroid disease (Rallison et al. 1974), although the prevalence of acute leukaemia in such children appeared to be elevated in those dying under 20 years of age during the period of greatest exposure to fallout (1952–1957) (Stevens et al. 1990).

Heritable effects

Heritable effects of irradiation, although well documented in other organisms, have yet to be observed in humans. Thus, intensive study of the more than 76 000 children of Japanese atomic bomb survivors, carried out over four decades, has failed to disclose any heritable effects of radiation in this population, as measured by untoward pregnancy outcomes, neonatal deaths, malignancies, balanced chromosomal rearrangements, sex-chromosome aneuploidy, alterations of serum or erythrocyte protein phenotypes, changes in sex ratio, or disturbances in growth and development (NAS 1990). Estimates of the risks of heritable effects of radiation to future generations rely heavily, therefore, on extrapolation from findings in laboratory animals.

From the available data, it is inferred that human germ cells are no more radiosensitive than those of the mouse and that the dose required to double the rate of heritable mutations in the human species must be at least 1.0 Sv (100 rem) (NAS 1990). Hence, on the basis of the existing evidence, it is estimated that less than 1 per cent of all genetically determined diseases in the human population is attributable to natural background irradiation (Table 30.6).

Table 30.6 Estimated frequencies of heritable disorders attributable to natural background ionizing irradiation[abc]

Type of Disorder	Natural prevalence	Contribution for natual background	
		First generation	Equilibrium Generations[d]
Autosomal dominant	180 000	20–100	300
X-linked	400	<1	<15
Recessive	2500	<1	Very slow increase
Chromosomal	4400	<20	Very slow increase
Congenital defects	20 000–30 000	30	30–300
Other disorders of complex aetiology			
Heart disease	600 000	Not estimated[e]	Not estimated[e]
Cancer	300 000	Not estimated[e]	Not estimated[e]
Selected others	300 000	Not estimated[e]	Not estimated[e]

[a] Based on NAS, 1990.

[b] Equivalent to ~1mSv (100 mrem) per year (Table 2), or ~30mSv (3 rem) per generation (30 years).

[c] Values rounded.

[d] After hundreds of generations, the addition of unfavourable radiation–induced mutations eventually becomes balanced by their loss from the population, resulting in a genetic 'equilibrium'.

[e] Quantitative risk estimates are lacking because of uncertainty about the mutational component of the disease(s) indicated.

The possibility that an excess of leukaemia and non-Hodgkin's lymphoma in young people residing in the village of Seascale, England, was caused by the occupational irradiation of their fathers at the Sellafield nuclear installation has been suggested by a case-control study (Gardner *et al.* 1990), as noted above. Conflicting with this interpretation, however, are: (1) the lack of any comparable excess in larger numbers of children born outside Seascale to fathers who had received similar, or even larger, occupational doses at the same nuclear plant (Wakeford *et al.* 1994*a*); (2) the lack of similar excesses in French (Hill and Laplanche 1990), Canadian (McLaughlin *et al.* 1993), or Scottish (Kinlen *et al.* 1993) children born to fathers with comparable occupational exposures; (3) the lack of excesses in the children of atomic bomb survivors (Yoshimoto *et al.* 1990); (4) the lack of excesses in United States counties containing nuclear plants (Jablon *et al.* 1991); and (5) the fact that the frequency of radiation-induced mutations implied by the interpretation is far higher than established rates (Wakeford *et al.* 1994*b*). On balance, therefore, the available data fail to support the paternal gonadal irradiation hypothesis (Doll *et al.* 1994).

Effects of prenatal irradiation

Throughout prenatal life, radiosensitivity is relatively high, the effects of a given dose varying markedly, depending on the developmental stage of the embryo or fetus at the time of exposure. During the pre-implantation period, the embryo is maximally susceptible to killing by irradiation. Subsequently, during critical stages in organogenesis, it is susceptible to the induction of malformations and other disturbances of development (UNSCEAR 1986), as exemplified by the dose-dependent increase in frequency

of mental retardation and the dose-dependent decrease in IQ test scores occurring in atomic bomb survivors who were irradiated between the 8th and 15th weeks (and, to a lesser extent, between the 16th and 25th weeks) after conception (UNSCEAR 1986).

Susceptibility to the carcinogenic effects of radiation also appears to be relatively high throughout the prenatal period, judging from the association between childhood cancer (including leukaemia) and prenatal exposure to diagnostic X-irradiation (NAS 1990). This association, although yet to be established as causal in nature, has been observed consistently in many case-control studies and is equally strong in twins (NAS 1990). While no excess of childhood cancer has been recorded in prenatally irradiated atomic bomb survivors, their numbers were relatively small (Yoshimoto *et al.* 1990). The results of the various case–control studies imply that prenatal irradiation causes a 4000 per cent per Sv (100 rem) increase in the risk of leukaemia and other childhood cancers (UNSCEAR 1986; NAS 1990), a risk far larger than that which is attributed to postnatal irradiation (UNSCEAR 1988; NAS 1990).

Prevention

In order to minimize the risks of injury , the following principles are recommended as guidelines to be observed in any activities involving exposure to ionizing radiation (ICRP 1991): (1) no such activity should be considered justifiable unless it produces a sufficient benefit to those who are exposed, or to society at large, to offset any harm it may cause; (2) in any such activity, the dose and/ or likelihood of exposure should be kept as low as is reasonably achievable (ALARA), all relevant economic and social factors being

Table 30.7 Recommended effective dose limits of ionizing radiation for occupationally exposed workers and members of the public[a]

Occupational exposure[b]

Annual	50 mSv (5 rem)
Cumulative	age ¥ 10 mSv (1 rem)

Public exposure[b]

Annual, continuous	1 mSv (100 mrem)
Annual, infrequent	5 mSv (500 mrem)

[a] From NCRP, 1993; ACGIH, 1993.
[b] Excluding medical and dental exposures.

taken into account; and (3) the radiation exposure of individuals resulting from any combination of such activities should be subject to dose limits (for example Table 30.7) that are far enough below the thresholds for non-stochastic effects to prevent such effects altogether, and that are also low enough to keep the risks of any resulting stochastic effects (which may have no thresholds) from exceeding socially acceptable levels.

Implicit in these guidelines are the requirements that any facility dealing with ionizing radiation: (1) be properly designed, (2) carefully plan and oversee its operating procedures, including dose calibration, (3) have in place a well-conceived radiation protection programme, (4) ensure that its workers are adequately trained and supervised, and (5) maintain a well-developed and well-rehearsed emergency preparedness plan, in order to be able to respond promptly and effectively in the event of a malfunction, spill, or other type of radiation accident (Shapiro 1990).

Since medical radiographic examinations and indoor radon constitute the most important controllable sources of exposure to ionizing radiation for members of the general public (Table 30.1), prudent measures to limit irradiation from these sources are called for (Upton *et al.* 1990). Other potential risks to human health and the environment calling for increased attention are those posed by the millions of cubic feet of radioactive and mixed wastes (mine and mill tailings, spent nuclear fuel, waste from the decommissioning of nuclear power plants, dismantled industrial and medical radiation sources, radioactive pharmaceuticals and reagents, heavy metals, polyaromatic hydrocarbons, and other contaminants) which are present in ever-growing quantities and which severely tax existing storage capacities at numerous sites (see for example NAS 1989; USEPA 1990, 1991; USNRC 1992; USDOE, 1993).

Non-ionizing radiation

Ultraviolet radiation

Nature, sources, and environmental levels

Ultraviolet radiations (UVR) comprise a spectrum (Fig. 30.1) of electromagnetic waves, subdivided for convenience into three bands: (1) UVA, 400 to 320 nm ('black light'); (2) UVB, 320 to 280

nm; and (3) UVC, 280 to 100 nm (which is germicidal). The chief source of UVR for members of the public is sunlight, which varies in intensity with latitude, elevation, and season (AMA 1989). Important man-made sources of high-intensity exposure include sun- and tanning-lamps, welding arcs, plasma torches, germicidal and black-light lamps, electric arc furnaces, hot-metal operations, mercury vapour lamps, and lasers. Common low-intensity sources include fluorescent lamps and certain laboratory equipment (NIOSH 1972).

Nature and mechanisms of injury

Since UVR does not penetrate deeply into human tissues, the injuries it causes are confined chiefly to the skin and eyes. Reactions of the skin to UVR, which are common among fair-skinned people, include: sunburn; skin cancers (basal cell and squamous cell carcinomas, and to a lesser extent melanomas); aging of the skin; solar elastoses; and solar keratoses. Injuries of the eye include photokeratitis, which may result from brief exposure to a high-intensity UVR source ('welder's flash') or from more prolonged exposure to intense sunlight ('snow blindness'); cortical cataract; and pterygium (Lerman 1988).

The effects of UVR result chiefly from its absorption in DNA, with the production of pyrimidine dimers, causing mutational changes in exposed cells. Sensitivity to UVR may be increased by DNA repair defects (for example xeroderma pigmentosum), by agents (such as caffeine) that inhibit the repair enzymes, and by photosensitizing agents (such as psoralens, sulphonamides, tetracyclines, nalidixic acid, sulphonylureas, thiazides, phenothiazines, furocumarins, and coal tar) which produce UVR-absorbing DNA photoproducts (Harper and Bickers 1989). The carcinogenic action of UVR is mediated primarily through direct effects on the exposed cells but may involve depression of local immunity as well (Kripke 1988). UVB, although far less intense than UVA in sunlight, plays a more important role in sunburn and skin carcinogenesis; UVA, however, contributes to the latter, as well as to tanning, some photosensitivity reactions, ageing of the skin, photokeratitis, and cortical lens opacities (AMA 1989).

Prevention

Excessive exposure to sunlight or other sources of UVR should be avoided, especially by fair-skinned individuals. In addition, protective clothing, UVR-screening lotions or creams, and UVR-blocking sunglasses should be used for the purpose when necessary. To protect occupationally exposed workers, it is recommended that exposure be limited to 1.0 mW/cm² for periods longer than 1000 seconds and 1000 mW/cm² (1.0 J/cm²) for periods of 1000 seconds or less (NIOSH 1972; ACGIH 1993).

From an environmental perspective, it is noteworthy that the protective layer of ozone in the stratosphere is being depleted by chlorofluorocarbons and other air pollutants, and that every 1 per cent decrease in ozone is expected to increase the UVR reaching the earth by 1 to 2 per cent, thereby increasing the rates of non-melanotic skin cancer by 2 to 6 per cent (Henriksen *et al.* 1990). The projected increase in cancer rates is, of course, only one of many adverse effects to be expected from increased intensities of UVR, the most serious, perhaps, being far-reaching impacts on vegetation and crop production.

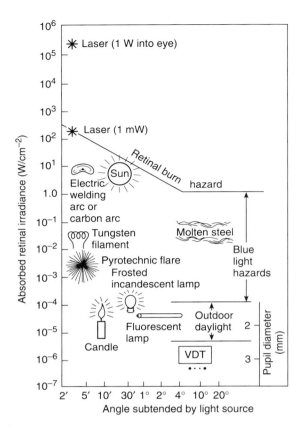

Fig. 30.4 Retinal irradiances (exposure dose rates) from representative light sources (reproduced from Sliney and Wolbarsht (1980), with permission).

Visible light
Nature, sources, and environmental levels
Visible light consists of electromagnetic waves varying in wavelength from 380 nm (violet) to 760 nm (red) (Fig. 30.1). Sources of visible light in the environment vary widely in the intensity of their emissions; common high-intensity sources other than the sun include lasers, electric welding or carbon arcs, and tungsten filament lamps (Fig. 30.4).

Nature and mechanisms of injury
Too bright a light can injure the eye through photochemical reactions in the retina; that is sustained exposure to intensities exceeding 0.1 mW/cm^2, such as can result from fixating a bright source of light, may produce photochemical blue-light injury, and brief exposure of the retina to intensities exceeding 10 W/cm^2, depending on image size, may cause a retinal burn (Fig. 30.4). The lens, iris, and cornea also are vulnerable to injury from the thermal effects of laser radiation (Sliney and Wolbarsht 1980). Too little illumination, conversely, also can be harmful, causing eye strain (Huer 1983) and/or seasonal affective disorder (SAD).

Prevention
Since bright, continuously visible light normally elicits an aversion response which acts to protect the eye against injury, few sources of light are large and bright enough to cause a retinal burn under normal viewing conditions. One must never look directly at a solar eclipse, and in situations involving potential exposure to such high-intensity sources as carbon arcs or lasers, appropriate training,

proper design of equipment, and protective eye shields are indicated (Sliney and Wolbarsht 1980; ANSI 1986; ACGIH 1993).

Infrared radiation
Nature, sources, and environmental levels
Infrared radiation (IR) consists of electromagnetic waves ranging in wavelength from 7 ¥ 10^{-5} m to 3 ¥ 10^{-2} m (Fig. 30.1). Some such radiation is emitted by all objects with temperatures above absolute zero, but potentially hazardous sources of IR include furnaces, ovens, welding arcs, molten glass, molten metal, and heating lamps.

Nature and mechanisms of injury
The injuries caused by IR are limited chiefly to burns of the skin and cataracts of the lens of the eye. The warning sensation of heat usually prompts aversion in time to prevent the skin from being burned by IR, but the lens of the eye is vulnerable in lacking both heat-sensing and heat-dissipating ability. As a result, glass blowers, blacksmiths, oven operators, and those working around heating and drying lamps are at risk of IR-induced cataracts (Lydahl and Philipson 1984).

Prevention
Control of IR hazards requires appropriate shielding of sources, proper training and supervision of potentially exposed persons, and use of protective clothing and goggles. It is also recommended that exposures to IR not exceed 10 mW/cm^2 (ACGIH 1993).

Microwave radiation
Nature, sources, and environmental levels
Microwave and radiofrequency radiation (MW/RFR) consists of electromagnetic waves ranging in frequency from about 3 kHz to 300 GHz (Fig. 30.1). Sources of MW/RFR occur widely in radar, television, radio, cellular phones, and other telecommunications systems, and are also used in various industrial operations (for example heating, welding, and melting of metals; processing of wood and plastic; high-temperature plasma), household appliances (such as microwave ovens), and medical applications (for example diathermy and hypothermia) (ILO 1986).

Nature and mechanisms of injury
The biological effects of MW/RFR are primarily thermal in nature, MW/RFR-induced injuries consist mainly of burns of the skin and other tissues. Burns have occasionally resulted from faulty or improperly used household microwave ovens and from the overexposure of patients in whom cutaneous pain and temperature senses that usually warn of impending injury are impaired. Because of the deep penetration of MW/RFR, the cutaneous burns it causes tend to involve dermal and subcutaneous tissues, and to heal slowly. Cataracts of the lens of the eye have been reported to result from high-intensity exposures (>1.5 kW/m^2) (McRee 1972), and even death from hyperthermia has been encountered in the industrial use of MW/RFR sources (McLaughlin 1957; Roberts and Michaelson 1985). Also well documented is the ability of MW/RFR to interfere with cardiac pacemakers and other medical devices (NCRP 1986; Michaelson 1991). Other effects reported in the literature, but as yet inconclusively documented, include impairment of fertility, developmental disturbances, neurobehavioural abnormalities, depression of immunity, and increased risks of cancer (Foster and Guy 1986; Michaelson 1991; Yost 1992).

Table 30.8 Threshold limit values for radiofrequency/microwave radiation

Frequency	Power density (mW/cm²)	Electric field strength squared (V²/m²)	Magnetic field strength squared (A²/m²)
30 kHz to 3MHz	100	377 000	2.65
3 MHz to 30 MHz	900/f²	3770(900/f²)	900(37.7 × f²)
30 MHz to 100 MHz	1	3770	0.027
100 MHz to 1000 MHz	f/100	3770(f/100)	f(37.7 × 100)
1 GHz to 300 GHz	10	37 700	0.265

From: ACGIH, 1993 (reproduced with permission); f denotes frequency in MHz.

Prevention

Proper design and shielding of MW/RFR sources are indicated, along with appropriate training and supervision of potentially exposed persons (especially those wearing cardiac pacemakers or other sensitive devices). Exposure to MW/RFR power densities exceeding the threshold limit values in Table 30.8 may cause detectable heating of tissue and should be avoided (NCRP 1986; ILO 1986; ACGIH 1993).

Extremely low-frequency electromagnetic fields

Nature, sources, and environmental levels

Extremely low-frequency (ELF) electromagnetic fields (EMFs) – that is time-varying magnetic fields with frequencies below 300 Hz – are present throughout the environment. The largest such fields arise intermittently from solar activity and thunderstorms, during which they may reach intensities on the order of 0.5 T (Grandolfo and Vecchia 1985). Far stronger than such naturally occurring EMFs are the localized 50 to 60 Hz fields that are generated by electric power lines, transformers, motors, household appliances, video display tubes (VDTs), and various medical devices, notably magnetic resonance imaging (MRI) systems (OTA 1989; Tenforde 1992). For example, the flux density on the ground beneath a 765 kV, 60 Hz power line carrying 1 kA per phase is of the order of 15 T, and close to common household appliances the flux density may range up to 2.5 mT (Tenforde 1992). Since the strength of such fields decreases rapidly with distance, however, the average ambient value in the household environment is less than 0.3 T (3 mG) (Silva et al. 1989). By the same token, while flux densities at video display terminals typically range up to 5 T, those at the location of the operator are generally less than 1 T (Tenforde 1992).

Nature and mechanisms of injury

Extremely-low-frequency EMFs induce electrical currents which can alter the properties of cell membranes and exert effects on electrically active tissues (nerves, neuromusculature, retina, heart) and on cardiac pacemakers. Induced current densities under 1 to 10 mA/m² produce few, if any, irreversible effects, which is not surprising in view of the fact that endogenous current densities of 0.1 to 10 mA/m² exist in many tissues. Induced current densities above 10 mA/m², on the other hand, although not genotoxic, reportedly produce various changes in the biochemistry and physiology of cells and tissues (for example alterations in metabo-

lism, growth rate, melatonin secretion, endocrine activity and immune response); and current densities above 1A can cause neural excitation and irreversible effects, such as cardiac fibrillation (Tenforde 1992).

In addition to the effects produced by strong EMFs, epidemiological data have suggested the possibility of severe effects from long-continued exposure to weaker EMFs; that is: (1) that the risks of leukaemia may be increased by residential exposure to household EMFs in children, (2) that the risks of brain cancer and leukaemia may be increased by occupational exposure to EMFs in utility workers , and (3) that the risks of having miscarriages or of bearing children with birth defects may be increased by chronic exposure to EMFs through the operation of VDTs in pregnant women (Bates 1991; Tenforde 1992). As yet, although the epidemiological data are inconclusive and their interpretation complicated by uncertainties in exposure assessment and by the lack of established biological mechanisms for the effects in question, the fact that such fields have been reported to influence cell growth, ion transport, melatonin secretion, and tumour promotion in some model systems (Adair 1991; Stuchly et al. 1991; Tenforde 1992) has contributed to public health concern (OTA 1989).

Prevention

Areas containing EMFs stronger than 0.1 mT, such as exist around transformers, accelerators, MRI systems, and other electric devices, should be posted with warning signs and should be avoided by persons wearing cardiac pacemakers. In addition, the strength of any 60 Hz time-varying magnetic field, such as typically exists around an MRI system, should be limited to 1 mT for occupational exposures and to 0.1 mT for those wearing cardiac pacemakers or for continuous exposures involving members of the general public (ACGIH 1993). To minimize the risks, if any, that may be associated with the use of electric blankets, wiring design changes have been introduced by some manufacturers to cancel the surface 60 Hz EMFs that such blankets would otherwise generate (Tenforde 1992).

Ultrasound

Nature, sources, and environmental levels

Although often classified for public health purposes with non-ionizing radiation, ultrasound is not a component of the electromagnetic spectrum but actually consists of mechanical vibrations at frequencies above the audible range (that is > 16 KHz) (NCRP 1983). Sources of high-power, low-frequency ultrasound are used widely in science and industry for cleaning, degreasing, plastic welding, liquid extracting, atomizing, homogenizing, and emulsifying operations, as well as in medicine for lithotripsy and other therapeutic applications. Low-power, high-frequency ultrasound is used widely in analytical work and in medical diagnosis (such as ultrasonography).

Nature and mechanisms of injury

The biological effects of ultrasound are similar in mechanism to those of mechanical vibration. High-power, low-frequency ultrasound, transmitted through the air or through bodily contact with a generating source, has been observed to cause a variety of effects in occupationally exposed workers, including headache, earache, tinnitus, vertigo, malaise, photophobia, hypercusia, peripheral neuritis, and autonomic polyneuritis, none of which appear to be irreversible. The possibility that it may cause adverse effects on the embryo also has been suggested (NCRP 1983).

Although excessive exposure to high-frequency ultrasound through bodily contact with the source may be expected, in principle, to cause complaints similar to those above, no adverse effects have been observed to result from exposure to high-frequency ultrasound at the low power levels used in medical ultrasonography (NCRP 1983).

Prevention

Protection against injury by ultrasound requires appropriate isolation and insulation of generating sources , as well as proper training and ear protective devices for those working around such sources. Yearly audiometric and neurological examinations of occupationally exposed workers also are recommended (WHO 1982).

Summary and conclusions

The adverse effects on human health caused by different forms of radiant energy are diverse, ranging from rapidly fatal injuries to cancers, birth defects, and hereditary disorders appearing months, years, or decades after exposure. The nature, frequency, and severity of effects depend on the type of radiant energy in question and the particular conditions of exposure. Most such effects are produced only by appreciable levels of exposure and can, therefore, be prevented completely by keeping any exposures from exceeding relevant thresholds. The genotoxic and carcinogenic effects of ionizing and ultraviolet radiations, in contrast, are presumed to increase in frequency as linear non-threshold functions of the dose and, therefore, not to be entirely preventable without eliminating all exposure to these two forms of radiation. Since it is not feasible to eliminate exposures to ionizing and ultraviolet radiations completely, protection against their mutagenic and carcinogenic effects requires that exposures to these agents be limited sufficiently to keep any associated risks from exceeding acceptable levels.

To achieve the desired level of protection against each of the different forms of radiation requires knowledge of the relevant exposure–risk relationships; appropriate design and operation of all radiation sources; proper training, equipment, and supervision of operating personnel; and education of members of the public in prudent measures for safeguarding their health. These requirements can be met satisfactorily in most situations involving radiation hazards, given the necessary commitment of effort and resources. Unresolved public health problems calling for particular attention at this time, however, include: (1) assessment of the risks associated with residential exposure to indoor radon, and of the pertinent remediation strategies; (2) development and implementation of measures for dealing with the hazards posed by the large and growing quantities of radioactive and mixed wastes; (3) assessment of the risks that may be associated with exposure to 60 Hz electromagnetic fields; and (4) further evaluation of stratospheric ozone depletion and its implications for ultraviolet-radiation-induced impacts on human health.

References

Adair, R.K. (1991). Constraints on biological effects of weak extremely-low-frequency electromagnetic fields. *Physical Review A*, **43**, 1039–48.

ACGIH (1993). *Threshold limit values and biological exposure indices for 1993–1994*. American Conference of Governmental Industrial Hygienists. ACGIH, Cincinnati.

AMA Council on Scientific Affairs (1989). Harmful effects of ultraviolet radiation. *Journal of the American Medical Association*, **262**, 380–4.

ANSI (1986). *Safe use of lasers*. American National Standards Institute, New York.

Bates, M.N. (1991). Extremely low frequency electromagnetic fields and cancer. The epidemiologic evidence. *Environmental Health Perspectives*, **95**, 147–56.

Doll, R., Evans, N.J., and Darby, S.C. (1994). Paternal exposure not to blame. *Nature*, **367**, 678–80.

Gardner, M.J., Hall, A., Snee, M.P., Downes, S., Powell, C.A., and Terell, J.D. (1990). Results of case–control study of leukaemia and lymphoma among young people near Sellafield nuclear plant in West Cumbria. *British Medical Journal*, **300**, 423–9.

Goodhead, D.J. (1988). Spatial and temporal distribution of energy. *Health Physios*, **55**, 231–40.

Grandolfo, M. and Vecchia, P. (1985). Natural and man-made environmental exposures to static and ELF electromagnetic fields. In *Biological effects and dosimetry of static and ELF electromagnetic fields* (ed. M. Grandolfo, S. M. Michaelson, and A. Rindi), pp. 49–70, Plenum, New York.

Hall, E.J. (1994). *Radiobiology for the radiologist* (4th edn). J. B. Lippincott, Philadelphia.

Harper, L.C. and Bickers, D.R. (1989). *Photosensitivity diseases. Principles of diagnosis and treatment* (2nd edn). B. C. Decker, Toronto.

Henriksen, T., Dahlback, A., Larsen, S., and Moan, J. (1990). Ultraviolet radiation and skin cancer. Effect of an ozone layer depletion. *Photochemistry and Photobiology*, **51**, 579– 82.

Hill, C. and Laplanche, A. (1990). Overall mortality and cancer mortality around French nuclear sites. A letter. *Nature*, **347**, 755–7.

Huer, H.H. (1983). Lighting. In *Encyclopaedia of occupational health and safety*, (ed. L. Parmeggiana), pp. 1225–31, International Labour Office, Geneva.

IAEA. (1986). *Biological dosimetry: chromosomal aberration analysis for dose assessment*, Technical report, No. 260. International Atomic Energy Agency, Vienna.

ICRP (International Commission on Radiological Protection) (1984). Non-stochastic effects of ionizing radiation. ICRP Publication, No. 41, *Annals of the ICRP* **14** (3), 1–33.

ICRP (International Commission on Radiological Protection) (1991). 1990 Recommendations of the International Commission on Radiological Protection. ICRP Publication, No. 60. *Annals of the ICRP* **21**, No. 1–3.

ILO (International Labour Office) (1986). *Protection of workers against radio-frequency and microwave radiation: a technical review*, Occupational safety and health series report No. 57, International Labour Office, Geneva.

Kasakov, V.S., Demidchik, E.P., and Astakhova, L.N. (1992). Thyroid cancer after Chernobyl. *Nature*, **359**, 21.

Jablon, S., Hrubec, Z., and Boice, J.D., Jr. (1991). Cancer in populations living near nuclear facilities. A survey of mortality nation-wide and incidence in two areas. *Journal of the American Medical Association*, **265**, 1403–8.

Kinlen, L.J. (1988). Evidence for an infective cause of childhood leukaemia: comparison of a Scottish New Town with nuclear reprocessing sites in Britain. *Lancet*, ii, 1323–7.

Kinlen, L.J., Clarke, K., and Balkwill, A. (1993). Paternal preconceptional radiation exposure in the nuclear industry and leukaemia and non-Hodgkin's lymphoma in young people in Scotland, *British Medical Journal*, **306**, 1153–8.

Kripke, M.L. (1988). Impact of ozone depletion on skin cancers. *Journal of Dermatological Surgery, Oncol.* **14**, 853–7.

Lerman, S.(1988). Ocular phototoxicity (editorial). *New England Journal of Medicine*, **319**, 1475–7.

Lubin, J.H. (1994). Invited commentary: lung cancer and exposure to residential radon. *American Journal of Epidemiology*, **140**, 323–32.

Lubin, J.H., Boice, J.D., Jr., Edling, C., *et al.* (1994). *Radon and lung cancer risk: a joint analysis of 11 underground miners studies*, NIH Publication, No. 94–3644. National Institutes of Health, Rockville, MD.

Lushbaugh, C.C., Fry, S.A., and Ricks, R.C. (1987). Nuclear reactor accidents: preparedness and consequences. *British Journal of Radiology*, **60**, 1159–83.

Lydahl, E. and Philipson, B. (1989). Infrared radiation and cataract. I. Epidemiologic investigation of iron and steel workers, II. Epidemiologic investigation of glass workers. *Cleta Ophthalmologica*, **62**, 976–92.

McLaughlin, J.T. (1957). Tissue destruction and death from microwave radiation (radar). *California Medicine*, **86**, 336.

McLaughlin, J.R., Clarke, E.A., Nishri, D., and Anderson, T.W.(1993). Childhood leukaemia in the vicinity of Canadian nuclear facilities. *Cancer Causes and Control* **4**, 51–8.

McRee, D.I. (1972). Environmental aspects of microwave radiation. *Environmental Health Perspectives*, **2**, 41–53.

Mettler, F.A. and Upton, A.C. (1995). *Medical effects of ionizing radiation*. Grune & Stratton, New York.

Mettler, F.A., Williamson, M.R., Royal, H.D., *et al.* (1992). Thyroid nodules in the population living around Chernobyl. *Journal of the American Medical Association*, **268**, 616–19.

Michaelson, S.M. (1991). Biological effects of radiofrequency radiation: concepts and criteria. *Health Physics*, **61**, 3–14.

NAS (National Academy of Sciences/National Research Council) (1989). *The nuclear weapons complex*. National Academy Press, Washington, DC.

NAS (National Academy of Sciences/National Research Council) (1990). *Health effects of exposure to low levels of ionizing radiation. BEIR V.* National Academy Press, Washington, DC.

NAS (National Academy of Sciences/National Research Council) (1994). *Health effects of exposure to radon. Time for reassessment?* National Academy Press, Washington, DC.

NCRP (National Council on Radiation Protection and Measurements) (1983). *Biological effects of ultrasound: mechanisms and clinical implications*, NCRP report, No. 74. NCRP, Bethesda, MD.

NCRP (National Council on Radiation Protection and Measurements) (1984). *Evaluation of occupational and environmental exposures to radon and radon daughters in the United States*, NCRP report, No. 78. NCRP, Bethesda, MD.

NCRP (National Council on Radiation Protection and Measurements) (1986). *Biological effects and exposure criteria for radiofrequency electromagnetic fields*, NCRP report, No. 86. NCRP, Bethesda, MD.

NCRP (National Council on Radiation Protection and Measurements) (1987). *Ionizing radiation exposure of the population of the United States*, NCRP report, No. 93. NCRP, Bethesda, MD.

NCRP (National Council on Radiation Protection and Measurements) (1989). *Exposure of the U.S. population from occupational radiation*, NCRP report, No. 101. NCRP, Bethesda, MD.

NCRP (National Council on Radiation Protection and Measurements) (1993). *Limitation of exposure to ionizing radiation*, NCRP report, No. 116. NCRP, Bethesda, MD.

NIH (National Institutes of Health) (1985). *Report of the National Institutes of Health Ad Hoc Working Group to Develop Radioepidemiological Tables*, NIH Publication No. 85–2748. US Government Printing Office, Washington, DC.

NIOSH (National Institute for Occupational Safety and Health) (1972). *Criteria for a recommended standard: occupational exposure to ultraviolet radiation*, DHEW publication, No. (NIOSH) HSM 73–11009. US Government Printing Office, Washington, DC.

OTA (Office of Technology Assessment, US Congress) (1989). *Biological effects of power frequency electric and magnetic fields – background paper*, OTA-BP-E–53. US Government Printing Office, Washington, DC.

Prisyazhiuk, A., Pjatak, O.A., Buzanov, V.A., *et al.* (1991). Cancer in the Ukraine, post-Chernobyl. *Lancet*, **338**, 1334–5.

Rallison, M., Dobyns, B., Keating, R., *et al.* (1974). Thyroid disease in children: a survey of subjects potentially exposed to fallout radiation. *American Journal of Medicine*, **56**, 457–63.

Robbins, J. and Adams, W. (1989). Radiation effects in the Marshall Islands. In: *Radiation and the thyroid* (ed. S. Nagataki) pp. 11–24. Exerpta Medica, Tokyo.

Roberts, N. J., Jr. and Michaelson, S.M. (1985). Epidemiological studies of human exposures to microwave radiation: a critical review. *International Archives of Occupational and Environmental Health*, **56**, 169–78.

Rubin, P. and Casarett, G.W. (1972). A direction for clinical radiation pathology: the tolerance dose. In: *Frontiers of radiation therapy and oncology* (ed. J. M. Vaeth), pp. 1–16. Univ. Park Press, Basel.

Shapiro, J. (1990). *Radiation protection: a guide for scientists and physicians*, (3rd edn). Harvard University Press, Cambridge, MA.

Silva, M., Hummon, N., Rutter, D., and Hooper, C. (1989). Power frequency magnetic fields in the home. *IEEE Transactions of Power Delivery*, **4**, 465–77.

Sliney, D. and Wolbarsht, M. (1980). *Safety with lasers*. Plenum, New York.

Stannard, J.N. (1988). *Radioactivity and health: a history*, US Department of Energy Report, DOE/RL/01830–T59. National Technical Information Services, US Department of Energy, Washington, DC.

Stevens, W., Till, J.E., Lyon, L., *et al.* (1990). Leukaemia in Utah and radioactive fallout from the Nevada test site. *Journal of the American Medical Association*, **264**, 585–91.

Stuchly, M.A., McLean, J.R.N., Burnett, R., Goddard, M., Lecuyer, D.W., and Mitchel, R.E.J. (1992). Modification of tumour promotion in the mouse skin by exposure to an alternating magnetic field. *Cancer Letters*, **65**, 1–7.

Tenforde, T.S. (1992). Biological interactions and potential health effects of extremely-low-frequency magnetic fields from power lines and other common sources. *Annual Reviews of Public Health*, **13**, 173–96.

UNSCEAR (United Nations Scientific Committee on the Effects of Atomic Radiation) (1982). *Ionizing Radiation: sources and biological effects*. Report to the General Assembly, with Annexes, United Nations, New York.

UNSCEAR (United Nations Scientific Committee on the Effects of Atomic Radiation) (1986). *Genetic and somatic effects of ionizing radiation*, Report to the General Assembly, with annexes. United Nations, New York.

UNSCEAR (United Nations Scientific Committee on the Effects of Atomic Radiation) (1988). *Sources, effects, and risks of ionizing radiation*, Report to the General Assembly, with annexes. United Nations, New York.

UNSCEAR (United Nations Scientific Committee on the Effects of Atomic Radiation) (1993). *Sources and effects of ionizing radiation*, Report to the General Assembly, with annexes. United Nations, New York.

Upton, A.C. (1986). Historical perspectives on radiation carcinogenesis. In: *Radiation carcinogenesis* (ed. A.C. Upton, R.E. Albert, F.J. Burns, and R.E. Shore, pp. 1–10. Elsevier, New York.

Upton, A.C., Shore, R.E., and Harley, N.H. (1990). The health effects of low-level ionizing radiation. *Annual Reviews of Public Health*, **13**, 127–50.

USDOE (US Department of Energy) (1987). *Health and environmental consequences of the Chernobyl nuclear power plant accident*, DOE/ER–0332. USDOE, Washington, DC.

USDOE (US Department of Energy) (1993). *US Department of Energy interim mixed waste inventory report: waste streams, treatment capacities, and technologies*, DOE/NBM–1100. USDOE, Washington, DC.

USEPA (US Environmental Protection Agency) (1990). *Medical waste management in the United States*, First interim report to Congress. US Environmental Protection Agency, Washington, DC.

USEPA (US Environmental Protection Agency) (1991). *Environmental radiation protection standards for the management and disposal of spent nuclear fuel, high-level, and transuranic radioactive waste*, Title 40, Part 191, Code of Federal Regulations (Draft Revised Standards). US Environmental Protection Agency, Washington, DC.

USEPA (US Environmental Protection Agency) (1992). *Technical support document for the 1992 citizen's guide to radon*, EPA 400–R–92–0ll. US Environmental Protection Agency, Washington, DC.

USNRC (US Nuclear Regulatory Commission) (1992). *National profile on commercially generated low-level radioactive waste*, NUREG/CR–5938. December, 1992.

Wakeford, R., Tawn, E.J., McElvenny, D.M., Scott, L.E., Binks, K., Parker, L., Dickinson, H., and Smith, J. (1994a). The descriptive statistics and health implications of occupational radiation doses received by men at the Sellafield nuclear installation before the conception of their children. *Journal of Radiological Protection*, **14**, 3–16.

Wakeford, R., Tawn, E.J., McElvenny, D.M., Binks, K., Scott, L.E., and Parker, L. (1994b). The Seascale childhood leukaemia cases – the mutation rates implied by paternal preconceptional radiation doses. *Journal of Radiological Protection*, **14**, 17–24.

Ward, J.F. (1988). DNA damage produced by ionizing radiation in mammalian cells: identities, mechanisms of formation, and repairability. *Progress Nucleic Acid Research and Molecular Biology*, **35**, 96–128.

WHO (World Health Organization) (1982). *Ultrasound environmental health criteria*, No. 22. World Health Organization, Geneva.

Yoshimoto, Y., Neel, J.V., Schull, W.J., Kato, H., Soda, M., Eto, R., and Mabuchi, K. (1990). Malignant tumours during the first two decades of life in the offspring of atomic bomb survivors. *American Journal of Human Genetics*, **46**, 1041–52.

Yost, M.G. (1992). Occupational health effects of nonionizing radiation. *Occupational Medicine: State of the Art Reviews*, **7**, 543–66.

31 Microbiology

Norman D. Noah

Introduction

Microbiological hazards predate those caused by other environmental contaminants and they remain serious and common causes of ill health, even though regulatory priority is often given to chemical or radiation hazards. The epidemiological methods used for the investigation of infectious disease are not substantially different from those used for any epidemiological investigation. Nevertheless, there are some investigative techniques which are particularly applicable to infectious diseases. They include the techniques of investigation of the host, agent, and environment, which are described in other chapters and techniques of surveillance and vaccine trials which are described in this chapter. The use of the microbiological laboratory in epidemiological studies is also discussed.

Population surveillance

The definition of population surveillance is 'Continuous analysis, interpretation, and feedback of systematically collected data, generally using methods distinguished by their practicality, uniformity and rapidity, rather than by accuracy or completeness' (Last 1995).

Thus surveillance is a type of observational study (Thacker *et al.* 1983). There are several key words in the definition provided by Last (1995, p. 163) which make his the preferred definition. 'Continuous' distinguishes surveillance from a survey. 'Practicality' is the essence of any workable surveillance system. 'Uniformity' ensures that the data can be interpreted sensibly, in particular as surveillance is all about trends. 'Rapidity' is important for the system to be useful. And the words 'rather than complete accuracy or completeness' sum up the rough and ready philosophy behind most surveillance systems which exist primarily for following trends in disease patterns. Many of these points, however, need to be qualified and are further discussed later in this section.

The word 'monitoring' should not be used interchangeably with surveillance: it is the ongoing evaluation of a control or management process (Eylenbosch and Noah 1988). The techniques of surveillance are usually necessary for efficient monitoring. Thus, monitoring the success or failure of a vaccine policy for a disease will involve surveillance of vaccine use and surveillance of the disease, although the overall process is one of monitoring. Monitoring can become a finely tuned measure in which outcome can be constantly evaluated to adjust the process.

Research is not an essential part of surveillance, although surveillance may facilitate research. Consequently there has been some discussion about the term 'epidemiological surveillance' and whether 'public health surveillance' is more valid (Thacker and Berkelman 1988).

Types of surveillance
Active and passive surveillance

In passive surveillance the recipient waits for the provider to report. In active surveillance routine checks of the provider are regularly made to ensure uniform and complete reporting. The globally successful smallpox eradication programme used active surveillance; each local health unit was 'coerced, persuaded, and cajoled' to report cases of smallpox each week, intensive further casefinding was undertaken when a case was notified, and sources of information other than medical—teachers, schoolchildren, civil servants, and so on—were used (Henderson 1976). The reporting of a negative return is an important but not an essential part of a surveillance system. For surveillance of very rare diseases, however, completeness becomes more important and 'negative reporting' becomes essential. Negative reporting has been used most effectively in the surveillance system for rare paediatric diseases, such as Reye's syndrome and Kawasaki disease, run by the British Paediatric Surveillance Unit in Britain (Hall and Glickman 1988).

Sentinel surveillance

Sentinel surveillance is essentially a type of 'sample surveillance' in which reporting sources are situated at various sites covering an area (which may be very large, for example a country), or a particular high-risk group such as commercial sex workers and may provide fairly complete reporting within the population covered by each reporting source. This ensures that resources are not wasted in a large unwieldy surveillance system. If the population (total or age and sex distributions) covered by each reporting centre is known, estimates of the disease or other indicator under surveillance can be made. Systems based on general practice reporting are the most common forms of sentinel surveillance and are discussed later in this chapter (see below).

Essentials of a surveillance system

The essential steps in any surveillance system are the collection of data, their analysis, their interpretation, and feedback of information.

These steps are similar to those taken in any scientific process. The collection of data is clearly the basic element of the system, but a failure of any of the other three steps in the process could also lead to failure of the system.

Collection of data

The collection of data has to be systematic, regular, uniform, and, in infectious diseases particularly, topical and relevant. For collection to be systematic, suppliers of information should understand clearly what needs to be reported, leaving little scope for value judgements in deciding what to report, such as only interesting or rare cases. For clinical reporting, case definitions are helpful, in particular for new or rare diseases and even for common and easily recognizable diseases, particularly if they become less common. An early case definition for AIDS was important in the initial surveillance of this infection. Measles is easily recognizable clinically, but a case definition became essential when the vaccine campaign in the United States and now in England was so successful that the infection became rare.

Case definitions may be rigid, but do not necessarily have to be highly specific. Careful consideration has to be given in individual instances as to whether sensitivity is more important than specificity. It may be important for example, to choose a high-sensitive, low-specific definition to encourage reporting and then to concentrate on encouraging high specificity as the surveillance system becomes established. For laboratory reporting, likewise, the criteria for what constitutes an acceptable report need to be understood clearly by the laboratory; for example isolation of the organism from particular sites or a 4-fold or greater rise in antibody titre or a single antibody titre above a certain level associated with a clinical feature characteristic of that infection, may all be acceptable. Nevertheless, in infectious disease there are often difficulties in associating a correctly identified organism with a particular illness, for example isolation of an echovirus from a patient with gastroenteritis. In these instances all laboratories should understand clearly whether every such isolation need be reported or only one where the isolate is considered to contribute to the symptoms (which may involve a value judgement). In the laboratory reporting system run by the Communicable Disease Surveillance Centre in England, all viral isolates are reported, although there is space on the form for the laboratory to indicate if the isolate is thought not to be relevant to the condition of the patient.

If feedback is to be regular, reporting must also be regular. The Communicable Disease Report for England and Wales is produced weekly and the laboratories report weekly. Regular reporting also helps to maintain discipline and routine, essential ingredients of any reporting system. The information received from providers must be relevant and topical, otherwise the interest of the participants is rapidly lost and their response will diminish. With infectious disease surveillance, serious infections, rare infections, or those against which a control measure is available or is being planned tend to be most worthwhile for surveillance.

Analysis of data

The analysis of data for infectious diseases is similar to that for any other type of epidemiological data. The basic principles of analysis by time, place, and person are fundamental.

Time Analysis by time is necessary if trends are to be discovered from surveillance data. In infectious disease in particular, temporal trends are helpful in predicting and planning for disease (Noah 1989). For infectious diseases there may be a significant delay of days or weeks between the time of acute illness and the date the infection is diagnosed and then reported. This is generally unavoid-

able. The time of onset of symptoms may be days or weeks before the illness is investigated. There will then be further delays before the disease is diagnosed and again a delay before it is reported to the surveillance unit. With serological diagnosis, because a rise in antibody occurs only during convalescence, the infection is only confirmed when the patient is better. Even with a weekly reporting system there will be further delay before the infection is finally recorded. The burden of reporting will be increased considerably by asking reporting laboratories to record the date of onset of illness, but the date the first specimen was received in the laboratory is usually readily available and often approximates to the time of acute illness. In the analysis of such data, the interval between this date and the date of reporting may need to be taken into account. Analysing laboratory data by the date of the first specimen may be less helpful for immediate detection of changes in incidence. The techniques of analysis by time and tests for seasonality or periodicity are outside the scope of this chapter.

Place The site of the reporting laboratory is normally taken to be the geographical location of the ill person. Except in the best organized of health-care systems however, this is not always true. In England and Wales, for example, the statutory notifications generally relate to the area of residence of the patient, but the local authority to which the infection is notified is not necessarily co-terminous with the health authority. There are rarely rigid boundaries or catchment areas for hospital or public health laboratories and their reports. It may be difficult or impossible to allow for these problems in the analysis of the data, although it may only rarely be necessary to do so.

Person The age and sex of cases reported are also important components of a surveillance report. It is possible to conduct a surveillance system based solely on the numbers and geographical location, but the sensitivity of the systems will be considerably reduced. Surveillance based on measles notifications in England and Wales has shown that, although the incidence in all age groups fell substantially following the introduction of the measles, mumps, rubella vaccine (MMR) in 1989 the proportion and incidence in people aged 10 to 24 years increased, as did the proportion in even older age groups (Fig. 31.1). In an outbreak of hepatitis B caused by a tattooist in one district of England (Limentani *et al.* 1979), simple analysis of notifications of 'infective jaundice' by time or place would not have uncovered the outbreak. An age and sex analysis however, would have revealed an increase in notified cases in males aged 15 to 29 years.

In the British laboratory surveillance system, some important and common organisms such as salmonellas were reported without the age and sex of the patient, as it would increase greatly the burden of reporting, collection, and analysis of such data to unmanageable levels. Reliance was placed on the ability to detect an increase in a rare salmonella serotype or phage type of a more common serotype. When this occurred, the age and sex of the cases were readily available from the reference laboratory and provided some aetiological clues: an increase in *Salmonella ealing* infections for example proved to be mainly in infants and was subsequently shown to be associated with powdered milk (Rowe *et al.* 1987).

Denominator data clearly are desirable, but they are not essential to an infectious disease surveillance system. In the United Kingdom only the Royal College of General Practitioners Research Unit has an in-built rate provided with its data outputs. In this

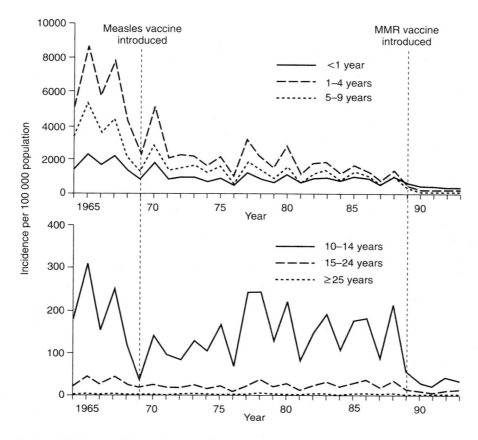

Fig. 31.1 Measles notifications in England and Wales, 1964–1994. (Reproduced from *Communicable Disease Report* (1994), **4**, 105, with permission.)

surveillance system, approximately 40 physicians in various parts of the country, covering approximately 200 000 patients, report new episodes of illness each week to the Central Research Unit (Fleming and Crombie 1985). As each general practitioner (**GP**) has an age and sex distribution available of their practice populations, consultation rates for the different illnesses can be calculated.

Interpretation

In the interpretation of surveillance data lies the skill of the epidemiologist. As Langmuir (1976) wrote of William Farr 'His weekly return was no archive for stale data, but with his facile pen became a literate weapon for effecting change. He presented his analysis with objectivity but then stated his own interpretations forcefully . . . '

In surveillance data a detailed understanding of the reporting system is necessary before a meaningful interpretation of the statistics can be made. Some knowledge of the size and demographic characteristics of the population covered by the surveillance system is also necessary. Every data source carries its own strengths and biases (Moro and McCormick 1988). With each data source, timeliness, completeness, representativeness, and accuracy (Thacker *et al.* 1983) should be considered. To these four qualities should be added that of significance (in its sense of 'importance'). Timeliness may be particularly important with laboratory statistics, where there may sometimes be a considerable delay between disease onset and laboratory diagnosis. Organisms need time to grow in

culture and acute and convalescent samples of sera are needed to demonstrate the 4-fold or greater rise in antibody necessary to substantiate a serological diagnosis. Rapid diagnostic methods for identification of an organism and the increasing use of IgM tests, however, have hastened considerably the diagnostic process for some infections. Notifications, although usually made on the basis of a clinical diagnosis, may not always be as prompt as one would expect and sentinel GP clinical reporting systems tend to be more timely (Tillett and Spencer 1982).

The need for completeness of reporting, particularly of common infections, is often exaggerated. Detection of disease trends by time, place, and person, sufficient for meaningful epidemiological interpretation, is possible with incomplete data. Striving for completeness may waste resources. For rare diseases, however or diseases that have become rare following a control programme, completeness grows in importance. Passive surveillance systems rarely achieve completeness; active systems are generally necessary.

The representativeness of the data collected needs thought and planning and the advantages of collecting data from more than one source may provide ways of validating one data source against another. In the surveillance system for infectious diseases in England and Wales conducted by the Communicable Disease Surveillance Centre, for example, the three main sources of data on meningococcal meningitis—hospital, notifications, and laboratory —showed similar trends over time (Fig. 31.2). Source data should be representative for time, place, and person.

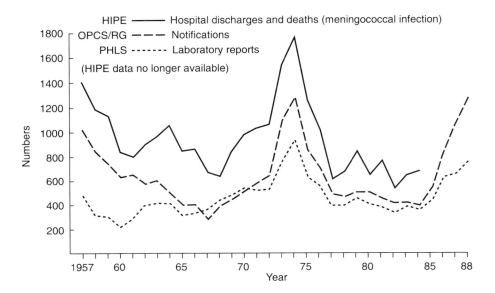

Fig. 31.2 Acute meningococcal meningitis—England and Wales 1957–88. (Prepared by CDSC.)

The significance of surveillance data should also be evaluated carefully in its interpretation and this can perhaps be best illustrated diagramatically, using laboratory reporting of influenza as an example.

If the population of a community affected by an outbreak of influenza is represented by the rectangular outline in Fig. 31.3, the number actually infected will be a proportion, represented by the circle (A). However, not all of these will have symptoms; those that do belong within circle (B). Only a small proportion of these will visit a doctor (C) (whether in hospital or general practice) and progressively smaller proportions will have a specimen sent for examination in a laboratory (D), specimens positive (E), and positive specimens reported to the surveillance unit (F). The biases and variables that occur during these steps also need to be considered. Those with symptomatic infections may be those never previously exposed to the particular influenza variant or subtype or the very young and the very old or those with a chronic disability,

such as a respiratory condition. Similarly, those who visit a doctor and those whom the doctor investigates may be influenced by several factors, including social class, age, severity of disease, and proximity to a laboratory. Laboratory success in its turn will depend on the availability and cost of reagents, the interest and expertise of the laboratory, and the age and severity of disease in the patient. Finally, the accuracy, completeness, and timeliness of reporting by the laboratory will be influenced by its motivation, organization, and efficiency, as well as by the usefulness of the surveillance system and the quality and value of its feedback. A similar progression can be worked out for notification, GP, hospital, and death certification data sources (Fig. 31.4).

The accuracy of the data provided by the laboratory will depend not only on its interest, expertise, and motivation, but also on the clarity of the instructions for reporting provided by the surveillance unit. These include acceptable diagnostic criteria for laboratory data; for antibody titre measurements, the levels acceptable to the

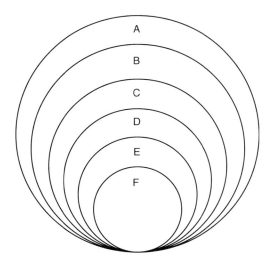

Fig. 31.3 Stages in the reporting of laboratory infection.

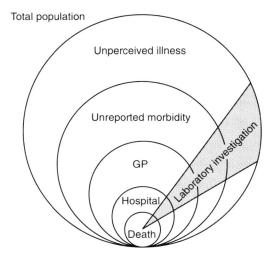

Fig. 31.4 Stages in the progression of disease.

collection unit should be clarified. For notification and GP data a clinical definition is used. A quality control scheme for participating laboratories is useful, as in the system run by the Public Health Laboratory Service in England and Wales, and the Centres for Disease Control and Prevention in the United States.

Dissemination of information and target groups

The logical end and indeed the purpose of any surveillance system, is the output and its quality and relevance are critical: not only must it be meaningful and intelligible, but it must also be directed at the appropriate targets, whether they be decision makers or research workers. Moreover, feedback to those who provide the reports has an important motivating role in any surveillance system. Some surveillance and monitoring systems may even improve performance, as in the COVER programme in England and Wales (see below).

For infectious disease surveillance systems, weekly or monthly reports are the most appropriate. The ability to adapt to changing patterns of infection—incorporating new diseases of importance, discarding outdated or useless data—needs to be in-built. Flexibility to provide urgent information is useful, as for outbreaks and as methods of communication continue to improve, this should make urgent dissemination easier.

The rapid development and availability of electronic methods of storing, analysing, and disseminating data and information have greatly facilitated the practice of surveillance. Powerful microcomputers and electronic networking have allowed data to be transmitted from source to surveillance centre without the use of post and paper—or indeed the tedious completion of surveillance forms. Data are not only stored in the computers but these by preprogrammed statistical analyses of the data can reveal changes in time, place, or person. The meaningful interpretation of such changes still requires the human element. Finally the dissemination of information has been revolutionized by the use of electronic methods. In the United Kingdom, the Communicable Disease Surveillance Centre provides rapid information to health authorities through its EPINET System. In France, the Minitel System is effective. In the United States, the Morbidity and Mortality Weekly Report (**MMWR**) is now available electronically.

Content and presentation

The summary report should contain not indigestible lists and tables, but easily understood analyses with appropriate evaluation of their significance. In particular for infectious disease, the reports need to be topical and relevant. Thus, short summaries of recent trends and changes, together with more detailed reviews of subjects and interests, are important ingredients of a surveillance report and these can be supplemented by reports of outbreaks and other items of general interest by reporter participants or other contributors.

'A successful report will educate and provide current scientific information for planning, prevention or change' (Eylenbosch and Noah 1988, p. 22).

Another function necessary for a successful surveillance system is the provision of an information service for individual enquiry. The organization of the surveillance unit and of the data collection system to provide information (as opposed to raw data) is as an important a part of any surveillance feedback service as the regular report. For a sporadic inquiry of this type, appropriate inter-

pretation of the information provided is necessary. Encouraging regular dialogue between providers, other interested parties, and the central surveillance unit is helpful in fostering a healthy relationship between them and the long-term usefulness of the surveillance system; it can also be regarded as a form of monitoring of the surveillance system.

Ideally, the content and presentation of the output of the surveillance system needs to be adapted so as to be made intelligible to each type of target group; lay politicians and decision makers, for example, might receive a different type of feedback from research workers and again from the public and media. This is rarely possible with the regular surveillance report, but an information section within the central unit could tailor the response appropriately to the *ad hoc* inquiry. The increasing interest in health by the lay public, media, and politicians makes it essential to provide accurate, relevant, and topical information with skill and flair.

Content of surveillance: sources of data

When discussing the epidemiology of infection or any other type of disease, it is useful to consider the different stages in the natural history of the disease process (Fig. 31.4). The figure is similar to that used for laboratory data (Fig. 31.3). The population again can be represented by the rectangular outline.

Within this population will be a subpopulation who will be infected asymptomatically or will be immune. A smaller proportion will develop symptomatic infection and progressively smaller proportions will have symptomatic unreported infections, visit a doctor, be admitted to hospital, or die. To have a true measure of the total impact of a disease on a population, information at all these levels is needed. In practice it is of course rarely possible, or perhaps necessary, to be so systematic, although information at most levels can often be obtained. Serological surveys will give information on asymptomatic infection or immunity levels and the taking of appropriate specimens or swabs from persons may detect asymptomatic carriers. Surveillance of predisposition to disease other than that determined by the absence of antibody is more difficult in the field of infectious disease, but surveillance of general functions such as growth, development, and nutritional status of children (Morley 1975; Irwig 1976; Carne 1984) may fall into this category, as will surveillance for infection in certain groups, such as tuberculosis in certain ethnic patients, HIV infection in haemophiliacs and homosexuals, and cytomegalovirus infections in the immunosuppressed or in those subjected to certain procedures, such as urinary catheterization. Unreported morbidity (Fig. 31.4) is not usually possible to place under passive surveillance. In a series of surveys conducted by the Office of Population Censuses and Surveys (**OPCS**) of England and Wales, the General Household Survey, information on unreported morbidity was obtained (Haskey and Birch 1985). Although each survey is finite, the collective information over many surveys constitutes a database suitable for surveillance.

A general practice surveillance system based on a sentinel reporting network was first successfully organized in the United Kingdom by the Royal College of General Practitioners in 1966 (Fleming and Crombie 1985) and since then in The Netherlands (Collette 1982) and Belgium (Thiers et al. 1979). General practice morbidity data are generally useful for providing information one tier in severity below that of hospital morbidity (Fig. 31.4). More specifically, in practice they produce information on clinical conditions with very low mortality not covered by notification, such as the common cold, chickenpox, or otitis media. In England and Wales, before mumps and rubella became notifiable in 1988, the Royal College of General Practitioners' (**RCGP**) clinical reporting system was an important source of information on these common infections; it remains an important source of information on clinical influenza, which is not notifiable. Sentinel reporting systems are generally inappropriate for rare diseases. When, as in the United Kingdom, the reporting GPs keep an age–sex register, a more accurate denominator is available than that used for notification, and indeed the RCGP data are published as rates. Most countries have a notification system which usually provides an essential source of information on the important communicable diseases; the characteristics of these systems are well known and will not be discussed in detail here. Notifications cover both general practice and hospital morbidity. It is often more useful to know what the notification rate is than to strive for completeness. Diseases that are perceived by the notifying doctors to be either a serious public health problem and communicable are often better notified than those that are not. Thus, tetanus is often poorly notified in countries such as England and Wales. It must be remembered that the primary objective of a notification system is not for surveillance but to provide an opportunity for local control, for which legal powers are usually available if necessary.

Surveillance systems using hospital admission data cover only a limited, though clearly important, phase in the natural history of an infection. Infections for which hospital data are ideal are those for which patients are usually admitted and admitted once only and in which the diagnosis can be confirmed. If the hospital reporting system is based on a sample, the disease should not be excessively less common. Meningococcal and other forms of bacterial meningitis are examples of infection which tend to be well documented in hospital data systems. Hospital data, on the other hand, may be available late, months or even years after the event.

Death certification is virtually a universal requirement in most countries. Death certificates are clearly important to any surveillance system, but for infectious diseases their value may be somewhat limited since infections are now rare as a primary cause of death. As infections remain an important cause of morbidity, death certifications need to be supplemented by one or more of the surveillance systems detailed above.

Other sources of data

Laboratory Laboratories provide important, perhaps essential, information for surveillance of infection Surveillance, supported by laboratory confirmation of clinical cases reported, showed that the malaria epidemics said to be occurring in the malarial southern states of the United States did not exist and the few cases confirmed microbiologically were imported or relapses (Langmuir 1963). In addition to this confirmatory role in surveillance that laboratories provide, they have an additional qualitative feature. Thus, laboratory data cannot only confirm the presence or absence of influenza, but the data can also show whether the virus is type A or type B, what the subtypes or variants are, and whether these have changed since the previous epidemic (Fig. 31.5). Similarly, atypical pneumonia may be caused by *Mycoplasma pneumoniae, Chlamydia*

psittaci or *Chlamydia pneumoniae, Coxiella burneti* (Q fever), several viruses, legionella, *Pneumocystis carinii*, and many other agents and usually only a laboratory can distinguish these successfully. In human infections, laboratories can provide data at all levels of the disease process shown in Fig. 31.4. Laboratory data often provide information on infection in vectors, animal, or other hosts or the environment, for example, salmonellosis.

Outbreaks Surveillance of laboratory-diagnosed infections can in itself lead to early recognition of outbreaks. Several examples of this have been reported, in particular with salmonellae (Gill *et al.* 1983; Rowe *et al.* 1987; Cowden *et al.* 1989) and with legionellas. Surveillance of outbreaks can also provide useful information and may be particularly worthwhile in countries where more sophisticated sources of data, such as laboratory data on individual infections, may not be available. Outbreak surveillance can be cheap and effective, although essentially an insensitive measure of disease trends.

Vaccine utilization Surveillance of vaccine utilization is an important component of the process of monitoring the effect of vaccine strategy on an infection. In England and Wales the COVER programme fulfils this function (Begg *et al.* 1989) and may have an additional effect in stimulating poorly performing districts to improve coverage. Serological surveillance can provide an indirect measure of the effectiveness of a vaccine strategy (Noah and Fowle 1988).

Sickness absence Sickness absence records may provide indications of major outbreaks in working populations. Influenza in particular produces measurable changes in sickness absence. Sickness absence can also be monitored in special groups, such as boarding schools and Post Office workers.

Disease determinants

Biological changes in agent, vector, and the reservoirs of infection can be placed under surveillance. Surveillance of changes in an agent, such as new subtypes or variants of influenza and antibiotic resistance in bacteria such as the gonococcus and *Staphylococcus* or protozoa, such as plasmodium, is regularly performed. Surveillance of biological vectors such as ticks and mosquitoes and of animal reservoirs of infections such as brucellosis and rabies, is an essential component of disease control in many countries.

Susceptibility to infection can be measured by skin testing or serological surveillance. In England and Wales, antibody profiles to current circulating influenza variants and to new variants are regularly performed in small samples of the population to assess the degree of susceptibility to a new variant. The degree of immunity to vaccinatable diseases is also regularly assessed (Morgan-Capner *et al.* 1988). The use of serum banks and immunological surveys in surveillance was persuasively argued by Raska (1971).

Other Other conditions that can be placed under surveillance include abortions, birth defects, injuries, behavioural risk factors, and occupational safety.

Objectives of surveillance

Many of the objectives of surveillance of infectious diseases have already been alluded to in the text and will be only summarized here. The main objectives of infectious disease surveillance are to monitor disease trends in time, place, and person, as illustrated below.

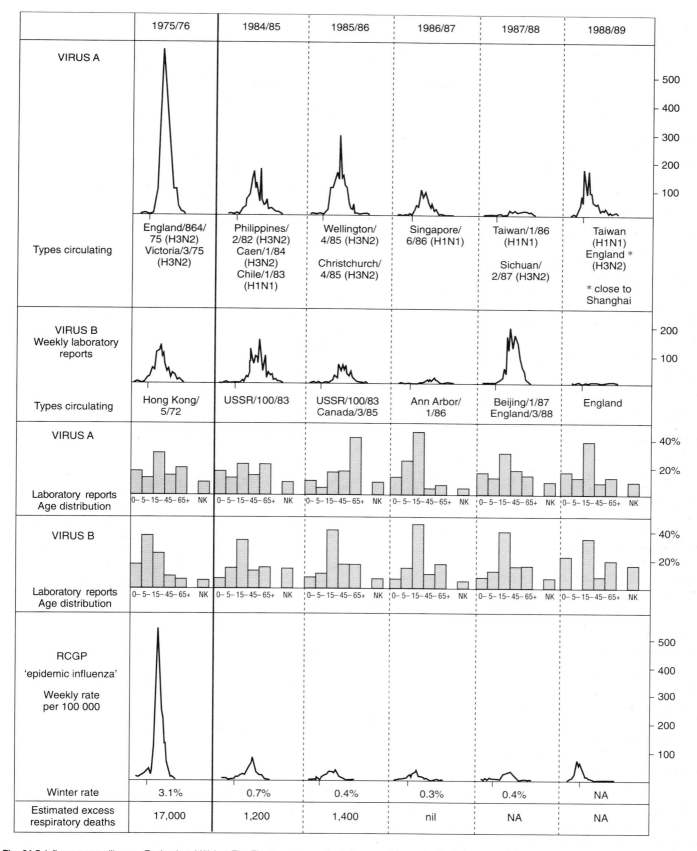

Fig. 31.5 Influenza surveillance—England and Wales. The Figure compares the indices used in monitoring influenza activity in England and Wales for the last major epidemic winter (1975/76) with the last five winters. (Reproduced from *Communicable Disease Report*, 1989, **44**, 3–4, with permission).

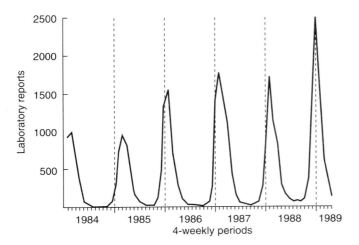

Fig. 31.6 Respiratory syncytial virus—England and Wales.

Anticipation of changes in incidence

Many infectious diseases follow regular patterns, both seasonal and secular. The respiratory syncytial virus follows a distinct seasonal pattern, causing epidemics every year with the peak incidence, in the Northern Hemisphere, almost invariably shortly after the New Year (Fig. 31.6). Minor variations in this pattern occur (Noah 1989). With some viruses, for example echovirus, a failure to return to the baseline by the end of its yearly cycle signifies that a resurgence will occur the following year (Figs. 31.7 and 31.8) (Epidemiology Research Laboratory 1975). Some organisms, for example *M. pneumoniae*, have long cycles extending over 4 years, but are particularly important as *M. pneumoniae* infection is treatable and early warning of an epidemic is of practical value (Fig. 31.9) (Monto 1974; Noah 1974). A review of cyclic variation in infections can be found in Noah (1989).

Early detection of outbreaks

Outbreaks of food poisoning which have been detected only because surveillance revealed an unexpected increase in a salmonella have already been noted and reports of some of these have been published (Gill *et al.* 1983; Rowe *et al.* 1987; Cowden *et al.* 1989). Occasionally, early detection of a new strain of an organism may lead to premature action which, with hindsight, turns out to have been inappropriate, as with the 1976 swine influenza episode

(Silverstein 1981). Surveillance may lead to the detection of new infections; for example, Lyme disease.

In an outbreak of hepatitis caused by a tattooist in England in 1978, surveillance by time alone would not have brought the outbreak to light; only the characteristic age and sex distribution (young adult males) would have shown a change (Limentani *et al.* 1979). Analysis of surveillance data by person, time, and place is more likely to reveal changes in pattern than analysis by one of these parameters alone.

Evaluation of effectiveness of preventive measures

Surveillance techniques are used to monitor the effects of a mass vaccination programme. Not only can changes in incidence be measured by time (Hinman *et al.* 1980), but also by person; for example, age changes in measles or mumps (Hinman *et al.* 1980; Cochi *et al.* 1988) have been recorded as a result of mass immunization. There have also been examples of monitoring changes in incidence by place (district) and correlating these changes with vaccination uptake rates (Pollard 1980). Effectiveness of a vaccination programme (Noah and Fowle 1988) can also be monitored by serological surveillance. The effect of withdrawing a source of infection, such as a contaminated food, from circulation can be monitored by surveillance, as with the *Salmonella napoli* outbreak caused by contaminated imported chocolate in England (Gill *et al.* 1983; Fig. 31.10).

Identification of vulnerable groups

Surveillance can expose vulnerable groups, for example by revealing ethnic or social differences in tuberculosis incidence. Appropriate action, such as BCG vaccination of neonates in such groups, can be taken. Serological surveillance can also identify susceptibility in particular groups of persons for selective vaccination.

Setting priorities for allocation of resources

From the examples above, it is clear that surveillance programmes can be used to provide information for setting priorities for resource allocation and, hence, for planning. This leads to more efficient use of health resources; although changes cannot always be anticipated in advance, their prompt detection can allow redistribution of resources at an early stage. Surveillance can also be useful in

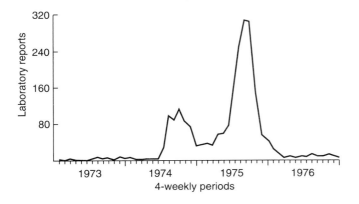

Fig. 31.7 Echovirus 19—England and Wales.

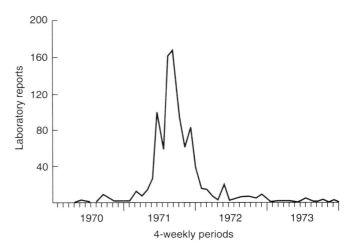

Fig. 31.8 Echovirus 4—England and Wales.

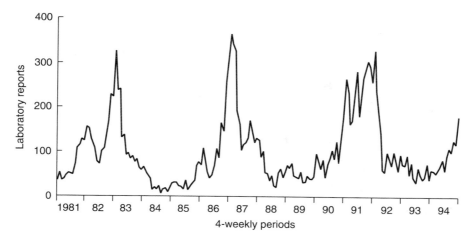

Fig. 31.9 Laboratory reports of *Mycoplasma pneumoniae* infections—England and Wales.

uncovering or monitoring changes in health practices, for example the increasing rate of caesarean sections in the United States between 1970 and 1988 (Thacker 1994).

Aetiological clues

Infectious disease patterns may help to generate hypotheses for the aetiology of chronic diseases. Secular variation compatible with certain infections has been noted with sudden infant death syndrome (Helweg-Larson *et al.* 1985), insulin-dependent diabetes (Gleason *et al.* 1982), deaths from asthma (Khot and Burn 1984), and anencephalus and spina bifida (Maclean and Macleod 1984).

Conclusion

'—probably most important, surveillance needs to be used more consistently and thoughtfully by policymakers' (Thacker 1994). It is up to public health physicians and epidemiologists to transform routine statistics into meaningful reliable and timely information so that health policy makers can be persuaded to act for change—for change is the ultimate goal of surveillance.

Setting up a surveillance system

In setting up a surveillance system, all the points discussed above need to be considered. It is important, in addition, to pilot the system first or to have a 'trial period' after which necessary adjustments can be made. In practice, as surveillance is essentially an ongoing process, adjustments may be made continually to 'fine tune' the system. Unnecessary extraneous or duplicate reporting should clearly be avoided and improvements always need to be made in the methods of flow of the information. Three attributes mentioned by Klaucke (1994) for an efficient surveillance system are simplicity, flexibility, and acceptability. Improving methods for the flow of information to and from the surveillance unit will enhance these three attributes. Electronic methods of reporting, obviating the use of paper, will not only simplify the system and reduce the effort involved, but will also increase its acceptability. Moreover, electronic systems make it easier for flexibility to be built in, so that conditions under surveillance can be added or deleted more easily. The surveillance system should be considered as a

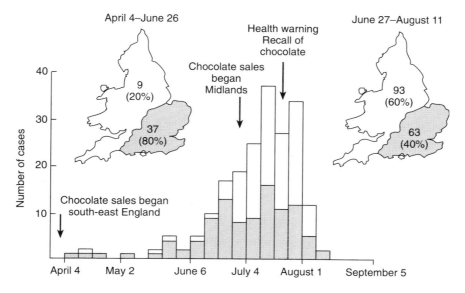

Fig. 31.10 *Salmonella napoli* outbreak 1982—England and Wales. Distribution of 202 primary household cases.

network of roads along which the types of consumer product sent can be changed according to need. In England and Wales, when rubella and mumps vaccines were introduced into the routine schedules, the two infections were placed under surveillance using the existing notification network and for legionnaires' and Lyme disease the laboratory network was used. Thus surveillance systems were put into operation rapidly, fairly painlessly, and at minimal extra cost.

Acceptability depends on simplicity and also on the perception by reporters of the importance of the data being collected. The quality of feedback, both in the initial stages of setting up the system and throughout the operation of the surveillance, affects acceptability.

The technology now available to facilitate surveillance is considerable. Electronic reporting in both directions—reporter to surveillance unit, surveillance unit to reporter and others—is now feasible. Details of the computer technology available are outside the scope of this chapter and in any case are rapidly changing.

The epidemiologist and the microbiology laboratory

Close collaboration between infectious disease epidemiologists and microbiologists is essential for effective outbreak investigation and control, for surveillance, and for vaccine use. Moreover, the microbiologist needs the epidemiologist and an understanding of epidemiology, as much as the epidemiologist needs the microbiologist and a knowledge of microbiology. Microbiology and epidemiology each have strengths and weaknesses that have to be acknowledged; a partnership between the two disciplines is essential in infectious disease epidemiology so that each can complement the other.

Outbreaks often cannot be effectively investigated without the use of epidemiology—in some food poisoning incidents for example, microbiological technology is still too limited to be able to identify the causal organism in the implicated food or in affected patients. In others, the implicated foods frequently are unavailable for microbiological testing. Similarly, some outbreak investigations will be unsuccessful without the use of microbiology. For surveillance of infectious disease, notifications based on clinical diagnosis alone, although useful if laboratory support is not available, are often lacking in precision and detail. In epidemiological studies and monitoring of vaccines, microbiological support is also essential. The use of the laboratory in epidemiological investigations of infectious disease will be explored in more detail below.

Understanding of microbiology by epidemiologists

Infectious disease epidemiologists require sound technical understanding of infection and micro-organisms to perform their work effectively. Knowledge of the ease or difficulty and expense of performing laboratory tests is most important. An understanding of what the tests mean and of their sensitivity and specificity is needed for informed interpretation of the results. The epidemiological significance of typing of organisms also has to be understood, as does the meaning of complex antibody tests, for example for hepatitis B virus. A working understanding of immunology is also necessary. Some clinical knowledge of infectious disease is essential for effective recognition and definition of cases and for their management. Epidemiologists are also responsible for reviewing the consistency and reasonableness of laboratory reports which are part of an investigation.

Epidemiology for microbiologists

Likewise microbiologists should have an understanding of the principles of epidemiology to be able to work in partnership with epidemiologists. This applies equally both to those microbiologists working in the community and in the hospital. Massive uncoordinated sampling of patients and/or food and the environment can usually be avoided in outbreak investigation. A knowledge of sensitivity and specificity, in particular applied to laboratory testing, is essential. For surveillance the importance of routine reporting following clearly defined rules must be recognized.

Aspects of the collaboration between epidemiologist and microbiologist are considered under the subjects of surveillance, outbreaks, and vaccines.

The laboratory in surveillance

Collaboration between microbiologist and epidemiologist undoubtedly leads to more sensitive and more refined surveillance, widening its scope considerably. Notifications of infectious disease, although essential, at best are usually fairly crude indicators of infection.

Confirmation of diagnosis

Clinical diagnoses, normally the basis for notifications, are not always accurate. Rubella is notoriously difficult to diagnose clinically; it is often confused with Fifth Disease an exanthem now known to be caused by parvovirus B19 and a laboratory surveillance system that includes both rubella virus and parvovirus B19 will distinguish between these. Clinical malaria in the south-eastern United States was shown by laboratory investigation not to be malaria when the Centers for Disease Control were first established in 1941; this early example underlined the importance of the laboratory in surveillance (Langmuir 1963). In a successful vaccine programme, as the disease reaches low levels, it is often necessary to confirm each notified case by using the laboratory. In the World Health Organization (**WHO**) programme for world eradication of poliomyelitis, the laboratory is essential for confirming the diagnosis even in this easily recognizable and characteristic disease. For eradication in a country to be ratified by the WHO (Wright *et al.* 1991), surveillance with laboratory back-up has to be continued for 3 years.

Reaching precision in diagnosis

Most notifiable diseases lack precision, which the laboratory can give. Influenza covers several types, subtypes, and variants (Table 31.1) which are generally indistinguishable clinically. Food poisoning covers not only several different types of infection, but often each of these infections can also be typed or subtyped further. Thus the causes of food poisoning include salmonellas, *Clostridium perfringens*, staphylococci, and *Escherichia coli*. All these organisms can be typed and the more common salmonellas further phage typed to afford even greater precision in diagnosis. Table 31.2 gives some examples of the precision and detail that laboratory surveillance can provide. Some of this detail is only useful for precision within outbreaks, for example phage typing of staphylococci and

Table 31.1 Examples of levels of diagnostic precision for surveillance

Disease for notification	Laboratory details		
Food poisoning	Salmonellas	*Salmonella typhimurium*	Phage typing
		Salmonella enteritidis	Phage typing
	Clostridium	*Clostridium perfringens*	Serotyping
	Staphylococci	*S. aureus*	Phage typing
			Enterotoxins in food
	Escherichia coli	O groups	
Influenza	Influenza A	Subtype (e.g. A/Hong Kong)	Variant, e.g. A/Johannesburg/ 33/94
	Influenza B		Variant, e.g. B/Beijing/184/93
Meningitis	*Bacterial*		
	Neisseria meningitids, Streptococcus pneumoniae Haemophilus influenzae, etc.	Group A, B, C, etc.	Serotyping/sulphonamide resistance
	Viral		
	Lymphocytic meningitis	Echo/coxsackie viruses	
Dysentery	*Shigella sonnei*	Types	
	Shigella flexneri, etc.	Types	
	Entamoeba histolytica		
Viral hepatitis	Types A, B, C, D, E, F	Limited typing for type B, but can differentiate between acute infection, 'high-risk' and 'low-risk' carriers, post-vaccination state	

C. perfringens; others are useful for surveillance —salmonellas, influenza, and meningococcal meningitis.

Increasing the scope of surveillance

There are many infections for which only laboratory surveillance is feasible—these include legionnaires' disease, psittacosis and Q fever, most adenoviral infections, and the enteroviruses (coxsackie A and B and echoviruses). Many are important public health problems, in particular in better developed countries in which the more traditional epidemic infections found in developing countries have become less common. Most of these infections are important enough to require surveillance to underpin outbreak investigation.

Table 31.2 Benefits of measles immunization over 10 years (United States)

Type of savings	Number
Cases averted	23 707 000
Lives saved	2 400
Cases of retardation averted	7 900
Additional years of normal and productive life by preventing premature death and retardation	709 000
School days saved	78 000 000
Physician visits saved	12 182 000
Hospital days saved	1 352 000
Net benefits	$1.3 billion

Source: Witte and Axnick (1975).

Psittacosis and Q fever are zoonoses and the enteroviruses cause outbreaks of lymphocytic meningitis, Bornholm disease, and other clinical conditions in the autumn season. The environmental sources of legionnaires' disease —water mainly—are well known.

International surveillance

Laboratory diagnosis is important for international surveillance. The spread of *Vibrio cholerae* el Tor across the world has been well documented (*Weekly Epidemiological Record* 1993). International surveillance of the subtypes and variants of influenza A virus is critical both for documenting spread and for early warning and for the formulation of vaccines.

Vectors and reservoirs of infection

The use of the laboratory in tracking the origin and spread of infection in animals and arthropods, as well as in water and soil, is important but will not be discussed here in detail. Influenza virus is of particular interest because of the interchanges and evolution of infection between a variety of animals and man. The possible origin of new influenza subtypes in the pig and duck agricultural environment of parts of China is still being studied (Webster *et al.* 1992) and the existence of a 'zoonotic pool' for viruses (Morse 1993) clearly needs close laboratory surveillance.

The laboratory in epidemiological investigation of vaccines

Technical microbiological expertise is clearly crucial to the development and preparation of vaccines and will not be considered further here. The use of the microbiological laboratory will be considered in the section on field investigation of vaccines in this chapter, so will only be considered in outline.

In phase 1 and 2 trials, efficacy is usually measured by measurement of antibody, which requires serological testing. In phase 2 trials in particular, phasing of vaccine doses will depend on antibody levels found. In field trials (phase 3) microbiology is usually required to confirm diagnosis of cases occurring in both case and control groups and this may be done by isolation and typing of the organism or by serology or both.

As a vaccine programme develops the overall incidence will fall, but cases will continue to occur for some time and microbiological confirmation of diagnosis becomes more important as the incidence diminishes to very low levels. In the present WHO initiative to eradicate poliomyelitis from the world, laboratory facilities worldwide needed strengthening to investigate every reported case of acute flaccid paralysis (**AFP**) (Wright *et al.* 1991) Only when every reported case of AFP proves not to be poliomyelitis over a period of 3 years can there be confidence that eradication has been achieved.

Assessment of vaccine success by serological testing of populations will be described in the section on the field investigations of vaccines.

The laboratory in outbreak investigation

In no other situation is the partnership between microbiologist and epidemiologist more important perhaps than in the investigation of an outbreak. Some outbreaks—such as foodborne outbreaks of small round structured virus (**SRSV**) infection or hepatitis A—can really only be solved by epidemiological techniques, as the causative organisms cannot be detected in food. In others, in particular those foodborne outbreaks in which the menu does not offer a choice, so that everyone usually eats everything on offer, the epidemiologist is considerably restricted and a microbiological solution is the only hope.

Inevitably, in many outbreaks no foods are available for testing, so that epidemiological analysis is essential. In other outbreaks too many foods are available for microbiological analysis: in a continuing outbreak of gastroenteritis on board ship, investigated by the Communicable Disease Surveillance Centre, London (O'Mahony *et al.* 1986) no particular meal was obviously at fault. More than 400 food items and ingredients were available for testing. Careful epidemiological analysis of the outbreak by time, place, and person showed that drinking water was the probable cause of the outbreak and subsequent investigation of the water tanks revealed a defect through which contamination of the water occurred from sewage outfall from the ship. In other food poisoning outbreaks, the epidemiological proof can be overwhelming, though the level of contamination in the offending food is so low that it is only confidence in the epidemiology that enables the laboratory to persist in ensuring 'microbiological proof'. In an outbreak of *S. ealing* infection caused by powdered infant milk, laboratories sampled more than 4000 unopened milk cartons before the organism was isolated (Rowe *et al.* 1987).

An outbreak of *Streptobacillus moniliformis* in a girls school in rural England illustrates well the need for microbiological and epidemiological expertise (McEvoy *et al.* 1987). Until the microbio-

logical diagnosis was made, the epidemiologists were attempting to analyse a large number of risk factors found in a rural and school environment. When the illness was diagnosed, a review of the literature revealed that one previous outbreak of the infection had been described in Haverhill, Massachusetts (hence the alternative name of Haverhill Fever for the illness), and had been attributed to raw milk. The girls in the school had indeed been exposed to raw milk. However, subsequent careful epidemiological analysis showed water to be even more significantly associated with illness. An examination of the water supply revealed that water from a pond in the school grounds, which was infested with rodents, was contaminating the school drinking water supply after it had been chlorinated.

Microbiology is useful for confirming foods and other sources of infection in outbreaks, such as water tanks (Campylobacter) and cooling towers (*Legionella pneumophila*), birds (psittacosis), and animals (rabies and plague). Increasing precision in microbiological diagnosis—typing of organisms such as phage typing and more recently molecular techniques, as well as typing of toxins—has been useful. In an outbreak of AIDS attributed to a dentist in Florida, molecular typing showed identical patterns in the virus obtained from patients and the primary case, thus confirming beyond reasonable doubt that he had indeed caused the infection in his patients (Hillis and Huelsenbeck 1994).

The epidemiologist can, on the other hand, aid the microbiologist in giving guidance on the number of patients to test in an outbreak and the foods or other items that need to be sampled. The pattern of the outbreak is also crucial to its management—in propagated or case-to-case outbreaks, for example a salmonella outbreak in a hospital, a planned epidemiological and microbiological approach to both investigation and management is the most efficient option. Point source outbreaks tend to create more publicity but are on the whole easier to control. The epidemiologist's role in differentiating between these two types of outbreaks is an essential one.

The work of the microbiologist in assessing levels of contamination in food is important to management and prevention. Levels of salmonella contamination in eggs have been shown to be extremely low and the organisms have been discovered in both the white and the yolk, either together or separately (Humphrey *et al.* 1989). This type of information ensures that correct advice on prevention can be given for handling and cooking eggs in the kitchen.

Field investigations of vaccines

Vaccines are a time-tested, highly efficient means of control for many infectious agents. In field investigations of transmissible disease, the epidemiological study of vaccines plays a major part. Epidemiological studies may be associated with vaccines in several different ways. First, the assessment of the need for a vaccine by undertaking surveillance or surveys will be necessary. Second, antibody and field trials to assess the efficacy and safety of the vaccine need to be conducted. Then follows the selection of an appropriate strategy and the implementation of the vaccine programme. Finally, the use of the vaccine and its effect on the population need to be closely monitored. These logical steps have not always been followed.

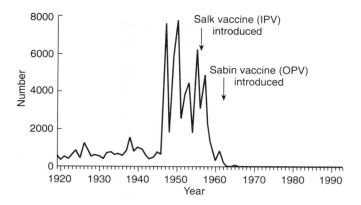

Fig. 31.11 Poliomyelitis notifications—England and Wales 1919—1993. (Prepared by CDSC.)

Assessment of the need for a vaccine
Morbidity and mortality of disease

The overall morbidity of the infection and its severity will usually be estimated from a surveillance programme. With measles the need for a preventive programme in the United Kingdom was first shown in 1963 (McCarthy and Taylor Robinson 1963). Miller (1964), by studying notifications of measles, was able to estimate the hospital admission rate (1 per cent), the respiratory and otitis media complication rate (6 to 9 per cent), and the neurological complication rate (0.7 per cent). Miller (1978) showed that these rates had changed little with time. Complication rates like these for an extremely common infection signified a serious health problem. Rey (1985) estimated that in France the total annual number of deaths from measles was 30, admissions to hospital was 6000, cases of encephalitis was 100 to 200, and subacute sclerosing pan-encephalitis (**SSPE**) was 10 to 20. Worldwide estimates tend to be cruder but none the less possible; using World Health statistics Cutting (1983) claimed that measles caused 1 to 1.5 million deaths in children in 1981. General practice surveillance systems may be useful in providing estimates of disease burdens, as for mumps in the United Kingdom (Research Unit of the Royal College of General Practitioners 1974). Serological studies are also used to assess the overall impact of an infection on a population and of the vulnerability of a target population. Studies on rubella in 1969 (Cockburn 1969) showed that by adulthood more than 80 per cent of a population had been infected, leaving 5 to 15 per cent of pregnant women susceptible and, hence, still vulnerable. In the United States the incidence of clinical rubella in pregnant women was found to vary from 4 to 8 per 10 000 in endemic periods to 20 per 10 000 in epidemic periods and subclinical infection could increase by up to 3-fold (Sever *et al.* 1969; White *et al.* 1969). Sometimes, as in polio, crude notification data on the most serious outcomes of poliovirus infection—paralysis and death—can be sufficient to point to a need for a vaccine (Fig. 31.11). For severe and very rare diseases only a selective vaccine policy can be considered, so these considerations do not apply.

Field studies

Field studies of vaccine efficacy (**VE**) and safety are clearly necessary before a vaccine is licensed for use. Postlicensing studies

are also important, but these require a different approach and will be considered separately.

Prelicensing vaccine trials

The earliest trial (phase 1) of a new vaccine usually involves a very small number (usually 20 to 50) of adult volunteers with a low level of risk of acquiring the disease. Efficacy is usually tested by measurement of antibody and adverse effects are closely monitored. Phase 1 tests the immunogenicity of the vaccine, following which the dose may be adjusted. Although only limited, preliminary information of safety is provided by a phase 1 trial; this is an important aspect of such a trial.

In the phase 2 trial a larger number of persons, between 100 and 200, constituting a target population are vaccinated. Their risk of acquiring the disease, again, should be low. Efficacy is again generally estimated by serological testing, and more precise information on dose–response and safety may be obtained, with some estimates of the rates of the more common side-effects. Information on contraindications may be available. The number of doses necessary may also become known after a phase 2 trial. If the phase 2 trial is satisfactory, a large field phase 3 trial of more than 500 high-risk subjects can begin. Vaccine protection is tested against disease acquisition. Questions that will need to be answered will include the efficacy of the vaccine, both in degree and duration, the rate of side-effects, both rare and common, the optimum age for giving vaccine, the dose, including how many and at what intervals, and the need for any adjuvants. Further contraindications to the vaccine may become apparent.

Vaccine efficacy can be assessed by measuring disease incidence, by serological test, or both. An important consideration in trials based on disease incidence is how much the two groups (case and control) vary in exposure to the infection and ascertainment of infection. If, as is generally believed, vaccinated groups tend to consist of those who are of higher social class and are thus groups which make better use of health services, diseases such as tuberculosis or whooping cough may be less common in them or less severe and, hence, less likely to be ascertained. While any such disease is more likely to be reported, these confounding factors may not cancel out each other. The allocation of persons to vaccine or control groups must be random and double blind to minimize the effect of such biases. This is generally known as random individual allocation. Group allocation—class, village, and factory—can also be used in vaccine trials; although the control group must also be matched carefully, it is not usually possible to allocate randomly or for the trial to be double blind. Detailed descriptions of how to conduct trials by individual or group allocation are given by Pollock (1966).

The disadvantages of a randomized controlled clinical trial are those of any longitudinal or cohort study: the necessity for large numbers of patients, the expense, the high drop-out rates that occur with long follow-up, and the fact that the vaccine is used under ideal but artificial conditions, the epidemiological equivalent of *in vitro*.

These limitations make postlicensing vaccine trials important (sometimes known as phase 4). Continued assessment or monitoring of vaccine use after licensing is mandatory (the equivalent of *in vivo*). The vaccine potency may change, either because of some change at the manufacturing level or along the chain which gets it to the user or in storage by the user, so that monitoring of vaccines at all levels of the chain is important, in particular as vaccines are often used in different climates and different population groups. Rare side-effects may become apparent. In postlicensing trials the populations immunized may be more or less responsive than in the prelicensing trials on account of differences in age, social class, or other factors. For these reasons, complacency is unwise after a successful large scale prelicensing trial.

Postlicensing monitoring

The success of any vaccine programme will depend on the overall population immunity level achieved. This is a function of efficacy × uptake of vaccine (Noah 1983). Vaccine efficacy is at its optimum when the vaccine leaves the manufacturer: factors that may influence efficacy after this include the age of the patient, the site of the injection, the immunological status of the patient, as well as the conditions under which the vaccine has been transported, stored, and made up. In addition, for unknown reasons (perhaps generic), some people may not be protected by the vaccine. Vaccine uptake is primarily influenced by the efficiency of the administrative processes in a country or province, but can also be affected by public perception of the vaccine itself (which may be rational or irrational) and of the disease. Factors influencing vaccine efficacy are also considered in more detail later in this chapter. Generally, a well-organized system for mass vaccination is much more efficient than sporadic vaccination campaigns. Thus postlicensing studies include not only continuous monitoring of vaccine efficacy, but also of uptake and implementation of the vaccine. Evaluation of outcome and of side-effects can also be studied.

Vaccine efficacy

Assessment by incidence The incidence of the disease in a population after vaccination is compared with that before vaccination. This is a simple, fairly universally undertaken, and useful method of assessing the impact of a mass vaccine programme on a population. Vaccine efficacy cannot usually be calculated from this method, only the effectiveness of the vaccine programme in broad terms. Moreover, demonstrations of a reduction in incidence following vaccination shows an association which may not be causal and the usual rules of Bradford Hill (1971) for assessing causality apply (see Chapter 15, Volume 2). Scarlet fever declined both in incidence and severity without a vaccine. Any change in incidence may have been caused by changing social circumstances, changes in the population, or a natural variation in the incidence of the disease. In England and Wales the use, first, of Salk poliovaccine in 1957, followed by Sabin vaccine in 1963, reduced the incidence of poliomyelitis to negligible numbers (Fig. 31.11), but the introduction of BCG vaccine in 1950 had a less than dramatic effect on an already declining disease (Fig. 31.12). This does not necessarily mean that the BCG vaccine was useless: a reduction in incidence could have been masked by more complete ascertainment or better diagnosis of cases and accompanying increase in transmission of or susceptibility to tuberculosis or a selective decrease in morbidity from a severe but rare form of tuberculosis, such as miliary tuberculosis or tuberculosis meningitis, too small to be detected by crude methods. Detailed surveillance would be necessary to detect such changes. In any event, with the threats of resurgence of tuberculosis, BCG vaccine may be all the more worthwhile now in the light of multiple drug-resistant tuberculosis.

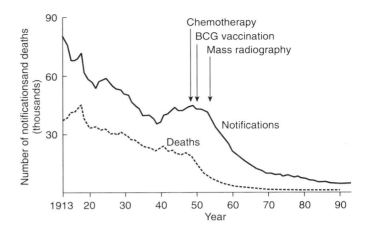

Fig. 31.12 Respiratory tuberculosis—England and Wales 1913–1990. (Prepared by CDSC.)

Assessment by immunological testing Immunological testing includes skin tests, such as tuberculin or Schick and serological testing. Tuberculin testing, generally using the Heaf or Mantoux tests, is performed to assess a person's immunity before vaccination. It has also been used to assess the quality of different strains of BCG. Schick tests for diphtheria are now rarely performed. The local reaction to smallpox vaccine was used to assess whether or not the vaccine had taken.

Serological testing can be performed using antitoxin (diphtheria and tetanus) or antibody (measles, rubella, etc.) levels. Serological tests first have to be shown to correlate with immunity to disease by disease incidence studies. Studies using such tests can be of two types, seroconversion or seroprevalence (Orenstein *et al.* 1985). *Seroconversion* Seroconversion studies are generally used in phases 1 and 2 and sometimes also in phase 3 of prelicensing trials. They are particularly useful for assessing vaccine response at different ages, as with measles vaccine and in different groups of persons; for example, healthy persons and those with immunosuppressive conditions respond differently to pneumococcal vaccine. Seroconversion studies are also useful for assessing vaccine efficacy for rare conditions in which antibody levels have already been shown to correlate with protection, as with tetanus, diphtheria, and polio. Moreover, seroconversion studies have the advantage that any change in antibody status can be attributed to the vaccine. Seroconversion studies require two blood samples and laboratory back-up, but these disadvantages can be weighed against the smaller number of subjects that need to be studied. A more serious disadvantage is the absence of a reliable serological test of immunity for some infections, such as whooping cough and meningococcal infections, although some tests are now available for these two infections.

Seroconversion studies and incidence studies can suffer from the same problems of having a case definition that is too specific (too high an antibody level), thus underestimating efficacy or one that is too sensitive (too low an antibody level), which will overestimate efficacy.

Seroprevalence Seroprevalence studies have the advantage of requiring only one blood test but the corresponding disadvantage is the difficulty of relating a 'positive' result to disease or vaccine.

Seroprevalence studies can be used to monitor the success of the vaccination programme, which is a function of both efficacy and uptake. Thus, the prevalence of poliovirus antibody in a highly immunized population with no wild virus disease will reflect the efficacy and uptake of the vaccine, whilst the prevalence of rubella antibody in pregnant women or women of childbearing age in a country with a selective rubella vaccine policy (so that the natural epidemics of rubella are virtually unaffected) will measure the overall immunity status of the target group, but will not easily distinguish how much of this is attributable to natural infection and how much to the success of the vaccine programme (Noah and Fowle 1988). If the expected seroprevalence of rubella antibody in this target group under conditions of natural rubella endemicity is known, then the gain in immunity attributable to vaccination of the target group can be calculated.

With seroprevalence studies the duration of protection can be evaluated also, but Marks et al. (1982) pointed out the importance of the timing of immunity measurements after vaccination and also the age of vaccination. In case–control studies using seroprevalence, these two parameters must be similar in cases and controls, that is the time lapse between vaccination and testing for immunity and the age of vaccination are crucial for matching.

In seroprevalence studies the same caveats apply about sensitivity and specificity of the antitoxin or antibody levels chosen to indicate immunity. In seroprevalence studies the choice of which class of antibody to measure can also be critical.

Seroprevalence studies related to previous vaccination require accurate records of previous vaccination (including timing and number of previous doses of vaccine) for meaningful interpretation (Orenstein et al. 1988). Absence of antibody may not always correlate with susceptibility.

Assessment by epidemiological studies

General comments For epidemiological studies of vaccine efficacy (VE) after licensing, a number of general comments need to be made. As with seroprevalence studies, the sensitivity and specificity of the case definition is important and has always to be a compromise. A highly sensitive case definition will include many spurious cases, leading to a falsely low VE, whereas too specific a case definition will lead to a falsely high VE. Case definition in both control and vaccinated groups should be undertaken with equal vigour, with due awareness of the tendency for case definition to be more specific in the vaccinated group. Exposure in the two groups should be similar: even if vaccinated and control groups have been closely matched by age, sex, social class, and geographical distribution, variations in exposure may still occur. The diagnosis should, if possible, be made 'blind' (Marks et al. 1982). In retrospective studies, ascertainment of vaccination history in the two groups must also be pursued with equal rigour and again should preferably be done 'blind'. Those with a previous history of the infection should not be included in either group of subjects.

Cohort studies

Outbreak investigations An outbreak often affords an opportunity to assess VE in a field setting (*in vivo*). The basic steps are to define the cohort under investigation, ascertain all cases according to an acceptable case definition, ascertain vaccination histories in the entire cohort, and calculate attack rates in vaccinated and unvaccinated persons, excluding those with a previous history of disease.

For very large cohorts sampling or cluster sampling (Henderson and Sundaresan 1982) can be used. In infections in which most cases occur in fairly well demarcated age groups, the cohort under study will usually exclude those outside these age groups, as well as those too young to have been vaccinated. The optimal age of vaccination can be ascertained from outbreak studies (Judelsohn et al. 1980).

Secondary attack rates in households Measuring the attack rates in members of a household (secondary cases) following the introduction of an infection by one member of the family (primary case) affords an attractive approach to VE studies because exposures in vaccinated and unvaccinated persons are similar, thus eliminating an important bias in these studies and also because the denominators (those exposed) can be fairly accurately determined. This type of study, however, needs more careful planning than most other postlicensing studies and it is usually better designed as a prospective study. They also need to be planned to take place during periods of high epidemicity of the infection. Studies on pertussis vaccine in England and Wales which used secondary attack rates in households suggested that the vaccines were ineffective (PHLS Whooping Cough Committee and Working Party 1973; PHLS Epidemiological Research Laboratory 1982). This was difficult to believe, because the incidence of whooping cough in the country at the time of the first study had been decreasing steadily and other studies (Noah 1976; Pollard 1980; PHLS Epidemiological Research Laboratory 1982) suggested that the vaccine was effective. The reasons for the failure of the household exposure studies to confirm efficacy were examined by Fine et al. (1988); they attributed the apparent lack of vaccine efficacy primarily to the inclusion of retrospectively ascertained cases and of households in which the primary cases constituted a vaccine failure.

Cluster sampling (Henderson and Sundaresan 1982) is a modified form of this method of estimating VE. It has the advantage of being cheaper and easier to conduct than a household study and is hence particularly suitable for developing countries, but it is also less rigorous (Orenstein et al. 1985).

Retrospective population cohort studies This type of study depends on the availability of fairly sophisticated disease reporting and vaccination recording systems. For each case of disease ascertained, the vaccination history is verified and from the number and percentage of those vaccinated in the base population, the attack rates in those vaccinated and unvaccinated can be calculated and the VE derived (Noah 1976; PHLS Epidemiological Research Laboratory and 21 Area Health Authorities 1982).

The effectiveness of vaccination, but not its efficacy, can sometimes be checked crudely by observing the correlation between the incidence of disease in separate districts with the vaccination rates in those districts (Sutherland and Fayers 1971; Pollard 1980; Noah and Fowle 1988). Sometimes chance plays a part in affording an opportunity to estimate the VE, as in 1970 to 1971 in Texarkana, a city straddling the Texas–Arkansas state line. The Texas side differed from the Arkansas side only in not having a measles vaccine policy, so that during the outbreak of measles, the attack rate in the Texas side of the city was 48.2 per cent compared with 4.2 per cent in the Arkansas side. The VE, based on attack rates of 105.9 per 1000 and 4.3 per 1000 in the unimmunized and in the immunized, respectively, was 95.9 per cent (Landrigan 1972).

Case–control studies   Case–control studies in vaccination issues are not common. The design of a case–control vaccine study is similar to that of any other case–control study. Each case of the disease is compared with one or more matched controls without the disease for a history of vaccination against the disease. As in all case–control studies, 'first cases must be representative of all cases in a specified population with respect to the exposure of interest, and controls must be similarly representative of all non-cases in the same specified population. Second information about exposures and other characteristics must be similar in quality for both cases and controls' (Comstock 1994). These specifications are extremely difficult to achieve in vaccine case–control studies. The advantages of a case–control study, on the other hand, are that it can be done more cheaply, quickly, and with fewer cases than for a cohort study. Moreover, the efficacy of vaccine given many years before can be assessed (Smith 1988). The method has been used recently in a study in the Gambia to assess the efficacy of three or more doses of trivalent oral poliovaccine (Deming *et al.* 1992). Nevertheless, bias can occur as the vaccines will not have been administered at random (as, for example, if those of higher socio-economic class have higher vaccination rates but lower expectancy of disease) and the vaccine histories in cases and controls may not be accurate (Smith 1988). The problems that need to be given attention in the design of case–control studies are similar to those in cohort vaccine studies. This subject has been dealt with recently in some detail by Comstock (1994).

The case–control method, nevertheless, lends itself well to BCG efficacy studies (Miceli *et al.* 1988; Smith 1988). First, when the overall incidence of the disease is low, the case–control approach can be used on existing cases of disease to evaluate a vaccine given many years earlier, making it cheaper and quicker. Second, because of the expense of large cohort studies and the time needed to assess the efficacy of BCG, the case–control approach is a more practical one. Third, the difficulty of a 'double-blind' approach to a vaccine such as BCG, and fourth, the large variation (from 100 to − 57 per cent) in estimates of efficacy of BCG with randomized controlled trials, further show the disadvantages of the cohort approach in trials of BCG.

Calculation of vaccine efficacy   Vaccine efficacy is the ratio of the observed diminution in attack rates (**AR**), that is the difference in ARs between vaccinated and unvaccinated groups, to the expected attack rate, that is, that in the unvaccinated group. Thus

$$\text{VE\%} = \frac{\text{AR unvaccinated} - \text{AR vaccinated}}{\text{AR unvaccinated}} \times 100 = (1 - \text{RR}) \times 100$$

where RR is the ratio of AR vaccinated to AR unvaccinated or relative risk.

In a case–control study, using unmatched controls and odds ratios (**ORs**), results can be arranged in a 2×2 table as follows:

	Case	Controls
Vaccinated	*a*	*b*
Unvaccinated	*c*	*d*

VE is $(1 - \text{OR}) \times 100$, where OR is *ad/bc*.

Refinements of these basic formulas can be found in Orenstein *et al.* (1985) and the impact of various types of bias on VE results in Orenstein *et al.* (1988).

Monitoring of side-effects of vaccines

Common side-effects   Monitoring side-effects of vaccines begins at the very first phase of vaccine trials, running in parallel with estimations of efficacy. With randomized control trials, evaluation of side-effects after vaccination is fairly straightforward, it being usually sufficient to compare the incidence of any reactions in vaccinees with that in controls. Where it is not practical, possible, or ethical to conduct a placebo-controlled study, some care is necessary in the interpretation of information on side-effects. In uncontrolled cohort studies, local side-effects (such as a stiff or painful arm) can still be evaluated successfully, but other symptoms, such as fever or convulsions which are non-specific to vaccines and may commonly occur from other causes in healthy children, are more difficult to evaluate without a control group. The time between the vaccination and the appearance of a side-effect also needs to be evaluated carefully. In the earliest trials of MMR vaccine, meningitis caused by the mumps component was not documented until the subjects were followed up for at least 28 days.

In the early measles vaccine trials in England (Measles Vaccine Committee of the Medical Research Council 1966) 9577 children aged 10 months to 2 years were immunized. Eighteen children developed convulsions, 11 of them between postvaccination days 6 and 9. Only five convulsions were reported in the control group of 16 327 children and none of them were between days 6 and 9. This study established not only that convulsions were a real side-effect of measles vaccine, but also that they characteristically occurred during a fixed interval after the vaccine. The need to compare this with the incidence of convulsions after natural disease became apparent and they were shown to be at least 10 times commoner after the disease than after the vaccine (Miller 1978). This was an extremely important finding in support of the vaccine and illustrates the value of careful epidemiological work in the study of vaccines.

Unlike drug trials, the side-effects of a vaccine can sometimes be evaluated by giving a combination of vaccines omitting the vaccine under trial instead of using a placebo in the control group. The side-effects of pertussis vaccine have been investigated by comparing symptoms in the case group after diphtheria–tetanus–pertussis vaccine (**DTP**) with those after diphtheria-tetanus (**DT**) vaccine in the controls (Pollock *et al.* 1984). Even in this controlled study it was found that adverse publicity to pertussis vaccine led to a reporting bias in the cases given DTP.

Rare side-effects   Various ingenious studies have been set up to investigate the incidence of rare side-effects after vaccination. In Denmark, Melchior (1977) compared the age-specific incidence of infantile spasms during the period when whooping cough vaccine was given at 5 months, 6 months, and 15 months with that during the period when it was given at 5 weeks, 9 weeks, and 10 months and found no difference. In England the alleged extremely rare side-effects of serious and permanent (but non-specific) brain damage after whooping cough vaccine (with quoted rates of 150 000 to 1 million) were difficult to refute and the publicity engendered by this led to a dramatic fall in the pertussis vaccine uptake rate from approximately 79 per cent in the early 1970s to 31 per cent in 1975. A carefully controlled case–control study, the National Childhood Encephalopathy Study, was conducted. In this study, the presence or absence of a history of recent vaccination was obtained in all cases of 'encephalopathy' reported to the study team and compared with controls. An association was shown between DTP given 3 to 7 days earlier and encephalopathy, but not between DT given at the same time and encephalopathy. It was possible to estimate from this study that the risk of persistent neurological damage in previously healthy children after pertussis vaccine was 1 : 1 310 000 immunizations; however the 95 per cent confidence limits were very wide, from 1 : 154 000 to 1 : 15 310 000. The reader is referred to the original study (Department of Health and Social Security 1981) for further details of the methodology, and to balanced reviews for details of the whooping cough vaccine controversy (Miller et al. 1982; Cherry 1992).

Other forms of side-effect evaluation include postmarketing surveillance which may be active or passive (Stetler et al. 1987). An active surveillance system is less prone to bias but is likely to be too expensive and unwieldy; the passive system is more prone to bias, but clearly simpler and cheaper.

Uptake and implementation of vaccines

> One has to be a stranger in Jerusalem not to realize that public acceptance of an immunization procedure determines its success or failure (Cohen 1978).

The need for field studies in vaccines does not cease at efficacy studies. The implementation of the vaccine is as important as its production and an effective safe vaccine with a poor uptake is of hardly greater benefit than no vaccine at all. In recent years this has been recognized and field studies to investigate the factors that influence uptake of vaccines are now common.

Studies on uptake may measure factors associated with social or service conditions. In one study (Jarman et al. 1988), social conditions associated with being underprivileged (such as over-crowding, unmarried, or single parents), living in high population density areas, being unskilled, and belonging to certain ethnic groups were found to be linked to low immunization uptake. Reasons given by family (Clarke 1980; Blair et al. 1985; Lakhani et al. 1987) or by clinic staff (Adjaye 1981; Lakhani et al. 1987) for refusal can also be investigated. Single-handed GPs, those aged over 65 years, or those with large list sizes and less than average expenditure on community health services were also associated with low uptake rates (Jarman et al. 1988). The efficiency of organization, quality of premises, and adequacy of staffing of three different types of immunization clinic—general practice, health centre, and child health clinic—were found to affect compliance (Alberman et al. 1986).

In another study the provision of individual performance indicators was enough to stimulate GPs to improve rates (Newlands and Davies 1988). An interesting phenomenon with an annual influenza vaccination programme in industry was noted by Smith et al. (1976): in successive years the uptake of vaccine fell considerably. The reasons for this were fairly complex and were probably associated with the need for giving vaccine yearly, the low incidence of influenza during the periods over which the vaccine was given, and the general perception by the target population that the vaccine was not very effective. The message that emanates from many of these studies, however, is that it is the administrative efficiency of the immunization programme and the motivation of the pro-fessionals that are the critical features in improving uptake (Noah 1982; Lakhani et al. 1987). Communication strategies can be designed to persuade people to attend immunization campaigns (Hingson 1974).

Evaluation of factors affecting vaccine programmes

The evaluation of the outcome of a vaccine programme can be conducted in several ways. Except with the most successful programmes reasons for non-acceptance of vaccine can be investigated. Reasons for failure/poor uptake may be because of social and professional attitudes to the vaccine, including the effect of the media or the administrative competence/managerial abilities of those responsible for the programme.

Social and professional attitudes to a vaccine or a vaccine programme may 'make or break' the programme. In the United Kingdom, reports by Kulenkampff et al. (1974) of alleged brain damage following whooping cough vaccine, fuelled by a television programme in the same year and by 'the writings in the lay press and medical journals and media interviews' of a professor who was a 'leading critic of the vaccination policy' (Cherry 1986) led to a catastrophic fall in pertussis vaccine uptake rates from approximately 79 per cent between 1967 and 1974 to a low of 30 per cent in 1978. Television programmes were found to be particularly influential (McKinnon 1979). The controversy had an effect on other routine vaccinations (DT and polio) which fortunately was transient and relatively slight. A survey of professional attitudes during the episode (Wilkinson et al. 1979) suggested that GPs, clinic doctors, or health visitors were ambivalent towards the pertussis vaccine. Most had noticed an increase in parental concern about the vaccine which was attributed to 'irresponsible', 'ill-controlled', or 'biased' publicity. This phenomenon occurred in the United Kingdom without the often cited problem of litigation risk in the United States.

Adjaye (1981), however, found that parental attitudes towards immunization were greatly influenced by medical and non-medical members of the health professions, while Berkeley (1983) in a study of attitudes to measles vaccine found that the professionals themselves were unsure about the contraindications to vaccine and to its value. In another study (Guest et al. 1986) many professionals offered invalid reasons for failure to give immunization.

Campbell (1983), in analysing reasons for poor uptake of measles vaccine in Britain, suggested that attitudes and ignorance, a cumbersome policy-making bureaucracy, the absence of legislation (which helped the United States programme) and of a standard record card for each child, and the initiative and motivation required by mothers towards a vaccine given some months after the primary course, were factors that accounted for the unpopularity of measles vaccine in Britain. Encouraging the health professionals to take a greater initiative was found to benefit uptake (Carter and Jones 1985). These and other studies (Bussey and Harris 1979; Pugh and Hawker 1986; Lakhani et al. 1987) suggested that the education of health professionals and an efficient administration with computerized recall and records were important factors in improving uptake rates. In the United States, school immunization laws were also a proven method of improving immunization uptake (Robbins et al. 1981).

Evaluation of outcome of immunization programmes

The case for long-term serological surveillance of immunization programmes has been forcefully advocated by Evans (1980) and Raska (1971). Evans argued that a surveillance system based on reporting of disease alone was insufficiently sensitive or specific to monitor a vaccine programme. An individual's history of immunization or disease correlated well with antibody presence in measles and mumps, but less well in rubella and poliomyelitis; moreover, for tetanus natural infection has virtually no bearing on antibody levels.

The reliability of a negative history of disease or immunization was, however, poor for measles, mumps, and rubella. The serological demonstration of satisfactory levels of durable antibody in immunized persons was a more reliable measure of vaccine effectiveness than monitoring the incidence of the disease itself and absence of antibody in particular communities or specific age groups could identify those who may need protection. Long-term surveillance of immunity after measles vaccination has also been advocated (*The Lancet* 1976). Serological studies have shown that vaccine failure and not waning vaccine-induced antibody accounted for most of the low or undetectable antibody titres in immunized children, in particular those immunized before 13 months of age (Yeager *et al.* 1977).

A study of measles vaccine on the survival pattern of 7- to 35-month-old children in Kasongo, Zaire (Kasongo Project Team 1981) used life-table analysis to evaluate outcome of the vaccination programme in a community with a high measles incidence and measles case–fatality rate. They found that, although the measles vaccine programme undoubtedly reduced the risk of measles death, the overall survival was less influenced by measles vaccine after 22 months of age.

Another study found that the success of a vaccine programme against measles, mumps, and rubella using MMR vaccine was reflected in the virtual disappearance of a common complication of all three infections (encephalitis) in their population of children (Koskiniemi and Vaheri 1989). Improved intellectual performance was an outcome noted in a cohort study in children who had been immunized against pertussis compared with those who had been hospitalized for the disease, even after allowing for social differences in the two groups (Butler *et al.* 1982).

Costing studies of vaccines

Costing studies are important both in assessing the need for a vaccine and in evaluating its efficiency. The detailed methodology of costing studies for infectious disease is considered elsewhere in this book. Costs include the costs of the vaccine and its administration. Costs of the vaccine may be influenced by factors as diverse as costs of development and market competition: the price of human-derived hepatitis B vaccine halved when the yeast-derived vaccine began to be marketed. Administration costs will include the cost of the syringes, personnel, and accommodation as well as costs of initiating and administering a record and follow-up programme. Benefits include savings on treatment costs, mortality, morbidity, the avoidance of intangibles such as pain and grief, and external benefits (Creese and Henderson 1980). It is debatable whether social benefits of successful intervention should be costed, because

the value of such benefits may not be convincing to pragmatic health care managers.

Patrick and Woolley (1981) pointed out that health managers may fail to be impressed by cost–benefit studies because the costs, which are health costs, have to be weighed against benefits which are usually social. Nevertheless, the benefits of providing supportive cost calculations are an important addition to the valuation of a vaccination programme.

A list of the benefits of immunization, simply and clearly stated, often cannot fail to convince as in one of the earliest such papers (Witte and Axnick 1975) describing the results of 10 years of measles immunization in the US in terms of lower morbidity and mortality and improved quality of life (Table 31.2).

Other studies (Creese and Henderson 1980; Koplan 1985) have amply shown the value for money of measles vaccine in terms of benefit–cost ratios for measles vaccine of 10 to 15 : 1. Cost studies can be successfully done in general practice (Binnie 1984). In this general practice, over a 20-year period, immunization not only brought about a small financial reward, but also reduced the number of consultations by 40 per cent, even though a home visit was often necessary to immunize a child. Examples of cost–benefit analysis of various immunizations which have demonstrated the benefit of vaccines and to which the reader is referred for details of methodology, include measles vaccine (Witte and Axnick 1975; Albritton 1978), pertussis vaccine (Koplan *et al.* 1979; Hinman and Koplan 1984, 1985), mumps vaccine (Koplan and Preblud 1982; White *et al.* 1985), polio (Fudenberg 1973), pneumococcal vaccine (Patrick and Woolley 1981), and hepatitis B in homosexuals (Adler *et al.* 1983). General articles on the cost–benefits of immunization programmes include Creese and Henderson (1980) and Koplan (1985). A formula has been developed for calculating vaccine profitability, defined as the economic yield, positive or negative, obtained per monetary unit invested in a campaign (Carvasco and Lardinois 1987).

References

Adjaye, N. (1981). Measles immunization. Some factors affecting non-acceptance of vaccine. *Public Health, London*, **95**, 185–8.

Adler, M.W., Belsey, E.M., McCutchan, J.A., and Mindel, A. (1983). Should homosexuals be vaccinated against hepatitis B? Cost and benefit assessment. *British Medical Journal*, **286**, 1621–4.

Alberman, E., Watson, E., Mitchell, P., and Day, S. (1986). The development of performance and cost indicators for preschool immunization. *Archives of Diseases in Childhood*, **61**, 251–6.

Albritton, R.B. (1978). Cost–benefits of measles eradication: effects of a federal intervention. *Policy Analysis*, **4**, 1.

Begg, N.T., Gill, O.N., and White, J. (1989). COVER (cover of vaccination evaluation rapidly): description of the England and Wales Scheme. *Public Health*, **103**, 81–9.

Berkeley, M.I.K. (1983). *Measles—the effect of attitudes on immunization.* Health Bulletin. Scottish Home and Health Department, Edinburgh, **41**, 141–7.

Binnie, G.A.C. (1984). Measles immunization profit and loss in a general practice. *British Medical Journal*, **289**, 1275–6.

Blair, S., Shave, N., and McKay, J. (1985). Measles matters, but do parents know? *British Medical Journal*, **290**, 623–4.

Bradford Hill, A. (1971). *Principles of medical statistics* (9th edn.). The Lancet Ltd, London.

Bussey, A.L. and Harris, A.S. (1979). Computers and effectiveness of the measles vaccination campaign in England and Wales. *Community Medicine*, **1**, 29–35.

Butler, N.R., Golding, J., Haslum, M., and Stewart-Brown S. (1982). Recent findings from the 1970 child health and education study: preliminary communication. *Journal of the Royal Society of Medicine*, **75**, 781–4.

Campbell, A.G.M. (1983). Measles immunization: why have we failed? *Archives of Diseases in Childhood*, **58**, 3–5.

Carne, S. (1984). Place of development surveillance in general practice. *Journal of the Royal Society of Medicine*, **77**, 819–20.

Carter, H. and Jones, I.G. (1985). Measles immunization: results of a local programme to increase vaccine uptake. *British Medical Journal*, **290**, 1717–19.

Carvasco, J.L. and Lardinois, R. (1987). Formula for calculating vaccine profitability. *Vaccine*, **5**, 123–7.

Cherry, J.D. (1986). The controversy about pertussis vaccine. *Current Clinical Topics in Infectious Diseases*, **7**, 216.

Cherry J.D. (1992). Pertussis: the trails and tribulations of old and new pertussis vaccines. *Vaccine*, **10**, 1033–8.

Clarke, S.J. (1980). Whooping cough vaccination: some reasons for non-completion. *Journal of Advanced Nursing*, **5**, 313–9.

Cochi, S.L., Preblud, S.R., and Orenstein, W.A. (1988). Perspectives on the relative resurgence of mumps in the United States. *American Journal of Diseases in Childhood*, **142**, 499–507.

Cockburn, W.C. (1969). World aspects of the epidemiology of rubella. *American Journal of Diseases in Childhood*, **118**, 112–22.

Cohen, H. (1978). Vaccination against pertussis, yes or no? In *International symposium on pertussis* (ed. C.R. Manclark and J.C. Hill), p. 249. National Institute of Health, Bethesda, MD.

Collete, B.J.A. (1982). The sentinel practices system in The Netherlands. In *Environmental epidemiology* (ed. P.E. Leaverton), p. 149. Praeger Publishers, New York.

Comstock, G.W. (1994). Evaluating vaccination effectiveness and vaccine efficacy by means of case–control studies. In *Epidemiologic reviews*; (ed. H.K Armenian). John Hopkins University School of Hygiene and Public Health, Baltimore, MD.

Cowden, J.M., O'Mahony, M., Bartlett, C.L.R. *et al.* (1989). A national outbreak of *Salmonella typhimurium* DT 124 caused by contaminated salami sticks. *Epidemiology and Infection*, **103**, 219–25.

Creese, A.L. and Henderson, R.H. (1980). Cost–benefit analysis and immunization programmes in developing countries. *Bulletin of the World Health Organization*, **58**, 491–7.

Cutting, W.A.M. (1983). Measles immunization. A review. *Journal of Tropical Pediatrics*, **29**, 246–7.

Deming, M., Jaiteh, K.O., Otten, M.W. *et al.* (1992). Epidemic poliomyelitis in The Gambia following the control of poliomyelitis as an endemic disease. II Clinical efficacy of trivalent oval polio vaccine. *American Journal of Epidemiology*, **135**, 393–408.

Department of Health and Social Security (1981). *Whooping cough*. Reports from Committee on Safety of Medicines and the Joint Committee on Vaccination and Immunization. HMSO, London.

Epidemiology Research Laboratory (1975). Echovirus 19 this summer? *British Medical Journal*, **2**, 346.

Evans, A.S. (1980). The need for serologic evaluation of immunization programs. *American Journal of Epidemiology*, **112**, 725–31.

Eylenbosch, W.J. and Noah, N.D. (ed.) (1988). *Surveillance in health and disease*. Oxford University Press.

Fine, P.E.M., Clarkson, J.A., and Miller, E. (1988). The efficacy of pertussis vaccines under conditions of household exposure. *International Journal of Epidemiology*, **17**, 635–42.

Fleming, D.M. and Crombie, D.L. (1985). The incidence of common infectious diseases: the weekly returns service of the Royal College of General Practitioners. *Health Trends*, **17**, 13–16.

Fudenberg, H.H. (1973). Fiscal returns of biomedical research. *Journal of Investigative Dermatology*, **61**, 321–9.

Gill, O.N., Bartlett, C.L.R., Sockett, P.N. *et al.* (1983). Outbreak of *Salmonella napoli* infection caused by contaminated chocolate bars. *The Lancet*, **i**, 574–7.

Gleason, R.E., Khan, C.B., Funk, I.B., and Craighead, J.E. (1982). Seasonal incidence of insulin dependent diabetes (IDDM) in Massachusetts 1964–1973. *International Journal of Epidemiology*, **11**, 39–45.

Guest, M., Horn, J., and Archer, L.N.J. (1986). Why some parents refuse pertussis immunization. *Practitioner*, **230**, 210.

Hall, S.M. and Glickman, M. (1988). The British paediatric surveillance unit. *Archives of Disease in Childhood*, **63**, 344–6.

Haskey, J.C. and Birch, D. (1985). Statistics from general practice: morbidity and its measurement using practice statistical reports. *Health Trends*, **17**, 32–39.

Helweg-Larsen, K., Bay, H., and Mac, F. (1985). A statistical analysis of the seasonality in sudden infant death syndrome. *International Journal of Epidemiology*, **14**, 566–74.

Henderson, D.A. (1976). Surveillance of smallpox. *International Journal of Epidemiology*, **5**, 19–28.

Henderson, R.H. and Sundaresan, T. (1982). Cluster sampling to assess immunization coverage: a review of experience with a simplified sampling method. *Bulletin of the World Health Organization*, **60**, 253–60.

Hillis, D.M. and Huelsenbeck, J.P. (1994). Support for dental HIV transmission. *Nature*, **369**, 24–5.

Hingson, R. (1974). Obtaining optimal attendance at mass immunization programs. *Health Services Reports*, **89**, 53–64.

Hinman, A.R. and Koplan, J.P. (1984). Pertussis and pertussis vaccine. Reanalysis of benefits, risk and costs. *Journal of the American Medical Association*, **251**, 3109–13.

Hinman, A.R. and Koplan, J.P. (1985). Pertussis and pertussis vaccine: further analysis of benefits, risks and costs. *Development in Biological Standardization*, **61**, 429–37.

Hinman, A.R., Brandling-Bennett, A.D., Bernier, R. *et al.* (1980). Current features of measles in the United States: feasibility of measles elimination. *Epidemiologic Reviews*, **2**, 153–70.

Humphrey, T.J., Baskerville, A., Mawer, S., Rowe, B., and Hopper, S. (1989). *Salmonella enteritidis* phage type 4 from the contents of intact eggs: a study involving naturally infected hens. *Epidemiological Infection*, **103**, 415–23.

Irwig, L.M. (1976). Surveillance in developed countries with particular reference to child growth. *International Journal of Epidemiology*, **5**, 57–61.

Jarman, B., Bosanquet, N., Rice, P., Dollimore, N., and Leese, B. (1988). Uptake of immunization in district health authorities in England. *British Medical Journal*, **296**, 1775–78.

Judelsohn, R.G., Pleissner, M.L., and O'Mara, D.J. (1980). School-based measles outbreaks: correlation of age at immunization with risk of disease. *American Journal of Public Health*, **70**, 1162–5.

Kasongo Project Team (1981). Influence of measles vaccination on survival pattern of 7–35 month-old children in Kasongo, Zaire. *The Lancet*, **i**, 764–7.

Khot, A. and Burn, R. (1984). Seasonal variation and time trends of deaths from asthma in England and Wales (1960–1982). *British Medical Journal*, **289**, 233–4.

Klaucke, D.N. (1994). Evaluating public health surveillance. In *Principles and practice of public health surveillance* (ed. S. M. Teutsch and R. E. Churchill). Oxford University Press.

Koplan, J.P. (1985). Benefits, risks and costs of immunization programmes. In *The value of preventive medicine* (ed. Ciba Foundation Symposium), pp. 55–680. Pitman, London.

Koplan, J.P. and Preblud, S.R. (1982). A benefit-cost analysis of mumps vaccine. *American Journal of Diseases in Childhood*, **136**, 362–4.

Koplan, J.P., Schoenbaum, S.C., Weinstein, M.C., and Fraser, D.W. (1979). Pertussis vaccine—an analysis of benefits, risks and costs. *New England Journal of Medicine*, **301**, 906–11.

Koskiniemi, M. and Vaheri, A. (1989). Effect of measles, mumps, rubella vaccination on pattern of encephalitis in children. *The Lancet*, **i**, 31–4.

Kulenkampff, M., Schwartzman, J.S., and Wilson, J. (1974). Neurological complications of pertussis inoculation. *Archives of Diseases in Childhood*, **49**, 46–9.

Lakhani, A.D.H., Morris, R.W., Morgan, M., Dale, C., and Vaile, M.S. (1987). Measles immunization: feasibility of a 90 per cent target uptake. *Archives of Diseases in Childhood*, **62**, 1209–14.

Landrigan, P.J. (1972). Epidemic measles in a divided city. *Journal of the American Medical Association*, **221**, 567–70.

Langmuir, A.D. (1963). The surveillance of communicable diseases of national importance. *New England Journal of Medicine*, **268**, 182–92.

Langmuir, A.D. (1976). William Farr: founder of modern concepts of surveillance. *International Journal of Epidemiology*. **5**, 13–18.

Last, J.M. (ed.) (1995). *A dictionary of epidemiology* (3rd edn). Oxford University Press.

Limentani, A.E., Elliott, L.M., Noah, N.D., and Lamborn, J. (1979). Outbreak of hepatitis B from tattooing. *The Lancet*, ii, 86–8.

McCarthy, K. and Taylor Robinson, C.H. (1963). Immunization against measles. *British Journal of Clinical Practice*, **17**, 650–9.

McEvoy, M.B., Noah, N.D., and Pilsworth, R. (1987). Outbreak of fever caused by *Streptobacillus moniliformis*, *The Lancet*, ii, 1361–3.

McKinnon, J.A. (1979). The impact of the media on whooping cough immunization. *Health Education Journal*, **37**, 198.

Maclean, M.H. and Macleod, A. (1984). Seasonal variation in the frequency of anencephalus and spina bifida births in the UK. *Journal of Epidemiology and Community Health*, **38**, 99–102.

Marks, J.S., Hayden, G.F., and Orenstein, W.A. (1982). Methodologic issues in the evaluation of vaccine effectiveness. *American Journal of Epidemiology*, **116**, 510–523.

Measles Vaccine Committee of the Medical Research Council (1966). Vaccination against measles. *British Medical Journal*, i, 441–6.

Melchior, J.C. (1977). Infantile spasms and early immunization against whooping cough: Danish survey from 1970 to 1975. *Archives of Diseases in Childhood*, **52**, 134–7.

Miceli, I., de Kantor, I., Colaiacovo, D. *et al.* (1988). Evaluation of the effectiveness of BCG vaccination using the case–control method in Buenos Aires, Argentina. *International Journal of Epidemiology*, **17**, 629–34.

Miller, C.L. (1978). Severity of notified measles. *British Medical Journal*, i, 1253.

Miller, D.L. (1964). Frequency of complications of measles, 1963. *British Medical Journal*, **2**, 75–78.

Miller, D.L., Alderslade, R., and Ross, E.M. (1982). Whooping cough and whooping cough vaccine: the risks and benefits debate. *Epidemiologic Reviews*, **4**, 1–24.

Monto, A.S. (1974). The Tecumseh study of respiratory illness. *American Journal of Epidemiology*, **100**, 458–68.

Morgan-Capner, P., Wright, J., Miller, C.L., and Miller, E. (1988). Surveillance of antibody to measles, mumps and rubella by age. *British Medical Journal*, **297**, 770–2.

Morley, D. (1975). Nutritional surveillance of young children in developing countries. *International Journal of Epidemiology*, **5**, 51–5.

Moro, M.L. and McCormick, A. (1988). Surveillance for communicable disease. In *Surveillance in health and disease* (ed. W.J. Eylenbosch and N.D. Noah), p. 166. Oxford University Press.

Morse, S.S (1993). Examining the origins of emerging viruses. In *Emerging viruses* (ed. S.S. Morse). Oxford University Press, New York and Oxford.

Newlands, M. and Davies, L. (1988). The use of performance indicators for immunization rates in general practice. *Public Health*, **102**, 269–73.

Noah, N.D. (1974). *Mycoplasma pneumoniae* infection in the United Kingdom, 1967–1973. *British Medical Journal*, **2**, 544–6.

Noah, N.D. (1976). Attack rates of notified whooping cough in immunized and unimmunized children. *British Medical Journal*, **1**, 128–9.

Noah, N.D. (1982). Measles eradication policies. *British Medical Journal*, **284**, 997–8.

Noah, N.D. (1983). The strategy of immunization. *Community Medicine*, **5**, 140–7.

Noah, N.D. (1989). Cyclical patterns and predictability in infection. *Epidemiology and Infection*, **102**, 175–90.

Noah, N.D. and Fowle, S.E. (1988). Immunity to rubella in women of childbearing age in the United Kingdom. *British Medical Journal*, **297**, 1301–4.

O'Mahony, M., Noah, N.D., Evans, B. *et al.* (1986) An outbreak of gastroenteritis on a passenger cruise ship. *Journal of Hygiene*, **97**, 229–36.

Orenstein, W.A., Bernier, R.H., Dondero, T. *et al.* (1985). Field evaluation of vaccine efficacy. *Bulletin of the World Health Organization*, **63**, l055.

Orenstein, W.A., Bernier, R.H., and Hinman, A.R. (1988). Assessing vaccine efficacy in the field. *Epidemiologic Reviews*, **10**, 212–41.

Patrick, K.M. and Woolley, F.R. (1981). A cost–benefit analysis of immunization for pneumococcal pneumonia. *Journal of the American Medical Association*, **245**, 473–7.

PHLS Epidemiological Research Laboratory and 21 Area Health Authorities (1982). Efficacy of pertussis vaccination in England. *British Medical Journal*, **285**, 357–9.

PHLS Whooping Cough Committee and Working Party (1973). Efficacy of whooping cough vaccines used in the United Kingdom before 1968: final report. *British Medical Journal*, **1**, 259–62.

Pollard, R. (1980). Relation between vaccination and notification rates for whooping cough in England and Wales. *The Lancet*, i, 1180–2.

Pollock, T.M. (1966). *Trials of prophylactic agents for the control of communicable diseases*. World Health Organization, Geneva.

Pollock, T.M., Miller, E., Mortimer, J.Y., and Smith, G. (1984). Symptoms after first immunization with DTP and DT vaccine. *The Lancet*, ii, 146–9.

Pugh, E.J. and Hawker, R. (1986). Measles immunization: professional knowledge and intention to vaccinate. *Community Medicine*, **8**, 340–7.

Raska, K. (1971). Epidemiological surveillance with particular reference to the use of immunological surveys. *Proceedings of the Royal Society of Medicine*, **64**, 684–8.

Research Unit of the Royal College of General Practitioners (1974). The incidence and complications of mumps. *Journal of the Royal College of General Practitioners*, **24**, 545–51.

Rey, M. (1985). Eradication of measles by widespread vaccination is beneficial and feasible. *Semaine des Hopitaux de Paris*, **61**, 21–5.

Robbins, K.B., Brandling-Bennett, A.D., and Hinman, A.R. (1981). Low measles incidence: association with enforcement of school immunization laws. *American Journal of Public Health*, **71**, 270–4.

Rowe, B., Hutchinson, D.N., Gilbert, R.J. *et al.* (1987). *Salmonella ealing* infections associated with consumption of infant dried milk. *The Lancet*, ii, 900–3.

Sever, J.L., Hardy, J.B., Nelson, K.B., and Gilkeson, M.R. (1969). Rubella in the collaborative perinatal research study. *American Journal of Diseases in Childhood*, **118**, 123–32.

Silverstein, A.M. (1981). *Pure politics and impure science: the swine flu affair*. Johns Hopkins University Press, Baltimore and London.

Smith, J.W.G., Fletcher, W.B., and Wherry, P.J. (1976). Vaccination in the control of influenza. *Postgraduate Medical Journal*, **52**, 399–404.

Smith, P.G. (1988). Epidemiological methods to evaluate vaccine efficacy. *British Medical Journal*, **44**, 679–90.

Stetler, H.C., Mullen, J.R., Brennan, J.P., Livengood, J.R., Orenstein, W.A., and Hinman, A.R. (1987). Monitoring system for adverse events following immunization. *Vaccine*, **5**, 169–74.

Sutherland, I. and Fayers, P.M. (1971). Effect of measles vaccination on incidence of measles in the community. *British Medical Journal*, **1**, 698–702.

Thacker, S.B. (1994). Historical development. In *Principles and practice of public health surveillance*, (ed. S.M. Teutsch and R.E. Churchill). Oxford University Press.

Thacker, S.B. and Berkelman, R.L. (1988). Public Health Surveillance in the United States *Epidemiologic Reviews*, **10**, 164–90.

Thacker, S.B., Choi, K., and Brachman, P.S. (1983). The surveillance of infectious diseases. *Journal of American Medical Association*, **249**, 1181–5.

The Lancet, (1976). Leading article: vaccination against measles. *Lancet*, ii, 132–4.

Thiers, G., Maes, R., van Lierde, R. *et al.* (1979). Surveillance van besmettelijke ziekten door een net van peilpraktijken. *Tijdschrift voor Geneeskunde*, **12**, 781.

Tillett, H.E. and Spencer, I.L. (1982). Influenza surveillance in England and Wales using routine statistics. *Journal of Hygiene (Cambridge)*, **88**, 83–94.

Webster, R.G., Bean, W.J., Gorman, O.T., Chambers, T.M., and Kawaoka, Y. (1992). Evolution and ecology of influenza A viruses. *Microbiological Reviews* **56**, 152–79.

Weekly Epidemiological Record (1993) Cholera—update end of 1993. *Weekly Epidemiological Record*, **69**, 13–20.

White, C.C., Koplan, J.P., and Orenstein, W.A. (1985). Benefits, risks and costs of immunization for measles, mumps and rubella. *American Journal of Public Health*, **75**, 739–44.

White, L.R., Sever, J.L., and Alepa, F.P. (1969). Maternal and congenital rubella before 1964: frequency, clinical features, and search for isoimmune phenomena. *Journal of Pediatrics*, **74**, 198–207.

Wilkinson, P., Tylden-Pattenson, L., and Gould, J. (1979). Professional attitudes towards vaccination and immunization within the Leeds Area Health Authority. *Public Health, London*, **93**, 11–5.

Witte, J.J. and Axnick, N.W. (1975). The benefits from 10 years of measles immunization in the United States. *Public Health Report*, **90**, 205–7.

Wright, P.F., Kim-Farley, R.J., de Quadros, C.A., Robertson, S.E., Scott, R.M., Ward, N.A., and Henderson, R.H. (1991). Strategies for the global eradication of poliomyelitis by the year 2000. *New England Journal of Medicine*, **325**, 1774–9.

Yeager, A.S., Davis, J.H., Ross, L.A., and Harvey, B. (1977). Measles immunization. Successes and failures. *Journal of the American Medical Association*, **237**, 347–51.

32 The analysis of human exposures to contaminants in the environment

Paul J. Lioy

Introduction

The presence of chemical and physical agents in the environments where people live, work, and play may cause illness. Therefore, it is essential to develop and employ reliable methods that define the intensity and duration of contact with such agents and assess the likelihood of any cause–effect relationship. The field of exposure analysis and its assessment is associated with epidemiology, risk assessment, and disease intervention and prevention (Lippmann and Lioy 1986; Graham *et al.* 1992; Sexton *et al.* 1992; Jayjock and Hawkins 1993) and the scientists and engineers who conduct these studies now are called exposure analysts (National Research Council 1985, 1991*b*, *c*). The kinds of exposures examined by the exposure analyst are illustrated in Fig. 32.1. The traditional term, industrial hygienist, refers specifically to those individuals who conduct exposure assessments in the workplace.

The exposure measurement techniques may be indirect or direct (National Research Council 1991*c*). Indirect techniques include sampling of locations (microenvironments) where contact may occur with a contaminant and administration of survey instruments; such as, time/activity questionnaires. Direct techniques include personal monitors worn by individuals, and samples of blood, urine, and other bodily fluids which permit measurements of exposure and dose for specific individuals.

The measurement of the concentration of physical, chemical, and/or biological agents in air, water and foods, and the estimation of human behaviours, using instruments such as time/activity pattern diaries, has led to the development of models that can predict exposure and dose. It is currently feasible to trace an agent from the source where it is produced and then follow its pathways and into the people exposed. Figure 32.2 illustrates the 'flow' of a contaminant through the points of contact, to the exposure, and to the dose that can appear inside the body. The domain of related scientific and professional disciplines—environmental science, exposure assessment, toxicology, and epidemiology—is also illustrated.

This chapter describes the features of exposure assessment, starting from concepts and theory. The types of exposure measurements and estimates needed for the applications to environmental health will be illustrated in varying detail, with information about lead, benzene, trihalomethanes, pesticides, airborne particulate matter, infectious agents, and alternate fuels. Finally, some observations will be made concerning the future of exposure assessment in public health practice.

Basic principles

Over the past 10 to 15 years, the theoretical and conceptual bases for exposure assessment have evolved from simple mathematical expressions that consider exposure and doses, to complex systems of exposure/dose equations and concepts that can describe multiple routes of contact with a toxic agent. The aim, as shown in Fig. 32.2, is to establish a relationship between an emitted contaminant and a dose which may cause a health outcome (Lioy 1990*a*).

Exposure to a contaminant is defined as the 'contact at a boundary between a human and the environment at a specific concentration over an interval of time'. The types of integral or summation equations needed to estimate or describe exposure are presented in Table 32.1 (National Research Council 1991*c*). The integral equation represents the actual exposure individuals will receive over the course of time, while the summation provides more practical representation of exposure that can be used to develop direct and indirect measurement techniques. More sophisticated versions of these equations can be used to estimate exposures in modelling studies (see Georgopoulos and Lioy 1994). Exposure

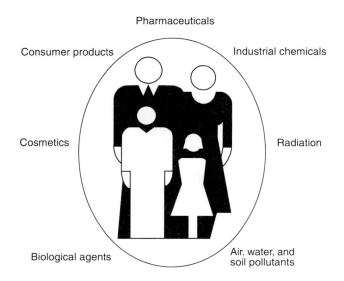

Fig. 32.1 Types of exposures that may be experienced by the general population.

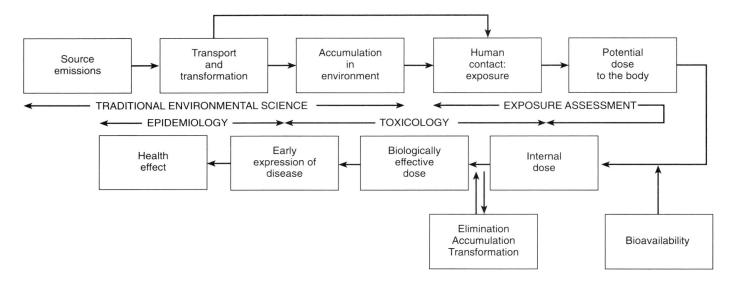

Fig. 32.2 Continuum for the emission of and exposure to a contaminant and the expression of a health effect. (Reproduced from Lioy (1990a), with permission.)

response to a contaminant after contact, including the time associated with elimination of that contaminant from the human body, or the retention of that contaminant or metabolized product in the body.

The definition of exposure provides logical locations for sampling. These occur at boundaries external to the body; thus, exposure is determined at the points of entry into the body, i.e. the nose, mouth, and skin. The data collected at these points of entry can then be used to establish criteria identifying exposure within a population and constructing predictive models (Sexton and Ryan 1988; Ott 1990; McKone 1991; Ryan 1991). Figure 32.3 illustrates three major routes of exposure: (a) inhalation of airborne agents; (b) ingestion of food and liquids; and (c) skin contact with air, soil, and all types of materials and products.

Once a contaminant has crossed a boundary and entered the body, it is then considered a dose, which is routinely described in one of three ways. Potential dose is the amount of material deposited on a surface which can potentially cause an effect on the surface or can be transferred to another organ or tissue; the entire mass (100 per cent) is assumed to cause a biological response.

Internal dose is the amount of material that is actually or estimated to be absorbed by an organ or tissue or absorbed into a surface and is available to undergo biological processes which can cause altered physiological function. Biologically effective dose is the amount of material that reaches the site of action (organ or tissue) in the body. It is the amount of the contaminant or metabolite that interacts with cellular macromolecules and alters physiological function (Lioy 1990a). The units most frequently encountered when calculating exposure and dose are shown in Table 32.2.

Biological markers of exposure/dose can be measured in body fluid specimens and then be associated with time of occurrence and/or persistence of the contaminant (National Research Council 1989a; Henderson et al. 1992). Henderson et al. published a conceptual framework for describing the persistence of the different types of markers in the body. The general time course of elimination of each type of marker is illustrated in Fig. 32.4. The results indicate that exhaled parent compounds yield the highest levels of biomarker concentrations relative to exposure concentration. Adducts spend the longest time in the body. The term 'markers of exposure' is currently used to describe most of the

---

Table 32.1 Equations governing exposure

Exposure

$$E_i = \int_{t_1}^{t_2} C_1(t)\,dt$$

When E_1 is the integrated exposure of an (ith) individual with a concentration (C_1) of a contaminant for time period t_1 to t_2 associated with a biological response

Microenvironmental increments of exposure

$$\Delta E_{ji} = C_{ji}(\Delta t)\Delta t_i$$

$\Delta E_{j,i}$ = The exposure of person i to a contaminant measured over an interval Δt associated with the jth activity (or location)

From this, a summation equation can be developed to represent an individual's exposure to all media, and to all chemicals that can cause the same effects

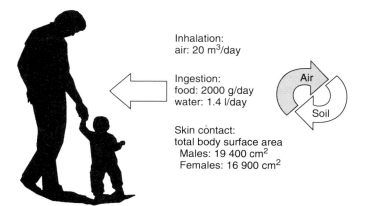

Inhalation:
air: 20 m³/day

Ingestion:
food: 2000 g/day
water: 1.4 l/day

Skin contact:
total body surface area
Males: 19 400 cm²
Females: 16 900 cm²

Fig. 32.3 Routes of exposure. A comprehensive exposure assessment invokes consideration of each possible route through which a chemical can enter the body.

Table 32.2 Examples of units used to express exposure

Variable	Typical units	
Concentration in media	mg/kg	(food)
	µg/l	(water)
	µg/m³ and fibres/m³	(air)
	mg/100 cm²	(contaminated surface)
	mg/g or %	(fraction by weight in consumer products or soil or dust):
Time increments	min, h, day, year, 70 years (lifetime)	
Rate of intake	l/day l/h, mg/kg body weight ingested per day (or per meal), mg inhaled per hour, min	
Quantity available for absorption (potential dose)	mg inhaled, total	
	mg inhaled/kg body weight	
	mg ingested, total	
	mg ingested/kg body weight	
	mg on skin, total	
	mg/cm² skin area	
	mg injected or implanted/kg body weight	
Concentration in body tissues	µg/ml blood	
	fibres/cm³ lung tissue	
Body burden	µg in bone (example)	
Organ dose	mg to liver (example)	

above, but in actuality the level of a contaminant or transformed product present in the body is defined as a dose (National Research Council 1989*b*).

Methodologies

The accurate measurement or estimation of exposure requires baseline information about the plausibility of human contact with the contaminant of concern and assists in establishing the data quality objectives for analysing any particular problem. In the

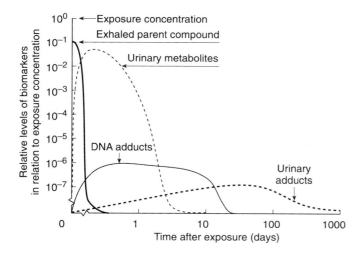

Fig. 32.4 Hypothetical relationships between different biological markers of exposure and time after a single exposure. (Reproduced from Henderson *et al.* (1989), with permission.)

selection of the appropriate measurement 'tools', the analyst needs also to account for factors such as the sensitivity and specificity of a technique for each medium or route studied and ease of sample handling and collection. In some situations simple techniques such as survey instruments are extremely valuable in acquiring semi-quantitative data for the characterization of exposure (Carpenter and Huston-Stein 1980; US Environmental Protection Agency 1988; Robinson *et al.* 1989; Freeman *et al.* 1991; National Research Council 1991*c*; Schwab *et al.* 1991). In other cases more complex techniques like microenvironmental or personal monitors are used to establish the primary route by which human contact occurs with a contaminant (Seifert and Abraham 1983; US Environmental Protection Agency 1988; National Research Council 1991*c*; Lioy 1993). It is important to note, however, that not all types of techniques have to be employed in a single study. Those selected would depend upon the data quality objectives and the hypotheses being tested for a particular study.

The issue of multimedia contact with contaminants has increased the awareness and the desire to obtain measurements on multiple routes of exposure, and to insure that exposure–response relationships are constructed for the media or routes of greatest concern (McKone 1991). The data gathered will improve the manager's ability to prioritize strategies for intervention and eventual reduction of exposure. Experience of exposure analysts with environmental health problems leads to a tacit point: it is not scientifically sound to prejudge which is the most important medium or route of concern for a particular contaminant (National Research Council 1991*c*; Lioy 1990*a*). Avoiding this pitfall will make it possible to obtain a broader view of a problem and improve the selection of measurement and analytical techniques. In the past, many studies have focused on a limited number of routes, and frequently have led to poorly identified exposures, and eventually selection of inappropriate remedial solutions.

One example of how a poorly designed assessment can lead to misclassification of exposure involves benzene (Wallace 1989). Two pie charts, shown in Fig. 32.5, apportion benzene exposure within the general population. The first pie chart identifies the emissions of benzene from major environmental sources and has been used in the past to define exposure reduction strategies. The second pie chart identifies the actual benzene exposure experienced by a statistically representative sample of the general population. The clear message from the emissions pie chart is that motor vehicles represent by far the major source of benzene to the ambient atmosphere and provide the greatest number of opportunities for members of the general population to experience benzene exposures in non-occupational settings. Thus, one is led to believe that the most important source of benzene is the automobile. In contrast, measurements made within personal monitoring studies, also in Fig 32.5, have shown that the predominant source contributing to benzene exposure (over 50 per cent) is cigarette smoke, with only 20 per cent of the exposures caused by automobile emissions. Thus, potentially high exposures to benzene would be misclassified or ignored in strategies to reduce benzene based primarily upon emissions data. Regulators or health officials would benefit from data collected on individual or population activities to help identify the 'true' major source of exposure.

Another example in which improved exposure assessment data provided better information on how commuters come into contact

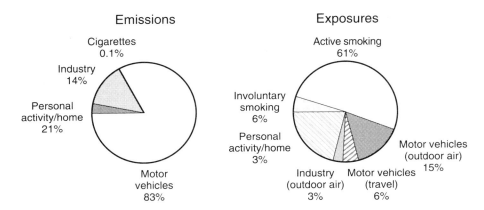

Fig. 32.5 Benzene emissions versus exposures. 'Personal activity/home' refers to benzene from materials such as paints, adhesives, and marking pens. For individuals who do not actively smoke, the 'active smoking' contribution to exposure is zero, and the other exposure categories increase proportionally. (Reproduced from Wallace (1989), with permission.)

with a contaminant is the fuel additive, methyl tert-butyl ether (**MTBE**). It is an oxygenate designed to reduce carbon monoxide and is representative of other chemicals found in new or reformulated fuels (Lioy *et al.* 1994). In this instance, many initial studies on oxygenated fuel were conducted to estimate the environmental levels of MTBE or other hydrocarbons caused by automobile tail pipe emissions. However, experience of the general public and gasoline station workers with gasoline oxygenated by MTBE at 15 per cent by volume have suggested that the highest exposures to the driver or passengers in an automobile, or garage workers, were derived from evaporative emissions released by the engine compartment or gas tank into the interior of a car or in microenvironments adjacent to gasoline service pumps. This is in contrast to the typical tail pipe emissions scenario used in exposure assessments for motor vehicle fuels. Experiments conducted using cars that followed a typical commuter route and then had the gasoline tank filled at some point during the trip are illustrated in Fig. 32.6. The results showed that the highest exposures to MTBE occurred during a tank refill. The approach used in the study demonstrated the importance of both personal and micro-

environmental analyses in providing insight on what can lead to high exposures to evaporative emissions. Other examples exist for dermal and ingestion exposure; however, the main point is not to demonstrate all misclassifications of exposure that can or have occurred, but to recognize that when you design a study, it must include flexibility to evaluate the possibility that a variety of sources and routes can affect exposure. This will improve the detection of and source apportionment of emissions, and how each affects the intensity of human contact with the contaminants of concern.

Approaches used in exposure analysis

Determination of human contact or potential contact with a contaminant is not an integral part of traditional environmental quality measurements. Usually there are criteria available for making environmental quality measurements, which establish a statistically representative sampling scheme for determining the areal extent of contamination and establishing long-term concentration trends within an environmental medium (Lodge 1989; Lioy 1990*b*; Anderson-Sprecher *et al.* 1994). Unfortunately, these measurements do not provide data which can be used to assess exposure directly. Historically, an assessment of exposure was based primarily on the concentration of a contaminant found in an environmental medium at a single sampling site for a prescribed sampling period. Little or no information was provided, however, on the duration of contact or the probability of contact with the contaminant by people spending time in the location where the measurements were being made. More representative historical examples of exposure measurements would be the breathing zone samples collected in occupational settings, where concentrations were much higher.

In many cases, environmental quality measurements continue to provide the only data available for calculating exposure–response relationships within various public health related studies, e.g. hazardous waste sites and air pollution (US Environmental Protection Agency 1989*a*). These data have been used in applications within epidemiology or risk assessment, and have yielded results with a high degree of uncertainty. Also, environmental quality measurements are rarely collected using strategies which ensure that the duration of the measurement is coupled with the relevant biological response time to the presence of a contaminant within

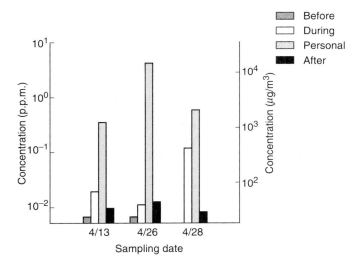

Fig. 32.6 MTBE exposure samples during commuter refuelling.

Table 32.3 Hierarchy of exposure measurements, estimates and surrogates

Type of metric	Approximation of human exposure
Quantified personal and biomarker monitoring	Accurate
Quantified area measurements in the vicinity of a person's activities	Accurate to precise
Quantified modelling estimates of contact with contaminants	Precise
Quantified ambient measurements in the vicinity of population of concern	Moderate
Surrogates of exposure source use, frequency of contact	Fair
Distance of a source from a residence (other locations) and duration of residence	Fair
Residence or employment in a geographical area in reasonable proximity to source or activity	Poor
Residence or employment in a defined geographical area containing a major source	Poor

Adapted from National Research Council 1991, with permission.

the body. As stated previously, the latter point is critical for exposure analysis. All too often environmental quality measurement programmes are based upon a regulatory requirement for determining compliance to a regulation, and/or the limits of detection and collection capacity of a sampler.

The major paradigm shift in framework for exposure analyses which started around 1990, has led to the expanded use of personal monitoring and/or microenvironmental monitoring for the development of exposure databases. Both types of monitors are more intrusive than the devices used for monitoring environmental quality since the sample is taken: (a) at or from the individual, (b) in an area occupied by the individual; or (c) from objects used, worn, or eaten by an individual. The samples also require the acquisition of time resolved data on where and how individuals spend their time (National Research Council 1991c).

A hierarchy of exposure measurements is presented in Table 32.3, and emphasizes that personal monitoring provides the best data for completing an exposure assessment (National Research Council 1991a). The table should be reviewed with some caution, however, since in some studies even weak metrics of exposure may be adequate for examining exposure–health effects relationships. The weak metrics are clearly useful in situations where an isolated source significantly affects a specific community, or a major event or episode has caused health effects. In addition, some techniques currently used for personal exposure could alter a person's usual activity patterns. For instance, personal samplers for particles are

usually bulky and cannot be worn comfortably during periods of outdoor and indoor exercise (Lioy 1993). Therefore, based upon the needs of a study, it can be safely stated that the exposure analyst has a virtual tool-box of techniques to ensure measurements can be used successfully to answer a public health question (Lioy 1992).

Another component critical to an exposure analysis is the identification of the study population. In contrast to studies on environmental quality, where minimal information is required on the population of concern, examination of exposure requires the selection of either a probability-based sample of the general population with possibilities for over-sampling of specific sub-groups, or a specific subgroup of the population that exhibits characteristics of susceptibility or is potentially at the high end of exposure to a contaminant. The latter is a major challenge because it is difficult a priori to select the high end exposure groups, i.e. those above the 90th percentile (US Environmental Protection Agency 1992a).

Typical sampling plans based on the general population or populations at risk are illustrated in Table 32.4. Selection of a susceptible subgroup is more difficult since detailed information is required on the physical or physiological characteristics of interest before selections are made for entry into a study. Some of the major questions that need to be addressed in proper selection of susceptible or sensitive individuals are shown in Table 32.5.

Media and routes of exposure

The preceding discussion generally described the environmental media and routes of entry to the body needed to characterize exposure. Each has been examined over the years to provide information on the magnitude and extent of environmental problems. For exposure assessment there is a special need to know how each medium or route is associated with the extent to which individuals or members of a population come into contact with a contaminant. Many types of sources that impact each medium, and some of the more common issues, are shown in Table 32.6. Clearly, inorganic and organic emissions can come from industrial processes, commercial activities, personal activities, disposal activities, and nature.

It is somewhat obvious that the environmental media which can lead to contact with a contaminant include air, water, soil, and food since people routinely come into contact with these each day. However, it may be somewhat of a surprise that all routes of entry to the body, except inadvertent or purposeful injection of a biological or chemical contaminant, may be directly or indirectly impacted by a contaminant originally released in one medium. This important point is illustrated in Table 32.7 for lead and pesticides.

Lead can be emitted by sources which directly impact the air, water, soil, and food and then transported to and deposited in another medium, indirectly causing exposures via multiple routes of entry to the body. From the standpoint of public health the situation is complicated because there is no easy formula available to determine the route of entry, or to apportion the sources contributing to lead burden. In the case of house dust, lead can be derived from indoor and outdoor sources, and ingestion occurs after dermal adhesion and transfer to the mouth or after the adhesion of the dust to a food or to toys (National Research Council 1993a). For pesticide exposures, there is an added source of

Table 32.4 Summary of sampling for exposure assessment

Sampling design	Condition for most useful application
Haphazard sampling	Only valid when target population and exposure are homogeneous in space and time; hence, not generally recommended
Purposive sampling	Target population well defined and homogeneous, so sample-selection bias is not a problem; or specific microenvironmental or personal samples selected for unique value and interest, rather than for making inferences to wider population
Probability sampling	
Simple random sampling	Homogeneous population
Stratified random sampling	Homogeneous population with strata (subregions); might consider strata as domains of study
Systematic sampling	Frequently most useful; trends over time and space must be quantified, can easily be adapted to total exposure
Multistage sampling	Target population large and homogeneous; simple random sampling used to select contiguous groups of population units
Cluster sampling	Economical when population units cluster (e.g. schools of fish); ideally, cluster means are similar in value, but concentrations within clusters should vary widely, and anticipate high end exposures
Double sampling	Must be strong linear relation between variable of interest and less expensive or more easily measured variable

Reproduced from National Research Council 1991c, with permission.

exposure—the direct application of a pesticide to surfaces by a homeowner or resident (this is in addition to any amount derived from the work of a professional exterminator or crop duster) (National Research Council 1993b).

The need to complete a source apportionment for lead, pesticides, and other chemicals provides a message for public health officials and the exposure assessor: the obvious answer (source) may not always provide the correct way to solve a problem. For instance, a person may live in a residence which has lead-based paint on the walls. The first thought would be that the lead paint was the major source of blood lead levels measured in the occupants. If the painted surface is isolated or intact, however, the source that could cause an increase in blood lead may be street dust and/or soil in the neighbourhood. Thus, source apportionment plays a crucial role in linking the point of emission through the route of exposure to an internal or biologically effective dose (see Fig. 32.2).

An example of how exposure and risk derived from multiple routes of entry can be underestimated is associated with regulations or public health advisories for potable water supplies. In the 1970s, potential exposures and health risks were based solely on the quantity of the contaminant ingested by drinking the water (US Environmental Protection Agency 1980) and assumed the consumption of 2 litres of water per day, which is unusually high for most members of the general population. Public health advisories on the use of contaminated water supplies, e.g. wells with water containing contaminants leached from hazardous waste sites, stated that individuals 'should not drink the water'. If scientists and regulators had seriously considered all the opportunities for contact with potable water prior to estimating the risk, they would have included two other routes of exposure: dermal and inhalation (Brown et al. 1984). Only after studies by Andelman (Andelman 1985), which focused on the shower as a route for inhalation exposure, and Jo et al. (1990) and Weisel et al. (1993), which demonstrated that significant human exposures to volatile organics occurred via inhalation and the dermal route during a showering or bathing, did the public health practice and environmental regulations embrace the concept of total exposure. The results have led to the concept that individuals should 'just not use contaminated water'. According to Jo et al. (1990) at least half of an individual's internal dose derived from chloroform found in a public water supply could be from just one 10-min shower per day. Obviously more and varied uses of the water would lead to higher or lower daily internal doses.

The importance of the dermal and inhalation routes is demonstrated in Fig. 32.7, for the concentration of chloroform found in exhaled breath after using a swimming pool. Integration of the area under the curve indicates the two routes made similar contributions to an internal dose, even though there is a much slower rate of chloroform accumulation via the dermal route (Georgopoulos *et al.* 1994).

Techniques

The measurement process used to establish the presence of a contaminant in one or more of the above media or routes can become complex and require the application of a variety of techniques. Two primary categories exist for exposure measurements: direct and indirect techniques (Fig. 32.8) (National Research Council 1991c). These categories correspond to the types of methods used to collect data or estimate exposure within field studies and modelling simulations, respectively. The main differences between these two types of techniques are associated with the proximity of the measurement or estimate of exposure to the

Table 32.5 Defining high exposure populations

Data collection methods
Choice of method
   Purposive exposure study
   Applied, or response, epidemiology
   Targeted case–control or cohorts
   Registries
   Reference population surveys
   Complete enumeration
Sampling design
   Representative
   Convenient
Detecting small populations or rare events

Defining subgroups of the population
Cultural characteristics
   Cultural identity
   Heterogeneity within categories
   Sensitive information
   Cultural habits or rituals
   Choice of appropriate indicator
Susceptibility characterizations
   Race
   Gender
   Age
   Disease state
   Population or family genetics
   Occupations (participation or avoidance)
Population
   Mobility
   Estimation of local population size
   Intermarriage
   Assimilation
   Daily living activities
   Proximity to a source or source region
   Observation of any effects

Table 32.6 Typical sources of contaminants that can be present in various media

Air (outdoor)
Smelters
Power plants
Petrochemical plants
Chemical manufacturing
Paper and pulp
Cement plants
Municipal incinerators
Degreasing operations
Atmosphere reactions
Space heating
Automobiles
Trucks
Transportation
Water treatment plants
Autobody repair
Mining operations

Air (indoor)
Passive smoking
Household products
Indoor combustion
Disinfectants
Paint, paint removers
Deodorizers
Rugs
Ventilation system
Water contaminants

Water
Landfills
Hazardous waste sites
Chemical plants
Pesticide production
Food process industry
Sewage treatment
Septic tank
Domestic waste
Agriculture
Agriculture run-off
Underground storage
Urban street run-off
Water system
Sealants

Soil
Hazardous wastes
Underground storage tanks
Domestic waste
Industrial dumping
Buried underground
Storage
Yard clean-up and maintenance
Spills and transportation

Food
Garden soil
Agricultural soil
Insufficient food cleaning
Insufficient food preparation
Pesticide residuals
Unapproved packaging

Injection
Contaminated needles and objects
Contaminated fluids
Contaminated products

individual, and the qualitative or quantitative nature of the information. At present, there is no uniformity in the quality and quantity of techniques available for any category of indirect or direct measurements. In fact, there are major instrumentation needs for each environmental medium and route of exposure. This is not to say there is a lack of sampling and analytical equipment to measure chemical, physical, and biological agents in various environmental media. However, many have been designed to provide environmental quality measurements rather than human exposure measurements. This important point is substantiated by the fact that many of the currently available techniques are too bulky to be used in applications requiring either microenvironmental and/or personal measurements (Lioy 1993).

Table 32.7 Example of multimedia chemicals and sources

Medium or pathway	Sources
Lead	
Outdoor air	Industrial
	Automobile
Indoor air	Infiltration of outdoor air
Outdoor soil	Air deposition
	Paint flaking
	Hazardous waste
Outdoor dust	Air deposition
	Paint flaking
	Soil resuspension
House dust	Tracked dust
	Paint flaking
	Air filtration
Food utensils/	Dust deposition
food preparation	Dust contact
	Pottery/glasses
Clothing	Surface contact
	Laundering of clothes
Water	Water pipes
	Water supply
Food	Grown in contaminated soil
	Preparation of Food
Pesticides	
Outdoor air	Spraying of crops in yards
Indoor air	Spraying of plants
	Outdoor air infiltration
Outdoor soil	Air deposition
	Direct spraying of plants/vegetation
Outdoor dust	Air deposition
	Resuspension of soil
House dust	Indoor spraying
	Tracked outdoor
	Dust/soil
	Outdoor air infiltration
Food	Surface deposition
	Fruit/vegetable
	Contamination
Food preparation	Surface dust
	Outdoor/house
Water	Run-off from soil
	Water supply

In many cases personal monitors require optimization for a number of parameters. A list of general technical criteria that must be met to develop these monitors is shown in Table 32.8 (National Research Council 1991*c*). It is apparent that the techniques must be compact, and each must have low detection limits and sufficient time resolution in order to obtain human exposures for the chemical(s) under consideration. These three features are difficult to achieve simultaneously in a single device. For example, as an instrument is miniaturized the substrate available for sample collection or the detection volume available for instrumental analyses (e.g. photo cell) is reduced. Consequently, the detection limits will rise and/or the time necessary to collect an adequate sample will increase, which can preclude their use in specific applications, e.g. low-level short-term exposure or acute exposures. Such incompatibilities can be eliminated only by conducting basic

research prior to the development of a sampling programme that will employ a device in any particular application. Sometimes there may be 'off the shelf' devices available for use in an application or study, but possibilities are limited for most media and routes of exposure. During the mid-1970s, because of the increased concern about health problems associated with indoor air pollution, micro-environmental and personal air measurement devices were developed for the detection of traditional contaminants (e.g. volatile organic substances, fine particles, and carbon monoxide). Others are being developed for agents such as microbiological aerosols. Some of the personal monitors are based on passive sampling techniques, while other sampling systems use an active pump (Seifert and Abraham 1983; Ryan *et al.* 1986; Samet *et al.* 1987, 1988).

Before the concept of total exposure became a starting point for the design of field studies and risk assessments, the following measurement issue received little attention: how comparable are the data collected by various techniques used across more than one medium or route of entry into the body? Unfortunately, there is no complete answer because of the many different types of physical, chemical, and biological agents that exist, and the nature of the emissions, transport, and accumulation and transformation processes that can affect the occurrence of biologically significant exposures. A summary of the types of techniques for collecting microenvironmental and personal samples is shown in Table 32.9. For microenvironmental studies of air pollution, for example, there exist both continuous and integrating monitors; the devices have high resolution and low detection limits for specific compounds, e.g. metals and volatile organics. The data can easily be used to estimate the direct inhalation exposure. However, for other media there are very few comparable, sophisticated and reliable samplers. In fact, there are no continuous monitors currently available for these sampling media that operate without the constant use of a technician as a personal shadow; for example, taking a surface soil sample at every location he or she came into contact with soil during the day (Hawley 1985).

For integrated samples, the situation is somewhat better. You can periodically obtain integrated samples from soil or dust

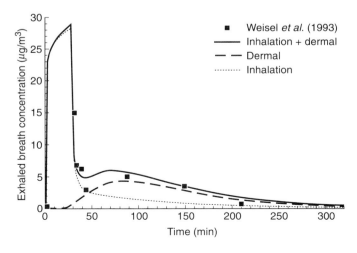

Fig. 32.7 Exhaled breath concentration of chloroform following inhalation and dermal absorption in a swimming pool (air concentration 100 μg/m³, water concentration 150 μg/l).

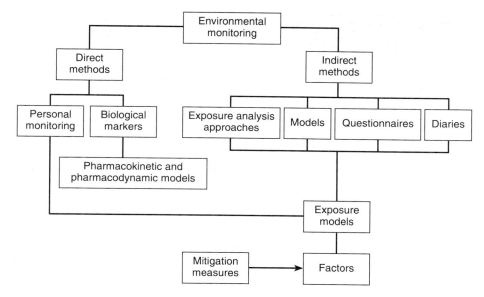

Fig. 32.8 Possible approaches for analysis of air contaminat exposures. (Reproduced from National Research Council 1991c, with permission.)

available for dermal contact or consumption, food available for consumption, and water or fluids for consumption. However, it is

Table 32.8 Methods criteria

Factor	Ideal condition
Sensitivity	Detects analytes at levels below those causing adverse health effect; sensitivity 0.1 times level of interest; range 0.1 – 10 times level of interest; precision and accuracy ± 5 per cent; easy and accurate calibration
Selectivity	No response to similar compounds that might be present simultaneously with the analyte of interest; can differentiate multiple compounds in single device
Rapidity	Short sampling and analysis times compared with biological response time or with significant changes in contaminant concentration; response time 90 per cent in less than 30 s; and output to a computer or computer compatible media (CD-ROM, Diskette)
Operation	Few complex components to change in the field, quick releases, low noise
Comprehensiveness	Sensitive to all contaminants that could result in a similar adverse health effect
Portability	Sampling and analysis device rugged, can be worn without modifying the normal behaviour of individual; lower power consumption; battery operated; stabilization time less than 15 min; temperature range -20° to 40°C; humidity range 0–100 per cent
Cost	Cost of sampling and analysis not prohibitive; device inexpensive; readily available components; few consumables; low maintenance

Reproduced from National Research Council (1991c), with permission.

still difficult to obtain integrated samples that represent the contact that can occur with water in all microenvironments and activities during a given day, e.g. swimming, bathing, cooking, etc.

At present the best means of obtaining comparable multimedia microenvironmental samples use periodic collection of integrated samples, as in studies estimating total exposure in a residential setting (Lioy and Pellizzari 1995; Pellizzari et al. 1995). The general concept involves capturing a day or week in the life of a statistically representative sample for a population or particular subgroup of a population at risk. Table 32.10 and Fig. 32.9 indicate the types of samples that can be collected to estimate a residential exposure for a week in the life of a family. The output from such a measurement study is a series of microenvironmental samples that are analysed for the chemicals of concern. The data are then used as input to exposure scenarios to specific environmental contaminants in residential settings. They can also be used to construct total exposure estimates using the summation equations found in Table 32.1.

One major component of this type of study is the application of questionnaires which must include a time/activity log that is completed by the members of the household during the time of the field sampling. The data are essential for reducing uncertainties that are inherent in the application of generic exposure scenarios to site-specific or person-specific assessments.

Activity logs have become customized to address the exposures that can occur for specific chemicals (Robinson et al. 1989; Freeman et al. 1991; Schwab et al. 1991). In addition logs address generic issues of contact with environmental contaminants (e.g. frequency of personal product use and contact with volatile components, frequency and duration of outdoor activities). For instance in a study of residential exposure to wastes laden with chromium, which was used as the fill prior to the construction of residences, typical questions for a week-long study of chromium exposure would include:

Table 32.9 General availability of monitors for measuring exposure

Route type	Personal	Microenvironmental	Environmental
Inhalation/gases			
Continuous monitor	Yes	Yes	Yes
Integrated monitor	Yes	Yes	Yes
Pesticides			
Continuous monitor	No	Yes	Yes
Integrated monitor	Yes	Yes	Yes
Ingestion			
Food			
Continuous monitor	No	No	No
Integrated monitor	Yes	Yes	Yes
Water			
Continuous monitor	No	No	No
Integrated monitor	No	Yes	Yes
Soil/dust			
Continuous monitor	No	No	No
Integrated monitor	No	Yes	Yes
Dermal			
Water			
Continuous monitor	No	No	No
Integrated monitor	No	Yes	Yes

No, not available; yes, available.

1. Were any of the following used in the house today?
   (a) vacuum; (b) carpet sweeper; (c) broom; (d) dust cloths/mops; (e) wet mops; (f) other house cleaning; (g) laundry.

2. Did you notice any green, yellow, red, or orange deposits or stains on the walls or floors of your home?

3. If you noticed these deposits, were you or members of your family in the room or rooms with these deposits for more than 10 min at a time?

Table 32.10 Sampling strategy

Types of samples	Location	Duration
Indoor air	Two high use rooms	1–7 days
Outdoor air	Breathing zone in yard	1–7 days
Soil	Yard surface: 0–2 cm gridded sweep yard; subsurface: 0–100 cm grided dig	Composited grab
Dust	Flat interior surface / Rugs on interior floor / Flat exterior walkways	Integrated wipe / Integrated vacuum / Integrated sweeps
Water	Drinking water / Shower water / Bath water	Daily tap water (1 l) / 10–30 min / Daily bath
Food	Kitchen prepared and consumed meals	1–7 day duplicate diet
Activity patterns	Residential actions or events	Daily diary

Results obtained by these types of methods can be validated by video records, technician observations, and fluorescent tracer studies, as in a study of residential exposure to wastes laden with chromium discussed above (Fenske *et al.* 1991).

Although not shown in Fig. 32.10, a residential microenvironmental study can easily be expanded to include personal monitoring and biological monitoring. Some of the more common are used to measure organic/inorganic chemicals in blood and urine. These samples will provide personal integrated or time series data for the duration of the sampling period, e.g. a day or a week. Biological monitoring data provides baseline information on the residents and can be used to determine if they have been 'truly' in contact with a contaminant. If a residential experiment is repeated one or more times, biological marker data can be valuable in pharmacokinetic model simulations for some contaminants. Follow-up biological monitoring samples can also allow the analyst to establish any incremental changes in dose.

Biological monitoring is currently being used to measure selected heavy metals in blood and urine, volatile organics in blood, and pesticides in blood and urine in studies at hazardous waste sites and within the National Human Exposure Assessment Survey (Pellizzari *et al.* 1995). There are some techniques available for measurement of metabolites and DNA adducts (Fiserova-Bergerova 1987; Perera *et al.* 1987; National Research Council 1989*a*, *b*, 1991*c*; Ashley *et al.* 1992), notably associated with the polycyclic aromatic hydrocarbons (Perera 1987). A first-order analysis of the data would be to determine the change in contaminant level for a bodily fluid which could be associated with a change in the type or intensity of exposure that occurred at the residence. A second-order analysis would involve the application of pharmacokinetic models (Gerlowsky and Jain 1983; Caudill and Pirkle 1992).

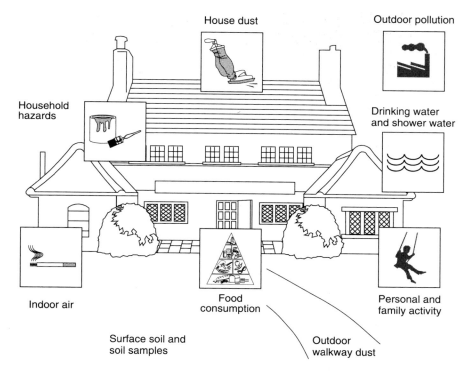

Fig. 32.9 Types of integrated microenvironmental sentinel for total home exposure to metals, pesticides, and/or volatile organics.

Data analysis and models

Once microenvironmental and/or personal exposure data have been acquired in a field study or estimated by a model, there are a number of analyses that can be used to place the data in a form that is helpful for examining a public health issue. The levels of analysis are dependent upon the types and amount of data available from a particular study or a series of companion or comparative studies (US Environmental Protection Agency 1989a). A parallel issue is the form of the data necessary for the application of interest, e.g. epidemiology or risk assessment. For instance the data can be reported as exposure using the units of concentration and time ($\mu g/m^3$ per h) or as a time weighted average ($\mu g/m^3$/per day). Then, depending upon the amount of data available, a distribution of exposure can be constructed and particular statistical quantities can be calculated. Information that is derived from a distribution of exposure are shown in Fig. 32.10, and include the mean exposure (50th percentile), the high end exposure (above 90th percentile), the form of the exposure distribution curve, and the worst possible case estimate (bounding estimate) of exposure (US Environmental Protection Agency 1992a).

If the database includes information that can be examined across pathways or routes of exposure, the result will be estimates of total exposure across each medium or each route of entry into the body. The data collected that represent a day or week of a family (Table 32.10 and Fig. 32.9), can be used to determine the micro-environmental increments to total exposure. Theoretically an integrated exposure can be derived from microenvironmental exposures by the summation formula found in Table 32.1.

Risk assessment applications require at least one further level of analysis: a dose calculated from the exposure level. The result can then be used in a risk characterization analysis; as stated earlier, these calculations can be in one of three forms: potential, internal, or biologically effective dose. The general form of the equations needed to calculate dose from exposure data is shown in Table 32.11. Based upon the ancillary information and parameters needed to complete such calculations (e.g. absorption rate), the value most frequently calculated is the potential dose. In rare instances the biologically effective dose can be calculated, but there are large uncertainties in the values used for factors to complete such calculations (Lioy 1990a).

A second reason for calculating a dose from the exposure data is to place units of measurement in a form that is consistent for

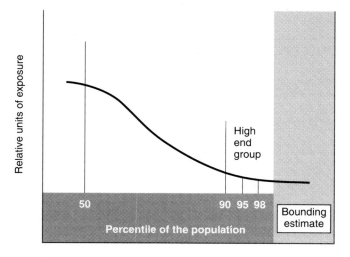

Fig. 32.10 Major parameters to be determined from a distribution (known/default) of population exposure.

Table 32.11 Generalized equations governing exposure and dose

Integrated exposure

$$E = \int_{t_1}^{t_2} C(t)\,dt$$

where E = exposure; $C(t)$ = time variant concentration; t_1, t_2 = time period of exposure associated with a specific biological response

Potential dose

$$D_p = \int_{t_2}^{t_1} C(t)f(x)\,dt;\ f(x) = CR$$

where D_p (mass or mass/body weight) = potential dose; $f(x)$ = contact rate

Internal dose

$$D_1 = \int_{t_1}^{t_2} f(x)g(ab)C(t)\,dt$$

D_1 = internal dose; $g(ab)$ = Absorption function (e.g. skin, lung membrane)

Biologically effective dose

$$D_{BE} = \int_{t_1}^{t_2} f(x)g(ab)p(as,rd,me,el)C(t)\,dt$$

where $p(as,rd,me,el)$ = a function based upon nature of assimilation, repair, metabolism elimination

comparisons among routes of entry. A typical form for dose is micrograms of contaminant per kilogram of body weight per unit of time. The format makes it easier to compare intensity of the contact with the amount that has been deposited within the body for different routes of entry. These data can also be used to determine which of the exposures encountered were at levels that may cause a biological effect.

As shown in Table 32.11 unless the investigator has acquired biological marker data, the determination of a dose requires information on a series of variables or factors that may only be measurable in detailed exposure assessment studies (US Environmental Protection Agency 1989*a*; American Industrial Health Council 1994). Examples of factors needed to complete dose calculations include rates of breathing, skin absorption, ingestion, internal absorption, elimination, and repair. Obviously, it is easier to acquire data on breathing or ingestion rate than on organic cellular repair mechanisms. In fact, there are no methods available at the current time which can quantify cellular repair.

A type of data that is usually not available for dose calculations, but could be obtained, is the bioavailability of a contaminant in the matrix that contains it (e.g. soil) (Umbreit *et al.* 1986; Kitsa *et al.* 1992; Ruby *et al.* 1993; Wainman *et al.* 1994). This value is dependent upon the amount of a contaminant that can be extracted from the matrix (e.g. soil) by bodily fluids found within the digestive system or the lung.

Since it is not possible to acquire data routinely in a field study on accumulation or elimination rates, or absorption factors, dose calculations employ what have been conventionally described as generic exposure factors (single values or a distribution of values). Based upon the type of dose calculation, the number of exposure factors selected could be minimal or extensive. These are driven by the data quality objectives, the amount of data available, the

anticipated variability of the activities affecting the dose, and the types of individual or population characteristics considered to be of importance. Once these types of information have been accumulated and the objectives of the analyses have been established, the analyst can complete either a point estimate of a dose or a distributional estimate of dose.

Point estimates of exposure require the application of an equation similar to those found in Table 32.11 for each route of exposure and each microenvironment that can lead to an individual having contact with chemicals. For example, selection of ingestion exposure, inhalation exposure, and dermal exposure scenarios can provide an estimate of the potential or, with additional data, an internal dose of a contaminant by completing a calculation similar to that illustrated in Table 32.12 (US Environmental Protection Agency 1989*a*). Results can then be summed for all microenvironments and media to obtain point estimates of exposure for a hypothetical or representative member of the local population.

Table 32.12 Point estimate of potential dose

Ingestion of chemicals in water or beverages

$$(mg/kg - day) = \frac{CW \times IR \times EF \times ED}{BW \times AT}$$

where CW = chemical concentration in water; IR = ingestion rate (litres/day); EF = exposure frequency (days/year); ED = exposure duration (years); BW = body weight (kg); AT = averaging time (period over which exposure is averaged – days)

Chemicals in soil

$$(mg/kg - day) = \frac{CS \times IR \times CV \times FI \times EF \times ED}{BW \times AT}$$

where CS = chemical concentration in soil (mg/kg); IR = ingestion rate (mg soil/day); CF = conversion factor (10^6 kg/mg); FI = fraction ingested from contaminated source (unitless); EF = exposure frequency (days/years); ED = exposure duration (years); BW = body weight (kg); AT = averaging time (period over which exposure is averaged – days)

Inhalation of airborne (vapour phase) chemicals

$$(\mu g/kg - day) = \frac{CA \times IR \times ET \times EF \times ED}{BW \times AT}$$

where CA = contaminant concentration in air ($\mu g/m^3$); IR = inhalation rate (m^3/h); ET = exposure time (h/day); EF = exposure frequency (days/year); ED = exposure duration (years); BW = body/weight (kg); AT = averaging time (period over which exposure is averaged – days)

Dermal contact with chemicals in soil

$$(mg/kg - day) = \frac{CS \times CF \times SA \times AF \times ABS \times EF \times ED}{BW \times AT}$$

where CS = chemical concentration in soil (mg/kg); CF = conversion factor (10^6 kg/mg); SA = skin to surface area available for contact (cm^2/event); AF = soil to skin adherence factor (mg/cm^2); ABS = absorption factor (unitless); EF = exposure/frequency (events/year); ED = exposure duration (years); BW = body weight (kg); AT = averaging time (period over which exposure is averaged – days)

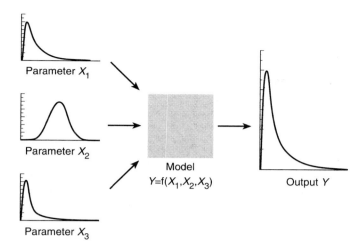

Fig. 32.11 Representation of Monte Carlo Analysis used to construct a dependent variable distribution Y.

One can also develop a distribution of dose point estimates based upon exposure measurements (e.g. personal monitoring) and/or estimates of exposure using exposure factors characteristic of the population of concern.

Recently, there has been a distinct move away from relying exclusively on point estimates of exposure and dose. This is done primarily to reduce the uncertainties that surround identifying a most exposed individual (US Environmental Protection Agency 1992*a*), which was frequently described as the person exposed to a compound throughout his or her lifetime. In fact, exposure assessors are now being encouraged to employ distributional analyses by the frequency distributions of all or selected factors needed to estimate particular exposures or doses. This has led to the use of Monte Carlo techniques for combining the selected distributions of parameters or variables (Rubinstein 1981; Marnicio *et al.* 1991; US Environmental Protection Agency 1992*a*; Hattis and Burmaster 1994). On the surface this appears to be a step forward in the development of exposure/dose databases especially for risk assessment applications. However, there are some 'land mines' buried in the analysis of distributions that employ the random selection of points to establish a distribution of exposure. Figure 32.11 illustrates the general concept of combining distributions of independent variables to establish an overall distribution of one dependent variable; in our case exposure or dose. At first glance this seems to be a relatively simple task, since Monte Carlo techniques, available in many computer programs, combine the points along each known or approximated variable distribution, and produce a final distribution that represents the exposure or dose. There are inherent statistical limitations to Monte Carlo analyses which must be examined prior to selecting the distributions used in applications of a particular set of exposure data. These have been outlined by numerous individuals (Rubinstein 1981; Marnicio *et al.* 1991; US Environmental Protection Agency 1992*a*; Hattis and Burmaster 1994). Beyond the statistical constraints, there are other informational issues which must be evaluated to ensure that the estimates are plausible and realistic. Included is the evaluation of the usefulness of the values combined across distributions to simulate either the high end exposures or low end exposures. An

example of a distribution of an exposure factor, fish ingestion, is shown in Fig. 32.12. It is clear that there is a tendency toward bimodality (American Industrial Health Council 1994). The shape of the curve indicates different consumption patterns for subgroups of a population. Thus, proper utilization of the data requires knowledge of consumption activities within a potentially affected population.

Evaluations of distributional data must also ascertain whether or not all projected exposures or doses can occur and do occur for the situation or activity under investigation. At a minimum, sensitivity analyses should be conducted on the tails of the variable distributions used to estimate the exposure/dose. For example, an acute toxin (e.g. cyanide or ozone) at sufficient concentration to induce a biological response (death or asthma attack, respectively) over a short period of time would not logically be coupled with a contact period equivalent to a week or more. An 82-year-old grandparent or non-athletic person would not be spending too much time engaging in activities with a ventilation rate as high as 1.5 m^3/h when the outdoor ozone concentrations exceed 150 p.p.b. Finally, a child would not be spending 24 h per day over a 12–year period sitting on the grounds of a hazardous waste site. These examples may seem somewhat absurd, but if the appropriate constraints are not placed on a distributional analysis of exposure, these types of results and worse could be propagated through a computer program and reported as part of the estimated distribution of exposure or dose.

Although distributional analyses are more likely to be conducted for risk assessments, they also are of value in epidemiological studies. A specific case is a comparison of a biological marker data for a contaminant or metabolite with a dose estimated from external exposure measurements. In intervention studies distributional data are of immense value for comparing a point measurement of exposure or dose (individual or affected subgroups) with the values observed and/or estimated for a much larger population (Lioy 1992).

Exposure assessment modelling

Predictions of an exposure or dose have been based on modelling of emissions, environmental transport, and fate (Thibodeaux 1979; Javandel *et al.* 1984; Cohen 1989; Georgopoulos 1990) and of population time/location and activity patterns combined with microenvironmental models (Ott 1980; Duan 1982, 1991; Schwab *et al.* 1991; Pardi 1992; Patrick 1994). This is called a prognostic assessment. Prediction of exposure can also be done based on modelling of biomarker information (Georgopoulos and Lioy 1994), which is called a diagnostic assessment.

Macro- and microenvironmental models can be improved by including physiologically based toxicokinetic models. Physiologically based models which relate exposure to internal and target tissue dose have been successfully applied to predict doses for a variety of toxicants. Both traditional 'lumped' parameter (ordinary differential equation) formulations, as well as 'refined' distributed parameter (partial and ordinary differential equation) schemes have been used for the inverse prediction from dose to exposure medium reconstruction (Georgopoulos and Lioy 1994; Georgopoulos *et al.* 1994). This approach utilizes time profiles following exposure to

Min.	Max.	4%	31%	44%	72%	95%
0.4	5.0	0.4	0.8	1.4	2.0	4.0

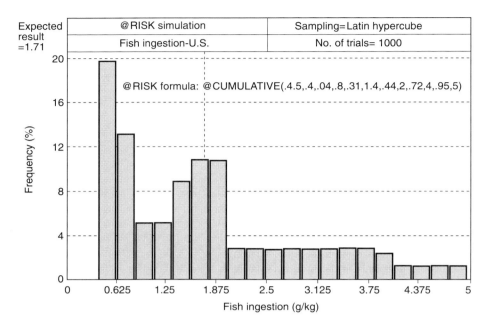

Fig. 32.12 Distribution of fish ingestion. (Reproduced from American Industrial Health Council (AIHC) (1994), with permission.)

biomarker concentrations found in excreted fluids to reconstruct the single and/or multimedia/multiroute exposures experienced by an individual, e.g. simultaneous inhalation and dermal absorption of a volatile organic substance present in air and water.

A detailed exposure assessment may also require resource-intensive data collection studies or model-based simulations to characterize one or more of the following: (a) source attributes; (b) toxicant properties; (c) geographical domain of influence attributes; (d) population composition/stratification; (e) population time/location pattern and activity patterns; (f) macroenvironmental media properties/concentrations; (g) microenvironmental media properties and concentrations; and (h) exposure routes and pathways. Consequently, the complexity of the exposure system and the wide range of information requirements necessitate simulation which can describe the exposure to dose or the dose to exposure. Finally, case-specific requirements of available mechanistic information must be available to link each component of the exposure continuum (Fig. 32.2), and then estimate doses potentially received by a particular population. The overall types of analyses and data needs required to complete an exposure simulation successfully are shown in Table 32.13 (Patrick 1994).

A general modelling framework can guide the collection and analysis of new data; conversely, the quality and quantity of available data limit the sophistication of any model. Priorities in data collection and model development must be established, and options must be explored for analysing available information and for modelling various components of the exposure system. Components of both single-medium and multimedia environmental and environmental exposure models, such as the human exposure model (HEM) II (US Environmental Protection Agency 1991)

used for assessment of population exposures from air releases and the STREAM model (Donigian and Mulkey 1992) used for exposure assessment of pesticide run-off, should be considered in the development and expansion of models.

Microenvironment models should be evaluated prior to their use in assessing exposure for the application under consideration (Ott *et al.* 1988; US Environmental Protection Agency 1989*b*). The relative advantages and limitations of stochastic simulation models (such as the simulation of human activity and pollution exposure or the benzene exposure assessment), cartesianization or convolution models, and the most general double covariance models have been summarized elsewhere (Georgopoulos and Lioy 1994).

An assumption of log normality for integrated exposures and doses provides a starting point for conducting probablistic exposure analyses (US Environmental Protection Agency 1992*a*). However, such an assumption, combined with the use of the off-the-shelf Monte Carlo simulation software, that typically assumes non-correlation among the variables, can lead to erroneous results. Log normal exposures are usually claimed as a direct result of log normality observed in ambient environmental concentrations; however, deviations to this assumption occur for the impact of isolated strong sources. Exponential concentration probability densities have been shown to apply in such systems. From a practical perspective a two- or three-parameter log normal distribution is flexible enough to fit the main range of most right-skewed data sets satisfactorily, a reason for its popularity in practice.

Potential problems are associated with the additional requirements for accuracy of data needed to describe high exposures and doses. It is exactly in that range where assumptions on independence (typical in Monte Carlo simulations) are less valid. One

Table 32.13 Exposure modelling: concepts and data

Analytical solution	Method for solving differential equations in a model using classical tools of algebra and calculus
Boundary conditions	Input values used to initialize the model
Calibration	The process of using a set of observed data to adjust the structure and/or internal coefficients of a model such that the output values are accurate with respect to a known value
Causation	The independent change in the value of one variable causes a predictable change in the value of dependent variables
Deterministic model	One in which the variations in the variables do not include a random component—there is one output for each set of inputs
Equilibrium	A system which is not exchanging energy or matter with its surrounding and is in equilibrium with the surroundings
Model	A theoretical construct attempts to relate an identified system to the data and information available to simulate the system
Numerical solution	Method for solving differential equations using numerical approximation techniques
Sensitivity analysis	The investigation of changes in dependent variable values resulting from changes in values in independent variables and in the posited relationships among variables
Stability	The ability of a numerical integration method to iterate to a solution
Steady state	The case where input to a system is balanced by output. A model in which no variables change for the time period under consideration
Stochastic model	One in which the variation in one or more variables includes a random component
Verification	Testing of a model following initial calibration

Source: adapted from Patrick 1994.

solution in any analysis is the use of asymptotic distributions of extremes, such as Gumbel's double exponential distribution, for the high ends ('distribution tails') of concentration and exposure time.

Practical application of exposure assessment has been mainly driven by generic or 'typical' assumptions (e.g. the person eating large quantities of waste all his or her life). However, as data evolve, management requirements for information obtained from large-scale, comprehensive exposure assessment programmes, such as the National Human Exposure Assessment Survey, will be overwhelming by comparison to current standards for routine exposure data management (Sexton 1994). Consequently, state-of-the-art information management tools must be evaluated and used to organize, utilize, and interpret efficiently exposure-related data. These include geographical information systems, interactive scientific visualization systems, distributed relational database management systems, and object oriented environments for data and model integration.

Exposure probabilities for individuals and populations

Exposure distributions (probability density functions and cumulative distribution functions of exposure) for individuals can be significantly different from the corresponding distributions within the entire population. For example, a bimodal distribution can be expected for those individuals exposed both in the workplace and at home. Consequently, population strata need to be characterized to achieve the data quality objectives. Exposure distributions which should be developed include individuals expected to experience the highest long-term exposures, individuals expected to experience the highest short-term exposures, and special or susceptible segments of the population.

As mentioned above, log normal distributions of integrated exposures are commonly employed, and they also have been suggested as a 'default' when case-specific information is not available (US Environmental Protection Agency 1992a). The log normal distribution has the correct right-skewed general shape for high exposures, is flexible and possesses mathematical properties that make its mathematical manipulation easy. However, its adoption in a particular study should be viewed with caution because log normality of a random variable implies certain assumptions regarding underlying physical processes. Other alternatives, such as asymptotic distributions for extreme values (e.g. bi-exponential), could potentially provide more appropriate information for risk analyses.

Attributes related to the potential target population and sensitive subpopulations should include: (a) plausible contact patterns with the contaminants for different routes of exposure; (b) spatial population distribution stratification by age and gender; and (c) identification of subgroups of people sharing potentially similar exposure patterns. As stated earlier, identification of time–activity patterns for potentially exposed populations, (schoolchildren versus adults, men versus women, office workers versus outdoor workers) and of spatial distributions of target population groups is essential for exposure assessments.

Uncertainties and variation

A key problem in exposure assessment is distinguishing between contributions to exposure which are uncertain due to a lack of knowledge, and those which vary from one element of a population to another over time and space (Mandel 1969; Bogen 1990; Frey 1992; Hoffman 1993). Uncertain quantities are modelled using probability distributions, while variable quantities are modelled using frequency distributions. In principle the frequency distribution for a population reflects true differences between individuals. From the variability of the population, a frequency distribution can be used to determine if the population should be separated into subgroups by age, gender, racial and ethnic groups, and by locating susceptible subgroups exposed to a contaminant.

In contrast, there may be uncertainty in identifying the characteristics of specific individuals within a population, due to systematic and random error in a measurement and analysis technique. In these cases, there is uncertainty about the variability of the frequency distribution. Thus, a population distribution of exposure can be variable and uncertain at the same time. Furthermore, variability can be misinterpreted as uncertainty in specific situations. Usually, there are distinctions between variability and uncertainty. Understanding variability guides the identification of subpopulations which may require the development of purposive studies (see Table 32.6). In contrast, knowing the degree of uncertainty of characteristic features of a population can be used to determine the research strategies needed to reduce uncertainty. Sorting out the differences between uncertainty and variability, however, requires independent characterizations.

Probability distribution models can be affected by a small sample size. In some cases only a few data points are available for quantities such as the mean, variance, and distribution. A confidence interval should be calculated only when the mean and variance of the distribution are well established with large numbers of samples or data. A small sample size will increase the uncertainty in the mean and the variance. Calculation of tolerance intervals is a method for identifying sources of uncertainty (Mandel 1969).

Uncertainty about the underlying distribution of a variable can limit the applicability of standard statistical tests. Most tolerance and confidence intervals assume a normal distribution for all measurements. In cases where measurement error dominates the observed variance, this assumption may be reasonable; however, when there is significant interindividual variability, a skewed distribution can result. In this case, tolerance and confidence intervals based on an assumption of normality will not provide valid information on error. Thus, it is important to view statistical tests as only one component in determining the accuracy of the exposure data.

Summary

The field of exposure analysis and its application to public health practices provide information and understanding of the variety of ways an individual or population comes into contact with a contaminant. The approach must be framed within a conceptual framework that can involve multiple disciplines and interdisciplinary studies. Calculations of exposure and dose are data intensive and many times require situation-specific or site-specific data to characterize exposure accurately. Finally, the scientific approaches employed to establish measurement and modelling procedures must incorporate information on biological mechanisms or health outcomes.

Acknowledgements

The author wishes to thank Roberta Salinger for typing the manuscript and Jason Lioy for graphics. The work is supported by an NIEHS Center Grant No. ES 05022 and the ATSDR Exposure Characterization Program No. ATU 298949.

References

American Industrial Health Council (AIHC) (1994). *Exposure factors handbook*, Sections 1–7. AIHC, Washington, DC.

Andelman, J.B. (1985). Inhalation exposure in the home to volatile organic contaminants of drinking water. *Science of the Total Environment*, **47**, 443–60.

Anderson-Sprecher, R., Flatman, G.T., and Borgman, L. (1994). Environmental sampling: a brief review. *Journal of Experimental Analysis and Environment Epidemiology*, **4**, 115–32.

Ashley, D.L., Bonin, M.A., Cardinali, F.L., *et al.* (1992). Determining volatile organic compounds in human blood from a large sample population by purse and trap gas chromatography\mass spectrometry. *Analytical Chemistry*, **64**, 1021–29.

Bogen, K.T. (1990) *Uncertainty in environmental risk assessment*. Garland Publishing, New York.

Brown, S.H., Bishop, O.R., and Rowan, C.A. (1984). The role of skin absorption as a route of exposure to volatile organic compounds in drinking water. *American Journal of Public Health*, **74**, 479–92.

Carpenter, G.J. and Huston-Stein, A. (1980). Activity, structure and sex-typed behavior in pre-school children. *Child Development*, **51**, 862–72.

Caudill, S.P. and Pirkle, J.L. (1992). Effects of measurement error on estimating biological half-life. *Journal of Experimental Analysis and Environmental Epidemiology*, **2**, 463–76.

Cohen, Y. (1989). Multimedia and intermedia transport modeling concepts in environmental monitoring. In *Intermedia pollutant transport: modelling and field measurements* (ed. D.T. Allen, I.R. Kaplan, and Y. Cohen). Plenum Press, New York.

Donigian, A.S. and Mulkey, L.A. (1992). STREAM, an exposure assessment methodology for agricultural pesticide runoff. In *Fate of pesticides and chemicals in the environment* (ed. J.L. Schnoor). Wiley, New York.

Duan, N. (1982). Models for human exposure to air pollution. *Environment International*, **8**, 805–9.

Duan, N. (1991). Stochastic microenvironment models for air pollution exposure. *Journal of Experimental Analysis and Environmental Epidemiology*, **1**, 235–57.

Fenske, R.A., Curry, P.B., Wandelmaier, F., and Ritter, L. (1991). Development of dermal and respiratory sampling procedures for human exposure to pesticides. *Indoor Environment*, **1**, 11–30.

Fiserova-Bergerova, V. (1987). Development of biological exposure indices (BEIs) and their implementation. *Applied Industrial Hygiene*, **2**, 87–92.

Freeman, N.C.G., Waldman, J., and Lioy, P.J. (1991). Design and evaluation of a location and activity log used for assessing personal exposure to air pollutants. *Journal of Experimental Analysis and Environmental Epidemiology*, **1**, 327–38.

Frey, H.C. (1992). *Quantitative analysis of uncertainty and variability in environmental policy making, AAAS/US EPA Environmental Science and Engineering Fellow Program*. American Association for the Advancement of Science, Washington, DC.

Georgopoulos, P.G. (1990). *The EOHSI compendium of air quality models—1990*. Ozone Research Center Technical Report ORC–TR901101. Environmental and Occupational Health Sciences Institute, Piscataway, New Jersey.

Georgopoulos, P. and Lioy, P.J. (1994) Conceptual and theoretical aspects of exposure and dose assessment. *Journal of Experimental Analysis and Environmental Epidemiology*, **4**, 253–85.

Georgopoulos, P.G., Roy, A., and Gallo, M. (1994). Reconstruction of exposure using physiologically based pharmacokinetic models. Exposure compounds analysis edition. *Environments and Epidemiology*, **4**, 1–20.

Gerlowsky, L.E. and Jain, R.K. (1983). Physiologically based pharmacokinetic models: principles and applications. *Journal of Pharmacological Science*, **72**, 1103–27.

Graham, J., Walker, K.D., Berry, M., *et al.* (1992). Role of exposure databases in risk assessment. *Archives of Environmental Health*, **47**, 408–21.

Hattis, D.B. and Burmaster, D.E. (1994) Some thoughts on choosing distributions for practical risk analyses. *Risk Analysis*.

Hawley, J.K. (1985). Assessment of health risk from exposure to contaminated soils, *Risk Analysis*, **5**, 282–302.

Henderson, R.F., Bechtold, W.E., and Maples, K.R. (1992). Biological markers as measure of exposure. *Journal of Experimental Analysis and Environmental Epidemiology*, **23** (Supplement 2), 1–14.

Hoffman, F.O. (1993). *Propagation of uncertainty in risk assessments: the need to distinguish between uncertainty due to lack of knowledge and uncertainty due to variability*. US PEA/University of Virginia Workshop on When and How Can You Specify a Probability Distribution When You Don't Know Much. University of Virginia, Charlottesville, Virginia.

Javandel, I., Doughty, C., and Tsang, C.F. (1984). *Groundwater transport: handbook of mathematical models*. AGU Water Resources Monograph 10, Washington, DC.

Jayjock, M.A. and Hawkins, N.C. (1993). A proposal for improving the role of exposure modelling in risk assessment. *American Industrial Hygiene Association Journal*, **54**, 733–41.

Jo, W.K., Weisel, C., and Lioy, P.J. (1990). Routes of exposure and body burden from showering with chlorinated tap water. *Risk Analysis*, **10**, 575–80.

Kitsa, V., Lioy, P.J., Chow, J.C., *et al.* (1992). Particle size distribution of total and hexavalent chromium in inspirable, thoracic and respirable soils from contaminated sites in New Jersey. *Aerosol Science and Technology*, **17**, 213–29.

Lioy, P.J. (1990*a*). The analysis of total human exposure for exposure assessment: a multi-discipline science for examining human contact with contaminants. *Environmental Science and Technology*, **24**, 938–45.

Lioy, P.J. (1990*b*) *Community air sampling strategies. Air sampling instruments*, 7th edn. (ed. S.S. Hering). ACGIH, Cincinnati, Ohio.

Lioy, P.J. (1992). Exposure analysis and the biological response to a contaminant: a melding necessary for environmental health sciences, *Journal of Experimental Analysis and Environmental Epidemiology*, **2**, (Supplement 1), 19–24.

Lioy, P.J. (1993). *Measurement of personal exposure to air pollution: status and needs, measurement challengers in atmospheric chemistry*, Advances in Chemistry Series No. 232, pp.373–92. American Chemical Society, Washington, DC.

Lioy, P.J. and Pellizzari, E. (1995) An approach to the design of a national survey of human exposure. *Journal of Experimental Analysis and Environmental Epidemiology*, **5**, 425–44.

Lioy, P.J., Weisel, C.P., Jo, W.K., Pellizzari, E., and Raymer, J.H. (1994) Microenvironmental and personal measurements of methyl-tertiary butyl ether (MTBE) associated with automobile use activities. *Journal of Experimental Analysis and Environmental Epidemiology*, **4**, 424–44.

Lippmann, M. and Lioy, P.J. (1986). Critical issues in air pollution epidemiology. *Environmental Health Perspectives*, **62**, 243–58.

Lodge, J.P. (1989). *Methods of air sampling and analysis*, 3rd edn, pp.1–763. Lewis Publishers, Chelsea, Michigan.

Mandel, J. (1969). *The statistical analysis of experimental data*. Wiley, New York.

Marnicio, R.J., Hakkinen, P.J., Lutkenhoff, S.D., Hertzberg, R.C., and Moskowitz, P.D. (1991). Risk analysis software and databases: review of riskware '90 conference and exhibition. *Risk Analysis*, **11**, 545–60.

McKone, T.E. (1991) Human exposure to chemicals from multiple media and through multiple pathways: research overview and comments. *Risk Analysis*, **11**, 5–10.

National Research Council (1989*a*). *Subcommittee report on biologic markers in pulmonary toxicology*, pp.1–1437. National Academy Press, Washington, DC.

National Research Council (1989*b*). *Subcommittee on Reproductive and Neurodevelopmental Toxicology Committee on Biological Markers, Report on biologic markers in reproductive toxicology*, pp.1–395. National Academy Press, Washington, DC.

National Research Council (1991*a*). *Environmental epidemiology*, Vol. 1. *Public health and hazardous wastes*, pp.1–282. National Academy Press, Washington, DC.

National Research Council (1991*b*). *Frontiers in assessing human exposures to environmental toxicants*, pp.1–65. National Academy Press, Washington, DC.

National Research Council (1991*c*). *Human exposure assessment for airborne pollutants: advances and opportunities*, pp.1–321. National Academy Press, Washington, DC.

National Research Council (1993*a*). *Measuring lead exposure in infants, children, and other sensitive populations*, pp.1–397. National Academy Press, Washington, DC.

National Research Council (1993*b*). *Pesticides in the diets of infants and children*, pp.1–386. National Academy Press, Washington, DC.

Ott, W. (1980). *Models of human exposure to air pollution*. Technical Report No. 32. Department of Statistics, Stanford University, California.

Ott, W.R. (1990). Total human exposure: basic concepts, EPA field studies, and future research needs. *Journal of Air and Waste Management Association*, **40**, 966–75.

Ott, W., Thomas, J., Mage, D., and Wallace, L. (1988). Validation of the simulation of human activity and pollution exposure (SHAPE) model using paired days from the Denver, Colorado, carbon monoxide field study. *Atmosphere Environment*, **22**, 2101–13.

Pardi, R.R. (1992). IMES: a system for identifying and evaluation computer models for exposure assessment. *Risk Analysis*, **11**, 319–21.

Patrick, D.R. (1994). *Toxic air pollution handbook*, pp.1–588. Van Nestrand, Reinhold, New York.

Pellizzari, E., Lioy, P.J., Witmore, R., *et al.* (in press). National Human Exposure Assessment Survey (NHEXAS): a pilot study in EPA region V. *Journal of Exposure Analysis and Environmental Epidemiology*, **5**, 327–58.

Perera, F.P., Santella, R.M., Brenner, D., *et al.* (1987). DNA adducts, protein adducts, sister chromatid exchange in cigarette smokers and non-smokers. *Journal of the National Cancer Institute*, **79**, 449–56.

Robinson, J.P., Wiley, J.A., Piazza, J., and Gerrett, K. (1989). *Activity patterns of California residents and their implications for potential exposure to pollution*, CARB-A6-177-33. California Air Resources Board, Sacramento, California.

Rubinstein, R.Y. (1981). *Simulation and the Monte Carlo methods*. Wiley, New York.

Ruby, M.V., Davis, A., Link, T.E., *et al.* (1993). Development of an '*in vitro*' screening test to evaluate the '*in vivo*' bioaccessibility of ingested mine-waste lead. *Environmental Science and Technology*, **27**, 2870–7.

Ryan, P.B. (1991) An overview of human exposure modelling. *Journal of Experimental Analysis and Environmental Epidemiology*, **1**, 453–74.

Ryan, P.B., Spengler, J.D., and Letz, R. (1986). Estimating personal exposures to NO_2. *Environment International*, **12**, 395–400.

Samet, J.M., Marbury, M.C., and Spengler, J.D. (1987). Health effects of sources of indoor air pollution I. *American Review of Respiratory Disease*, **136** 1466.

Samet, J.M., Marbury, M.C., and Spengler, J.D. (1988). Health effect of sources of indoor air pollution II. *American Review of Respiratory Disease*, **137**, 221.

Schwab, M., Teiblanche, A.P.S., and Spengler, J.D. (1991). Self reported exertion levels on time/activity diaries. *Application to Exposure Assessment*, **1**, 339–56.

Seifert, B. and Abraham, H.J. (1983). Use of passive samplers for the determination of gaseous organic substances in indoor air at low concentration levels. *International Journal of Environmental Analytical Chemistry*, **13**, 237–54.

Sexton, K. (1995). Overview and introduction to the National Human Exposure Assessment Survey (NHEXAS): the value of human exposure information. *Journal of Experimental Analysis and Environmental Epidemiology*, **5**, 229–32.

Sexton, K. and Ryan, P.B. (1988). *Assessment of human exposure to air pollution: methods, measurements and models, air pollution: the automobile and public health*, pp. 207–38. National Academy Press, Washington, DC.

Sexton, K., Seleven, S.G., Wagener, D.K., and Lybarger, J.A. (1992). Estimating human exposure to environmental pollutants: availability and utility of existing databases. *Archives of Environmental Health*, **47**, 398–407.

Thibodeaux, L.J. (1979). *Chemodynamics: environmental movement of chemicals in air, water, and soil*, Wiley, New York.

Umbreit, T.H., Hesse, E.J., and Gallo, M.A. (1986). Bioavailability of dioxin in soil from a 2, 4, 5, 8 TCDD manufacturing site. *Science*, **232**, 945–7.

US Environmental Protection Agency (1980). *Federal register* 79318–79379.

US Environmental Protection Agency (1988). *Total Human Exposure Research Council (THERC). Research needs in human exposure: a 5-year comprehensive assessment (1990–1994)*. Office of Research and Development, Washington, DC.

US Environmental Protection Agency (1989*a*). *Exposure factors handbook*, EPA/600/08–89/043. Office of Health and Environmental Assessment, Washington, DC.

US Environmental Protection Agency (1989*b*). *Interim on benzene exposure assessment model* (BEAM), EPA 600/X89/015. EMSL, Las Vegas, Nevada.

US Environmental Protection Agency (1991). *Human exposure model, II. User's guide (draft)*. Office of Air Quality Planning and Standards, US EPA, Research Triangle Park, North Carolina.

US Environmental Protection Agency (1992a). *Guidelines for exposure assessment*, FRL–4129. Federal Register, Washington DC.

US Environmental Protection Agency (1992b). *A Monte Carlo approach to simulating residential occupancy periods and its applications to the general population*. EPA–450/3–92–011. Office of Air Quality Planning and Standards, USECA, Research Triangle Park, NC.

Wainman, T., Hazen, R., and Lioy, P. (1994) The extractability of CR(VI) from contaminated soil in synthetic sweat. *Journal of Experimental Analysis and Environmental Epidemiology*, **4**, 171–81.

Wallace, L.A. (1989). Major sources of benzene exposure. *Environmental Health Perspectives*, **82**, 165–9.

Weisel, C.P., Jo, W.K. and Lioy, P.J. (1993). Utilization of breath analysis for exposure and dose estimates of chloroform. *Journal of Exposure Analysis and Environmental Epidemiology*, **2** (Supplement 1), 55–69.

33 Risk assessment, risk communication, and risk management

Gilbert S. Omenn and Elaine M. Faustman

Introduction

Risk assessment as an organized activity of the federal agencies in the United States began in the 1970s. Earlier, the American Conference of Governmental Industrial Hygienists had set threshold limited values for exposures of workers and the Food and Drug Administration (**FDA**) had set acceptable daily intakes for dietary pesticide residues and food additives. In the 'Delaney Clause' of 1958, Congress instructed the FDA to prohibit substances found to cause cancer in animals (or humans, of course) from being used as food additives that could reach humans through the food supply. For some time, it was pragmatic to declare safe any food sources in which standard tests found no evidence of these chemicals (Albert 1994). Advances in analytical chemistry, however, exposed the fact that 'not detectable' was not the same as 'not present' or 'zero risk'. The agencies had to develop 'tolerance levels' and 'acceptable risk levels'.

In the mid–1970s the US Environmental Protection Agency (**EPA**) and the FDA issued guidance for estimating risks from low-level exposures to potentially carcinogenic chemicals (Albert 1994). Their guidance made estimated risks of one extra cancer lifetime per 100 000 people (EPA, at first) or per 1 000 000 people (FDA) action levels for regulatory attention. These estimated incremental risks represent very conservative acceptable or negligible risk levels, since cancers claim the lives of 230 000 of every 1 million people in the United States. Thus, the regulatory agencies sought to prevent an increase from a countable 23 per cent of deaths due to cancers to an estimated risk of 23.0001 per cent. Furthermore, as explained later, these estimates represent worst-case or 'upper bound' estimates, not actuarial counts like the 230 000 cancer deaths per million deaths in the general population. A safety-factor approach, for example, generating an 'acceptable daily intake', is more commonly used in other countries.

During the 1977 to 1980 period, an Interagency Regulatory Liaison Group was actively engaged in bridging scientific, statutory, and policy responsibilities and the activities of the EPA and the FDA, the Occupational Safety and Health Administration (**OSHA**), and the Consumer Product Safety Commission (**CPSC**). The White House Office of Science and Technology Policy participated in the scientific discussions supporting risk assessment and risk management (Calkins *et al.* 1980). A framework was developed for identifying potential hazards, characterizing the risks

and managing the risks, usually by reduction of use or reduction of exposures (see Table 33.1).

A National Research Council (1983) report on 'Risk assessment in the Federal Government: managing the process', subsequently called *The red book*, helped the regulatory agencies set in gear a common framework for assessing risks from chemicals. *The red book* provided a framework (Table 33.2) for the hazard identification and risk characterization components of the risk assessment/risk management framework in Table 33.1. A strong research base is an essential aspect (Office of Technology Assessment 1992; Faustman and Omenn 1996).

Table 33.1 Framework for regulatory decision making about potential hazards to health and the environment: risk assessment and risk management

1. Identification of hazard	Epidemiology Toxicology *In vitro* tests Structure–activity relationships
2. Characterization of risk	Potency Exposures Susceptibility
3. Control of risk	Information Regulation Substitution

Based on Calkins *et al.* (1980) and Omenn (1984).

Table 33.2 Framework for risk assessment from "*The red book*" (NRC 1983)

Hazard identification: can the agent cause the adverse effect?

Dose–response assessment: what is the relationship between dose and incidence of adverse effects in humans or in animals?

Exposure assessment: what exposures are currently experienced or can be anticipated under various circumstances?

Risk characterization: what is the estimated incidence of the adverse effect in a given population or subpopulation? What is the nature of the effect? What is the strength of the evidence?

Definitions

Risk assessment is the systematic scientific characterization of potential adverse health effects resulting from human exposures to hazardous agents or situations (National Research Council 1983; Faustman and Omenn 1996). Risk is defined as the probability of an adverse outcome. The term 'hazard' is used by North Americans to refer to intrinsic toxic properties; internationally, this term is defined as the probability of an adverse outcome. This chapter presents risk assessment approaches for both cancer and non-cancer hazards. Analogous approaches can be applied to ecological risks (National Research Council, Committee on Risk Assessment Methodology 1993). The objectives of risk assessment are outlined in Table 33.4 (see below).

Both qualitative assessment of the nature of effects and strength of the evidence and quantitative estimation of the risk are essential components of the risk characterization (Tables 33.1 and 33.2). We want to emphasize the importance of the phrase 'characterization of risk', since many public health practitioners, environmentalists, and regulators tend to equate risk assessment with quantitative risk assessment, getting a number (or a number with uncertainty bounds), and ignoring crucial information about the strength of the evidence, the nature of the health effect, and the means of avoiding or reversing effects of exposure.

Risk management refers to the process by which policy actions are chosen to deal with hazards identified in the risk assessment/risk characterization process. Risk managers consider the scientific evidence and risk estimates together with statutory, engineering, economic, social, and political factors in evaluating alternative regulatory options, selecting among the options, and discussing those options with interested parties, the stakeholders. Risk communication is the challenging process of making risk assessment and risk management information comprehensible to community groups, lawyers, politicians, judges, business people, labour, and environmentalists. Often these people have important inputs for various stages of this process, so listening is a crucial, too-often-neglected aspect of risk communication. Sometimes the decision-makers and stakeholders simply want to know the 'bottom line': is a substance or a situation 'safe' or not? Others will be interested in knowing why the risk estimates are uncertain and complicated and may be eager to challenge underlying assumptions. Risk management decisions are reached under diverse statutes in the United States (Table 33.3) and analogous statutes or regulations in other countries.

Some statutes specify reliance on risk alone, while others require a balancing of risks and benefits of the product or activity (Table 33.4). Risk assessment has provided a valuable framework for priority setting within regulatory and health agencies, in the development process within companies, and in resource allocation in environmental organizations. Similar statutes and regulatory regimes have been developed in many other countries and through such international organizations as the International Programme for Chemical Safety (**IPCS**) of the World Health Organization (**WHO**). There is growing interest in the harmonization of testing protocols and assessment of risks and standards.

A major challenge for risk assessment, risk communication, and better risk management is to demonstrate the biological plausibility and clinical significance of the conclusions from epidemiological,

Table 33.3 Major toxic chemical laws in the US and agency responsible

EPA	Air pollutants	Clean Air Act 1970, 1977, 1990
	Water pollutants	Federal Water Pollution Control Act 1972, 1977
	Drinking water	Safe Drinking Water Act 1974
	Pesticides	Fungicides, Insecticides, & Rodenticides Act (**FIFRA**) 1972
	Ocean dumping	Marine Protection Research, Sanctuaries Act 1972
		Ocean Radioactive Dumping Ban Act 1995
	Toxic chemicals	Toxic Substances Control Act (**TSCA**) 1976
	Hazardous wastes	Resource Conservation & Recovery Act (**RCRA**) 1976
	Abandoned hazardous wastes	Superfund (**CERCLA**) 1980, 1986
CEQ	Environmental impacts	National Environmental Policy Act (**NEPA**) 1969
OSHA	Work-place	Occupational Safety and Health (**OSH**) Act 1970
FDA	Foods, drugs, and cosmetics	FDC Acts 1906, 1938, 1962, 1977
CPSC	Dangerous consumer products	Consumer Product Safety Act
DOT	Transport of hazardous materials	THM Act 1975, 1976, 1978, 1979, 1984, 1990 (×2)

EPA, Environmental Protection Agency; CEQ, Council for Environmental Quality (now Office of Environmental Policy); OSHA, Occupational Safety of Health Administration; FDA, Food and Drug Administration; CPSC, Consumer Product Safety Commission; DOT, Department of Transportation.

lifetime animal, short-term, and structure–activity studies of chemicals thought to have potential adverse effects on human health and the environment. Biomarkers of exposure, effect, or

Table 33.4 Objectives of risk assessment

Balance risks and benefits

    Drugs
    Pesticides

Set target levels of risk

    Food contaminants
    Water pollutants

Set priorities for programme activities

    Regulatory agencies
    Manufacturers
    Environmental/consumer organizations

Estimate residual risks and extent of risk reduction after steps are taken to reduce risks individual susceptibility can link the presence of a chemical in various environmental compartments to specific sites of action in target organs and to host responses (National Research Council 1989a,b, 1992a,b). Mechanistic investigations of the actions of specific chemicals can help us penetrate the black box approach of simply counting tumours in exposed animals and better appreciation of the mechanisms and extent of individual variation in susceptibility between humans can help us better protect subgroups of people and better relate findings in animals to risk estimates in humans. Individual behavioural risk factors and social risk factors are important too and can be brought into this characterization. In public policy and public health practice, public and media attitudes toward the local polluters, other apparently responsible parties, and responsible government agencies may be critically important, reflecting what has been labelled 'the outrage factor' by Sandman (1993). Thus, all of the public health sciences are needed for comprehensive risk assessment and risk management.

Effective two-way communication with stakeholders and thoughtful justification of the policy implications arising from choices of assumptions in weighing the evidence, extrapolating beyond actual observations, and estimating the variability and uncertainties must be combined with the 'best science'. This concept was captured in the title of the National Research Council, Committee on Risk Assessment of Hazardous Air Pollutants (1994) report 'Science and judgment in risk assessment'.

This chapter reviews the status of certain facets of the framework approach and its application to environmental health problems. For details about the contributing scientific fields, please see the preceding chapters in the environmental health sciences section of the textbook and other relevant chapters on epidemiologic approaches, determinants of health and disease, and public health functions.

Hazard identification: epidemiology, lifetime rodent bioassay, short-term tests, and structure-activity relationships

Epidemiology

The most convincing evidence for human risk is a well-conducted epidemiologic study in which a positive association between exposure and disease has been observed. Epidemiologic approaches are basically opportunistic. Studies begin with known or presumed exposures, comparing exposed versus non-exposed individuals or with known cases, compared with persons lacking the particular diagnosis. There are important limitations. When the study is exploratory, hypotheses are often weak. Exposure estimates are often crude and retrospective, in particular for conditions with a long latency before clinical manifestations appear. Generally, there are multiple exposures, in particular when a full week or a full lifetime is considered. Lifestyle factors, such as smoking and diet, may be important and are difficult to sort out. There is always a trade-off between detailed information on relatively few persons and very limited information on large numbers of persons. Humans are highly outbred, so the method must consider variation in susceptibility between people who are exposed. Finally, the expression of results (odds ratios, relative risks, and confidence intervals) may be unfamiliar to non-epidemiologists and the caveats self-effacing epidemiologists cite often discourage risk managers (Omenn 1993).

Epidemiology is in the midst of a transformation. Biomarkers and mechanistic hypotheses are helping us 'get inside the black box' of statistical associations to gain an understanding that enhances biological plausibility and clinical relevance (National Research Council 1989a,b; 1992a,b) and some hypotheses of causative relationships are being tested with prevention clinical trials, like CARET, the B-Carotene and Retinol Efficacy Trial to prevent lung cancer in high-risk smokers and asbestos-exposed workers (Omenn et al. 1994). Environmental exposure reduction actions should be considered analogues of such prevention trials.

As noted in The red book, many questions arise in the assessment of results from epidemiologic studies, for example the following:

1. What relative weights should be given to studies with differing results? Should positive results override negative results? Should a study be weighted in accord with its statistical power? Its quality? Are there certain kinds of flaws, such as in choice of the control or comparison group, that should make a study be disregarded altogether?

2. What relative weights should be given to the results from different types of epidemiological studies? Should the findings of a prospective study supersede those of a case–control study or case–control findings supersede ecological findings?

3. What statistical significance should be required for results to be considered positive? Should that criterion be different for the primary hypothesis than for correlations which arise from massaging the data afterward?

4. What is the significance of a positive finding in a study in which the route of exposure is different from that under analysis?

5. Should evidence for different types of tumour responses be combined (for example, different tumour sites or benign versus malignant tumours)? What about cancer and non-cancer endpoints?

Lifetime rodent bioassays

Bioassays have been developed as standardized, experimental protocols to identify chemicals capable of causing cancers, birth defects, neurotoxicity, or other toxicity in laboratory animals. Typically, one chemical is tested at a time in rats and mice, both sexes, with 50 animals per dose group and near lifetime exposure to 90, 50, and 10 to 25 per cent of what is determined in preliminary studies to be the maximally tolerated dose. Based on results from 379 long-term carcinogenicity studies, Haseman and Lockhart (1993) concluded that most target sites showed a strong correlation (65 per cent) between males and females, in particular for forestomach, liver, and thyroid tumours; in fact, for efficiency they suggested that bioassays could rely on a combination of male rats and female mice, thereby cutting in half the number of animals required for a lifetime rodent bioassay—and assuming that other uses would be found for the female rats and male mice! Estimation and use of the maximally tolerated dose is a vexing problem, not at all resolved by a recent panel on the subject (National Research Council, Committee on Risk Assessment Methodology 1993) or by others troubled by toxicity or cell proliferation responses at maximal dose that may be not at all representative of responses at lower doses (Ames and Gold 1990).

Results must be extrapolated from high dose to low dose, and then from animals to humans. Such extrapolations require numerous choices, most importantly the choice of data set, plus assumptions about the dose–response curve from observations in the 10 to 100 per cent range down to 10^{-6} risk estimates at the upper confidence limit or use of a bench-mark or reference dose approach (see below). Lifetime bioassays can be enhanced by investigations of mechanisms and assessment of multiple endpoints in the same study. It is feasible and desirable to tie these bioassays together with mechanistically oriented, short-term tests and biomarker and genetic studies in epidemiology. *The red book* questions here remain important:

1. Is a positive result from a single animal study sufficient or should positive results from two or more animal studies be required? Should studies be weighted according to their quality and statistical power? Should negative results of similar quality be given less weight?

2. How should evidence of different metabolic pathways or very different metabolic rates between animals and humans be factored into a risk assessment? Substantial advances in the past decade are discussed later in this chapter.

Short-term tests

Many chemicals in widespread commerce have not been tested adequately for risk assessment purposes (National Research Council 1984) and the costs of $1 to $2 million and 3 to 5 years' work per chemical tested are prohibitive in the aggregate. Thus, there is a major interest in devising inexpensive, short-term tests for screening chemicals. These tests can also yield important information about mechanisms, distinguishing genotoxic from non-genotoxic effects between carcinogens, for example. The *Salmonella* reverse mutation test ('Ames test') and certain cytogenetic tests, especially of bone marrow following *in vivo* exposure, seem useful and robust. Nevertheless, progress has been slow and frustrating. Many years have been spent trying to make the mouse lymphoma test and the sister chromatid exchange assay interpretable for risk assessment purposes. In recent years, short-term tests for non-cancer endpoints such as developmental toxicity, reproductive toxicity, neurotoxicity, and immunotoxicity have become available (Atterwill *et al.* 1992; Harris *et al.* 1992; Shelby *et al.* 1993; Whittaker and Faustman 1994; Faustman and Omenn 1996). Mechanistic information from these systems has been applied to risk assessment (Abbott *et al.* 1992; EPA 1994*a*; Leroux *et al.* 1995).

An emerging class of short-term tests utilizes transgenic mouse models. Tennant *et al.* (1995) have shown that mutagenic carcinogens can be identified with high sensitivity and specificity using hemizygous p53 (+/−) mice in which one allele of the *p53* gene has been inactivated. A TG.AC transgenic mouse carrying a *V-Ha-ras* gene construct developed papillomas and malignant tumours in response to mutagenic and non-mutagenic carcinogens and tumour promoters, but not in response to non-carcinogens. It is likely that these animal models will supplant at least part of the two-species, two-sex rodent bioassay in the next decade.

Structure–activity relationships

A chemical's structure, solubility, stability, pH sensitivity, electrophilicity, chemical reactivity, and pathways of metabolism can be important information for hazard identification by inference. Historically, certain key molecular structures have provided regulators with some of the most readily available information on which to assess hazard potential. For example, the majority of the first 14 occupational carcinogens regulated by the OSHA belonged to the aromatic amine chemical class. The US EPA Office of Toxic Substances relies on structure–activity relationships (**SARs**) to meet deadlines for responses to premanufacturing notices for new chemicals under Toxic Substances Control Act (TSCA) (see Table 33.3). *N*-Nitroso, aromatic amine, amino azo, and phenanthrene structures are alerts to prioritize chemicals for additional evaluation as potential carcinogens. Chemicals with structures related to valproic acid or retinoic acid are suspected as developmental toxicants (Faustman and Omenn 1996).

Structure–activity relationships can be used in assessing the relative toxicity of chemically related compounds. A prominent example was the EPA's reassessment of health risks associated with 2,3,7,8-tetrachlorodibenzo-*p*-dioxin and related chlorinated and brominated dibenzo-*p*-dioxins, dibenzofurans, and planar biphenyls, using toxicity equivalence factors (**TEFs**), based on induction of the *Ah* receptor (EPA 1994*c*). The estimated toxicity of environmental mixtures containing these chemicals is the sum of the product of the concentration of each multiplied by its TEF value.

Integrating hazard identification information

A remarkable collegial effort to relate the findings of short-term tests to the presumed gold standard of the lifetime rodent cancer bioassay result was conducted between 1989 and 1994 under the aegis of the National Toxicology Program (**NTP**) and the National Institute of Environmental Health Sciences. For a set of 44 consecutive chemicals entered into the NTP lifetime bioassay programme, Tennant *et al.* (1990) predicted the results, based upon knowledge of the structural features of the chemicals, results from short-term tests, and (sometimes) previous bioassay data. In response to their Carcinogen Prediction Challenge, nine other groups of scientists made predictions for the same set of chemicals, based on their own criteria. At the conclusion, an international workshop was held at which the NTP lifetime rodent bioassay results for 40 chemicals were revealed: 20 had clear or some evidence of carcinogenicity in one or more of the four species/sex groups of rats and mice, of whom 14 were clear positives and nine were positive in more than one organ site (National Institute of Environmental Health Sciences 1993; Ashby and Tennant 1994). Tennant *et al.* (1990) correctly predicted 75 per cent of the carcinogens (17 out of 20 carcinogens and 13 out of 20 non-carcinogens); thus, they had a ratio of false positives to false negatives of 2.3 (seven out of three), a sensitivity of 0.85 (17 out of 20), and a specificity of 0.65 (13 out of 20). None of the other groups did as well; some did no better than chance (National Institute of Environmental Health Sciences 1993; Omenn *et al.* 1995). They used combinations of computerized structural alerts or structure–activity relationships and results from *in vitro* and *in vivo* tests. The results reveal very different approaches to balancing false-negative versus false-positive outcomes, apparently with different implicit 'cut-points'.

Social cost analytical approaches have been published, relying upon short-term tests, lifetime rodent bioassays, or a combination of testing strategies to guide risk management for potentially hazardous chemicals. In the Lave–Omenn value-of-information model (Lave and Omenn 1986; Lave *et al.* 1988; Omenn and Lave 1988), 'cost effective' means that the costs of testing plus the social costs of false positives (loss of the economic value of the chemical) and of false negatives (economic value of the disease burden incurred as a result of use of the chemical) are less than the costs of misclassification by simply treating all chemicals as carcinogenic and avoiding exposures to the extent feasible. For example, we might set the cost/consequences of a false negative at $10 million, 10 times the social cost of a false positive, on the average. Then, for the Tennant *et al.* (1990) correct prediction of 30 out of 40 of the NTP results, the social cost of misclassification would be $7 million for the seven false positives plus $30 million for the three false negatives (Omenn *et al.* 1995). In the Lave–Omenn (1986) estimation, if the bioassay were used at $1 million per chemical tested and the true proportion of rodent carcinogens is assumed to be 10 per cent among tested chemicals, the testing ($40 million for 40 chemicals) would have to be 100 per cent accurate just to break even against the alternative of simply calling all chemicals carcinogenic for rodents. Such an alternative practice would require instituting general approaches to minimize exposures. If regulatory decisions could be based on interpretation of far less expensive short-term tests, the margin for cost-effective decision-making would be much greater (Omenn and Lave 1988). Thus, there is still considerable incentive to come up with more reliable, more predictive, short-term biological and structural approaches.

Risk characterization: dose–response, exposure analysis, variation in susceptibility, and relation of effects in rodents to risk in humans

As noted above, the characterization of risk involves more than quantitative estimation of the risk (with or without uncertainty bounds). Crucial information about the nature of health (and ecologic) risks, the strength of the evidence, the feasibility of prevention or treatment of the adverse effects, and the variation of risk in the population cannot be captured in a number; these attributes require careful qualitative and descriptive characterization that can be used in health advisories.

Dose–response

Analyses of dose–response relationships must start with the determination of the critical effect. Many chemicals have more than one adverse effect on health and/or ecological endpoints. We commonly choose the most strikingly positive data set, even if not representative, in order for the usual extrapolation models to function well in our computer models. Linearized multistage models or bench-mark dose approaches, depending on the endpoint, are used to estimate 'virtually safe doses', generally far below the observable range. We continue to use maximally tolerated dose regimens in animals, while awaiting better understanding of the

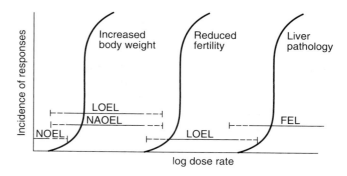

Fig. 33.1 Dose–Response curves with thresholds. Idealized dose–response curves for three different endpoints or effects. The parentheses indicate the ranges for experimental results categorized according to NOEL, NOAEL, LOEL, LOAEL, and FEL. Depending upon the quality of the data, some of these categories (for example, NOAEL and LOEL may overlap). Based on Hartung (1987).

underlying mechanisms on an organ site-by-organ site or a chemical-by-chemical basis.

The fundamental basis of the quantitative relationships between exposure to an agent and the incidence of an adverse response is the dose–response assessment. Approaches for characterizing dose–response relationships include effect levels such as LD_{50}, ED_{10}, and no observed adverse effect levels (NOAELs), margins of safety and therapeutic indexes, and various models for extrapolation to very low doses (National Research Council 1983).

For risk assessment purposes, human exposure data for the prediction of human response are usually quite limited. The risk assessor is interested in low environmental exposures of humans, which are way below the experimentally observable range of responses from animal assays. Thus, high- to low-dose extrapolation and animal to human risk extrapolation methods are required and comprise major aspects of dose–response assessment.

Figure 33.1 presents the concept of threshold and indicates that each response to an agent can have a separate threshold dose. In this example, progressively adverse responses are modelled, from changes in body weight, to reduced fertility, to liver pathology, with increasing dose. A 5 per cent increase in body weight would not be considered an adverse effect, only an effect level, hence the use of the no observed effect level (**NOEL**) and then lowest observed effect level (**LOEL**), as well as **NOAELs**, to describe this first curve. As doses increase and reduced fertility is observed, the NOAELs and then the lowest observed adverse effect levels (**LOAELs**) are noted. At higher doses, a frank effect level (**FEL**) signifies that signs of liver necrosis are observed.

The highest dose level that does not produce a significantly elevated increase in adverse response is called the NOAEL. Significance usually refers to both biological and statistical criteria (Faustman *et al.* 1994) and is dependent upon the number of dose levels tested, the number of animals tested at each dose, and the background incidence of the adverse response in the non-exposed control groups. The NOAEL should not be perceived as risk free; NOAELs for continuous endpoints average 5 per cent risk and NOAELs based on quantal endpoints can be associated with a risk of greater than 10 per cent (Allen 1994*a,b*; Faustman *et al.* 1994).

NOAELs can be used as a basis for risk assessment calculations, such as reference doses or acceptable daily intake values (Renwick and Walker 1993). Reference doses (**RfD**s) or concentrations (**RfC**s) are estimates of a daily exposure to an agent that is assumed to have no adverse health impact on the human population. Acceptable daily intake (**ADI**) values used by the WHO for pesticides and food additives define the daily intake of chemical, which during an entire lifetime appears to be without appreciable risk on the basis of all known facts at that time (WHO 1962). RFDs and ADI values are typically calculated from NOAEL values by dividing by uncertainty (**UF**) and/or modifying (**MF**) factors (EPA, 1991):

$$RfD = NOAEL / (UF \times MF)$$

$$ADI = NOAEL / (UF \times MF)$$

These safety factors allow for interspecies (animal to human) and intraspecies (human) variation with default values of 10 each. An additional 10-fold uncertainty factor is used to extrapolate from short-exposure duration studies to a situation more relevant for effects study or to account for inadequate numbers of animals or other experimental limitations. MFs can be used to adjust the uncertainty factors if data on mechanisms, pharmacokinetics, or relevance of the animal response to human risk justify such modification.

If only a LOAEL value is available, then an additional 10-fold factor is used routinely to arrive at a value more comparable to a NOAEL. Allen *et al.* (1994*a*) have shown for developmental toxicity endpoints that application of the 10-fold factor for LOAEL to NOAEL conversion is too large.

Another way the NOAEL values have been utilized for risk assessment is to evaluate a 'margin of exposure' (**MOE**) or 'margin of safety' (**MOS**), where the ratio of the NOAEL determined in animals and expressed as mg/kg/day is compared with the level to which a human may be exposed. For example, if human exposures are calculated to be via drinking water and the water supply in the equation contains 1 p.p.m. of the chemical, then the exposure per day would be 1 mg/l × 2 l/day − 50 kg = 0.04 mg/kg/day for a 50 kg woman. If the NOAEL for neurotoxicity is 100 mg/kg/day, then the MOE would be 2500 for the oral exposure route for neurotoxicity from the drinking water. Such a large value is reassuring for public health officials.

Low values of the MOE indicate that the human levels of exposure are close to levels for the NOAEL in animals. There is no factor included in this calculation for differences in human or animal susceptibility or animal to human extrapolation. Thus, MOE values of less than 100 have been used by regulatory agencies as flags for requiring further evaluation.

Some important common human exposures are so close to LOAELs—such as lead, particulates, sulphur oxides, ozone, and carbon monoxide, among air pollutants—that regulatory agencies use an informal margin of safety approach, heavily weighted with consideration of technical feasibility.

The NOAEL approach has been criticized on several points: the NOAEL must, by definition, be one of the experimental doses tested, once identified, the rest of the dose–response curve is ignored, experiments that test fewer animals often result in higher NOAELs and thus larger reference doses, despite greater uncertainty, and the NOAEL approach does not identify the actual

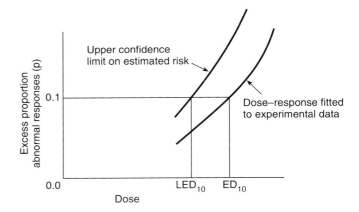

Fig. 33.2 Illustration of BMD approach. The LED_{10} is the lower confidence limit of the dose associated with a 10 per cent incidence of adverse effect. Based on Kavlock *et al.* (1995).

responses at the NOAEL and will vary based on experimental design, resulting in regulatory limits set at varying levels of risk.

Because of these limitations, an alternative to the NOAEL approach, the bench-mark dose (**BMD**) method, was proposed by Crump (1984) and extended by Kimmel and Gaylor (1988). In this approach the dose–response is modelled and the lower confidence bound for a dose at a specified response level is calculated. Figure 33.2 shows how a BMD is calculated using a 10 per cent bench-mark response and a 95 per cent lower confidence bound on dose. In this case, the RFD would be

$$RfD = BMD_{10} / UF \times MF$$

The values to be used for the uncertainty factors and modifying factors for BMDs can be the same factors as for the NOAEL or lower values due to use of the full dose–response curve and of a lower confidence bound on the dose (Barnes *et al.* 1995).

The BMD approach has been applied to non-cancer endpoints, including developmental (Allen *et al.* 1994*a,b*) and reproductive toxicity (Auton *et al.* 1994). BMD_5 values were similar to NOAELs for a wide range of developmental toxicity endpoints. A generalized log logistic dose–response model has advantages in dealing with litter size and intralitter correlations (Allen *et al.* 1994*b*).

The BMD approach has four advantages: it uses the full dose–response curve, as opposed to focusing on a single test dose, as in the NOAEL approach, it includes a measure of variability (lower confidence limit on dose associated with upper confidence limit on risk), it uses responses within the experimental range versus extrapolation of responses to low doses not tested experimentally (but then divides by those uncertainty factors), and it facilitates comparisons of a consistent bench-mark response level for RfD calculations across studies and agents.

Non-threshold approaches

Numerous dose–response curves can be proposed in the low-dose region of the dose–response curve if a threshold assumption is not made. Because the risk assessor generally needs to extrapolate far below the region of the dose–response curve for which experimentally observed data are available, the choice of models to generate curves in this region of the dose–response curve has received lots of

---

Table 33.5 Models used in risk extrapolation

Statistical or distribution models

    Log-probit
    Logit
    Weibull

Mechanistic models

    One hit
    Multihit
    Multistage
    Linearized multistage
    Stochastic two-stage model (Moolgavkar–Venson–Knudson)

Model enhancement

    Time-to-tumour response
    Physiologically based toxicokinetic models
    Biologically based dose–response models

---

attention. Two general types of dose–response model exist: statistical probability distribution models and mechanistic models (Krewski and Van Ryzin 1981). Table 33.5 lists common models that have been used in risk extrapolation.

The distribution models are based on the assumption that each individual has a tolerance level for a response test agent, a variable following a specific probability distribution for the cumulative dose–response function (Faustman and Omenn 1996).

The mathematical modelling approach to dose–response relationships tries to take account of the postulated biological mechanisms of response. Radiation research has spawned a series of 'hit models' for cancer modelling, where a 'hit' is defined as a critical cellular event that must occur before a toxic effect is produced. These models assume that an infinitely large number of targets exists, for example, in the DNA, the organism responds with a toxic response only after a minimum number of targets has been modified, a critical target is altered if a sufficient number of hits occurs, and the probability of a hit in the low-dose range of the dose–response curve is proportional to the dose of the toxicant (Brown 1984).

The simplest mechanistic model is the one-hit (one-stage) linear model in which only one hit or critical cellular interaction is required for a cell to be altered. For example, based on somatic mutation theory, a single mutational change would be sufficient for a cell to become neoplastic through a transformational event and dose-independent clonal expansion. The probability statement for these models is $(d) = 1 - \exp^{(-\lambda d)}$ where λd equals the number of hits occurring during a time period. A single molecule of a genotoxic carcinogen would have a minute but finite chance of causing a mutational event.

Armitage and Doll (1957) developed a multistage model for carcinogenesis based on the hypothesis that a series of ordered stages was required for a cell to undergo mutation, initiation, transformation, and progression to form a tumour. This relationship was generalized by Crump (1980) by maximizing the likelihood function over polynomials so that the probability statement is

$$P(d) = 1 - \exp\left[-\lambda_0 + \lambda d_1 + \lambda d_2 + \dots \lambda_1 d^k\right]$$

If the true value of λ_1 is replaced with λ_1^* (the upper confidence limit of λ_1), then a linearized multistage model can be derived where the expression is dominated by $(\lambda d^*)d$ at low doses. The slope on this confidence interval, q_1^*, is used by the EPA for quantitative cancer assessment. To obtain an upper 95 per cent confidence interval on risk, the q_1^* value (Δ risk/Δ dose in mg/kg/day) is multiplied by the amount of exposure (mg/kg/day). Thus, the upper bound estimate on risk (R) is calculated as

$$R = q_1^* \text{ risk(mg/kg/day)}^{-1} \times \text{exposure (mg/kg/day)}$$

This relationship has been used to calculate a 'virtually safe dose' (**VSD**) which represents the lower 95 per cent confidence limit on a dose that gives an 'acceptable level' of risk (for example, an upper confidence limit for 10^{-6} excess risk). Since both the q_1^* and VSD values are calculated using 95 per cent confidence intervals, the values are believed to represent conservative estimates.

The US EPA utilizes the linearized multistage (**LMS**) model to calculate 'unit risk estimates', for example, the increased individual lifetime risks of cancer over a 70 year lifespan for a 70 kg human breathing 1 μg/m^3 of contaminated air or drinking 2 litres of water contaminated at 1 p.p.m. (1 mg/l per day).

Toxicological enhancements of the models

Table 33.5 lists three areas of research that have improved the application of models used in risk extrapolation. Physiologically based toxicokinetic (**PBTK**) modelling generates 'internal effective doses' at target organ sites, rather than relying on single-value external exposure estimates. Biologically based dose–response (**BBDR**) modelling connects the generalized mechanistic models discussed in the previous section to specific biological processes. Measured rates are incorporated into the mechanistic equations to replace default or computer-generated values. For example, the Moolgavkar–Venson–Knudson (**MVK**) model is based on a two-stage model for carcinogenesis; two mutations are required for carcinogenesis and birth and death rates of cells are modelled through clonal expansion and tumour formation. This model has been applied to human epidemiologic data on retinoblastoma and to animal data of kidney and liver tumours in the 2–acetylaminofluorene (**2–AAF**) 'mega mouse' study, bladder cancer in saccharin-exposed rats, rat lung tumours following radiation exposure, rat liver tumours following N-nitrosomorpholine exposure, respiratory tract tumours following benzo[a]pyrene exposure, and mouse liver tumours following chlordane exposure (Cohen and Ellwein 1990; Moolgavkar and Luebeck 1990; National Research Council, Council on Risk Assessment Methodology 1993). Additional applications are needed to continue validation of the model. Kohn *et al.* (1993) and Anderson (1983) used PBPK and BBDR information to improve dioxin risk assessment. EPA relied on Ah receptor binding in its dioxin risk reassessment (EPA 1994*c*).

Development of biologically based dose–response models for endpoints other than cancer are limited; several approaches are being explored in developmental toxicity, utilizing cell cycle kinetics, enzyme activity, litter effects, and cytotoxicity as critical endpoints (Faustman *et al.* 1989; Shuey *et al.* 1994; Leroux et al. 1995). Unfortunately, there is a lack of specific, quantitative biological information for most toxicants and for most endpoints.

Table 33.6 Exposure scenarios for dioxin via ingestion of contaminated recreational fish

Central exposure estimate[b]

$$
LADD^{a} = \frac{\dfrac{3 \times 10^{-9} \text{ mg dioxin}}{\text{g fish}} \times \dfrac{150 \text{ g fish}}{\text{meal}} \times \dfrac{3 \text{ meals}}{\text{year}} \times \dfrac{1.0 \text{ contact}}{\text{fraction}}}{70 \text{ kg body weight} \times \dfrac{70 \text{ years}}{\text{lifetime}} \times \dfrac{365 \text{ days}}{\text{year}}}
$$

$$
LADD = 5.3 \times 10^{-11} \text{ mg/kg/day}
$$

High-end exposure estimate[c]

$$
LADD = 1.2 \times 10^{-9} \text{ mg/kg/day}
$$

[a] EPA (1994d); LADD = lifetime average daily dose.

[b] Daily ingestion is calculated using 3 p.p.t. for dioxin level in fish tissue, 150 g of fish consumed per meal, for three meals per year, averaged over 365 days/year. The rate of ingestion for central estimates is 1.2 g of fish per day.

[c] The high-end exposure estimate uses 200 g fish per meal for 10 meals per year and 15 p.p.t. for dioxin contaminant level in the fish tissue based on a study downstream from 104 pulp mills. The rate of ingestion for this high-end exposure estimate is 4.1 g fish per day.

Exposure analysis

Exposure assessment is a crucial element of the risk assessment process, because there is no risk in the absence of exposure. Careful assessment of sources, pathways, environmental transformations, routes of entry, time course of exposure, total exposure from all sources and activities, and translation from ambient levels to target tissue effective dose is essential for exposure assessment. A good example is the work of the Electric Power Research Institute (1994) on emissions from electric utility boilers. Multiple chemical exposures and chemical–physical–biological agent interactions (Mumtaz *et al.* 1993) and exposure-specific sources of uncertainty (Bailar 1991) still need to be addressed.

The key step in making an exposure assessment is determining what exposure pathways are relevant for the risk scenario under development. The subsequent steps quantitate each pathway identified as a potentially relevant exposure and then summarize these pathway–specific exposures for calculation of the overall exposure. The EPA has published guidelines for determining such exposures (EPA 1989a,b, 1992). Such calculations can include an estimation of total exposures for a specified population as well as calculation of exposure for highly exposed individuals. The use of a hypothetical maximally exposed individual (**MEI**) is no longer favoured in exposure assessment, due to its extremely conservative assumptions at each step of the estimation. High end exposure estimates (**HEEEs**) and theoretical upper-bound estimates (**TUBEs**) are now recommended by the EPA.

HEEE calculations are designed to represent 'a plausible estimate' of exposure of individuals in the upper 90th percentile of the exposure distribution. TUBE estimations are 'bounding calculations' designed to represent exposures at a level that exceeds the exposures experienced by all individuals in the exposure distribution and are calculated by assuming limits for all exposure variables.

A calculation for individuals exposed at levels near the middle of the exposure distribution is a central estimate. A lifetime average daily dose (**LADD**) is calculated as follows:

$$
LADD = \frac{\begin{array}{c}\text{concentration of the toxicant}\\ \text{in the exposure media}\end{array} \times \begin{array}{c}\text{contact}\\ \text{rate}\end{array} \times \begin{array}{c}\text{contact}\\ \text{fraction}\end{array} \times \begin{array}{c}\text{exposure}\\ \text{duration}\end{array}}{(\text{body weight}) \, (\text{lifetime})}
$$

Table 33.6 illustrates an application of this exposure calculation. This figure gives a central estimate and an HEEE for a potential dioxin exposure from recreational fish (EPA 1994d). These estimates differ in the estimates for the amount of fish ingested, the contamination level in the fish, and the frequency of eating meals of recreationally captured fish. Obviously such estimates would differ even more if the full range of potential toxicant containment levels were used. Utilizing better estimates for the distribution of containment levels is a major focus of recent risk assessment research. To obtain such estimates, several techniques such as generating subjective uncertainty distributions and Monte Carlo composite analyses of parameter uncertainty have been applied, as described in detail elsewhere (National Research Council, Committee on Risk Assessment of Hazardous Air Pollutants 1994). The recent health assessment documents for the US EPA on tetrachlorodibenzo-*p*-dioxin (TCDD) and related compounds (EPA 1994c) also provide detailed examples of how to approach exposure uncertainties. These approaches can provide a reality check useful in generating more realistic exposure estimates.

Several endpoint-specific exposure considerations need to be mentioned. In general, estimates of cancer risk use averages over a lifetime. In a few cases, short-term exposure limits (STELs) are required (for example, ethylene oxide) and characterization of short, but high levels of exposure are required. In these cases exposures are not averaged over the lifetime. With developmental

Table 33.7 Reference values for dose calculations: lifespan, body weight, food and water intake, and nominal air intake for adults

Species	Sex	Lifespan (year)	Body weight (kg)	Food intake (wet weight) (g/day)	Water intake (m/day)	Air intake (m³/day)
Human	M	70	75	1500	2500	20
	F	78	60	1500	2500	20
Mouse	M	2	0.03	5	5	0.04
	F	2	0.025	5	5	0.04
Rat	M	2	0.5	20	25	0.2
	F	2	0.35	18	20	0.2
Hamster	M	2	0.125	12	15	0.09
	F	2	0.110	12	15	0.09

See Faustman and Omenn (1996), for details and references.

toxicity it is assumed that a single exposure can be sufficient to produce an adverse developmental effect and there is time-dependent specificity of many adverse developmental outcomes (EPA 1991). Thus, daily doses are used rather than lifetime weighted averages. Table 33.7 provides useful reference values for exposure dose calculations.

Finley *et al.* (1994) recommended distributions for exposure factors frequently used in health risk assessments, based on Monte Carlo simulations. Such age-specific distributions for soil ingestion rates, inhalation rates, body weights, skin surface area, soil-on-skin adherence, tap water ingestion, fish consumption, residential occupancy, and occupational tenure, can be refined with additional data and can replace point estimates.

Variation in susceptibility

Both toxicology and epidemiology have been slow to recognize the marked variation in susceptibility among humans and to pay attention to outliers. Assay results and toxicokinetic modelling generally utilize means and standard deviations, or even standard errors of the mean, making the range seem smaller. In occupational and environmental medicine, physicians are often asked, 'Why me, Doc?' when they inform the patient that hazards on the job might explain a clinical problem. The EPA and OSHA are expected, under the Clean Air Act and the Occupational Safety and Health Act, to promulgate standards that protect the most susceptible subgroups or individuals in the population. By focusing investigations on the most susceptible individuals, there might be a better chance of elucidating the underlying mechanisms (Omenn *et al.* 1990). Nevertheless, this work is still in its infancy. New methods and specific biomarkers of biotransformation and sites of action of chemicals could permit rapid advances.

Host factors that influence susceptibility to environmental exposures are several: genetic traits (including sex and age), pre-existing diseases, behavioural traits (including most importantly smoking), co-existing exposures, medications/vitamins, and protective measures (including respirators, gloves, and other barriers). Genetic studies are of two kinds.

1. Investigations of the effects of chemicals and radiation on the

genes and chromosomes, which constitute 'genetic toxicology': tests measure evidence of mutations (Ames test, and adduct formation between chemicals and DNA or chemicals and proteins), chromosomal aberrations, sister chromatid exchange, DNA repair, and oncogen activation.

2. Ecogenetic studies, identifying inherited variation in susceptibility (predisposition and resistance) to specific exposures, ranging across pharmaceuticals ('pharmacogenetics'), pesticides, inhaled pollutants, foods, food additives, sensory stimuli, allergic and sensitizing agents, and infectious agents.

Variation in susceptibility has been demonstrated for all of these kinds of external agents (Omenn and Motulsky 1978; Omenn *et al.* 1990; Nebert 1991, National Research Council 1993). The ecogenetic variation may affect either the biotransformation systems (enzymes that activate or detoxify chemicals) or the sites of action in target tissues.

Extrapolation from rodents to humans

Some of the most important scientific advances in the past decade and some of the most promising work for the future provide mechanism-based information for the critical question of relating rodent results to human risks. For all endpoints, it is essential to know more about the similarities and differences across species. Detailed knowledge of molecular mechanisms and cellular and organ system responses can guide us to make better decisions about which chemicals that produce cancers, neurotoxicity, birth defects, or other adverse effects in rodents really represent significant risks of doing the same in humans. Nearly all of our predictions about carcinogenicity risks for humans are based on the results from lifetime rodent bioassays. These bioassays are hardly themselves a 'gold standard', given their statistical and biological limitations and the observation that congruence of results between rats and mice is only 70 per cent (Lave *et al.* 1988; Haseman and Lockhart 1993). It is unlikely that rodent–human congruence would be higher. As summarized by McClain (1994), we now can cite several rodent

Table 33.8 Rodent carcinogenic responses not likely to apply in humans

Tumour site	Illustrative chemical agents
Male rat kidney	D-Limonene, unleaded gasoline
Male bladder	Saccharin, nitrilotriacetic acid
Rat thyroid	Ethyl bis dithiocarbamate (EBDC) fungicides, goitrogens
Forestomach only (after gavage)	Butyl hydroxyanisole (BHA), propionic acid, ethyl acrylate
Lung	Various particles
Mouse liver	Certain classes of liver carcinogens

carcinogenic responses that are candidates for no similar effect in humans (Table 33.8).

Briefly, the male rat kidney has been demonstrated to respond with a nephropathy mediated by an $\alpha 2$ euglobulin for which there is no significant counterpart in humans or in other animals. The EPA action has recognized this distinction. The thyroid and other hormone-dependent tumours in rodents reflect marked species differences in the stimulating and feedback systems; sustained, excessive levels of thyroid-stimulating hormone (**TSH**) and lack of serum thyroid-binding globulin are the key elements in the hyperplasia and tumours of the rat thyroid (McClain and Harbison 1992). The incidence of spontaneous thyroid follicular cell neoplasia is also much higher in rats in the laboratory (for example Fischer 344) and among animals in endemic areas of iodine deficiency where many people have goitres, but rarely is thyroid cancer found in humans there. Local necrosis and reactive hyperplasia in the bladder and in the forestomach represent responses to high local concentrations of the cytotoxic agent. On the other hand, many chemicals do cause tumours or other adverse effects in other parts of the body when administered (conveniently) by gavage, so the point here applies only to those chemicals whose effects are limited to the local point of application. Lung tumours have occurred with a variety of essentially inert particles, including titanium dioxide and carbon black, when the clearance capacity is markedly exceeded. The mouse liver cancer picture is considerably more complicated, with half a dozen different mechanisms, some of which seem to have definite counterparts in humans. Other mechanisms, involving induction of peroxisomes, cytotoxicity, and microsomal enzyme induction, seem much less likely to represent a significant risk in humans (McClain 1994).

Information resources

There has been a figurative explosion of toxicology information now available on-line. HazDat can be accessed through the world-wide web by using the following address: http:\\/atsdr1.atsdr.cdc-.gov: 8080\atsdrhome.html. This database contains information on hazardous substance releases and contaminants, as well as over 160 public health statements from the Agency for Toxic Substances and Disease Registry (ATSDR) chemical-specific toxicology profiles. EXTOXNET (http:\\www.oes.orst.edu:70/1\ext) provides information on the environmental chemistry and toxicology of pesti-

cides, food additives, natural toxicants, and environmental contaminants. It is a product of an *ad hoc* consortium of university toxicologists and environmental chemists.

Other key sources of information for toxicologists are available through large databases such as RTECS, Toxline, and Medline. Scientific publications from the International Agency for Research on Cancer (**IARC**) are useful. The US EPA provides health hazard information on over 500 chemicals and includes the most current oral RfDs, inhalation RfCs, and carcinogen unit risk estimates (q_1^*) on the Integrated Risk Information System (**IRIS**). There are complaints about long lags in updating IRIS information. To access IRIS, call the IRIS Risk Information Hotline (513) 569–7254.

Integrating qualitative and quantitative aspects of risk assessment: classification schemes

Qualitative assessment of hazard information should include consideration of the concordance of toxicological findings across species and target organs, of consistency across duplicate experimental conditions, and of adequacy of the experiments to detect the adverse endpoints of interest.

The National Toxicology Program (**NTP**) uses several categories to classify bioassay results. The NTP's evaluation guidelines allow for categories of clear, some, equivocal, and no evidence, as well as inadequate study. The category 'clear evidence of carcinogenicity' includes dose-related increases in malignant or combined malignant and benign neoplasms seen across all doses and significant increases in at least two of the four species/sex test groups.

Qualitative assessment of animal or human evidence is done by many agencies including the EPA and IARC. Similar classifications are used for both the animal and human evidence categories by both agencies. These classifications include levels of sufficient, limited, inadequate, and no evidence (EPA 1994b) while the IARC classifications are sufficient, limited, inadequate, evidence suggesting lack of carcinogenicity, and no evidence (IARC 1987). Table 33.9 presents IARC's list of human carcinogens, of which 20 are chemical, 13 are pharmaceutical (mostly cancer chemotherapy agents), and 11 are manufacturing processes, as summarized through 1987 (IARC 1987).

These evidence classifications are used for the overall weight of evidence in carcinogenicity classification schemes. Although differing group number or letter categories are used, striking similarities exist between the EPA and IARC approaches. The EPA's proposed changes to their risk assessment guidelines for carcinogenic substances include relabelled categories described as 'known', 'likely', or 'not likely' to be carcinogenic to humans (EPA 1996). Another category, 'cannot evaluate', comprises inadequate data and incomplete or inconclusive data.

So far we have discussed approaches for evaluating cancer endpoints. Similar weight of evidence approaches for reproductive risk assessment utilize 'sufficient' and 'insufficient' evidence categories (EPA 1994d). The Institute for Evaluating Health Risks has defined an 'evaluative process' by which reproductive and developmental toxicity data can be evaluated consistently and integrated to ascertain their relevance for human health risk assessment (Moore *et al.* 1995).

Table 33.9 Chemicals and related exposures with sufficient evidence for carcinogenicity in humans

Chemicals	Pharmaceuticals	Manufacturing processes
Aflatoxins	Analgesic mixtures w/phenacetin	Aluminium
4-Amino-biphenyl	Azathioprine	Auramine
Arsenic and arsenic compounds	Chlornaphazine	Betel quid with tobacco
Asbestos	Chlorambucil	Coal gasification
Benzene	CCNU (nitrosoureas)	Coke production
Benzidine	Cyclophosphamide	Furniture/cabinet making
Bis(chloromethyl)ether	Oestrogen(steroidal/non-steroidal)	Haematite (radon)
Chromium (VI) compounds	Melphalan	Iron/steel founding
Coal tar/pitches	Methoxsalen + UVR	Isopropyl alcohol
Erionite	MOPP (alkylating combinations)	Magenta
Mineral oils	Myleran	Rubber
Mustard gas	Oral contraceptives	
2-Naphthylamine	Treosulphan	
Nickel and nickel compounds		
Shale oils		
Soots		
Talc with asbestiform fibres		
Tobacco products		
Tobacco smoke		
Vinyl chloride		

From IARC (1987, Table 1, pp. 56–74).

Ethylene oxide: an example of chemical-specific risk assessment

Ethylene oxide (**EtO**) is a colourless gas that is used as a chemical intermediate in the manufacture of industrial products such as ethylene glycol, polyester fibres, and detergents. Ethylene oxide is also used as a pesticide fumigant. Over 75 000 hospital workers are exposed via its use as an antimicrobial sterilant. EtO is one of the 25 chemicals of highest production volume in the United States, with over 5 billion pounds produced in 1987. There is evidence from animal tests and human exposure studies that EtO is a carcinogen, mutagen, reproductive toxicant, and neurotoxicant. We will focus on assessment of its carcinogenic effects. EtO has been regulated under OSHA, CPSC, EPA, and FDA statutes.

Short-term assay information

Ethylene oxide has been shown, like many reactive epoxides, to be a direct-acting (genotoxic) mutagen. It has been evaluated in bacterial, plant, drosophila germ cells, and rodent and human cell assays. EtO causes chromosomal aberrations and point mutations. In fact, EtO is frequently used as a positive control in assays of other potentially mutagenic agents.

Rodent bioassays

All three rodent bioassays conducted with EtO by inhalation found dose-related increases in tumours in both rats and mice, both male and female. Increased rates for mononuclear cell leukaemia, peritoneal mesothelioma, mixed brain tumours, alveolar/bronchiolar carcinomas and adenomas, lymphomas, papillary cystadenoma of the harderian gland, uterine adenocarcinomas, and mammary gland tumours were observed (Snellings *et al.* 1984*a,b*). Exposure levels tested include 0, 10, 33, 50 and 100 p.p.m. for 6 to 7 h/day for 5 days per week for 2 years.

Epidemiology

Published studies of EtO-exposed workers are positive for cancer risk. The standardized mortality rates for chemical plant workers were approximately 9 for stomach oesophageal cancers and leukaemia (Hogstedt *et al.* 1986). This study, as well as others on chemical plant workers, was complicated by exposure to multiple chemicals besides EtO and by relatively small cohort sizes (700 to 3000 participants). Studies of 20 000 EtO sterilizer-exposed workers found significant increases in haematopoietic cancers in male workers (Steenland *et al.* 1991); these increases might have been complicated by other exposure factors such as HIV infection. Molecular biomarker studies correlating EtO exposure, levels of hydroxyethyl adducts in haemoglobin, and cancer incidence failed to establish a direct correlation of adducts and cancer but did show a good dose–response relationship for the adducts and EtO exposures (Hagmar *et al.* 1991).

Qualitative assessment

Both the US EPA and IARC have concluded that EtO is a probable human carcinogen (EPA–B2 classification and IARC–2A classification). They determined that there is sufficient animal, but limited bordering on inadequate human evidence to base this qualitative assessment.

Exposure assessment

Occupational exposures to EtO are primarily via inhalation. For chemical plant workers, a 7 h/day, 5 day/week, 50 weeks per year exposure scenario is appropriate. An appropriate model of exposure for EtO sterilizer workers in hospitals should include multiple short-term exposure peaks spread throughout the work day, reflecting cycles of EtO sterilizer operation. Both the time weighted average (**TWA**) and short-term exposure limits (**STELs**) would be particularly important for genotoxic carcinogens such as EtO, since DNA repair systems are known to be saturable at higher exposure levels.

Susceptible populations

Because EtO is a genotoxic carcinogen, individuals with compromised DNA repair pathways would be at greater risk than other individuals. Other susceptible populations include the unborn children of workers. EtO is already a reactive epoxide, not requiring activation; no variation has been related to detoxification pathways.

Quantitative risk assessment and standard setting

The OSHA has used the rodent mesothelioma and leukaemia data to model upper bound estimates on risk (Snellings *et al.* 1984*a, b*; National Toxicology Program 1987). The current q_1^* (upper 95 per cent confidence limit on cancer risk) for EtO is 3.4×10^{-1} per mg EtO/kg body weight/day based on the EPA's evaluation of the Snellings *et al.* (1984*a*) study of incidence of mononuclear cell leukaemia and brain tumours in female rats. The current OSHA TWA for EtO is 1 p.p.m. exposure averaged over an 8-h day. The initially proposed STEL value of 5 p.p.m. was not upheld by the courts.

Regulatory risk management/control of exposures

One of the key regulatory needs to improve the safe use of EtO in occupational settings is the establishment of the STEL values. Our review of the options supports the establishment of a 15 min exposure limit that must not exceed five times the 8-h TWA.

Improved ventilation controls for the EtO sterilization units in hospitals can continue to offer an excellent solution for the safe use of this sterilization process. The OSHA currently provides several recommended engineering options. These include use of non-recirculating exhaust hoods built directly over the sterilizer door, a capture box built over the floor drains for the sterilizers, and extended vacuum purges of the sterilizer chamber with 'door locked' phases that prevent premature entry.

Substitutes

Few of the alternatives to EtO sterilization are effective or appropriate. Chemical disinfecting requires long soaking times (11 h) for comparable levels of sterilization, costs more due to personnel time in processing, and results in alternative exposures (glutaraldehyde is the chemical disinfectant of choice). Other less favourable alternatives do not provide adequate sterilization.

Comparing international approaches to carcinogen risk assessment

For many years there has been an information-sharing process aimed at harmonization of chemical-testing regimes and clinical trials methodologies, so that data might be accepted in multiple countries that are members of the Organization for Economic Cooperation and Development (**OECD**). The United Nations (**UN**) Conference on the Environment in Rio de Janeiro, Brazil in 1992 established harmonization of risk assessment as one of its goals, with a coordinating role for the International Programme on Chemical Safety. The negotiation in 1994 of the General Agreement on Trade and Tariffs (**GATT**) and establishment of a World Trade Organization made harmonization of various aspects of testing, risk assessment, labelling, registration, and standards potentially important elements in trade, not just in regulatory science.

Moolenaar (1994) summarized the carcinogen risk assessment methodologies used by various countries as a basis for regulatory actions. He tabulated the risk characterization, carcinogen identification, risk extrapolation, and chemical classification schemes of the US EPA, the US Public Health Service, the WHO/IARC, the American Conference of Governmental Industrial Hygienists (**ACGIH**), Australia, the European Economic Community (**EEC**), Germany, The Netherlands, Norway, and Sweden. The approach of the EPA to estimate an upper bound to human risk is unique; all other countries estimate human risk values based on the expected incidence of cancer from the exposures under review. The United Kingdom follows a case-by-case approach to risk evaluations for both genotoxic and non-genotoxic carcinogens, with no generic procedures. Denmark, the EEC, the United Kingdom, and The Netherlands all divide carcinogens into genotoxic and non-genotoxic agents and use different extrapolation procedures for each. Norway does not extrapolate data to low doses, using instead the TD_{50} to divide category I carcinogens into tertiles by probable potency. The United Kingdom, EEC, and The Netherlands all treat non-genotoxic chemical carcinogens as threshold toxicants. A NOAEL and safety factors are used to set acceptable daily intake (**ADI**) values. It may be time for the United States. to consider applying the BMD method to non-genotoxic carcinogens, instead of the linearized multistage model.

The OECD countries have a well-established process of comparing economies of member countries for various bench-mark parameters. An effort has been initiated to stimulate similar thinking about sentinel measures for comparisons of country performance in environmental protection (Lykke 1992). The UN Conference in Rio and other international forums now seek international consensus on reductions of emissions of global (carbon dioxide) or regional (sulphur dioxide) importance.

Table 33.10 Congressional mandate for US Commission on Risk Assessment and Risk Management

1. The uses and limitations of risk assessment in establishing emissions and effluent standards, ambient standards, exposure standards, acceptable concentration levels, tolerances, or other environmental criteria for hazardous substances that present a risk of carcinogenic effects or other chronic health effects.

2. The most appropriate exposure scenarios for describing and estimating cancer risks or risks of other chronic health effects from hazardous substances.

3. Methods to reflect uncertainties in measurement and estimation techniques, the existence of synergistic or antagonistic effects among hazardous substances, and the variability in susceptibility within human populations.

4. Risk management policy issues, including the use of lifetime cancer risks to individuals in communicating about risks, comparisons of similar and dissimilar risks, cost–benefit and cost-effectiveness analyses of exposure reduction measures, and choices of standards for 'how clean is clean?'.

5. The degree to which it is possible or desirable to develop a consistent standard of acceptable risk across the various Federal programmes and agencies and as part of efforts for international cooperation and harmonization of the regulation of hazardous chemicals.

The United States Commission on Risk Assessment and Risk Management

The 1990 Clean Air Act Amendments (Title III) established a long-term plan for the EPA to determine whether additional controls on emissions of 189 named hazardous air pollutants will be required to reduce the estimated residual risks after the implementation of maximum achievable control technologies. The National Academy of Sciences was called upon to review the methods used by the EPA to determine the carcinogenic risk associated with exposures to hazardous air pollutants from sources subject to regulation and to evaluate risk assessment methods for non-cancer health effects, as well. The title of the report 'Science and judgment in risk assessment' (National Research Council, Committee on Risk Assessment of Hazardous Air Pollutants 1994) reflects the interplay of scientific methods and social/political/cultural values. This report is a major input to the Presidential Commission mandated by the same section of the 1990 amendments. The commission was launched in May 1994 with 10 members appointed, according to the statute, as follows: three by the President, three by the Senate, three by the House of Representatives, and one by the National Academy of Sciences. The commission's mandate is summarized in Table 33.10.

The commission is reviewing carefully the risk assessment approaches and risk communication needs related to cancer and non-cancer health effects and will focus much of its effort on the risk-based decision-making processes which good science can assist. Although ecological risks were not made part of the mandate by Congress, the commission has noted that a similar framework approach to that used in this chapter for health risks can, in fact, be applied productively to ecological risks (see also National Research Council, Committee on Risk Assessment Methodology 1993). The

commission's work is conducted in public meetings around the country. The deliberations are not limited to the Clean Air Act or the EPA, since issues about appropriate uses of risk assessment, the extrapolation to 'acceptable risk' levels, the explanation of findings to stakeholders and decision makers, the incorporation of parameters important to local citizens, Indian Nations, and environmental organizations, and the sorting out of overlapping statutes and regulations apply to numerous other laws and many other federal and state agencies. A leading example is the Environmental Restoration and Waste Management Program of the US Department of Energy (**DOE**), which is responsible for the clean up of the DOE's nuclear weapons production sites (Omenn 1994).

Risk perception

Individuals respond differently to hazardous situations, as do societies. An event that is accepted by one individual may be unacceptable to another (Fischhoff 1981; Fischhoff et al. 1993). Understanding these behavioural responses is critical in developing risk management options. Experts and lay persons commonly disagree. In a classic study, students, League of Women Voters members, active club members, and scientific experts were asked to rank 30 activities or agents in order of their annual contribution to deaths (Slovic et al. 1979). The lay groups all ranked motorcycles and handguns as highly risky and vaccinations, home appliances, power mowers, and football as relatively safe. Club members viewed pesticides, spray cans, and nuclear power as safer than did other lay persons. Students ranked contraceptives and food preservatives as riskier and mountain climbing as safer than did the others. The experts, however, ranked electric power, surgery, swimming, and X-rays as more risky and nuclear power and police work as less risky than did lay persons. Perceptions of risk by toxicologists in academia, industry, and government also have been studied (Neil et al. 1994); there were group differences in responses involving chemical hazards.

Figure 33.3 illustrates the relationship of psychological factors such as dread, perceived uncontrollability, and involuntary exposure (horizontal axis) to factors that represent the extent to which a hazard is familiar, observable, and 'essential' (vertical axis) (Morgan 1993). For example, the upper right sector of risk space includes pesticide use, radioactive waste, DNA technology, electromagnetic fields, asbestos insulation, and mercury. Risks that have these features are good candidates for public demand for government regulations and are less likely to be 'acceptable' (Lowrance 1976).

Comparative analyses of risks

This aspect of risk assessment, risk communication, and risk management is so logical that it may be surprising to learn that comparisons of risks are extremely controversial. Public health practitioners practice comparative risk assessment, at least intuitively, on a routine basis when deciding how to allocate their own time, their staff's time, and other resources. They must make judgements about what and how to advise their local communities about potential and definite risks.

Most people routinely and intuitively compare risks of alternative activities—on the job, in recreational pursuits, in interpersonal interactions, in investments. From 1993 the United States Congress has pressed for the systematic use of comparisons of

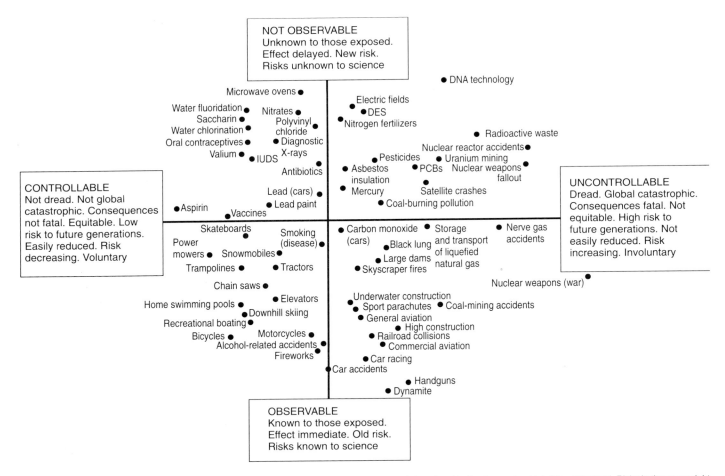

Fig. 33.3 Risk space, risk perception. The axes correspond approximately to a hazard's 'dreadfulness' and to the degree to which it is understood. Risks in the upper right quadrant of this space are most likely to provoke calls for government regulation. From Morgan (1993).

similar and dissimilar risks by federal regulatory agencies. The aim was to make the benefits and costs of health, safety, and environmental protection actions more explicit, more comprehensible, and, hopefully, more cost-effective. However, determining how best to conduct comparative risk analyses and do so efficiently has proved difficult, due to the great variety of health and environmental benefits, the uncertainties about cost estimates, and the differing distributions of benefits and costs across the population.

A new concept, environmental justice, has arisen to reflect the ethical guidance that poor, disenfranchised neighbourhoods should be protected as much as well-to-do suburban neighbourhoods (Rios *et al.* 1993). In fact, the poor may need greater protection due to their coexisting higher risk factors for poor pregnancy outcomes, impaired growth and development, smoking-related cancers, asthma, and lead toxicity, among other health problems. On the other hand, poor rates of prenatal care and childhood immunization, acute lead toxicity from bullets, poor housing, lack of education, and joblessness may make hypothetical or long-term estimated risks from chemical pollutant exposures relatively less salient.

Several formal analyses to compare risks have been developed. One method estimates the contribution of a particular activity or exposure to deaths in the general population, combining reports of actual deaths and estimates of likely or worst-case effects of various

risk factors. McGinnis and Foege (1993) compiled the 10 leading reported causes for the 2.1 million American deaths in 1990 and then listed the real causes of death, beginning with smoking (430 000 excess deaths), then poor diet and inactivity, and then alcohol (see Table 33.11). The message here is clear: almost one-half of deaths and a higher proportion of premature deaths, are caused by preventable risk factors, mostly individual behaviours. They estimate 60 000 deaths per year in the United States from exposure to toxic substances.

Another approach determines the average estimated loss of life expectancy due to various causes (Crouch and Wilson 1982). For example, male smokers lose an estimated 2250 days of life expectancy, persons 20 per cent overweight lose 900 days, alcohol users lose 130 days, persons of low socio-economic class lose 700 days, and those impaired by occupational hazards lose 30 to 300 days. Yet a third approach estimates the exposure required to increase the annual death rate by 1 death per 1 million deaths. Estimates for different exposures include smoking 1.4 cigarettes (heart disease and cancer deaths), drinking 0.5 litres of wine (cirrhosis of the liver), or eating 40 tablespoons of peanut butter (liver cancer caused by aflatoxin contamination of the peanuts per day).

All of these approaches have serious limitations due to inadequate information on the variability of the statistics, uncertainty about the size of the population at risk due to specific exposures, complex exposures, multiple additional risk factors, and complicated aetiology of deaths.

People clearly vary in their perceptions of risk—on both technical and emotional grounds; Sandman (1993) classified these aspects as 'hazard' and 'outrage', respectively. A different kind of risk comparison is conducted at the programme planning level across diverse types of risks. The US EPA published its landmark review *Unfinished business* in 1987, ranking EPA programmes in priority for more investment, compared with current funding levels and technical progress. In 1990, the EPA's Science Advisory Board published *Reducing risks*, categorizing the relative risks of cancers, non-cancer endpoints, and various ecological impacts (EPA 1990). Meanwhile, the EPA has sponsored or encouraged comparative risk analysis forums or projects in 18 states. Vermont and Colorado had particularly productive experiences with considerable public involvement. The state of Washington generated a public process and report called *Washington 2010*; a mayoral task force produced a report on *Seattle's environmental priorities* that has guided budget decisions and public understanding. A highly publicized project in California yielded a draft report just before the 1994 state elections which remained in limbo many months later, due to controversial statements about 'environmental justice' and social welfare aspects. Its array of high, medium, and low priorities among health and ecological risks was not controversial and may still be utilized in state planning. Local governments, faced with unfunded regulatory mandates and limited budgets, are seeking rational and cost-effective options. One approach has been called 'community risk profiles' (Wernick 1995). Philosophies of regulation are outlined in Table 33.12.

Economic analyses

In 1995 the United States Congress moved aggressively to try to make the cost–benefit analysis the basis for regulatory decisions in the health, safety, and environmental arena. Cost–benefit analysis requires conversion of all benefits—cancers, birth defects, and habitat destruction averted, for example—to a monetary value and reliable estimates of costs. There are huge uncertainties in each

Table 33.12 Philosophies of regulation

1. Regulation of only proven human toxicants: 'count the bodies'
2. Best available technology (BAT) approach: engineering solutions
3. Protect all citizens with equal effectiveness: uniform risk/equal rights
4. Cost-effectiveness or cost–benefit
5. If any evidence suggests harm, eliminate hazard: 'Delaney' approach

type of estimate. In addition, there is no simple way of weighing the consequences to poor communities, big manufacturers, and other subsets of the population. No-one has clarified what should be the decision-making metric and who will enforce its decisions, except to invite even more litigation! Nevertheless, it is certainly logical to require government agencies to affirm to taxpayers and consumers that the expected benefits of actions they mandate will 'justify' the direct and indirect costs to society.

Cost-effectiveness analysis is less controversial. It specifies benefits as lives saved, life years gained, cancer deaths averted, tons of emissions reduced, or habitats protected. Then the estimated costs of various means of achieving specified benefits can be compared. Cost-effectiveness analyses, like comparisons of risks, can be conducted for specific regulations or to contrast whole classes of actions. In the latter category, Tengs *et al.* (1995), summarized published reports of costs per year of life gained (saved) from various medical, public health, occupational safety, and environmental protection interventions. Childhood immunizations and prenatal care save more than they cost in dollars. For examples, influenza immunization costs approximately $6000 per life year gained, chloridination of drinking water costs approximately $4000, annual breast cancer screening age 40 to 64 years costs approximately $17 000, construction safety rules cost approximately $38 000, home radon control costs approximately $140 000, and proposed additional environmental asbestos and radiation controls cost more than a million dollars per life year estimated to be gained. These differences are dramatic. It is not simple to compare risk management options without reference to detailed data, various specific statutory requirements and intent, and the salience of these different services and risks to the public.

Risk communication

Public health agencies and officials regularly engage in communication with the public and with public officials and private sector parties about health risks. It is a primary mission of public health to investigate the causes of health problems and the ways to reduce the incidence and consequences of such problems. Actions must include environmental controls, such as protection of air, water, and food from chemical and microbiological contamination and protection against radioactive exposures in medical care, industry, and the general environment. For inactive (abandoned) hazardous waste sites, the federal Superfund law requires the ATSDR to assess and issue a public health advisory statement for each of the 1300+ National Priorities List Sites.

Table 33.11 Causes of death

Listed causes		'Real causes'	
Heart disease	720 000	Tobacco	400 000
Cancers	505 000	Diet/activity patterns	300 000
Cerebrovascular disease	144 000	Alcohol	100 000
'Accidents'	92 000	Microbial agents	90 000
Chronic lung disease	87 000	Toxic agents	60 000
Pneumonia and influenza	80 000	Firearms	35 000
Diabetes mellitus	48 000	Sexual behaviour	30 000
Suicide	31 000	Motor vehicles	25 000
Cirrhosis/liver disease	26 000	Illicit use of drugs	20 000
HIV infection	25 000		
Total US 1990	2 148 000	Total	1 060 000

Based on McGinnis and Foege (1993).

Actions also must include health education to promote healthy behaviours and reduce unhealthy behaviours—smoking, violence, alcohol and other drug abuse, sexually transmitted diseases, physical inactivity, and social isolation. Clinical preventive services of immunizations, counselling, and screening are important medical contributions to individual patients and public health services are important to the health status of communities. Finally, communication about risks and risk reduction must mobilize public policy in the form of incentives and disincentives for health promotion and against pollution and unhealthy behaviours. In the United States, reports from all Surgeons General since 1979 have sustained a campaign called 'Healthy People', which embraces health protection, health promotion, and clinical preventive services (Oberle *et al.* 1994). Local communities increasingly take part in the risk communication process. Their knowledge of exposure pathways in the past and of apparent health and ecological effects can redirect the technical assessments. Their views on future uses of contaminated sites can be crucial to deciding how stringent must be the clean up. All of these programmes must be integrated to achieve a reinforcing strategy for disease and injury prevention and for health promotion (Commission on Risk Assessment and Risk Management 1996; National Research Council 1996).

Conclusion

The scientific community has come a long way in the past 10 to 20 years in expanding the science base, in better defining our questions about assumptions and models, and in helping regulators to make risk-based decisions for protection of human health and the environment. The period ahead should have an acceleration of knowledge from the public health sciences and important inputs from our constituencies—legislators, regulators, manufacturers, environmentalists, media, and affected communities—throughout the global commons.

References

Abbott, B.D., Harris, M.W., and Birnbaum, L.S. (1992). Comparisons of the effects of TCDD and hydrocortisone on growth factor expression provide insight into their interaction in the embryonic mouse palate. *Teratology*, **45**, 35–53.

Albert, R.E. (1994). Carcinogen risk assessment in the US Environmental Protection Agencies. *Critical Reviews in Toxicology*, **24**, 75–85.

Allen, B.C., Kavlock, R.J., Kimmel, C.A., and Faustman, E.M. (1994*a*). Dose response assessments for developmental toxicity: II. Comparison of generic benchmark dose estimates with NOAELs. *Fundamental Applied Toxicology*, **23**, 487–95.

Allen, B.C., Kavlock, R.J., Kimmel, C.A., and Faustman, E.M. (1994*b*). Dose response assessment for developmental toxicity: III. Statistical models. *Fundamental Applied Toxicology*, **23**, 496–509.

Ames, B.N. and Gold, L.S. (1990). Too many rodent carcinogens: mitogenesis increases mutagenesis. *Science*, **249**, 970–1.

Anderson, E.L. (1983). Quantitative approaches in use to assess cancer risk. *Risk Analysis*, **3**, 277–95.

Armitage, P. and Doll, R. (1957). A two-stage theory of carcinogenesis in relation to the age distribution of human cancer. *British Journal of Cancer*, **11**, 161–9.

Ashby, J. and Tennant, R.W. (1994). Prediction of rodent carcinogenicity for 44 chemicals: results. *Mutagenesis*, **9**, 7–15.

Atterwill, C.K., Johnston, H., and Thomas, S.M. (1992). Models for the *in vitro* assessment of neurotoxicity in the nervous system in relation to xenobiotic and neurotrophic factor-mediated events. *Neurotoxicology*, **13**, 39–53.

Auton, T.R. (1994). Calculation of benchmark doses from teratology data. *Regulatory Toxicology and Pharmacology*, **19**, 152–67.

Bailar, J. C., III (1991). Scientific inferences and environmental health problems. *Chance: New Directions for Statistics and Computing*, **4**, 27–38.

Barnes, D.G., Daston G.P., Evans J.S., Jarbek, A.M., Kavlock R.J., Kimmel C.A. (1995). Benchmark dose workshop. *Regulatory Toxicology and Pharmacology*, **21**, 296–306.

Brown, C.C. (1984). High–to low-dose extrapolation in animals. In *Assessment and management of chemical risks* (ed. J.V. Rodricks, and R.G. Tardiff), pp. 57–79. American Chemical Society, Washington, DC.

Calkins, D. R., Dixon, R.L., Gerber, C.R., Zarin, D., and Omenn, G.S. (1980). Identification, characterization, and control of potential human carcinogens: a framework for federal decision-making. *Journal of the National Cancer Institute*, **61**, 169–75.

Cohen, S.M. and Ellwein, L.B. (1990). Proliferative and genotoxic cellular effects in 2–acetylaminofluorene bladder and liver carcinogenesis: biological modeling of the EDO1 study. *Toxicology and Applied Pharmacology*, **104**, 79–93.

Commission on Risk Assessment and Risk Management. (June 13, 1996). *Risk Assessment and Risk Management in Regulatory Decision-Making: Draft Report for Public Review and Comment*.

Crouch, E.A.C. and Wilson, R. (1982). *Risk/benefit analysis*. Ballinger, Cambridge, MA.

Crump, K.S. (1980). An improved procedure for low-dose carcinogenic risk assessment from animal data. *Journal of Environmental Pathology and Toxicology*, **5**, 675–84.

Crump, K.S. (1984). A new method for determining allowable daily intakes. *Fundamental Applied Toxicology*, **4**, 854–71.

EPA (1989*a*). *Risk assessment guidance for Superfund. Human health evaluation manual*, Part A. EPA Office of Policy Analysis, Washington, DC.

EPA (1989*b*). *Exposure factors handbook, final report*. EPA Office of Health and Environmental Assessment, Washington, DC.

EPA (1990). *Reducing risk: setting priorities and strategies for environmental protection*. EPA Science Advisory Board, Washington, DC.

EPA (1991). *Alpha2 euglobulin: association with chemically-induced renal toxicity and neoplasia in the male rat*. EPA, Washington, DC.

EPA (1992). Guidelines for developmental toxicity risk assessment. *Federal Register*, **57**, 22888–938.

EPA (1994*a*). *Guidelines for reproductive toxicity risk assessment*. EPA Office of Research and Development, Washington, DC.

EPA (1994*b*). *Draft revisions to the guidelines for carcinogen risk assessment*. EPA Office of Research and Development, Washington, DC.

EPA (1994*c*). *Health assessment document for 2,3,7,8–tetrachlorodibenzo–p–dioxin (TCDD) and related compounds*, Vol I–III. EPA Office of Research and Development, Washington, DC.

EPA (1994*d*). *Estimating exposure to dioxin-like compounds*. Office of Health and Environmental Assessment, Exposure Assessment Group, Washington, DC.

EPA (1996). *Risk Assessment Guidelines*. EPA Office of Research and Development, Washington, DC.

Electric Power Research Institute (EPRI) (1994). *Electric utility trace substances synthesis report*. Electric Power Research Institute, Palo Alto, CA.

Faustman, E.M., Kimmel, C., and Wellington, D. (1989). Characterization of a developmental toxicity dose–response model. *Environmental Health Perspectives*, **79**, 229–41.

Faustman, E.M. and Omenn, G.S. (1996). Risk assessment. In *Casarett and Doull's toxicology*, (5th edn) (ed. C.D. Klaassen). pp. 75–88. McGraw-Hill, Inc., New York.

Faustman, E.M., Allen, B.C., Kavlock, R.J., and Kimmel, C.A. (1994). Dose–response assessment of developmental toxicity: I. Characterization of data base and determination of NOAELs. *Fundamental and Applied Toxicology*, **79**, 229–41.

Finley, B., Proctor, D., Scott, P., Harrington, N., Paustenbach D., and Price, P. (1994). Recommended distributions for exposure factors frequently used in health risk assessment. *Risk Analysis*, **14**, 533–53.

Fischhoff, B. (1981). Cost–benefit analysis: an uncertain guide to public policy. *Annals of the New York Academy of Science*, **363**, 173–88.

Fischhoff, B.B., Bostrom, A., and Quadrel, M.J. (1993). Risk perception and communication. *Annual Review of Public Health*, 14, 183–203.

Hagmar, L., Welinder, H., Linden, K., Attewell, R., Osterman-Golkar, S., and Torndqvist, M. (1991). An epidemiological study of cancer risk among workers exposed to ethylene oxide using hemoglobin adducts to validate environmental exposure assessments. *International Archives of Occupational and Environmental Health*, 63, 271–7.

Harris, M.W., Chapin, R.E., Lockhart, A.C., and Jokinen, M.P. (1992). Assessment of a short-term reproductive and developmental toxicity screen. *Fundamental and Applied Toxicology*, 19, 186–96.

Hartung, R. (1987). Dose–response relationships. In *Toxic substances and human risk: principles of data interpretation* (ed. R. G. Tardiff and J.V. Rodricks), pp. 29–46. Plenum Press, New York.

Haseman, J.K. and Lockhart, A.M. (1993). Correlations between chemically related site–specific carcinogenic effects in long-term studies in rats and mice. *Environmental Health Perspectives* 101, 50–4.

Hogstedt, C., Aringer, L., and Gustavsson, A. (1986). Epidemiologic support for ethylene oxide as a cancer-causing agent. *Journal of the American Medical Association*, 225, 1575–8.

IARC (1987). *IARC monographs on the evaluation of carcinogenic risks to humans*, (Suppl. 7). International Agency for Research on Cancer, Lyon, France.

Kavlock, R.J., Allen, B.C., Faustman, E.M., and Kimmel, C.A. (1995). Dose response assessments for developmental toxicity: IV. Benchmark doses for fetal weight changes. *Fundamental and Applied Toxicology*, 26, 211–22.

Kimmel, C.A. and Gaylor, D.W. (1988). Issues in qualitative and quantitative risk analysis for developmental toxicology. *Risk Analysis*, 8, 15–20.

Kohn, M.C., Lucier, G.W., Clark, G.C., Sewall, C., Tritscher, A.M., and Portier, C.J. (1993). A mechanistic model of effects of dioxin on gene expression in the rat liver. *Toxicology and Applied Pharmacology*, 120, 138–54.

Krewski, D. and Van Ryzin, J. (1981). Dose response models for quantal response toxicity data. In *Statistics and related topics*, (ed. M. Csorgo, D.A. Dawson, J.N.K. Rao, and A.K. Seleh), pp. 201–229. North-Holland, Amsterdam.

Lave, L.B. and Omenn, G.S. (1986). Cost-effectiveness of short-term tests for carcinogenicity. *Nature*, 334, 29–34.

Lave, L.B., Ennever, F., Rosenkranz, H.S., and Omenn G.S. (1988). Information value of the rodent bioassay. *Nature*, 336, 631–3.

Leroux, B.G., Leisenring, W.M., Moolgavkar, S.H., and Faustman, E.M. (1996). A biologically based dose-response model for development. *Risk Analysis*. (In press.)

Lowrance, W.W. (1976). *Of acceptable risk*, pp. 180. William Kaufmann, Inc., Los Altos, CA.

Lykke, E. (ed.) (1992). *Achieving environmental goals: the concept and practice of environmental performance review*. Pinter Publishers, London.

McClain, R.M. and Harbison, M.L. (1992). Receptor mediated cell proliferation and thyroid neoplasia. *BGA Schriften*, 3, 49–59.

McClain, R.M. (1994). Mechanistic considerations in the regulation and classification of chemical carcinogens. In *Nutritional toxicology* (ed. F.N. Kotsonis, M. Mackey, and J. Hijele), pp. 278–304. Raven Press Ltd, New York, NY.

McGinnis, J.M. and Foege, W.H. (1993). Actual causes of death in the United States. *Journal of the American Medical Association*, 270, 2207–12.

Moolenar, R.J. (1994). Carcinogen risk assessment: international comparison. *Regulatory Toxicology and Pharmacology*, 20, 302–36.

Moolgavkar, S.H. and Luebeck, G. (1990). Two–event model for carcinogenesis: biological, mathematical, and statistical considerations. *Risk Analysis*, 10, 323–41.

Moore, J.A., Daston, G.P., Faustman, E.M., Golub, M.S., Hart, W.L., and Hughes, C.Jr., (1995). An evaluative process for assessing human reproductive and developmental toxicity of agents. *Reproductive Toxicology*, 9, 61–95.

Morgan, G.M. (1993). Risk analysis and management. *Scientific America*, 269, 32–5, 38–41.

Mumtaz, M.M., Sipes I.G., Clewell H.J., and Yang R.S. (1993). Risk assessment of chemical mixtures: biologic and toxicologic issues. *Fundamental and Applied Toxicology*, 21, 258–69.

National Institute of Environmental Health Sciences (NIEHS) (1993). *Predicting chemical carcinogenesis in rodents, an international workshop, 24–25 May, 1993*. National Institute of Environmental Health Sciences, Research Triangle Park, NC.

National Research Council (NRC) (1983). *Risk assessment in the federal government: managing the process*. National Academy Press, Washington, DC.

National Research Council (NRC) (1984). *Toxicity testing: strategies to determine needs and priorities*. National Academy Press, Washington, DC.

National Research Council (NRC) (1989a). *Biological markers in pulmonary toxicology*. National Academy Press, Washington, DC.

National Research Council (NRC) (1989b). *Biological markers in reproductive toxicology*. National Academy Press, Washington, DC.

National Research Council (NRC) (1992a). *Biological markers in immunotoxicology*. National Academy Press, Washington, DC.

National Research Council (NRC) (1992b). *Environmental neurotoxicology*. National Academy Press, Washington, DC.

National Research Council (NRC) (1993). *Pesticides in the diets of infants and children*. National Academy Press, Washington, DC.

National Research Council (NRC) Committee on Risk Assessment Methodology (CRAM) (1993). *Issues in risk assessment, use of the maximum tolerated dose in animal bioassays for carcinogenicity*. National Academy Press, Washington, DC.

National Research Council (NRC), Committee on Risk Assessment of Hazardous Air Pollutants. (1994). *Science and judgment in risk assessment*. National Academy Press, Washington, DC.

National Research Council (NRC). (1996). *Understanding Risk*. National Academy Press, Washington, DC.

National Toxicology Program (NTP) (1987). *Toxicology and carcinogenesis studies of ethylene oxide in B6C3F1 mice*. US Department of Health and Human Services, Public Health Services, National Institutes of Health, Research Triangle Park, N.C.

Nebert, D.W. (1991). Role of genetics and drug metabolism in human cancer risk. *Mutation Research*, 247, 267–81.

Neil, N., Malmfors, T. and Slovic, P. (1994). Intuitive toxicology: expert and lay judgments of chemical risks. *Toxicologic Pathology*, 22, 198–201.

Oberle, M.W., Baker, E.L., and Magenheim, M.J. (1994). Healthy People 2000 and community health planning. *Annual Review of Public Health*, 15, 259–75.

Office of Technology Assessment (OTA) (1992). *Centralized risk assessment research*. National Academy Press, Washington, DC.

Omenn, G.S. (1984). Characterizing risks: utilizing knowledge about mechanisms. In *Molecular and cellular approaches to understanding mechanisms of toxicity* (ed. A.H. Tashjian, Jr), pp. 224–45. Harvard School of Public Health, Boston, MA.

Omenn, G.S. (1993). Commentary: the role of environmental epidemiology in public policy. *Annals of Epidemiology*, 3, 319–22.

Omenn, G.S. (1994). Can systematic, integrated risk assessment with full stakeholder participation enhance clean-up at DOE's sites? The 1994 Herbert H. Parker Lecture. In *33rd Hanford Symposium on Health and the Environment. In-situ remediation: scientific basis for current and future technologies*, Part I, (ed. G.W.Gee and R.Wing) pp. xv–xxx, Battelle Press, Columbus.

Omenn, G.S. and Lave, L. B. (1988). Scientific and cost-effectiveness criteria in selecting batteries of short-term tests. *Mutation Research*, 205, 41–9.

Omenn, G.S. and Motulsky, A.G. (1978). Ecogenetics: genetic variation in susceptibility to environmental agents. In *Genetic issues in public health and medicine* (ed. B.H. Cohen, A.M. Lilienfeld and P.C. Huang), pp. 83–111. C.C. Thomas, Springfield, IL.

Omenn, G.S., Omiecinski, C.J., and Eaton D.L. (1990). Ecogenetics of chemical carcinogens. In *Biotechnology and human genetic predisposition to disease* (ed. C.R. Cantor, C.T. Caskey, L.E. Hood, D. Kamely, and G.S. Omenn), pp. 81–93. Wiley, New York.

Omenn, G.S., Goodman, G., Thornquist, M., Grizzle, J., Rosenstock, L., Barnhart, S. *et al.* (1994). The β–Carotene and Retinol Efficacy Trial (CARET) for chemoprevention of lung cancer in high risk populations: smokers and asbestos-exposed workers. *Cancer Research*, 54, 2038s–43s.

Omenn, G.S., Stuebbe, S., and Lave, L. (1995). Predictions of rodent carcinogenicity testing results: interpretation in light of the Lave-Omenn value-of-information model. *Molecular Carcinogenesis*, **14**, 37–45.

Renwick, A.G. and Walker, R. (1993). An analysis of the risk of exceeding the acceptable or tolerable daily intake. *Reg. Toxicology Pharmacology*, **18**, 463–80.

Rios, R., Poje, G.V., and Detels, R. (1993). Susceptibility to environmental pollutants among minorities. *Toxicology and Industrial Health*, **9**, 797–820.

Sandman, P.M. (1993). *Responding to community outrage: strategies for effective risk communication.* American Industrial Hygiene Association, Fairfax, VA.

Shelby, M.D., Bishop, J.B., Mason, J.M., and Tindall, K.R. (1993). Fertility, reproduction and genetic disease: studies on the mutagenic effects of environmental agents on mammalian germ cells. *Environmental Health Perspectives*, **100**, 283–91.

Shuey, D.L., Lau, C., Logsdon, T.R., Zucker, R.M., Elstein, K.H., Narotsky, M.G. (1994). Biologically based dose–response modeling in developmental toxicology: biochemical and cellular sequelae of 5–fluorouracil exposure in the developing rat. *Toxicology and Applied Pharmacology*, **126**, 129–44.

Slovic, P., Fischhoff, B., and Lichtenstein, S. (1979). Rating the risks. *Environment*, **21**, 1–20, 36–9.

Snellings, W.M., Weill, C.S., and Maronpot, R.R. (1984*a*). A two-year inhalation study of the carcinogenic potential of ethylene oxide in Fischer 344 rats. *Toxicology and Applied Pharmacology*, **75**, 105–17.

Snellings, W.M., Weill, C.S., and Maronpot, R.R. (1984*b*). A subchronic inhalation study on the toxicologic potential of ethylene oxide in B6C3F1 mice. *Toxicology and Applied Pharmacology*, **76**, 510–18.

Steenland, K., Stayner, L., Greife, A., Halperin, W., Hayes, R., Hornung, R., and Nowlin, S. (1991). Mortality among workers exposed to ethylene oxide. *New England Journal of Medicine*, **324**, 1402–7.

Tengs, O.T., Adams, M.E., Pliskin, J.S., Safran, D.G., Siegel, J.E., Weinstein, M.C., and Graham, J.D. (1995). Five-hundred life-saving interventions and their cost-effectiveness. *Risk Analysis*, **15**, 369–90.

Tennant, R.W., Spalding, J.W., Stasiewicz, S., and Ashby, J. (1990). Prediction of the outcome of rodent carcinogenicity bioassays currently being conducted on 44 chemicals by the National Toxicology Program. *Mutagenesis* **5**, 3–14.

Tennant, R.W., French, J.E., and Spalding, J.W. (1995) Identifying chemical carcinogens and assessing potential risk in short-term bioassays using transgenic mouse models. *Environmental Health Perspectives*, **103**, 942–50.

Wernick, I.K. (ed.) (1995). *Community risk profiles: a tool to improve environment and community health.* The Rockefeller University, New York.

Whittaker, S.G. and Faustman, E.M. (1994). *In vitro* assays for developmental toxicity. In *In vitro toxicology* (ed. S.C. Gad), pp. 97–122. Raven Press, New York.

WHO (1962). *WHO: Principles in governing consumer safety in relation to pesticide residues.* WHO, Geneva.

34 Risk perception and communication

Baruch Fischhoff, Ann Bostrom, and Marilyn Jacobs Quadrel

Introduction

Role of risk perceptions in public health

Many health risks are the result of deliberate decisions by individuals consciously trying to make the best choices for themselves and for those important to them. Some of these choices are private. They include decisions such as whether to wear bicycle helmets and seatbelts, whether to read and follow safety warnings, whether to buy and use condoms, and how to select and cook food. Other choices involve societal issues. They include such decisions as whether to protest the siting of hazardous waste incinerators and half-way houses, whether to vote for fluoridation and 'green' candidates, and whether to support sex education in schools.

In some cases, single choices can have a large effect on health risks (for example, buying a car with airbags, taking a dangerous job, or getting pregnant). In other cases, the effects of individual choices are small, but can accumulate over multiple decisions (for example, repeatedly ordering broccoli, wearing a seatbelt, or using the escort service in parking garages). In still other cases, choices intended to affect health risks do nothing at all or the opposite of what is expected (for example, responses to baseless cancer scares or subscription to quack treatments).

In order to make health decisions wisely, individuals need to understand the risks and the benefits associated with alternative courses of action. They also need to understand the limits to their own knowledge and to the advice proffered by various experts. This chapter reviews the research base for systematically describing people's degree of understanding about health risk issues. We also consider some fundamental topics in designing and evaluating messages for improving that understanding. Following convention, these pursuits will be called risk perception and risk communication research, respectively.

The role of perceptions about risk perceptions in public health

The fundamental assumption of this chapter is that statements about other people's understanding must be disciplined by systematic data. People can be hurt by inaccuracies in their risk perceptions. They can also be hurt by inaccuracies in what various other people believe about those perceptions. Particularly significant others include physicians, nurses, public health officials, legislators, regulators, and engineers—all of whom have some say in what risks

Preparation of this chapter was supported by the National Institute of Alcohol Abuse and Alcoholism.

are created, what is communicated about them, and what role lay-people have in determining their own fates.

If their understanding is overestimated, people may be thrust into situations that they are ill prepared to handle (for example, choosing between complex medical procedures). If their understanding is underestimated, people may be disenfranchised from decisions that they could and should make. The price of such misperceptions of risk perceptions may be exacted in the long-term as well as in individual decisions. The outcomes of health risk decisions partly determine people's physical and financial resources. The processes by which health risk decisions are made partly determine people's degree of autonomy in managing their own affairs and in shaping their society.

In addition to citing relevant research results, this chapter will emphasize research methods. One conventional reason for doing so is improving access to material that is scattered over specialist literatures or is part of the implicit knowledge conveyed in professional training. A second conventional reason is to help readers evaluate the substantive results reported here, by giving a feeling for how they were produced.

A less conventional reason is to make the point that method matters. We are routinely struck by the strong statements made about other people's competence to manage risks, solely on the basis of anecdotal observation and intuition. These statements appear directly in pronouncements about, for example, why people mistrust various technologies or fail to 'eat correctly'. Such claims appear more subtly in the myriad of health advisories, advertisements, and warnings directed at the public without any systematic evaluation. These practices assume that the communicator knows what people currently know, what they need to learn, what they want to hear, and how they will interpret a message.

Even casual testing with a focus group shows a willingness to have those (smug) assumptions challenged. Focus groups are a popular technique in market research. In them, survey questions, commercial messages, political postures or consumer products are discussed by groups of lay people. Although they can generate unanticipated alternative interpretations, focus groups create a very different situation than that faced by an individual trying to make sense out of a question, message, or product. Indeed, Merton (1987), the primary inventor of focus groups as a technique for uncovering possible hypotheses, has repudiated them as a technique for testing (even those) hypotheses. The research methods presented here show the details needing attention and, conversely, the pitfalls to casual observation. We also show the limits to such research, in terms of how far current methods can go and how quickly they can get there. It has been our experience that, once the case has been made for conducting behavioural research, it is expected to produce results immediately. That is, of course, a prescription for failure and for undermining the perceived value of future behavioural research. Furthermore, the cumulative attack on public competence can lead to its disenfranchisement and the transfer of authority to technical experts, be they physicians or technology managers. Indeed, some attacks seem designed to effect such a change in the balance of political power. In particular, in matters of environmental policy, there are those who would just as soon have no research (or ambiguous research) regarding public perceptions of risk—so that they can fill the void with their own punditry (Fischhoff *et al.* 1983; Fischhoff 1990).

Overview

The next section on quantitative assessment treats the most obvious question about lay people's risk perceptions: do they understand how big (or small) risks are? It begins with representative results regarding the quality of lay people's quantitative judgments, along with some relevant psychological theory. It continues with issues in survey design, focused on how design choices can affect respondents' apparent competence. Some of these methodological issues reveal substantive aspects of lay risk perceptions.

The following section shifts the focus from summary estimates of risk to judgments about qualitative features of the events being considered. It begins with the barriers to communication created when experts and lay people unwittingly use terms differently. For example, when experts tell (or ask) people about the risks of drinking and driving, what do people think is meant regarding the kinds and amounts of 'drinking' and of 'driving'? We then ask how people believe that risks are created and controlled, as a basis for generating and evaluating action options.

The final section provides a general process for developing communications about health risks. That process begins by identifying the information to be communicated, based on a descriptive study of what recipients know already and a formal analysis of what they need to know in order to make informed decisions. The process continues by selecting an appropriate format for presenting that information. It concludes with an explicit, empirical evaluation of the resulting communication, with the process being iterated if the results are wanting. The process is illustrated with examples taken from several case studies, looking at such diverse health risks as those posed by radon, Lyme disease, electromagnetic fields, carotid endarterectomy, and nuclear energy sources in space.

This chapter will not address several issues that belong in a fuller account. These include the roles of emotion, individual differences, culture, and social processes in decisions about risk. This set of restrictions suits the chapter's focus on how individuals think about risks. It may also suit a public health perspective, where it is often necessary to 'treat' populations (with information) in fairly uniform ways. Access to missing topics might begin with Jasanoff (1986), Weinstein (1987), Heimer (1988), Krimsky and Plough (1988), National Research Council (1989), Otway and Wynne (1989), Douglas (1992), Krimsky and Golding (1992), Royal Society (1992), Yates (1992), and Leiss and Chociolko (1994).

Quantitative assessment
Estimating the size of risks

A common presenting symptom in experts' complaints about lay decision making is that 'they (the public) do not realize how small (or large) the risk is'. If that were the case, then the mission of risk communication would be conceptually simple (although still technically challenging): transmitting credible estimates of the magnitude of risks. The need for such communication can be seen in research showing that lay estimates of risk are, indeed, subject to biases (Kahneman *et al.* 1982; Slovic 1987; Weinstein 1987; Stallen and Tomas 1988). Rather less evidence directly implicates these biases in inappropriate risk decisions or substantiates the idealized notion of people waiting for crisp risk estimates so that they can 'run' decision-making models in their heads. Such estimates are necessary, but not sufficient, for effective decisions. Accurate estimates alone cannot tell people what actions are possible or what goals are worth pursuing. They might not even show what risks are worth worrying about—in so far as there may be nothing to do about large risks, while small risks might be expeditiously handled. None the less, some notion of risk size is needed just to begin focusing one's attention.

In one early attempt to evaluate lay estimates of the size of risks, Lichtenstein *et al.* (1978) asked people to estimate the number of deaths in the United States from 30 causes (for example, botulism, tornadoes, and motor vehicle accidents). The 'people' in this study were members of the League of Women Voters and their spouses. Generally speaking, the people in the studies described here have been students paid for participation (hence, typically older than the proverbial college sophomores of some psychological research) or convenience samples of adults recruited through diverse civic groups (for example, garden clubs, parent-teacher associations, and bowling leagues). These groups have been found to differ more in what they think than in how they think. That is, their respective experiences have created larger differences in specific beliefs than in thought processes. Fuller treatment of sampling issues must await another opportunity.) Lichtenstein *et al.* used two different response modes, allowing a check for the consistency of responses. One task presented pairs of causes; subjects chose the more frequent and then estimated the ratio of frequencies. The second task asked subjects to estimate the number of deaths in an average year. These subjects were told the answer for one cause, as an anchor, providing an order of magnitude feeling for the kinds of answers that were expected; a pretest had found that many subjects lacked a good idea of how many people live or die in the United States, in an average year. The study reached several conclusions which have been borne out by subsequent studies (for example, Vlek and Stallen 1980).

Internal consistency
Estimates of relative frequency were quite consistent, both within and across the response mode. Thus, people seemed to have a moderately well-articulated internal risk scale, which they were able to express even in the unfamiliar response modes used in these studies—in life, they had probably never been asked any question as explicit as these quantitative estimates of risk.

Anchoring bias

Direct estimates were influenced by the anchor given. Subjects who were told that 50 000 people die annually from motor accidents produced estimates two to five times higher than did subjects who were told that 1000 die from electrocution. Thus, people seem to have less of a feel for absolute frequency, rendering them sensitive to the implicit cues in how questions are asked (Poulton 1989).

Compression

Subjects' estimates showed less dispersion than did the statistical estimates. While the statistical estimates varied over six orders of magnitude, the typical subject's estimates ranged over three to four. In this case, the result was overestimation of small frequencies and underestimation of large ones. However, the anchoring bias suggests that this overall pattern might have changed with different procedures, making the compression of estimates the more fundamental result. For example, using an even lower anchor (for example, the average annual toll of botulism deaths) would have reduced the overestimation of small frequencies and increased the underestimation of large ones. If these responses reflect subjects' actual feeling for the relative size of different risks, then people may have difficulty appreciating the enormous range in the frequencies of life's risks. That would not be surprising, considering how rare it is for media reports to include explicit quantitative estimates.

Availability bias

At each level of statistical frequency, some causes of death (for example, homicide, tornadoes, and flood) consistently received higher estimates than others. Additional analyses showed these to be causes that are disproportionately visible (for example, as reported in the news media and as experienced in subjects' lives). This bias seemed to reflect a special case of a general tendency to estimate the frequency of events by the ease with which they are remembered or imagined—while failing to realize what a fallible index such availability is (Tversky and Kahneman 1973; Kahneman *et al.* 1982). These results are consistent with those in experimental psychology, showing that people are generally quite proficient at tracking how frequently events are observed, but not so good at detecting systematic biases in those observations (for example, Hasher and Zacks 1984; Koriat 1993).

Miscalibration of confidence judgments

In a subsequent study (Fischhoff *et al.* 1977), subjects were asked how confident they were in their ability to choose the more frequent in a pair of causes of death (for example, tornado and asthma). They tended to be overconfident. For example, they chose correctly only 75 per cent of the time when they were 90 per cent confident of having done so. This result is a special case of the general tendency to be inadequately sensitive to the extent of one's knowledge (Lichtenstein *et al.* 1982; Yates 1989).

Figure 34.1 shows typical results from such a calibration test. In this case, subjects expressed their confidence in having chosen the correct answer to two alternative questions regarding health risks (for example, alcohol is (1) a depressant and (2) a stimulant). In the figure, each point reflects the proportion of correct responses associated with answers assigned a particular probability of being correct. Thus, in the lowest curve, subjects were correct approximately 70 per cent of the time when 100 per cent certain of being correct. The two upper curves reflect a group of middle-class

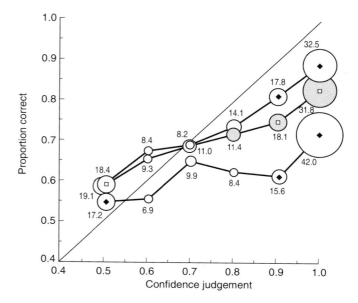

Fig. 34.1 Calibration curves for adults (top, white: n = 45), not-at-risk teenagers (middle, dark: n = 43), and at-risk teenagers (bottom, white: n = 45). Each point indicates the proportion of correct answers among those in which subjects expressed a particular confidence level and the size of each circle indicates the percentage of answers held with that degree of confidence. Source: Quadrel (1990).

adults and some of their adolescent children, recruited through school organizations. As in other studies of cognitive ability, the judgemental processes of these groups are quite similar (Keating 1988). The lowest curve reflects at-risk teenagers, recruited from group homes and treatment centres. They knew less about these risk issues, but were just as confident; indeed, over 40 per cent of their responses indicated complete confidence in the associated answer. One possible explanation of this overconfidence is that their personal experiences with risks create an illusion of understanding, leading them to feel inappropriately like experts. A second is that high-risk teenagers have less ability to think critically about the bases of their beliefs or less willingness to do so. Effective decision making requires not just having knowledge, but also recognizing the limits to one's understanding.

Response mode problems

One recurrent obstacle to assessing or improving lay people's estimates of risk is a reliance on verbal quantifiers for both communicating and eliciting risk estimates. It is hard for people to know what experts mean when a risk is described as 'very likely' or 'rare'. It is equally difficult for experts to evaluate lay perceptions expressed in those terms. Such terms mean different things to different people and even to the same person in different contexts (for example, likely to be fatal versus likely to rain, rare disease versus rare Cubs baseball championship). Such ambiguity has been found even within communities of professionals, such as physicians and intelligence officers (Lichtenstein and Newman 1967; Beyth-Marom 1982). The criticality of such ambiguity depends, of course, on how the estimates are used. Sometimes, inferred probabilities of 1 and 10 per cent will lead to the same choice; sometimes not. The variability of interpretations should increase with the diversity of individuals and decisions.

Table 34.1 Comparison of numerical verbal and statistical risk estimates ('Please estimate your personal risk to the following events in the next 3 years')

Risk	Quantitative response scale (% median probability)	Verbal response scale		Statistical risk estimate (% probability)
		Median	Mean	
Electrocution	0.1	1.0	1.67	0.015
Cancer	0.3	2.0	2.09	0.06
Influenza	55.0	5.0	4.72	86.2
Car injury	10.0	3.0	3.38	4.7
Herpes	0.1	1.0	1.73	4.1
AIDS virus/sexual	0.02	1.0	1.41	0.2

Source: Linville *et al.* (1993).

Table 34.1 shows the results of asking a fairly homogeneous group of subjects (undergraduates at an Ivy League college) to judge seven risks in both quantitative and qualitative terms, with reported statistical rates. The quantitative estimates used a response scale that explicitly offered probabilities as low as 0.01 per cent (or 1 in 10 000). The qualitative scale used typical labels (converted to interval-scale equivalents in the data analyses: 1 = very unlikely; 2 = unlikely, 3 = somewhat unlikely, 4 = somewhat likely, 5 = likely, and 6 = very likely). Comparing the two response scales revealed a non-linear relationship between the two. Specifically, the median probabilities (column 1) associated with the median qualitative estimates (column 2) were very unlikely (0.01 per cent), unlikely (0.5 per cent), somewhat unlikely (5 per cent), somewhat likely (25 per cent), likely (60 per cent), and very likely (96 per cent). Budescu and Wallsten (1995) reviewed the evidence on the predictability of such equivalencies across tasks and what they reveal about experiences with risks.

The Lichtenstein *et al.* (1978) study provided anchors in order to give subjects a feeling for how to answer. The anchors should have improved subjects' performance by drawing responses to the correct range, within which subjects were drawn to higher or lower values depending on the value of the anchor that they received. Most of the study's conclusions were relatively insensitive to these anchoring effects—except for the critical question of how much people overestimate or underestimate the risks that they face.

Perceived lethality

A study by Fischhoff and MacGregor (1983) provides another example of the dangers of relying on a single response mode. They used four different response modes to ask about the chances of dying, conditional on being afflicted with each of various maladies: how many people die out of each 100 000 who get influenza, how many people died out of the 80 million who caught influenza last year, for each person who dies of influenza, how many have it and survive, and 800 people died of influenza last year, how many survived? Again, there was strong ordinal consistency across response modes, while absolute estimates varied over one to two orders of magnitude. A follow-up study looked for independent evidence of the relative suitability of these different response modes. It found that subjects liked one format much less than the others. They were also least able to remember statistics reported in that format. This was also the format that produced the most

discrepant results—estimating the number of survivors for each person who succumbed to a problem.

Perceived invulnerability

Estimating the accuracy of risk estimates requires not only an appropriate response mode, but also a standard against which responses can be compared. The studies just described asked about population risks in situations where credible statistical estimates were available to the investigators. People's performance might be different (and harder to evaluate) with risks whose magnitude is less readily calculated. Furthermore, for many decisions, people's understanding of population risks is less relevant than their understanding of personal risks. Unfortunately, personalized risk statistics are usually hard to come by.

In order to circumvent these problems, some investigators have asked subjects to judge whether they are more or less at risk than others in (more or less) similar circumstances (Svenson 1981; Weinstein 1989). They find that most people in most situations see themselves as facing less risk than average others; that could, of course, be true for only half a population. A variety of processes could account for such a bias, including both cognitive ones (for example, the greater availability of the precautions that one takes—than those taken by others) and motivational ones (for example, wishful thinking). Such an optimism bias could prompt unwanted risk taking (for example, because warnings seem more applicable to other people than to oneself). In a recent study (Quadrel *et al.* 1993), we asked subjects to judge the probability of various misfortunes befalling them and several target others (a close friend, an acquaintance, a parent, and a child).

The events involved 'a death or injury requiring hospitalization over the next 5 years', from sources such as motor accidents, drug addiction, and explosions. Subjects were most likely to see each person's risks similarly, meaning that perceived invulnerability was the exception, rather than the rule. However, when they did make a distinction, they were twice as likely to see themselves as the person facing less risk. This perception of relative personal invulnerability was particularly large for risks seen as under some personal control. Here, too, adults and adolescents responded similarly, despite the common belief that teenagers take risks, in part, because of a unique perception of invulnerability (Elkind 1967).

A log-linear response mode

Figure 34.2 shows the response mode used in this study. It uses a linear scale for probabilities between 1 and 100 per cent and six cycles of a log scale for smaller ones. The scale was explained to subjects in groups and introduced with a few examples having obvious and extreme values (for example, being hit by lightning and catching a cold), in order to help subjects to understand it. Quadrel *et al.* (1993) found similar scale usage, not to mention similar beliefs (as noted above), among groups of middle-class adults, their high-school children, and high-risk teenagers, recruited from group homes and treatment centres. The statistical risk estimates of Table 34.1 were elicited with a variant of this scale. Comparison between columns 1 and 4 allows a quantitative assessment of the accuracy of the risk estimates. Formal analysis might show whether errors of this magnitude would be large enough to influence decisions relying on them, (see the section on Value of information analysis below).

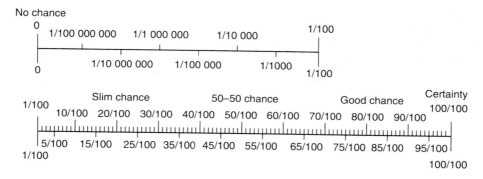

Fig. 34.2 Log-linear response scale for eliciting probability assessments, facilitating the expression of very small probabilities. Source: Quadrel *et al.* (1993).

The critical question in considering the usefulness of such a response mode is whether the additional information that it provides compensates for the extra demands that it imposes on subjects. For example, does it inspire enough confidence that one is willing to infer that the young adults in Table 34.1 moderately underestimate their risk of herpes infection (over the next 3 years), while moderately overestimating their risk of acquired immune deficiency syndrome (**AIDS**) (although recognizing that it is still very small)? Is it helpful to know that subjects assigned a probability of less than 1 in 10 million approximately 10 per cent of the time and a probability of less than 1 in 10000 approximately one-third of the time?

In our experience, the limiting factor on using this kind of scale is not the subjects' ability to understand quantitative probabilities. Rather, it is whether they have the reading ability needed to process the instructions on just how it is to be used. In our administration, the instructions were read aloud to circumvent any problems. Given the highly limited usefulness of verbal quantifiers, we believe that little is lost by using quantitative response scales. Using responses to quantitative scales, Viscusi (1992) was able to argue that the public health establishment has more than succeeded in convincing adults of the risks of smoking. If that is the case, then communications should be focused on teenagers or on the risks of addiction.

Realizing the potential of precise response scales requires applying them to precisely defined events. Some years ago, the US National Weather Service considered abandoning quantitative probability of precipitation forecasts because of reported consumer confusion. Murphy *et al.* (1980) discovered that the confusion was actually about the event being predicted. For example, did a 70 per cent chance of rain refer to the portion of the area to be covered, the percentage of time that it would rain, the chance of measurable rain at any spot in the area, or the chance at the weather station? (It is the last.) Event ambiguity is treated further below and in Fischhoff (1994).

Defining risk

These studies provide measures of risk perceptions, if one assumes that people define 'risk' as 'probability of death'. However, observation of scientific practice shows that, even among professionals, 'risk' can have a variety of meanings (Crouch and Wilson 1982; Fischhoff *et al.* 1984; Royal Society 1992; National Research Council 1996). For some experts, 'risk' equals expected loss of life expectancy, for other risk analysts, it is expected probability of

premature fatality, while for still others, it is the total number of deaths or deaths per person exposed or per hour of exposure or loss of ability to work (Starr 1969; Inhaber 1979; Wilson 1979; Zentner 1979).

Unwitting use of different definitions can lead to controversy and confusion, in so far as the relative riskiness of different jobs, avocations, technologies, and diseases depends on the choice of definition. Although often left to the conventions of technical experts, the choice of definition is a political/ethical decision which can significantly affect a society's allocation of resources. For example, hazards producing deaths by injury become relatively 'riskier' if one counts the total years lost rather than weighting all deaths equally. That measure of risk places a greater premium on deaths among young people, because more years of life are lost with them. Some of the apparent disagreement between experts and lay-people regarding the magnitude of risks in society seems due to differing definitions of 'risk' (Slovic *et al.* 1979; Vlek and Stallen 1980; Fischhoff *et al.* 1983).

Catastrophic potential

One early study asked experts and lay people to estimate the 'risk of death' faced by society as a whole from 30 activities and technologies (Slovic *et al.* 1979). The experts' judgements were much more highly correlated with statistical estimates of average year fatalities than were the lay people's estimates. When lay people were asked to estimate average year fatalities, they responded much like the experts. However, when lay people estimated 'risk of death', they also seemed to consider (what they saw as) the catastrophic potential of the technology (that is, its ability to cause large numbers of deaths in non-average years). Thus, experts and lay people agreed about routine death tolls (for which scientific estimates are relatively uncontroversial) and disagreed about the possibility of anomalies (for which the science is typically much weaker). This seemingly reasonable pattern would be obscured by the casual observation that experts and lay people disagree about 'risk' or by the assumption that any disagreement means that the experts are right and the lay people are wrong.

Sensing that there was something special about catastrophic potential, some risk experts have suggested that social policy pay special attention to the regulation of hazards carrying that kind of threat. One experimental study found, however, that people did not care more for losing many lives in a single incident than for losing the same number of lives in separate incidents (Slovic *et al.* 1984). (When incidents involving large numbers of fatalities are easy to

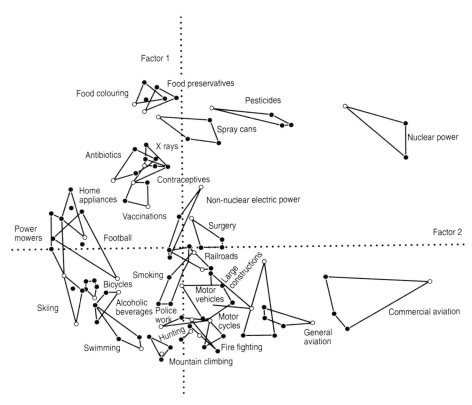

Fig. 34.3 Location of 30 hazards within the two-factor space obtained from League of Women Voters and student, active club and expert groups. Respondents evaluated each activity or technology on each of nine features. Ratings were subjected to principal components factor analysis, with a varimax rotation. Connected lines join or enclose the loci of four group points for each hazard. Open circles represent data from the expert group. Unattached points represent groups that fall within the triangle created by the other three groups. Source: Slovic *et al.* (1985).

imagine, catastrophic potential can be rated high because of availability, even when estimates of average year fatalities are relatively low, as was the case for nuclear power in this study.) Rather catastrophic potential worries people because a technology posing such threats may prove to be out of control, despite its promoters' promises. Such 'surprise potential' is strongly correlated with 'catastrophic potential' in people's judgments; the same is presumably true in scientific estimates (Funtowicz and Ravetz 1990). The two features represent, however, rather different ethical bases for distinguishing among risks.

Dimensions of risk

Uncertainty and catastrophic potential are not the only dimensions of risk that might influence how they are judged. Much research and speculation has been devoted to these features of risk (for example, Lowrance 1976; Slovic *et al.* 1980; Vlek and Stallen 1980; Green and Brown 1981; Cole and Withey 1982), with the set of proposed features running to several dozen. This is an unwieldy number of features for a descriptive theory of risk perceptions, a prescriptive guide to risk decisions, or a scheme for predicting public responses to new hazards or hazard-reduction schemes. As a result, various empirical studies have attempted both to check these speculations and to reduce the number of considerations. Most have followed (and elaborated on) a correlation scheme offered by Fischhoff *et al.* (1978). In it, members of a liberal civic organization rated 30 environmental hazards on nine hypothesized aspects of risk; factor analysis reduced the mean ratings of nine aspects to two

'dimensions', which accounted for 78 per cent of the variance. Similar patterns were found with students, members of a conservative civic organization, members of a liberal women's organization, and technical risk assessors. Figure 34.3 shows the factor scores for 30 hazards within the common factor space for these four groups.

Hazards at the high end of the vertical factor (for example, food colouring and pesticides) tended to be new, unknown, involuntary, and delayed in their effects. High (right-side) scores on the horizontal factor (for example, nuclear power and commercial aviation) mean that consequences are seen as certain to be fatal and affecting large numbers of people, should something go wrong. The vertical factor was labelled unknown risk and the horizontal factor dread risk. They might be seen as capturing the cognitive and emotional bases of people's concern, respectively.

Other studies, employing variants on this 'psychometric paradigm', have yielded results that are similar in many respects. For example, despite changes in elicitation mode, scaling techniques, items rated, and subject population, two or three dimensions have proved adequate. Where a third dimension emerges, it typically refers to the absolute number of lives exposed to the threat in present or future generations; catastrophic potential has been used as a label. The position of particular technologies in this space proves to be highly robust. Moreover, that position is correlated strongly with various attitudes, including the desired stringency of regulation. Such analyses of mean responses are most suitable for predicting aggregate responses to hazards. The international and intercultural comparison of such risk spaces has proven to be a fruitful area, with a standard methodology revealing local differences (and similarities) (for example, Kuyper and Vlek 1984; Englander et al. 1986; Goszczyska et al. 1991; Karpowicz-Lazreg and Mullet 1993; Vaughan 1993; Jianguang 1994; Rohrmann 1994).

Risk comparisons

The multidimensional character of risk means that hazards that are similar in many ways may still evoke quite different responses. This fact is neglected in appeals to accept one risk because one accepts another risk that is similar to it in some ways (Fischhoff et al., 1981; Crouch and Wilson 1982). The most ambitious of these appeals present elaborate lists of hazards, exposure to which is adjusted so that they pose equivalent statistical risks (for example, consuming one tablespoonful of peanut butter and living for 50 years at the boundary of a nuclear power plant both create a 1 in 1 million risk of premature death). Recognizing that such comparisons are often perceived as self-serving, the Chemical Manufacturers Association commissioned a guide to risk comparisons (Covello et al. 1988), which presents many such lists, along with the attached caution, 'Warning! Use of data in this table for risk comparison purposes can damage your credibility'. The guide also offers advice on how to make risk comparisons, if one feels the compulsion, along with examples of more and less acceptable comparisons. Although the advice was derived logically from risk-perception research, it was not tested empirically. In such a test, we found little correlation between the authors' predicted degree of acceptability and that judged by several diverse groups of subjects (Roth et al. 1990; MacGregor 1991).

One possible reason for the failure of these predictions is that the manual's authors knew too much (from their own previous research) to produce truly unacceptable comparisons. More important than identifying the specific reasons for this failure is the general cautionary message: because we all have experience in dealing with risks, it is tempting to assume that our intuitions are shared by others. Often, they are not. Effective risk communication requires careful empirical research. Poor risk communication can often cause more public health (and economic) damage than the risks that it attempts to describe. One should no more release an untested communication than an untested medical device. The need for research is further magnified when one crosses cultural or national boundaries.

Qualitative assessment

Event definitions

Scientific estimates of the magnitude of a risk require detailed specification of the conditions under which it is to be observed. For example, a fertility counsellor estimating a woman's risk of an unplanned pregnancy would consider the frequency and timing of intercourse, the kinds of contraceptive used (and the diligence of their application), her physiological condition (and that of her partner), and so on. If lay people are to make accurate assessments, they require the same level of detail. That is true whether they are estimating risks for their own sake or for the benefit of an investigator studying risk perceptions.

When investigators omit needed details, they create adverse conditions for subjects. In order to respond correctly, subjects must

first guess the question and then know the answer to it. Consider, for example, the question 'what is the probability of pregnancy with unprotected sex?' A well-informed subject who understood this to mean a single exposure would be seen as underestimating the risk—by an investigator who intended the question to mean multiple exposures.

Such ambiguous 'events' are common in surveys of public risk perceptions. For example, a National Center for Health Statistics (**NCHS**) survey (Wilson and Thornberry 1987) question asked, 'How likely do you think it is that a person will get the AIDS virus from sharing plates, forks, or glasses with someone who has AIDS?' Fischhoff (1989) asked a relatively homogeneous group of subjects to answer this question, then to say what they thought was meant regarding the amount and kind of sharing that it implied. For their responses to be interpretable, subjects must spontaneously assign the same value to each missing detail and investigators must guess what value subjects have chosen. These subjects generally agreed about the kind of sharing (82 per cent interpreted it as sharing during a meal), but not about the frequency (a single occasion, 39 per cent; several occasions 20 per cent; routinely, 28 per cent; uncertain, 12 per cent). Thus, these subjects were answering a variety of different questions, rendering their responses ambiguous. In this case, the response mode was also ambiguous (very likely, unlikely, and so on), so that even precise questions would have revealed little. A survey question about the risks of sexual transmission evoked similar disagreement.

Interestingly, all of the subjects who reported uncertainty about the frequency and intensity of sharing (or of sexual activity) still made likelihood judgments. If people are willing to respond to survey questions that they do not understand, any relationship between their reported beliefs and behaviors would tend to be blurred. That could, in turn, lead an observer to think, for example, that 'information does not work with teenagers', in so far as their actions seem unrelated to their beliefs. If so, that would be a special case of the general tendency for poor measurement to reduce the power of research designs. An important role of the NCHS study, one of an annual series, is to guide national policy on AIDS. No-one has studied what readers of the NCHS survey's results believed about subjects' interpretations of its questions. However, if they misunderstood subjects' beliefs, then they may have produced ineffective and misdirected communications.

Supplying details

Aside from their methodological importance, the details that subjects infer can be substantively interesting. People's intuitive theories of risk are revealed in the variables that they note and the values that they supply. In a systematic evaluation of these theories, Quadrel (1990) asked adolescents to think aloud as they estimated the probability of several deliberately ambiguous events (for example, being involved in a motor accident after drinking and driving and getting AIDS through sex).

These subjects typically wondered (and made assumptions) about a large number of features. In this sense, subjects arguably showed more sophistication than the investigators who created the surveys from which these simplistic questions were taken or adapted. Generally speaking, these subjects were interested in variables that could figure in scientific risk analyses. That is, they wanted relevant information that had been denied them by the investigators. There were, however, some interesting exceptions. Although subjects wanted to know the 'dose' involved with most risks, they did not ask about the amount of sex in a question about the risks of pregnancy or in another question about the risks of human immunodeficiency virus (HIV) transmission. They seemed to believe that an individual either is or is not susceptible to the risk, regardless of the amount of the exposure. In other cases, subjects asked about variables with a less clear connection to risk level (for example, how well members of the couple knew one another).

In a follow-up study, Quadrel (1990) presented richly specified event descriptions to teenagers drawn from the same populations (school organizations and substance abuse treatment homes). Subjects initially estimated the probability of a risky outcome on the basis of some 12 details. Then they were asked how knowing each of three additional details would change their estimates. One of those details had been identified as relevant by subjects in the preceding study, while two had not. Subjects in this study were much more sensitive to changes in the relevant details than to changes in the irrelevant ones. Thus, at least in these studies, teenagers did not balk at making quantitative judgments regarding complex stimuli. When they did so, they revealed consistent intuitive theories in rather different tasks.

Cumulative risk: a case in point

As knowledge accumulates about people's intuitive theories of risk, it will become easier to predict which details subjects know and ignore, as well as which omissions they will notice and rectify. In time, it might become possible to infer the answers to questions that are asked from ones that are not—as well as the inferences that people make from risks that are described explicitly to risks that are not. The invulnerability results reported above show the need for empirical research to discipline extrapolations from one setting to another. Asking people about the risks to other people like themselves is not the same as asking them about their personal risk. Nor can it be assumed that hearing about others' risk levels will lead people to draw personal conclusions.

One common and seemingly natural extrapolation is across settings differing in the number of exposures to a risk. Telling people about the risk from a single exposure should allow them to infer the risk from the number of exposures they expect to face; asking subjects what risk they expect from one number of exposures should allow one to infer what they expect from other numbers. Unfortunately, for both research and communication, teenagers' insensitivity to the amount of intercourse in determining the risks of pregnancy or HIV transmission proves to be a special case of a general problem. Several reviews (Cvetkovich et al. 1975; Morrison 1985) have concluded that between one-third and one-half of sexually active adolescents explain not using contraceptives with variants of, 'I thought I (or my partner) could not get pregnant'.

In another study, Shaklee and Fischhoff (1990) found that adults greatly underestimated the rate at which the risk of contraceptive failure accumulates through repeated exposure—even after eliminating (from the data analysis) the 40 per cent or so of subjects who saw no relationship between risk and exposure. One corollary of this bias is not realizing the extent to which seemingly small differences in annual failure rates (the statistic that is typically reported) can lead to large differences in cumulative risk. Bar-Hillel (1974) and Cohen and Hansel (1958) found underaccumulation in simple clearly described gambles. Wagenaar and Sagaria (1975) found it in estimating cumulative environmental degradation.

After providing practice with a response mode facilitating the expression of small probabilities, Linville et al. (1993) asked college students to estimate the probability of HIV transmission from a man to a woman as the result of one, 10, or 100 cases of protected sex. For one contact, the median estimate was 0.10, a remarkably high value, compared to public health estimates (Fineberg 1988; Kaplan 1989). For 100 contacts, the median estimate was 0.25, which is a more reasonable value; however, it is also quite inconsistent with the single-exposure estimate. Assuming their independence, 100 exposures should provide a near-certainty of transmission. Very different pictures of people's risk perceptions would emerge if a study asked just one of these questions. Conversely, risk communicators could achieve quite different effects if they chose to relate the risk of just one exposure or just 100. Communicators might create confusion if they chose to communicate both risks, leaving recipients to reconcile the seeming inconsistency.

Mental models of risk decisions

Each of these studies brought one element of a decision to subjects' attention. A more comprehensive research strategy asks respondents to judge each element in a standard representation of their decision-making situation. Perhaps the most common such models have an expectancy value form (Feather 1982). In them, decisions are assumed to be determined by a multiplicative combination of the rated likelihood and (un)desirability of various prespecified consequences. Health-belief and theory-of-reasoned-action models fall into this general category. For example, Bauman (1980) had seventh graders evaluate 54 possible consequences of using marijuana, in terms of their importance, likelihood, and valence (that is, whether each is positive or negative). A 'utility structure index', computed from these three judgments, predicted approximately 20 per cent of the variance in subjects' reported marijuana usage. Related studies have had similar success in predicting other teen risk behaviours.

The experience of these studies resembles that of earlier studies of 'clinical judgement', which successfully predicted expert decision making with multiple regression models applied to experts' ratings of standard variables. Initially, investigators interpreted the regression coefficients as reflecting the weights that people give to different concerns (Hoffman 1960; Hammond et al. 1964; Goldberg 1968). However, formal analyses eventually showed that many weighting schemes would produce similar predictions, so long as they contained the same variables (or correlated surrogates) (Wilks, 1938; Dawes and Corrigan 1974). The good news in this result is that any linear combination of relevant variables will have some predictive success. The bad news is that it can be very difficult to distinguish alternative models, in terms of their relative accuracy as descriptions of decision-making processes. Thus, linear models can have considerable practical value in predicting choices, while still having limited ability to clarify how choices are made (Camerer 1981; Dawes et al. 1989). As a result, linear models provide a sort

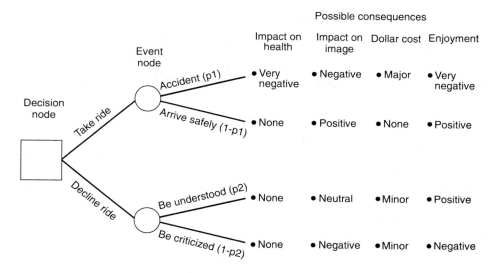

Fig. 34.4 Decision tree for whether to take or decline a ride from friends who have been drinking. Source: Fischhoff and Quadrel (1991).

of cognitive task analysis, identifying the kinds of factors that might be involved in people's choices. Other procedures are needed to clarify the finer structure of how decisions are made.

One such procedure was used by Beyth-Marom *et al.* (1993), who asked teenagers drawn from low-risk settings (for example, sports teams and service clubs) and their parents to produce the possible consequences of several decisions (for example, you decided to smoke marijuana which was passed around at a party). Some subjects were asked to consider the act of accepting the offer, while others considered the consequences of rejecting it, in order to see whether these formally complementary options would elicit complementary perceptions. In almost all respects, the teenagers and parents responded quite similarly. On average, they produced approximately six consequences, with a somewhat higher number for accepting the risky offer than for rejecting it (suggesting that the thought of doing something is more evocative than the thought of not doing it). Respondents produced many more bad than good consequences of performing the focal behavior, but fairly equal numbers for not performing it; thus, avoiding the risk was not as attractive as accepting it was unattractive. Most of the consequences that respondents mentioned were social reactions and personal effects. The social reactions of peers were particularly salient as consequences of rejecting the risk behavior (for example, more subjects said 'they will laugh at me if I decline the offer' than 'they will like me if I accept'). The thought of performing a behaviour once and of performing it regularly evoked somewhat different consequences. For example, the social reactions of peers were mentioned more frequently as consequences of 'accepting an offer to smoke marijuana at a party', while decreased mental function was mentioned more frequently for 'using marijuana'. These open-ended questions produced quite different consequences than the ones that appeared in earlier studies which required respondents to evaluate each item in a fixed list (for example, the proportion of positive consequences was lower here). It would seem hard to understand lay perceptions or to improve them without understanding such details, which seem to require an open-ended approach to be observed. For example, one might

waste time and credibility trying to bring adolescents to adult's level of awareness about consequences, something that they already seem to have.

Another study further weakened the degree of imposed task structure by letting teenagers choose three recent difficult decisions in their lives, to be described in their own terms (Fischhoff 1996). These descriptions were coded in terms of their content (what's on teenagers' minds) and structure (how those issues are formulated). Figure 34.4 shows a moderately well-structured choice about drinking and driving. None of the decisions that the 105 teenagers chose dealt with drinking and driving, although quite a few dealt with drinking. For those decisions that were mentioned, few had an option structure as complicated as that in the simple decision tree of Fig. 34.4. Rather, most were described in terms of a single option (for example, whether to go to a party where alcohol would be served).

In a two-option decision, as in Fig. 34.4, the consequences of the alternative option are logically implied. However, that need not mean that they are intuitively obvious to the decision maker. Indeed, Beyth-Marom *et al.* (1993) found that the consequences produced for engaging in a risky behaviour were not the mirror image of the consequences of rejecting that opportunity. This asymmetry is also seen in experimental results showing that foregone benefits of decisions (their 'opportunity costs') are much less visible than their direct costs. The differential visibility of such consequences can, in turn, be associated with ineffective decision making. For example, the direct risks of vaccinating one's children loom disproportionately large relative to the indirect risks of failing to vaccinate them (Harding and Eiser 1984; Ritov and Baron 1990).

We believe that a mix of structured and unstructured studies is needed to piece together a full account of lay decisions—as a prelude to predicting or aiding them. Normative decision theory provides a conceptual framework for determining which topics to study. Descriptive decision theory provides methodological and theoretical tools for pursuing that study. All are imperfect. However, in combination, they can begin to provide the sort of complex descriptions that people's decisions about complex topics deserve. Attention to methodological detail always is critical. Decision variables will explain little if they are poorly measured. People whose behaviour seems unpredictable may lose the respect of observers and, thereby, become the target of manipulation if others conclude that this is the only way to get them to behave responsibly—for their own good.

Mental models of risk processes

The role of mental models

As noted, people often have flawed intuitive theories of how risks accumulate over repeated exposure, not realizing how risks mount up through repeated exposure—and perhaps neglecting the long-term perspective altogether. Such research can improve the communication of quantitative probabilities. Those probabilities are of greatest direct use to individuals who face well-formulated decisions in which quantitative estimates of a health risk (or benefit) play clearly defined roles. For example, a couple explicitly planning their family size needs to know the probability of success and of side-effects for whichever contraceptive strategies they will consider. Alternatively, a homeowner poised to decide whether to test for radon needs quantitative estimates of the cost and accuracy of tests, the health risks of different radon levels, the cost and efficacy of ways to mitigate radon problems, and so on (Svenson and Fischhoff 1985).

Often, however, people are not poised to decide anything. Rather, they just want to know what the risk is and how it works. Such substantive knowledge is essential for following an issue in the news media, for participating in public discussions, for feeling competent to make decisions, and for generating options among which to decide. In these situations, people's objective is to have intuitive theories that correspond to the main elements of the reigning scientific theories (emphasizing those features relevant to control strategies).

The term mental model is often applied to intuitive theories that are sufficiently well elaborated to generate predictions in diverse circumstances (Galotti 1989). Mental models have a long history in psychology (Craik 1943; Oden 1987), having been used in such diverse settings as uncovering how people understand physical processes (Gentner and Stevens 1983), international tensions (Means and Voss 1985), complex equipment (Rouse and Morris 1986), energy conservation (Kempton 1987), psychological interactions (Furnham 1988), and the effects of drugs (Jungermann *et al.* 1988; Slovic *et al.* 1989).

If these mental models contain critical 'bugs', they can lead to erroneous conclusions, even among people who are otherwise well informed. For example, not knowing that repeated sex increases the associated risks could undermine much other knowledge. Bostrom *et al.* (1992) found that many people know that radon is a colourless, odourless, radioactive gas. Unfortunately, people also associate radioactivity with permanent contamination. However, this property of (widely publicized) high-level waste is not shared by radon. Not realizing that the relevant radon by-products have short half-lives, homeowners might not even bother to test (believing that there was nothing that they could do, should a problem be detected). They might also not appreciate the risk in minute concentrations, which release their energy quickly.

Eliciting mental models

In principle, the best way to detect such misconceptions would be to capture people's entire mental model on a topic. Doing so would also identify those correct beliefs upon which communications could be built (and which should be reinforced). The critical methodological threat to capturing mental models is reactivity, changing responses as a result of the elicitation procedure. One wants neither to induce nor to dispel misconceptions, either through leading questions or subtle hints. The interview should neither preclude the expression of unanticipated beliefs nor inadvertently steer subjects around topics (Ericsson and Simon 1980; Galotti 1989; Hendrickx 1991).

Bostrom *et al.* (1992) offered one possible compromise strategy, which has been used for a variety of risks (Morgan *et al.* 1990; Maharik and Fischhoff 1992; see also Kempton 1991). Their interview protocol begins with very open-ended questions, asking subjects what they know about a topic, then prompting them to consider exposure, effects, and mitigation issues. These basic categories seemed so essential that mentioning them would correct an oversight, rather than introduce a foreign concept. Subjects are asked to elaborate on every topic that they mention. Once these minimally structured tasks are exhausted, subjects sort a large stack of diverse photographs according to whether each seems related to the topic, explaining their reasoning as they go. When previously unmentioned beliefs appear at this stage, they are likely to represent latent portions of people's mental models—the sort that might emerge in everyday life if people had cause to consider specific features of their own radon situation. For example, when shown a picture of a supermarket produce counter, some respondents told us that plants might become contaminated by taking up radon from the air or soil. Some also inferred that their houseplants would not be so healthy if they had a radon problem.

Once transcribed, interviews are coded into an expert model of the risk. This is a directed network or influence diagram (Howard 1989), showing the different factors affecting the magnitude of the risk. The expert model is created by pooling the knowledge of a diverse group of experts. It might be thought of as an expert's mental model, although it would be impressive for any single expert to produce it all in a single session. Figure 34.5 shows a portion of our influence diagram for radon, focused on reducing the risks in a house with a crawl space. An arrow between nodes indicates that the value of the variable at its head depends on the value of the variable at its tail. Thus, for example, the lungs' particle clearance rate depends on an individual's smoking history. Influence diagrams are convenient ways to display the functional relationships between variables. Their structure allows one, in principle, to substitute quantitative estimates of these relationships and to compute risk levels. Influence diagrams can also be mapped into decision trees, showing the relevance of various information for decision making (which can, in turn, provide guidance on the critical question of which risk information is most worth communicating—see below).

No lay person would have this mental model. Indeed, few experts would view a problem in its full complexity (for example, knowing the factors involved in both lung clearance building materials emissions). However, it provides a template for characterizing a lay person's mental model. That characterization can be performed in terms of the appropriateness of people's beliefs, their

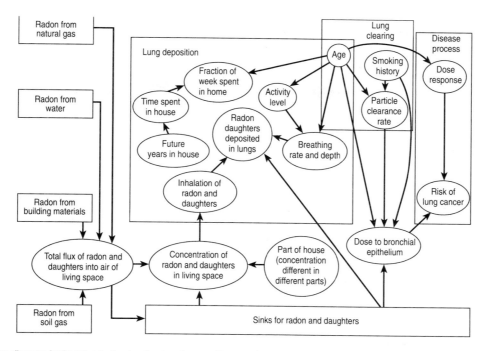

Fig. 34.5 Expert influence diagram for health effects of radon in a home with a crawl space. This diagram was used as a standard and as an organizing device to characterize the content of lay mental models. Source: Morgan *et al.* (1992).

specificity (that is, level of detail), and the category of knowledge that they represent. For most risks, beliefs can be categorized as pertaining to exposure processes, effects processes (that is, health and physiology), and mitigation behaviours—the basic components of risk analysis. Other beliefs provide background information, which influences interpreting many of the relations in the diagram (for example, radon is a gas). In evaluating appropriateness, we characterized beliefs as accurate, erroneous, peripheral (correct, but not relevant), or indiscriminate (too imprecise to be evaluated). Bostrom *et al.* (1992) found that most subjects knew that radon concentrates indoors (mentioned by 92 per cent), is detectable with a test kit (96 per cent), is a gas (88 per cent), and comes from underground (83 per cent). Most knew that radon causes cancer (63 per cent). However, many also believed erroneously that radon affects plants (58 per cent), contaminates blood (38 per cent), and causes breast cancer (29 per cent). Only two subjects (8 per cent) mentioned that radon decays. (Subjects were drawn from civic groups in the Pittsburgh area, which had had a moderate degree of radon publicity.) The robustness of these beliefs was examined (and generally confirmed) in subsequent studies using more easily administered structured questionnaires derived from the open-ended interviews.

Creating communications
Selecting information

The first step in designing communications is to select the information that they should contain. In many existing communications, this choice seems arbitrary, reflecting some expert's notion of 'what people ought to know'. Poorly chosen information can have several negative consequences: it can waste recipients' time, it can be seen as wasting their time (indicating insensitivity to their situation), it can take up the place (in the media or school) that

could be filled with pertinent information (imposing an opportunity cost), and it can lead them to misunderstand the extent of their knowledge. In addition, recipients may be judged unduly harshly if they are uninterested in information that seems irrelevant to them, but has been deemed significant by the experts. The Institute of Medicine's (1986) important report, *Confronting AIDS*, despaired after a survey showed that only 41 per cent of the public knew that AIDS was caused by a virus. Yet, one might ask what role that information could play in any practical decision (as well as what those subjects who answered correctly meant by 'a virus').

The information in a communication should reflect a systematic theoretical perspective, capable of being applied objectively. Here are three candidates for such a perspective, suggested by the research cited above.

Mental model analysis

Communications could attempt to convey a comprehensive picture of the processes creating (and controlling) a risk. Bridging the gap between lay mental models and expert models would require adding missing concepts, correcting mistakes, strengthening correct beliefs, and de-emphasizing peripheral ones. Following the mental model procedure outlined above has several potential advantages: it allows the emergence of lay beliefs that never would have occurred to an expert (for example, plants are sensitive to radon concentrations) and it increases the chances of revealing the terms in which lay people express their beliefs.

Calibration analysis

Communications could attempt to give recipients the appropriate degree of confidence in their beliefs. They would focus on cases where people confidently hold incorrect beliefs that could lead to inappropriate actions or lack the confidence in correct beliefs needed to act on them. For example, only 45 per cent of the high-risk teenagers in Quadrel's (1990) study knew that having a beer would affect their driving as much as drinking a shot of vodka. However, they were, on average, very confident in their (usually wrong) answers. For this particular question, the adults were just as overconfident as the high-risk youth, whereas the low-risk teenagers judged their chances of a correct response more realistically. Such local misconceptions or 'bugs' can undermine otherwise correct beliefs that deserve focused attention in communications

Those who provide information have an obligation to communicate how much confidence should be placed in it. For example, Fortney (1988) reported the results of a meta-analysis on all then-available studies of the health effects of oral contraceptives. She concluded, with great confidence, that, for a non-smoking woman, using the contraceptive pill throughout her reproductive career would do something between increasing her life expectancy by 4 days and decreasing it by 80 days. In addition, she was able to say that it was highly unlikely that this forecast would change greatly because the existing database was so large that no conceivable additional study could materially alter the conclusions. Such an explicit estimation of uncertainty is much more valuable than any verbal summary. Unfortunately, individuals are all too likely to be left guessing at the implicit claims of definitiveness in the typical newspaper account of a hot new medical study.

Value of information analysis

Communications could attempt to provide the pieces of information having the largest possible impact on pending decisions. Value-of-information analysis is the general term for techniques determining the sensitivity of decisions to different information (Raiffa 1968; von Winterfeldt and Edwards 1986).

Merz *et al.* (1993) applied value-of-information analysis to a well-specified medical decision, whether to undergo carotid endarterectomy. Both this procedure, which involves scraping out an artery leading to the brain and its alternatives have a variety of possible positive and negative effects. These effects have been the topic of extensive research, providing quantitative risk estimates of varying precision. Merz (1991) created a simulated population of patients, varying in their physical conditions and preferences for different health states. He found that knowing about a few, but only a few, of the possible side-effects would change the preferred decision for a significant portion of patients. He argued that communications should focus on these few side-effects; doing so would make better use of patients' limited attention than the usual laundry lists of possibilities (although none of those should be hidden). He also argued that his procedure could provide an objective criterion for identifying the information that must be transmitted (and understood) in order to insure medical informed consent.

Between the time that Merz (1991) submitted his dissertation and its defence, the results of a major clinical trial were released. Incorporating them in his model made little difference to its conclusions (Merz *et al.* 1993). That is, from this perspective, information produced by the trial had little practical importance for determining the advisability of the surgery. This is not to say that the study did not contribute to the understanding of fundamental physiological processes or that it might not have produced other results that would have been more useful to patients. However, the results do give pause for thought regarding the allocation of

research resources. Thus, value-of-information analysis can be used for prioritizing the scientific information to be collected as well as that to be transmitted. It has, for example, been applied to the testing of chemicals for carcinogenicity (Lave and Omenn 1986; Omenn *et al.* 1995).

The choice between these approaches would depend on, among other things, how much time is available for communication, how well the decisions are formulated, and what scientific risk information exists. For example, value-of-information analysis might be particularly useful for identifying the focal facts for public service announcements. Calibration analysis may be used to identify surprising facts, of the sort that might both grab recipients' attention and change their behaviour. A mental model analysis might be better suited to the preparation of explanatory brochures or curricula.

Formatting information

Once information has been selected, it must be presented in a comprehensible way. That means taking into account the terms that recipients use for understanding individual concepts and the mental models that they use for integrating those concepts. It also means building on the results of research on text comprehension. That research shows, for example, that comprehension improves when text has a clear structure and, in particular, when that structure conforms to recipients' intuitive representation of a topic; that critical information is more likely to be remembered when it appears at the highest level of a clear hierarchy; and that readers benefit from 'adjunct aids', such as highlighting, advanced organizers (showing what to expect), and summaries. Such aids might even be better than full text for understanding, retaining, and being able to look up information. Fuller treatment can be found in sources such as Reder (1985), Kintsch (1986), Garnham (1987), Ericsson (1988) and Schriver (1989).

In a given application, several formats may meet these general constraints. Recently, we created two brochures, using clear but different structures for explaining the risks of radon (Atman *et al.*, 1994). One was organized around a decision tree, showing the options facing homeowners, the probabilities of possible consequences, and the associated costs or benefits. The second was organized around a directed network, representing, in effect, a simplified version of the expert model partially depicted in Fig. 34.5. Both brochures were compared with the Environmental Protection Agency's (**EPA**) widely distributed '*Citizen's guide to radon*', built around a question-and-answer format, with little attempt to summarize or impose a general structure. All three brochures substantially increased readers' understanding of the material presented in them. However, the structured brochures did better (and similar) jobs of enabling readers to make inferences about issues that were not mentioned explicitly and to give advice to others who had not read the material. To the EPA's great credit, its brochure was much more extensively evaluated than the vast majority of public health communications—although without the benefit of these procedures from applied cognitive psychology (Desvousges *et al.* 1989; Smith *et al.* 1995).

Evaluating communications

Effective risk communications can help people to reduce their health risks or to obtain greater benefits in return for those risks

Table 34.2 Data collection options for reader-based evaluations of risk communications

	Strengths	Weaknesses
Concurrent		
Think-aloud protocol	Protocols identify problems with text content and organization, can produce surprises	Costly, time-consuming, difficult to analyse, samples usually small
Retrospective		
Open-ended interview	Least reactive—avoids structuring answers for respondents Identifies how reader structures knowledge, is less reactive than most methods	Coding scheme necessary—data potentially difficult to analyse Costly, time-consuming, samples usually small
Short questions, recall	Measures what 'sticks' in readers' minds, can measure how readers assign importance	May not elicit information used in actual decision making, responses driven by context, difficult to analyse
Problem solving (scenarios)	Elicits decision-making information and strategies	Frames problems for respondents—may be reactive
Closed-ended	Data structured, easier, and less expensive to collect and analyse, large samples more feasible	Potentially reactive—may misrepresent respondents' knowledge and attitudes
Knowledge tests (true–false, multiple choice)	Can verify specific misconceptions and beliefs, data readily comparable	Costly, difficult to design valid questions and response scales

Source: Bostrom *et al.* (1994).

that they take. Ineffective communications cannot only fail to do so, but also incur opportunity costs, in the sense of occupying the place (in recipients' lives and society's functions) that could be taken up by more effective communications. Even worse, misdirected communications can prompt wrong decisions by omitting key information or failing to contradict misconceptions, create confusion by prompting inappropriate assumptions or emphasizing irrelevant information, and provoke conflict by eroding recipients' faith in the communicator. By causing undue alarm or complacency, poor communications can have greater public health impact than the risks that they attempt to describe. Because communicators' intuitions about recipients' risk perceptions cannot be trusted, there is no substitute for empirical validation (Fischhoff *et al.* 1983; Fischhoff 1987; Slovic 1987; National Research Council 1989; Rohrmann 1990).

The most ambitious evaluations ask whether recipients follow the recommendations given in the communication (Lau *et al.* 1980; Weinstein 1987). However, that standard requires recipients not only to understand the message, but also to accept it as relevant to their personal circumstances. For example, homeowners without the resources to address radon problems might both understand and ignore a communication advocating testing; women might hear quite clearly what actions an 'expert' recommends for reducing their risk of sexual assault, yet reject the political agenda underlying that advice (Fischhoff 1992). Judging a programme's effectiveness according to its behavioural effects requires great confidence that one knows what is right for others.

A more modest but ethically simpler evaluation criterion is to ensure that recipients have understood what a message was trying to say. That necessary condition might prove sufficient if the recommended action is obviously appropriate—once one knows the facts. Unfortunately, formal evaluations seem to be remarkably rare,

among the myriad of warning labels, health claims and advisories, public service announcements, operating instructions, and so on, that one encounters in everyday life and work (Laughery *et al.* 1994).

Evaluating what people take away from communications faces the same methodological challenges as measuring their ambient risk perceptions. The evaluator wants to avoid changing people's beliefs through the cues offered by how questions and answers are posed, restricting the expression of non-expert beliefs and suppressing the expression of inconsistent beliefs, over a series of questions.

For example, in the course of evaluating its radon risk communications, the US EPA (Desvousges *et al.* 1989) posed the following question: 'What kinds of problems are high levels of radon exposure likely to cause? (a) Minor skin problems (b) Eye irritations (c) Lung cancer'. This question seems to risk inflating subjects' apparent level of understanding in several ways. Subjects who know only that radon causes cancer might deduce that it causes lung cancer. The words 'minor' and 'irritation' might imply that these are not the effects of 'high levels' (of anything). Moreover, there is no way for subjects to express other misconceptions, such as that radon causes breast cancer or other lung problems (which emerged with some frequency in our open-ended interviews) (Bostrom *et al.* 1992).

Table 34.2 summarizes approaches in reader-based evaluation. In principle, open-ended interviews provide the best way to reduce such threats. Performing them to the standards of scientific publication is labour-intensive. It involves conducting, transcribing, and coding interviews, with suitable reliability checks (in addition to the effort of producing an expert model and determining explicit communication goals). The stakes riding on many risk communications should justify that investment, considering the costs of dissemination and of the ensuing ineffective choices. Realistically speaking, the needed time and financial resources will not always be available. In some such cases, a small number of open-ended, one-on-one interviews might still provide valuable stepping stones to structured tests, suitable for mass administration. Those quizzes will cover the critical topics in the expert model, express questions in terms familiar to subjects, and estimate the prevalence of misconceptions. Even if systematic study is impractical, one-on-one interviews, using think-aloud protocols, can be administered quickly, purely for their heuristic value. It is depressing how often this rudimentary precaution is not taken. One occasional developmental tool is focus groups. However, group pressure can suppress uncertainty, as well as the expression of idiosyncratic beliefs and interpretations. Group testing is best suited to situations where communications will be received and processed in circumstances like those of the group.

Conclusions

Understanding risk perception and risk communication is a complicated business, perhaps as complicated as assessing the magnitude of the risks being considered. A chapter of this length can, at best, indicate the dimensions of this complexity and the directions of plausible solutions. In this treatment, we have emphasized methodological issues because we believe that these topics often seem deceptively simple. Because we ask questions in everyday life, eliciting others' beliefs may seem straightforward; because we talk everyday, it may seem simple to communicate about health risks. Unfortunately, there are many pitfalls to such amateurism, some of which emerge in the research described here. Hints at these problems can be found in those occasions in life where we have misunderstood or been misunderstood, particularly when discussing unfamiliar topics with strangers.

Research on these topics is fortunate in being able to draw on well-developed collections of literature in such areas as cognitive, health, and social psychology, psycholinguistics, psychophysics, and behavioural decision theory. It is unfortunate in having to face the particularly rigorous demands of assessing and improving complex beliefs about health risks. These often involve unfamiliar topics, surrounded by unusual kinds of uncertainty, for which individuals and groups lack stable vocabularies. Health risk decisions also raise difficult and potentially threatening trade-offs. Even the most carefully prepared and evaluated communications may not be able to eliminate the anxiety and frustration that such decisions create. However, systematic preparation can keep communications from adding to the problem. At some point in complex decisions, we 'throw up our hands' and go with what seems right. Good risk communications can help people get farther into the problem before that happens.

Health risk decisions are not just about cognitive processes and coolly weighed information. Emotions play a role, as do social processes. None the less, it is important to get the cognitive part right, lest people's ability to think their way to decisions be underestimated and underserved.

References

Atman, C.J., Bostrom, A., Fischhoff, B., and Morgan, M.G. (1994). Designing risk communications: completing and correcting mental models of hazardous processes, Part 1. *Risk Analysis*, **14**, 779–88.

Bar-Hillel, M. (1974). Similarity and probability. *Organizational Behavior and Human Performance*, **11**, 277–82.

Bauman, K.E. (1980). *Predicting adolescent drug use: utility structure and marijuana*. Praeger, New York.

Beyth-Marom, R. (1982). How probable is probable? Numerical translation of verbal probability expressions. *Journal of Forecasting*, **1**, 257–69.

Beyth-Marom, R., Austin, L., Fischhoff, B., Palmgren, C., and Quadrel, M.J. (1993). Perceived consequences of risky behaviours. *Developmental Psychology*, **29**, 549–63.

Bostrom, A., Fischhoff, B., and Morgan, M.G. (1992). Characterizing mental models of hazardous processes: a methodology and an application to radon. *Journal of Social Issues*, **48(4)**, 85–100.

Bostrom, A., Atman, C.J., Fischhoff, B., and Morgan, M.G. (1994). Evaluating risk communications: completing and correcting mental models of hazardous processes. Part 2. *Risk Analysis*, **14**, 789–98.

Budescu, D.F. and Wallsten, T.S (1995). Processing linguistic probabilities: general principles and empirical evidence. In *Decision making: a cognitive perspective* (ed. J.R. Busemeyer, R. Hastie, and D.L. Medin). pp. 275–318 New York: Academic Press.

Camerer, C. (1981). General conditions for the success of bootstrapping models. *Organizational Behavior and Human Performance*, **27**, 411–22.

Cohen, J. and Hansel, C.E.M. (1958). The nature of decisions in gambling. *Acta Psychologica*, **13**, 357–70.

Cole, G. and Withey, S. (1982). Perspectives in risk perceptions. *Risk Analysis*, **1**, 143–63.

Covello, V.T., Sandman, P.M., and Slovic, P. (1988). *Risk communication, risk statistics, and risk comparisons: a manual for plant managers*. Chemical Manufacturers Association, Washington, DC.

Craik, K. (1943). *The nature of explanation*. Cambridge University Press, Cambridge.

Crouch, E.A.C. and Wilson, R. (1982). *Risk/benefit analysis*. Ballinger, Cambridge, MA.

Cvetkovich, G., Grote, B., Bjorseth, A., and Sarkissian, J. (1975). On the psychology of adolescents' use of contraceptives. *Journal of Sex Research*, **11**, 256–70.

Dawes, R.M. and Corrigan, B. (1974). Linear models in decision making. *Psychological Bulletin*, **81**, 95–106.

Dawes, R.M., Faust, D., and Meehl, P. (1989). Clinical versus actuarial judgement. *Science*, **243**, 1668–74.

Desvousges, W.H., Smith, V.K., and Rink, H.H., III (1989). *Communicating radon risk effectively: radon testing in Maryland*. US Environmental Protection Agency, Office of Policy, Planning and Evaluation, Washington, DC.

Douglas, M. (1992). *Risk and blame*. Routledge, London.

Elkind, D. (1967). Egocentrism in adolescence. *Child Development*, **38**, 1025–34.

Englander, T., Farago, K., Slovic, P., and Fischhoff, B. (1986). A comparative analysis of risk perception in Hungary and the United States. *Social Behaviour*, **1**, 55–6.

Ericsson, K.A. (1988). Concurrent verbal reports on text comprehension: a review. *Text*, **8**, 295–325.

Ericsson, K.A. and Simon, H.A. (1980). Verbal reports as data. *Psychological Review*, **87**, 215–51.

Feather, N. (ed.) (1982). *Expectancy, incentive and action*. Erlbaum, Hillsdale, NJ.

Fineberg, H.V. (1988). Education to prevent AIDS. *Science*, **239**, 592–6.

Fischhoff, B. (1987). Treating the public with risk communications: a public health perspective. *Science, Technology, and Human Values*, **12(3/4)**, 13–9.

Fischhoff, B. (1989). Making decisions about AIDS. In *Primary prevention of AIDS* (ed. V. Mays, G. Albee, and S. Schneider), pp. 168–205, Sage, Newbury Park, CA.

Fischhoff, B. (1990). Psychology and public policy: tool or tool maker? *American Psychologist*, **45**, 57–63.

Fischhoff, B. (1992). Giving advice: decision theory perspectives on sexual assault. *American Psychologist*, **47**, 577–88.

Fischhoff, B. (1994). What forecasts (seem to) mean. *International Journal of Forecasting*, **10**, 387–403.

Fischhoff, B. (1996). The real world: what good is it? *Organizational Behaviour and Human Decision Processes*, in press.

Fischhoff, B. and MacGregor, D. (1983). Judged lethality: how much people seem to know depends upon how they are asked. *Risk Analysis*, 3, 229–36.

Fischhoff, B. and Quadrel, M.J. (1991). Adolescent alcohol decisions. *Alcohol Health & Research World*, 15, 43–51.

Fischhoff, B., Slovic, P., and Lichtenstein, S. (1977). Knowing with certainty: the appropriateness of extreme confidence. *Journal of Experimental Psychology: Human Perception and Performance*, 3, 552–64.

Fischhoff, B., Slovic, P., Lichtenstein, S., Read, S., and Combs, B. (1978). How safe is safe enough? A psychometric study of attitudes towards technological risks and benefits. *Policy Sciences*, 8, 127–52.

Fischhoff, B., Lichtenstein, S., Slovic, P., Derby, S.L., and Keeney, R.L. (1981). *Acceptable risk*. Cambridge University Press, New York.

Fischhoff, B., Slovic, P., and Lichtenstein, S. (1983). The 'public' vs. the 'experts': perceived vs. actual disagreement about the risks of nuclear power. In *Analysis of actual vs. perceived risks* (ed. V. Covello, G. Flamm, J. Rodericks and R. Tardiff), pp. 235–49. Plenum, New York.

Fischhoff, B., Watson, S., and Hope, C. (1984). Defining risk. *Policy Sciences*, 17, 123–39.

Fortney, J. (1988). Contraception: a life-long perspective. In *Dying for love*. (pp. 33–8) National Council for International Health, Washington, DC.

Funtowicz, S.O. and Ravetz, J.R. (1990). *Uncertainty and quality in science for policy*. Kluwer, Boston.

Furnham, A.F. (1988). *Lay theories*. Pergamon, Oxford.

Galotti, K.M. (1989). Approaches to studying formal and everyday reasoning. *Psychological Bulletin*, 105, 331–51.

Garnham, A. (1987). *Mental models as representations of discourse and text*. Halsted Press, New York.

Gentner, D. and Stevens, A.L. (ed.) (1983). *Mental models*. Erlbaum, Hillsdale, NJ.

Goldberg, L.R. (1968). Simple models or simple processes? *American Psychologist*, 23, 483–96.

Goszczynska, M., Tyszka, T., and Slovic, P. (1991). Risk perception in Poland: a comparison with three other countries. *Journal of Behavioural Decision Making*, 4, 179–93.

Green, C.H. and Brown, R.A. (1981). *The perception and acceptability of risk*. Duncan of Jordanstone School of Architecture, Dundee, UK.

Hammond, K.R., Hursch, C.J., and Toddy, F.J. (1964). Analyzing the components of clinical inference. *Psychological Review*, 71, 438–56.

Harding, C.M. and Eiser, J.R. (1984). Characterizing the perceived risks and benefits of some health issues. *Risk Analysis*, 4, 131–41.

Hasher, L. and Zacks, R.T. (1984). Automatic processing of fundamental information. *American Psychologist*, 39, 1372–88.

Heimer, C.A. (1988). Social structure psychology, and the estimation of risk. *Annual Review of Sociology*, 14, 491–519.

Hendrickx, L.C.W.P. (1991). 'How versus how often: the role of scenario information and frequency information in risk judgement and risky decision making.' Doctoral dissertation. Rijksuniversiteit Groningen.

Hoffman, P.J. (1960). Paramorphic models representation of clinical judgment. *Psychological Bulletin*, 57, 116–31.

Howard, R.A. (1989). Knowledge maps. *Mananagement Science*, 35, 903–22.

Inhaber, H. (1979). Risk with energy from conventional and non-conventional sources. *Science*, 203, 718–23.

Institute of Medicine (1986). *Confronting AIDS*. National Academy Press, Washington, DC.

Jasanoff, S. (1986). *Risk management and political culture*. Russell Sage Foundation, New York.

Jianguang, Z. (1994). Environmental hazards in the Chinese public's eyes. *Risk Analysis*, 14, 163–9.

Jungermann, H., Schutz, H., and Thüring, M. (1988). Mental models in risk assessment: informing people about drugs. *Risk Analysis*, 8, 147–55.

Kahneman, D., Slovic, P., and Tversky, A. (ed.) (1982). *Judgment under uncertainty: Heuristics and biases*. Cambridge University Press, New York.

Kaplan, E.H. (1989). What are the risks of risky sex? *Operations Research*, 37, 198–209.

Karpowicz-Lazreg, C. and Mullet, E. (1993). Societal risk as seen by the French public. *Risk Analysis*, 13, 253–8.

Keating, D.P. (1988). *Cognitive processes in adolescence*. Ontario Institute for Studies in Education, Toronto.

Kempton, W. (1987). Variation in folk models and consequent behaviour. *American Behavioural Scientist*, 31 (2), 203–18.

Kempton, W. (1991). Lay perspectives on global climate change. *Global Environmental Change*, 1, 183–208.

Kintsch, W. (1986). Learning from text. *Cognition and Instruction*, 3, 87–108.

Koriat, A. (1993). How do we know that we know? *Psychological Review*, 100, 609–39.

Krimsky, S. and Golding, D. (ed.) (1992). *Theories of risk*. Praeger, New York.

Krimsky, S. and Plough, A. (1988). *Environmental hazards*. Auburn House, Dover, MA.

Kuyper, H. and Vlek, C. (1984). Contrasting risk judgements among interest groups. *Acta Psychological*, 56, 205–18.

Lau, R., Kaine, R., Berry, S., Ware, J., and Roy, D. (1980). Channeling health: a review of the evaluation of televised health campaigns. *Health Education Quarterly*, 7, 56–89.

Laughery, K.S., Wogalter, M.S., and Young, S.L. (ed.) (1994). *Human factors perspectives on warnings*. Human Factors and Ergonomics Society, Santa Monica, CA.

Lave, L.B. and Omenn, G.S. (1986). Cost effectiveness of short-term tests for carcinogenicity. *Nature*, 324, 29–34.

Leiss, W. and Chociolko, C. (1994). *Risk and responsibility*. McGill-Queens University Press, Montreal and Kingston.

Lichtenstein, S. and Newman, J.R. (1967). Empirical scaling of common verbal phrases associated with numerical probabilities. *Psychonomic Science*, 9, 563–4.

Lichtenstein, S., Slovic, P., Fischhoff, B., Layman, M. and Combs, B. (1978). Judged frequency of lethal events. *Journal of Experimental Psychology: Human Learning and Memory*, 4, 551–78.

Lichtenstein, S., Fischhoff, B., and Phillips, L.D. (1982). Calibration of probabilities: state of the art to 1980. In *Judgment under uncertainty: heuristics and biases* (ed. D. Kahneman, P. Slovic, and A. Tversky), pp. 306–34. Cambridge University Press, New York.

Linville, P.W., Fischer, G.W., and Fischhoff, B. (1993). AIDS risk perceptions and decision biases. In *The social psychology of HIV infection* (ed. J.B. Pryor and G.D. Reeder), pp. 5–38. Erlbaum, Hillsdale, NJ.

Lowrance, W. (1976). *Of acceptable risk*. Kaufmann, San Francisco.

MacGregor, D. (1991). Worry over technological activities and life concerns. *Risk Analysis*, 11, 315–25.

Maharik, M. and Fischhoff, B. (1992). The risks of nuclear energy sources in space: some activists' perceptions. *Risk Analysis*, 12, 383–92.

Means, M.L. and Voss, J.F. (1985). Star wars: a developmental study of expert and novice knowledge studies. *Journal of Memory and Language*, 24, 746–57.

Merton, R.F. (1987). The focused interview and focus groups. *Public Opinion Quarterly*, 51, 550–66.

Merz, J.F. (1991). Toward a standard of disclosure for medical informed consent: development and demonstration of a decision-analytic methodology. PhD dissertation. Carnegie Mellon University.

Merz, J., Fischhoff, B., Mazur, D.J., and Fischbeck, P.S. (1993). Decision-analytic approach to developing standards of disclosure for medical informed consent. *Journal of Toxics and Liability*, 15, 191–215.

Morgan, M.G., Florig, H.K., Nair, I., Cortes, C., Marsh, K., and Pavlosky, K. (1990). Lay understanding of power-frequency fields. *Bioelectromagnetics*, 11, 313–35.

Morgan, M.G., Fischhoff, B., Bostrom, A., Lave, L., and Atman, C.J. (1992). Communicating risk to the public. *Environmental Science and Technology*, 26, 2048–56.

Morrison, D.M. (1985). Adolescent contraceptive behaviour: a review. *Psychological. Bulletin*, 98, 538–68.

Murphy, A.H., Lichtenstein, S., Fischhoff, B., and Winkler, R.L. (1980). Misinterpretations of precipitation probability forecasts. *Bulletin of the American Meteorological Society*, 61, 695–701.

National Research Council (1989). *Improving risk communication*. National Academy Press, Washington, D.C.

National Research Council (1996). *Understanding risk*. National Academy Press, Washington, DC.

Oden, G.C. (1987). Concept, knowledge, and thought. *Annual Review of Psychology*, **38**, 203–27.

Omenn, G.S., Stuebbe, S., and Lave, L. (1995) Predictions of rodent carcinogenicity testing results: interpretation in light of the Lave-Omenn value-of-information model. *Molecular Carcinogenesis*, **14**, 35–7.

Otway, H.J. and Wynne, B. (1989). Risk communication: paradigm and paradox. *Risk Analysis*, **9**, 141–5.

Poulton, E.C. (1989). *Bias in quantifying judgement*. Lawrence Erlbaum, Hillsdale, NJ.

Quadrel, M.J. (1990). Elicitation of adolescents' risk perceptions: qualitative and quantitative dimensions. PhD dissertation. Carnegie Mellon University.

Quadrel, M.J., Fischhoff, B., and Davis, W. (1993). Adolescent (in)vulnerability. *American Psychologist*, **48**, 102–16.

Raiffa, H. (1968). *Decision analysis: introductory lectures on choices under uncertainty*. Addison-Wesley, Reading, MA.

Reder, L.M. (1985). Techniques available to author, teacher, and reader to improve retention of main ideas of a chapter. In *Thinking and learning skills: volume 2, research and open questions*, (ed. S.F. Chipman, J.W. Segal, and R. Glaser), pp. 37–64). Lawrence Erlbaum Associates, Hillsdale, NJ.

Ritov, I. and Baron, J. (1990). *Status quo* and omission bias. Reluctance to vaccinate. *Journal of Behavioural Decision Making*, **3**, 263–77.

Rohrmann, B. (1990). Analyzing and evaluating the effectiveness of risk communication programs. Unpublished manuscript, University of Mannheim.

Rohrmann, B. (1994). Risk perception of different societal groups: Australian findings and cross-national comparisons. *Australian Journal of Psychology*, **46**, 151–163.

Roth, E., Morgan, G., Fischhoff, B., Lave, L. and Bostrom, A. (1990). What do we know about making risk comparisons? *Risk Analysis*, **10**, 375–87.

Rouse, W.B. and Morris, N.M. (1986). On looking into the black box: prospects and limits in the search for mental models. *Psychological Bulletin*, **100**, 349–63.

Royal Society (1992). *Risk analysis, perception and management*. Royal Society, London.

Schriver, K.A. (1989). *Plain language for expert or lay audiences: designing text using protocol-aided revision*. Communications Design Center, Carnegie Mellon University.

Shaklee, H. and Fischhoff, B. (1990). The psychology of contraceptive surprises: judging the cumulative risk of contraceptive failure. *Journal of Applied Psychology*, **20**, 385–403.

Slovic, P. (1987). Perceptions of risk. *Science*, **236**, 280–5.

Slovic, P., Fischhoff, B., and Lichtenstein, S. (1979). Rating the risks. *Environment*, **21(4)**, 14–20, 36–9.

Slovic, P., Fischhoff, B., and Lichtenstein, S. (1980). Facts and fears: understanding perceived risk. *In Societal risk assessment: how safe is safe enough?* (ed. R. Schwing and W.A. Albers, Jr), pp. 181–214. Plenum Press, New York.

Slovic, P., Lichtenstein, S., and Fischhoff, B. (1984). Modelling the societal impact of fatal accidents. *Management Science*, **30**, 464–74.

Slovic, P., Fischhoff, B., and Lichtenstein, S. (1985). Characterizing perceived risk. In *Perilous progress: technology as hazard* (ed. R.W. Kates, C. Hohenemser, and J. Kasperson), pp. 91–123. Westview, Boulder, CO.

Slovic, P., Kraus, N.N., Lappe, H., Letzel, H., and Malmfors, T. (1989). Risk perception of prescription drugs: report on a survey in Sweden. *Pharmaceutical Medicine*, **4**, 43–65.

Smith, V.K., Desvousges, W.H., and Payne, J.W. (1995). Do risk information programs promote mitigating behaviour? *Journal of Risk and Uncertainty*, **10**, 203–21.

Stallen, P.J.M. and Tomas, A. (1988). Public concerns about industrial hazards. *Risk Analysis*, **8**, 235–45.

Starr, C. (1969). Societal benefit versus technological risk. *Science*, **165**, 1232–38.

Svenson, O. (1981). Are we all less risky and more skillful than our fellow drivers? *Acta Psychologica*, **47**, 143–8.

Svenson, O. and Fischhoff, B. (1985). Levels of environmental decisions. *Journal of Environmental Psychology*, **5**, 55–68.

Tversky, A. and Kahneman, D. (1973). Availability: a heuristic for judging frequency and probability. *Cognitive Psychology*, **4**, 207–32.

Vaughan, E. (1993). Individual and cultural differences in adaptation to environmental risks. *American Psychologist*, **48**, 1–8.

Viscusi, K. (1992). *Smoking: making the risky decision*. Oxford University Press, New York.

Vlek, C. and Stallen, P.J. (1981). Judging risks and benefits in the small and in the large. *Organizational Behaviour and Human Performance*, **28**, 235–71.

Vlek, C. and Stallen, P.J. (1980). Rational and personal aspects of risk. *Acta Psychologica*, **45**, 273–300.

von Winterfeldt, D. and Edwards, W. (1986). *Decision analysis and behavioral research*. Cambridge University Press, New York.

Wagenaar, W.A. and Sagaria, S.D. (1975). Misperception of exponential growth. *Perception and Psychophysics*, **18**, 416–22.

Weinstein, N. (1987). *Taking care: understanding and encouraging self-protective behaviour*. Cambridge University Press, New York.

Weinstein, N.D. (1989). Effects of personal experience on self-protective behaviour. *Psychological Bulletin*, **105**, 31–50.

Wilks, S.S. (1938). Weighting systems for linear functions of correlated variable where there is no dependent variable. *Psychometrika*, **8**, 23–40.

Wilson, R. (1979). Analyzing the risks of everyday life. *Technology Review*, **81(4)**, 40–6.

Wilson, R.W. and Thornberry, O.T. (1987). Knowledge and attitudes about AIDS: provisional data from the National Health Interview Survey, August 10–30, 1987. *Advance Data*, No. 146.

Yates, J.F. (1989). *Judgment and decision making*. Prentice Hall, Englewood Cliffs, NJ.

Yates, J.F. (ed.) (1992). *Risk taking*. Wiley, Chichester.

Zentner, R.D. (1979). Hazards in the chemical industry. *Chemical and Engineering News*, **57(45)**, 25–7, 30–4.

35 What is ergonomics?

Åsa Kilbom

Brief history

Ergonomics is a 'young' area of scientific research and applications, which uses knowledge of human capacities and limitations to design work systems and environments. It was first defined and described in 1949 with the establishment of the Ergonomics Society in the United Kingdom (Murrell 1965). One important impetus was the large problems encountered during the Second World War when advanced technology, especially new weapons, were introduced. These new 'man–machine' systems were found to perform poorly because of a mismatch between humans and technology. Previously attempts had been made to fit humans to new technology by means of training and information, but neither humans nor technology could be used to their full capacity with this approach. When knowledge of human capabilities was employed, the overall efficiency was vastly improved.

Thus, the first applications of ergonomics were in the defence industry both in the United States and in the United Kingdom. However, research in the area had already started in England around 1915 with the establishment of the Industrial Fatigue Research Board. Fatigue was to be prevented through proper allocation of breaks and suitable working hours, and thereby improved efficiency of production would be achieved. During the First World War the productivity of the British ammunition factories was shown to increase in parallel with a reduction of weekly working hours (Vernon 1921).

While productivity, safety, and health were always the main goals of ergonomics, the focus of research and applications has shifted considerably over the years. After the Second World War, the concepts of ergonomics were gradually introduced into the manufacturing industry and in other physically strenuous jobs. From the 1970s human–computer interaction and health consequences of poor ergonomics, especially in the occupational setting, grew in importance. At present, much attention is given to work organization issues (macroergonomics) and techniques for implementing ergonomic improvements through worker participatory processes.

Geographically too there have been substantial differences in focus. Psychological aspects of ergonomics, especially cognitive and sensory issues, dominated research in the United States for many years and are often referred to as 'human factors'. Manufacturing systems and consumer issues have received much attention in research from the United Kingdom and Japan. Work physiology has dominated research in the rest of Europe, especially in the Nordic countries. In some degree these differences in focus reflect differences in scientific traditions, partly in industrial structures and legislation related to occupational injuries.

In the 1990s the advantages of good ergonomics can be seen in occupational settings, in public life, and in homes. Reduction of heavy lifting and handling of objects through lifting devices, the introduction of ergonomically designed furniture and computers in offices, and the design of transportation systems are examples that bear witness to these advances. Much remains to be done, however, to ensure safe, healthy, and productive workplaces, homes, and public spaces.

Definition

Ergonomics, according to the International Ergonomics Association, 'integrates knowledge derived from the human sciences to match jobs, systems, products and environments to the physical and mental abilities and limitations of people.' According to Clark and Corlett (Clark and Corlett 1984) 'ergonomics is the study of human abilities and characteristics which affect the design of equipment, systems and jobs and its aims are to improve efficiency, safety and well-being'. There are a number of additional definitions with somewhat different phrasing.

A system designed according to ergonomic principles is thus easy to use, results in less fatigue and ill health, is more satisfying to the user, and is safer and more productive. In exceptional cases high productivity, safety, and health may not be parallel outcomes in the short term. In most cases, however, high productivity, health, and safety go hand in hand in the short term as well as in the long term.

Characteristics of ergonomics

One important characteristic of ergonomics is that it is both a scientific area of research and a practical area of application. Another important characteristic is that ergonomics is multidisciplinary and requires knowledge in three main areas: (a) anatomy and physiology; (b) psychology; and (c) technology. Although it is impossible to have extensive knowledge in all these fields, the ergonomist must be able to integrate knowledge from areas other than that of his or her own basic training. In large ergonomic projects a teamwork approach, with representatives of several disciplines with a common ergonomics perspective, may be the most successful.

When solving ergonomic problems in real life it is obvious that a multidisciplinary approach is needed. In research, some of the

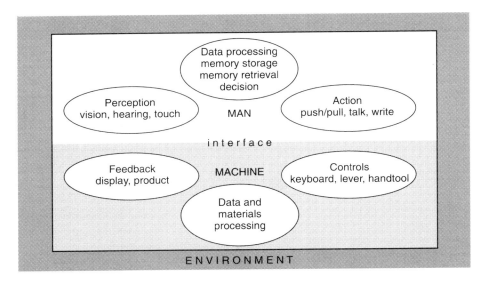

Fig. 35.1 The 'man–machine' system.

basic research questions have to be tackled separately by psychologists, physiologists, and engineers in order to expand existing knowledge. However, most ergonomic research is applied, and therefore requires a truly multidisciplinary approach. The multidisciplinary research approach needs to be strengthened; this requires a more intense collaboration between research groups, in order to establish common frames of reference. Joint training in ergonomics, where students with varying backgrounds can meet and develop a common outlook on ergonomics, is a key link to multidisciplinary applications and research in ergonomics.

The 'man–machine' system

Ergonomics concerns interaction with the environment in a way that maximizes safety, efficiency, and health. Traditionally, this interaction has been conceptualized as the 'man–machine system' (Fig. 35.1). In reality humans interact not only with technical devices ('machines'), but also with their social environment and with other humans. Nevertheless, since the first applications were aimed at machines and other technical equipment, the term has remained though it is now used with a wider definition. In this system, the 'machine' presents information to human often via displays, information is perceived by the operator's sensory apparatus, the operator then uses his or her cognitive capacity and memory to decide on a suitable response, which is transferred to the 'machine' as a motor activity—pushing buttons or handling objects. With the wider definition the 'machine' can be either another human being who feeds his or her response back via talk, signs (sign interpretation), or touch, or alternatively it can be society, which feeds its response back via road traffic signs, books or in other ways. The human response can then be via another form of motor activity, like talking, writing, or steering a car.

One important feature of the man–machine concept is that humans do not perform their actions in isolation, but as part of a system. The aim of the system is to perform efficiently, which requires an optimization of the interface between the person and the 'machine'. Thus the feedback from the machine must be presented in a way that is perceived quickly and without mistakes,

and the controls must be designed to comply with the person's strength and body dimensions. Efficiency also implies an optimal allocation of tasks between humans and 'machines', so that each component of the system performs the task he/she/it performs best (Chapanis 1965; Oborne *et al.* 1993; Mital *et al.* 1994). For example, humans are superior to machines in recognition of subtle patterns and decision-making requiring experience, while machines are superior in activities that require precision and endurance.

This system can be seen as a closed loop where deviations from the desired 'state' of the system are corrected. Humans (or operators) are seen as elements of the system, whose task is to respond to the feedback from the 'machine'. The quality of the response depends, of course, on their individual physiological, anatomical, sensory, and cognitive capacity. In a high-tech system designed for extreme demands on safety, like a nuclear power plant or a chemical process industry, it is crucial that the operator does not deviate from the predicted performance. Nevertheless, in modern thinking on ergonomics it is acknowledged that the individual has a more central role, and also brings his or her own goals into the system, and can also bring about changes and improvements to it. This 'person-centred' philosophy within ergonomics sees the operator as the one who controls and dominates the system, bringing into it his or her own concepts of the purpose of the system, as well as anticipation and prediction of the system (Oborne, *et al.* 1993).

Future of ergonomics

In a short period of time ergonomics has grown to become an important area of applied science and practical applications. This is especially true for working life, but gradually special ergonomic applications for consumers, for people with physical or mental disabilities and older people, for leisure and sports, and for developing countries are emerging. Thus ergonomics, through its effects on health, safety, and well-being, has a large impact on public health.

The International Ergonomics Association, which was formed by a number of national societies, recently issued minimum requirements for training and practical experience in ergonomics, to be fulfilled by those researchers, consultants, and others who wish to be approved as 'European Ergonomist'. Similar requirements have been developed for the United Kingdom, the United States, and Australia. Professional qualifications like these are likely to raise the quality of ergonomic work still further.

Human characteristics pertaining to ergonomics

Human capacity for work varies widely among children, young and old people, between the genders, and between individuals with different nutritional and educational background. Even among the individuals of a certain subset of the population, the capacity varies with heredity, health, training, and previous experience. Therefore work tasks, both in occupational and private life, must be designed to fit the capacities of a large range of people. This applies to body size, strength and fitness, and sensory as well as cognitive capacity. For working life, checklists have been developed to ensure a good fit between capacity and demands. If demands on human capacity are too high, then reduced comfort, fatigue, disease, or injuries occur. Human capacity is seldom taxed up to 100 per cent; the only exceptions are in all-out life-saving operations. Commonly, levels of a few per cent up to as much as 50 per cent of capacity are taxed in physically demanding jobs. No similar figures are available for sensory and mental capacity. A strong association exists between the relative capacity available for a task and its duration. Thus the longer a certain demand has to be met, the lower is the relative capacity that can be used without fatigue.

Anatomy

When designing good work stations, tools, and machines, care must be taken to make them adjustable to individual differences in body size, in order not to exclude parts of the population from work. Anthropometric data for use in work-station design are available for most parts of the body and for some subsets of the population (Pheasant 1986). It is common to design work stations and tools to fit the 5th to the 95th percentile of the grown-up male and female population. In Fig. 35.2 those anthropometric measures most commonly used for design of work stations are defined.

There are large variations in body size and body proportions between ethnic groups, and also for limb length among individuals with similar body height. With the increased mobility of population groups around the world, it is no longer acceptable to design work stations only, for instance, for Caucasians in Europe and for the Japanese population in Japan. The wider range of work-station requirements caused by this mixture of population groups must be taken into account. This calls for continuous revisions of anthropometric data.

In addition to the static anthropometric body measures available for work-station and tool design, there is also a need to consider functional or dynamic measures of the human capacity to reach, bend, and stretch (Pheasant 1986). Dynamic anthropometric data have been obtained when subjects were allowed to adopt natural postures and movements to perform a certain task. Such measures are scarce, and the generalizability of the data is questionable. Therefore they usually have to be collected for each specific work situation, for example, for sitting in a driver cabin.

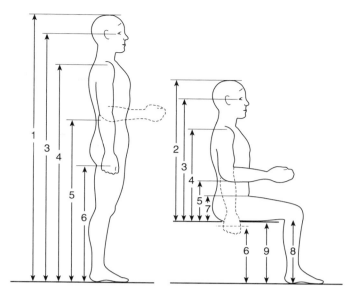

Fig. 35.2 Commonly used anthropometric measures and their definitions (from Hansson 1987). 1, body height; 2, sitting height; 3, eye height; 4, shoulder height; 5, elbow height; 6, knuckle height; 7, thigh height; 8, knee height; 9, height of seat. (Reprinted from Hansson 1987, with permission from Almqvist & Wiksell.)

Physical working capacity

Physical working capacities relevant for ergonomics include cardio-vascular, aerobic, and muscular capacities for maximal and sub-maximal, dynamic, and sustained (static) activity. Most physical capacities demonstrate a peak at age 20 to 30 years and a gradual decline by about 30 per cent up to the age of 60 (Åstrand and Rodahl 1986). Women usually have on average a 30 per cent lower aerobic power (expressed in litres of maximal oxygen uptake per minute) than men, and about 30 to 50 per cent lower maximal muscle strength. However, at a given level of relative submaximal exertion, there is no gender difference. Very large interindividual differences in capacity have been described related to heredity, physical training, and health status.

In general, the occupationally active population demonstrates higher capacities then the general population. There are also differences between occupational groups, with those performing physically demanding tasks usually demonstrating higher values (Åstrand 1967a, 1988). This difference appears to be caused mainly by selection, since physically demanding jobs do not usually contain work tasks strenuous enough to introduce a training effect. Moreover, differences between occupations are most obvious in young age groups. In fact, muscle strength has been shown to decrease more with age in blue collar groups than in white collar groups, which may be attributed to a combination of musculoskeletal trauma and 'wear and tear' among those performing physically heavy work (Era et al. 1992).

Physically fit workers exhibit higher productivity and less fatigue in strenuous jobs than less fit workers (Åstrand 1967b). Conversely, it is still an open question whether strong individuals run a lower risk of acquiring musculoskeletal disorders than weaker ones. This may be true for jobs requiring high force exertion in, for example, manual handling tasks, but it could not be demonstrated among women performing electronics assembly work (Chaffin et al. 1978; Jonsson et al. 1988). Pre-employment strength testing as a method to select only those less likely to develop work-related musculoskeletal disorders cannot be recommended on the basis of scientific studies, because the predictive power of such testing is either weak or non-existent, depending on the job in question. Individual factors like muscle strength are considered of minor importance for work-related musculoskeletal disorders in comparison with work-related risk factors (Hagberg *et al.* 1995).

Neuromuscular function in precision tasks and the effect of motor skill training are areas under rapid development, possibly with high relevance for musculoskeletal disorders.

Sensory capacity

Vision, hearing and touch are all-important factors in our perception of the environment, such as for a relevant response to cues from machines, displays, warning signs and other signs, and information received from other people. Taste and smell are less important for ergonomics but may be life-saving in toxic environments.

In order to enable humans to respond to sensory stimuli without missing information or overreacting, the contrast between the relevant information and the 'noise' caused by irrelevant visual and hearing stimuli, that is the signal to noise ratio, must be high. One common example of inadequate signal to noise ratios is trying to read texts on computer screens with too little contrast, or with bright lights surrounding the screen. In leisure time activities like jogging and cycling, music from earphones will camouflage important safety information from the traffic.

Frequently the sensory input from vision is overemphasized in ergonomic design, when sound or touch stimuli might have filled the same purpose. Handicap ergonomics has many examples of successful switches from vision to hearing (e.g. traffic signals) and from vision to touch (Braille).

With advancing age the sensitivity of the eye to light and of the ear to sound is reduced: therefore, the elderly require even higher signal to noise ratios in order to perceive important information. Work with poorly presented sensory information requires a high level of attention and therefore leads to stress and/or fatigue.

Cognitive capacity

In accordance with the man–machine system, information is perceived through the sensory organs and then processed in the brain, leading to a decision on a line of action. The capacity to process information and make decisions (cognitive capacity) requires a short-term (working) memory for processing and a long-term memory, for storage of relevant experience and knowledge.

The quality of information processing can be improved by presenting information in a form that makes it easy for the brain to code in the short-term memory. Information should be organized in such a way that it is easy to compare and relate to previous experience, and so that it can be stored in the long-term memory and retrieved in a suitable form for use later (Sanders and McCormick 1992).

The capacity for information processing is gradually reduced with age, but it is usually not until the age of around 65 years that a noticeable change occurs (Rabbitt 1991). With increasing age the variation around mean values of cognitive capacities appears to increase, probably because of the training effects of different life styles and jobs (Salthouse 1990; Rabbitt 1991). Neurophysiological and psychological research indicates that it is the brain's 'hardware' (number of brain cells) that decline with age, rather than the 'software' (quality of processing). Even though the memory deteriorates slowly, experience can compensate for reduced capacity, especially in complex decision-making.

Work design

Work-station and equipment design

Work stations, equipment, tools, and other objects handled must be designed in a way that facilitates their use, permits variations in work routines, does not give fatigue, and leads to a high efficiency rate. Common effects of poor work-station design are twisted and bent neck and trunk postures, and elevated arms leading to fatigue and musculoskeletal disorders. In the office this applies to its furniture and to the computer, in industry it applies to machines and tools as well as to supports, and at home it applies to the design of the kitchen and the usability of cleaning equipment.

Standing work

The advantage of a standing posture is that the combined mobility of the trunk and arms permits a much larger reach and work area than is possible in the sitting position. Another advantage is that much larger forces can be exerted, especially if the work area is relatively low so that the arms can be held straight and the trunk weight can be used. Conversely, standing work is tiring for the legs, especially for older people and for those with peripheral circulatory problems in the legs. The work area should be at different heights dependent on the character of the work (Grandjean 1988). For precision work the hands must be held relatively close to the eyes to allow sufficient accuracy. Working with elevated arms is tiring, though, so a good supporting work surface must be provided. For light work, on an assembly line, the working area should be close to the elbow height. When heavy work is performed the working height should be even lower (Fig. 35.3). The horizontal area in front of a standing person that is optimal for arm work is small (Hansson 1987) (Fig. 35.4). When work is performed standing and walking it can be made less fatiguing if shoes are changed a few times a day and if the floor is not hard—concrete floors are extremely tiring.

Sitting work

Sitting work is preferred by most because it is not tiring for the legs. Conversely, sitting in many jobs implies confined and static postures with elevated shoulders and arms, and frequent or sustained twisting and bending of the neck. The optimal horizontal area in front of a seated person is even smaller than for standing work. In general, commonly occurring work tasks should not be performed beyond forearm reach. Work outside this area should only be performed occasionally because it requires elevated arms and therefore becomes tiring. In addition, in work outside the optimal area much less force can be exerted. The basic posture in sitting requires that (Hansson 1987)

- the shoulders are lowered, the upper arms are nearly vertical, and the forearms are flexed about 100° in relation to the upper arms
- the forearm and hand form a straight line, or alternatively the hand can be slightly extended

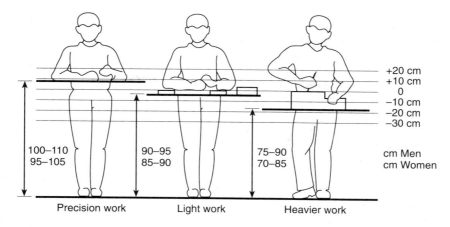

Fig. 35.3 Recommended height for benches for standing work (from Grandjean 1988). The reference Line (± 0) is the height of the elbows above the floor which averages 1050 mm for men and 98 mm for women. (Reprinted from Grandjean 1988, with permission from Taylor & Francis.)

- the forearm is held at about a 10 to 20° angle towards the table.

The head posture in seated work is frequently static, mainly because so many current work tasks are performed at the computer. The line of vision should be horizontal or somewhat below horizontal, and, especially for prolonged work at the visual display terminal, the screen must be of high quality with good contrast, no flicker, and adjustable height. The seated workplace must also provide sufficient leg space, because sitting with the trunk twisted requires static muscle exertion and is very tiring. No seated posture—even with good furniture—can be maintained for prolonged periods. Frequent changes between sitting, standing, and walking reduces fatigue, and many modern workplaces therefore have work surfaces where the height can be adjusted for both standing and sitting. A minimum requirement is that the height can be adjusted to fit both a tall man and a small woman.

Manual handling

Manual handling—lifting, lowering, holding, carrying, pushing, and pulling—is an important risk factor for low back disorders. Over the years much effort has been spent on trying to establish maximum limits for manual handling. In the National Institute of Occupational Safety and Health equation the acceptability of two-handed lifting is estimated, based on the weight of the object, its horizontal distance from the body, the degree of asymmetrical lifting, the height of the object and the vertical distance that it is to be moved, and the frequency of lifting (Waters *et al.* 1993). Although this equation does not apply to all lifting situations, its development and presentation has increased the awareness among ergonomists about the importance of reducing manual handling. Apart from the reduction in object weight and distances from the body, manual handling tasks should be designed to eliminate trunk bending and twisting, remove obstructions, provide good coupling of the load and the worker, and eliminate uneven or slippery surfaces.

Case study on manual handling in nursing (Ljungberg *et al.* 1989) The importance of work-station design, technical lifting aides, and work organization was studied among nursing aides in two geriatric wards in different hospitals. One of the wards was traditional with cramped work spaces, narrow corridors, and small lavatories where there was only room for one nursing aide to help the patient. Mobile hoists were available but the space was so cramped that they were seldom used. In the modern ward both corridors and rooms were spacious, and about 50 per cent of the beds had motorized overhead hoists for lifting patients. Moreover, the modern ward had a new work organization incorporating 'group-care', that is, a senior nurse and two nursing aides shared the responsibility for 12 patients, whereas work at the traditional ward was more like an 'assembly line'.

Work in lifting and carrying was compared between the two wards. The vertical force in each lifting and carrying manoeuvre, as well as the time for each lift, was measured using wooden shoes instrumented with strain gauges. The work performed in lifting was considerably less in the modern ward, whether expressed as total kilograms lifted per hour, the duration of each lift, or proportion of lifts performed with uneven distribution of weight between right and left leg (Table 35.1).

It is not possible to tell in this case if it was the differences in work organization, use and availability of technical aids, or work-station layout that most accounted for these large differences. It is most likely to be a combination of all three. This case demonstrates clearly that it is possible to reduce physical stresses due to manual handling substantially.

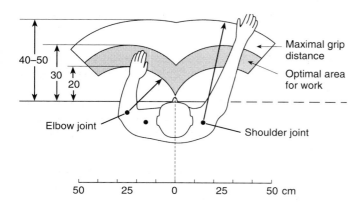

Fig. 35.4 Optimal work area for the hands in standing work (Hansson 1987). (Reprinted from Hansson 1987, with permission from Almqvist & Wiksell.)

Table 35.1 Workload in lifting and carrying. A comparison between two geriatric hospital wards

	Traditional ward	Modern ward
Number of lifts/h	30	14
Number of lifts/h with asymmetric uplift	14.8	7.5
Cumulated vertical force per hour (N)	2880	1660
Average duration of each lift (s)	10.5	4.8
Time for lifting (% of working day)	8.6	1.9

Repetitive work, breaks, and pauses

Lack of time for recovery after sustained or repetitive work is believed to be an important factor in the aetiology of work-related musculoskeletal disorders predominantly of the forearm and wrist. In the design of work, repetitive tasks should be avoided by providing frequent breaks and alternative tasks that do not tax the same tissues. Repetitive tasks should not be machine-paced, and the individual should be allowed to set his or her own pace. Tasks that require precision, force exertion, and speed in combination with repetitiveness especially imply very high risks for disorders (Kilbom 1994).

Presentation and communication of information

Several large-scale accidents have brought to the attention of decision-makers that information, both at workplaces and in public places, must be presented in a way that is easily understandable and compatible with human comprehension (see case study on haemo-dialysis accident below). Warning signs must use symbols and icons familiar to people; the colour red signifies something forbidden and green means acceptable, and the symbol for radioactivity is well known for everybody. Deficiencies in this conceptual compatibility are especially noteworthy in the design of computer programmes. Movement compatibility implies that there is a concordance between the movement of a control or a lever, and the ensuing movement of a machine or tool; you turn the wheel to the right when you want to make a right turn (Sanders and McCormick 1992). Spatial compatibility reflects human expectations with regard to the relative positioning of displays and controls and the understanding of 'high' versus 'low' measurements; high values are expected to be at the top of, or at the right-handed side of, a display, whereas low values are expected to be represented at the bottom or the left end.

The information on a display or a warning sign (auditory or visual) needs to be coded in a way that accentuates the crucial information, while redundant information is suppressed. Recommendations for the design of warning signs and labels have been given by Lehto (Lehto 1992). The schematic representation of the very complex London subway is a good example of a simplified, schematic, yet easily understandable system.

The quality of information processing can be further improved by giving undivided attention to the task and improving motivation. Therefore care should be taken when presenting information so that the attention is not divided between simultaneous or conflicting demands.

Environment

Adverse climatic conditions, poor lighting, vibrations, noise, low frequency sound, and slippery or unstable ground conditions, all can severely influence working capacity, endurance, and reliability. This is partly because these factors require additional physiological resources in addition to the work task; for instance, heat reduces blood circulation available for working muscles, cold reduces motor precision, and vibrations and slippery ground require muscle exertion for stabilizing the body. Poor lighting, noise and low frequency sound divert attention and reduce the signal to noise ratio. Standards are available from the International Standards Organization for hot climates and for vibrations, but their main aim is to prevent ill health, and they are not intended for safety purposes or to maintain well-being and high productivity.

Organizational design and management

The organization of work, that is, the leadership style (democratic or authoritarian), the hierarchical structure of the organization (flat or high pyramid), the influence of employees on decision-making, the distribution of work tasks among employees, the industrial relations within the organization, the wage/salary negotiating system, and the level of technology have been shown to influence productivity, well-being, and health in an organization. These organizational issues are often referred to as organizational design and management or macroergonomics (Hendricks 1986).

Organizations which promote employee initiatives, support development of skills and experience, and lets employees exert their own control over quality and quantity of work, adapt more easily to structural changes in society and appear to maintain a higher level of innovations. The underlying philosophy is that humans not only need bread and clothing for satisfaction and full development; when the above additional demands are met people can contribute more to the aims of the organization.

The full consequences of work organized along these lines are not yet fully realized—some disadvantages may follow, for example, for persons with little initiative. Moreover, stress levels may increase above acceptable levels when every individual strains to be as creative and productive as possible. There is no doubt, however, that work organization has a profound influence on productivity and health.

Areas of application

Occupational work

Many early applications of ergonomics were concerned with physically strenuous jobs like mining, forestry, and heavy tasks in industry. High aerobic demands and heavy manual handling characterize these jobs, and problems with general fatigue, accidents and low back pain were encountered at an early stage.

In the last decades manufacturing industry has mechanized many heavy tasks, and work reorganization and the use of robotic technology has further reduced aerobic demands in traditionally strenuous jobs. This implies increased demands on work postures and repetitive movements, and the pattern of complaints now also includes musculoskeletal problems of the shoulder, neck, hand, and arm regions. Similar problems are encountered in the office environment, especially among people performing data entry work (Bergqvist et al. 1995). However, a large proportion of the working population still performs physically strenuous work. Thus in an interview study of about 10 000 people from the Swedish working population, 38 per cent reported physical demands exceeding normal standing and walking, and 20 per cent of the men and 9 per cent of the women had heavy physical demands, causing breathlessness, at work. This applies especially to employees in mining, agriculture, transportation, and building work, and in so-called service jobs in health care, catering, and cleaning. Many employees in these jobs are middle-aged and elderly women performing work tasks that require a large proportion of their aerobic power.

Poor health and discomfort are common outcomes of badly designed work systems. The most common symptoms are musculoskeletal, yet general discomfort, stomach trouble, headaches, and a multitude of other psychosomatic symptoms are common unspecific signs of poor work design.

Work-related musculoskeletal disorders

In most countries employees with work-related musculoskeletal disorders are eligible for compensation, and employers are required to insure employees against such disorders. Musculoskeletal disorders constitute a major part of all registered occupational diseases in many countries. Criteria for considering a musculoskeletal disorder as an occupational condition very between different countries, making comparison of disease figures difficult. Even in countries with relatively strict criteria, musculoskeletal disorders are the largest group of diseases, representing a third of all registered occupational diseases (Vaaranen et al. 1994). The costs of musculoskeletal disorders have been estimated to range from 2.7 to 5.2 per cent of the gross national product in the Nordic countries in 1991, at a time when all costs due to illness were estimated to range from 15.8 to 22.2 per cent of the gross national product (Hansen 1993). An attempt to evaluate the aetiological fraction of musculoskeletal disorders due to work resulted in an estimate ranging from 15 to 49 per cent. Using an assumption of an aetiological fraction of 32 per cent, the cost of work-related musculoskeletal disorders can be estimated to be approximately 1 per cent of the gross national product in the Nordic countries.

Work-related musculoskeletal disorders cover a wide range of inflammatory and degenerative diseases and include some less well-known states of pain and functional impairment. Body regions most commonly involved are the low back, neck, shoulder, forearm, and hand. Clinically, the most common disease entities are tendinitis, tenosynovitis, peritendinitis, myalgia, nerve entrapment syndromes, low back pain, sciatica, and arthrosis.

Work-related disorders of the shoulder and arm are in some countries referred to as repetition strain injury, cumulative trauma disorders, or occupational cervicobrachial disorders (Maeda 1977; McDermott 1986; Putz-Anderson 1988). These umbrella terms indicate that the disorders are caused by repetitive work, cumulative trauma, and occupation, respectively, whereas it is generally acknowledged that the causality is more complex and that several risk factors, on and off jobs, contribute to the conditions. Moreover, there is a great deal of overlapping between repetition strain injury, cumulative trauma disorders, and occupational cervicobrachial disorders, and these terms are imprecise, cover a large range of clinical conditions and often lack clear diagnostic criteria. Therefore musculoskeletal disorders at the workplace are more accurately described as work-related disorders. A work-related disorder is, according to the World Health Organization (WHO) definition, multifactorial, and the work environment and the performance of work contribute significantly, in varying magnitude, to the causation of the disease (WHO 1985). Work-related disorders must therefore be separated from specific occupational disorders where one factor is sufficient to cause the disease. The work-relatedness of many musculoskeletal disorders has been discussed extensively by Hagberg et al. (Hagberg et al. 1995).

Inflammations of tendons and surrounding tissues (tendinitis, peritendinitis, and tenosynovitis), especially in the forearm and wrist, elbow, and shoulder have a high prevalence and incidence in occupations with prolonged periods of repetitive and static work loads (Kurppa et al. 1991). Tendon disorders may have an acute or insidious onset. Workers usually recover, but they may in some cases develop chronic disorders.

Myalgias, that is pain and functional impairment of muscles, occur predominantly in the shoulder and neck region in occupations with large static demands, when performing precision work with the hands or work with elevated arms (Kilbom et al. 1986; Winkel and Westgaard 1992b).

Nerve entrapment syndromes occur especially in the wrist and forearm, causing pain and loss of sensibility and strength. They occur in work tasks that require prolonged, repetitive and forceful handgrips and wrist movements often combined with exposure to local vibration. With continued exposure, functional impairment may remain for life. The most common work-related nerve entrapment syndrome is carpal tunnel syndrome (Hagberg et al. 1992).

Degenerative disorders commonly occur in the spine, usually in the neck and low back region, as well as in the hip and knee joints. Such disorders are common in the general population at older ages. However, several factors at work, especially heavy physical work, manual handling of objects and forward bending/twisting of the trunk interact with ageing and accelerate the degenerative joint process (Riihimäki 1991; Vingård 1991). The course of these disorders is chronic, and usually exposure to risk factors at work has lasted for many years before symptoms occur.

The risk factors for work-related musculoskeletal disorders are thus static work especially as encountered in fatiguing postures, heavy manual handling, vibrations, traumas, and repetitive work, in combination with psychological and social factors like high demands and low degree of control over one's own work (International Commission for Occupational Health, Musculoskeletal Committee 1996).

Cultural differences in disorders manifestations (repetitive strain injury in Australia, connective tissue disorder in North

Table 35.2 Distribution (%) and average sick-leave due to cases of reported occupational accidents in Sweden 1992 by some important 'principal external agencies'. Total number of reported accidents 67 000

Principal external agency	All reported accidents (%)	Average sick-leave (days)
Hand-held tools and implements	10.9	16
Lifting machines and appliances	14.1	34
Other machines	10.1	29
Construction parts, interior fittings, scaffolding, ladders	21.7	32
Materials, goods, packaging, containers	21.9	29
Chemicals, physical or biological factors	14.9	25

America) exist, perhaps related to medical traditions and the circumstances under which the disorders were first noted. The occupational health legislation and compensation systems influence the pattern of reporting. Nevertheless, there is a core of severe musculoskeletal disorders that could be prevented by improved work design. Ergonomics has an important role in prevention.

Occupational accidents

A high incidence of occupational accidents in some branches of industry was the original impetus for occupational health and safety legislation in many countries. Table 35.2 summarizes official statistics on occupational accidents in Sweden by 'principal external agency' and consequences (sick-leave) (Statistics Sweden 1994). A very large proportion of the accidents occurs while handling machines, tools, and other technical devices, and are costly because of relatively long periods of sick-leave. Accidents have also been subdivided by 'main event', that is by the circumstances surrounding the accident. The two most common 'main events' are 'fall on same level' and 'overexertion of body part' which have an annual incidence of 3.2 and 2.7 per 1000 men and 2.1 and 2.5 per 1000 women, respectively, in Sweden.

It is obvious that poor machine and tool design, lack of maintenance and house-keeping, and lack of work procedures contribute to most occupational accidents. Instructions and warning signs are often not designed in accordance with ergonomic principles. Prevention therefore requires attention to all aspects of ergonomics, technical redesign, consideration to cognitive ergonomics, and reorganization of work procedures.

Despite today's deficiencies much has happened. Over the past 10 to 20 years the incidence of occupational accidents has been reduced in many western countries. For example, in Sweden the incidence of reported occupational accidents per 1000 men in the workforce has come down from 40 in 1980 to 16 in 1992. Corresponding figures for women are 11.5 and 7.5.

Cost–benefit of ergonomics

Well-designed ergonomic systems usually improve efficiency and productivity in industry, both directly and as an effect of improved health and reduced sick-leave (Simpson 1988; Oxenburgh 1991). The costs for ergonomic improvements like re-engineering of work stations and tools, introduction of new production methods and work reorganization can be compared with the costs of keeping a poor work system unchanged. Factors that should be balanced against the costs for improvements are high sick-leave absences and

high staff turnover in combination with low quality production, often including a large proportion of rejected products.

Case study from a railway maintenance workshop   (Oxenburgh 1991) In this workshop where diesel engines were maintained and repaired, problems with low productivity and unacceptably high injury rates were encountered. The work stations required awkward postures because of problems with access, reach and visibility, and the risk of accidents was high because of temporary, makeshift support for the engine parts during repair.

The solution chosen was via adoption of a new management style that encouraged worker participation in the change process. The improvements were introduced via consultative teams consisting of workers and engineers who used their own experience but also drew on information gathered from visits to other workshops. Quality control was improved by allowing workers to take responsibility for their work and encouraging customer feedback as to the acceptability of the work. Work practices and work systems were improved in collaboration with ergonomic consultants. The cost for the physical improvements was about 6 per cent of the yearly labour costs. The injury rate did not decrease, but the severity of injuries was reduced and absenteeism due to injury was halved. The productivity gain was very high and the throughput of diesel engines increased by 80 per cent. Altogether the costs of improvements were paid back in 4 months.

Ergonomics and public health

Consumer applications

This area is becoming increasingly important, partly as a consequence of the product liability legislation now introduced in many Western countries. The manufacturer of any product can be made economically responsible if it can be demonstrated the disease or accidents ensued when the product was used. Therefore ergonomic considerations must influence the compilation of instructions and design of warning signs, as well as the design of the product itself.

The ergonomic design of products, implements, and entire systems for use by the general population covers a wide area. Some important examples that may influence public health are the design of

- transport systems (see below)
- furniture and kitchen utensils
- floor covers
- commonly used tools
- containers for carrying and storing products.

Designs must often fit the anthropometry, strength, and endurance of the entire population. Information and warning signs must, in a similar way, be understandable to populations with large variations in sensory and cognitive capacity, cultural background, and level of schooling. All areas of design must be considered: a product or an implement must be shaped and marked in a way that explains its function; safety devices must be designed without demands on previous training and experience; and size, weight, and grips must fit a wide variety of human body sizes. Design for the public therefore requires even more sophisticated considerations than design for working life, where the user population is better defined in terms of physical and psychological capacities, and where additional training can be given to selected groups.

While disorders of muscles and joints are common consequences of poor ergonomic design in occupational settings, the public health consequences are more often in the nature of accidents. The main difference is that the public is seldom exposed to very prolonged and/or repeated use of systems and implements designed without consideration to ergonomics, whereas it often encounters unexpected events or unfamiliar devices. Accidents often happen as a consequence of a combination of several deficient design details; consider slipping and falling due to a combination of slippery floors and manual transport of bulky, wobbly objects that obscure vision. Kitchen accidents may happen due to a combination of unsuitable working heights, poor lighting, and ambiguous labelling of stove controls.

Poor ergonomic design of consumer products not only leads to accidents with consequences for public health, it frequently affects quality of life by introducing annoyance and fatigue. Some examples are; carrying food from the supermarket in plastic bags that cut into your fingers, trying to open containers that require more than your grip strength, or sorting money of different denominations. In all these cases a better design would reduce discomfort and fatigue, make the task less time-consuming, and reduce the risk of mistakes.

Ergonomic applications in transportation systems

Traffic accident is one of the leading causes of death and disability today. In the United States, traffic injury is second only cancer in the total financial cost to the community of major disabilities and deaths. Even in some developing countries where infectious disease is still a significant cause of death, traffic injury accounts for a percentage of all deaths similar to that in some highly motorized countries (Trinca et al. 1988).

Traffic accidents are often blamed on 'human error'. The car driver 'disregarded' the warning sign, the truck driver stepped on the breaks 'too late', the signal box attendant 'forgot' the coming train, and so on. What if the warning sign was obscured because of the car design and the position of the sign, the truck driver was just entering a tunnel with sudden (relative) darkness, and the signal box attendant was tired because of having to work double shifts? Transportation systems can be designed in a way that takes human limitations into consideration, instead of relying on unrealistic instructions, rules, and regulations that do not comply with human capacity.

Traffic accidents have a complex causality, and ergonomics can play an important role for prevention through the design of vehicles and traffic signs, and the engineering of roads and railways. Because of the high speed of movement in traffic, the design of transportation systems has special requirements. The speed places excessive demands on reaction time, short-term memory and vision of both drivers and pedestrians, although these demands can be moderated by the design of the system (Lay 1986; Ogden 1990).

Reaction time can be reduced by encouraging familiarity, because drivers react faster to a familiar situation, and by reducing the number of alternatives. For example, unusual intersection layouts, and a large number of exits from a roundabout, require longer response times.

Short-term memory is crucial for driver performance because most of the driving task is performed by processing information that never leaves the short-term memory. Therefore, warning signs should require an immediate response, drivers should be frequently reminded of control information which varies along the road (for example speed limits), and the driver must be allowed to respond to one stimulus before the next is imposed.

Of all information required by a vehicle driver 90 per cent is supplied by vision. As the amount of visual information is nearly without limit, the driver must continuously select the most important cues to help in his or her driving. As the demands increase the driver tends to be overloaded and misses some information, or sheds part of it. This situation occurs typically when the data processing demands increase, but it also takes place immediately after a situation of overload. Thus the departure side of an intersection may be more accident prone than the approach side, which also implies that pedestrian crossings and bus stops should not be placed after intersections. Only 1 to 1.5 fixations of vision per second are realistic in driving. Road traffic signs must therefore be separated in time and space and must only be used for the most necessary information. They must be within the field of vision of the driver which, when moving at a certain speed, implies a narrower field both horizontally and vertically than for a stationary observer. Delineation, that is markings of road alignment immediately ahead, is important for road traffic safety since it helps the driver to keep within the traffic lane and also helps to plan the route forwards. It is especially important at the approach to curves and crests, and for elderly drivers whose visual capacity is often reduced.

The design of the driver cabin directly influences traffic safety by the degree of visibility that it affords to the driver. But the preventive effect of cabin design is also indirect, by providing a comfortable seated posture protected from vibration. These aspects of driving have been discussed by Pheasant (for example Pheasant 1991). Apart from these factors, traffic safety is influenced by a large number of circumstances like fatigue, medication, and ill health of the driver, training of drivers and pedestrians, legislation, traffic density, and weather conditions (Ogden 1990; Sanders and McCormick 1992).

The public as victims in technological environments—two case studies

Most people have read about disasters in high-tech environments like Three Mile Island or Chernobyl. Such disasters can be ascribed to the combined effects of design defects, conflicts between safety and productivity goals, poor operating and maintenance procedures, and inadequate training (Reason 1990). Ergonomics is central in the causality of many of these accidents because of poor system design which is not compatible with human capacity and its limitations. The operators or workers involved are often victims, but the reason these disasters are widely publicized and analysed is that the public—the third party—is exposed to risks without the ability to protect itself. The following two case studies illustrate that serious accidents can—and will—happen when technical systems have not been designed and implemented with consideration to human limitations.

The tram accident   In a recent tram accident in Sweden, 13 people died and 29 were taken to hospital when a tram raced downhill along the track with the brakes disconnected. All those killed or injured were waiting at the next stop, or were pedestrians or car passengers happening to pass further down. The tram had been taken out of service because of a breakdown in the overhead power supply. As the electric power had been cut, the normal electrodynamic breaks did not function and mechanical breaks had automically taken over. The traffic supervisor in charge of the removal of the tram decided to use the downslope to move the tram further down where the power was intact. However, the mechanical breaks first had to be released, which could be done by a simple handgrip from the outside of each carriage. The intention was to use the mechanical breaks again further down. However, for the mechanical breaks to be functional again they had to be refilled with pressurized air which could only be done when under electrical power. As a consequence, the tram driver had no possibility of stopping the tram from racing down the track.

This accident appears to be a typical example of so-called 'human error'. However, the subsequent investigation revealed several errors in the design of the system (Haverikommission 1992). The drivers and supervisors knew that the mechanical breaks must not be released unless the tram was secured by other means, but they did not know why; neither did they know how the breaks were constructed or what the consequences might be of disconnecting the mechanical breaks. Moreover, they had been given no formal training in emergency procedures of this nature. The mechanical breaks had been designed with an external release mechanism that was easily accessible but without any cautioning signs. This case is an unfortunate example of the combined effects of deficiencies in technical design and training and emergency procedures that could have been avoided by the application of ergonomics.

The haemodialysis accident   In 1983, three patients died and 12 others were exposed to severe threats to their lives when they were undergoing haemodialysis in a Swedish hospital. They were regularly treated with haemodialysis without severe complications but on this occasion the haemodialysis unit, used for all these patients, fed sterile water instead of physiological saline into the patients. The nurse on duty was charged and later sentenced for negligence, since she had switched off the alarm system of the haemodialysis unit.

In order to understand the sequence of events it is necessary to know how the alarm panel of the haemodialysis unit was designed (Fig. 35.5). It had six horizontal rows of lamps and switches, for the conductivity (ion concentration) of the haemodialysis fluid, for its temperature, for the level of fluid in the tanks, and for the amount

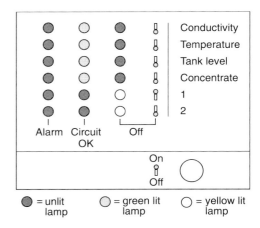

Fig. 35.5 Control panel of the haemodialysis unit before it was disconnected (revised from Lundberg 1992).

of concentrated saline available for diluting with water to create the haemodialysis fluid. Two more rows (1 and 2) were available but not in use. The vertical row of switches was for turning the alarm system on or off, and the first column of lamps (from the right) had yellow warning lamps that were lit when the alarm was in the 'off' position. Since rows 1 and 2 were not in use their alarms had been turned off, and therefore the corresponding lamps were lit yellow, that is they were constantly indicating a warning. The second vertical column of lamps had green lamps that were lit when the alarm was on and when conductivity, temperature, and so on were within given acceptable levels. The vertical column of lamps to the extreme left had red lamps that were lit when the ion concentration, temperature, tank level, or amount of concentrate were below or above the set 'safe' levels. The main switch at the bottom of the panel was connected to an acoustic alarm that was common for all four alarm functions.

In a retrospective attempt to analyse the accident, the most likely series of events seems to have been as follows (Lundberg 1992): the nurse was experienced in the use of the system and in the treatment of haemodialysis patients. The day of the accident was different, though, because the nurse demonstrated the haemodialysis unit to a visitor and explained its function. Normally the nurses did not have to use the six alarm switches; they had been left on the panel because the unit had needed occasional adjustments by technicians, and the system had to be opeational even when one of the circuits was out of function (albeit with intensified surveillance). The apparatus had been in use for several years and had undergone several improvements. On this occasion, however, the nurse noted that the main switch was 'on', that is, turned up; whereas the four top switches were turned down, that is, they appeared to be turned off (see Fig. 35.5). Consequently, she turned up the four top switches, believing that she had turned the alarms on. She did not know, however, that the main switch and the other switches had their 'on' and 'off' positions in different directions, and that she was actually disconnecting the alarms! Neither did she know that she not only disconnected the alarms but that the emergency stop of the system was disconnected with the same switch. The haemodialysis unit continued working even though the alarms were disconnected. When the concentrated saline solution ran out, it continued with mere distilled water, with disastrous consequences for the patients. The nurse might have taken warning from the fact that the four yellow warning lamps lit up when the alarms were turned off; however, she was used to two of the yellow lights always being on, and said, during the trial, that she thought they should be on.

Sentencing this nurse on duty caused considerable discussion and was widely considered unjust. Obviously the design of the haemodialysis unit, as well as the nurse's understanding of its function, were poor. Insufficient oral information about the system had been given. The surveillance of the system was done by technicians for whom its function was obvious but they did not convey their understanding to the nurses operating the system. The case emphasizes the need for unambiguous designs of control panels with consistent markings, for proper training, and for clear, written procedures both for routines and emergencies. Why then blame only one person? Were not the designers at fault, and the head of the haemodialysis unit for not providing instruction and training? The application of ergonomic principles in the design of this haemodialysis system, as well as for similar surveillance systems used in hospitals, is necessary for the avoidance of accidents.

Ergonomics for special interest groups
Sport and leisure
Although usually not described in ergonomic terms, many implements and tools used in leisure time and in various sports have been developed with the multidisciplinary approach of ergonomics, emphasizing high levels of achievement and absence of accidents and injuries. Some examples of ergonomic development are hand-grip fit in golf clubs and tennis rackets to improve force output and reduce the risk of epicondylitis, and the development of sport shoes to reduce impact forces and periostial and tendon inflammation.

Physical or mental disability, rehabilitation, and the elderly
These areas have advanced greatly in recent years. Design for rehabilitation and for people with physical or mental disabilities concentrates on compensating for reduced muscle strength and precision, hearing defects, reduced vision, and mobility. In the future, more emphasis should also be put on compensating for longer reaction times and reduced cognitive capacity. Computer use, for example, is often out of reach for both people with disabilities and elderly people because of poor visibility, demands on rapid information processing, and the introduction of unfamiliar symbols. In the same way as a handicap may affect only one out of several functional capacities, an elderly person may have most functions well preserved. There is therefore no need to distinguish between ergonomics for people with physical or mental disabilities and the elderly. In fact, it would make more economic sense if products were designed for use by those with limited abilities, as well as by the more able-bodied (Haigh 1993).

In a recent survey of commercially available products intended for elderly people, it was found that many of them were inappropriate or inadequate to perform the task for which they were intended (Gardner *et al.* 1993). Some did not perform the intended job; others introduced hazards that could have led to serious accidents, but which could have been avoided after simple consumer trials and redesign. One group of ergonomists and designers

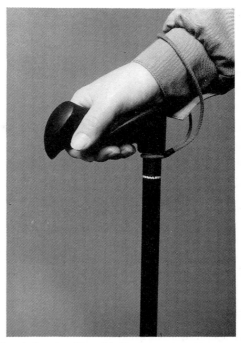

Fig. 35.6 New design of walking stick (Benktzon 1993). Note the large contact area between hand and handle and the small forearm to hand angle. (Reproduced from Benktzon 1993, with permission from Butterworth-Heinemann.)

in Sweden, Ergonomi-Design Gruppen, have successfully designed a range of products for people with disabilities and the elderly (Benktzon 1993). Modification of products such as knives, walking sticks, and cutlery have made people with reduced strength and mobility of the hand or arm more self-sufficient in their everyday life (Fig. 35.6).

The design process is stepwise, via thorough studies of the functional ability of groups of people with disabilities, preparing a range of test tools, prototype testing, and finally manufacturing. The same approach has been used in the redesign of products for craftsmen and other occupational groups who have repeated and prolonged use of tools and implements. Small design details can be of vital importance for the safety, comfort, and usability for craftsmen as well as for people with disabilities. Pliers, screwdrivers, and butcher's knives with improved grip surface and grip diameter, and a coffee pot with its centre of gravity closer to the hand, are other commercial products developed by the group. They all reduce the load on the forearm and hand thus reducing the risk of musculoskeletal disorders and are therefore used widely. Solutions originally created for the elderly or for people with physical or mental disabilities have frequently been found acceptable to a broader range of users (Benktzon 1993).

Ergonomics in developing countries
In developing countries with high rates of unemployment it is tempting for employers who build up small and middle-sized industries to disregard safety and health (Kogi and Sen 1987). Labour inspectors are scarce and have limited resources, and surveillance of occupational conditions is often lacking. Ergonomics must therefore be promoted not only as a means to improve

safety, but also to fulfil other management goals, especially high productivity, and must stem from local initiatives.

According to Kogi, support from international organizations and states should be organized so as to enable people to identify priority problems and effective solutions using locally available materials and skills (Kogi 1991). The support should provide for

(1) practical advice on how to identify priority problems and how to find solutions;

(2) practical guidance, particularly through learning-by-doing, about ways to implement immediate improvements.

Because of the great need for improvements and the scarcity of ergonomists in developing countries, the International Labour Organization has developed a training programme targeting entrepreneurs and workers of small and medium-sized enterprises (Louzine 1982). The training programme focuses on the simultaneous improvement of working conditions and productivity, and encourages low-cost, voluntary measures using a participatory approach. Eight themes have been selected for the programme, because of their importance for both working conditions and productivity:

- materials storage and handling
- work-station design
- machine safety
- control of hazardous substances
- lighting
- welfare facilities and services
- work premises
- work organization

During the programme, local examples are used and the participants are encouraged to find practical improvements by means of self-help and sharing of experience. If managers and workers do not see any likelihood of a productivity gain and do not learn to use their own ideas and skills, they will quickly lose interest.

Implementing change
Legislation, standards, guidelines
National legislation concerning ergonomic factors varies widely between different countries. Traditionally, legislation in occupational health focused on quantitative data, for example heights, weights, and other minimum physical requirements to improve safety. The validity of strict quantitative data is difficult to prove, and therefore a more modern approach is to develop functional requirements, for example a certain work process must not produce injuries and must comply with safe handling (Kilbom 1995). Intense work is under way in the European Community to develop directives relevant for ergonomics, and some have already been presented for machine work, manual handling (EEC/90/269 Directive), and work at visual display terminals (Dul and de Flaming 1994). In the United States an ergonomics standard has recently been proposed but has not yet been accepted.

In the public sector intensification of product liability legislation has given better tools for consumers in pursuing safety.

Standards are being developed nationally and internationally but are usually not legally binding. The International Standardization Organization issues standards complementary to the European Community standards. Other examples are the proposed American National Standards Institute standards on upper limb disorders (ANSI Z–365).

Large manufacturing or scientific organizations often develop codes of practice or guidelines for the specific area of their activity. These can be made more precise, relating to the conditions at hand at a certain organization, and are therefore useful for the practitioner (for example Mital and Kilbom 1992; Winkel and Westgaard 1992a; Kilbom 1994).

Training
The labour inspectorate is, in most countries, the organization responsible for the follow-up of ergonomics legislation. Since inspectors are usually poorly trained in ergonomics, this surveillance is often ineffective. In countries with a well-developed occupational health service (e.g. the Nordic countries) physiotherapists and safety engineers are usually well trained in ergonomics and perform valuable work.

Sometimes the occupational health service is unable to sufficiently influence the development of new work stations—the work is reactive rather than proactive. For improved ergonomic conditions, both at workplaces and for the public, those responsible for developing technical systems need more training in ergonomics. Thus production engineers, designers, architects, and systems engineers (in computing) and also personnel managers need more training which is seldom provided by technical universities. Since few universities provide postgraduate degrees in ergonomics there is so far an unfulfilled need for training, which is even more pronounced in developing countries.

Participatory approaches
In recent years it has been proved repeatedly that improvements of ergonomic conditions are most efficiently achieved when all those using a particular system are also involved in its improvement. 'Expert' advice, for example, a short-term consultant frequently results in failure, unless supported by the experience of those manufacturing or using the product. The knowledge of the consumer or the worker is often unspoken but can be used for product and system improvement in practical trials. The group of people involved can be expanded further; in a manufacturing industry it should include not only the product designer and manufacturing engineer, but also the workers, the occupational health staff, those who sell and promote the product, and its users (Noro and Imada 1991). However, such participatory approaches must be used with some caution since, for example, it is not easy for the worker or consumer to predict new hazards that may arise from a change in design.

References
American Journal of Preventive Medicine (1989). *Injury Prevention: Meeting the Challenge*, 5, 1–303.
Åstrand, I. (1967a). Aerobic working capacity in men and women in some professions. *Försvarsmedicin*, 3, 163–70.
Åstrand, I. (1967b). Degree of strain during building work as related to individual aerobic work capacity. *Ergonomics*, 10, 293–303.

Åstrand, I. (1988). Physical demands in worklife. *Scandinavian Journal of Work Environment and Health*, **14**, 10–13.

Åstrand, P.O. and Rodahl, K. (1986). *Textbook of work physiology.* McGraw-Hill, New York.

Benktzon, M. (1993). Designing for our future selves: the Swedish experience. *Applied Ergonomics*, **24**, 19–27.

Bergqvist, U., Wolgast, E., Nilsson, B., and Voss, M. (1995). The influence of VDT work on musculoskeletal disorders. *Ergonomics*, **38**, 754–62.

Chaffin, D., Herrin, G., and Keyserling, W.M. (1978). Preemployment strength testing – an updated position. *Journal of Occupational Medicine*, **6**, 403–8.

Chapanis, A. (1965). On the allocation of functions between men and machines. *Occupational Psychology*, **39**, 1–11.

Clark, T.S. and Corlett, E.N. (1984). *The Ergonomics of Workspaces and Machines – A design manual.* Taylor & Francis, London.

Dul, J. and de Flaming, P. (1994). A review of ISO and CEN standards on ergonomics. In: *Proceedings of the 12th Triennial Congress of the International Ergonomics Association.* Human Factors Association of Canada, Toronto, Canada, pp. 131–133.

Era, P., Lyyra, A.L., Viitasalo, J.T., and Heikkinen, E. (1992) Determinants of isometric muscle strength in men of different ages. *European Journal of Applied Physiology*, **64**, 84–91.

Gardner, L., Powell, L., and Page, M. (1993). An appraisal of a selection of products currently available to older consumers. *Applied Ergonomics*, **24**, 35–9.

Grandjean, E. (1988). *Fitting the task to the man. A textbook of occupational ergonomics.* Taylor & Francis, London.

Hagberg, M., Morgenstern, H., and Kelsh, M. (1992). Impact of occupations and job tasks on the prevalence of carpal tunnel syndrome: a review. *Scandinavian Journal of Work Environment and Health*, **18**, 337–45.

Hagberg, M., Hendricks, H., Silverstein, B., Smith, M., Welsh, R., and Caryon, P. (1995). *Work related musculoskeletal disorders (WMSDs): a reference book for prevention.* Taylor & Francis, London.

Haigh, R. (1993). The ageing process: a challenge for design. *Applied Ergonomics*, **24**, 9–14.

Hansen, S.M. (1993). *Arbeidsmiljø og samfundsøkonomi.* Nordisk Ministerråd, Nord 1993:22.

Hansson, J.-E. (1987). Funktionell anatomi, antropometri och biomekanik. In *Människan i arbete.* (ed. N. Lundgren, G., Luthman, and K. Elgstrand) pp. 92–118. Almqvist & Wiksell, Stockholm.

Haverikommissionen (1992). *Spårvagnsolycka 1992–03–12.* Swedish Board of accident investigation Report no J 1992:1, Stockholm.

Hendricks, H.W. (1986). Macroergonomics: a conceptual model for integrating human factors with organizational design. In *Proceedings of the Human factors in organizational design and management 11.* (ed. O. Brown and H. Hendricks). pp. 467–77. North Holland, London.

Jonsson, B.G., Persson, J., and Kilbom, Å. (1988). Disorders of the cervicobrachial region among female workers in the electronics industry. A two-year follow up. *International Journal of Industrial Ergonomics*, **3**, 1–12.

Kilbom, Å. (1994). Repetitive work of the upper extremity: Part 1 – Guidelines for the practitioner. Part II – The scientific basis (knowledge base) for the guide. *International Journal of Industrial Ergonomics*, **14**, 51–86.

Kilbom, Å. (1995). Prevention of musculoskeletal disorders through standards and guidelines: possibilities and limitations. In *From Research to Prevention.* (ed. J. Rantanen, S. Lehtinen, S. Hernberg, K. Lindström, M. Sorsa, J. Starck, and E. Viikari-Juntura), pp. 178–86. Finnish Institute of Occupational Health, Helsinki.

Kilbom, Å., Persson, J., and Jonsson, B.G. (1986). Disorders of the cervicobrachial region among female workers in the electronics industry. *International Journal of Industrial Ergonomics*, **1**, 37–47.

Kogi, K., 1991. Patricipatory training for low-cost improvements in small enterprises in developing countries. In *Participatory Ergonomics.* (ed. K. Noro and A. Imada). pp. 73–80. Taylor & Francis, London.

Kogi, K. and Sen, R. (1987). Third world ergonomics. *International Reviews of Ergonomics*, **1**, 77–118.

Kurppa, K., Viikari-Juntura, E., Kuosma, E., Huuskonen, M., and Kivi, P.

(1991). Incidence of tenosynovitis or peritendinitis and epicondylitis in a meat-processing factory. *Scandinavian Journal of Work Environment and Health*, **17**, 32–7.

Lay, M. (1986). *Handbook of road technology.* Gordon and Breach, London.

Lehto, M. (1992). Designing warning signs and warning labels. Part I: Guidelines for the practitioner. Part II: The scientific basis for the guide. *International Journal of Industrial Ergonomics*, **10**, 78–95.

Ljungberg, A.-S., Kilbom, Å., and Hägg, G. (1989). Occupational lifting by nursing aides and warehouse workers. *Ergonomics*, **32**, 59–78.

Louzine, A. (1982). Improving working conditions in small enterprises in developing countries. *International Labour Review*, **121**, 443–54.

Lundberg, A. (1992). *Dialysmålet—ett öppet sår i svensk tättskipning.* Private Report.

Maeda, K. (1977). Occupational cervicobrachial disorders and its causative factors. *Journal of Human Ergology*, **6**, 193–202.

McDermott, F. (1986). Repetition strain injury: a review of current understanding. *Medical Journal of Australia*, **144**, 196–200.

Mital, A. and Kilbom, Å. (1992). Design, selection and use of hand tools to alleviate trauma of the upper extremities. *International Journal of Industrial Ergonomics*, **10**, 1–21.

Mital, A., Motorwala, A., Kulkarni, M., Sinclair, M., and Siemieniuch, C. (1994). Allocation of functions to humans and machines in a manufacturing environment. Part I – Guidelines for the practitioner. *International Journal of Industrial Ergonomics*, **14**, 3–29.

Murrell, K.F.H. (1965). *Ergonomics – Man in his working environment.* Chapman & Hall, London.

Oborne, D.J., Branton, R., Leal, F., Shipley, P., and Stewart, T. (1993). *Person-Centred Ergonomics. A Brantonian View of Human Factors.* Taylor & Francis, London.

Ogden, K. (1990). Human factors in traffic engineering. *Institute of Transportation Engineers Journal*, **60**, 41–6.

Oxenburgh, M. (1991). *Increasing productivity and profit through health and safety.* CCH Australia, Chicago.

Pheasant, S. (1986). *Bodyspace.* Taylor & Francis, London.

Pheasant, S. (1991). *Ergonomics, work and health.* Macmillan Academic and Professional Ltd, London.

Putz-Anderson, V. (1988). *Cumulative Trauma Disorders: A manual for musculoskeletal diseases of the upper limbs.* Taylor & Francis, London.

Rabbitt, P. (1991). Management of the working population. *Ergonomics*, **34**, 775–90.

Reason, J. (1990). *Human error.* Cambridge University Press, Cambridge.

Riihimäki, H., 1991. Low-back pain, its origin and risk indicators. *Scandinavian Journal of Work Environment and Health*, **17**, 81–90.

Salthouse, T.A. (1990). Influence of experience on age differences in cognitive functioning. *Human Factors*, **32**, 551–69.

Sanders, M. and McCormick, E. (1992). *Human factors in engineering and design.* McGraw-Hill, New York.

Scientific Committee for Musculoskeletal Disorders of the International Commission on Occupational Health (1996). Musculoskeletal disorders – work-related risk factors and prevention. *International Journal of Occupational and Environmental Health*, in press.

Simpson, G. (1988). The economic justification for ergonomics. *International Journal of Industrial Ergonomics*, **2**, 157–63.

Statistics Sweden (SCB) (1994). *Arbetssjukdomar och arbetsolyckor 1992.* Sveriges Officiella Statistik, Stockholm.

Trinca, G., Johnston, I., Campbell, F., *et al.* (1988). *Reducing traffic injury – A global challenge.* Royal Australasian College of Surgeons, Melbourne.

Vaaranen, V., Vasama, M., Toikkanen, J., Jolanki, R. and Kaupinen, T. (1994). *Ammattitaudit 1993 (Occupational diseases in Finland 1993).* Institute of Occupational Health, Helsinki.

Vernon, H.M. (1921). *Industrial fatigue and efficiency.* Routledge, London.

Vingård, E., 1991. *Work, sports, overweight and osteoarthrosis of the hip.* Ph. D thesis, Karolinska Institute, Stockholm.

Waters, T.W., Putz-Anderson, V., Garg, A., and Fine, L.J. (1993). Revised NIOSH equation for the design and evaluation of manual lifting tasks. *Ergonomics*, **36**, 749–76.

Winkel, J. and Westgaard, R. (1992*a*). Occupational and individual risk factors for shoulder-neck complaints: Part I – Guidelines for the practitioner. *International Journal of Industrial Ergonomics*, **10**, 79–83.

Winkel, J. and Westgaard, R.H. (1992*b*). Occupational and individual risk factors for shoulder-neck complaints: Part II – The scientific basis (literature review) for the guide. *International Journal of Industrial Ergonomics*, **10**, 85–104.

WHO (1985). *Identification and control of work related diseases*. World Health organisation, Technical Report Series no 714, Geneva.

Index

Page numbers in **bold** refer to major sections of the text.

vs denotes differential diagnosis or comparisons.

Since the major subject of this title is public health, entries have been kept to a minimum under this keyword and readers are advised to seek more specific references. Entries under specific countries have been limited to major topics. Additional statistics may be found within the text

Indexing style/conventions used

Alphabetical order. This index is in letter-by-letter order, whereby hyphens, en-rules and spaces within index headings are ignored in the alphabetization. Terms in brackets are excluded from initial alphabetization.

Cross-references. Cross-reference terms in *italics* are either general cross-references, or refer to subentry terms within the same main entry (the main entry term is not repeated, in order to save space) i.e. they are not main entry terms.

Abbreviations used in subentries (without explanation):

AIDS	Acquired immunodeficiency syndrome	HIV	Human immunodeficiency virus
CDC	Centers for Disease Control and Prevention (US)	IDDM	Insulin dependent diabetes mellitus
GDP	Gross domestic product	NIDDM	Non-insulin dependent diabetes mellitus
GNP	Gross national product	STDs	Sexually transmitted diseases

A

ABO blood group 150
abortion
  Canada 266
  illegal/restricted 362
  induced 1362
  Japan 98, 487
  legislation 361, 362
  on medical grounds 362
  problems 361
    access and authorization 362
  publications on data 468
  ratio 834
  sex-selective 88–9
  spontaneous 1362
    caffeine intake and 552
  UK statistics 468
  unsafe and risk of death 1362
  US 110
Abortion Act (1967 - UK) 468
absenteeism 741
abstracting, US hospital discharge survey 444
abuse 1495
  see also alcohol abuse; child neglect/ abuse; drug abuse; sexual abuse; substance abuse
'academic skills disorders' 1451
acceptable daily intake (ADI) 974, 980
accidents 1291, 1322
  consumer products 439, 440
  Health of the Nation (White Paper) target 252
  Japan 65
  mortality 97
  occupational *see* occupational accidents
  prevention *see* injury control
  see also injuries; motor vehicle injuries/ accidents
accuracy
  risk quantification 990
  surveillance data 932–3
  technical/semantic, of communication system 420
acetyltransferase 150
Acheson Report (1988 - UK) 391, 1151

acid aerosols 204, 1096
acidity, atmospheric 204
acid rain 63, 207
acid water 207
acquired immunodeficiency syndrome
  see AIDS
Actinomyces 189
activities of daily living (ADL) 1434, 1435, 1446
  instrumental (IADL) 1434, 1446
activity logs, total exposure estimates 959
acupuncturists, licensing in Japan 56
acute flaccid paralysis (AFP) 940
acute medical care *see* emergency care
adaptation
  environmental hazard reduction 1611
  undernutrition 164
adaptation/aids *see* aids/adaptations
adducts 956
adenotonsillectomy 778
Adenoviridae 180
adenoviruses 180
adenylate cyclase 185
adhesins 187
adjustment (covariate control) methods 599, 613
adjustment disorders 1150
administration
  Japan *see under* Japan
  national health systems 1641
  public, approach to management 890–1
  social *see* social administration
  UK public health 29–30, 32–3
  US public health *see* United States of America (USA)
administrative prevalence, mild learning disability 1459
adolescent medicine 1407–8, 1410
adolescents/adolescence 1397–413
  alcohol abuse 1497
  antiauthority/antisocial behaviour 1403–4
  behaviour 1399, 1403, 1404
    health promotion relationship 1408–9
  behavioural disorders 1146
  chronic illness/hospitalization, response 1400–1
  clinical significance of maturation 1399

adolescents/adolescence *(continued)*
  crime rate in US 1323
  definition 1397–8
  demography 1397–8
  drug abuse 1392, 1402–3, 1497
  eating disorders 1404–5
  ethical and legal issues 1406
  growth and development 1398–9
  health care services 1406–8, 1410
    disabled adolescents 1408
    primary care 1407
    psychiatric services 1408
    specialist services 1407–8
  health concerns and knowledge 1399–400
  health education 1400, 1405, 1409
  health and family 1406
  health promotion/prevention programme 1408–9, 1410
  high-risk behaviour 1399
  homelessness 1404
  homicide in US 1321
  maturational stress 1399
  medical disorders 1400–1
  mental health problems 1401–5
    emotional 1401–2
  mortality/mortality rates 1323, 1399
    causes 1399
  parent estrangement 1404
  parenthood 1405–6
  parenting difficulties 1399
  pregnancy in 839–40, 1397, 1405–6
    rates 110, 839, 1340–1
  problems in school 1404
  sexually-related problems 1405–6
  sexual offences 1406
  smoking and substance abuse 1402–3
  social alienation 1404
  social value attached 1398, 1410
  suicidal behaviour 1402
  suicide 1324, 1347, 1397, 1410
  surgery 1406
  teaching/training of health care staff for 1409, 1410
  US national health objective 1550–1
  violence *see under* interpersonal violence
    see also children

β-adrenoreceptor blockers *see* beta-blockers
adults
  alcohol and drug abuse 1497
  genetic screening 1583
  undernutrition in 163–4
adverse drug reactions (ADR)
  in elderly 1490
  genetic variability 150
  schizophrenia treatment 1157
advertising
  alcohol/cigarette bans 9, 363
  restraints in motor vehicles 1309
  see also media
Advisory Committee on Immunization Practices (ACIP) 1271
Advisory Group on the Medical Aspects of Air Pollution Episodes (AGMEAPE) 1619
advocacy 1468
aerosols 1094
aetiological fraction 564
aetiological heterogeneity, principle 145
aetiological studies
  case–control studies 547, 549, 554
  cross-sectional studies 530–1
aetiology of disease *see* causation; disease; *specific diseases*
affective disorders *see* anxiety disorders; depression; mood disorders
aflatoxin B1 1058, 1616
Africa
  AIDS
    case definition 1268
    case number 1280, 1282
    clinical features 1267
    control and prevention 1277
    costs 1283
    impact 1282, 1283
    transmission 1272
  health education and STD prevention 1254, 1277
  HIV infection transmission 1272
  migraine headache prevalence 1199
  mortality decline 86

discrimination
  HIV-positive patients 358
  protection of women at work 1371
  race 99, 110
  sex 99
disease
  advanced societies 574, 1568
  aetiology
    generalized assumption to specific
      causes 30
    sanitarianism and 22
    social patterning and 776–7
  assessment of burden, in surveillance
    planning 737
  carrier, control in Victorian England 30
  chronic *see* chronic disease
  'civilization' 574, 1566
  determinants 526
  end-points 502
  frequency/co-occurrence with risk
    factors 505
  global burden in terms of DALYs 407
  health relationship *see* epidemiology
  induction period 621
  latent period 621
  natural history, epidemiology role in 503
  poverty relationship *see under* poverty
  predisposition, surveys 933
  prevalence
    cross-sectional surveys 525
    see also prevalence; *specific diseases*
  prevention *see* prevention of disease
  registers/registries
    assessment of medical care benefits
      215
    impact of medical care 225–30
    see also cancer, registries; registries
  risk 563
    epidemiology role in identification
      503, 504
    public perception 1621
  risk factors *see* risk factors of disease
  spectrum, epidemiology use in
    description 502–3
  stages in progression 932, 933
  surveillance *see* surveillance
  temporal relationship with exposure 505
  transmission mechanisms, epidemiology
    role 503
  trend prediction by epidemiology 503
disinfectant, bleach effectiveness 1507
disinfection 1605
disk drives 722
dislocations, injury statistics in US
  1296–7
dispensarization 1649
dispersion, measures 659–60
disposal of waste *see* waste
distance learning, computer application
  732
distortion, communication system
  problem 420
distributional analyses, exposures to
  contaminants 963
distribution models, dose–response
  relationships 975
distributions *see under* statistical methods
District Health Authorities (UK) 1151
district nurses, care of elderly 1480
diverticular disease of colon 1236–7
  epidemiology 1237
divorce
  economic/social/psychological impact
    1341–2
  effects on adolescents 1342, 1404
  mortality and 116
  rates 82, 91, 842
    increase 1341–2
  records, in Japan 479
**DMFT (decayed, missing and filled
  permanent teeth) values** 1161,
  1163

DNA
  analysis, Down's syndrome 1462
  damage, dose–response curve for toxins/
    chemicals 908
  methods to study 141
  polymorphism 141, 150
  radiation-induced damage 151, 916, 923
  ultraviolet radiation injury 923
DNA viruses 177, 180
doctor(s)
  Japan *see* Japan, doctors
  numbers, Japan 58, 67, 68, 484–5
  patient commitment to advice 795
  Philippines 1644
  position, public health management
    891–2, 897
  remuneration, in Japan 60
  school 60
  tobacco smokers and cancer 1054
  US number 303–4
  see also general practitioners (GPs);
    physicians
doctor–patient interaction
  communication failure 794, 795, 798
  compliance or conflict? 797
  disparity of power 797–8
  interactionist perspective 769
  interpersonal skills and 797
  non-compliance and 795–6, 798
  Parsonian perspective 767, 768, 797
  patient dissatisfaction 797
domestic violence 1299, 1355, 1372
  types 1372
  US 1299, 1324
domiciliary care homes, US survey 444
dose–response
  non-threshold approaches 974–5
  in risk characterization 973–5
  thresholds 973
dose–response curves 973–5
  cancer prevention 1058–9
  toxicology 907–8
dose–response models 975
  mechanistic 975
  multistage 975
  probability distribution 975
doses
  biologically effective 952, 962
  in exposure analysis 976–7
  exposure to environmental contaminants
    952, 953, 961–2, 963, 976–7
  internal 952, 962
  potential 952, 962
    point estimate 962
  reference values for calculations 977
  in risk characterization 973–4
double-blind clinical trials *see under*
  clinical trials
double counting, costs/benefits 855
doughnut principle in management
  898
Down's syndrome (trisomy 21) 142,
  1461, 1462–3
  case–control study and information bias
    552–3
  chromosomal studies 153
  detection 142
  education 1470
  features 1462–3
  fetal diagnosis 1462
  incidence 1455
  mental retardation 1454, 1457
  prevalence 1461, 1462
    maternal age and 1384, 1461, 1462
  stimulation and training programmes
    1458
  survival, life-tables 1458
  UK register 1390
dracunculiasis 1602
  eradication goal 1606
  eradication measures 1606–7
Dracunculus medinensis 194
'drift hypothesis' 131

drink driving laws 363, 1302, 1310
drinking
  legal age for 1299, 1302
  see also alcohol
drinking-water, pollution 8–9, 957, 1057,
  1615
driving, dangerous
  by adolescents 1399
  see also motor vehicle injuries/accidents
drowning
  prevention 1314
  swimming pool 1302
drug(s) 398
  adverse effects *see* adverse drug reactions
    (ADR)
  carcinogenic 979
  child-proof containers 851, 1314
  as commodity of national health system
    1640
  control *see* drug control
  costs 355
  global approach 405
  importing, national policies 355
  inflammatory bowel disease and 1233
  inventories, operational research in 879
  metabolism, genetic variability 150
  pancreatitis due to 1239
  patent protection 267
  prescribing
    Canada 267
    cost-effective initiatives, UK 250
    for elderly 1490–1
  prices, regulation 355
  product liability and compensation
    issues 355
  promotion, ethical issues 394
  public health relationship in US 42–3
  reactions, genetic variability 150
  regulation 354–5, 380
    see also drug control
  social goal 377
  trials *see* clinical trials
  US disasters 311
  users *see* drug abuse
drug abuse 1495–515
  adolescents 1392, 1402–3, 1497
  aetiology 1498–9
  assessment and severity 1496
  bleach sterilisation of equipment 1504,
    1505, 1509
    absence of harmful effects 1505
    effectiveness as disinfectant 1507
    effectiveness of programme 1505–6
  cessation/initiation data 1498–9
  consequences 1498
  data in US 436
  definitions 1495–6
  dependence 1145, 1147
  epidemiology 1317, 1496–8
    adults 1497–8
    consequence of changes to family
      1347
    youth *see* drug abuse, adolescents
  harm reduction perspective 1511
  hepatitis B/C infections in 1508
  HIV/AIDS with *see* drug abuse and
    HIV/AIDS *(below)*
  injury incidence 1299
  intravenous
    behavioural change to prevent
      infections 1597
    equipment sterilisation *see above*
    prevalence 1498
    'shooting galleries' 1273, 1501
  prevention 1403, 1499–500, 1601
    intervention programmes 1499–500
    see also drug abuse and HIV/AIDS
  social/economic costs 1498
  syringe-exchange programmes 1276,
    1277, 1504–5, 1597
    absence of harmful effects 1505
    effectiveness 1505–6
    HIV incidence and 1506–8

drug abuse *(continued)*
  syringe-exchange programmes
    (continued)
      integration with other programmes
        1509
      see also drug abuse and HIV/AIDS
    treatment 1500–1
      approaches/programmes 1500
      effectiveness 1500–1
    private programmes 1300
drug abuse and HIV/AIDS 1272–3,
  1495, 1496, **1501–11**
  costs 1498
  face-to-face education 1502
  harm reduction 1511
  incidence/seroprevalence 1273, 1281,
    1501, 1506–7
    after syringe-exchange 1507–8
  means for behaviour change 1504–9,
    1600
  prevention programmes
    evolution 1502
    high seroprevalence areas 1510
    integrating multiple programmes 1509
    New York 1502, 1504, 1505
    outreach/bleach distribution 1505–6,
      1507, 1509
    see also drug abuse, syringe-exchange
  prevention theories 1502–4
    psychological theories of behaviour
      1503
    social change theories 1503–4
  problematic issues 1509–10
  provision of prevention services 1277,
    1509
  response to health education 125
  sexual transmission 1277, 1281, 1509–10
  transmission mechanism 1273, 1501
  voluntary counselling/testing 1510
Drug Abuse Warning Network (DAWN)
  436–7
drug control 354–5
  FDA's 'drug lag' and approval
    acceleration 355
  legislation 354
    examples 354–5
    issues in 355
  programmes, Australia 354–5
drug dependence 1145, 1147
Drug Enforcement Administration 436
'drug lag' 355
dual-record systems 79
dual X-ray absorptiometry (DEXA)
  scanning 1181–2
Duchenne muscular dystrophy,
  screening 155
Duffy factor 191
duodenal ulcer, treatment 589
duration effects, demographic data
  analysis 79
dust
  occupational lung disease 1089
  volcano 203
dynamic programming 876
dysentery
  amoebic *see* amoebiasis
  bacillary *see* shigellosis
  diagnostic precision for surveillance 939
dysmenorrhoea 1360

E

**Early Breast Cancer Trialists'
  Collaborative Group** 219
Earth, warming of 207, 208
Eastern Europe
  abortion law 362
  disadvantaged
    initiatives for 1531
    Western Europe comparison 1525
  environmental legislation 353
  private medicine 356